Meyler's Side Effects of Drugs

The International Encyclopedia of Adverse Drug Reactions and Interactions

Complementary to this volume

Side Effects of Drugs Annuals 24–29 (1999–2006)
Edited by Jeffrey K. Aronson (Earlier annuals are no longer available in print)

Drugs During Pregnancy and Lactation, Second edition (2006)
Edited by Christof Schaefer et al.

The Law and Ethics of the Pharmaceutical Industry (2005)
By Graham Dukes

Introduction to Clinical Pharmacology, Fifth edition (2006)
By Marilyn Edmunds

Principles of Clinical Pharmacology, Second edition (2006)
Edited by Arthur Atkinson et al.

Writing Clinical Research Protocols (2006)
By E. De Renzo

A Pharmacology Primer (2003)
By Terry Kenakin

Publishing history of *Meyler's Side Effects of Drugs*

*Volume**	*Date of publication*	*Editors*
First published in Dutch	1951	L Meyler
First published in English	1952	L Meyler
First updating volume	1957	L Meyler
Second volume	1958	L Meyler
Third volume	1960	L Meyler
Fourth volume	1964	L Meyler
Fifth volume	1966	L Meyler, C Dalderup, W Van Dijl, and HGG Bouma
Sixth volume	1968	L Meyler and A Herxheimer
Seventh volume	1972	L Meyler and A Herxheimer
Eighth volume	1975	MNG Dukes
Ninth edition	1980	MNG Dukes
Tenth edition	1984	MNG Dukes
Eleventh edition	1988	MNG Dukes
Twelfth edition	1992	MNG Dukes
Thirteenth edition	1996	MNG Dukes
Fourteenth edition	2000	MNG Dukes & JK Aronson
Fifteenth edition	2006	JK Aronson

*The first eight volumes were updates; the ninth edition was the first encyclopedic version and updating continued with the Side Effects of Drugs Annual (SEDA) series.

At various times, full or shortened editions of volumes in the Side Effects series have appeared in French, Russian, Dutch, German, and Japanese.
The website of *Meyler's Side Effects of Drugs* can be viewed at:
http://www.elsevier.com/locate/Meyler.

Meyler's Side Effects of Drugs

The International Encyclopedia of Adverse Drug Reactions and Interactions

Fifteenth edition

Editor
JK Aronson, MA, DPhil, MBChB, FRCP, FBPharmacol S
Oxford, United Kingdom

Honorary Editor
MNG Dukes, MA, DPhil, MB, FRCP
Oslo, Norway

ELSEVIER
AMSTERDAM • BOSTON • HEIDELBERG • LONDON • NEW YORK • OXFORD
PARIS • SAN DIEGO • SAN FRANCISCO • SINGAPORE • SYDNEY • TOKYO

Elsevier
Radarweg 29, PO Box 211, 1000 AE Amsterdam, The Netherlands

Fifteenth edition 2006
Reprinted 2007

British Library Cataloguing in Publication Data
A catalogue record for this book is available from the British Library

Library of Congress Cataloging-in-Publication Data
A catalog record for this book is available from the Library of Congress

ISBN: 978-0-444-50998-7 (Set)
ISBN: 978-0-444-52251-1 (Volume 1)
ISBN: 978-0-444-52252-8 (Volume 2)
ISBN: 978-0-444-52253-5 (Volume 3)
ISBN: 978-0-444-52254-2 (Volume 4)
ISBN: 978-0-444-52255-9 (Volume 5)
ISBN: 978-0-444-52256-6 (Volume 6)

For information on all Elsevier publications
visit our website at books.elsevier.com

Printed and bound in *Great Britain*

07 08 09 10 10 9 8 7 6 5 4 3 2

Contents

Contributors

In this list the main contributors to the Encyclopedia are identified according to the original chapter material to which they made the most contribution. Most have contributed the relevant chapters in one or more editions of the *Side Effects of Drugs Annuals* 23-27 and/or the 14th edition of *Meyler's Side Effects of Drugs*. A few have contributed individual monographs to this edition.

M. Allwood
Derby, United Kingdom
Intravenous infusions—solutions and emulsions

M. Andersen
Odense, Denmark
Antihistamines

M. Andrejak
Amiens, France
Drugs affecting blood coagulation, fibrinolysis, and hemostasis

J.K. Aronson
Oxford, United Kingdom
Antiepileptic drugs
Antiviral drugs
Positive inotropic drugs and drugs used in dysrhythmias

S. Arroyo
Milwaukee, Wisconsin, USA
Antiepileptic drugs

I. Aursnes
Oslo, Norway
Drugs that affect lipid metabolism

H. Bagheri
Toulouse, France
Radiological contrast agents

A.M. Baldacchino
London, United Kingdom
Opioid analgesics and narcotic antagonists

D. Battino
Milan, Italy
Antiepileptic drugs

Z. Baudoin
Zagreb, Croatia
General anesthetics and therapeutic gases

A.G.C. Bauer
Rotterdam, The Netherlands
Antihelminthic drugs
Dermatological drugs, topical agents, and cosmetics

M. Behrend
Deggendorf, Germany
Drugs acting on the immune system

T. Bicanic
London, United Kingdom
Antiprotozoal drugs

L. Biscarini
Perugia, Italy
Anti-inflammatory and antipyretic analgesics and drugs used in gout

J. Blaser
Zurich, Switzerland
Various antibacterial drugs

C. Bokemeyer
Tübingen, Germany
Cytostatic drugs

S. Borg
Stockholm, Sweden
Antidepressant drugs

J. Bousquet
Montpellier, France
Antihistamines

P.J. Bown
Redhill, Surrey, United Kingdom
Opioid analgesics and narcotic antagonists

C.N. Bradfield
Auckland, New Zealand
General anesthetics and therapeutic gases

C.C.E. Brodie-Meijer
Amstelveen, The Netherlands
Metal antagonists

P.W.G. Brown
Sheffield, United Kingdom
Radiological contrast agents

A. Buitenhuis
Amsterdam, The Netherlands
Sex hormones and related compounds, including hormonal contraceptives

H. Cardwell
Auckland, New Zealand
Local anesthetics

A. Carvajal
Valladolid, Spain
Antipsychotic drugs

R. Cathomas
Zurich, Switzerland
Drugs acting on the respiratory tract

A. Cerny
Zurich, Switzerland
Various antibacterial drugs

G. Chevrel
Lyon, France
Drugs acting on the immune system

C.C. Chiou
Bethesda, Maryland, USA
Antifungal drugs

N.H. Choulis
Attika, Greece
Metals
Miscellaneous drugs and materials, medical devices, and techniques not dealt with in other chapters

L.G. Cleland
Adelaide, Australia
Corticotrophins, corticosteroids, and prostaglandins

P. Coates
Adelaide, Australia
Miscellaneous hormones

J. Costa
Badalona, Spain
Corticotrophins, corticosteroids, and prostaglandins

P. Cottagnoud
Bern, Switzerland
Various antibacterial drugs

P.C. Cowen
Oxford, United Kingdom
Antidepressant drugs

S. Curran
Huddersfield, United Kingdom
Hypnosedatives and anxiolytics

H.C.S. Daly
Perth, Western Australia
Local anesthetics

A.C. De Groot
Hertogenbosch, The Netherlands
Dermatological drugs, topical agents, and cosmetics

M.D. De Jong
Amsterdam, The Netherlands
Antiviral drugs

A. Del Favero
Perugia, Italy
Anti-inflammatory and antipyretic analgesics and drugs used in gout

P. Demoly
Montpellier, France
Antihistamines

J. Descotes
Lyon, France
Drugs acting on the immune system

A.J. De Silva
Ragama, Sri Lanka
Snakebite antivenom

H.J. De Silva
Ragama, Sri Lanka
Gastrointestinal drugs

F.A. De Wolff
Leiden, The Netherlands
Metals

S. Dittmann
Berlin, Germany
Vaccines

M.N.G. Dukes
Oslo, Norway
Antiepileptic drugs
Antiviral drugs
Metals
Sex hormones and related compounds, including hormonal contraceptives

H.W. Eijkhout
Amsterdam, The Netherlands
Blood, blood components, plasma, and plasma products

E.H. Ellinwood
Durham, North Carolina, USA
Central nervous system stimulants and drugs that suppress appetite

C.J. Ellis
Birmingham, United Kingdom
Drugs used in tuberculosis and leprosy

P. Elsner
Jena, Germany
Dermatological drugs, topical agents, and cosmetics

T. Erikkson
Lund, Sweden
Thalidomide

E. Ernst
Exeter, United Kingdom
Treatments used in complementary and alternative medicine

M. Farré
Barcelona, Spain
Corticotrophins, corticosteroids, and prostaglandins

P.I. Folb
Cape Town, South Africa
Cytostatic drugs
Intravenous infusions—solutions and emulsions

J.A. Franklyn
Birmingham, United Kingdom
Thyroid hormones and antithyroid drugs

M.G. Franzosi
Milan, Italy
Beta-adrenoceptor antagonists and antianginal drugs

J. Fraser
Glasgow, Scotland
Cytostatic drugs

H.M.P. Freie
Maastricht, The Netherlands
Antipyretic analgesics

C. Fux
Bern, Switzerland
Various antibacterial drugs

P.J. Geerlings
Amsterdam, The Netherlands
Drugs of abuse

A.H. Ghodse
London, United Kingdom
Opioid analgesics and narcotic antagonists

P.L.F. Giangrande
Oxford, United Kingdom
Drugs affecting blood coagulation, fibrinolysis, and hemostasis

G. Gillespie
Perth, Australia
Local anaesthetics

G. Girish
Sheffield, United Kingdom
Radiological contrast agents

V. Gras-Champel
Amiens, France
Drugs affecting blood coagulation, fibrinolysis, and hemostasis

A.I. Green
Boston, Massachusetts, USA
Drugs of abuse

A.H. Groll
Münster, Germany
Antifungal drugs

H. Haak
Leiden, The Netherlands
Miscellaneous drugs and materials, medical devices, and techniques not dealt with in other chapters

F. Hackenberger
Bonn, Germany
Antiseptic drugs and disinfectants

J.T. Hartmann
Tübingen, Germany
Cytostatic drugs

K. Hartmann
Bern, Switzerland
Drugs acting on the respiratory tract

A. Havryk
Sydney, Australia
Drugs acting on the respiratory tract

E. Hedayati
Auckland, New Zealand
General anesthetics and therapeutic gases

E. Helsing
Oslo, Norway
Vitamins

R. Hoigné
Wabern, Switzerland
Various antibacterial drugs

A. Imhof
Seattle, Washington, USA
Various antibacterial drugs

L.L. Iversen
Oxford, United Kingdom
Cannbinoids

J. W. Jefferson
Madison, Wisconsin, USA
Lithium

D.J. Jeffries
London, United Kingdom
Antiviral drugs

M. Joerger
St Gallen, Switzerland
Drugs acting on the respiratory tract

G.D. Johnston
Belfast, Northern Ireland
Positive inotropic drugs and drugs used in dysrhythmias

P. Joubert
Pretoria, South Africa
Antihypertensive drugs

A.A.M. Kaddu
Entebbe, Uganda
Antihelminthic drugs

C. Koch
Copenhagen, Denmark
Blood, blood components, plasma, and plasma products

H. Kolve
Münster, Germany
Antifungal drugs

H.M.J. Krans
Hoogmade, The Netherlands
Insulin, glucagon, and oral hypoglycemic drugs

M. Krause
Scherzingen, Switzerland
Various antibacterial drugs

S. Krishna
London, United Kingdom
Antiprotozoal drugs

M. Kuhn
Chur, Switzerland
Drugs acting on the respiratory tract

R. Latini
Milan, Italy
Beta-adrenoceptor antagonists and antianginal drugs

T.H. Lee
Durham, North Carolina, USA
Central nervous system stimulants and drugs that suppress appetite

P. Leuenberger
Lausanne, Switzerland
Drugs used in tuberculosis and leprosy

M. Leuwer
Liverpool, United Kingdom
Neuromuscular blocking agents and skeletal muscle relaxants

G. Liceaga Cundin
Guipuzcoa, Spain
Drugs that affect autonomic functions or the extrapyramidal system

P.O. Lim
Dundee, Scotland
Beta-adrenoceptor antagonists and antianginal drugs

H.-P. Lipp
Tübingen, Germany
Cytostatic drugs

C. Ludwig
Freiburg, Germany
Drugs acting on the immune system

T.M. MacDonald
Dundee, Scotland
Beta-adrenoceptor antagonists and antianginal drugs

G.T. McInnes
Glasgow, Scotland
Diuretics

I.R. McNicholl
San Francisco, California, USA
Antiviral drugs

P. Magee
Coventry, United Kingdom
Antiseptic drugs and disinfectants

A.P. Maggioni
Firenze, Italy
Beta-adrenoceptor antagonists and antianginal drugs

J.F. Martí Massó
Guipuzcoa, Spain
Drugs that affect autonomic functions or the extrapyramidal system

L.H. Martín Arias
Valladolid, Spain
Antipsychotic drugs

M.M.H.M. Meinardi
Amsterdam, The Netherlands
Dermatological drugs, topical agents, and cosmetics

D.B. Menkes
Wrexham, United Kingdom
Hypnosedatives and anxiolytics

R.H.B. Meyboom
Utrecht, The Netherlands
Metal antagonists

T. Midtvedt
Stockholm, Sweden
Various antibacterial drugs

G. Mignot
Saint Paul, France
Gastrointestinal drugs

S.K. Morcos
Sheffield, United Kingdom
Radiological contrast agents

W.M.C. Mulder
Amsterdam, The Netherlands
Dermatological drugs, topical agents, and cosmetics

S. Musa
Wakefield, United Kingdom
Hypnosedatives and anxiolytics

K.A. Neftel
Bern, Switzerland
Various antibacterial drugs

A.N. Nicholson
Petersfield, United Kingdom
Antihistamines

L. Nicholson
Auckland, New Zealand
General anesthetics and therapeutic gases

I. Öhman
Stockholm, Sweden
Antidepressant drugs

H. Olsen
Oslo, Norway
Opioid analgesics and narcotic antagonists

I. Palmlund
London, United Kingdom
Diethylstilbestrol

J.N. Pande
New Delhi, India
Drugs used in tuberculosis and leprosy

J.K. Patel
Boston, Massachusetts, USA
Drugs of abuse

J.W. Paterson
Perth, Australia
Drugs acting on the respiratory tract

K. Peerlinck
Leuven, Belgium
Drugs affection blood coagulation, fibrinolysis, and hemostasis

E. Perucca
Pavia, Italy
Antiepileptic drugs

E.H. Pi
Los Angeles, California, USA
Antipsychotic drugs

T. Planche
London, United Kingdom
Antiprotozoal drugs

B.C.P. Polak
Amsterdam, The Netherlands
Drugs used in ocular treatment

T.E. Ralston
Worcester, Massachusetts, USA
Drugs of abuse

P. Reiss
Amsterdam, The Netherlands
Antiviral drugs

H.D. Reuter
Köln, Germany
Vitamins

I. Ribeiro
London, United Kingdom
Antiprotozoal drugs

T.D. Robinson
Sydney, Australia
Drugs acting on the respiratory tract

Ch. Ruef
Zurich, Switzerland
Various antibacterial drugs

M. Schachter
London, United Kingdom
Drugs that affect autonomic functions or the extrapyramidal system

A. Schaffner
Zurich, Switzerland
Various antibacterial drugs
Antifungal drugs

S. Schliemann-Willers
Jena, Germany
Dermatological drugs, topical agents, and cosmetics

M. Schneemann
Zürich, Switzerland
Antiprotozoal drugs

S.A. Schug
Perth, Australia
Local anesthetics

G. Screaton
Oxford, United Kingdom
Drugs acting on the immune system

J.P. Seale
Sydney, Australia
Drugs acting on the respiratory tract

R.P. Sequeira
Manama, Bahrain
Central nervous system stimulants and drugs that suppress appetite

T.G. Short
Auckland, New Zealand
General anesthetics and therapeutic gases

D.A. Sica
Richmond, Virginia, USA
Diuretics

G.M. Simpson
Los Angeles, California, USA
Antipsychotic drugs

J.J. Sramek
Beverly Hills, California, USA
Antipsychotic drugs

A. Stanley
Birmingham, United Kingdom
Cytostatic drugs

K.J.D. Stannard
Perth, Australia
Local anesthetics

B. Sundaram
Sheffield, United Kingdom
Radiological contrast agents

J.A.M. Tafani
Toulouse, France
Radiological contrast agents

M.C. Thornton
Auckland, New Zealand
Local anesthetics

B.S. True
Campbelltown, South Australia
Corticotrophins, corticosteroids, and prostaglandins

C. Twelves
Glasgow, Scotland
Cytostatic drugs

W.G. Van Aken
Amsterdam, The Netherlands
Blood, blood components, plasma, and plasma products

C.J. Van Boxtel
Amsterdam, The Netherlands
Sex hormones and related compounds, including hormonal contraceptives

G.B. Van der Voet
Leiden, The Netherlands
Metals

P.J.J. Van Genderen
Rotterdam, The Netherlands
Antihelminthic drugs

R. Verhaeghe
Leuven, Belgium
Drugs acting on the cerebral and peripheral circulations

J. Vermylen
Leuven, Belgium
Drugs affecting blood coagulation, fibrinolysis, and hemostasis

P. Vernazza
St Gallen, Switzerland
Antiviral drugs

T. Vial
Lyon, France
Drugs acting on the immune system

P. Vossebeld
Amsterdam, The Netherlands
Blood, blood components, plasma, and plasma products

G.M. Walsh
Aberdeen, United Kingdom
Antihistamines

T.J. Walsh
Bethesda, Maryland, USA
Antifungal drugs

R. Walter
Zurich, Switzerland
Antifungal drugs

D. Watson
Auckland, New Zealand
Local anesthetics

J. Weeke
Aarhus, Denmark
Thyroid hormones and antithyroid drugs

C.J.M. Whitty
London, United Kingdom
Antiprotozoal drugs

E.J. Wong
Boston, Massachusetts, USA
Drugs of abuse

C. Woodrow
London, United Kingdom
Antiprotozoal drugs

Y. Young
Auckland, New Zealand
General anesthetics and therapeutic gases

F. Zannad
Nancy, France
Antihypertensive drugs

J.-P. Zellweger
Lausanne, Switzerland
Drugs used in tuberculosis and leprosy

A. Zinkernagel
Zürich, Switzerland
Antiprotozoal drugs

M. Zoppi
Bern, Switzerland
Various antibacterial drugs

O. Zuzan
Hannover, Germany
Neuromuscular blocking agents and skeletal muscle relaxants

Foreword

My doctor is
A good doctor
He made me no
Iller than I was

Willem Hussem (The Netherlands) 1900–1974
Translation: Peter Raven

"*Primum non nocere*"—in the first place, do no harm—is often cited as one of the foundation stones of sound medical care, yet its origin is uncertain. Hippocrates? There are some who will tell you so;[1] but the phrase is not a part of the Hippocratic Oath, and the Father of Medicine wrote in any case in his native Greek.[2] It could be that the Latin phrase is from the Roman physician Galenius, while others attribute it to Scribonius Largus, physician to one of the later Caesars,[3] and there is a lot of reason to believe that it actually originated in 19th century England.[4] Hippocrates himself, in the first volume of his *Epidemics*, put it at all events better in context: "When dealing with diseases have two precepts in mind: to procure benefit and not to harm."[5] One must not become overly obsessed by the safety issue, but it is a necessary element in good medical care.

The ability to do good with the help of medicines has developed immensely within the last century, but with it has come the need to keep a watchful eye on the possibility of inflicting harm on the way. The challenge is to recognize at the earliest possible stage the adverse effects that a valuable drug may induce, and to find ways of containing them, so that risk never becomes disproportionate to benefit. The process of drug development will sometimes result in methods of treatment that are more specific to their purpose than were their predecessors and hence less likely to produce unwanted complications; yet the more novel a therapeutic advance the greater the possibility of its eliciting adverse effects of a type so unfamiliar that they are not specifically looked for and long remained unrecognized when they do occur. The entire process of keeping medicines safe today involves all those concerned with them, whether as researchers, manufacturers, regulators, prescribers, dispensers, or users, and it demands an effective and honest flow of information and thought between them.

For several decennia, concerned by its own errors in the past, the science of therapeutics put unbounded faith in the ability of well-planned clinical trials to arrive at the truth about the properties of medicines. Insofar as efficacy was concerned that was and remains a sound move, closing the door to charlatanism as well as to well-meant amateurism. Therapeutic trials with a new medicine were also able to delineate those adverse effects that occurred in a fair proportion of users. If serious, they would bar the drug from entry to the market altogether, while if transient and reasonably tolerable they would form the basis for warnings and precautions as well as the occasional contraindication. The problem lay with those adverse drug reactions that occurred rather less commonly or not at all in populations recruited for therapeutic trials, yet which could soon arise in the much broader spectrum of patients exposed to the drug once it was marketed across the world. The influence of race or climate might explain some of them; others might reflect interactions with foods, alcohol, or other drugs; yet others could only be explained, if at all, in terms of the particular susceptibility of certain individuals. Scattered across the globe, these effects might readily be overlooked, regarded as coincidental, or at worst dismissed contemptuously as "merely anecdotal".

The seriousness of the adverse effects issue became very apparent even as the reputation of controlled trials deservedly grew, and it touched on both newer and older drugs. The thalidomide calamity, involving several thousand cases of drug-induced phocomelia, was fortunately recognized by Widukind Lenz and others in the light of individual case reports within two years of the introduction of the product. On the other hand, generations elapsed between the patenting of aspirin in 1899 and the realization in 1965 that it might induce Reye's syndrome when used to treat fever in children. Such events, and many less spectacular, showed that, however vital well-controlled studies had become, there was good reason to remain alert for signals emerging from individual cases. Unanticipated events occurring during drug treatment might indeed reflect mere coincidence, but again they might not; and for many of the patients who suffered in consequence there was nothing in the least anecdotal about them.

Fortunately, the 1950s and 1960s of the 20th century saw the first positive reactions to the adverse reaction issue. Effective drug regulation emerged in one country after another. In 1952, Prof. Leo Meyler of The Netherlands produced his first "Side Effect of Drugs" to pull together data from the world literature. A number of national adverse reaction monitoring bureaux were established to gather data from the field and examine carefully reports of suspected side effects of medicines, creating the basis for the World Health Organization to establish its global reporting system. The pharmaceutical industry has increasingly realized its duty to collect and pass on the information that comes into its possession through its wide contacts with the health professions. Later years have seen the emergence, notably in Sweden and in Britain, of systems through which patients themselves can report possible adverse effects to the medicines they have taken. All these processes fit together in what the French language so appropriately terms "pharmacovigilance", with vigilance as the watchword for all concerned.

In this continuing development, the medical literature provides a resource with vast potential. The world is believed to have some 20 000 medical journals, of which a nuclear group of a thousand or so can be relied upon to publish reports and analyses of adverse effects—not only in the framework of formal investigations but also in letters, editorials, and reports of meetings large and small. Much of that information comprises not so much firm facts as emergent knowledge, based directly on experience in the field and calling urgently for attention. The book that Leo Meyler created has, in the course of fifteen editions and with the support of an ever-larger team of professionals, provided the means by which that attention can be mobilized. It has become the world's principal tool in bringing together, encyclopedically but critically, the evidence on the basis of which adverse drug effects and interactions can be recognized, discussed, and accommodated into medical practice. Together with its massive database and its complementary *Side Effects of Drugs Annuals*, it has evolved into a vital instrument in ensuring that drugs are used wisely and well and with due caution, in the light of all that is known about them. There is nothing else like it, nor need there be; across the world, *Meyler* has become a pillar of responsible medical care.

M.N. Graham Dukes
Honorary Editor, *Meyler's Side Effects of Drugs*
Oslo, Norway

Notes

1. Lichtenhaeler C. Histoire de la Médicine, Fayard, Paris, 1978:117.
2. Smith CM. Origin and uses of *Primum non nocere*. J Clin Pharmacol 2005;45:371–7.
3. Albrecht H. Primum nil nocere. Die Zeit, 6 April, 2005.
4. Notably in a book by Inman T. *Foundation for a New Theory and Practice of Medicine*. London, 1860.
5. I am indebted to Jeffrey Aronson for his own translation of the Greek original from Hippocrates *Epidemics*, Book I, Section XI, which seems to convey the meaning of the original [ἀσκεῖν περὶ τὰ νοσημάτα δῦο, ὠφελειν ἤ μὴ βλάπτειν] rather better than the published translations of his work.

Preface

This is a completely new edition of what has become the standard reference text in the field of adverse drug reactions and interactions since Leopold Meyler published his first review of the subject 55 years ago. Although we have retained the old title, *Meyler's Side Effects of Drugs*, the subtitle of this edition, *The Encyclopedia of Adverse Drug Reactions and Interactions*, reflects both modern terminology and the scope of the review. The structure of the book may have changed, but the *Encyclopedia* remains the most comprehensive reference source on adverse drug reactions and interactions and a major source of informed discussion about them.

Scope

The scope of the *Encyclopedia* remains wide. It covers not only the vast majority of prescription drugs, old and new, but also non-prescribed substances (such as anesthetics, antiseptics, lifestyle compounds, and drugs of abuse), herbal medicines, devices (such as blood glucose meters), and methods in alternative and complementary medicine. For this edition, entries on some substances that were regarded as obsolete, such as thalidomide and smallpox vaccine, have been rewritten and restored. Other compounds, such as diethylstilbestrol, although no longer in use, continue to cast their shadow and are included. Yet others, currently regarded as obsolete, have been retained, both for historical reasons and because one can never be sure when an old compound may once more become relevant or provide useful information in relation to another compound. Some drugs have been withdrawn from the market in some countries since the last edition of *Meyler* was published; rofecoxib, cisapride, phenylpropanolamine, and kava (see Piperaceae) are examples. Nevertheless, detailed monographs have been included on these substances because of the lessons that they can teach us and in some cases because of their relevance to other compounds in their classes that are still available; it is also not possible to predict whether these compounds will eventually reappear in some other form or for some new indication.

In the last 15 years there has been increasing emphasis on the use of high-quality evidence in therapeutic practice, principally as obtained from large, randomized clinical trials and from systematic reviews of the results of many such trials. However, while it has been possible to obtain useful information about the beneficial effects of interventions in this way, evidence about harms, including adverse drug reactions, has been more difficult to obtain. Even trials that yield good estimates of benefits are poor at providing evidence about harms for several reasons:

- benefits are usually single, whereas harms are usually multiple;
- the chance of any single form of harm is usually smaller than the chance of benefit and therefore more difficult to detect; however, multiple harms can accumulate and affect the benefit-to-harm balance;
- benefits are identifiable in advance, whereas harms are not or not always;
- the likely time-course of benefits can generally be predicted, while the time-course of harms often cannot and may be much delayed by comparison with the duration of a trial.

For all these reasons, larger and sometimes longer studies are needed to detect harms. In recent years attempts have been made to conduct systematic reviews of adverse reactions, but these have also been limited by several problems:

- harms are in general poorly collected in randomized trials and trials may not last long enough to detect them all;
- even when they are well collected, as is increasingly happening, they are often poorly reported;
- even when they are well reported in the body of a report, they may not be mentioned in titles and abstracts;
- even when they are well reported in the body of a report, they may be poorly indexed in large databases.

All this means that it is difficult to collect information on adverse drug reactions from randomized, controlled trials for systematic review. This can be seen from the evidence provided in Table 1, which shows the proportion of different types of information that have been used in the preparation of two volumes of the *Side Effects of Drugs Annual*, proportions that are likely be the same in this *Encyclopedia.*

Wherever possible, emphasis in this *Encyclopedia* has been placed on information that has come from systematic reviews and clinical trials of all kinds; this is reflected in new headings under which trial results are reported (observational studies, randomized studies, placebo-controlled studies). However, because many reports of adverse drug reactions (about 30%) are anecdotal, with evidence from one or just a few cases, many individual case studies (see below) have also been included. We need better methods to make use of the information that this large body of anecdotes provides.

Structure

The first major change that readers will notice is that the chapter structure of previous editions has given way to a monographic structure. That is because some of the information about individual drugs has previously been scattered over different chapters in the book; for example ciclosporin was previously covered in Chapter 37 and in scattered sections throughout Chapter 45; it is now dealt with in a single monograph. The monographs are arranged in alphabetical order, with cross-referencing as required. For example, if you turn to the monograph on cetirizine, you will be referred to the complementary general monograph on antihistamines, where much information that is relevant to cetirizine is given; the monograph on cetirizine itself contains information that is relevant only to cetirizine and not to other antihistamines. Within each monograph the material is arranged in the same way as in the *Side Effects of Drugs Annuals* (see "How to use this book").

Case Reports

A new feature, recognizable from the Annuals, but not incorporated into previous editions, is the inclusion of case reports of adverse effects. This feature reflects the fact that about 30% of all the literature that is reported and discussed in the Annuals derives from such reports (see Table 1). In some cases the only information about an adverse effect is contained in an anecdotal report; in other cases the report illustrates a variant form of the reaction. A case report also gives more immediacy to an adverse reaction, allowing the reader to appreciate more precisely the exact nature of the reported event.

Classification of Adverse Drug Reactions

Another new feature of this edition is the introduction of the DoTS method of classifying adverse drug reactions, based on the **Dose** at which they occur relative to the beneficial dose, the **Time-course** of the reaction, and individual **Susceptibility factors** (see "How to use this book"). This has been done for selected adverse effects, and I hope that as volumes of SEDA continue to be published and the *Encyclopedia's* electronic database is expanded, it will be possible to classify increasing numbers of adverse reactions in this way.

References

Because all the primary and secondary literature is thoroughly surveyed in the Annuals, the *Encyclopedia* has become increasingly compact relative to the amount of information available (even though it has increased in absolute size), with many unreferenced statements and cross-references to the Annuals, on the assumption that all the information would be readily available to the reader, although that may not always be the case. To restore all the reference material on which the *Encyclopedia* has been based as it has evolved over so many years would be a gargantuan task, but in this edition a major start has been made. Many references to original material have been restored, and there is now hardly a statement that is not backed up by at least one reference to primary literature. In addition, almost all of the material that was published in Annuals 23 to 27 (SEDA-23 to SEDA-27) has been included, complete with citations. This has resulted in the inclusion of more than 40 000 references in this edition. Readers will still have to refer to earlier editions of the Annual (SEDA-1 to SEDA-22) and occasionally to earlier editions of *Meyler's Side Effects of Drugs* for more detailed descriptions, but now that the *Encyclopedia* is available electronically this will be repaired in future editions.

Methods and Contributors

I initially prepared the text of the *Encyclopedia* by combining text from the 14th edition of *Meyler's Side Effects of Drugs* and the five most recent annuals (SEDA-23 to SEDA-27). [Later literature is covered in SEDA-28 and the forthcoming SEDA-29.] I next restored missing references to the material and extended it where important information had not been included. The resulting monographs were then sent to experts for review, and their comments were incorporated into the finished monographs. I am grateful to all those, both authors of chapters in previous editions and Annuals and those who have reviewed the monographs for this edition, for their hard work and for making their expertise available.

Acknowledgements

This 15th edition of *Meyler's Side Effects of Drugs* was initiated and carefully planned with Joke Jaarsma at Elsevier, who has provided unstinting support during the production of several previous editions of *Meyler's Side Effects of Drugs* and the *Side Effects of Drugs Annuals*. Early discussions with Dieke van Wijnen at Elsevier about the structure of the text were invaluable. Professor Leufkens from the Faculty of Pharmacy at the University of Utrecht was instrumental in helping us to assemble the preliminary content for this edition; pharmacy students in his department entered the text

Table 1 Types of articles on adverse drug reactions published in 6576 papers in the world literature during 1999 and 2003 (as reviewed in SEDA-24 and SEDA-28)

Type of article	Number of descriptions* (%)
An anecdote or set of anecdotes (that is reported case histories)	2084 (29.9)
A major, randomized, controlled trial or observational study	1956 (28.1)
A minor, randomized, controlled trial or observational study or a non-randomized study (including case series)	1099 (15.8)
A major review, including non-systematic statistical analyses of published studies	951 (13.7)
A brief commentary (for example an editorial or a letter)	362 (5.19)
An experimental study (animal or in vitro)	263 (3.77)
A meta-analysis or other form of systematic review	172 (2.47)
Official statements (for example by Governmental organizations, the WHO, or manufacturers)	75 (1.07)
Total no. of descriptions*	6962
Total no. of articles	6576

* Some articles are described in more than one way

electronically into templates under the guidance of Joke Zwetsloot from Elsevier. Christine Ayorinde provided excellent assistance while I expanded and edited the material. The International Non-proprietary Names were checked by Renée Aronson. At Elsevier the references were then checked and collated by Liz Perill, who also copyedited the material, with Ed Stolting, and shepherded it through conversion to different electronic formats. Bill Todd created the indexes. Stephanie Diment oversaw the project and coordinated everyone's efforts.

The History of Meyler

The history of *Meyler's Side Effects of Drugs* goes back 55 years; a full account can be found at http://www.elsevier.com/locate/Meyler and the various volumes are listed before the title page of this set. When Leopold Meyler, a physician, experienced unwanted effects of drugs that were used to treat his tuberculosis, he discovered that there was no single text to which medical practitioners could turn for information about the adverse effects of drug therapy; Louis Lewin's text *Die Nebenwirkungen der Arzneimittel* ("The Untoward Effects of Drugs") of 1881 had long been out of print (SEDA-27, xxv–xxix). Meyler therefore surveyed the current literature, initially in Dutch as *Schadelijke Nevenwerkingen van Geneesmiddelen* (Van Gorcum, 1951), and then in English as *Side Effects of Drugs* (Elsevier, 1952). He followed up with what he called surveys of unwanted effects of drugs. Each survey covered a period of two to four years and culminated in Volume VIII (1976), edited by Graham Dukes (SEDA-23, xxiii-xxvi), Meyler having died in 1973. By then the published literature was too extensive to be comfortably encompassed in a four-yearly cycle, and an annual cycle was started instead; the first *Side Effects of Drugs Annual* (SEDA-1) was published in 1977. The four-yearly review was replaced by a complementary critical encyclopaedic survey of the entire field; the first encyclopaedic edition of *Meyler's Side Effects of Drugs*, which appeared in 1980, was labeled the ninth edition.

Since then, *Meyler's Side Effects of Drugs* has been published every four years, providing an encyclopaedic survey of the entire field. Had the cycle been adhered to, the 15th edition would have been published in 2004, but over successive editions the quantity and nature of the information available in the text has changed. In the new millennium it was clear that for this edition a revolutionary approach was needed, and that has taken a little longer to achieve, with a great deal of effort from many different individuals.

We have come a long way since Meyler published his first account in a book of 192 pages. I think that he would have approved of this new *Encyclopedia.*

J. K. Aronson
Oxford, October 2005

How to use this book

In a departure from its previous structure, this edition of *Meyler's Side Effects of Drugs* is presented as individual drug monographs in alphabetical order. In many cases a general monograph (for example Antihistamines) is complemented by monographs about specific drugs (for example acrivastine, antazoline, etc.); in that case a cross-reference is given from the latter to the former.

Monograph Structure

Within each monograph the information is presented in sections as follows:

GENERAL INFORMATION
Includes, when necessary, notes on nomenclature, information about the results of observational studies, comparative studies, and placebo-controlled studies in relation to reports of adverse drug reactions, and a general summary of the major adverse effects.

ORGANS AND SYSTEMS
Cardiovascular (includes heart and blood vessels)
Respiratory
Ear, nose, throat
Nervous system (includes central and peripheral nervous systems)
Neuromuscular function
Sensory systems (includes eyes, ears, taste)
Psychological, psychiatric
Endocrine (includes hypothalamus, pituitary, thyroid, parathyroid, adrenal, pancreas, sex hormones)
Metabolism
Nutrition (includes effects on amino acids, essential fatty acids, vitamins, micronutrients)
Electrolyte balance (includes sodium, potassium)
Mineral balance (includes calcium, phosphate)
Metal metabolism (includes copper, iron, magnesium, zinc)
Acid–base balance
Fluid balance
Hematologic (includes blood, spleen, and lymphatics)
Mouth and teeth
Salivary glands
Gastrointestinal (includes esophagus, stomach, small bowel, large bowel)
Liver
Biliary tract
Pancreas
Urinary tract (includes kidneys, ureters, bladder, urethra)
Skin
Hair
Nails
Sweat glands
Serosae (includes pleura, pericardium, peritoneum)
Musculoskeletal (includes muscles, bones, joints)
Sexual function
Reproductive system (includes uterus, ovaries, breasts)
Immunologic (includes effects on the immune system and hypersensitivity reactions)
Autacoids
Infection risk
Body temperature
Multiorgan failure
Trauma
Death

LONG-TERM EFFECTS
Drug abuse
Drug misuse
Drug tolerance
Drug resistance
Drug dependence
Drug withdrawal
Genotoxicity
Mutagenicity
Tumorigenicity

SECOND-GENERATION EFFECTS
Fertility
Pregnancy
Teratogenicity
Fetotoxicity
Lactation

SUSCEPTIBILITY FACTORS (relates to features of the patient)
Genetic factors
Age
Sex
Physiological factors
Cardiac disease
Renal disease
Hepatic disease
Thyroid disease
Other features of the patient

DRUG ADMINISTRATION
Drug formulations
Drug additives
Drug contamination (includes infective agents)
Drug adulteration
Drug dosage regimens (includes frequency and duration of administration)
Drug administration route
Drug overdose

DRUG–DRUG INTERACTIONS
FOOD–DRUG INTERACTIONS
SMOKING
OTHER ENVIRONMENTAL INTERACTIONS
INTERFERENCE WITH DIAGNOSTIC TESTS
DIAGNOSIS OF ADVERSE DRUG REACTIONS
MANAGEMENT OF ADVERSE DRUG REACTIONS
MONITORING THERAPY

Classification of Adverse Drug Reactions

Selected major reactions are classified according to the DoTS system (BMJ 2003;327:1222–5). In this system adverse reactions are classified according to the **Dose** at which they usually occur relative to the beneficial dose, the **Time-course** over which they occur, and the **Susceptibility factors** that make them more likely, as follows:

1 **Relation to dose**
- *Toxic reactions* (reactions that occur at supratherapeutic doses)
- *Collateral reactions* (reactions that occur at standard therapeutic doses)
- *Hypersusceptibility reactions* (reactions that occur at subtherapeutic doses in susceptible patients)

2 **Time-course**
- *Time-independent reactions* (reactions that occur at any time during a course of therapy)
- *Time-dependent reactions*
  - Immediate reactions (reactions that occur only when a drug is administered too rapidly)
  - First-dose reactions (reactions that occur after the first dose of a course of treatment and not necessarily thereafter)
  - Early reactions (reactions that occur early in treatment then abate with continuing treatment)
  - Intermediate reactions (reactions that occur after some delay but with less risk during longer- term therapy, owing to the "healthy survivor" effect)
  - Late reactions (reactions the risk of which increases with continued or repeated exposure), including withdrawal reactions (reactions that occur when, after prolonged treatment, a drug is withdrawn or its effective dose is reduced)
  - Delayed reactions (reactions that occur some time after exposure, even if the drug is withdrawn before the reaction appears)

3 **Susceptibility factors**
- *Genetic*
- *Age*
- *Sex*
- *Physiological variation*
- *Exogenous factors* (for example drug–drug or food–drug interactions, smoking)
- *Diseases*

Drug Names And Spelling

Drugs are usually designated by their recommended or proposed International Non-proprietary Names (rINN or pINN); when these are not available, chemical names have been used. If a fixed combination has a generic combination name (for example co-trimoxazole for trimethoprim + sulfamethoxazole) that name has been used; in some cases brand names have been used.

Spelling

Where necessary, for indexing purposes, American spelling has been used, for example anemia rather than anaemia, estrogen rather than oestrogen.

Cross-references

The various editions of *Meyler's Side Effects of Drugs* are cited in the text as SED-13, SED-14, etc.; the *Side Effects of Drugs Annuals* 1-22 are cited as SEDA-1, SEDA-2, etc. This edition includes most of the contents of SEDA-23 to SEDA-27. SEDA-28 and SEDA-29 are separate publications, which were prepared in parallel with the preparation of this edition.

Indexes

Index of drug names
An index of drug names provides a complete listing of all references to a drug for which adverse effects and/or drug interactions are described. The monograph on herbal medicines contains tabulated cross-indexes to the plants that are covered in separate monographs.

Index of adverse effects
This index is necessarily selective, since a particular adverse effect may be caused by very large numbers of compounds; the index is therefore mainly directed to adverse effects that are particularly serious or frequent, or are discussed in special detail; before assuming that a given drug does not have a particular adverse effect, consult the relevant monograph.

Alphabetical list of drug monographs

The number in parentheses after each heading is the number of the corresponding chapter in the Side Effects of Drug Annuals (SEDA-28 and later) in which the item is usually covered.

C

C1 esterase inhibitor concentrate

General Information

Hereditary angioedema, which is characterized by episodic bouts of swelling of submucosal and subcutaneous tissue, is due to a hereditary abnormality of C1 esterase inhibitor, either a deficiency of the normal enzyme or more rarely the presence of an abnormal enzyme. If C1 esterase inhibitor deficiency can be demonstrated, infusion of concentrated C1 esterase inhibitor is effective in treating the attack. In three studies, no adverse effects were recorded (1–3).

Organs and Systems

Immunologic

Allergic reactions to C1 esterase inhibitor concentrate have been observed, including possible exacerbation of angioedema (4).

Infection risk

The use of C1 esterase inhibitor concentrate has been associated with transmission of hepatitis C, but this can be prevented by heat treatment (5).

References

1. Bork K, Witzke G. Long-term prophylaxis with C1-inhibitor (C1 INH) concentrate in patients with recurrent angioedema caused by hereditary and acquired C1-inhibitor deficiency. J Allergy Clin Immunol 1989;83(3):677–82.
2. Kunschak M, Engl W, Maritsch F, Rosen FS, Eder G, Zerlauth G, Schwarz HP. A randomized, controlled trial to study the efficacy and safety of C1 inhibitor concentrate in treating hereditary angioedema. Transfusion 1998;38(6): 540–9.
3. Visentin DE, Yang WH, Karsh J. C1-esterase inhibitor transfusions in patients with hereditary angioedema. Ann Allergy Asthma Immunol 1998;80(6):457–61.
4. Nomura S, Hashimoto J, Osawa G. Can C1 esterase inhibitor concentrate be a cause of the exacerbation of hereditary angioneurotic oedema? Vox Sang 1995;69(1):85.
5. Cicardi M, Mannucci PM, Castelli R, Rumi MG, Agostoni A. Reduction in transmission of hepatitis C after the introduction of a heat-treatment step in the production of C1-inhibitor concentrate. Transfusion 1995;35(3):209–12.

Cabergoline

General Information

Cabergoline is an ergoline derivative that has been used in patients with hyperprolactinemia (SEDA-15, 133), but is used nowadays in patients with Parkinson's disease. Its adverse effects include nausea, hypotension, headache, gastric pain, dizziness, and weakness, which as a rule resolve over time.

It is almost universally accepted that directly acting dopamine receptor agonists have less efficacy than levodopa, although the reasons are not clear. Neurologists from London have sought to question this assumption by using cabergoline ($n = 11$) and pergolide ($n = 7$) at considerably higher doses than recommended (1). The actual mean doses were 8.8 and 9.4 mg/day, compared with recommended maxima of 6 and 5 mg/day respectively. The high doses were tolerated by the patients for 2.3–2.5 years; mild dyskinesias ($n = 7$), ankle edema ($n = 3$), and hallucinations ($n = 1$) were the only reported adverse effects. The authors concluded that the therapeutic window for these drugs is apparently much greater than is generally accepted, and that higher doses can be given safely with potentially enhanced efficacy.

Organs and Systems

Respiratory

- Interstitial pneumonitis occurred in a 65-year-old man who had taken cabergoline in a low dose (1 mg/day) for 4 months (2). He was given no specific therapy, but withdrawal of the drug resulted in clinical recovery after 3 weeks and radiological resolution within 2 months.

Nervous system

When cabergoline is used in patients with Parkinson's disease, the same spectrum of dyskinesias and psychiatric complications as with bromocriptine is observed (3).

The successful use of ergot derivatives to shrink macroprolactinomas can have unwanted neurological consequences, and this has been described in two case reports.

Three Italian men aged 39, 42, and 53 years with invasive prolactinomas took cabergoline 1.0–3.0 mg/week and all developed CSF rhinorrhea after 2–7 months (4). This was clearly a consequence of loss of the "stopper" effect of the tumor, owing to shrinkage, and in each case was successfully treated by endoscopic trans-sphenoidal surgery.

- A 42-year-old Spanish man took cabergoline (up to 3 mg/day) for a large prolactinoma causing hypopituitarism and symptomatic chiasmal compression (5). After 18 months there was only a minimal tumor remnant on the floor of the sella turcica, but there was chiasmal herniation. However, there were no clinical effects of this, and in particular the visual fields were normal.

Serosae

Some patients who developed retroperitoneal or pleural fibrosis from bromocriptine experienced aggravation of the condition when they switched to cabergoline. Cabergoline may share this risk with bromocriptine (SEDA-17, 169).

- A 76-year-old man taking cabergoline 10 mg/day developed constrictive pericarditis after 11 months (6). He required pericardiectomy, but cabergoline was continued and a few months later he was found to have pleuropulmonary fibrosis, which did not resolve on drug withdrawal.

References

1. Navan P, Bain PG. Long term tolerability of high dose ergoline derived dopamine agonist therapy for the treatment of Parkinson's disease. J Neurol Neurosurg Psychiatry 2002; 73(5):602–3.
2. Frank W, Moritz R, Becke B, Pauli R. Low dose cabergoline induced interstitial pneumonitis. Eur Respir J 1999; 14(4):968–70.
3. Clarke CE, Deane KD. Cabergoline versus bromocriptine for levodopa-induced complications in Parkinson's disease. Cochrane Database Syst Rev 2001;(1):CD001519.
4. Cappabianca P, Lodrini S, Felisati G, Peca C, Cozzi R, Di Sarno A, Cavallo LM, Giombini S, Colao A. Cabergoline-induced CSF rhinorrhea in patients with macroprolactinoma. Report of three cases. J Endocrinol Invest 2001;24(3):183–7.
5. Marcos L, De Luis DA, Botella I, Hurtado A. Tumour shrinkage and chiasmal herniation after successful cabergoline treatment for a macroprolactinoma. Clin Endocrinol (Oxf) 2001;54(1):126–7.
6. Ling LH, Ahlskog JE, Munger TM, Limper AH, Oh JK. Constrictive pericarditis and pleuropulmonary disease linked to ergot dopamine agonist therapy (cabergoline) for Parkinson's disease. Mayo Clin Proc 1999;74(4):371–5.

Cadmium

General Information

Cadmium is a bluish-white metallic element (symbol Cd; atomic no. 48). It is found as cadmium sulfate in a mineral called greenockite.

Cadmium is an environmental and occupational pollutant that is associated with nephrotoxicity (1) and bone toxicity (2); even low concentrations can impair renal function and/or increase bone fragility. Cadmium is also an adulterant in infant formulas and weaning foods.

Cadmium concentrations were determined in 59 baby food samples, including milk-based cereals and milk-based and soya-based formulas, recommended from 0–18 months of age. The mean weekly intake of dietary cadmium was estimated to be 0.1–3.1 μg/kg. Exposure to dietary cadmium from weaning diets can be up to 12 times higher in children fed infant formulas than in breast-fed children (3).

References

1. Fels LM. Risk assessment of nephrotoxicity of cadmium. Ren Fail 1999;21(3–4):275–81.
2. Staessen JA, Roels HA, Emelianov D, Kuznetsova T, Thijs L, Vangronsveld J, Fagard R. Environmental exposure to cadmium, forearm bone density, and risk of fractures: prospective population study. Public Health and Environmental Exposure to Cadmium (PheeCad) Study Group. Lancet 1999;353(9159):1140–4.
3. Eklund G, Oskarsson A. Exposure of cadmium from infant formulas and weaning foods. Food Addit Contam 1999; 16(12):509–19.

Caffeine

General Information

Caffeine is a methylxanthine used to stimulate the central nervous system in combating fatigue and drowsiness. Caffeine stimulates the central nervous system, skeletal muscle contraction and gastric secretion. It acts to a lesser extent on the kidney, producing a diuresis. Most of its adverse effects result from accentuated pharmacological actions, including those described above, and they may become especially evident in pathologically or genetically predisposed individuals. Differences in the activity of *N*-acetylases in the liver, secondary to genetic polymorphism lead to differential susceptibility to caffeine (xanthine toxicity) (1). A certain degree of tolerance develops to some of the pharmacological actions of caffeine, but there is little or no tolerance to its central stimulatory effects; however, some kind of psychic habituation can develop after prolonged consumption.

The term "caffeinism" refers to a state of acute or chronic toxicity resulting from the ingestion of high doses of caffeine. An average intake of 500–600 mg/day of caffeine (about 7–9 cups of tea or 4–7 cups of coffee) is currently regarded as representing a significant health risk. The symptoms of caffeinism include behavioral, psychophysiological, and affective manifestations. They include restlessness, anxiety, irritability, agitation, muscle tremor, insomnia, headache, sensory disturbances, diuresis, cardiovascular symptoms, and gastrointestinal complaints (SEDA-10, 5). At very high doses caffeine can even produce epileptiform convulsions. Acute overdosage can occur and produce severe CNS excitation in sensitive individuals and small children (SEDA-15, 1). Tonic-clonic seizures have been reported postpartum. Maternal use of caffeine in pregnancy can cause dysrhythmias in the neonate (SEDA-14, 1). Because of a significant abuse potential and potential toxicity, formulations that contain a high content of caffeine have been made available by prescription only in some European countries.

Workers in the coffee industry often develop allergic reactions, in the form of dermatitis, rhinitis, and bronchial asthma, on exposure to dust in the process of stripping the chaff from raw beans before roasting (2). This may or may not be a reaction to caffeine itself.

The ability of caffeine to catalyse the formation of *N*-nitrosamine in the digestive tract has raised the question of its being carcinogenic (see "Pancreas" below). Caffeine has been associated with fibrocystic breast disease (3). However, a study of benign proliferative endothelial disorder of the breast did not show any association with methylxanthine consumption (SEDA-15, 1).

Organs and Systems

Cardiovascular

There is debate over the association between caffeine intake and cardiovascular disease. Increases in mean blood pressure, blood glucose and free fatty acid concentrations, and urinary catecholamine excretion have been found after acute ingestion of 150 mg of caffeine (SEDA-4, 4). While not particularly potent, caffeine appears to produce cardiac dysrhythmias, including ventricular tachycardia. Furthermore, in non-smokers, daily consumption of five cups of percolated coffee per day (about 680 mg of caffeine) was associated with a modestly increased risk of having a cardiac arrest without a prior history of cardiovascular disease (4). In patients with pre-existing heart disease, caffeine lowers the effective and functional refractory period of the atrioventricular node (SEDA-4, 5). A two-fold increased risk of myocardial infarction has been suggested for women who drink six or more cups of coffee a day (5), and in two studies, men who drank five or more cups of coffee a day had an approximately two-fold increase in the risk of myocardial infarction (6) or coronary artery disease (7). However, prospective studies of the relation between caffeine consumption and an increased risk of coronary artery disease (or stroke) have been negative (SEDA-15, 1) or inconclusive (8,9), as has been the association between the consumption of coffee and serum cholesterol concentration assessed in 24 cross-sectional epidemiological studies (SEDA-15, 1). However, a Finnish study did show a positive-dose relation with serum cholesterol after adjustment for confounding variables, in men but not in women. It has also been suggested that the relation is seen only with boiled and not instant or filter coffee.

Guaraná is produced from the guaraná plant (*Paullina cupana*), the seeds of which contain 3.6–5.8% caffeine.

- A 25-year-old woman, who had pre-existing mitral valve prolapse and a history of having had bouts of palpitation with caffeine, developed intractable ventricular fibrillation after consuming a "natural energy" guaraná health drink containing a high concentration of caffeine (10). At autopsy, she was found to have sclerosis and myxoid changes in the mitral valve leaflets. The caffeine concentration in her aortic blood was 19 μg/ml.

This case highlights the need for more careful regulation of "natural" products, including warning patients with underlying health problems, and clear labeling to document the presence of any constituents with potentially adverse effects. It also shows the need for medical practitioners to be familiar with the more widely used "natural remedies" and their toxicological profiles. Following the death of this patient, the Western Australian Coroner recommended that Race 2005 Energy Blast should be removed from the local market, and the product was recalled nationally in August 1999.

Nervous system

Insomnia, anxiety, tachycardia, and tremor are among the symptoms most commonly reported with caffeine (11). Tenseness and irritability also occur and, with high intake, symptoms resembling those of anxiety neurosis (12). A case of "caffeine psychosis" has also been reported (13). Dose–response associations have not been particularly well studied, but some are known (SEDA-7, 6). Paradoxically, six cases have been reported of pathological sleepiness induced by caffeine (14). Tonic-clonic seizures occurred postpartum in a woman who had received 500 mg of caffeine sodium benzoate for headache after lumbar puncture; a prolonged half-life was implicated (SEDA-17, 1).

Consumption of methylxanthine-containing products can aggravate the neurological symptoms associated with the glucose transporter type 1 (Glut 1 deficiency syndrome). The human erythrocyte and the brain glucose transporters are identical, and the erythrocyte transporter has been used in four patients with individual mutations in the Glut 1 gene to demonstrate that caffeine and theophylline inhibit glucose transport (15). The Glut 1 deficiency syndrome represents impaired glucose transport across the blood–brain barrier caused by partial Glut 1 deficiency, which results in hypoglycorrhachia, seizures, and developmental delay. Identifying potential inhibitors of Glut 1 is essential in preventing further impairment of glucose transport in these patients. In addition to phosphodiesterase inhibition and adenosine A_1 receptor antagonism by methylxanthines, it is likely that inhibition of glucose transport also contributes to the convulsive effects of methylxanthines in high doses.

Psychological, psychiatric

Red Bull, a mixture of caffeine, taurine, and inositol, a widely consumed "power drink," affects mental performance and mood.

- A 36-year-old man with bipolar-I disorder had a second manic episode, after having been in remission for 5 years while taking lithium to maintain a serum lithium concentration of 0.8–1.1 mmol/l (16). One week before this episode, he drank three cans of Red Bull at night, as he needed less sleep; 3 days later he drank three more cans. After 4 days he was feeling euphoric, hyperactive, and insomniac. He gradually became more hyperactive and had increased libido and irritability. He took no more Red Bull and improved within 7 days.

Based on this report, the authors suggested that stimulant beverages that contain caffeine might cause cognitive and behavioral changes, especially in vulnerable patients with bipolar illness.

Metabolism

The major metabolic effects of caffeine are increase in free fatty acids and blood glucose concentration (17,18).

Electrolyte balance

Hypokalemia and myopathy are known effects of caffeine toxicity, and severe hypokalemia and fatigue and hypokalemia with myopathy have been described before (19).

Gastrointestinal

Large doses of caffeine can cause nausea and vomiting. Caffeine is a potent stimulant of hydrochloric acid secretion (20) and has been incriminated in exacerbating duodenal ulcers. However, decaffeinated coffee has also been reported to be as potent as instant coffee in stimulating gastric acid secretion (20).

Pancreas

A relation between coffee consumption and pancreatic cancer was originally reported in a case-control study (SEDA-7, 8), with an unexpected increase in pancreatic cancer in coffee drinkers (relative risk in men 2.6). The same group studied differences in mortality from pancreatic cancer in different countries in relation to differences in coffee consumption and found a significant relation between increases in coffee consumption and increases in mortality from pancreatic cancer. However, the data on which the findings were based were crude.

Although the results of published epidemiological studies are compatible with a small effect of coffee consumption on pancreatic carcinogenesis, the interpretation of these findings is not clear, because of the possibility of residual confounding and other sources of bias (21). In two large cohort studies of 1 907 222 person-years of follow-up, there were 288 cases of pancreatic cancer with no evidence of an association between coffee and pancreatic cancer (22). Furthermore, there is no association between folate intake, caffeine consumption, and the risk of pancreatic cancer (23).

The relation between coffee drinking and the presence of the K-*ras* mutation in patients with exocrine pancreas cancer has been investigated in Spain in 121 cases in which tissue specimens were available (24). In exocrine pancreatic cancer, the K-*ras* gene may be activated less often among regular coffee drinkers, suggesting that caffeine, or other compounds present in coffee, or other factors with which coffee drinking is associated, may modulate K-*ras* activation. While the results of this study may have mechanistic and pathogenic relevance, they have no clinical or health policy implications.

Urinary tract

Large doses of caffeine cause diuresis. Daily consumption of caffeine citrate increased the mean urinary excretion rate of tubular cells and erythrocytes in volunteers (25). The nephrotoxicity of analgesic antipyretic drug combinations may result from a combined effect, in which aspirin, phenacetin, and caffeine all play a role (SEDA-4, 5). In 10 asymptomatic women and 20 women with confirmed detrusor instability, caffeine caused a significant increase in detrusor pressure on bladder filling in the latter, but no difference in volume at first contraction, height of contraction, or bladder capacity (26).

As up to 10% of about 42 000 dialysis patients have suffered from renal insufficiency due to analgesic nephropathy (in the postphenacetin era), German nephrologists have demanded that medications that contain fixed combinations of analgesics (paracetamol, aspirin, or propyphenazone plus caffeine) be withdrawn from the market, following the example of their US colleagues in the National Kidney Foundation (27).

Skin

Urticaria as an allergic response to caffeine has been reported (SEDA-4, 5).

Musculoskeletal

Caffeine toxicity is an uncommon cause of myopathy, but a history of excessive dietary and pharmaceutical consumption of caffeine should be sought in any patient with unexplained myopathy, particularly if there is concomitant hypokalemia (28).

- A 21-year-old woman with a 12-month history of progressive muscle weakness, nausea, vomiting, diarrhea, and weight loss had significant worsening of muscle weakness over 2 weeks, associated with exercise-induced muscle stiffness and pain. She had severe hypokalemia and metabolic acidosis. For the past 1–2 years she had been consuming about 8 liters of cola every day. She stopped drinking cola and took potassium supplements, after which her hypokalemia and muscle weakness resolved and the serum creatine kinase activity fell. Based on the concentration of caffeine in the cola, it was estimated that she had been consuming at least 1 g/day of caffeine for more than 12 months.

Long-Term Effects

Drug abuse

Abuse of analgesic combinations has been thought to be especially facilitated if they contain caffeine or codeine, reinforcing abuse. However, this has not been confirmed in an expert review, in which it was concluded that the available evidence does not support the claim that analgesics co-formulated with caffeine, in the absence of phenacetin, stimulate or sustain overuse (29). Caffeine has a synergistic effectiveness with analgesics, but although it can cause dependence, the risk is low. Withdrawal is not likely to cause increased need of analgesics. However, there is strong dependence behavior in patients using formulations containing phenacetin, antipyretics/analgesics, and caffeine. This finding may have led to the impression that caffeine stimulates overuse of analgesics.

Drug withdrawal

Restlessness, irritability, and headache are withdrawal effects attributable to caffeine. These and other symptoms can occur with lower doses of caffeine than generally supposed (30). The caffeine withdrawal headache may be responsible for the widespread practice of taking caffeine-containing analgesics habitually, since a withdrawal headache could create a vicious cycle of drug use (SEDA-5, 6).

Tumorigenicity

A possible association between the use of methylxanthine consumption and the occurrence of fibrocystic breast disease has been suggested (SEDA-6, 8) (3). It was concluded that in women who are predisposed to fibrocystic disease, methylxanthines are factors in its development. The mechanism of this effect might be an inhibitory action on the activity of cyclic AMP and cyclic GMP phosphodiesterases.

Second-Generation Effects

Fertility

It has been suggested that the use of caffeine to improve the mobility of human sperm used in artificial insemination may be very risky, owing to the potential for chromosome damage and also possible damage to the fertilized ovum (SEDA-5, 32).

Another study suggested that a high daily intake of caffeine may predispose women to reproductive difficulties (SEDA-9, 2). Although delayed mitosis and excessive chromatid breaks have been noted in human lymphocytic cultures to which caffeine was added (31), the rapid and almost complete metabolism of caffeine in man may protect against the various deleterious effects found in human cell culture studies and animal studies.

Epidemiological studies requiring further verification have suggested a relation between caffeine intake and reduced fertility, even at a consumption as low as the caffeine equivalent of more than one cup of brewed coffee a day (SEDA-14, 1). A more recent study has suggested that this reduction in fertility is limited to non-smokers; possible acceleration of caffeine metabolism in smokers has been offered as a possible explanation for the apparent effect of smoking (32).

Fetotoxicity

In two studies (SEDA-6, 9), there was a relation between caffeine consumption and fetotoxicity. In one, a high rate of spontaneous abortions, stillbirths, and prematurity at birth was associated with ingestion of more than 600 mg of caffeine per day by either the mother or the father. In the other, a daily intake of more than eight cups of coffee by the mother increased the frequency of congenital malformations.

Concern about the possible harmful effects of caffeine on the outcome of pregnancy has evolved mainly from studies of animals which have shown a reduction in intrauterine fetal growth. However, the implications of these data for men are unclear, because of the differences in mode of exposure to caffeine, the amounts consumed, and caffeine metabolism. The possible effects of caffeine intake on the human fetus have been reviewed (SEDA-7, 8); the conclusion was that the scientific data currently available could not answer the question. In an analysis of interview and medical record data in 12 205 non-asthmatic women to evaluate the relation between coffee consumption and adverse outcomes in pregnancy, the findings were negative.

In eight pregnant women at 32–36 weeks of gestation, two cups of caffeinated or decaffeinated coffee were associated with an increase in the incidence of fetal breathing activity, and the caffeinated coffee was associated with a significant fall in baseline fetal heart rate (33). Three cases of fetal dysrhythmias resulting from excessive intake of caffeine by the mother during pregnancy have been reported (SEDA-14, 1).

Some studies have reported that a caffeine consumption of over 150 mg/day during pregnancy may be associated with a small but statistically significant increase in the risks of spontaneous abortion and low birth weight, although the authors could not rule out contributions of maternal age, smoking, ethanol use, or other confounders (34). Careful evaluation of these confounders may at least partly resolve the controversy surrounding possible adverse effects of caffeine on pregnancy outcome.

Whether the consumption of caffeine during pregnancy increases the risk of spontaneous abortion is controversial. In a nested case-control study, 591 women who had a spontaneous abortion before 140 days of gestation were compared with 2558 matched women from the same clinic who gave birth to live infants at 28 weeks' gestation and who had serum drawn on the same day of gestation as the women who had abortions (35). The women were enrolled in the Collaborative Perinatal Project from 1959 to 1966, and the serum paraxanthine concentration was measured 30 years later. Moderate consumption of caffeine was unlikely to increase the risk of spontaneous abortion; only extremely high serum paraxanthine concentrations were associated with spontaneous abortion.

Lactation

The relation between serum and breast milk concentrations of caffeine has been studied (SEDA-6, 8). Caffeine accumulation in the infant would depend on the average concentration in maternal serum and breast milk over time, the volume of milk ingested, and particularly the infant's clearance rate of caffeine.

Susceptibility Factors

Age

Infants

Xanthines have been given to infants at the risk of sudden infant death syndrome or idiopathic apnea of prematurity (see monograph on Theophylline). About 50% of 30 infants treated with caffeine (and 12 of 18 infants treated with theophylline) had significant increases in episodes of gastroesophageal reflux (36). The authors stressed that screening for reflux should precede the administration of caffeine (and theophylline) to infants at the risk of sudden infant death syndrome. As expected, the frequency of adverse effects such as tachycardia and gastroesophageal reflux is lower with lower doses of caffeine; for example 2.5 mg/kg qds (SEDA-17, 1).

Children

In healthy boys, there were increases in subjective anxiety in long-term low-caffeine users, and withdrawal symptoms in high-caffeine users. No beneficial effects of caffeine use were found (37). It has been recommended that children should take caffeine only in analgesic products and in a dose related to their age (SEDA-5, 6).

Other features of the patient

In patients who are susceptible to cardiac dysrhythmias, restriction of caffeine may be indicated. Caffeine can also add to the rise in renin and noradrenaline that occur in hepatic cirrhosis and can also considerably aggravate diarrhea in patients with irritable bowel syndrome (SEDA-15, 1).

Drug Administration

Drug overdose

Excessive amounts (1 g or more) of caffeine can cause untoward central nervous effects, including psychotic organic brain syndrome (SEDA-5, 6).

Oral route

Oral doses that cause death are said to range from 3 to 50 g of caffeine, but death from excessive caffeine ingestion is rare, perhaps owing to its emetic effect. Death may be due to cardiovascular shock, but chronic potentially lethal toxicity, even for heavy coffee or tea drinkers, is very unlikely since 60–100 cups a day would be required.

Intravenous route

In two instances in which caffeine was given intravenously, convulsions and death were recorded at doses of 400 mg and 3.2 g (38).

The elimination of caffeine has been described in a neonate weighing 1860 g, born at 31 weeks of gestation, after the accidental administration of 160 mg/kg. The first serum concentration was 218 mg/l at 36.5 hours after dosing. The half-life was 81 hours, the clearance 0.01 l/hour (0.17 ml/minute), and the volume of distribution 1.17 liters. Toxic manifestations were hypertonia, sweating, tachycardia, cardiac failure, pulmonary edema, and metabolic disturbances such as metabolic acidosis, hyperglycemia, and raised creatine kinase activity. An unusual feature of this infant's illness was gastric dilatation. These signs resolved by day 7 at a serum concentration of 60–70 mg/l (39).

Confirmed reports of caffeine overdose are rare. Postmortem concentrations of caffeine measured in femoral blood were 220 and 190 mg/l in two adults who took unknown doses (40). In view of the extensive use of caffeine, the authors emphasized the forensic importance of measuring caffeine.

Drug–Drug Interactions

General

A comprehensive textbook has listed more than 40 drugs that interact with caffeine (41). See also the monograph on Theophylline.

Caffeine has been included in a wide variety of fixed drug combinations (for example, with non-steroidal anti-inflammatory drugs or antihistamines). The purpose of including caffeine is to increase systemic availability (for example, antipyrine), to counteract adverse effects of the other drug (for example, sedation induced by antihistamines), or to provide additional therapeutic efficacy (aspirin). The use of combination formulations complicates evaluation of caffeine's adverse effects.

Aspirin

In a comparison of a caffeine-free formulation containing aspirin 650 mg plus citric acid 60 mg and a formulation containing aspirin 650 mg plus caffeine citrate 120 mg (equivalent to 60 mg of anhydrous caffeine), caffeine significantly increased the rate of appearance as well as the maximum concentration of the salicylate in plasma by about 31 and 15% respectively; the AUC of salicylate was also significantly higher (42). The authors concluded that caffeine can increase the systemic availability of aspirin in man without any other effects on the salicylate disposition.

However, in a systematic review and meta-analysis of published randomized controlled trials, it was found that caffeine did not enhance the analgesic effect of aspirin (43).

Benzodiazepines

Caffeine and other central stimulants can reverse daytime sedation from benzodiazepine use. There was a positive effect of caffeine 250 mg on early morning performance after placebo, and flurazepam 30 mg given the night before (44,45), particularly in terms of subjective assessment of mood and sleepiness. However, one cannot assume that the alerting effect of caffeine necessarily reverses the amnestic, disinhibiting, or insight-impairing effects of benzodiazepines. Indeed, caffeine may actually worsen learning and performance already impaired by lorazepam (46).

Carbamazepine

In five children, due to receive carbamazepine for epilepsy, the caffeine breath test was carried out before the administration of carbamazepine 200–600 mg and after a minimum of 2–3 weeks therapy (47). The results suggested that carbamazepine induces the metabolism of caffeine by CYP1A2.

Clozapine

In an open, randomized, crossover study in 12 non-smoking healthy volunteers, caffeine 400–1000 mg/day reduced clozapine clearance, probably by inhibiting CYP1A2 (48). Differences in habitual caffeine intake can, therefore, explain some of the large variability in the kinetics of clozapine (49), and should be taken into consideration when clozapine is used. An earlier case report (50) also suggested that caffeine increases plasma concentrations of clozapine, causing toxic symptoms.

In seven schizophrenic patients taking clozapine monotherapy, caffeine was withdrawn for 5 days; clozapine plasma concentrations fell by 50% (51). The authors suggested that schizophrenic patients treated with clozapine should have their caffeine intake supervised, and that monitoring of concentrations of clozapine and its metabolite may be warranted.

Ephedrine

Even low doses of caffeine can, in sensitive patients, cause tremor, insomnia, and anxiety, and such problems are much more marked if ephedrine is given together with caffeine, as it sometimes is for appetite control (SEDA-17, 161).

Idrocilamide

The pharmacokinetics of caffeine is greatly altered by concomitant administration of the myorelaxant, idrocilamide, which inhibits the biotransformation of caffeine and prolongs its half-life nine-fold (SEDA-5, 7). Consequently, when idrocilamide is prescribed, partial or total abstinence from caffeine-containing products should be enforced.

Lithium

Caffeine increases renal lithium clearance, and it is conceivable that drastic curtailment of caffeine intake could result in an increase in serum lithium concentration.

Mexiletine

Mexiletine reduces the clearance of theophylline, and this combination has been reported to cause ventricular tachycardia (52). A similar interaction with caffeine has been reported (53).

Neuroleptic drugs

Caffeine can alter the plasma concentrations of neuroleptic drugs (SEDA-5, 6).

Excess caffeine can stimulate the CNS, which can worsen psychosis and thus interfere with the effects of neuroleptic drugs (54). Neuroleptic drugs can precipitate from solution when mixed with coffee or tea (55), but the clinical significance of this interaction is unknown (56).

Oral contraceptives

The clearance of both theophylline and caffeine is reduced in oral contraceptive users, and their half-lives are increased, probably because of inhibition of hepatic metabolism by cytochrome P450 isozymes (57). Again, caution in dosage is advisable.

Phenylpropanolamine

Phenylpropanolamine, which is available over the counter for weight loss, inhibits caffeine metabolism, leading to excessive stimulation; for example, manic psychosis (SEDA-17, 1).

Interference with Diagnostic Tests

Dexamethasone suppression test

A false-positive dexamethasone-suppression test has been associated with ingestion of caffeine equivalent to 4–5 cups of coffee (58).

References

1. Benet LZ, Kroetz DL, Sheiner LB. Pharmacokinetic: the dynamics of drug absorption, distribution, and elimination. In: Hardman JG, Limbird LE, Molinoff PB, Ruddon RW, Gilman AG, editors. Goodman and Gilman's The Pharmacological Basis of Therapeutics. 9th ed. New York: McGraw-Hill, 1996:28.
2. Berrens L. The chemistry of atopic allergens. Monogr Allergy 1971;7:1–298.
3. Boyle CA, Berkowitz GS, LiVolsi VA, Ort S, Merino MJ, White C, Kelsey JL. Caffeine consumption and fibrocystic breast disease: a case-control epidemiologic study. J Natl Cancer Inst 1984;72(5):1015–19.
4. Weinmann S, Siscovick DS, Raghunathan TE, Arbogast P, Smith H, Bovbjerg VE, Cobb LA, Psaty BM. Caffeine intake in relation to the risk of primary cardiac arrest. Epidemiology 1997;8(5):505–8.
5. Mann JI, Thorogood M. Coffee-drinking and myocardial infarction. Lancet 1975;2(7946):1215.
6. International Coffee Organization. United States of America: Coffee Drinking Study; 1989.
7. LeGrady D, Dyer AR, Shekelle RB, Stamler J, Liu K, Paul O, Lepper M, Shryock AM. Coffee consumption and mortality in the Chicago Western Electric Company Study. Am J Epidemiol 1987;126(5):803–12.
8. Hemminki E, Pesonen T. Regional coffee consumption and mortality from ischemic heart disease in Finland. Acta Med Scand 1977;201(1–2):127–30.
9. Yano K, Rhoads GG, Kagan A. Coffee, alcohol and risk of coronary heart disease among Japanese men living in Hawaii. N Engl J Med 1977;297(8):405–9.
10. Cannon ME, Cooke CT, McCarthy JS. Caffeine-induced cardiac arrhythmia: an unrecognised danger of healthfood products. Med J Aust 2001;174(10):520–1.
11. Mellinger GD, Balter MB, Uhlenhuth EH. Insomnia and its treatment: prevalence and correlates. Arch Gen Psychiatry 1985;42(3):225–32.
12. Greden JF. Anxiety or caffeinism: a diagnostic dilemma. Am J Psychiatry 1974;131(10):1089–92.
13. McManamy MC, Schube PG. Caffeine intoxication: report of a case the symptoms of which amounted to psychosis. N Engl J Med 1936;215:616.
14. Regestein QR. Pathologic sleepiness induced by caffeine. Am J Med 1989;87(5):586–8.
15. Ho YY, Yang H, Klepper J, Fischbarg J, Wang D, De Vivo DC. Glucose transporter type 1 deficiency syndrome (Glut1DS): methylxanthines potentiate Glut1 haploinsufficiency in vitro. Pediatr Res 2001;50(2):254–60.
16. Machado-Vieira R, Viale CI, Kapczinski F. Mania associated with an energy drink: the possible role of caffeine, taurine, and inositol. Can J Psychiatry 2001;46(5):454–5.
17. Bellet S. Caffeine and serum cholesterol. JAMA 1966; 196:229.
18. Jankelson OM, Beaser SB, Howard FM, Mayer J. Effect of coffee on glucose tolerance and circulating insulin in men with maturity-onset diabetes. Lancet 1967;1(7489):527–9.
19. Benowitz NL. Clinical pharmacology of caffeine. Annu Rev Med 1990;41:277–88.
20. Cohen S, Booth GH Jr. Gastric acid secretion and lower-esophageal-sphincter pressure in response to coffee and caffeine. N Engl J Med 1975;293(18):897–9.
21. La Vecchia C, Liati P, Decarli A, Negri E, Franceschi S. Coffee consumption and risk of pancreatic cancer. Int J Cancer 1987;40(3):309–13.
22. Michaud DS, Giovannucci E, Willett WC, Colditz GA, Fuchs CS. Coffee and alcohol consumption and the risk of pancreatic cancer in two prospective United States cohorts. Cancer Epidemiol Biomarkers Prev 2001; 10(5):429–37.
23. Skinner HG, Michaud DS, Giovannucci EL, Rimm EB, Stampfer MJ, Willett WC, Colditz GA, Fuchs CS. A prospective study of folate intake and the risk of pancreatic cancer in men and women. Am J Epidemiol 2004; 160(3):248–58.
24. Porta M, Malats N, Guarner L, Carrato A, Rifa J, Salas A, Corominas JM, Andreu M, Real FX. Association between coffee drinking and K-*ras* mutations in exocrine pancreatic cancer. PANKRAS II Study Group J Epidemiol Community Health 1999;53(11):702–9.
25. Prescott LF. Effects of acetylsalicylic acid, phenacetin, paracetamol, and caffeine on renal tubular epithelium. Lancet 1965;19:91–5.
26. Creighton SM, Stanton SL. Caffeine: does it affect your bladder? Br J Urol 1990;66(6):613–14.
27. Tuffs A. German nephrologists demand painkiller ban. Lancet 1996;348(9032):952.

28. Rice JE, Faunt JD, Warren JE. Excessive cola consumption as a cause of hypokalaemic myopathy. Intern Med J 2001;31(5):317–18.
29. Feinstein AR, Heinemann LA, Dalessio D, Fox JM, Goldstein J, Haag G, Ladewig D, O'Brien CP. Do caffeine-containing analgesics promote dependence? A review and evaluation. Clin Pharmacol Ther 2000;68(5):457–67.
30. Griffiths RR, Evans SM, Heishman SJ, Preston KL, Sannerud CA, Wolf B, Woodson PP. Low-dose caffeine physical dependence in humans. J Pharmacol Exp Ther 1990;255(3):1123–32.
31. Jensen TK, Henriksen TB, Hjollund NH, Scheike T, Kolstad H, Giwercman A, Ernst E, Bonde JP, Skakkebaek NE, Olsen J. Caffeine intake and fecundability: a follow-up study among 430 Danish couples planning their first pregnancy. Reprod Toxicol 1998;12(3):289–95.
32. Mulvihill JJ. Caffeine as teratogen and mutagen. Teratology 1973;8(1):69–72.
33. Salvador HS, Koos BJ. Effects of regular and decaffeinated coffee on fetal breathing and heart rate. Am J Obstet Gynecol 1989;160(5 Part 1):1043–7.
34. Fernandes O, Sabharwal M, Smiley T, Pastuszak A, Koren G, Einarson T. Moderate to heavy caffeine consumption during pregnancy and relationship to spontaneous abortion and abnormal fetal growth: a meta-analysis. Reprod Toxicol 1998;12(4):435–44.
35. Klebanoff MA, Levine RJ, DerSimonian R, Clemens JD, Wilkins DG. Maternal serum paraxanthine, a caffeine metabolite, and the risk of spontaneous abortion. N Engl J Med 1999;341(22):1639–44.
36. Vandenplas Y, De Wolf D, Sacre L. Influence of xanthines on gastroesophageal reflux in infants at risk for sudden infant death syndrome. Pediatrics 1986;77(6):807–10.
37. Rapoport JL, Elkins R, Neims A, Zahn T, Berg CJ. Behavioral and autonomic effects of caffeine in normal boys. Dev Pharmacol Ther 1981;3(2):74–82.
38. Jokela S, Vartiainen A. Caffeine poisoning. Acta Pharmacol Toxicol (Copenh) 1959;15:331–4.
39. Anderson BJ, Gunn TR, Holford NH, Johnson R. Caffeine overdose in a premature infant: clinical course and pharmacokinetics. Anaesth Intensive Care 1999; 27(3):307–11.
40. Riesselmann B, Rosenbaum F, Roscher S, Schneider V. Fatal caffeine intoxication. Forensic Sci Int 1999;103(Suppl 1):S49–52.
41. Stockley IH. Drug Interactions: a Source Book of Adverse Interactions Their Mechanisms, Clinical Importance and Management, 3rd ed. London: Blackwell Scientific, 1994.
42. Thithapandha A. Effect of caffeine on the bioavailability and pharmacokinetics of aspirin. J Med Assoc Thai 1989;72(10):562–6.
43. Zhang WY, Po AL. Do codeine and caffeine enhance the analgesic effect of aspirin? A systematic overview. J Clin Pharm Ther 1997;22(2):79–97.
44. Johnson LC, Spinweber CL, Gomez SA. Benzodiazepines and caffeine: effect on daytime sleepiness, performance, and mood. Psychopharmacology (Berl) 1990;101(2):160–7.
45. Johnson LC, Spinweber CL, Gomez SA, Matteson LT. Daytime sleepiness, performance, mood, nocturnal sleep: the effect of benzodiazepine and caffeine on their relationship. Sleep 1990;13(2):121–35.
46. Rush CR, Higgins ST, Bickel WK, Hughes JR. Acute behavioral effects of lorazepam and caffeine, alone and in combination, in humans. Behav Pharmacol 1994;5(3): 245–54.
47. Parker AC, Pritchard P, Preston T, Choonara I. Induction of CYP1A2 activity by carbamazepine in children using the caffeine breath test. Br J Clin Pharmacol 1998; 45(2):176–8.
48. Hagg S, Spigset O, Mjorndal T, Dahlqvist R. Effect of caffeine on clozapine pharmacokinetics in healthy volunteers. Br J Clin Pharmacol 2000;49(1):59–63.
49. Jerling M, Merle Y, Mentre F, Mallet A. Population pharmacokinetics of clozapine evaluated with the nonparametric maximum likelihood method. Br J Clin Pharmacol 1997;44(5):447–53.
50. Odom-White A, de Leon J. Clozapine levels and caffeine. J Clin Psychiatry 1996;57(4):175–6.
51. Carrillo JA, Herraiz AG, Ramos SI, Benitez J. Effects of caffeine withdrawal from the diet on the metabolism of clozapine in schizophrenic patients. J Clin Psychopharmacol 1998;18(4):311–16.
52. Kessler KM, Interian A Jr, Cox M, Topaz O, De Marchena EJ, Myerburg RJ. Proarrhythmia related to a kinetic and dynamic interaction of mexiletine and theophylline. Am Heart J 1989;117(4):964–6.
53. Joeres R, Richter E. Mexiletine and caffeine elimination. N Engl J Med 1987;317(2):117.
54. Bezchlibnyk KZ, Jeffries JJ. Should psychiatric patients drink coffee? Can Med Assoc J 1981;124(4):357–8.
55. Kulhanek F, Linde OK, Meisenberg G. Precipitation of antipsychotic drugs in interaction with coffee or tea. Lancet 1979;2(8152):1130.
56. Bowen S, Taylor KM, Gibb IA. Effect of coffee and tea on blood levels and efficacy of antipsychotic drugs. Lancet 1981;1(8231):1217–18.
57. Patwardhan RV, Desmond PV, Johnson RF, Schenker S. Impaired elimination of caffeine by oral contraceptive steroids. J Lab Clin Med 1980;95(4):603–8.
58. Lee MA, Flegel P, Cameron OG, Greden JF. Chronic caffeine consumption and the dexamethasone suppression test in depression. Psychiatry Res 1988;24(1):61–5.

Calcipotriol

General Information

Topical calcipotriol (a vitamin D analogue) is an effective and safe treatment for mild to moderate psoriasis vulgaris. Its mode of action is identical to that of 1,25-dihydroxycolecalciferol (calcitriol).

Organs and Systems

Nervous system

Calcipotriol can cause headache (SEDA-20, 157).

Mineral balance

With the use of doses larger than the recommended maximum of 100 g/week, a few reports have documented hypercalcemia and hypercalciuria (SEDA-18, 176) (SEDA-22, 172) (1,2). However, hypercalcemia has also been reported in a few patients using no more than the recommended doses (3,4). Calcipotriol exerts its effects on systemic calcium homeostasis by increasing intestinal absorption of calcium and probably phosphate. This results in suppression of parathyroid hormone and 1,25-dihydroxycolecalciferol (5).

Skin

At recommended doses, the adverse effects of calcipotriol are limited to skin reactions. Lesional and perilesional irritation occurs in about 20% of patients (6). Contact dermatitis is rare. Photosensitization can occur when calcipotriol is used in patients undergoing UVB phototherapy.

Contamination of the facial skin can result in frank irritant contact dermatitis. Allergic contact dermatitis has been observed in some patients (7–10).

Hyperpigmentation due to local application of vitamin D in combination with photochemotherapy has been described. Calcipotriol may have the same potential.

- In one case, there was profound hyperpigmentation during UVB 311 nm phototherapy in combination with local calcipotriol, applied after the UVB irradiation (11). Calcipotriol-treated areas, and not the surrounding normal skin, started to show increased pigmentation after six sessions of irradiation, stabilized during therapy, and slightly decreased in intensity during the 6 months after photochemotherapy had ended. No photoallergy tests were performed.

Calcipotriol can occasionally convert psoriasis vulgaris into pustular psoriasis (SEDA-19, 165).

Immunologic

Contact allergic reactions to calcipotriol are rare. In one case patch tests with Psorcutan Salbe and calcipotriol (its active ingredient) were both positive (10).

References

1. Fogh K, Kragballe K. Vitamin D3 analogues. Clin Dermatol 1997;15(5):705–13.
2. Berth-Jones J, Bourke JF, Iqbal SJ, Hutchinson PE. Urine calcium excretion during treatment of psoriasis with topical calcipotriol. Br J Dermatol 1993;129(4):411–14.
3. Russell S, Young MJ. Hypercalcaemia during treatment of psoriasis with calcipotriol. Br J Dermatol 1994;130(6):795–6.
4. Kawahara C, Okada Y, Tanikawa T, Fukusima A, Misawa H, Tanaka Y. Severe hypercalcemia and hypernatremia associated with calcipotriol for treatment of psoriasis. J Bone Miner Metab 2004;22(2):159–62.
5. Bourke JF, Mumford R, Whittaker P, Iqbal SJ, Le Van LW, Trevellyan A, Hutchinson PE. The effects of topical calcipotriol on systemic calcium homeostasis in patients with chronic plaque psoriasis. J Am Acad Dermatol 1997; 37(6):929–34.
6. Guilhou JJ. Le calcipotriol. [Calcipotriol.] Ann Dermatol Venereol 2001;128(3 Pt 1):229–37.
7. de Groot AC. Contact allergy to calcipotriol. Contact Dermatitis 1994;30(4):242–3.
8. Park YK, Lee JH, Chung WG. Allergic contact dermatitis from calcipotriol. Acta Derm Venereol 2002;82(1):71–2.
9. Krayenbuhl BH, Elsner P. Allergic and irritant contact dermatitis to calcipotriol. Am J Contact Dermat 1999;10(2):78–80.
10. Frosch PJ, Rustemeyer T. Contact allergy to calcipotriol does exist. Report of an unequivocal case and review of the literature. Contact Dermatitis 1999; 40(2):66–71.
11. Rutter A, Schwarz T. Ausgeprägte Hyperpigmentierung in psoriatischen Plaques als Folge einer Kombinationsbehandlung mit UVB-311 nm und Calcipotriol. [Market hyperpigmentation in psoriatic plaque as a sequelae of combination therapy with UVB-311 and calcipotriol.] Hautarzt 2000;51(6):431–3.

Calcitetracemate

General Information

The use of calcitetracemate in the treatment of lead poisoning has been described (1). Between 1993 and 2000, 45 adult patients consulted the Poison Centre of Marseilles, France after lead exposure (9 women, 36 men, average age 44, range 22–76 years). In 22 patients, a calcitetracemate provocation test was negative. Six patients with a positive test refused to be treated; the other 16 were treated with a total of 58 courses of calcitetracemate by infusion 500 mg bd for 5 days. The mean blood lead concentration in these 16 patients was 566, range 320–943 ng/ml; the mean urinary lead excretion was 3011, range 789–7229 μg/day. The mean amount of lead eliminated in the urine during chelation therapy was 30 912 μg. In 12 patients in whom lead exposure ended after the diagnosis of lead poisoning, chelation therapy reduced the blood lead concentration by 69%. In four patients in whom exposure continued during treatment, the blood lead concentration fell by only 7%. In the 16 treated patients, there was clinical improvement and no adverse effects of chelation therapy.

Drug Administration

Drug administration route

Lead poisoning in a six-week-old child was treated by adding disodium calcitetracemate to the peritoneal dialysis fluid (2).

References

1. de Haro L, Prost N, Gambini D, Bourdon JH, Hayek-Lanthois M, Valli M, Jouglard J, Arditti J. Le saturnisme des adultes: experience du Centre antipoison de Marseille de 1993 à 2000. [Lead poisoning in adults. Experience of the Poison Control Center of Marseille from 1993 to 2000.] Presse Méd 2001;30(37):1817–20.
2. Buneaux F, Protin P, Besson-leaud M, Fabiani P. Rôle du laboratoire dans le diagnostic et la traitement d'une intoxication par le plomb. [Role of the laboratory in the diagnosis and treatment of lead poisoning.] Eur J Toxicol Environ Hyg 1976;9(3):165–70.

Calcitonin

General Information

Calcitonin inhibits osteoclastic bone resorption, increases the urinary excretion of calcium and phosphate, and reduces serum calcium. It is established in the treatment of disorders of high bone turnover, including Paget's disease and postmenopausal osteoporosis, but is less effective than the bisphosphonates. Calcitonin is less effective than other therapeutic measures in the treatment of acute hypercalcemia. Long-term administration of calcitonin reduces morbidity in cases of osteogenesis imperfecta and algoneurodystrophy (SEDA-13, 1307) (1,2). The role of calcitonin in treating acute pain due to osteoporotic crush fractures has been reviewed, but the mechanism of its analgesic effect is not known (3).

When used continuously in high doses, the therapeutic effect of calcitonin is sustained for only a few months, probably because of down-regulation of osteoclast receptors. The duration of the response to calcitonin can be extended by periodically interrupting treatment. A number of regimens, ranging from cycles of a few days to several months, are effective both as prophylaxis in healthy postmenopausal women and in women with established osteoporosis; however, the risk of fractures is not reduced (4). Calcitonin also has a potent analgesic effect independent of its effect on bone, possibly mediated through endogenous opioids (5). It appears to be more effective when given intranasally than subcutaneously for this indication.

Salmon- and eel-derived calcitonins are more potent than the human and porcine forms. Intranasal calcitonin has a systemic availability of only 3% of the subcutaneous form but is associated with fewer adverse effects, probably because of lower systemic availability. Antibodies against calcitonin are often found after prolonged treatment, more commonly with salmon (30–69%) or eel calcitonin than with human calcitonin. Antibodies do not usually affect the clinical effect of calcitonin and have not been reported to cause any harm to the patient. Antibody-mediated resistance is exceptional.

The adverse effects of calcitonin, although common, are usually mild and are dose-related in the therapeutic range. They include gastrointestinal effects (nausea, cramps, and vomiting), dizziness and flushing, and local reactions either at the injection site (rash, pruritus) or in the nose (rhinitis, dryness, sneezing, and rarely epistaxis). In 40 patients there was nausea and dizziness in 37% of those given rectal salmon calcitonin compared with 6% of those given placebo (6).

Observational studies

The usefulness of intranasally administered salmon calcitonin for 2 years has been evaluated in 44 glucocorticoid-dependent asthmatics (SEDA-19, 378) (7). All were taking calcium supplements (1000 mg/day), but one group also took calcitonin 100 IU every other day. Calcitonin increased spinal bone mass during the first year of treatment, and maintained bone mass in a steady state during the second year. However, the rate of vertebral fractures was similar in the two groups. The addition of salmon calcitonin did not increase the efficacy of calcium plus vitamin D in the prevention of bone loss in 48 newly diagnosed patients taking glucocorticoids for giant cell arteritis and polymyalgia rheumatica in a double-blind, randomized, placebo-controlled trial (SEDA-21, 418) (8).

Placebo-controlled studies

Salmon calcitonin nasal spray prevented bone loss in the lumbar spine of 31 patients treated with prednisone for polymyalgia rheumatica (SEDA-22, 448) (9). They were randomized to salmon calcitonin nasal spray 200 IU/day or matched placebo for 1 year. Both groups were treated with calcium supplements if their dietary intake was below 800 mg/day. With calcitonin the mean bone mineral density in the lumbar spine fell by 1.3% and with placebo by 5% after 1 year. There were no differences in the hip, including the femoral neck and trochanter, or in total body bone density.

Organs and Systems

Cardiovascular

Flushing occurs soon after administration of calcitonin in up to 20% of patients and usually settles within several minutes (10).

Respiratory

When salmon calcitonin 100 IU was given intravenously to 18 patients with atopic asthma in a randomized, double-blind, crossover study, to assess any potential anti-inflammatory effect, it significantly reduced FEV1 and FVC, but the effect lasted less than 1 hour (11). Three subjects had dyspnea that did not require specific treatment.

Ear, nose, throat

In a randomized, placebo-controlled trial 22% of 1255 postmenopausal women taking calcitonin compared with 15% of women taking placebo had rhinitis (nasal congestion, discharge, or sneezing) (12). Almost all cases were of mild to moderate severity.

Gastrointestinal

Nausea is common with calcitonin, and vomiting or diarrhea occur more rarely. These symptoms usually settle without treatment if the drug is continued and may also be reduced by giving the dose at bedtime.

In 46 patients with Paget's disease given synthetic salmon thyrocalcitonin 80 IU/day for 3 months, there were hot flushes in 35% and nausea in 24%; in only one case was it necessary to stop treatment because of intractable diarrhea (13).

Urinary tract

In postmenopausal osteoporosis treatment with calcitriol plus etidronate or calcitonin produced improvement in spinal bone mineral density, but a high rate of nephrotoxic adverse events (14).

Skin

Rash and pruritus can occur at the site of subcutaneous injections of calcitonin (15).

Immunologic

Calcitonin allergy is very rare.

- A 60-year-old woman tolerated daily intranasal calcitonin for 6 months of the year for 4 years (16). She developed nasal watering, nasal and ocular pruritus, and sweating immediately after the administration of nasal calcitonin when she restarted after a 6-month break. These symptoms recurred 2 years later, with abdominal pain and hypotension, after 10 months of intramuscular calcitonin, and were again reproduced by a lower dose intramuscularly.

- A 65-year-old woman, who had previously tolerated calcitonin nasal spray, developed eye and nose congestion, an itchy nose, and sneezing minutes after using intranasal salmon calcitonin (17). She was later given intramuscular salmon calcitonin and developed generalized urticaria and nasal itching within minutes. Skin testing was positive with eel and salmon calcitonins but not human calcitonin, and she was treated with human calcitonin without adverse effects.

Drug Administration

Drug formulations

Intranasal calcitonin is associated with fewer adverse effects than parenteral formulations, probably because of low systemic availability. However, a meta-analysis has confirmed that adverse events are poorly reported in clinical trials (18). The pooled relative risk for rhinitis from four trials ($n = 1663$) was 1.72, but this did not reach statistical significance.

Drug–Drug Interactions

Lithium

In four women serum lithium concentrations fell significantly within 3 days of starting calcitonin (19) because of increased renal clearance of lithium (19,20). Serum lithium concentrations should therefore be monitored in patients who start to take calcitonin.

References

1. Nishi Y, Hamamoto K, Kajiyama M, Ono H, Kihara M, Jinno K. Effect of long-term calcitonin therapy by injection and nasal spray on the incidence of fractures in osteogenesis imperfecta. J Pediatr 1992;121(3):477–80.
2. Gobelet C. Place de la calcitonine dans le traitement de l'algoneurodystrophie. [The role of calcitonin in the treatment of algoneurodystrophy.] Schweiz Rundsch Med Prax 1986;75(1–2):7–9.
3. Maksymowych WP. Managing acute osteoporotic vertebral fractures with calcitonin. Can Fam Physician 1998;44:2160–6.
4. Meunier PJ. Evidence-based medicine and osteoporosis: a comparison of fracture risk reduction data from osteoporosis randomised clinical trials. Int J Clin Pract 1999; 53(2):122–9.
5. Lyritis GP, Paspati I, Karachalios T, Ioakimidis D, Skarantavos G, Lyritis PG. Pain relief from nasal salmon calcitonin in osteoporotic vertebral crush fractures. A double blind, placebo-controlled clinical study. Acta Orthop Scand Suppl 1997;275:112–14.
6. Lyritis GP, Ioannidis GV, Karachalios T, Roidis N, Kataxaki E, Papaioannou N, Kaloudis J, Galanos A. Analgesic effect of salmon calcitonin suppositories in patients with acute pain due to recent osteoporotic vertebral crush fractures: a prospective double-blind, randomized, placebo-controlled clinical study. Clin J Pain 1999; 15(4):284–9.
7. Luengo M, Pons F, Martinez de Osaba MJ, Picado C. Prevention of further bone mass loss by nasal calcitonin in patients on long term glucocorticoid therapy for asthma: a two year follow up study. Thorax 1994; 49(11):1099–102.
8. Healey JH, Paget SA, Williams-Russo P, Szatrowski TP, Schneider R, Spiera H, Mitnick H, Ales K, Schwartzberg P. A randomized controlled trial of salmon calcitonin to prevent bone loss in corticosteroid-treated temporal arteritis and polymyalgia rheumatica. Calcif Tissue Int 1996;58(2):73–80.
9. Adachi JD, Bensen WG, Bell MJ, Bianchi FA, Cividino AA, Craig GL, Sturtridge WC, Sebaldt RJ, Steele M, Gordon M, Themeles E, Tugwell P, Roberts R, Gent M. Salmon calcitonin nasal spray in the prevention of corticosteroid-induced osteoporosis. Br J Rheumatol 1997;36(2):255–9.
10. Gennari C, Fischer JA. Cardiovascular action of calcitonin gene-related peptide in humans. Calcif Tissue Int 1985; 37(6):581–4.
11. Kawalski H, Polanowicz U, Jonderko G, Kucharz EJ, Krol W, Klimmek K, Gina AR, Pieczyrak R, Slifirski J, Shani J. Immunological parameters and respiratory functions in patients suffering from atopic bronchial asthma after intravenous treatment with salmon calcitonin. Immunol Lett 1999;70(1):15–19.
12. Chesnut CH 3rd, Silverman S, Andriano K, Genant H, Gimona A, Harris S, Kiel D, LeBoff M, Maricic M, Miller P, Moniz C, Peacock M, Richardson P, Watts N, Baylink D. A randomized trial of nasal spray salmon calcitonin in postmenopausal women with established osteoporosis: the prevent recurrence of osteoporotic fractures study. PROOF Study Group. Am J Med 2000;109(4):267–76.
13. Bouvet JP. Traitement de la maladie de Paget par la thyrocalcitonine de saumon. Etude cooperative en double insu. [Treatment of Paget's disease with salmon thyrocalcitonin. Cooperative double-blind study.] Nouv Presse Méd 1976;6(17):1447–50.
14. Gurlek A, Bayraktar M, Gedik O. Comparison of calcitriol treatment with etidronate–calcitriol and calcitonin–calcitriol combinations in Turkish women with postmenopausal osteoporosis: a prospective study. Calcif Tissue Int 1997; 61(1):39–43.
15. Siminoski K, Josse RG. Prevention and management of osteoporosis: consensus statements from the Scientific Advisory Board of the Osteoporosis Society of Canada. 9. Calcitonin in the treatment of osteoporosis. CMAJ 1996;155(7):962–5.
16. Porcel SL, Cumplido JA, de la Hoz B, Cuevas M, Losada E. Anaphylaxis to calcitonin. Allergol Immunopathol (Madr) 2000;28(4):243–5.
17. Rodriguez A, Trujillo MJ, Herrero T, Baeza ML, de Barrio M. Allergy to calcitonin. Allergy 2001;56(8):801.
18. Cranney A, Tugwell P, Zytaruk N, Robinson V, Weaver B, Shea B, Wells G, Adachi J, Waldegger L, Guyatt G. Osteoporosis Methodology Group and The Osteoporosis Research Advisory Group. Meta-analyses of therapies for postmenopausal osteoporosis. VI. Meta-analysis of calcitonin for the treatment of postmenopausal osteoporosis Endocr Rev 2002;23(4):540–51.
19. Passiu G, Bocchetta A, Martinelli V, Garau P, Del Zompo M, Mathieu A. Calcitonin decreases lithium plasma levels in man. Preliminary report. Int J Clin Pharmacol Res 1998;18(4):179–81.
20. Bachofen M, Bock H, Beglinger C, Fischer JA, Thiel G. Calcitonin, ein proximal tubular wirkendes Diuretikum: Lithium-Clearance-Messungen am Menschen. [Calcitonin, a proximal-tubular-acting diuretic: lithium clearance measurements in humans.] Schweiz Med Wochenschr 1997;127(18):747–52.

Calcium carbimide

General Information

Calcium carbimide has effects and uses similar to those of disulfiram, and has been used in the treatment of chronic alcoholism (1). Its alternative name, cyanamide, has also been used to designate carbimide, which is used in veterinary medicine.

Organs and Systems

Hematologic

Calcium carbimide has been linked to granulocytopenia (2) (SEDA-22, 525).

Liver

Calcium carbimide has been linked to liver damage (3) (SED-12, 1244), but caution is needed in attributing liver damage in alcoholic patients to drugs.

Skin

Calcium carbimide has been linked to skin reactions (4).

- A 37-year-old man developed itchy erythema on his trunk and legs after taking calcium carbimide (dose not specified) for 3 days. He had an eosinophilia of 22%. Patch-testing with calcium carbimide was positive. The eruption subsided after withdrawal.
- A 60-year-old man developed keratotic erythema on his trunk and extremities after taking calcium carbimide (dose not specified) for 1 month. Patch-testing with calcium carbimide was positive. The eruption subsided after withdrawal, but itch and redness persisted for 9 months.

References

1. Peachey JE. A review of the clinical use of disulfiram and calcium carbimide in alcoholism treatment. J Clin Psychopharmacol 1981;1(6):368–75.
2. Ajima M, Usuki K, Igarashi A, Okazaki R, Hamano K, Urabe A, Totsuka Y. Cyanamide-induced granulocytopenia. Intern Med 1997;36(9):640–2.
3. Yokoyama A, Sato S, Maruyama K, Nakano M, Takahashi H, Okuyama K, Takagi S, Takagi T, Yokoyama T, Hayashida M, et al. Cyanamide-associated alcoholic liver disease: a sequential histological evaluation. Alcohol Clin Exp Res 1995; 19(5):1307–11.
4. Kawana S. Drug eruption induced by cyanamide (carbimide): a clinical and histopathologic study of 7 patients. Dermatology 1997;195(1):30–4.

Calcium channel blockers

See also Individual agents

General Information

The calcium channel blockers block the movement of calcium across L-type calcium channels. The main drugs that share this action are verapamil (a phenylalkylamine), diltiazem (a benzthiazepine), and the dihydropyridines, which include amlodipine, darodipine, felodipine, isradipine, lacidipine, lercanidipine, manidipine, nicardipine, nifedipine, nimodipine, nisoldipine, and nitrendipine. Other agents, for example prenylamine and lidoflazine, are now rarely used, and perhexiline, having failed to reach the market at all in some countries, was withdrawn in the UK after continuing concerns about its safety (1). Mibefradil blocks T type calcium channels; it was withdrawn within 1 year of marketing because of multiple drug interactions, emphasizing the need for rigorous drug assessment before release and the importance of postmarketing surveillance of new drugs (2).

Although they are chemically heterogeneous, many adverse effects are common to all calcium channel blockers, predictable from their pharmacological actions. Calcium plays a role in the functions of contraction and conduction in the heart and in the smooth muscle of arteries; drugs that interfere with its availability (of which there are many, the calcium channel blockers being the most specific) will therefore act in all these tissues. A few idiosyncratic and hypersensitivity reactions have also been reported with individual calcium channel blockers.

The properties of these drugs vary widely (3). Nifedipine is said to have little negative inotropic effect and no effect on the atrioventricular node; verapamil is a potent cardiac depressant, with a marked effect on the atrioventricular node; and diltiazem has less cardiac depressant effect but inhibits atrioventricular nodal activity.

Controversy has surrounded the use of calcium channel blockers in the treatment of hypertension (4) and ischemic heart disease (5), with evidence for an association with unfavorable coronary outcomes compared with other therapies. Most of the evidence comes from the use of short-acting formulations, especially short-acting nifedipine. The hypothesis put forward to explain these findings was that short-acting formulations cause reflex activation of the sympathetic nervous system (6). Further observational studies showed that these drugs were also associated with gastrointestinal hemorrhage (7) and cancer (8). Claims of conflicts of interests amongst authors were published (9), often amid heated debate. Further evidence against the short-acting calcium channel blockers in hypertension has been forthcoming (10,11) and a worse than expected outcome with respect to coronary outcomes in diabetic patients has fuelled the debate (12). Further evidence of gastrointestinal bleeding has been published (13), but there is evidence against a link with cancer (14). All these scares have undoubtedly reduced the standing of this class of drugs in the eyes of physicians.

That calcium channel blockers are effective in relieving the symptoms of angina pectoris is beyond doubt. However, the Angina and Silent Ischemia Study (15), in which nifedipine, diltiazem, and propranolol were compared with placebo in a crossover study, produced conflicting results. Only diltiazem improved treadmill exercise time and only propranolol convincingly reduced the number of silent ischemic episodes during ambulatory monitoring. These findings are hard to explain (16). Beta-blockers may be cardioprotective and therefore preferable to calcium channel blockers (17). The clinically significant deterioration seen in patients with impaired left ventricular function taking calcium channel blockers is important, as many patients with angina have previously had a myocardial infarction or have poor left ventricular function. Calcium channel blockers cannot be assumed to be safe second-line drugs for angina in patients with poor cardiac reserve, although newer agents may prove to be safer (18).

Calcium channel blockers are very effective in controlling variant angina, and are often used during coronary angioplasty and after coronary artery surgery. They are also useful in patients who are intolerant of beta-blockers (19), or who have a poor response to nitrates, or who have concurrent hypertension.

General adverse effects

Throbbing headache, facial warmth and flushing, and dizziness are minor complaints associated with the use of calcium channel blockers; these effects are believed to be caused by inhibitory actions on smooth muscle (20). Palpitation, muscle cramps, and pedal edema also occur (21–27). Dizziness, facial flushing, leg edema, postural hypotension, and constipation have been reported in up to one-third of patients. They are rarely severe and often abate on continued therapy. More serious adverse effects, mainly those affecting cardiac conduction, are much less common, and only rarely is withdrawal necessary.

Organs and Systems

Cardiovascular

Cardiac failure

Although acute hemodynamic studies have suggested that calcium channel blockers can be beneficial in cardiac failure (28), long-term treatment has been associated with clinical deterioration. Calcium channel blockers should therefore be prescribed with caution for patients with impaired cardiac function, who should be regularly reassessed; treatment should be withdrawn if the signs or symptoms of cardiac failure appear. In some cases heart failure is predictable, as in the case of a patient with aortic stenosis who developed left ventricular failure after treatment with nifedipine (29). Increased sympathetic activity can also compensate for the myocardial suppressant effects of calcium channel blockers, and the combination of these drugs (particularly verapamil) with beta-adrenoceptor antagonists has therefore given cause for concern in the past, although this combination is now considered relatively safe for the majority of patients with normal cardiac function (30–32).

Myocardial ischemia

There have been many studies of the efficacy of calcium channel blockers in early and late intervention in myocardial infarction (33). These studies have failed to show convincing benefits. Indeed, in the nifedipine intervention studies there was a consistent trend towards higher mortality in the treated patients than in those taking placebo. A study in which patients were randomized to placebo or nifedipine within 48 hours of admission was terminated after 1358 patients had been recruited, because mortality at 6 months was 15.4% on nifedipine and 13.3% on placebo (34).

It has been argued that dihydropyridine calcium channel blockers, which increase heart rate, can all increase the risk of death and reinfarction (35,36). Early beneficial results with diltiazem in patients with non-Q-wave infarction (37) were not confirmed in the Multicenter Diltiazem Postinfarction Trial (38). In patients with pulmonary congestion, diltiazem was associated with an increase in cardiac events, and there was a similar result in patients with low ejection fractions. However, verapamil does appear to reduce reinfarction (39), a benefit that is more marked in those without heart failure (40). Nifedipine may also have a detrimental effect in unstable angina; it certainly appears to offer no benefit (41).

A retrospective case-control study (4) has sparked controversy concerning the use of short-acting calcium channel blockers in treating hypertension. The study involved 623 cases of fatal and non-fatal myocardial infarction over a period of 8 years, and 2032 age- and sex-matched controls. The risk of myocardial infarction in patients taking calcium channel blockers was 16 per 1000, compared with 10 per 1000 in patients taking beta-blockers or thiazides. However, this result may have been an example of confounding by indication, since patients exposed to calcium channel blockers will have been more likely to have had peripheral vascular disease, lung disease (a low forced expiratory volume being a risk factor for cardiovascular disease), higher serum cholesterol concentrations, and diabetes mellitus. Careful statistical analysis was carried out in an attempt to control for some of the confounding factors, but such confounding can only be properly controlled for in a randomized study. A meta-analysis of 16 randomized secondary prevention studies in patients with coronary heart disease showed that the use of short-acting nifedipine is associated with an increased mortality in a dose-related manner (dose, risk: 30–50 mg, 1.06; 60 mg, 1.18; 80 mg, 2.83) (5). However, the event rates in this study were relatively small. A prospective cohort study in 906 elderly hypertensive patients showed that short-acting nifedipine is associated with a relative mortality risk of 1.7 compared with beta-blockers (42). After the publication of these studies, the FDA recommended that short-acting nifedipine should no longer be used in hypertension or unstable angina (43).

Disturbances of cardiac rhythm

Calcium channel blockers differ in their effects on the myocardial conduction system. Both verapamil and diltiazem have significant inhibitory effects on both sinoatrial and atrioventricular nodal function, whereas nifedipine has little or no effect. Nevertheless, nifedipine can on occasion cause troublesome bradydysrhythmias (44,45).

Severe conduction disturbances can also occur if calcium channel blockers are used in hypertrophic cardiomyopathy (46), but these drugs are used in this condition (47).

Hypotension

There are many case reports of symptomatic hypotension, usually in hypertensive patients treated with large dosages of calcium channel blockers (48,49) or in patients with myocardial infarction (50). These may represent injudicious prescribing rather than true adverse drug effects. In the DAVIT II study, 1.9% of the verapamil-treated group versus 1.6% of the placebo-treated group developed hypotension or dizziness (40); the frequency of hypotension in a randomized study of diltiazem after infarction was 0.6% in the drug-treated group and 0.2% in the placebo-treated group (37).

Respiratory

Adverse respiratory effects are uncommon with calcium channel blockers. However, three cases of acute bronchospasm accompanied by urticaria and pruritus have been reported in patients taking verapamil (51), and a patient with Duchenne-type muscular dystrophy developed respiratory failure during intravenous verapamil therapy for supraventricular tachycardia (52). Recurrent exacerbations of asthma occurred in a 66-year-old lady with hypertension and bronchial asthma given modified-release verapamil (53).

In pulmonary hypertension, both verapamil and nifedipine increase mean right atrial pressure in association with hypotension, chest pain, dyspnea, and hypoxemia; the severe hemodynamic upset resulted in cardiac arrest in two patients after verapamil and death in another after nifedipine (54). A patient with pulmonary hypertension also developed pulmonary edema whilst taking nifedipine (55) and another seems to have developed this as an allergic reaction (56).

Nervous system

Calcium channel blockers can cause parkinsonism. Of 32 patients with this complication, only three had made a full recovery 18 months after withdrawal; patients under 73 years of age tended to have a better prognosis (57). It is not known if these patients would have developed parkinsonism in any case, and whether the drugs merely act as precipitants.

Calcium channel blockers can worsen myasthenic syndromes. Myasthenia gravis can deteriorate with oral verapamil (58). A patient with Lambert–Eaton syndrome and a small-cell carcinoma of the lung developed respiratory failure within hours of starting treatment with verapamil for atrial flutter, and required assisted ventilation (59). Only after verapamil had been withdrawn did breathing improve. Verapamil affects calcium channels in nerve membranes in animals, but the experimental concentrations used exceeded those found in clinical practice (59). Thus, the evidence for a drug-related effect is circumstantial. In another case, diltiazem triggered Lambert–Eaton syndrome, which improved with drug withdrawal (60).

Sensory systems

Eyes

Painful eyes occurred in 14% of patients taking nifedipine compared with 9% in captopril-treated patients in a postmarketing surveillance study (61). The mechanism is unknown but is not via ocular vasodilatation (62).

Taste

Transient disturbances of taste and smell, without other signs of neurological deficit, have been reported after nifedipine and diltiazem. The time to the onset of symptoms after nifedipine varied from days to months, and symptoms regressed within 24 hours of withdrawal (63). With diltiazem the effect gradually abated over 10 weeks, despite continuation of therapy (64).

Psychological, psychiatric

A patient taking diltiazem developed the signs and symptoms of mania (65) and another developed mania with psychotic features (66). There have also been reports that nifedipine can cause agitation, tremor, belligerence, and depression (67), and that verapamil can cause toxic delirium (68). Nightmares and visual hallucinations have been associated with nifedipine (69). Depression has been reported as a possible adverse effect of nifedipine (70).

Some reports have suggested that calcium channel blockers may be associated with an increased incidence of depression or suicide. However, there is a paucity of evidence from large-scale studies. A study of the rates of depression with calcium channel blockers, using data from prescription event monitoring, involved gathering information on symptoms or events in large cohorts of patients after the prescription of lisinopril, enalapril, nicardipine, and diltiazem by general practitioners (71). The crude overall rates of depression during treatment were 1.89, 1.92, and 1.62 per 1000 patient-months for the ACE inhibitors, diltiazem, and nicardipine respectively. Using the ACE inhibitors as the reference group, the rate ratios for depression were 1.07 (95% CI = 0.82, 1.40) and 0.86 (0.69, 1.08) for diltiazem and nicardipine respectively. This study does not support the hypothesis that calcium channel blockers are associated with depression.

Endocrine

In six hypertensive patients given nitrendipine 20 mg/day for 30 days, there was inhibition of aldosterone response but no significant change in ACTH secretion in response to corticotrophin-releasing hormone (72).

The calcium-dependent pathway of aldosterone synthesis in the zona glomerulosa is blocked by calcium channel blockers, producing a negative feedback increase in the pituitary secretion of ACTH, which in turn causes hyperplasia of the zona glomerulosa. This leads to increased production of androgenic steroid intermediate products and subsequently testosterone, which acts on gingival cells and matrix, giving rise to gingival hyperplasia (see the section on Mouth and teeth).

Metabolism

Calcium transport is essential for insulin secretion, which is therefore inhibited by calcium channel blockers (73).

Despite this, calcium channel blockers generally have minimal effects on glucose tolerance in both healthy and diabetic subjects. Oral glucose tolerance is not affected by verapamil, and basal blood glucose concentrations were not altered during long-term verapamil administration (74). Similarly, neither nifedipine nor nicardipine produced significant hyperglycemic effects in either diabetic or non-diabetic patients (75–77). In 117 hypertensive patients nifedipine caused a significant rise in mean random blood glucose of only 0.3 mmol/l (78), an effect that was clearly of no clinical relevance. In the Treatment of Mild Hypertension Study, 4 years of monotherapy with amlodipine maleate caused no change compared with placebo in the serum glucose of 114 hypertensive patients (79). In a review (80) it was concluded that in usual dosages calcium channel blockers do not alter glucose handling. However, in a few patients diabetes appeared de novo or worsened considerably on starting nifedipine (78,81), so there may be a small risk in some individuals.

Fluid balance

Edema of the legs is a well-recognized reaction to nifedipine and also occurs with verapamil, diltiazem, and the long-acting dihydropyridines (82,83), suggesting that this is a class effect of calcium channel blockers.

Hematologic

Calcium channel blockers rarely cause hematological effects. A hemorrhagic diathesis, including impaired platelet function, develops in chronic renal insufficiency, in which calcium channel blockers are used widely as antihypertensive agents. In 156 patients with moderate to severe chronic renal insufficiency not on hemodialysis calcium channel blockers prolonged the bleeding time (OR = 3.52; 95% CI = 1.01, 12.3) (84). However, despite this effect, there were no clinically serious hemorrhagic events during the study. Among those taking calcium channel blockers, 21 patients with prolonged bleeding times were randomly assigned to two groups; in one group treatment was withdrawn and bleeding time shortened; in those who continued to take the treatment the bleeding time was unchanged.

Nifedipine has been reported to cause agranulocytosis (85) and leukopenia was attributed to diltiazem; the latter patient had scleroderma, active rheumatoid disease, and pulmonary fibrosis, but the white cell count fell after 3 weeks of diltiazem, recovered on withdrawal, and fell on rechallenge (86). Diltiazem has also been reported to cause immune thrombocytopenia in a 68-year-old man with angina (87).

Mouth and teeth

Gingival hyperplasia, similar to that seen with phenytoin and ciclosporin, is a rare but well-recognized adverse effect of nifedipine (88). It has also been reported in patients taking felodipine (89,90), nitrendipine (SEDA-16, 200), and verapamil (91), suggesting that this adverse effect is a class effect. Only one case of gingival hyperplasia related to calcium channel blockers was reported to the Norwegian Adverse Drug Reaction Committee up to 1991, despite their widespread use (92). However, subclinical gingival hyperplasia on tissue histology was found in 83 and 74% of patients taking nifedipine and diltiazem respectively (93). The reaction generally occurs within a few months of starting treatment, and in some cases drug withdrawal produces marked regression of clinical hyperplasia. The mechanism of this adverse effect is unclear, but has been proposed to involve a hormonal imbalance in the hypothalamic–pituitary–adrenal axis (94).

Periodontal disease has been assessed in 911 patients taking calcium channel blockers, of whom 442 were taking nifedipine, 181 amlodipine, and 186 diltiazem, and in 102 control subjects (95). There was significant gingival overgrowth in 6.3% of the subjects taking nifedipine, while the prevalence induced by amlodipine or diltiazem was not significantly different than in the controls. The severity of overgrowth in the nifedipine group was related to the amount of gingival inflammation and also to sex, men being three times as likely to develop overgrowth than women.

Gastrointestinal

Because of effects on smooth muscle, the calcium channel blockers (particularly verapamil (96) but also diltiazem) can cause constipation. This may be due to colonic motor activity inhibition (97). Gastroesophageal reflux can also occur, and the calcium channel blockers should be avoided in patients with symptoms suggestive of reflux esophagitis (98). Calcium channel blockers (verapamil, diltiazem, and nifedipine) can also be associated with an increased incidence of gastrointestinal bleeding, as reported in a prospective cohort study in 1636 older hypertensives, with a relative risk of 1.86 (95% CI = 1.22, 2.82) compared with beta-blockers (7). However, this finding was not confirmed in other retrospective studies (13,99,100).

Liver

Mild hepatic reactions have been observed in association with verapamil, nifedipine (101–104), and diltiazem (105,106). In some cases fever, chills, and sweating have been associated with right upper quadrant pain, hepatomegaly, and mild increases in serum bilirubin and transaminase activity; in others, patients have remained asymptomatic. One patient had granulomatous hepatitis with diltiazem (107); another had a periportal infiltrate rich in eosinophils while taking verapamil (108). The increase in liver enzyme activities is generally transient, although mild persistent abnormalities have been seen. Occasionally, extreme increases in hepatic enzyme activities have been reported (85,105). Their frequency appears to be low, and since the symptoms and signs are mild they could easily be overlooked.

Skin

Apart from minor flushing and leg erythema associated with edema, skin reactions with calcium channel blockers are infrequent; the frequency has been estimated at 1.3% for diltiazem (109).

An erythematous rash with painful edema has been described with nifedipine (110) and also with diltiazem, but without the edematous element (109).

Mild erythema multiforme and Stevens–Johnson syndrome have been reported as probable reactions to diltiazem (85) and long-acting nifedipine (111).

Nifedipine, verapamil, and diltiazem have all been implicated as possible causes of erythema multiforme and its variants, Stevens–Johnson syndrome and toxic epidermal necrolysis, and/or exfoliative dermatitis from FDA data (112).

Psoriasiform eruptions have been reported in patients taking verapamil and nicardipine (SEDA-16, 199).

Photo-induced annular or papulosquamous eruptions due to subacute cutaneous lupus erythematosus with positive antinuclear, anti-Ro, and anti-La antibodies have been reported with verapamil, nifedipine, and diltiazem (113).

Reproductive system

Calcium channel blockers can occasionally cause menorrhagia (114) and gynecomastia (115).

Immunologic

Verapamil, nifedipine, and diltiazem have all been associated with allergic reactions, including skin eruptions and effects on liver and kidney function. Nifedipine has also been reported to cause a febrile reaction (116), and diltiazem was associated with fever, lymphadenopathy, hepatosplenomegaly, an erythematous maculopapular rash, and eosinophilia in a 50-year-old man (117).

Long-Term Effects

Drug withdrawal

The possibility of a calcium antagonist withdrawal syndrome has been raised (118–127), as it has been reported that withdrawal of verapamil, nifedipine, and diltiazem can worsen angina or even cause myocardial infarction. However, in a randomized, double-blind study of withdrawal of nifedipine in 81 patients before coronary artery bypass surgery, angina at rest occurred only in patients who had experienced similar symptoms previously, and there were no early untoward effects of drug withdrawal (120). If a withdrawal syndrome does exist, it could be due to rebound coronary vasospasm, but the present weight of evidence suggests that withdrawal results in no more than the loss of a useful therapeutic effect or the unmasking of progressive disease (127).

Tumorigenicity

A retrospective cohort study in 5052 elderly subjects, of whom 451 were taking verapamil, diltiazem, or nifedipine, showed that these drugs were associated with a cancer risk of 1.72 (95% CI = 1.27, 2.34), and there was a significant dose–response relation (8). A small risk of cancer (RR = 1.27; 95% CI = 0.98, 1.63) with calcium channel blockers was reported in a nested case-control retrospective study involving 446 cases of cancers in hypertensive patients (128). However, the authors concluded that this finding may have been spurious, as there was no relation between the cancer risk and the duration of drug use. Another study did not show any excess cancer risk with short-acting nifedipine after myocardial infarction in patients followed up for 10 years, although there were only 22 cancer deaths in 2607 patients (129). Neither did the much larger Bezafibrate Infarction Prevention (BIP) Study, which reported cancer incidence data in 11 575 patients followed for a mean period of 5.2 years, with 246 incident cancer cases, 129 among users (2.3%) and 117 (2.1%) among non-users of calcium channel blockers (130). Others also failed to find a positive link between calcium channel blockers and cancer (14,131). However, elderly women taking estrogens and short-acting calcium channel blockers had a significantly increased risk of breast carcinoma (hazard ratio = 8.48; 95% CI = 2.99, 24) (132). This controversy can perhaps only be resolved by prospective studies with longer follow-up periods (133), although ideal studies are unlikely ever to be conducted.

Second-Generation Effects

Pregnancy

The calcium channel blockers have had very limited use in pregnancy. The absence of reports of fetal deaths, malformations, or other maternal or neonatal adverse effects cannot therefore be construed as indicating safety. However, a comparison of nifedipine and hydralazine in 54 patients with severe pre-eclampsia showed that nifedipine is more effective, allowing delivery of more mature infants (134).

- Modified-release nifedipine 40 mg tds caused marked hypotension when used to delay preterm labor in a previously healthy 29-year-old woman who started contracting at 29 weeks; the hypotension may have precipitated an uncomplicated non-Q-wave myocardial infarction (135).

When nifedipine is combined with intravenous magnesium to delay preterm labor, colonic pseudo-obstruction can occur (136).

Lactation

Both verapamil (137) and diltiazem (138) are excreted in breast milk, but the risk to the suckling infant is unclear.

Susceptibility Factors

Patients with impaired function of the sinus node or impaired atrioventricular conduction can develop sinus bradycardia, sinus arrest, heart block, hypotension and shock, and even asystole, with verapamil (139) or diltiazem. These drugs should not be given to patients with aberrant conduction pathways associated with broad-complex tachydysrhythmias, and they can cause severe conduction disturbances in hypertrophic cardiomyopathy.

Similarly, verapamil should be used with caution in patients with heart failure, and both diltiazem and nifedipine can cause problems in patients with poor cardiac reserve. However, the PRAISE study (18) suggested that amlodipine may be used safely, even in the presence of severe heart failure optimally treated with diuretics, digoxin, and ACE inhibitors. In this study, amlodipine significantly reduced cardiac mortality by more than a third in non-ischemic dilated cardiomyopathy, without significantly affecting mortality in ischemic cardiomyopathy (140).

Calcium antagonists should be avoided when possible in the peri-infarction period.

The use of calcium channel blockers in patients with pulmonary hypertension has been associated with cardiac arrest and sudden death.

Caution should be exercised in using verapamil in patients with hepatic cirrhosis, as its metabolism is reduced, leading to high plasma concentrations and potential toxicity (SEDA-16, 198). Similarly, lower starting and maintenance doses of other calcium channel blockers should be used in the presence of liver impairment. This also applies to patients with chronic renal insufficiency, especially those taking the modified-release formulation of verapamil (SEDA-17, 238).

Drug Administration

Drug overdose

The treatment of overdosage with calcium channel blockers has been reviewed (141); other reports have reviewed poisoning with verapamil (142–144), and other calcium channel blockers (145,146).

The features appear to be arterial hypotension, bradycardia due to sinus node depression and atrioventricular block, and congestive cardiac failure and angina (147–149). Although the therapeutic effects are different according to the drug, in overdosage the effects are similar (145). Severe metabolic acidosis (usually lactic acidosis) and generalized convulsions can also occur (150) and hypoglycemia has been reported (151). Non-cardiogenic pulmonary edema has been reported with diltiazem (152) and verapamil (153). Several deaths have occurred with verapamil.

- An overdose of nifedipine 280 mg produced marked vasodilatation in a young patient with advanced renal insufficiency; it was successfully treated with intravenous calcium (154).

Treatment consists of gastric lavage, activated charcoal, and cathartics. Contrary to popular belief, significant overdosage of immediate-release verapamil can be associated with delayed absorption, as suggested by a case report, the authors of which suggested the use of repeated doses of activated charcoal (142). In severe cases total gut lavage should be considered. Intravenous calcium gluconate (155), glucagon (156), pressor amines (isoprenaline, adrenaline, or dobutamine), artificial ventilation, and cardiac pacing may all be required. Hemoperfusion does not appear to influence the clinical course, but 4-aminopyridine reversed the features of a modest accidental overdose of verapamil in a patient on maintenance hemodialysis (157). The rationale for the use of aminopyridine, an antagonist of non-depolarizing neuromuscular blocking agents, supported by prior animal experiments, was the enhancement of transmembrane calcium flux and the facilitation of synaptic transmission. This is of potential value, in view of the apparent unresponsiveness of some patients to supportive measures.

Five cases of overdose of calcium channel blockers have been reported (158):

- a 34-year-old woman who took amlodipine 0.86 mg/kg;
- a 48-year-old man who took an unknown amount of modified-release diltiazem;
- a 5-month-old girl inadvertently given nifedipine 20 mg;
- a 14-year-old girl who took modified-release verapamil 30 mg/kg;
- a 31-year-old man who took modified-release verapamil 71 mg/kg.

All were successfully treated with hyperinsulinemia/euglycemia therapy. The authors described the mechanism of action of this form of therapy, which is mainly related to improvement in cardiac contractility and peripheral vascular resistance and reversal of acidosis. They proposed indications and dosing for this therapy consisting in most cases of intravenous glucose with an intravenous bolus dose of insulin 1 U/kg followed by an infusion of 0.5–1 U/kg/hour until the systolic blood pressure is over 100 mm/Hg and the heart rate over 50/minute. Hyperinsulinemia/euglycemia therapy is currently reserved as an adjunct to conventional therapy and is recommended only after an inadequate response to fluid resuscitation, high-dose calcium salts, and pressor agents.

Drug–Drug Interactions

Beta-adrenoceptor antagonists

The greatest potential for serious mishap arises from interactions between calcium channel blockers (especially verapamil and related compounds) and beta-adrenoceptor antagonists (159,160). This combination can cause severe hypotension and cardiac failure, particularly in patients with poor myocardial function (161–163). The major risk appears to be associated with the intravenous administration of verapamil to patients who are already taking a beta-blocker (164), but a drug-like tiapamil, which closely resembles verapamil in its pharmacological profile, might be expected to carry a similar risk (165). Conversely, intravenous diltiazem does not produce deleterious hemodynamic effects in patients taking long-term propranolol (166). However, there have been instances when the combination of diltiazem with metoprolol caused sinus arrest and atrioventricular block (167).

The concurrent use of oral calcium channel blockers and beta-adrenoceptor antagonists in the management of angina pectoris or hypertension is less likely to result in heart block or other serious adverse effects (168), and these two drug groups are commonly used together. However, caution is still advised, and nifedipine or other dihydropyridine derivatives would be preferred in this type of combination (26,169,170). Nevertheless, the combination of nifedipine with atenolol in patients with stable intermittent claudication resulted in a reduction in walking distance and skin temperature, whereas either drug alone produced benefits (171).

Carbamazepine

A pharmacokinetic interaction has been described between carbamazepine and the calcium channel blockers verapamil (172) and diltiazem (173). With both drugs, inhibition of the hepatic metabolism of carbamazepine resulted in increased serum carbamazepine concentrations and neurotoxicity, with dizziness, nausea, ataxia, and diplopia. Adding nifedipine to carbamazepine was not associated with alterations in steady-state carbamazepine concentrations (173).

Cardiac glycosides

Calcium channel blockers interact with cardiac glycosides. The main mechanism is inhibition of digoxin renal tubular secretion by inhibition of P glycoprotein. In a review of the interactions of calcium channel blockers with digoxin, in which their clinical relevance was assessed, it was concluded that serious consequences can be prevented by careful monitoring, especially in patients whose serum digoxin concentration is already near the upper end of the therapeutic range (174).

Verapamil suppresses renal digoxin elimination acutely, but this suppression disappears over a few weeks (175). However, inhibition of the extrarenal clearance of digoxin persists, and the result of this complex interaction is an increase in steady-state plasma digoxin concentrations of less than 100%. Patients taking both drugs should be carefully monitored. However, the pharmacodynamic effects of digoxin are apparently reduced by verapamil (176), so that dosage adjustment may be unnecessary. Cardiovascular collapse and/or asystole has followed the use of intravenous verapamil in patients taking oral digoxin alone (177) or in combination with quinidine, propranolol, or disopyramide (165).

The interaction of digoxin with nifedipine increases plasma digoxin concentrations by only about 15% (178,179) and is less important.

Diltiazem increases digoxin concentrations by 20–50% (180,181).

Interactions of digoxin with nitrendipine (182) and bepridil (183) have also been described.

Verapamil and diltiazem, but not nifedipine, increase steady-state plasma digitoxin concentrations (184).

Ciclosporin

Calcium channel blockers are given to transplant patients for their protective effect against ciclosporin-induced nephrotoxicity and to optimize ciclosporin immunosuppression in order to reduce early rejection of renal grafts. Nifedipine has been used to treat ciclosporin-induced hypertension, although amlodipine may be just as effective (185).

However, some calcium channel blockers have pharmacokinetic interactions: diltiazem, verapamil, nicardipine, and amlodipine increase ciclosporin concentrations, whereas nifedipine, felodipine, and isradipine do not (SED-14, 604) (SEDA-21, 210) (SEDA-21, 212) (SEDA-22, 216). Two confirmations of these observations have been published. In a retrospective study of 103 transplant patients verapamil and diltiazem, but not nifedipine or isradipine, caused a significant increase in plasma ciclosporin concentrations (186). The effect of verapamil and diltiazem on ciclosporin concentrations was independent of dosage. In a crossover comparison between verapamil, felodipine, and isradipine in 22 renal transplant recipients, verapamil interacted pharmacokinetically with ciclosporin but felodipine and isradipine did not (187).

Nine kidney transplant recipients had an increase in trough whole blood ciclosporin concentrations of 24–341% after introduction of nicardipine (188). A similar interaction has been reported with diltiazem (189) and verapamil (190).

Cimetidine

The histamine H_2 receptor antagonist cimetidine increases plasma concentrations of nifedipine and delays its elimination by inhibition of hepatic mono-oxygenases. Maximum plasma nifedipine concentrations and AUC can be increased by as much as 80%, and this results in a significant increase in the antihypertensive and antianginal effects of nifedipine and also toxicity (191,192).

Cimetidine also increases plasma concentrations of nitrendipine and nisoldipine (182,193).

Ranitidine, which inhibits the microsomal mono-oxygenase system only slightly, does not alter plasma dihydropyridine concentrations to the same extent (194).

Combinations of calcium channel blockers

Paralytic ileus has been attributed to the combined use of diltiazem and nifedipine (195).

- A 62-year-old man with chest pain underwent cardiac catheterization. The diagnosis was vasospastic angina and he was given nifedipine 20 mg bd; when his angina attacks persisted he was also given oral diltiazem 100 mg bd. After 2 days, although his angina was well controlled, abdominal distension and vomiting occurred, and an X-ray suggested intestinal ileus. The drugs were withdrawn and the ileus resolved. It recurred when the treatment was resumed and gradually resolved again after withdrawal.

The disorder was suspected to be due to enhanced pharmacodynamic effects caused by the combination of the two calcium channel blockers. However, plasma concentrations of nifedipine have also been reported to increase about three-fold when it is combined with diltiazem (196).

Dantrolene

Dantrolene interacts with verapamil and with diltiazem, causing myocardial depression and cardiogenic shock (SEDA-16, 199).

Grapefruit juice

The ability of grapefruit to increase the plasma concentrations of some drugs was accidentally discovered when grapefruit juice was used as a blinding agent in a drug interaction study of felodipine and alcohol (197). It was noticed that plasma concentrations of felodipine were much higher when the drug was taken with grapefruit juice than those previously reported for the dose of drug administered. In other studies concurrent administration of grapefruit juice and felodipine increased the AUC, causing increased heart rate, and reduced diastolic blood pressure (198), or caused increased blood pressure and heart rate, headaches, flushing, and light-headedness (199). Grapefruit increases plasma concentrations of nifedipine (200) and nisoldipine (201) by increasing their systemic availability (202); with nisoldipine or nitrendipine there was an increase in heart rate.

Prazosin

An interaction of prazosin with nifedipine or verapamil resulted in acute hypotension (203,204). The mechanism appears to be partly kinetic (the systemic availability of prazosin increasing by 60%) and partly dynamic.

Theophylline

Theophylline toxicity has been reported in several patients, apparently stabilized on theophylline, after the introduction of verapamil (205) or nifedipine (206).

References

1. Committee on Safety of Medicines. Perhexiline maleate (Pexid): adverse reactions. Curr Probl 1983;11.
2. Po AL, Zhang WY. What lessons can be learnt from withdrawal of mibefradil from the market? Lancet 1998;351(9119):1829–30.
3. Wood AJ. Calcium antagonists. Pharmacologic differences and similarities. Circulation 1989;80(Suppl 6):IV184–8.
4. Psaty BM, Heckbert SR, Koepsell TD, Siscovick DS, Raghunathan TE, Weiss NS, Rosendaal FR, Lemaitre RN, Smith NL, Wahl PW, et al. The risk of myocardial infarction associated with antihypertensive drug therapies. JAMA 1995;274(8):620–5.
5. Furberg CD, Psaty BM, Meyer JV. Nifedipine. Dose-related increase in mortality in patients with coronary heart disease. Circulation 1995;92(5):1326–31.
6. Grossman E, Messerli FH. Calcium antagonists in cardiovascular disease: a necessary controversy but an unnecessary panic. Am J Med 1997;102(2):147–9.
7. Pahor M, Guralnik JM, Furberg CD, Carbonin P, Havlik R. Risk of gastrointestinal haemorrhage with calcium antagonists in hypertensive persons over 67 years old. Lancet 1996;347(9008):1061–5.
8. Pahor M, Guralnik JM, Ferrucci L, Corti MC, Salive ME, Cerhan JR, Wallace RB, Havlik RJ. Calcium-channel blockade and incidence of cancer in aged populations. Lancet 1996;348(9026):493–7.
9. Stelfox HT, Chua G, O'Rourke K, Detsky AS. Conflict of interest in the debate over calcium-channel antagonists. N Engl J Med 1998;338(2):101–6.
10. Alderman MH, Cohen H, Roque R, Madhavan S. Effect of long-acting and short-acting calcium antagonists on cardiovascular outcomes in hypertensive patients. Lancet 1997;349(9052):594–8.
11. McMurray J, Murdoch D. Calcium-antagonist controversy: the long and short of it? Lancet 1997;349(9052):585–6.
12. Estacio RO, Jeffers BW, Hiatt WR, Biggerstaff SL, Gifford N, Schrier RW. The effect of nisoldipine as compared with enalapril on cardiovascular outcomes in patients with non-insulin-dependent diabetes and hypertension. N Engl J Med 1998;338(10):645–52.
13. Garcia Rodriguez LA, Cattaruzzi C, Troncon MG, Agostinis L. Risk of hospitalization for upper gastrointestinal tract bleeding associated with ketorolac, other non-steroidal anti-inflammatory drugs, calcium antagonists, and other antihypertensive drugs. Arch Intern Med 1998;158(1):33–9.
14. Rosenberg L, Rao RS, Palmer JR, Strom BL, Stolley PD, Zauber AG, Warshauer ME, Shapiro S. Calcium channel blockers and the risk of cancer. JAMA 1998;279(13):1000–4.
15. Stone PH, Gibson RS, Glasser SP, DeWood MA, Parker JD, Kawanishi DT, Crawford MH, Messineo FC, Shook TL, Raby K, et al. Comparison of propranolol, diltiazem, and nifedipine in the treatment of ambulatory ischemia in patients with stable angina. Differential effects on ambulatory ischemia, exercise performance, and anginal symptoms. The ASIS Study Group. Circulation 1990;82(6):1962–72.
16. Maseri A. Medical therapy of chronic stable angina pectoris. Circulation 1990;82(6):2258–62.
17. Psaty BM, Koepsell TD, LoGerfo JP, Wagner EH, Inui TS. Beta-blockers and primary prevention of coronary heart disease in patients with high blood pressure. JAMA 1989;261(14):2087–94.
18. Packer M, O'Connor CM, Ghali JK, Pressler ML, Carson PE, Belkin RN, Miller AB, Neuberg GW, Frid D, Wertheimer JH, Cropp AB, DeMets DL. Effect of amlodipine on morbidity and mortality in severe chronic heart failure. Prospective Randomized Amlodipine Survival Evaluation Study Group. N Engl J Med 1996; 335(15):1107–14.
19. Vetrovec GW, Parker VE. Alternative medical treatment for patients with angina pectoris and adverse reactions to beta blockers. Usefulness of nifedipine. Am J Med 1986;81(4A):20–7.
20. Andersson KE. Effects of calcium and calcium antagonists on the excitation-contraction coupling in striated and smooth muscle. Acta Pharmacol Toxicol (Copenh) 1978;43(Suppl 1):5–14.
21. Jones RI, Hornung RS, Sonecha T, Raftery EB. The effect of a new calcium channel blocker nicardipine on 24-hour ambulatory blood pressure and the pressor response to isometric and dynamic exercise. J Hypertens 1983; 1(1):85–9.
22. Stoepel K, Deck K, Corsing C, Ingram C, Vanov SK. Safety aspects of long-term nitrendipine therapy. J Cardiovasc Pharmacol 1984;6(Suppl 7):S1063–6.
23. Dubois C, Blanchard D, Loria Y, Moreau M. Clinical trial of new antihypertensive drug nicardipine: efficacy and tolerance in 29,104 patients. Curr Ther Res 1987;42:727.
24. Sorkin EM, Clissold SP. Nicardipine. A review of its pharmacodynamic and pharmacokinetic properties, and therapeutic efficacy, in the treatment of angina pectoris, hypertension and related cardiovascular disorders. Drugs 1987;33(4):296–345.
25. Sundstedt CD, Ruegg PC, Keller A, Waite R. A multicenter evaluation of the safety, tolerability, and efficacy of isradipine in the treatment of essential hypertension. Am J Med 1989;86(4A):98–102.
26. DeWood MA, Wolbach RA. Randomized double-blind comparison of side effects of nicardipine and nifedipine in angina pectoris. The Nicardipine Investigators Group. Am Heart J 1990;119(2 Pt 2):468–78.
27. Cheer SM, Mc Clellan K. Manidipine: a review of its use in hypertension. Drugs 2001;61(12):1777–99.
28. Matsumoto S, Ito T, Sada T, Takahashi M, Su KM, Ueda A, Okabe F, Sato M, Sekine I, Ito Y. Hemodynamic effects of nifedipine in congestive heart failure. Am J Cardiol 1980;46(3):476–80.
29. Gillmer DJ, Kark P. Pulmonary oedema precipitated by nifedipine. BMJ 1980;280(6229):1420–1.
30. Subramanian B, Bowles MJ, Davies AB, Raftery EB. Combined therapy with verapamil and propranolol in chronic stable angina. Am J Cardiol 1982;49(1):125–32.
31. Bassan M, Weiler-Ravell D, Shalev O. Additive antianginal effect of verapamil in patients receiving propranolol. BMJ (Clin Res Ed) 1982;284(6322):1067–70.

32. Terry RW. Nifedipine therapy in angina pectoris: evaluation of safety and side effects. Am Heart J 1982; 104(3):681–9.
33. Yusuf S, Wittes J, Friedman L. Overview of results of randomized clinical trials in heart disease. I. Treatments following myocardial infarction. JAMA 1988; 260(14):2088–93.
34. Goldbourt U, Behar S, Reicher-Reiss H, Zion M, Mandelzweig L, Kaplinsky E. Early administration of nifedipine in suspected acute myocardial infarction. The Secondary Prevention Reinfarction Israel Nifedipine Trial 2 Study. Arch Intern Med 1993;153(3):345–53.
35. Held PH, Yusuf S, Furberg CD. Calcium channel blockers in acute myocardial infarction and unstable angina: an overview. BMJ 1989;299(6709):1187–92.
36. Held PH, Yusuf S. Effects of beta-blockers and calcium channel blockers in acute myocardial infarction. Eur Heart J 1993;14(Suppl F):18–25.
37. Gibson RS, Boden WE, Theroux P, Strauss HD, Pratt CM, Gheorghiade M, Capone RJ, Crawford MH, Schlant RC, Kleiger RE, et al. Diltiazem and reinfarction in patients with non-Q-wave myocardial infarction. Results of a double-blind, randomized, multicenter trial. N Engl J Med 1986;315(7):423–9.
38. The Multicenter Diltiazem Postinfarction Trial Research Group. The effect of diltiazem on mortality and reinfarction after myocardial infarction. N Engl J Med 1988; 319(7):385–92.
39. The Danish Study Group on Verapamil in Myocardial Infarction. Verapamil in acute myocardial infarction. Eur Heart J 1984;5(7):516–28.
40. The Danish Verapamil Infarction Trial II—DAVIT II. Effect of verapamil on mortality and major events after acute myocardial infarction. Am J Cardiol 1990; 66(10):779–85.
41. Lubsen J, Tijssen JGP, Kerkkamp HJJ. Early treatment of unstable angina in the coronary care unit: a randomised, double blind, placebo controlled comparison of recurrent ischaemia in patients treated with nifedipine or metoprolol or both. Report of The Holland Interuniversity Nifedipine/Metoprolol Trial (HINT) Research Group. Br Heart J 1986;56(5):400–13.
42. Pahor M, Guralnik JM, Corti MC, Foley DJ, Carbonin P, Havlik RJ. Long-term survival and use of antihypertensive medications in older persons. J Am Geriatr Soc 1995;43(11):1191–7.
43. Barnett AA. News. Lancet 1996;347:313.
44. Zangerle KF, Wolford R. Syncope and conduction disturbances following sublingual nifedipine for hypertension. Ann Emerg Med 1985;14(10):1005–6.
45. Villani GQ, del Giudice S, Arruzzoli S, Dieci G. Blocco seno-atriale dopo somministrazione orale di nifedipina. Descrizione di un caso. [Sinoatrial block after oral administration of nifedipine. Description of a case.] Minerva Cardioangiol 1985;33(9):557–9.
46. Epstein SE, Rosing DR. Verapamil: its potential for causing serious complications in patients with hypertrophic cardiomyopathy. Circulation 1981;64(3):437–41.
47. Hopf R, Rodrian S, Kaltenbach M. Behandlung der hypertrophen Kardiomyopathie mit Kalziumantagonisten. Therapiewoche 1986;36:1433.
48. Wachter RM. Symptomatic hypotension induced by nifedipine in the acute treatment of severe hypertension. Arch Intern Med 1987;147(3):556–8.
49. Schwartz M, Naschitz JE, Yeshurun D, Sharf B. Oral nifedipine in the treatment of hypertensive urgency: cerebrovascular accident following a single dose. Arch Intern Med 1990;150(3):686–7.
50. Shettigar UR, Loungani R. Adverse effects of sublingual nifedipine in acute myocardial infarction. Crit Care Med 1989;17(2):196–7.
51. Graham CF. Intravenous verapamil-isotopin (Calan): acute bronchospasm. ADR Highlights 1982;868:82.
52. Zalman F, Perloff JK, Durant NN, Campion DS. Acute respiratory failure following intravenous verapamil in Duchenne's muscular dystrophy. Am Heart J 1983;105(3):510–11.
53. Ben-Noun L. Acute asthma associated with sustained-release verapamil. Ann Pharmacother 1997;31(5):593–5.
54. Packer M, Medina N, Yushak M. Adverse hemodynamic and clinical effects of calcium channel blockade in pulmonary hypertension secondary to obliterative pulmonary vascular disease. J Am Coll Cardiol 1984; 4(5):890–901.
55. Batra AK, Segall PH, Ahmed T. Pulmonary edema with nifedipine in primary pulmonary hypertension. Respiration 1985;47(3):161–3.
56. Hasebe N, Fijikana T, Wantanabe M, et al. A case of respiratory failure precipitated by injecting nifedipine. Kokya To Junkan 1988;36:1255.
57. Garcia-Ruiz PJ, Garcia de Yebenes J, Jimenez-Jimenez FJ, Vazquez A, Garcia Urra D, Morales B. Parkinsonism associated with calcium channel blockers: a prospective follow-up study. Clin Neuropharmacol 1992;15(1):19–26.
58. Swash M, Ingram DA. Adverse effect of verapamil in myasthenia gravis. Muscle Nerve 1992;15(3):396–8.
59. Krendel DA, Hopkins LC. Adverse effect of verapamil in a patient with the Lambert–Eaton syndrome. Muscle Nerve 1986;9(6):519–22.
60. Ueno S, Hara Y. Lambert–Eaton myasthenic syndrome without anti-calcium channel antibody: adverse effect of calcium antagonist diltiazem. J Neurol Neurosurg Psychiatry 1992;55(5):409–10.
61. Coulter DM. Eye pain with nifedipine and disturbance of taste with captopril: a mutually controlled study showing a method of postmarketing surveillance. BMJ (Clin Res Ed) 1988;296(6629):1086–8.
62. Kelly SP, Walley TJ. Eye pain with nifedipine. BMJ (Clin Res Ed) 1988;296(6633):1401.
63. Levenson JL, Kennedy K. Dysosmia, dysgeusia, and nifedipine. Ann Intern Med 1985;102(1):135–6.
64. Berman JL. Dysosmia, dysgeusia and diltiazem. Ann Intern Med 1985;103:154.
65. Brink DD. Diltiazem and hyperactivity. Ann Intern Med 1984;100(3):459–60.
66. Ahmad S. Nifedipine-induced acute psychosis. J Am Geriatr Soc 1984;32(5):408.
67. Palat GK, Hooker EA, Movahed A. Secondary mania associated with diltiazem. Clin Cardiol 1984;7(11):611–12.
68. Jacobsen FM, Sack DA, James SP. Delirium induced by verapamil. Am J Psychiatry 1987;144(2):248.
69. Pitlik S, Manor RS, Lipshitz I, Perry G, Rosenfeld J. Transient retinal ischaemia induced by nifedipine. BMJ (Clin Res Ed) 1983;287(6408):1845–6.
70. Eccleston D, Cole AJ. Calcium-channel blockade and depressive illness. Br J Psychiatry 1990;156:889–91.
71. Dunn NR, Freemantle SN, Mann RD. Cohort study on calcium channel blockers, other cardiovascular agents, and the prevalence of depression. Br J Clin Pharmacol 1999;48(2):230–3.
72. Rocco S, Mantero F, Boscaro M. Effects of a calcium antagonist on the pituitary–adrenal axis. Horm Metab Res 1993;25(2):114–16.
73. Malaisse WJ, Sener A. Calcium-antagonists and islet function-XII. Comparison between nifedipine and chemically related drugs. Biochem Pharmacol 1981; 30(10):1039–41.
74. Giugliano D, Gentile S, Verza M, Passariello N, Giannetti G, Varricchio M. Modulation by verapamil of

insulin and glucagon secretion in man. Acta Diabetol Lat 1981;18(2):163–71.
75. Donnelly T, Harrower AD. Effect of nifedipine on glucose tolerance and insulin secretion in diabetic and non-diabetic patients. Curr Med Res Opin 1980;6(10):690–3.
76. Abadie E, Passa PH. Diabetogenic effect of nifedipine. BMJ (Clin Res Ed) 1984;289(6442):438.
77. Collings WCJ, Cullen MJ, Feely J. The effect of therapy with dihydropyridine calcium channel blockers on glucose tolerance in non-insulin dependent diabetes. Br J Clin Pharmacol 1986;21:568P.
78. Zezulka AV, Gill JS, Beevers DG. Diabetogenic effects of nifedipine. BMJ (Clin Res Ed) 1984;289(6442):437–8.
79. Neaton JD, Grimm RH Jr, Prineas RJ, Stamler J, Grandits GA, Elmer PJ, Cutler JA, Flack JM, Schoenberger JA, McDonald R, et al. Treatment of Mild Hypertension Study. Final results. Treatment of Mild Hypertension Study Research Group. JAMA 1993; 270(6):713–24.
80. Trost BN. Glucose metabolism and calcium antagonists. Horm Metab Res Suppl 1990;22:48–56.
81. Bhatnagar SK, Amin MMA, Al-Yusuf AR. Diabetogenic effects of nifedipine. BMJ (Clin Res Ed) 1984;289:19.
82. Lindenberg BS, Weiner DA, McCabe CH, Cutler SS, Ryan TJ, Klein MD. Efficacy and safety of incremental doses of diltiazem for the treatment of stable angina pectoris. J Am Coll Cardiol 1983;2(6):1129–33.
83. Petru MA, Crawford MH, Sorensen SG, Chaudhuri TK, Levine S, O'Rourke RA. Short- and long-term efficacy of high-dose oral diltiazem for angina due to coronary artery disease: a placebo-controlled, randomized, double-blind crossover study. Circulation 1983; 68(1):139–47.
84. Hayashi K, Matsuda H, Honda M, Ozawa Y, Tokuyama H, Okubo K, Takamatsu I, Kanda T, Tatematsu S, Homma K, Saruta T. Impact of calcium antagonists on bleeding time in patients with chronic renal failure. J Hum Hypertens 2002;16(3):199–203.
85. Voth AJ, Turner RH. Nifedipine and agranulocytosis. Ann Intern Med 1983;99(6):882.
86. Quigley MA, White KL, McGraw BF. Interpretation and application of world-wide safety data on diltiazem. Acta Pharmacol Toxicol (Copenh) 1985;57(Suppl 2):61–73.
87. Baggott LA. Diltiazem-associated immune thrombocytopenia. Mt Sinai J Med 1987;54(6):500–4.
88. Ramon Y, Behar S, Kishon Y, Engelberg IS. Gingival hyperplasia caused by nifedipine—a preliminary report. Int J Cardiol 1984;5(2):195–206.
89. Lombardi T, Fiore-Donno G, Belser U, Di Felice R. Felodipine-induced gingival hyperplasia: a clinical and histologic study. J Oral Pathol Med 1991;20(2):89–92.
90. Young PC, Turiansky GW, Sau P, Liebman MD, Benson PM. Felodipine-induced gingival hyperplasia. Cutis 1998;62(1):41–3.
91. Cucchi G, Giustiniani S, Robustelli F. Gengivite ipertrofica da verapamil. [Hypertrophic gingivitis caused by verapamil.] G Ital Cardiol 1985;15(5):556–7.
92. Lokken P, Skomedal T. Kalsiumkanalblokkerindusert gingival hyperplasi. Sjelden, eller tusener av tilfeller i Norge? [Gingival hyperplasia induced by calcium channel blockers. Rare or frequent in Norway?] Tidsskr Nor Laegeforen 1992;112(15):1978–80.
93. Fattore L, Stablein M, Bredfeldt G, Semla T, Moran M, Doherty-Greenberg JM. Gingival hyperplasia: a side effect of nifedipine and diltiazem. Spec Care Dentist 1991; 11(3):107–9.
94. Nyska A, Shemesh M, Tal H, Dayan D. Gingival hyperplasia induced by calcium channel blockers: mode of action. Med Hypotheses 1994;43(2):115–18.
95. Ellis JS, Seymour RA, Steele JG, Robertson P, Butler TJ, Thomason JM. Prevalence of gingival overgrowth induced by calcium channel blockers: a community-based study. J Periodontol 1999;70(1):63–7.
96. Hedback B, Hermann LS. Antihypertensive effect of verapamil in patients with newly discovered mild to moderate essential hypertension. Acta Med Scand Suppl 1984;681:129–35.
97. Bassotti G, Calcara C, Annese V, Fiorella S, Roselli P, Morelli A. Nifedipine and verapamil inhibit the sigmoid colon myoelectric response to eating in healthy volunteers. Dis Colon Rectum 1998;41(3):377–80.
98. Gaginella TS, Maxfield DL. Calcium-channel blocking agents and chest pain. Drug Intell Clin Pharm 1988; 22(7–8):623–5.
99. Smalley WE, Ray WA, Daugherty JR, Griffin MR. No association between calcium channel blocker use and confirmed bleeding peptic ulcer disease. Am J Epidemiol 1998;148(4):350–4.
100. Suissa S, Bourgault C, Barkun A, Sheehy O, Ernst P. Antihypertensive drugs and the risk of gastrointestinal bleeding. Am J Med 1998;105(3):230–5.
101. Rotmensch HH, Roth A, Liron M, Rubinstein A, Gefel A, Livni E. Lymphocyte sensitisation in nifedipine-induced hepatitis. BMJ 1980;281(6246):976–7.
102. Davidson AR. Lymphocyte sensitisation in nifedipine-induced hepatitis. BMJ 1980;281(6251):1354.
103. Centrum Voor Geneesmiddelenbewaking. Nifedipine en hepatitis. Folia Pharmacother 1981;8:7.
104. Stern EH, Pitchon R, King BD, Wiener I. Possible hepatitis from verapamil. N Engl J Med 1982;306(10):612–13.
105. Tartaglione TA, Pepine CJ, Pieper JA. Diltiazem: a review of its clinical efficacy and use. Drug Intell Clin Pharm 1982;16(5):371–9.
106. McGraw BF, Walker SD, Hemberger JA, Gitomer SL, Nakama M. Clinical experience with diltiazem in Japan. Pharmacotherapy 1982;2(3):156–61.
107. Sarachek NS, London RL, Matulewicz TJ. Diltiazem and granulomatous hepatitis. Gastroenterology 1985;88(5 Pt 1):1260–2.
108. Guarascio P, D'Amato C, Sette P, Conte A, Visco G. Liver damage from verapamil. BMJ (Clin Res Ed) 1984;288(6414):362–3.
109. Wirebaugh SR, Geraets DR. Reports of erythematous macular skin eruptions associated with diltiazem therapy. DICP 1990;24(11):1046–9.
110. Grunwald Z. Painful edema, erythematous rash, and burning sensation due to nifedipine. Drug Intell Clin Pharm 1982;16(6):492.
111. Barker SJ, Bayliff CD, McCormack DG, Dilworth GR. Nifedipine-induced erythema multiforme. Can J Hosp Pharm 1996;49:160.
112. Stern R, Khalsa JH. Cutaneous adverse reactions associated with calcium channel blockers. Arch Intern Med 1989;149(4):829–32.
113. Crowson AN, Magro CM. Subacute cutaneous lupus erythematosus arising in the setting of calcium channel blocker therapy. Hum Pathol 1997;28(1):67–73.
114. Rodger JC, Torrance TC. Can nifedipine provoke menorrhagia? Lancet 1983;2(8347):460.
115. Clyne CAC. Unilateral gynaecomastia and nifedipine. BMJ (Clin Res Ed) 1986;292:380.
116. Carraway RD. Febrile reaction following nifedipine therapy. Am Heart J 1984;108(3 Pt 1):611.
117. Scolnick B, Brinberg D. Diltiazem and generalized lymphadenopathy. Ann Intern Med 1985;102(4):558.
118. Offerhaus L, Dunning AJ. Angina pectoris: variaties op het thema nifedipine. [Angina pectoris; variations on the nifedipine theme.] Ned Tijdschr Geneeskd 1980; 124(45):1928–32.

119. Pedersen OL, Mikkelsen E, Andersson KE. Paradoks angina pectoris efter nifedipin. [Paradoxal angina pectoris following nifedipine.] Ugeskr Laeger 1980;142(29):1883–4.
120. Gottlieb SO, Gerstenblith G. Safety of acute calcium antagonist withdrawal: studies in patients with unstable angina withdrawn from nifedipine. Am J Cardiol 1985; 55(12):E27–30.
121. Gottlieb SO, Ouyang P, Achuff SC, Baughman KL, Traill TA, Mellits ED, Weisfeldt ML, Gerstenblith G. Acute nifedipine withdrawal: consequences of preoperative and late cessation of therapy in patients with prior unstable angina. J Am Coll Cardiol 1984;4(2):382–8.
122. Kay R, Blake J, Rubin D. Possible coronary spasm rebound to abrupt nifedipine withdrawal. Am Heart J 1982;103(2):308.
123. Engelman RM, Hadji-Rousou I, Breyer RH, Whittredge P, Harbison W, Chircop RV. Rebound vasospasm after coronary revascularization in association with calcium antagonist withdrawal. Ann Thorac Surg 1984; 37(6):469–72.
124. Lette J, Gagnon RM, Lemire JG, Morissette M. Rebound of vasospastic angina after cessation of long-term treatment with nifedipine. Can Med Assoc J 1984;130(9):1169–74.
125. Mysliwiec M, Rydzewski A, Bulhak W. Calcium antagonist withdrawal syndrome. BMJ (Clin Res Ed) 1983; 286(6381):1898.
126. Schick EC Jr, Liang CS, Heupler FA Jr, Kahl FR, Kent KM, Kerin NZ, Noble RJ, Rubenfire M, Tabatznik B, Terry RW. Randomized withdrawal from nifedipine: placebo-controlled study in patients with coronary artery spasm. Am Heart J 1982;104(3):690–7.
127. Subramanian VB, Bowles MJ, Khurmi NS, Davies AB, O'Hara MJ, Raftery EB. Calcium antagonist withdrawal syndrome: objective demonstration with frequency-modulated ambulatory ST-segment monitoring. BMJ (Clin Res Ed) 1983;286(6364):520–1.
128. Jick H, Jick S, Derby LE, Vasilakis C, Myers MW, Meier CR. Calcium-channel blockers and risk of cancer. Lancet 1997;349(9051):525–8.
129. Jonas M, Goldbourt U, Boyko V, Mandelzweig L, Behar S, Reicher-Reiss H. Nifedipine and cancer mortality: ten-year follow-up of 2607 patients after acute myocardial infarction. Cardiovasc Drugs Ther 1998;12(2):177–81.
130. Braun S, Boyko V, Behar S, Reicher-Reiss H, Laniado S, Kaplinsky E, Goldbourt U. Calcium channel blocking agents and risk of cancer in patients with coronary heart disease. Benzafibrate Infarction Prevention (BIP) Study Research Group. J Am Coll Cardiol 1998;31(4):804–8.
131. Hole DJ, Gillis CR, McCallum IR, McInnes GT, MacKinnon PL, Meredith PA, Murray LS, Robertson JW, Lever AF. Cancer risk of hypertensive patients taking calcium antagonists. J Hypertens 1998;16(1):119–24.
132. Fitzpatrick AL, Daling JR, Furberg CD, Kronmal RA, Weissfeld JL. Use of calcium channel blockers and breast carcinoma risk in postmenopausal women. Cancer 1997;80(8):1438–47.
133. Howes LG, Edwards CT. Calcium antagonists and cancer. Is there really a link? Drug Saf 1998;18(1):1–7.
134. Fenakel K, Fenakel G, Appelman Z, Lurie S, Katz Z, Shoham Z. Nifedipine in the treatment of severe preeclampsia. Obstet Gynecol 1991;77(3):331–7.
135. Oei SG, Oei SK, Brolmann HA. Myocardial infarction during nifedipine therapy for preterm labor. N Engl J Med 1999;340(2):154.
136. Pecha RE, Danilewitz MD. Acute pseudo-obstruction of the colon (Ogilvie's syndrome) resulting from combination tocolytic therapy. Am J Gastroenterol 1996;91(6):1265–6.
137. Inove H. Excretion of verapamil in human milk. BMJ (Clin Res Ed) 1984;288(6417):645.
138. Okada M, Inoue H, Nakamura Y, Kishimoto M, Suzuki T. Excretion of diltiazem in human milk. N Engl J Med 1985;312(15):992–3.
139. Hagemeijer F. Verapamil in the management of supraventricular tachyarrhythmias occurring after a recent myocardial infarction. Circulation 1978;57(4):751–5.
140. O'Connor CM, Carson PE, Miller AB, Pressler ML, Belkin RN, Neuberg GW, Frid DJ, Cropp AB, Anderson S, Wertheimer JH, DeMets DL. Effect of amlodipine on mode of death among patients with advanced heart failure in the PRAISE trial. Prospective Randomized Amlodipine Survival Evaluation. Am J Cardiol 1998;82(7):881–7.
141. Kenny J. Treating overdose with calcium channel blockers. BMJ 1994;308(6935):992–3.
142. Buckley CD, Aronson JK. Prolonged half-life of verapamil in a case of overdose: implications for therapy. Br J Clin Pharmacol 1995;39(6):680–3.
143. Sauder P, Kopferschmitt J, Dahlet M, Tritsch L, Flesch F, Siard P, Mantz JM, Jaeger A. Les intoxications aiguës par le verapamil. A propos de 6 cas. Revue de la litterature. [Acute verapamil poisoning. 6 cases. Review of the literature.] J Toxicol Clin Exp 1990;10(4):261–70.
144. McMillan R. Management of acute severe verapamil intoxication. J Emerg Med 1988;6(3):193–6.
145. Ramoska EA, Spiller HA, Myers A. Calcium channel blocker toxicity. Ann Emerg Med 1990;19(6):649–53.
146. Howarth DM, Dawson AH, Smith AJ, Buckley N, Whyte IM. Calcium channel blocking drug overdose: an Australian series. Hum Exp Toxicol 1994;13(3):161–6.
147. Perkins CM. Serious verapamil poisoning: treatment with intravenous calcium gluconate. BMJ 1978;2(6145):1127.
148. Candell J, Valle V, Soler M, Rius J. Acute intoxication with verapamil. Chest 1979;75(2):200–1.
149. Kenney J. Calcium channel blocking agents and the heart. BMJ (Clin Res Ed) 1985;291:1150.
150. Borkje B, Omvik P, Storstein L. Fatal verapamilforgiftning. [Fatal verapamil poisoning.] Tidsskr Nor Laegeforen 1986;106(5):401–2.
151. Zogubi W, Schwartz JB. Verapamil overdose: report of a case and review of the literature. Cardiovasc Rev Rep 1984;5:356.
152. Humbert VH Jr, Munn NJ, Hawkins RF. Noncardiogenic pulmonary edema complicating massive diltiazem overdose. Chest 1991;99(1):258–9.
153. Brass BJ, Winchester-Penny S, Lipper BL. Massive verapamil overdose complicated by noncardiogenic pulmonary edema. Am J Emerg Med 1996;14(5):459–61.
154. Schiffl H, Ziupa J, Schollmeyer P. Clinical features and management of nifedipine overdosage in a patient with renal insufficiency. J Toxicol Clin Toxicol 1984;22(4):387–95.
155. Pearigen PD, Benowitz NL. Poisoning due to calcium antagonists. Experience with verapamil, diltiazem and nifedipine. Drug Saf 1991;6(6):408–30.
156. Walter FG, Frye G, Mullen JT, Ekins BR, Khasigian PA. Amelioration of nifedipine poisoning associated with glucagon therapy. Ann Emerg Med 1993;22(7):1234–7.
157. ter Wee PM, Kremer Hovinga TK, Uges DR, van der Geest S. 4-Aminopyridine and haemodialysis in the treatment of verapamil intoxication. Hum Toxicol 1985; 4(3):327–9.
158. Boyer EW, Duic PA, Evans A. Hyperinsulinemia/euglycemia therapy for calcium channel blocker poisoning. Pediatr Emerg Care 2002;18(1):36–7.
159. Klieman RL, Stephenson SH. Calcium antagonists–drug interactions. Rev Drug Metab Drug Interact 1985; 5(2–3):193–217.
160. Pringle SD, MacEwen CJ. Severe bradycardia due to interaction of timolol eye drops and verapamil. BMJ (Clin Res Ed) 1987;294(6565):155–6.

161. Opie LH, White DA. Adverse interaction between nifedipine and beta-blockade. BMJ 1980;281(6253):1462.
162. Staffurth JS, Emery P. Adverse interaction between nifedipine and beta-blockade. BMJ (Clin Res Ed) 1981;282(6259):225.
163. Anastassiades CJ. Nifedipine and beta-blocker drugs. BMJ 1980;281(6250):1251–2.
164. Young GP. Calcium channel blockers in emergency medicine. Ann Emerg Med 1984;13(9 Pt 1):712–22.
165. Saini RK, Fulmor IE, Antonaccio MJ. Effect of tiapamil and nifedepine during critical coronary stenosis and in the presence of adrenergic beta-receptor blockade in anesthetized dogs. J Cardiovasc Pharmacol 1982;4(5):770–6.
166. Rocha P, Baron B, Delestrain A, Pathe M, Cazor JL, Kahn JC. Hemodynamic effects of intravenous diltiazem in patients treated chronically with propranolol. Am Heart J 1986;111(1):62–8.
167. Kjeldsen SE, Syvertsen JO, Hedner T. Cardiac conduction with diltiazem and beta-blockade combined. A review and report on cases. Blood Press 1996;5(5):260–3.
168. Leon MB, Rosing DR, Bonow RO, Lipson LC, Epstein SE. Clinical efficacy of verapamil alone and combined with propranolol in treating patients with chronic stable angina pectoris. Am J Cardiol 1981;48(1):131–9.
169. Sorkin EM, Clissold SP, Brogden RN. Nifedipine. A review of its pharmacodynamic and pharmacokinetic properties, and therapeutic efficacy, in ischaemic heart disease, hypertension and related cardiovascular disorders. Drugs 1985;30(3):182–274.
170. Goa KL, Sorkin EM. Nitrendipine. A review of its pharmacodynamic and pharmacokinetic properties, and therapeutic efficacy in the treatment of hypertension. Drugs 1987;33(2):123–55.
171. Solomon SA, Ramsay LE, Yeo WW, Parnell L, Morris-Jones W. Beta blockade and intermittent claudication: placebo controlled trial of atenolol and nifedipine and their combination. BMJ 1991;303(6810):1100–4.
172. Macphee GJ, McInnes GT, Thompson GG, Brodie MJ. Verapamil potentiates carbamazepine neurotoxicity: a clinically important inhibitory interaction. Lancet 1986;1(8483):700–3.
173. Brodie MJ, MacPhee GJ. Carbamazepine neurotoxicity precipitated by diltiazem. BMJ (Clin Res Ed) 1986;292(6529):1170–1.
174. De Vito JM, Friedman B. Evaluation of the pharmacodynamic and pharmacokinetic interaction between calcium antagonists and digoxin. Pharmacotherapy 1986; 6(2):73–82.
175. Pedersen KE, Dorph-Pedersen A, Hvidt S, Klitgaard NA, Pedersen KK. The long-term effect of verapamil on plasma digoxin concentration and renal digoxin clearance in healthy subjects. Eur J Clin Pharmacol 1982;22(2):123–7.
176. Schwartz JB, Keefe D, Kates RE, Kirsten E, Harrison DC. Acute and chronic pharmacodynamic interaction of verapamil and digoxin in atrial fibrillation. Circulation 1982;65(6):1163–70.
177. Kounis NG. Asystole after verapamil and digoxin. Br J Clin Pract 1980;34(2):57–8.
178. Kleinbloesem CH, van Brummelen P, Hillers J, Moolenaar AJ, Breimer DD. Interaction between digoxin and nifedipine at steady state in patients with atrial fibrillation. Ther Drug Monit 1985;7(4):372–6.
179. Kirch W, Hutt HJ, Dylewicz P, Graf KJ, Ohnhaus EE. Dose-dependence of the nifedipine–digoxin interaction? Clin Pharmacol Ther 1986;39(1):35–9.
180. Oyama Y, Fujii S, Kanda K, Akino E, Kawasaki H, Nagata M, Goto K. Digoxin–diltiazem interaction. Am J Cardiol 1984;53(10):1480–1.
181. D'Arcy PF. Diltiazem–digoxin interactions. Pharm Int 1985;6:148.
182. Kirch W, Hutt HJ, Heidemann H, Ramsch K, Janisch HD, Ohnhaus EE. Drug interactions with nitrendipine. J Cardiovasc Pharmacol 1984;6(Suppl 7):S982–5.
183. Belz GG, Wistuba S, Matthews JH. Digoxin and bepridil: pharmacokinetic and pharmacodynamic interactions. Clin Pharmacol Ther 1986;39(1):65–71.
184. Kuhlmann J. Effects of verapamil, diltiazem, and nifedipine on plasma levels and renal excretion of digitoxin. Clin Pharmacol Ther 1985;38(6):667–73.
185. Venkat-Raman G, Feehally J, Elliott HL, Griffin P, Moore RJ, Olubodun JO, Wilkinson R. Renal and haemodynamic effects of amlodipine and nifedipine in hypertensive renal transplant recipients. Nephrol Dial Transplant 1998;13(10):2612–16.
186. Jacob LP, Malhotra D, Chan L, Shapiro JI. Absence of a dose-response of cyclosporine levels to clinically used doses of diltiazem and verapamil. Am J Kidney Dis 1999;33(2):301–3.
187. Yildiz A, Sever MS, Turkmen A, Ecder T, Turk S, Akkaya V, Ark E. Interaction between cyclosporine A and verapamil, felodipine, and isradipine. Nephron 1999;81(1):117–18.
188. Bourbigot B, Guiserix J, Airiau J, Bressollette L, Morin JF, Cledes J. Nicardipine increases cyclosporin blood levels. Lancet 1986;1(8495):1447.
189. Pochet JM, Pirson Y. Cyclosporin–diltiazem interaction. Lancet 1986;1(8487):979.
190. Citterio F, Serino F, Pozzetto U, Fioravanti P, Caizzi P, Castagneto M. Verapamil improves Sandimmune immunosuppression, reducing acute rejection episodes. Transplant Proc 1996;28(4):2174–6.
191. Kirch W, Janisch HD, Heidemann H, Ramsch K, Ohnhaus EE. Einfluss von Cimetidin und Ranitidin auf Pharmakokinetik und antihypertensiven Effect von Nifedipin. [Effect of cimetidine and ranitidine on the pharmacokinetics and anti-hypertensive effect of nifedipine.] Dtsch Med Wochenschr 1983;108(46):1757–61.
192. Dylewicz P, Kirch W, Benesch L, Ohnhaus EE. Influence of nifedipine with and without cimetidine on exercise tolerance in patients after myocardial infarction. In: Proceedings 6th International Adalat Symposium, Geneva, 1985. ICS 71. Amsterdam: Excerpta Medica, 1986.
193. van Harten J, van Brummelen P, Lodewijks MT, Danhof M, Breimer DD. Pharmacokinetics and hemodynamic effects of nisoldipine and its interaction with cimetidine. Clin Pharmacol Ther 1988;43(3):332–41.
194. Kirch W, Kleinbloesem CH, Belz GG. Drug interactions with calcium antagonists. Pharmacol Ther 1990;45(1):109–36.
195. Harada T, Ohtaki E, Sumiyoshi T, Hosoda S. Paralytic ileus induced by the combined use of nifedipine and diltiazem in the treatment of vasospastic angina. Cardiology 2002;97(2):113–14.
196. Toyosaki N, Toyo-oka T, Natsume T, Katsuki T, Tateishi T, Yaginuma T, Hosoda S. Combination therapy with diltiazem and nifedipine in patients with effort angina pectoris. Circulation 1988;77(6):1370–5.
197. Bailey DG, Spence JD, Edgar B, Bayliff CD, Arnold JM. Ethanol enhances the hemodynamic effects of felodipine. Clin Invest Med 1989;12(6):357–62.
198. Rodvold KA, Meyer J. Drug–food interactions with grapefruit juice. Infect Med 1996;13:868–912.
199. Feldman EB. How grapefruit juice potentiates drug bioavailability. Nutr Rev 1997;55(11 Pt 1):398–400.
200. Hashimoto Y, Kuroda T, Shimizu A, Hayakava M, Fukuzaki H, Morimoto S. Influence of grapefruit juice on plasma concentration of nifedipine. Jpn J Clin Pharmacol Ther 1996;27:599–606.
201. Azuma J, Yamamoto I, Wafase T, Orii Y, Tinigawa T, Terashima S, Yoshikawa K, Tanaka T, Kawano K.

Effects of grapefruit juice on the pharmacokinetics of the calcium channel blockers nifedipine and nisoldipine. Curr Ther Res Clin Exp 1998;59:619–34.
202. Bailey DG, Spence JD, Munoz C, Arnold JM. Interaction of citrus juices with felodipine and nifedipine. Lancet 1991;337(8736):268–9.
203. Jee LD, Opie LH. Acute hypotensive response to nifedipine added to prazosin in treatment of hypertension. BMJ (Clin Res Ed) 1983;287(6404):1514.
204. Pasanisi F, Meredith PA, Elliott HL, Reld JL. Verapamil and prazosin: pharmacodynamic and pharmacokinetic interactions in normal man. Br J Clin Pharmacol 1984; 18:290P.
205. Burnakis TG, Seldon M, Czaplicki AD. Increased serum theophylline concentrations secondary to oral verapamil. Clin Pharm 1983;2(5):458–61.
206. Parrillo SJ, Venditto M. Elevated theophylline blood levels from institution of nifedipine therapy. Ann Emerg Med 1984;13(3):216–17.

Calcium dobesilate

General Information

Calcium dobesilate is an antioxidant that has been used to treat diabetic retinopathy, in which it slows progression of the disease during long-term oral treatment by reducing microvascular permeability, leading to improved visual acuity (1). It not only acts as an antioxidant but also stimulates endothelial production of nitric oxide.

In early studies the most common adverse effects of calcium dobesilate after oral administration were gastrointestinal disturbances and, occasionally, nervousness and fever (SEDA-3, 181) (SEDA-16, 204).

In a systematic review of the published literature from 1970 to 2003, a postmarketing surveillance report covering the period 1974–1998, and periodic safety update reports covering the period 1995–2003 from the French regulatory authorities pharmacovigilance database, the following adverse effects were reported: fever (26%), gastrointestinal disorders (12.5%), skin reactions (8.2%), arthralgia (4.3%), and agranulocytosis (4.3%) (2).

Organs and Systems

Hematologic

Agranulocytosis associated with calcium dobesilate has occasionally been reported (3). Although the risk has been calculated at 121 cases per million per year from case-control and case-population studies (4), there have been many fewer spontaneous reports than are consistent with this relatively high figure, and the true incidence is unknown (5).

Drug Administration

Drug administration route

Intramuscular calcium dobesilate can be painful (SEDA-3, 181).

References

1. Berthet P, Farine JC, Barras JP. Calcium dobesilate: pharmacological profile related to its use in diabetic retinopathy. Int J Clin Pract 1999;53(8):631–6.
2. Allain H, Ramelet AA, Polard E, Bentue-Ferrer D. Safety of calcium dobesilate in chronic venous disease, diabetic retinopathy and haemorrhoids. Drug Saf 2004; 27(9):649–60.
3. Garcia Benayas E, Garcia Diaz B, Perez G. Calcium dobesilate-induced agranulocytosis. Pharm World Sci 1997;19(5):251–2.
4. Ibanez L, Ballarin E, Vidal X, Laporte JR. Agranulocytosis associated with calcium dobesilate clinical course and risk estimation with the case-control and the case-population approaches. Eur J Clin Pharmacol 2000;56(9–10):763–7.
5. Zapater P, Horga JF, Garcia A. Risk of drug-induced agranulocytosis: the case of calcium dobesilate. Eur J Clin Pharmacol 2003;58(11):767–72.

Calcium salts

General Information

Calcium is a soft grayish-white metallic element, one of the alkaline earth metals (symbol Ca; atomic no. 20). It is found in sources such as lewisite (calcium antimonate), colemanite and pandermite (calcium borates); ankerite, aragonite, calcite, chalk, dolomite, and stromatolite (calcium carbonates); hydrophilite (calcium chloride); powellite (calcium molybdate); whewellite (calcium oxalate); autunite (calcium phosphate); anorthite, apophyllite, chabazite, datolite, epidote, eudialite, feldspar, gyrolite, hornblende, margarite, melilite, monticellite, nephrite, pectolite, phillipsite, piedmontite, prehnite, scapolite, scawtite, scolecite, thaumasite, titanite, vesuvianite, wollastonite, and zeolite (calcium silicates); glauberite, gypsum, and polyhalite (calcium sulfates); perovskite (calcium titanate); and scheelite (calcium tungstate). Calcium phosphate is a major constituent of bones (apatite).

Uses

Salts of calcium are used as a source of calcium:

- to treat hypocalcaemia (for example calcium gluconate);
- to treat hyperphosphatemia (for example calcium acetate, calcium carbonate);
- to treat hyperkalemia (calcium polystyrene sulfonate; see monograph on Polystyrene sulfonates);
- to treat and prevent osteomalacia and osteoporosis (in combination with vitamin D or a bisphosphonate);
- as antacids (for example calcium hydroxide and calcium carbonate).

However, although calcium salts can produce short-term relief from dyspepsia, calcium ions stimulate antral gastrin release, and hence gastric acid secretion, making them unsuitable for long-term treatment of peptic disorders (1).

Other uses of calcium salts incidental to the calcium they contain include:

- in wound dressings (calcium alginate);
- to prevent methotrexate toxicity (calcium folinate and levofolinate);
- in lead poisoning (sodium calcium edetate).

Organs and Systems

Mineral balance

In one study of the use of calcium carbonate as a phosphate binder in patients on chronic hemodialysis, there was a low incidence of hypercalcemia at daily doses below 6 g (2), whereas in another report on 26 dialysis patients who used calcium carbonate for 3 years, 42% developed new calcification (3).

Calcium edetate can cause mild transient hypercalcemia (4) and hypercalciuria (5).

Acid–base balance

Long-term use of calcium salts can cause the milk-alkali syndrome and alkalosis in conjunction with hypercalcemia and renal insufficiency (6). It presents acutely with headache, nausea, irritability, and weakness, or chronically with uremia, alkalosis, and hypercalcemia. Sustained high dosage and/or concurrent renal disease are common antecedents (7).

Gastrointestinal

There is an unsubstantiated belief that calcium-containing antacids cause a rebound increase in gastric acid secretion that is more intense than with other antacids. This was thought to be due to absorption of calcium, the resultant hypercalcemia leading to increased acid secretion. This has been investigated in two trials. One (8) was an open, randomized, crossover study in 12 healthy volunteers who were given calcium carbonate and magnesium carbonate (Rennie) and hydrotalcite (Talcid). The other (9) was a double-blind, crossover trial in 12 healthy volunteers who were given placebo, Maalox liquid, and Rennie liquid. All the antacids had similar efficacy and there was no evidence of acid rebound with calcium carbonate.

Urinary tract

In general, there is an increased risk of nephrolithiasis with prolonged high calcium intake. Studies aimed at determining whether high calcium intake increases the risk of nephrolithiasis have shown that in patients at risk of nephrolithiasis or with a history of nephrolithiasis, calcium can be safely given for osteoporosis, provided there is careful monitoring (10,11).

In a French analysis of 22 510 urinary calculi performed by infrared spectroscopy, drug-induced urolithiasis was divided into two categories: first, stones with drugs physically embedded ($n = 238$; 1.0%), notably indinavir monohydrate ($n = 126$; 53%), followed by triamterene ($n = 43$; 18%), sulfonamides ($n = 29$; 12%), and amorphous silica ($n = 24$; 10%); secondly, metabolic nephrolithiasis induced by drugs ($n = 140$; 0.6%), involving mainly calcium/vitamin D supplementation ($n = 56$; 40%) and carbonic anhydrase inhibitors ($n = 33$; 24%) (12). Drug-induced stones are responsible for about 1.6% of all calculi in France. Physical analysis and a thorough drug history are important elements in the diagnosis.

Second-Generation Effects

Pregnancy

In a pregnant woman, calcium-containing antacids raised the calcium concentration to the point where hemodialysis was required (SEDA-17, 413).

References

1. Levant JA, Walsh JH, Isenberg JI. Stimulation of gastric secretion and gastrin release by single oral doses of calcium carbonate in man. N Engl J Med 1973;289(11):555–8.
2. Malberti F, Surian M, Poggio F, Minoia C, Salvadeo A. Efficacy and safety of long-term treatment with calcium carbonate as a phosphate binder. Am J Kidney Dis 1988;12(6):487–91.
3. Sperschneider H, Gunther K, Stein G, Marzoll I, Kirchner E. Untersuchungen zum Einsatz von Calciumcarbonat als Phosphatbinder bei Dialysepatienten im Langzeitverlauf uber 3 Jahre. [Use of calcium carbonate (CaCO3) as phosphate binder in dialysis patients in long-term follow-up over 3 years.] Z Urol Nephrol 1990;83(8):449–58.
4. Emmett M, Sirmon MD, Kirkpatrick WG, Nolan CR, Schmitt GW, Cleveland MB. Calcium acetate control of serum phosphorus in hemodialysis patients. Am J Kidney Dis 1991;17(5):544–50.
5. Adachi JD, Ioannidis G. Calcium and vitamin D therapy in corticosteroid-induced bone loss: what is the evidence? Calcif Tissue Int 1999;65(4):332–6.
6. Vanpee D, Delgrange E, Gillet JB, Donckier J. Ingestion of antacid tablets (Rennie) and acute confusion. J Emerg Med 2000;19(2):169–71.
7. Muldowney WP, Mazbar SA. Rolaids–yogurt syndrome: a 1990s version of milk–alkali syndrome. Am J Kidney Dis 1996;27(2):270–2.
8. Simoneau G. Absence of rebound effect with calcium carbonate. Eur J Drug Metab Pharmacokinet 1996;21(4):351–7.
9. Hurlimann S, Michel K, Inauen W, Halter F. Effect of Rennie Liquid versus Maalox Liquid on intragastric pH in a double-blind, randomized, placebo-controlled, triple cross-over study in healthy volunteers. Am J Gastroenterol 1996;91(6):1173–80.
10. Pak CY, Sakhaee K, Hwang TI, Preminger GM, Harvey JA. Nephrolithiasis from calcium supplementation. J Urol 1987;137(6):1212–13.
11. Ringe JD. The risk of nephrolithiasis with oral calcium supplementation. Calcif Tissue Int 1991;48(2):69–73.
12. Cohen-Solal F, Abdelmoula J, Hoarau MP, Jungers P, Lacour B, Daudon M. Les lithiases urinaires d'origine médicamenteuse. [Urinary lithiasis of medical origin.] Therapie 2001;56(6):743–50.

Campanulaceae

See also Herbal medicines

General Information

The genera in the family of Campanulaceae (Table 1) include lobelia and Venus' looking glass.

Table 1 The genera of Campanulaceae

Asyneuma (harebell)
Brighamia (brighamia)
Campanula (bell flower)
Campanulastrum (bell flower)
Canarina (canarina)
Clermontia (clermontia)
Cyanea (cyanea)
Delissea (delissea)
Downingia (calico flower)
Gadellia (gadellia)
Githopsis (bluecup)
Heterocodon (heterocodon)
Hippobroma (hippobroma)
Howellia (howellia)
Jasione (jasione)
Legenere (false Venus' looking glass)
Legousia (legousia)
Lobelia (lobelia)
Nemacladus (threadplant)
Parishella (parishella)
Platycodon (platycodon)
Porterella (porterella)
Rollandia (rollandia)
Trematolobelia (false lobelia)
Triodanis (Venus' looking-glass)
Wahlenbergia (wahlenbergia)

Lobelia inflata

Lobelia inflata (Indian tobacco) contains lobeline and other pyridine alkaloids. It has been used as an emetic, antidepressant, respiratory stimulant, an aid to smoking cessation, and a treatment for metamfetamine abuse (1).

Adverse effects

Lobeline has peripheral effects similar to those of nicotine, whereas its central activity may be different. It has been associated with nausea, vomiting, headache, tremors, and dizziness. Symptoms caused by overdosage include profuse sweating, paresis, tachycardia, hypertension, Cheyne-Stokes respiration, hypothermia, coma, and death. Large doses are convulsant.

Reference

1. Dwoskin LP, Crooks PA. A novel mechanism of action and potential use for lobeline as a treatment for psychostimulant abuse. Biochem Pharmacol 2002;63(2):89–98.

Camphor

General Information

The symptoms of systemic camphor poisoning have been reviewed (1).

Organs and Systems

Nervous system

Systemic nervous system adverse reactions after cutaneous contact with camphor have been reported (2).

- A 15-month-old child had crawled through spirits of camphor containing 10% camphor. Over the next 48 hours he became progressively ataxic and had several brief generalized motor seizures. The seizures persisted for 2 days despite appropriate therapy. Over 15 days he slowly improved; recovery in motor and mental function was eventually complete. The child had no further seizures until 1 year later, when a camphorated vaporizer containing 4.81% camphor was administered by the mother. During inhalation there was a brief major motor seizure.

Breathing difficulties, convulsions, and coma have been reported after repeated topical application of camphor-containing agents (3).

Skin

- A woman developed severe eczema of the ears, neck, and upper chest after having applied Earex ear drops. Patch tests with rectified camphor oil were positive on days 2 and 4 (4).

References

1. American academy of Pediatrics. Committee on Drugs. Camphor: who needs it? Pediatrics 1978;62(3):404–6.
2. Skoglund RR, Ware LL Jr, Schanberger JE. Prolonged seizures due to contact and inhalation exposure to camphor. A case report. Clin Pediatr (Phila) 1977;16(10):901–2.
3. Gossweiler B. Kampfervergiftungen heute. [Poisoning by camphor today.] Schweiz Rundsch Med Prax 1982; 71(38):1475–8.
4. Stevenson OE, Finch TM. Allergic contact dermatitis from rectified camphor oil in Earex ear drops. Contact Dermatitis 2003;49(1):51.

Candesartan cilexetil

See also Angiotensin II receptor antagonists

General Information

Candesartan cilexetil is the prodrug of candesartan, an angiotensin II type 1 (AT_1) receptor antagonist. Absorbed candesartan cilexetil is completely metabolized to candesartan. Candesartan has a half-life of about 9 hours (slightly longer in elderly people).

In an open study of 4531 hypertensive patients, the total incidence of adverse effects of candesartan was 6.1% (1). Individual adverse effects did not occur in more than 0.8% and were mainly dizziness and headache.

Susceptibility Factors

Renal disease

In patients undergoing chronic hemodialysis, the safety profile did not differ from that reported in other populations, except for some rare cases of hypotension during hemodialysis. Hemodialysis does not affect the kinetics of candesartan. Because of the variability of oral clearance and the pronounced influence of hemodialysis-induced volume contraction on the hemodynamic effects of candesartan, careful monitoring is recommended (2).

References

1. Schulte KL, Fischer M, Lenz T, Meyer-Sabellek W. Efficacy and tolerability of candesartan cilexetil monotherapy or in combination with other antihypertensive drugs. Results of the AURA study. Clin Drug Invest 1999;18:453–60.
2. Pfister M, Schaedeli F, Frey FJ, Uehlinger DE. Pharmacokinetics and haemodynamics of candesartan cilexetil in hypertensive patients on regular haemodialysis. Br J Clin Pharmacol 1999;47(6):645–51.

Cannabaceae

See also Herbal medicines

General Information

The family of Cannabaceae contains two genera:

1. *Cannabis* (hemp)
2. *Humulus* (hop).

The cannabinoids are covered in a separate monograph.

Humulus lupulus

Humulus lupulus (hop) contains a variety of sesquiterpenoids, diterpenoids, and triterpenoids, phytoestrogens, and the flavonoid xanthohumol, which has some in vitro anti-HIV activity (1). Apart from their use in brewing beer, hops have been used for sedative purposes, but evidence of efficacy is poor.

Adverse effects

Hop farmers are exposed to air that can contain dust, endotoxin, and micro-organisms. In one study of 19 farms in Poland Gram-positive bacteria formed 22–96% of the total count; among them, corynebacteria and endospore-forming bacilli were prevalent (2). Fungi constituted 3.7–65% of the total count; the dominant species were *Penicillium citrinum*, *Alternaria alternata*, and *Cladosporium epiphyllum*. Thermophilic actinomycetes and Gram-negative bacteria were detected in the air of only 10 and six farms respectively. The concentrations of endotoxin were 313–6250 μg/g. The hop growers seem to be exposed to lower concentrations of dust, micro-organisms, and endotoxin than other branches of agriculture, which the authors partly attributed to antimicrobial properties of *H. lupulus*.

Eight of twenty-three hops farmers, who had been exposed to organic dust from *H. lupulus*, reported symptoms of chronic bronchitis and five reported work-related symptoms, including dry cough and dyspnea (3).

After 30 years of working with hop without any health problems a 46-year-old farmer developed erythema of the face, neck, and upper chest, edema of the eyelids, conjunctivitis, and dermatitis of the hands (4). Her symptoms were provoked by both fresh and dried hops, appeared after half-an-hour of working, and persisted over 1–2 days. Skin tests yielded the following results: hop leaves (saline extract)—prick positive, patch negative; hop leaves (glycerol extract)—prick positive, patch negative; hop cones (saline extract)—prick positive, patch negative; hop cones (glycerol extract)—prick negative, patch positive after 48 and 72 hours. Despite discontinuing work, the patient had several relapses attributed to other sources of hop allergens: a beauty cream, a herbal sedative, and her husband, also a hop farmer.

Systemic urticaria has been reported in patients who had been exposed to *H. lupulus* (5), in one case with arthralgia and fever (6).

Flavonoids in hops that persist in beer can inhibit certain isoforms of cytochrome P450 in vitro (7). At a concentration of 10 μmol/l xanthohumol almost completely inhibited CYP1A1 and other hop flavonoids inhibited it by 27–91%. At a concentration of 10 μmol/l xanthohumol completely inhibited CYP1B1 and other hop flavonoids inhibited it by 2–99%. The most effective inhibitors of CYP1A2 were the two prenylated flavonoids, 8-prenylnaringenin and isoxanthohumol, which produced over 90% inhibition in concentrations of 10 μmol/l. However, the flavonoids were poor inhibitors of CYP2E1 and CYP3A4 and so in vivo drug interactions are unlikely to be of importance.

References

1. Wang Q, Ding ZH, Liu JK, Zheng YT. Xanthohumol, a novel anti-HIV-1 agent purified from Hops *Humulus lupulus* Antiviral Res 2004;64(3):189–94.
2. Gora A, Skorska C, Sitkowska J, Prazmo Z, Krysinska-Traczyk E, Urbanowicz B, Dutkiewicz J. Exposure of hop growers to bioaerosols. Ann Agric Environ Med 2004; 11(1):129–38.
3. Skorska C, Mackiewicz B, Gora A, Golec M, Dutkiewicz J. Health effects of inhalation exposure to organic dust in hops farmers. Ann Univ Mariae Curie Sklodowska [Med] 2003;58(1):459–65.
4. Spiewak R, Dutkiewicz J. Occupational airborne and hand dermatitis to hop (*Humulus lupulus*) with non-occupational relapses. Ann Agric Environ Med 2002;9(2):249–52.
5. Estrada JL, Gozalo F, Cecchini C, Casquete E. Contact urticaria from hops (*Humulus lupulus*) in a patient with previous urticaria-angioedema from peanut, chestnut and banana Contact Dermatitis 2002;46(2):127.

6. Pradalier A, Campinos C, Trinh C. Urticaire systemique induite par le houblon. [Systemic urticaria induced by hops.] Allerg Immunol (Paris) 2002;34(9):330–2.
7. Henderson MC, Miranda CL, Stevens JF, Deinzer ML, Buhler DR. In vitro inhibition of human P450 enzymes by prenylated flavonoids from hops, *Humulus lupulus*. Xenobiotica 2000;30(3):235–51.

Cannabinoids

General Information

Cannabis is the abbreviated name for the hemp plant *Cannabis sativa*. The common names for cannabis include marijuana, grass, and weed. Other names for cannabis refer to particular strains; they include bhang and ganja. The most potent forms of cannabis come from the flowering tops of the plants or from the dried resinous exudate of the leaves, and are referred to as hashish or hash.

Cannabis is one of the oldest and most widely used drugs in the world. In different Western countries the possible therapeutic use of cannabinoids as antiemetics in patients with cancer or in patients with multiple sclerosis has become an issue, because of the prohibition of cannabis, and has polarized opinion about the seriousness of its adverse effects (1,2).

Pharmacology

The primary active component of cannabis is Δ9-tetrahydrocannabinol (THC), which is responsible for the greater part of the pharmacological effects of the cannabis complex. Δ8-THC is also active. However, the cannabis plant contains more than 400 chemicals, of which some 60 are chemically related to Δ9-THC, and it is evident that the exact proportions in which these are present can vary considerably, depending on the way in which the material has been harvested and prepared. In man, Δ9-THC is rapidly converted to 11-hydroxy-Δ9-THC (3), a metabolite that is active in the central nervous system. A specific receptor for the cannabinols has been identified; it is a member of the G-protein-linked family of receptors (4). The cannabinoid receptor is linked to the inhibitory G-protein, which is linked to adenyl cyclase in an inhibitory fashion (5). The cannabinoid receptor is found in highest concentrations in the basal ganglia, the hippocampus, and the cerebellum, with lower concentrations in the cerebral cortex.

When cannabis is smoked, usually in a cigarette with tobacco, the euphoric and relaxant effects occur within minutes, reach a maximum in about 30 minutes, and last up to 4 hours. Some of the motor and cognitive effects can persist for 5–12 hours. Cannabis can also be taken orally, in foods such as cakes (for example "space cake") or sweetmeats (for example hashish fudge) (6).

Many variables affect the psychoactive properties of cannabis, including the potency of the cannabis used, the route of administration, the smoking technique, the dose, the setting, the user's past experience, the user's expectations, and the user's biological vulnerability to the effects of the drug.

Animal and in vitro toxicology

Δ9-tetrahydrocannabinol, the active component in herbal cannabis, is very safe. Laboratory animals (rats, mice, dogs, monkeys) can tolerate doses of up to 1000 mg/kg, equivalent to some 5000 times the human intoxicant dose. Despite the widespread illicit use of cannabis, there are very few, if any, instances of deaths from overdose (7).

Long-term toxicology studies with THC were carried out by the National Institute of Mental Health in the late 1960s (8). These included a 90-day study with a 30-day recovery period in both rats and monkeys and involved not only Δ9-THC but also Δ8-THC and a crude extract of marijuana. Doses of cannabis or cannabinoids in the range 50–500 mg/kg caused reduced food intake and lower body weight. All three substances initially depressed behavior, but later the animals became more active and were irritable or aggressive. At the end of the study the weights of the ovaries, uterus, prostate, and spleen were reduced and the weight of the adrenal glands was increased. The behavioral and organ changes were similar in monkeys, but less severe than those seen in rats. Further studies were carried out to assess the damage that might be done to the developing fetus by exposure to cannabis or cannabinoids during pregnancy. Treatment of pregnant rabbits with THC at doses up to 5 mg/kg had no effect on birth weight and did not cause any abnormalities in the offspring (8).

A similarly detailed toxicology study was carried out with THC by the National Institute of Environmental Health Sciences in the USA, in response to a request from the National Cancer Institute (9). Rats and mice were given THC up to 500 mg/kg five times a week for 13 weeks; some were followed for a period of recovery over 9 weeks. By the end of the study more than half of the rats treated with the highest dose (500 mg/kg) had died, but all of the remaining animals appeared to be healthy, although in both species the higher doses caused lethargy and increased aggressiveness. The THC-treated animals ate less food and their body weights were consequently significantly lower than those of untreated controls at the end of the treatment period, but returned to normal during recovery. During this period the animals were sensitive to touch and some had convulsions. There was a trend towards reduced uterine and testicular weights.

In further studies rats were treated with doses of THC up to 50 mg/kg and mice with up to 500 mg/kg 5 times a week for 2 years in a standard carcinogenicity test (9). After 2 years, more treated animals had survived than controls, probably because the treated animals ate less and had lower body weights. The treated animals also had a significantly lower incidence of the various cancers normally seen in aged rodents in testes, pancreas, pituitary gland, mammary glands, liver, and uterus. Although there was an increased incidence of precancerous changes in the thyroid gland in both species and in the mouse ovary after one dose (125 mg/kg), these changes were not dose-related. The conclusion was that there was "no evidence of carcinogenic activity of THC at doses up to 50 mg/kg." This was also supported by the failure to detect any genetic toxicity in other tests designed to identify drugs capable of causing chromosomal damage. For example, THC was negative in the so-called "Ames test," in which bacteria are exposed to very high concentrations of a drug to see whether it causes mutations. In another test, hamster ovary cells were exposed to high concentrations of the drug in tissue culture; there were no effects on cell division that might suggest chromosomal damage.

By any standards, THC must be considered to be very safe, both acutely and during long-term exposure. This probably partly reflects the fact that cannabinoid receptors are virtually absent from those regions at the base of the brain that are responsible for such vital functions as breathing and blood pressure control. The available animal data are more than adequate to justify its approval as a human medicine, and indeed it has been approved by the FDA for certain limited therapeutic indications (generic name = dronabinol) (7).

Respiratory

There have been several attempts to address this question by exposing laboratory animals to cannabis smoke. After such exposure on a daily basis for periods of up to 30 months, extensive damage has been observed in the lungs of rats (10), dogs (11), and monkeys (12), but it is very difficult to extrapolate these findings to man, as it is difficult or impossible to imitate human exposure to cannabis smoke in any animal model.

Nervous system

Animal studies on neurotoxicity have yielded conflicting results. Treatment of rats with high doses of THC given orally for 3 months (13) or subcutaneously for 8 months (14) produced neural damage in the hippocampal CA3 zone, with shrunken neurons, reduced synaptic density, and loss of cells. But in perhaps the most severe test of all, rats and mice treated on 5 days each week for 2 years had no histopathological changes in the brain, even after 50 mg/kg/day (rats) or 250 mg/kg/day (mice) (9). Although claims were made that exposure of a small number of rhesus monkeys to cannabis smoke led to ultrastructural changes in the septum and hippocampus (15,16), subsequent larger-scale studies failed to show any cannabis-induced histopathology in monkey brain (17).

Studies of the effects of cannabinoids on neurons in vitro have also yielded inconsistent results. Exposure of rat cortical neurons to THC shortened their survival: twice as many cells were dead after exposure to THC 5 μmol/l for 2 hours than in control cultures (18). Concentrations of THC as low as 0.1 μmol/l had a significant effect. The effects of THC were accompanied by release of cytochrome c, activation of caspase-3, and DNA fragmentation, suggesting an apoptotic mechanism. All of the effects of THC could be blocked by the antagonist AM-251 or by pertussis toxin, suggesting that they were mediated through CB1 receptors. Toxic effects of THC have also been reported in hippocampal neurons in culture, with 50% cell death after exposure to THC 10 μmol/l for 2 hours or 1 μmol/l for 5 days (19). The antagonist rimonabant blocked these effects, but pertussis toxin did not. The authors proposed a toxic mechanism involving arachidonic acid release and the formation of free radicals. On the other hand, other authors have failed to observe any damage in rat cortical neurons exposed for up to 15 days to THC 1 mmol/l, although they found that this concentration killed rat C6 glioma cells, human astrocytoma U373MG cells, and mouse neuroblastoma N18TG12 cells (20). In a remarkable study, injection of THC into solid tumors of C6 glioma in rodent brain led to increased survival times, and there was complete eradication of the tumors in 20–35% of the treated animals (21). A stable analogue of anandamide also produced a drastic reduction in the tumor volume of a rat thyroid epithelial cell line transformed by K-ras oncogene, implanted in nude mice (22). The antiproliferative effect of cannabinoids has suggested a potential use for such drugs in cancer treatment (23).

Some authors have reported neuroprotective actions of cannabinoids. WIN55,212-2 reduced cerebral damage in rat hippocampus or cerebral cortex after global ischemia or focal ischemia in vivo (24). The endocannabinoid 2AG protected against damage elicited by closed head injury in mouse brain, and the protective effects were blocked by rimonabant (25). THC had a similar effect in vivo in protecting against damage elicited by ouabain (26). Rat hippocampal neurons in tissue culture were protected against glutamate-mediated damage by low concentrations of WIN55,212-2 or CP-55940, and these effects were mediated through CB1 receptors (27). But not all of these effects seem to require mediation by cannabinoid receptors. The protective effects of WIN55,212-2 did not require either CB1 or CB2 cannabinoid receptors in cortical neurons exposed to hypoxia (24), and there were similar findings for the protective actions of anandamide and 2-AG in cortical neuronal cultures (28). Both THC and cannabidiol, which is not active at cannabinoid receptors, protected rat cortical neurons against glutamate toxicity (29) and these effects were also independent of CB1 receptors. The authors suggested that the protective effects of THC might be due to the antioxidant properties of these polyphenolic molecules, which have redox potentials higher than those of known antioxidants (for example ascorbic acid).

Pregnancy

In animals, THC can cause spontaneous abortion, low birth weight, and physical deformities (30). However, these were only seen after treatment with extremely high doses of THC (50–150 times higher than human doses), and only in rodents and not in monkeys.

Tolerance and dependence

Many animal studies have shown that tolerance develops to most of the behavioral and physiological effects of THC (31). Dependence on cannabinoids in animals is clearly observable, because of the availability of CB_1 receptor antagonists, which can be used to precipitate withdrawal. Thus, a behavioral withdrawal syndrome was precipitated by rimonabant in rats treated for only 4 days with THC in doses as low as 0.5–4.0 mg/kg/day (32). The syndrome included scratching, face rubbing, licking, wet dog shakes, arched back, and ptosis, many of the signs that are seen in rats undergoing opiate withdrawal. Similar withdrawal signs occurred when rats treated chronically with the synthetic cannabinoid CP-55940 were given rimonabant (33). Rimonabant-induced withdrawal after 2 weeks of treatment of rats with the cannabinoid HU-120 was accompanied by a marked increase in release of the stress-related neuropeptide corticotropin-releasing factor in the amygdala, a result that also occurred in animals undergoing heroin withdrawal (34). An electrophysiological study showed that precipitated withdrawal was also associated with reduced firing of dopamine neurons in the ventral tegmental area of rat brain (35).

These data clearly show that chronic administration of cannabinoids leads to adaptive changes in the brain, some of which are similar to those seen with other drugs of dependence. The ability of THC to cause selective release of dopamine from the nucleus accumbens (36) also suggests some similarity between THC and other drugs in this category.

Furthermore, although many earlier attempts to obtain reliable self-administration behavior with THC were unsuccessful (31), some success has been obtained recently. Squirrel monkeys were trained to self-administer low doses of THC (2 μg/kg per injection), but only after the animals had first been trained to self-administer cocaine (37). THC is difficult to administer intravenously, but these authors succeeded, perhaps in part because they used doses comparable to those to which human cannabis users are exposed, and because the potent synthetic cannabinoids are far more water-soluble than THC, which makes intravenous administration easier. Mice could be trained to self-administer intravenous WIN55212-2, but CB_1 receptor knockout animals could not (38).

Another way of demonstrating the rewarding effects of drugs in animals is the conditioned place preference paradigm, in which an animal learns to approach an environment in which it has previously received a rewarding stimulus. Rats had a positive THC place preference after doses as low as 1 mg/kg (39).

Some studies have suggested that there may be links between the development of dependence to cannabinoids and to opiates (40). Some of the behavioral signs of rimonabant-induced withdrawal in THC-treated rats can be mimicked by the opiate antagonist naloxone (41). Conversely, the withdrawal syndrome precipitated by naloxone in morphine-dependent mice can be partly relieved by THC (42) or endocannabinoids (43). Rats treated chronically with the cannabinoid WIN55212-2 became sensitized to the behavioral effects of heroin (44). Such interactions can also be demonstrated acutely. Synergy between cannabinoids and opiate analgesics has been described above. THC also facilitated the antinociceptive effects of RB 101, an inhibitor of enkephalin inactivation, and acute administration of THC caused increased release of Met-enkephalin into microdialysis probes placed into the rat nucleus accumbens (45).

The availability of receptor knockout animals has also helped to illustrate cannabinoid–opioid interactions. CB_1 receptor knockout mice had greatly reduced morphine self-administration behavior and less severe naloxone-induced withdrawal signs than wild type animals, although the antinociceptive actions of morphine were unaffected in the knockout animals (38). The rimonabant–precipitated withdrawal syndrome in THC-treated mice was significantly attenuated in animals with knockout of the pro-enkephalin gene (46). Knockout of the μ opioid (OP_3) receptor also reduced rimonabant-induced withdrawal signs in THC-treated mice, and there was an attenuated naloxone withdrawal syndrome in morphine-dependent CB_1 knockout mice (47,48).

These findings clearly point to interactions between the endogenous cannabinoid and opioid systems in the CNS, although the neuronal circuitry involved is unknown. Whether this is relevant to the so-called "gateway" theory is unclear. In the US National Household Survey of Drug Abuse, respondents aged 22 years or over who had started to use cannabis before the age of 21 years were 24 times more likely than non-cannabis users to begin using hard drugs (49). However, in the same survey the proportion of cannabis users who progressed to heroin or cocaine use was very small (2% or less). Mathematical modeling using the Monte Carlo method suggested that the association between cannabis use and hard drug use need not be causal, but could relate to some common predisposing factor, for example "drug-use propensity" (50).

Tumorigenicity

THC does not appear to be carcinogenic, but there is plenty of evidence that the tar derived from cannabis smoke is. Bacteria exposed to cannabis tar develop mutations in the standard Ames test for carcinogenicity (51), and hamster lung cells in tissue culture develop accelerated malignant transformations within 3–6 months of exposure to tobacco or cannabis smoke (52).

General adverse effects

A review has summarized the evidence related to the adverse effects of acute and chronic use of cannabis (53). The effects of acute usage include anxiety, impaired attention, and increased risk of psychotic symptoms. Probable risks of chronic cannabis consumption include bronchitis and subtle impairments of attention and memory.

The adverse effects of cannabis can be considered under two main headings, reflecting psychoactive and autonomic effects, in addition to which there are direct toxic effects. The most frequently reported psychoactive effects include enhanced sensory perception (for example a heightened appreciation of color and sound). Cannabis intoxication commonly heightens the user's sensitivity to other external stimuli as well, but subjectively slows the appreciation of time. In high doses, users may also experience depersonalization and derealization. Various forms of psychomotor performance, including driving, are significantly impaired for 8–12 hours after using cannabis. The most serious possible consequence of cannabis use is a road accident if a user drives while intoxicated.

Adverse reactions have been reported at relatively low doses and principally affect the psyche, leading to anxiety states, panic reactions, restlessness, hallucinations, fear, confusion, and rarely toxic psychosis. These effects appear to be reversible (54). Ingestion of cake with cannabis by people who seldom use or have never used cannabis before can result in mental changes, including confusion, anxiety, loss of logical thinking, fits of laughter, hallucinations, hypertension, and/or paranoid psychosis, which can last as long as 8 hours.

The autonomic effects of cannabis lead to tachycardia, peripheral vasodilatation, conjunctival congestion, hyperthermia, bronchodilatation, dry mouth, nystagmus, tremor, ataxia, hypotension, nausea, and vomiting, that is a spectrum of effects that closely resembles the consequences of overdosage with anticholinergic agents. Some individuals have sleep disturbances. Increased appetite and dry mouth are other common effects of cannabis intoxication.

Hypersensitivity reactions are rare, but a few have been reported after inhalation. Delayed hypersensitivity reactions, particularly affecting vascular tissue, have been recorded with chronic systemic administration. Tumor-inducing effects are difficult to attribute to cannabis alone. Animal studies have shown neoplastic pulmonary lesions superimposed on chronic inflammation, but such pathology may be primarily associated with the "tar" produced by burning marijuana. The most serious potential adverse effects of cannabis use come from the inhalation of the same carcinogenic hydrocarbons that are present in tobacco, and some data suggest that heavy cannabis users are at risk of chronic respiratory diseases and lung cancer.

The effects of oral cannabinoids (dronabinol or *Cannabis sativa* plant extract) in relieving pain and muscle spasticity have been studied in 16 patients with multiple sclerosis (mean age 46 years, mean duration of disease 15 years) in a double-blind, placebo-controlled, crossover study (55). The initial dose was 2.5 mg bd, increasing to 5 mg bd after 2 weeks if the dose was well tolerated. The plant extract was more likely to cause adverse events; five patients had increased spasticity and one rated an adverse event of acute psychosis as severe. All physical measures were in the reference ranges. There were no significant differences in any measure of efficacy score that would indicate a therapeutic benefit of cannabinoids. This study is the largest and longest of its kind, but the authors acknowledged some possible shortcomings. The route of administration could affect subjective ratings, since the gastrointestinal tract is a much slower and more inefficient route than the lungs. Another possibility is that the dose was too small to have the desired therapeutic effects.

Organs and Systems

Cardiovascular

Marijuana has several effects on the cardiovascular system, and can increase resting heart rate and supine blood pressure and cause postural hypotension. It is associated with an increase in myocardial oxygen demand and a decrease in oxygen supply. Peripheral vasodilatation, with increased blood flow, orthostatic hypotension, and tachycardia, can occur with normal recreational doses of cannabis. High doses of THC taken intravenously have often been associated with ventricular extra beats, a shortened PR interval, and reduced T wave amplitude, to which tolerance readily develops and which are reversible on withdrawal. While the other cardiovascular effects tend to decrease in chronic smokers, the degree of tachycardia continues to be exaggerated with exercise, as shown by bicycle ergometry.

Marijuana use is most popular among young adults (18–25 years old). However, with a generation of post-1960s smokers growing older, the use of marijuana in the age group that is prone to coronary artery disease has increased. The cardiovascular effects may present a risk to those with cardiovascular disorders, but in adults with normal cardiovascular function there is no evidence of permanent damage associated with marijuana (54,56,57), and it is not known whether marijuana can precipitate myocardial infarction, although mixed use of tobacco and cannabis make the evaluation of the effects of cannabis very difficult.

Ischemic heart disease

Investigators in the Determinants of Myocardial Infarction Onset Study recently reported that smoking marijuana is a rare trigger of acute myocardial infarction (58). Interviews of 3882 patients (1258 women) were conducted on an average of 4 days after infarction. Reported use of marijuana in the hour preceding the first symptoms of myocardial infarction was compared with use in matched controls. Among the patients, 124 reported smoking marijuana in the previous year, 37 within 24 hours, and 9 within 1 hour of cardiac symptoms. The risk of myocardial infarction was increased 4.8 times over baseline in the 60 minutes after marijuana use and then fell rapidly. The authors emphasized that in a majority of cases, the mechanism that triggered the onset of myocardial infarction involved a ruptured atherosclerotic plaque secondary to hemodynamic stress. It was not clear whether marijuana has direct or indirect hemodynamic effects sufficient to cause plaque rupture.

Cardiac dysrhythmias

Paroxysmal atrial fibrillation has been reported in two cases after marijuana use (59).

- A healthy 32-year-old doctor, who smoked marijuana 1–2 times a month, had paroxysmal tachycardia for several months. An electrocardiogram was normal and a Holter recording showed sinus rhythm with isolated supraventricular extra beats. He was treated with propranolol. He later secretly smoked marijuana while undergoing another Holter recording, which showed numerous episodes of paroxysmal atrial tachycardia and atrial fibrillation lasting up to 2 minutes. He abstained from marijuana for 12 months and maintained stable sinus rhythm.
- A 24-year-old woman briefly lost consciousness and had nausea and vomiting several minutes after smoking marijuana. She had hyporeflexia, atrial fibrillation (maximum 140/minute with a pulse deficit), and a blood pressure of 130/80 mmHg. Echocardiography was unremarkable. Within 12 hours, after metoprolol, propafenone, and intravenous hydration with electrolytes, sinus rhythm was restored.

The authors discussed the possibility that Δ9-THC, the active ingredient of marijuana, can cause intra-atrial re-entry by several mechanisms and thereby precipitate atrial fibrillation.

Sustained atrial fibrillation has also been attributed to marijuana (60).

- A 14-year-old African-American man with no cardiac history had palpitation and dizziness, resulting in a fall, within 1 hour of smoking marijuana. After vomiting several times he had a new sensation of skipped heartbeats. The only remarkable finding was a flow murmur. The electrocardiogram showed atrial fibrillation. Echocardiography was normal. Serum and urine toxicology showed cannabis. He was given digoxin, and about 12 hours later his cardiac rhythm converted to sinus rhythm. Digoxin was withdrawn. He abstained from marijuana over the next year and was symptom free.

The authors noted that marijuana's catecholaminergic properties can affect autonomic control, vasomotor reflexes, and conduction-enhancement of perinodal fibers in cardiac muscle, and thus lead to an event such as this.

Arteritis
A case of progressive arteritis associated with cannabis use has been reported (61).

- A 38-year-old Afro-Caribbean man was admitted after 3 months of severe constant ischemic pain and numbness affecting the right foot. The pain was worse at night. He also had intermittent claudication after walking 100 yards. He had a chronic history of smoking cannabis about 1 ounce/day, mixed with tobacco in the early years of usage. However, at the time of admission, he had not used tobacco in any form for over 10 years. He had patchy necrosis and ulceration of the toes and impalpable pulses in the right foot. The serum cotinine concentrations were consistent with those found in non-smokers of tobacco. Angiography of his leg was highly suggestive of Buerger's disease (thromboangiitis obliterans).

Remarkably, this patient, despite having abstained from tobacco for more than 10 years, developed a progressive arteritis leading to ischemic changes. While arterial pathology with cannabis has been reported before, it has been difficult to dissociate the effects of other drugs.

Respiratory

Acute inhalation of marijuana or THC causes bronchodilatation, but with chronic use resistance in the bronchioles increases (62,63). Prolonged use of cannabis by inhalation can cause chronic inflammatory changes in the bronchial tree, in part related to the inhalants that accompany the smoke. In some cases attacks of asthma and glottal and uvular angioedema can occur. Reduced respiratory gas exchange has been reported in long-term smokers, and under experimental conditions THC can depress respiratory function slightly and act as a respiratory irritant. In fact, chronic marijuana cigarette smoking and chronic tobacco cigarette smoking produce very similar changes, but these occur after smoking fewer cigarettes when marijuana is smoked, compared with tobacco-smoking. With marijuana inhalation, when a filter is never used, inhalation is deeper and the smoke is held in the lungs for longer than when smoking commercially produced tobacco-based cigarettes (64). There is therefore a greater build-up of carbon monoxide, reduction in carboxyhemoglobin saturation, and alveolar cellular irritation with depression of macrophages (SEDA-13, 25). Pneumothorax, pneumopericardium, and pneumomediastinum have been reported when positive pulmonary pressure is applied or a Valsalva maneuver used, as often happens (65,66).

A possible role of marijuana use in the formation of large lung bullae has been discussed (67). Four men, who smoked both tobacco and marijuana, developed large, multiple, bilateral, peripheral bullae at their lung apices, with normal parenchymal tissue elsewhere. Three patients with large bullae in the upper lung lobe have been reported (68). All had been heavy marijuana smokers over 10–24 years. However, they all had at least nine pack-years of cigarette exposure and so marijuana may not have been the only cause of their lung bullae. Nevertheless, the authors recommended that all those who present with upper lung bullae should be screened for cannabis use.

While Δ9-THC may not contribute directly to lung bullae, it is possible that the respiratory dynamics of smoking the drug explains it. Typically, a draw on a marijuana joint has, on average, a depth of inspiration that is one-third greater, a volume two-thirds greater, and a breath-holding time four times longer than a draw on a cigarette. The marijuana joint lacks a filter tip, and the practice of smoking "leads to a fourfold greater delivery of tar and a five times greater increase in carboxyhemoglobin per cigarette smoked" (62). Smoking three to four joints of marijuana per day is reported to produce a symptom profile and damage to the respiratory airways similar to that caused by smoking 20 tobacco cigarettes daily.

Nervous system

Marijuana can interact with the neurotransmitter dopamine, and the effects of marijuana on the brain in schizophrenia have been studied by single photon emission computerized tomography (SPECT) (69).

A 38-year-old man with schizophrenia secretively smoked marijuana during a neuroimaging study. A comparison of two sets of images, before and after marijuana inhalation, showed a 20% reduction in the striatal dopamine D_2 receptor binding ratio, suggestive of increased synaptic dopaminergic activity.

On the basis of this in vivo SPECT study, the authors speculated that marijuana may interact with dopaminergic systems in brain reward pathways.

Sensory systems

Eyes
No consistent effects of cannabinoids on the eyes have been reported, apart from a reduction in intraocular pressure (70). The initial reduction in intraocular pressure is followed by a rebound increase associated with increased prostaglandin concentrations.

Ears
The effect of THC, 7.5 mg and 15 mg, on auditory functioning has been investigated in eight men in a double-blind, randomized, placebo-controlled, crossover trial (71). Blood concentrations of THC were measured for up to 48 hours after ingestion, and audiometric tests were carried out at 2 hours. There were no significant differences across treatments, suggesting that cannabis does not affect the basic unit of auditory perception.

Psychological, psychiatric

The psychological effects of cannabis vary with personal and social factors. However, some guidance to the essential effects of the drug can be derived from investigations with THC and marijuana in non-user volunteers. Blood concentrations of THC over 75 μg/ml under these conditions are associated with euphoria, and somewhat higher concentrations with dissociation of events and memory and impairment of psychomotor tasks lasting over 24 hours (54).

Through random urine testing of draftees to the Italian army, 133 marijuana users were identified, tested, and interviewed (72). Among these marijuana users, 83% of those with cannabis dependence, 46% with cannabis abuse, and 29% of occasional users had at least one DSM-IIIR psychiatric diagnosis. With greater cannabis use, the risk of associated psychiatric disabilities tended to increase progressively.

Occasional and regular users can suffer panic attacks, paranoia, hallucinations, or feelings of unreality (depersonalization and derealization).

Psychosis

The causal relation between cannabis abuse and schizophrenia is controversial. Cannabis abuse, and particularly heavy abuse, can exacerbate symptoms of schizophrenia and can be considered as a risk factor eliciting relapse in schizophrenia (74). Chronic cannabis use can precipitate schizophrenia in vulnerable individuals (75).

Four cases in which psychosis developed after relatively small amounts of marijuana were smoked for the first time have been reported (76). All required hospitalization and neuroleptic drug treatment. Each had a mother with manic disorder and two had psychotic features. The authors noted that marijuana is a dopamine receptor agonist, and mania may be associated with excessive dopaminergic neurotransmission. The use of marijuana may precipitate psychosis or mania in subjects who are genetically vulnerable to major mental illness.

Marijuana abuse and its possible associated risks in reinforcing further use, causing dependence, and producing withdrawal symptoms among adolescents with conduct symptoms and substance use disorders has been investigated in 165 men and 64 women selected and then interviewed from a group of 255 consecutive admissions to a university-based adolescent substance abuse treatment program (77). All had DSM-IIIR substance dependence, 82% had conduct disorder, 18% had major depression, and 15% had attention-deficit/hyperactivity disorder. Most (79%) met the criteria for cannabis dependence. Two-thirds of the cannabis-dependent individuals admitted serious drug-related problems and reported associated drug withdrawal symptoms according to the Comprehensive Addiction Severity Index in adolescents (CASI). For the majority, progression from first to regular cannabis use was as rapid as tobacco progression and more rapid than that of alcohol.

Cognitive effects

Long-term heavy use of cannabis impairs mental performance, causes defects in memory (especially short-term memory), and leads to impairment of memory, attention, and organization and integration of complex information (78). Adolescents with pre-existing disabilities in learning and cognition have experienced serious aggravation of their problem from regular use of cannabis (79).

The effects of chronic marijuana smoking on human brain function and cognition have been further investigated (62). Normalized regional brain blood flow and regional brain metabolism, measured using PET scanning with ^{15}O, were compared in 17 frequent marijuana users and 12 non-users. Testing was performed after at least 26 hours of monitored abstinence in all subjects. Marijuana users had hypoactivity or reduced brain blood flow in a large region of the posterior cerebellum compared with controls. This is consistent with what was reported in the only previous PET study of chronic marijuana use (80). The cerebellum is hypothesized to have input to aspects of cognition, specifically timing, the processing of sensory information, and attention and prediction of real-time events. Users often report that marijuana smoking is followed by alterations in the sense of time and less efficient cognitive processing.

The safety and possible benefits of long-term marijuana use have been studied in four seriously ill patients in the Missoula Chronic Clinical Cannabis Use Study with a quality-controlled sample of marijuana (73). They were evaluated using an extensive neurocognitive battery.

- A 62-year-old woman with congenital cataracts smoked marijuana illicitly for 12 years (current use 3–4 g/day smoked and 3–4 g/day orally). She had mild-to-moderate difficulty with attention and concentration and minimal-to-mild difficulty with acquisition and storage of very complex new verbal material. Her executive functioning was not affected.
- A 50-year-old man with hereditary osteo-onychodysplasia had smoked marijuana since 1974 to alleviate muscle spasms and pain (current use 7 g/day of 3.75% THC). He had mild-to-moderate impairment of attention and concentration and reduced ability to acquire new verbal material. He scored poorly on the California Verbal Learning Test (CVLT), a measure of short-term memory recall, and had difficulty with motor tasks.
- A 48-year-old man with multiple congenital cartilaginous exostoses had smoked marijuana since the late 1970s (current use 9 g/day of 2.7% THC). His neurocognitive scores suggest mild difficulty in sustaining attention and a minimal-to-mild deficit in the acquisition of new verbal material.
- A 45-year-old woman with multiple sclerosis had smoked cannabis since 1990 to control pain and muscle spasms (current use marijuana cigarettes containing 3.5% THC 10/day). She had impairment of concentration, learning, and memory efficiency. Her ability to acquire new verbal information was also impaired.

The authors attributed these cognitive deficits not to marijuana use but rather to the patients' illnesses, arguing that it is difficult for patients with painful debilitating diseases to concentrate on neurocognitive tasks. Any abnormalities in MRI imaging and electroencephalography were attributed to age-related brain deterioration. There were no significant abnormalities of respiratory function, apart from a "slight downward trend in FEV_1 and FEV_1/FVC ratios, and perhaps an increase in FVC" in three patients, interpretation of these findings being complicated by concomitant tobacco smoking. One patient had mild polycythemia and a raised white cell count. None had abnormal endocrine tests. This was a comprehensive study of the long-term effects of cannabis, but concomitant illnesses and use of tobacco made the results difficult to interpret.

Concerns have been raised about the possible adverse effects of acute as well as chronic medicinal and recreational use of cannabis on cognition and the body (81). The author, while acknowledging the therapeutic role of cannabinoids in the management of pain and other conditions, expressed concern that in recent years the prevalence of recreational cannabis use (especially in the young) and the potency of the available products have markedly increased in the UK.

An unusual account of transient amnesia after marijuana use has been reported from Europe (82).

- A 40-year-old healthy man with a long history of cannabis use was hospitalized with an acute memory disturbance after smoking for several hours a strong type of marijuana called "superskunk." After smoking, he had difficulty recollecting recent events and would ask the same questions repeatedly. While his routine laboratory results were within the reference ranges, his urine and blood toxic screens had very high concentrations of cannabinoids (and no other drugs). He was alert and oriented to his name, address, date, and place of birth, but could not recall his marital status, whether he had children, or the nature of his job. He was disoriented in time. He performed normally in tests of general cognitive functioning (for example Raven's matrices, word fluency, Rey's complex figurecopy) and short-term memory (for example digit span, verbal cues), but showed severe impairment in verbal and non-verbal long-term components of anterograde memory tests. He had a severe retrograde memory defect mainly affecting autobiographical memory, with a temporal gradient such that remote facts were preserved. These memory impairments lasted 4 days and then rapidly improved, leaving amnesia for the acute episode. Electroencephalography during the amnestic episode was normal, except for brief trains of irregular slow activity in the frontal areas bilaterally. A SPECT scan of his brain was normal. A week later, repeat neuropsychological examination showed normal memory and a normal electroencephalogram and MRI scan of the brain with enhancement. One year later, he had stopped using marijuana and had no further amnestic episodes.

The authors found similarities between the memory disorder seen here and transient global amnesia, which consists of anterograde amnesia and a variably graded retrograde amnesia. Such amnesia has been previously reported with a number of substances and medications, but not with marijuana. The authors stated that although memory impairment has been reported with marijuana before, it has never involved retrieval of already learned material. They wondered if the memory impairment was due to marijuana-induced changes in cerebral blood flow and ischemia through vasospasm. However, their SPECT data did not support this theory. They considered the possibility that cannabinoid receptors, which are dense in the hippocampus, could have been occupied by marijuana, resulting in such memory loss. They cautioned that the effects of marijuana on memory may be more severe than previously thought.

Endocrine

In animals (particularly monkeys), cannabis depresses ovarian and testicular function. In man, chronic use has been associated with reduced serum FSH and LH concentrations in a few people, often accompanied by reduced serum testosterone, oligospermia, reduced sperm motility, and gynecomastia (83). There is no evidence of impairment of male fertility; no studies have been carried out on female fertility. There is evidence of slightly shortened gestation periods in chronic users (84). There are variable non-specific effects on serum prolactin and growth hormone and a rise in plasma cortisol concentrations has been recorded in one study.

Hematologic

Of the hematological changes very occasionally noted, polycythemia appears to be secondary to reduced pulmonary oxygen exchange (see the Respiratory section in this monograph).

Immunologic

Tetrahydrocannabinol depresses lymphocyte and macrophage activity in cell cultures, while in rats in vivo it directly suppresses natural killer cell activity and impairs T lymphocyte transformation by phytohemagglutinin in concentrations of cannabinoids achievable with the usual doses (85). Variable results have been obtained in man in tests of circulating T cells and hormonal immunity (86).

In animals and man, chronic use often suppresses the immune system's response to inhaled bacterial or fungal material. In this connection it is relevant to note that a contaminant mould (*Aspergillus*) found in cannabis can predispose immunocompromised cannabis smokers to infection. It has been suggested that baking the cannabis (at 300°F for 15 minutes) before smoking will kill the fungus and reduce the potential risk (87).

The effects of marijuana on immune function have been reviewed (88). The studies suggest that marijuana affects immune cell function of T and B lymphocytes, natural killer cells, and macrophages. In addition, cannabis appears to modulate host resistance, especially the secondary immune response to various infectious agents, both viral and bacterial. Lastly, marijuana may also affect the cytokine network, influencing the production and function of acute-phase and immune cytokines and modulating network cells, such as macrophages and T helper cells. Under some conditions, marijuana may be immunomodulatory and promote disease.

A severe allergic reaction after intravenous marijuana has been reported (89).

- A 25-year-old man with intermittent metamfetamine use developed facial edema, pruritus, and dyspnea 45 minutes after injecting a mixture of crushed marijuana leaves and heated water. He was anxious, and had tachypnea, respiratory stridor, wheezing, edema of the face and oral mucosa, and truncal urticaria. There was mild pre-renal uremia and urine toxicology was positive for metamfetamine and marijuana. Skin testing was not done. With appropriate medical intervention there was resolution of symptoms within a day.

The authors noted that marijuana may have contaminants, including *Aspergillus*, *Salmonella*, herbicides, and mercury, which can trigger allergic reactions.

Long-Term Effects

Drug tolerance

Tolerance develops with heavy chronic use in individuals who report problems in controlling their use and who continue to use cannabis despite adverse personal consequences (53).

Drug withdrawal

Withdrawal symptoms occur after chronic heavy use (53). Abrupt withdrawal of high-level use of cannabinoids causes irritability, restlessness, and insomnia, with a rebound increase in REM sleep, tremor, and anorexia lasting up to a week (90–92). Occasional use does not appear to be associated with major consequences.

Second-Generation Effects

Pregnancy

Behavioral anomalies have been identified in the offspring of monkeys and women exposed to cannabis during pregnancy (93,94). These include reduced visual responses, increased auditory responses, and reduced quietude. Most of the effects resolved within 4–5 weeks postpartum and there were no abnormalities at 1 year.

Teratogenicity

In animals, THC crosses the placenta and is excreted in breast milk. There is conflicting evidence concerning teratogenicity in animals, but no definitive evidence in man. However, there have been many anecdotal reports of abnormalities. Although these were without consistent characteristics, the descriptions would readily fit the fetal alcohol syndrome (95–98) and clinical evaluation of the use of cannabis during pregnancy is complicated by the frequent concomitant use of alcohol and tobacco.

Fetotoxicity

The effect of maternal and prenatal marijuana exposure on offspring from birth to adolescence is being investigated (99). The Ottawa Prenatal Prospective Study (OPPS), a longitudinal project begun in 1978, recently reported its findings in 146 low-risk, middle-class children aged 9–12 years. Their performances on neurobehavioral tasks that focus on visuoperceptual abilities (ranging from basic skills to those requiring integration and cognitive manipulation of such skills) were analysed. Performance outcomes were different in children with prenatal exposure to cigarette smoking and those with prenatal exposure to marijuana. Maternal cigarette smoking affected fundamental visuoperceptual functioning. Prenatal marijuana use had a negative effect on performance in visual problem-solving, which requires integration, analysis, and synthesis. In a second prospective study, the effects of prenatal marijuana exposure and child behavior problems were studied in 763 subjects aged 10 years (100). Prenatal maternal marijuana exposure was associated with increased hyperactivity, impulsivity, and inattention in the children. There was also increased delinquency and externalizing problems. The authors suggested a possible pathway between prenatal marijuana exposure and delinquency, which may be mediated by the effects of marijuana exposure on symptoms of inattention.

Susceptibility Factors

Age

Children

In young children, accidental ingestion leads to the rapid onset of drowsiness, hypotonia, dilated pupils, and coma. Fortunately, gradual recovery occurs spontaneously, barring accidents. Passive inhalation of marijuana in infants can have serious consequences.

- A 9-month-old girl presented with extreme lethargy and a modified Glasgow coma scale of 10, after having been exposed to cigarette and cannabis smoke at the home of her teenage sister's friend (101). The physical examination and laboratory results were unremarkable. Cannabinoids were detected in a urine screen.

While chronic adult users can display apathy and impaired concentration, these effects are possibly in part associated with other factors. No permanent organic brain damage has been demonstrated (101,102).

Other features of the patient

People with pre-existing coronary artery disease may have an increased incidence of attacks of angina (103). In individuals who are vulnerable to schizophrenia, cannabis can precipitate psychoses or aggravate schizophrenia. The control of epilepsy may be impaired. Users undergoing anesthesia may react unexpectedly and may have enhanced nervous system depression. Because of impairment of judgement and psychomotor performance, users should not drive or operate machinery for at least 24 hours after administration.

Drug–Drug Interactions

Alcohol

Additive psychoactive effects sought by users may be achieved by combinations of cannabis and alcohol, but at the same time the ability of THC to induce microsomal enzymes will increase the rate of metabolism of alcohol and so reduce the additive effects (90).

Anticholinergic drugs

The anticholinergic effects of cannabis (90) may result in interactions with other drugs with anticholinergic effects, such as some antidysrhythmic drugs.

Barbiturates, short-acting

Additive psychoactive effects sought by users may be achieved by combinations of cannabis and short-acting barbiturates, but at the same time the ability of THC to induce microsomal enzymes will increase the rate of metabolism of barbiturates and so reduce the additive effects (90).

Disulfiram

Concurrent administration with disulfiram is associated with hypomania (104).

Lysergic acid diethylamide

"Flashbacks," or the return of hallucinogenic effects, occur in almost a quarter of those who have used LSD, particularly if they have also used other CNS stimulants, such as alcohol or marijuana. They can experience distortions of perception of objects, space, or time, which intrude without warning into reality, resulting in delusions, panic, and unusual images. A "trailing phenomenon" has also been reported, in which the visual perception of objects is reduced to a series of interrupted pictures rather than a constant view. The frequency of these events may slowly abate over several years, but in a significant number their incidence later increases (105,106).

Psychotropic drugs

Cannabis alters the effects of psychotropic drugs, such as opioids, anticholinergic drugs, and antidepressants, although variably and unpredictably (90).

Sildenafil

Myocardial infarction has been attributed to the combination of cannabis and sildenafil.

- A 41-year-old man developed chest tightness radiating down both arms (107). He had taken sildenafil and cannabis recreationally the night before. His vital signs were normal and he had no signs of heart failure. However, electrocardiography showed an inferior evolving non-Q-wave myocardial infarct and his creatine kinase activity was raised (431 U/l).

Cannabis inhibits CYP3A4, which is primarily responsible for the metabolism of sildenafil, increased concentrations of which may have caused this cardiac event.

References

1. Caswell A. Marijuana as medicine. Med J Aust 1992;156(7):497–8.
2. Voelker R. Medical marijuana: a trial of science and politics. JAMA 1994;271(21):1645–8.
3. Woody GE, MacFadden W. Cannabis related disorders. In: Kaplan HI, Sadock B, editors. Comprehensive Textbook of Psychiatry. Baltimore: Williams & Wilkins, 6th ed, vol. 1. 1995:810–17.
4. Herkenham M. Cannabinoid receptor localization in brain: relationship to motor and reward systems. Ann NY Acad Sci 1992;654:19–32.
5. Childers SR, Fleming L, Konkoy C, Marckel D, Pacheco M, Sexton T, Ward S. Opioid and cannabinoid receptor inhibition of adenylyl cyclase in brain. Ann NY Acad Sci 1992;654:33–51.
6. Aronson J. When I use a word...: Sloe gin. BMJ 1997;314:1106.
7. Iversen LL. The Science of Marijuana. New York: Oxford University Press, 2000.
8. Braude MC. Toxicology of cannabinoids. In: Paton WM, Crown J, editors. Cannabis and its Derivatives. Oxford: Oxford University Press, 1972:89–99.
9. Chan PC, Sills RC, Braun AG, Haseman JK, Bucher JR. Toxicity and carcinogenicity of delta 9-tetrahydrocannabinol in Fischer rats and B6C3F1 mice. Fundam Appl Toxicol 1996;30(1):109–17.
10. Fleischman RW, Baker JR, Rosenkrantz H. Pulmonary pathologic changes in rats exposed to marihuana smoke for 1 year. Toxicol Appl Pharmacol 1979;47(3):557–66.
11. Roy PE, Magnan-Lapointe F, Huy ND, Boutet M. Chronic inhalation of marijuana and tobacco in dogs: pulmonary pathology. Res Commun Chem Pathol Pharmacol 1976;14(2):305–17.
12. Fligiel SE, Beals TF, Tashkin DP, Paule MG, Scallet AC, Ali SF, Bailey JR, Slikker W Jr. Marijuana exposure and pulmonary alterations in primates. Pharmacol Biochem Behav 1991;40(3):637–42.
13. Scallet AC, Uemura E, Andrews A, Ali SF, McMillan DE, Paule MG, Brown RM, Slikker W Jr. Morphometric studies of the rat hippocampus following chronic delta-9-tetrahydrocannabinol (THC). Brain Res 1987;436(1):193–8.
14. Landfield PW, Cadwallader LB, Vinsant S. Quantitative changes in hippocampal structure following long-term exposure to delta 9-tetrahydrocannabinol: possible mediation by glucocorticoid systems. Brain Res 1988;443(1–2):47–62.
15. Harper JW, Heath RG, Myers WA. Effects of *Cannabis sativa* on ultrastructure of the synapse in monkey brain. J Neurosci Res 1977;3(2):87–93.
16. Heath RG, Fitzjarrell AT, Fontana CJ, Garey RE. *Cannabis sativa*: effects on brain function and ultrastructure in rhesus monkeys. Biol Psychiatry 1980;15(5):657–90.
17. Scallet AC. Neurotoxicology of cannabis and THC: a review of chronic exposure studies in animals. Pharmacol Biochem Behav 1991;40(3):671–6.
18. Downer E, Boland B, Fogarty M, Campbell V. Delta 9-tetrahydrocannabinol induces the apoptotic pathway in cultured cortical neurones via activation of the CB_1 receptor. Neuroreport 2001;12(18):3973–8.
19. Chan GC, Hinds TR, Impey S, Storm DR. Hippocampal neurotoxicity of Δ9-tetrahydrocannabinol. J Neurosci 1998;18(14):5322–32.
20. Sanchez C, Galve-Roperh I, Canova C, Brachet P, Guzman M. Δ9-tetrahydrocannabinol induces apoptosis in C6 glioma cells. FEBS Lett 1998;436(1):6–10.
21. Galve-Roperh I, Sanchez C, Cortes ML, del Pulgar TG, Izquierdo M, Guzman M. Anti-tumoral action of cannabinoids: involvement of sustained ceramide accumulation and extracellular signal-regulated kinase activation. Nat Med 2000;6(3):313–19.
22. Bifulco M, Laezza C, Portella G, Vitale M, Orlando P, De Petrocellis L, Di Marzo V. Control by the endogenous cannabinoid system of ras oncogene-dependent tumor growth. FASEB J 2001;15(14):2745–7.
23. Guzman M, Sanchez C, Galve-Roperh I. Control of the cell survival/death decision by cannabinoids. J Mol Med 2001;78(11):613–25.
24. Nagayama T, Sinor AD, Simon RP, Chen J, Graham SH, Jin K, Greenberg DA. Cannabinoids and neuroprotection in global and focal cerebral ischemia and in neuronal cultures. J Neurosci 1999;19(8):2987–95.
25. Panikashvili D, Simeonidou C, Ben-Shabat S, Hanus L, Breuer A, Mechoulam R, Shohami E. An endogenous cannabinoid (2-AG) is neuroprotective after brain injury. Nature 2001;413(6855):527–31.

26. van der Stelt M, Veldhuis WB, Bar PR, Veldink GA, Vliegenthart JF, Nicolay K. Neuroprotection by △9-tetrahydrocannabinol, the main active compound in marijuana, against ouabain-induced in vivo excitotoxicity. J Neurosci 2001;21(17):6475–9.
27. Shen M, Thayer SA. Cannabinoid receptor agonists protect cultured rat hippocampal neurons from excitotoxicity. Mol Pharmacol 1998;54(3):459–62.
28. Sinor AD, Irvin SM, Greenberg DA. Endocannabinoids protect cerebral cortical neurons from in vitro ischemia in rats. Neurosci Lett 2000;278(3):157–60.
29. Hampson AJ, Grimaldi M, Axelrod J, Wink D. Cannabidiol and (-)△9-tetrahydrocannabinol are neuroprotective antioxidants. Proc Natl Acad Sci USA 1998;95(14):8268–73.
30. Zimmer L, Morgan JP. Marijuana Myths, Marijuana Facts. New York: Lindesmith Centre, 1997.
31. Pertwee RG. Tolerance to and dependence on psychotropic cannabinoids. In: Pratt J, editor. The Biological Basis of Drug Tolerance. London: Academic Press, 1991:232–65.
32. Aceto MD, Scates SM, Lowe JA, Martin BR. Dependence on delta 9-tetrahydrocannabinol: studies on precipitated and abrupt withdrawal. J Pharmacol Exp Ther 1996; 278(3):1290–5.
33. Rubino T, Patrini G, Massi P, Fuzio D, Vigano D, Giagnoni G, Parolaro D. Cannabinoid-precipitated withdrawal: a time-course study of the behavioral aspect and its correlation with cannabinoid receptors and G protein expression. J Pharmacol Exp Ther 1998;285(2):813–19.
34. Rodriguez de Fonseca F, Carrera MR, Navarro M, Koob GF, Weiss F. Activation of corticotropin-releasing factor in the limbic system during cannabinoid withdrawal. Science 1997;276(5321):2050–4.
35. Diana M, Melis M, Muntoni AL, Gessa GL. Mesolimbic dopaminergic decline after cannabinoid withdrawal. Proc Natl Acad Sci USA 1998;95(17):10269–73.
36. Tanda G, Pontieri FE, Di Chiara G. Cannabinoid and heroin activation of mesolimbic dopamine transmission by a common mu1 opioid receptor mechanism. Science 1997;276(5321):2048–50.
37. Tanda G, Munzar P, Goldberg SR. Self-administration behavior is maintained by the psychoactive ingredient of marijuana in squirrel monkeys. Nat Neurosci 2000; 3(11):1073–4.
38. Ledent C, Valverde O, Cossu G, Petitet F, Aubert JF, Beslot F, Bohme GA, Imperato A, Pedrazzini T, Roques BP, Vassart G, Fratta W, Parmentier M. Unresponsiveness to cannabinoids and reduced addictive effects of opiates in CB_1 receptor knockout mice. Science 1999;283(5400):401–4.
39. Lepore M, Vorel SR, Lowinson J, Gardner EL. Conditioned place preference induced by delta 9-tetrahydrocannabinol: comparison with cocaine, morphine, and food reward. Life Sci 1995;56(23–24):2073–80.
40. Manzanares J, Corchero J, Romero J, Fernandez-Ruiz JJ, Ramos JA, Fuentes JA. Pharmacological and biochemical interactions between opioids and cannabinoids. Trends Pharmacol Sci 1999;20(7):287–94.
41. Kaymakcalan S, Ayhan IH, Tulunay FC. Naloxone-induced or postwithdrawal abstinence signs in △9-tetrahydrocannabinol-tolerant rats. Psychopharmacology (Berl) 1977;55(3):243–9.
42. Hine B, Friedman E, Torrelio M, Gershon S. Morphine-dependent rats: blockade of precipitated abstinence by tetrahydrocannabinol. Science 1975;187(4175):443–5.
43. Yamaguchi T, Hagiwara Y, Tanaka H, Sugiura T, Waku K, Shoyama Y, Watanabe S, Yamamoto T. Endogenous cannabinoid, 2-arachidonoylglycerol, attenuates naloxone-precipitated withdrawal signs in morphine-dependent mice. Brain Res 2001;909(1–2):121–6.
44. Pontieri FE, Monnazzi P, Scontrini A, Buttarelli FR, Patacchioli FR. Behavioral sensitization to heroin by cannabinoid pretreatment in the rat. Eur J Pharmacol 2001;421(3):R1–3.
45. Valverde O, Maldonado R, Valjent E, Zimmer AM, Zimmer A. Cannabinoid withdrawal syndrome is reduced in pre-proenkephalin knock-out mice. J Neurosci 2000;20(24):9284–9.
46. Valverde O, Noble F, Beslot F, Dauge V, Fournie-Zaluski MC, Roques BP. △9-tetrahydrocannabinol releases and facilitates the effects of endogenous enkephalins: reduction in morphine withdrawal syndrome without change in rewarding effect. Eur J Neurosci 2001;13(9):1816–24.
47. Lichtman AH, Fisher J, Martin BR. Precipitated cannabinoid withdrawal is reversed by △(9)-tetrahydrocannabinol or clonidine. Pharmacol Biochem Behav 2001;69(1–2):181–8.
48. Lichtman AH, Sheikh SM, Loh HH, Martin BR. Opioid and cannabinoid modulation of precipitated withdrawal in △(9)-tetrahydrocannabinol and morphine-dependent mice. J Pharmacol Exp Ther 2001;298(3):1007–14.
49. US Department of Health and Human Services. National Household Survey on Drug Abuse, 1982–94. Computer Files (ICPSR Version). Ann Arbor, MI: Inter-University Consortium for Political Social, 1999.
50. Morral AR, McCaffrey DF, Paddock SM. Reassessing the marijuana gateway effect. Addiction 2002;97(12):1493–504.
51. Wehner FC, van Rensburg SJ, Thiel PG. Mutagenicity of marijuana and Transkei tobacco smoke condensates in the Salmonella/microsome assay. Mutat Res 1980; 77(2):135–42.
52. Leuchtenberger C, Leuchtenberger R. Cytological and cytochemical studies of the effects of fresh marihuana smoke on growth and DNA metabolism of animal and human lung cultures. In: Braude MC, Szara S, editors. The Pharmacology of Marijuana. New York: Raven Press, 1976:595–612.
53. Hall W, Solowij N. Adverse effects of cannabis. Lancet 1998;352(9140):1611–16.
54. Institute of Medicine. Marijuana and Health. Washington, DC: National Academy Press, 1982.
55. Killestein J, Hoogervorst EL, Reif M, Kalkers NF, Van Loenen AC, Staats PG, Gorter RW, Uitdehaag BM, Polman CH. Safety, tolerability, and efficacy of orally administered cannabinoids in MS. Neurology 2002; 58(9):1404–7.
56. Avakian EV, Horvath SM, Michael ED, Jacobs S. Effect of marihuana on cardiorespiratory responses to submaximal exercise. Clin Pharmacol Ther 1979;26(6):777–81.
57. Relman AS. Marijuana and health. N Engl J Med 1982;306(10):603–5.
58. Mittleman MA, Lewis RA, Maclure M, Sherwood JB, Muller JE. Triggering myocardial infarction by marijuana. Circulation 2001;103(23):2805–9.
59. Kosior DA, Filipiak KJ, Stolarz P, Opolski G. Paroxysmal atrial fibrillation following marijuana intoxication: a two-case report of possible association. Int J Cardiol 2001;78(2):183–4.
60. Singh GK. Atrial fibrillation associated with marijuana use. Pediatr Cardiol 2000;21(3):284.
61. Schneider HJ, Jha S, Burnand KG. Progressive arteritis associated with cannabis use. Eur J Vasc Endovasc Surg 1999;18(4):366–7.
62. Wu TC, Tashkin DP, Djahed B, Rose JE. Pulmonary hazards of smoking marijuana as compared with tobacco. N Engl J Med 1988;318(6):347–51.
63. Tashkin DP, Calvarese BM, Simmons MS, Shapiro BJ. Respiratory status of seventy-four habitual marijuana smokers. Chest 1980;78(5):699–706.

64. Tashkin DP. Pulmonary complications of smoked substance abuse. West J Med 1990;152(5):525–30.
65. Douglass RE, Levison MA. Pneumothorax in drug abusers. An urban epidemic? Am Surg 1986;52(7):377–80.
66. Tashkin DP, Coulson AH, Clark VA, Simmons M, Bourque LB, Duann S, Spivey GH, Gong H. Respiratory symptoms and lung function in habitual heavy smokers of marijuana alone, smokers of marijuana and tobacco, smokers of tobacco alone, and nonsmokers. Am Rev Respir Dis 1987;135(1):209–16.
67. Johnson MK, Smith RP, Morrison D, Laszlo G, White RJ. Large lung bullae in marijuana smokers. Thorax 2000;55(4):340–2.
68. Thompson CS, White RJ. Lung bullae and marijuana. Thorax 2002;57(6):563.
69. Voruganti LN, Slomka P, Zabel P, Mattar A, Awad AG. Cannabis induced dopamine release: an in-vivo SPECT study. Psychiatry Res 2001;107(3):173–7.
70. Dawson WW, Jimenez-Antillon CF, Perez JM, Zeskind JA. Marijuana and vision—after ten years' use in Costa Rica. Invest Ophthalmol Vis Sci 1977;16(8):689–99.
71. Mulheran M, Middleton P, Henry JA. The acute effects of tetrahydrocannabinol on auditory threshold and frequency resolution in human subjects. Hum Exp Toxicol 2002;21(6):289–92.
72. Troisi A, Pasini A, Saracco M, Spalletta G. Psychiatric symptoms in male cannabis users not using other illicit drugs. Addiction 1998;93(4):487–92.
73. Russo E, Mathre ML, Byrne A, Velin R, Bach PJ, Sanchez-Ramos J, Kirlin KA. Chronic cannabis use in the compassionate investigational new drug program: an examination of benefits and adverse effects of legal clinical cannabis. J Cannabis Ther 2002;2:3–57.
74. Linszen DH, Dingemans PM, Lenior ME. Cannabis abuse and the course of recent-onset schizophrenic disorders. Arch Gen Psychiatry 1994;51(4):273–9.
75. Andreasson S, Allebeck P, Engstrom A, Rydberg U. Cannabis and schizophrenia. A longitudinal study of Swedish conscripts. Lancet 1987;2(8574):1483–6.
76. Bowers MB Jr. Family history and early psychotogenic response to marijuana. J Clin Psychiatry 1998; 59(4):198–9.
77. Crowley TJ, Macdonald MJ, Whitmore EA, Mikulich SK. Cannabis dependence, withdrawal, and reinforcing effects among adolescents with conduct symptoms and substance use disorders. Drug Alcohol Depend 1998;50(1):27–37.
78. Solowij N. Cannabis and Cognitive Functioning. Cambridge: Cambridge University Press, 1998.
79. Schwartz RH, Gruenewald PJ, Klitzner M, Fedio P. Short-term memory impairment in cannabis-dependent adolescents. Am J Dis Child 1989;143(10):1214–19.
80. Volkow ND, Gillespie H, Mullani N, Tancredi L, Grant C, Valentine A, Hollister L. Brain glucose metabolism in chronic marijuana users at baseline and during marijuana intoxication. Psychiatry Res 1996;67(1):29–38.
81. Ashton CH. Adverse effects of cannabis and cannabinoids. Br J Anaesth 1999;83(4):637–49.
82. Stracciari A, Guarino M, Crespi C, Pazzaglia P. Transient amnesia triggered by acute marijuana intoxication. Eur J Neurol 1999;6(4):521–3.
83. Kolodny RC, Masters WH, Kolodner RM, Toro G. Depression of plasma testosterone levels after chronic intensive marihuana use. N Engl J Med 1974;290(16):872–4.
84. Fried PA, Watkinson B, Willan A. Marijuana use during pregnancy and decreased length of gestation. Am J Obstet Gynecol 1984;150(1):23–7.
85. Klein TW, Newton C, Friedman H. Inhibition of natural killer cell function by marijuana components. J Toxicol Environ Health 1987;20(4):321–32.
86. Pillai R, Nair BS, Watson RR. AIDS, drugs of abuse and the immune system: a complex immunotoxicological network. Arch Toxicol 1991;65(8):609–17.
87. Levitz SM, Diamond RD. Aspergillosis and marijuana. Ann Intern Med 1991;115(7):578–9.
88. Klein TW, Friedman H, Specter S. Marijuana, immunity and infection. J Neuroimmunol 1998;83(1–2):102–15.
89. Perez JA Jr. Allergic reaction associated with intravenous marijuana use. J Emerg Med 2000;18(2):260–1.
90. Jones RT. Cannabis and health. Annu Rev Med 1983; 34:247–58.
91. Carney MW, Bacelle L, Robinson B. Psychosis after cannabis abuse. BMJ (Clin Res Ed) 1984;288(6423):1047.
92. Liakos A, Boulougouris JC, Stefanis C. Psychophysiologic effects of acute cannabis smoking in long-term users. Ann NY Acad Sci 1976;282:375–86.
93. Fried PA. Marihuana use by pregnant women: neurobehavioral effects in neonates. Drug Alcohol Depend 1980; 6(6):415–24.
94. Abel EL. Prenatal exposure to cannabis: a critical review of effects on growth, development, and behavior. Behav Neural Biol 1980;29(2):137–56.
95. Qazi QH, Mariano E, Milman DH, Beller E, Crombleholme W. Abnormalities in offspring associated with prenatal marihuana exposure. Dev Pharmacol Ther 1985;8(2):141–8.
96. Fried PA. Marihuana use by pregnant women and effects on offspring: an update. Neurobehav Toxicol Teratol 1982;4(4):451–4.
97. Greenland S, Staisch KJ, Brown N, Gross SJ. Effects of marijuana on human pregnancy, labor, and delivery. Neurobehav Toxicol Teratol 1982;4(4):447–50.
98. Nahas G, Frick HC. Developmental effects of cannabis. Neurotoxicology 1986;7(2):381–95.
99. Fried PA, Watkinson B. Visuoperceptual functioning differs in 9- to 12-year olds prenatally exposed to cigarettes and marihuana. Neurotoxicol Teratol 2000; 22(1):11–20.
100. Goldschmidt L, Day NL, Richardson GA. Effects of prenatal marijuana exposure on child behavior problems at age 10. Neurotoxicol Teratol 2000;22(3): 325–36.
101. Wert RC, Raulin ML. The chronic cerebral effects of cannabis use. II. Psychological findings and conclusions. Int J Addict 1986;21(6):629–42.
102. Wert RC, Raulin ML. The chronic cerebral effects of cannabis use. I. Methodological issues and neurological findings. Int J Addict 1986;21(6):605–28.
103. Aronow WS, Cassidy J. Effect of marihuana and placebo-marihuana smoking on angina pectoris. N Engl J Med 1974;291(2):65–7.
104. Lacoursiere RB, Swatek R. Adverse interaction between disulfiram and marijuana: a case report. Am J Psychiatry 1983;140(2):243–4.
105. Watson SJ. Hallucinogens and other psychotomimetics: biological mechanisms. In: Barchas JD, Berger PA, Cioranello RD, Elliot GR, editors. Psychopharmacology from Theory to Practise. New York: Oxford University Press, 1977.
106. Strassman RJ. Adverse reactions to psychedelic drugs. A review of the literature. J Nerv Ment Dis 1984; 172(10):577–95.
107. McLeod AL, McKenna CJ, Northridge DB. Myocardial infarction following the combined recreational use of Viagra and cannabis. Clin Cardiol 2002;25(3):133–4.

Capparaceae

See also Herbal medicines

General Information

The genera in the family of Capparaceae (Table 1) include caper and stinkweed.

Capparis spinosa

The leaf and fruit of *Capparis spinosa* (caper plant) both contain isothiocyanates, in addition to the flavonoid rutinoside and the quaternary alkaloid stachydrine.

Adverse effects

Allergic contact dermatitis can follow the application of *C. spinosa* in the form of wet compresses (1).

Table 1 The genera of Capparaceae

Atamisquea (atamisquea)
Capparis (caper)
Cleome (spiderflower)
Cleomella (stinkweed)
Forchhammeria (forchhammeria)
Koeberlinia (allthorn)
Morisonia (morisonia)
Oxystylis (oxystylis)
Polanisia (clammyweed)
Wislizenia (wislizenia)

Reference

1. Angelini G, Vena GA, Filotico R, Foti C, Grandolfo M. Allergic contact dermatitis from *Capparis spinosa* L. applied as wet compresses. Contact Dermatitis 1991; 24(5):382–3.

Capreomycin

See also Antituberculosis drugs

General Information

Capreomycin has been abandoned for the treatment of tuberculosis and replaced by first-choice drugs. In rare cases, it has been administered in infections with non-tuberculous mycobacteria when there is multiple drug resistance to the first-line antituberculosis drugs (1).

Organs and Systems

Electrolyte balance

Marked renal loss of sodium, chloride, potassium, and magnesium with progressive metabolic alkalosis and hyper-reninemia have been reported (2).

Urinary tract

A Bartter-like syndrome has been reported in a 25-year-old man taking prolonged capreomycin for drug-resistant pulmonary tuberculosis (2).

Drug–Drug Interactions

Streptomycin

Capreomycin should never be combined with streptomycin or other aminoglycosides because of nephrotoxicity and ototoxicity (3).

References

1. Mandell GL, Sande MA. Antimicrobial agents: drugs used in the chemotherapy of tuberculosis and leprosy. In: Goodman Gilman A, Rall TW, Nies AS, Taylor P, editors. Goodman and Gilman's The Pharmacological Basis of Therapeutics. 8th ed. Chapter 49. New York: Pergamon Press, 1990:1146.
2. Steiner RW, Omachi AS. A Bartter's-like syndrome from capreomycin, and a similar gentamicin tubulopathy. Am J Kidney Dis 1986;7(3):245–9.
3. Hugues FC, Moore N, Julien D. Les interactions observées avec les médicaments antituberculeux. [Interactions of antitubercular drugs.] Rev Pneumol Clin 1988; 44(6):278–85.

Captopril

See also Angiotensin converting enzyme inhibitors

General Information

Captopril is a sulfhydryl-containing ACE inhibitor used in the management of hypertension and heart failure, after myocardial infarction, and in diabetic nephropathy.

Organs and Systems

Respiratory

Two cases of alveolitis have been reported with captopril, one associated with eosinophilia (1) and the other with a lymphocytic pulmonary infiltrate (2).

Sensory systems

A report from the Australian Drug Evaluation Committee has confirmed that dysgeusia (taste disturbance and taste loss) is more likely to complicate treatment with captopril than with other ACE inhibitors; captopril accounted for more than half the cases of taste loss (3). Taste loss was dose-related, in that more than 90% of reports detailed a daily dose of 50 mg or more. Most cases recovered on withdrawal, although the sense of taste had not returned 7 months after withdrawal in one case, and in two of the reports there was associated anosmia. Although there was no significant difference between captopril and lisinopril

(4), it appears that captopril, presumably via its sulfhydryl group, is more likely to provoke dysgeusia.

Hematologic

Anecdotal reports of a bone-marrow suppressant effect of captopril have been published, but not since 1989. Cases of neutropenia and agranulocytosis (5–8) have also been reported, although in some of these there were complicating issues, making a clear association difficult to establish. Usually the incidence is higher in patients with renal insufficiency or collagen vascular disease. In few cases the white cell count returned to normal when captopril was withdrawn. Although agranulocytosis has been attributed to the presence of the sulfhydryl group in captopril, it has also been reported with enalapril (9).

Agranulocytosis has also been reported in association with toxic epidermal necrolysis (10).

- A 59-year-old woman with long-standing hypertension took captopril 200 mg bd plus hydrochlorothiazide 50 mg od and 3 days later developed nausea, vomiting, malaise, and a severe, pruritic, erythematous rash, with severe dehydration and orthostatic hypotension. The diuretic was withdrawn and intravenous fluids and diphenhydramine were given. She recovered within 1 week and remained asymptomatic for 4 weeks. She then developed fever, malaise, a new rash, orthostatic hypotension, and diffuse erythroderma. Her posterior pharynx was erythematous. She had neutropenia (900×10^6/l) and captopril was withdrawn. She was treated empirically with antibiotics and intravenous fluids and subcutaneous granulocyte colony-stimulating factor (G-CSF) for 5 days. The erythroderma progressed to large coalescing blisters, which then ruptured, producing large areas of weeping skin over all her limbs. The bone-marrow and skin recovered fully within 2 weeks.

Autoimmune thrombocytopenia, gradually reversible on withdrawal of captopril, was reported in three patients taking captopril (11).

Pancreas

Two new cases of pancreatitis with captopril have been reported (12,13). It has been suggested that early detection of raised serum amylase and lipase activities can prevent the development of full-blown pancreatitis (13).

Urinary tract

Acute renal insufficiency with tubular necrosis has been described (14). It occurred within 24 hours of the first dose of captopril and required hemodialysis for 8 weeks. The diagnosis of ischemic tubular necrosis was confirmed by renal biopsy. Few previous cases of ACE inhibitor-induced nephropathy have been documented by renal biopsy.

Immunologic

Lupus–like syndrome has been reported with captopril (15). The authors believed their patient to be the fifth such published case.

- A 54-year-old Caucasian man presented with a 4-week history of chills, fever, malaise, and generalized arthralgia. Following an aortic valve replacement, he had taken aspirin, coumadin, and captopril 25 mg tds for 1 year. He was febrile (temperature 39.4°C), normotensive, with diffuse livedo reticularis, and the physical signs of aortic valve disease. Infective endocarditis was ruled out by appropriate investigations. He had a raised erythrocyte sedimentation rate (142 mm/hour) and a positive antinuclear antibody test (FANA 1:2560) with a negative antinative DNA test. Captopril was withdrawn and he was given prednisone for 5 days. His symptoms resolved rapidly and the livedo reticularis cleared within 2 days. The FANA and ESR returned to normal and remained so at follow-up 6 months later.

During early drug development, the occurrence of antinuclear antibodies in 10 of 37 patients taking high doses of captopril was described (16).

Drug–Drug Interactions

General anesthesia

The hazards of general anesthesia in the presence of ACE inhibitors have been recognized and reviewed (17). It has generally been accepted that ACE inhibitors should be continued up to the time of surgery. Patients should be monitored aggressively and hemodynamic instability treated appropriately.

- An 86-year-old man, who was taking captopril 25 mg bd and bendroflumethiazide 25 mg/day for hypertension, had a transurethral resection of the prostate under spinal anesthesia, and developed profound bradycardia and hypotension with disturbances of consciousness during transfer to the recovery room (18). Initial treatment with atropine produced rapid improvement in cardiovascular and cerebral function. A further hypotensive episode, without bradycardia, occurred about 1 hour later, but responded rapidly to methoxamine. He made a full recovery overnight.

The authors suggested that the concomitant administration of captopril may have contributed to the adverse effect, since the renin–angiotensin system is important in maintaining blood pressure during anesthesia. Because of a protective effect of angiotensin II in the presence of sympathetic blockade by presynaptic stimulation of adrenergic neurons, the authors hypothesized that hypotension and bradycardia in this patient may have been magnified by suppression of the renin–angiotensin system, resulting in an enhanced negative Bainbridge effect.

Iron and other transition metals

Captopril has been reported to react with iron and other transition metals. This interaction has been investigated in vivo in seven healthy adults (19). Co-administration of ferrous sulfate and captopril resulted in a 37% decrease in the AUC of unconjugated captopril, with no significant changes in C_{max} or t_{max}. The plasma AUC of total captopril was not altered. The authors suggested that the interaction may be specific to captopril among ACE inhibitors, because it contains a sulfhydryl group. Therefore, if iron salts were to be taken by a patient requiring an ACE inhibitor, an agent other than captopril might be considered.

Interference with Diagnostic Tests

Legal reaction

Like other sulfhydryl-containing compounds, captopril can cause false-positive ketonuria when assessed with the Legal reaction (sodium nitroprusside reacting with acetoacetic acid and possibly with acetone). It has therefore been suggested that in patients with diabetes taking such drugs ketonuria should be assessed with the Acetest (20). Alternatively, a blood ketone test with Acetest and/or enzymatic detection of beta-hydroxybutyric acid can be performed for confirmation.

References

1. Schatz PL, Mesologites D, Hyun J, Smith GJ, Lahiri B. Captopril-induced hypersensitivity lung disease. An immune-complex-mediated phenomenon. Chest 1989;95(3):685–7.
2. Kidney JC, O'Halloran DJ, FitzGerald MX. Captopril and lymphocytic alveolitis. BMJ 1989;299(6705):981.
3. Boyd I. Captopril-induced taste disturbance. Lancet 1993;342(8866):304.
4. Neil-Dwyer G, Marus A. ACE inhibitors in hypertension: assessment of taste and smell function in clinical trials. J Hum Hypertens 1989;3(Suppl 1):169–76.
5. Lacueva J, Enriquez R, Bonilla F, Cabezuelo JB. Agranulocitosis por captopril en insufficienca renal. Nefrologia 1992;12:76–7.
6. Ortega G, Molina Boix M, Vidal JB, de Paco M, del Bano MD, Ruiz F. Tratamiento con captopril de la hipertension arterial en la nefropatia lupica. [Treatment of arterial hypertension with captopril in lupus nephropathy.] An Med Interna 1992;9(2):72–5.
7. Fernandez Seara J, Dominguez Alvarez LM, Rodriguez Perez R, Pereira Jorge JA, Rodriguez Canal A. Agranulocitosis inducida por captopril tras cuarto mese de tratamiento. [Agranulocytosis induced by captopril after 4 months of treatment.] An Med Interna 1991; 8(8):398–400.
8. Ortega G, Molina M, Rivera MD, Serrano C. Neutropenia inducida porbajas dosis de captopris en pacientes hipertensos sin enfermedad autoimmune asociada. [Neutropenia induced by low doses of captopril in hypertensive patients without associated autoimmune disease.] An Med Interna 1999; 16(8):436.
9. Elis A, Lishner M, Lang R, Ravid M. Agranulocytosis associated with enalapril. DICP 1991;25(5):461–2.
10. Winfred RI, Nanda S, Horvath G, Elnicki M. Captopril-induced toxic epidermal necrolysis and agranulocytosis successfully treated with granulocyte colony-stimulating factor. South Med J 1999;92(9):918–20.
11. Pujol M, Duran-Suarez JR, Martin Vega C, Sanchez C, Tovar JL, Valles M. Autoimmune thrombocytopenia in three patients treated with captopril. Vox Sang 1989;57(3):218.
12. Iliopoulou A, Giannakopoulos G, Pagoy H, Christos T, Theodore S. Acute pancreatitis due to captopril treatment. Dig Dis Sci 2001;46(9):1882–3.
13. Borgia MC, Celestini A, Caravella P, Catalano C. Angiotensin-converting-enzyme inhibitor administration must be monitored for serum amylase and lipase in order to prevent an acute pancreatitis: a case report. Angiology 2001;52(9):645–7.
14. Al Shohaib S, Raweily E. Acute tubular necrosis due to captopril. Am J Nephrol 2000;20(2):149–52.
15. Ratliff NB 3rd, Pieranna F, Manganelli P. Captopril induced lupus. J Rheumatol 2002;29(8):1807–8.
16. Reidenberg MM, Case DB, Drayer DE, Reis S, Lorenzo B. Development of antinuclear antibody in patients treated with high doses of captopril. Arthritis Rheum 1984;27(5):579–81.
17. Mets B. The renin angiotensin system and ACE inhibitors in the perioperative period. In: Skarvan K, editor. Arterial Hypertension. London: Bailliere Tindall, 1997:581–604.
18. Williams NE. Profound bradycardia and hypotension following spinal anaesthesia in a patient receiving an ACE inhibitor: an important "drug" interaction? Eur J Anaesthesiol 1999;16(11):796–8.
19. Schaefer JP, Tam Y, Hasinoff BB, Tawfik S, Peng Y, Reimche L, Campbell NR. Ferrous sulphate interacts with captopril. Br J Clin Pharmacol 1998;46(4):377–81.
20. Csako G, Elin RJ. Spurious ketonuria due to captopril and other free sulfhydryl drugs. Diabetes Care 1996;19(6):673–4.

Carbachol

General Information

Carbachol is a quaternary ammonium compound that shares both the muscarinic and nicotinic actions of acetylcholine but is much more slowly deactivated. Carbachol has been used topically in ophthalmology and systemically (subcutaneously, for example in doses of 2 mg/day) for urinary retention. Severe cholinergic effects can result. In one instance they primarily involved the gastrointestinal tract and the patient died of esophageal rupture (1). In other cases patients have experienced extreme bradycardia with hypotension, requiring treatment with intravenous atropine. As carbachol is not destroyed by cholinesterase, a cumulative effect is possible in patients who receive regular doses at short intervals; in one case, hypotension only developed on the third treatment day (2).

References

1. Cochrane P. Spontaneous oesophageal rupture after carbachol therapy. BMJ 1973;1(5851):463–4.
2. van der Meer FJ, van der Vijver JC. Bradycardie en cardiogene shock veroorzaakt door carbachol. [Bradycardia and cardiogenic shock caused by carbachol.] Ned Tijdschr Geneeskd 1982;126(22):1010–12.

Carbamazepine

See also Antiepileptic drugs

General Information

Carbamazepine is usually regarded as the drug of choice for partial seizures (with or without secondary generalization) and it can also be valuable in preventing primary generalized tonic-clonic seizures.

General adverse reactions

Cerebellovestibular and oculomotor dysfunction (with dizziness, diplopia, nystagmus, ataxia), fatigue, and sedation (usually transient) are relatively common. Nausea, vomiting, cognitive dysfunction, headache, myoclonus (including non-epileptic myoclonus), exacerbation of seizures, movement disorders, behavioral or psychiatric disturbances, hyponatremia, and altered cardiac conduction are less common.

Hypersusceptibility reactions

Hypersusceptibility reactions to carbamazepine are relatively common and range from cutaneous reactions (including Stevens–Johnson syndrome and toxic epidermal necrolysis, severe forms of erythema multiforme) to systemic reactions with fever, lymphadenopathy, and/or involvement of the bone marrow, the liver, the heart, the gastrointestinal system, the lungs, and other organs.

In ten children with chorea (eight girls and two boys; aged 7–16 years), nine with rheumatic fever, carbamazepine (4–10 mg/kg/day; plasma concentrations 12–34 μmol/l) produced improvement within 2–14 days (1). The chorea disappeared within 2–12 weeks. There were no adverse effects.

Organs and Systems

Cardiovascular

Carbamazepine can depress the cardiac conducting system (SEDA-16, 71). There have been a few reports of reversible atrioventricular block (SED-12, 130) (2–4), and asystole has been described in a patient with Guillain–Barré syndrome (SEDA-18, 62).

In one patient carbamazepine caused pacemaker failure until the pacemaker was adjusted, no doubt because of its effects on cardiac conduction (SEDA-18, 62).

Three cases of carbamazepine-induced Stokes–Adams attacks caused by intermittent total atrioventricular block, sinoatrial block with functional escape rhythm, and intermittent asystole have been described; it was suggested that cardiac conduction should be assessed if syncope or changes in seizure type occur in patients taking carbamazepine (5).

Bradydysrhythmias of different types and severity have also been reported, especially in the elderly, but they do not seem to be common.

There has been a report of carbamazepine-induced hypertension (6).

- A 33-year-old man with complex partial seizures was switched from phenytoin to carbamazepine. His blood pressure was 118/70, but 4 months later, while he was taking carbamazepine 600 mg bd, his blood pressure was 150/112 and 1 month later 142/110. He was taking no medications beside carbamazepine. Secondary causes of hypertension were ruled out. Carbamazepine was withdrawn and gabapentin prescribed. One month later his blood pressure was normal, and it remained so at subsequent follow-up appointments over the next 2 years.

A case of congestive heart failure possibly caused by carbamazepine has been described (SED-12, 130) (7), but there have been no subsequent reports.

Potentially fatal eosinophilic myocarditis may be a manifestation of carbamazepine hypersensitivity (SEDA-22, 86).

Four additional cases of carbamazepine-induced sinus node dysfunction ($n = 3$) and atrioventricular block ($n = 1$) were described in elderly Japanese women taking 200–600 mg/day. In two of the three patients rechallenged, sinus arrest recurred within 48 hours (8).

In 12 patients in whom carbamazepine was withdrawn, power-spectrum analysis of RR interval variability was used to investigate changes in sympathetic/parasympathetic autonomic equilibrium (9). Abrupt withdrawal of carbamazepine altered the sympathovagal balance during non-REM sleep, shifting the sympathovagal balance toward sympathetic predominance. However, analysis of the before and after withdrawal cardiac Holter recordings showed no serious cardiac dysrhythmias in any patient.

Respiratory

Acute hypersensitivity reactions involving the lung or the bronchi have been reported, but are rare (SEDA-16, 71) (SEDA-18, 62).

Nervous system

Most central nervous system adverse effects are mild, transient, and reversible on dosage adjustment. Those reported more commonly (in 10–50% of patients, depending on dosage and assessment method) include somnolence, which is usually transient, diplopia, nystagmus, dizziness, fatigue, headache, ataxia, and cognitive dysfunction. These effects may be intermittent and related to high peak concentrations of the drug. Dividing the total daily dose or switching to a modified-release formulation can minimize these effects (SEDA-19, 64). Patients with MRI evidence of cerebellar atrophy may be more prone to nystagmus, dizziness, and ataxia when they take carbamazepine (SEDA-21, 69).

Carbamazepine can precipitate or aggravate myoclonic, atonic, and absence seizures, especially in children and adolescents with a history of bilaterally synchronous spike-and-wave discharges in the electroencephalogram; both generalized and partial seizures can be worsened (10). In children, the new appearance of generalized paroxysmal discharges after treatment may be predictive of seizure exacerbation or suboptimal control (11). Tonic seizures are occasionally aggravated by carbamazepine (SEDA-22, 85). Non-epileptic myoclonus occurs rarely.

A mild reduction in motor and sensory conduction velocities, possibly related to folate deficiency, has been found in patients taking long-term treatment (SED-13, 146) (12), but symptoms of peripheral neuropathy are uncommon.

Asterixis, dystonias, and dyskinesias (including motor tics, orofacial and lingual dyskinesias, and oculogyric crises) are uncommon, as are auditory disturbances (SED-13, 146) (13–15), (SEDA-20, 60) (SEDA-21, 69).

Neuroleptic malignant syndrome occurred in a middle-aged man who had previously experienced the same reaction to tiotixene (SEDA-17, 72). A 54-year-old man who had been taking neuroleptic drugs for about 30 years developed neuroleptic malignant syndrome within 3 days of taking add-on carbamazepine (400 mg/day) (16). It was speculated that the pathogenesis could have involved rebound cholinergic activity after a reduction in plasma neuroleptic drug concentrations by carbamazepine.

Aseptic meningitis reversible on drug withdrawal has been described at least three times (17).

Retrospective studies have suggested that antiepileptic drugs can be associated with peripheral nerve dysfunction. This has been prospectively studied in 81 patients (aged 13–67 years) without polyneuropathy who took sodium valproate ($n = 44$) or carbamazepine ($n = 37$) as monotherapy in standard daily doses (18). After 2 years one patient had clinical signs of polyneuropathy and six had symptoms of polyneuropathy, but electrophysiology did not show significant changes or trends. Only one patient had abnormal electrophysiological findings, which were only subclinical, and eight patients had abnormal values at two subsequent visits. There were no consistent patterns, and the data were unaffected when the drugs were examined separately or when patients were grouped according to whether or not they had symptoms of polyneuropathy. The authors concluded that previously untreated young to middle-aged patients who take valproic acid or carbamazepine for 2 years are not at risk of polyneuropathy.

Combined phonic and motor tics occurred in a 7-year-old boy with Down's syndrome when he took carbamazepine 19 mg/kg for suspected focal epilepsy (19). Carbamazepine concentrations were within the usual target range. The symptoms resolved completely after withdrawal.

Carbamazepine can cause altered visual evoked potentials and brainstem evoked potentials (20). In 100 epileptic patients aged 8–18 years taking carbamazepine in a modified-release formulation, interpeak latencies of I-III and III-V of brainstem evoked potentials were significantly delayed and N75/P100 and P100/N145 amplitudes in the visual evoked potentials were reduced.

Relatively low doses of carbamazepine (300–600 mg/day) have been reported to cause serious worsening of disability in five patients with multiple sclerosis (21). The authors suggested that this effect was due to blockade of sodium channels by carbamazepine.

Sensory systems

There was abnormal color perception in 28% of 18 patients taking carbamazepine monotherapy; in one case there was an abnormality in the blue-yellow (tritan) axis (22). In the same patients carbamazepine had no effect on contrast sensitivity or glare sensitivity (23).

Auditory disturbance is rarely associated with carbamazepine.

- A 25-year-old woman had falsely higher pitch perception after starting carbamazepine for schizoaffective disorder (24). Her serum carbamazepine concentration was in the usual target range. The symptom resolved on withdrawal.

Psychological, psychiatric

Behavioral and psychiatric disturbances are less common with carbamazepine than with other anticonvulsants.

- A 9-year-old boy with seizures developed intermittent complex visual hallucinations during therapy with fosphenytoin and, on a separate occasion, carbamazepine (25).

In 10 children with rolandic epilepsy, carbamazepine impaired memory and possibly visual search tasks (26). Evaluation of individual data suggested that some children were especially vulnerable to the adverse effects of carbamazepine on cognition. The authors did not comment on the fact that rolandic epilepsy is regarded as a syndrome for which treatment in most cases is not indicated.

The cognitive effects of carbamazepine and gabapentin have been compared in a double-blind, crossover, randomized study in 34 healthy elderly adults, of whom 19 withdrew (15 while taking carbamazepine, probably because of excessively rapid dosage titration) (27). The primary outcome measures were standardized neuropsychological and mood state tests, yielding 17 variables. Each subject had cognitive testing at baseline (before drug treatment), at the end of the first drug phase, the end of the second drug phase, and 4 weeks after completion of the second drug phase. Adverse events were frequently reported with both anticonvulsants, although they were more common with carbamazepine. There were significant differences between carbamazepine and gabapentin for only one of 11 cognitive variables, with better attention/vigilance for gabapentin, although the effect was modest. Both carbamazepine and gabapentin can cause mild cognitive deficits in elderly subjects, and gabapentin has a slightly better profile.

Endocrine

Carbamazepine therapy in eight women was associated with increased serum concentrations of sex hormone binding globulin (SHBG) and a reduced serum ratio of 17-α-estradiol and estradiol to SHBG. Of 56 women who had been taking carbamazepine for over 5 years, 14 had menstrual disturbances, which tended to be associated with raised SHBG and reduced serum concentrations of 17-α-estradiol (28). Carbamazepine may also reduce serum LH, progesterone, dehydroepiandrosterone, and the free androgen index (29,30), and some of these changes may be associated with anovulatory cycles and menstrual irregularities.

Men taking carbamazepine had mean low serum concentrations of dehydroepiandrosterone and a high SHBG concentration. Moreover, 18% of men taking carbamazepine for epilepsy reported reduced libido, impaired potency, or both.

Metabolism

Changes in body weight have been evaluated in 349 patients taking carbamazepine, phenytoin, or tiagabine. Carbamazepine add-on therapy caused significant mean weight gain of 1.5% (31). Tiagabide add-on therapy caused no significant weight change when added to either phenytoin or carbamazepine.

Some antiepileptic drugs have been associated with low serum and erythrocyte folate concentrations and high total plasma homocysteine concentrations in some patients. The concentrations of folate and homocysteine have been measured in 42 patients taking carbamazepine and 42 matched healthy controls (32). Patients taking carbamazepine had significantly lower serum and erythrocyte folate concentrations. There was hyperhomocystinemia (over 15 μmol/l) in 24% of the patients and 5% of the controls.

Nutrition

Concentrations of plasma homocysteine, plasma pyridoxal 5′-phosphate (active vitamin B6), serum folate, erythrocyte folate, and serum vitamin B12 have been measured both during fasting and after methionine in 60 epileptic patients (aged 14–18 years) and 63 sex- and age-matched controls before therapy and after 1 year of therapy with valproate or carbamazepine (33). After 1 year the patients who took valproate and carbamazepine had significantly increased plasma homocysteine concentrations compared with both baseline and control values and there was a significant fall in serum folate and plasma pyridoxal 5′-phosphate. Serum vitamin B12 and erythrocyte folate were unchanged.

The genetic determinants of this effect on homocysteine have been determined in 136 epileptic children taking carbamazepine or valproate as monotherapy (34). Nutritional determinants (folate and vitamins B6 and B12) and genetic determinants (MTHFR 677CT) of plasma homocysteine were studied in a random sample of 59 of those children. Total homocysteine concentrations were significantly increased and folate and vitamin B6 concentrations were significantly reduced. Carbamazepine lowered folate concentrations in association with hyperhomocysteinemia, which seemed to be related to the homozygous MTHFR 677CT mutation. Valproate, although also associated with hyperhomocysteinemia, only reduced vitamin B6 concentrations, independent of the MTHFR genotype.

Electrolyte balance

Carbamazepine can cause hyponatremia due to stimulation of antidiuretic hormone secretion (35,36). In a boy who developed hyponatremia it also seems to have caused fluid retention and cardiomegaly (SEDA-18, 62).

Symptomatic cases are relatively rare, but two cases have been reported (37).

- A 72-year-old woman developed somnolence and continuous sharp waves over the left hemisphere when carbamazepine was added to primidone and a diuretic. Her serum sodium concentration was initially 130 mmol/l and fell further to 100 mmol/l.
- In a 65-year-woman, carbamazepine-induced hyponatremia (127–130 mmol/l) led to serial tonic-clonic seizures, somnolence, confusion, and an electroencephalographic misdiagnosis of non-convulsive status.

Both patients recovered with normalization of the serum sodium when the carbamazepine dose was tapered.

In 117 patients with chronic epilepsy taking carbamazepine in residential care the retrospective prevalence of hyponatremia was 42% compared with 9.4% in controls (38). Higher doses and serum concentrations of carbamazepine were associated with a higher risk of hyponatremia.

Hematologic

In view of the very low incidence of serious blood dyscrasias, such as pancytopenia and agranulocytosis, indiscriminate continuous hematological monitoring is of little value (SED-13, 145) (39). Leukopenia occurs in up to 21% of patients, usually during the first 3 months of treatment, with a higher risk in those with a low or low-normal pretreatment white blood cell count. Although it may reverse during continuation of treatment (SED-12, 131) (40), (SEDA-20, 60), high-risk cases should be monitored. Bone-marrow aspirates need not be performed routinely in patients with chronic leukopenia and continuation of treatment is probably safe, although caution is required if the neutrophil count is consistently below 1.0×10^9/l (SEDA-19, 66). Other authors have recommended a reduction in dose or withdrawal of treatment if white cell counts are below 3.0×10^9/l or if neutrophil counts are below 1.0×10^9/l.

Some 15 cases of thrombocytopenia, reversible after withdrawal of carbamazepine, have been published (SED-13, 147) (41,42). There have also been single case reports of reticulocytosis (SED-13, 147) (43), leukopenia with thrombocytopenia with Henoch-Schönlein purpura (SEDA-18, 63), hemolytic anemia, and pure red cell aplasia (SED-13, 147) (44).

Serious blood dyscrasias from carbamazepine can be accompanied or preceded by a rash.

- A 66-year-old man had severe leukopenia a few days after a generalized rash appeared on the 36th day after he started to take carbamazepine (45).
- A 69-year-old woman had severe leukopenia and thrombocytopenia about a month after the onset of a rash and 2 months after she started to take carbamazepine (45).

In both patients, the abnormalities resolved after withdrawal, except for the platelet count, which increased but did not fully normalize over 6 weeks. This report suggests that patients developing a rash on carbamazepine should be monitored for the possible risk of associated blood dyscrasias.

Increased concentrations of PIVKA-II (prothrombin-induced by vitamin K absence for factor II) were found in four of six samples of cord blood collected at parturition from the placenta in 12 mothers exposed to carbamazepine during pregnancy (46). Prothrombin concentrations were also reduced in the whole group. High PIVKA-II concentrations were also recorded in cord blood from a newborn exposed prenatally to phenytoin and vigabatrin, but not in two exposed to phenytoin alone and one exposed to valproate alone. These results are consistent with evidence that enzyme-inducing anticonvulsants, particularly carbamazepine, interfere with vitamin K metabolism during pregnancy and can result in bleeding disorders in the newborn. Administration of vitamin K is recommended in these newborns at time of birth or in the mother toward the end of pregnancy. The authors also discussed the possibility that vitamin K supplementation in early pregnancy might reduce the risk of fetal facial dysmorphisms caused by enzyme-inducing anticonvulsants.

Gastrointestinal

Nausea, vomiting, and gastric intolerance are relatively uncommon and mild. However, there have been reports of severe diarrhea requiring drug withdrawal. Eosinophilic colitis (47) and lymphocytic colitis (SEDA-22, 85) are rare reactions.

A report of two cases has suggested that carbamazepine can cause colitis as part of the anticonvulsant hypersensitivity syndrome (48).

- A 47-year-old man developed fever, lymphadenopathy, flu-like symptoms, facial edema, a skin rash, and diarrhea after taking carbamazepine 200 mg/day for 3 weeks. Laparotomy because of severe abdominal pain 2 weeks later showed severe colitis with perforations.
- A 41-year-old woman had diarrhea, fever, and a skin rash after taking carbamazepine 300 mg/day for 4 weeks. Colitis was confirmed at colonic biopsy.

Both patients also had raised liver enzymes, peripheral eosinophilia, and eosinophils in the colonic infiltrate. Persistent recovery occurred after carbamazepine was withdrawn.

Lymphocytic colitis has been attributed to carbamazepine in a 77-year-old man, who had taken it for 6 months (49).

Liver

There have been several reports of fatal hepatic failure (SED-12, 132) (50), granulomatous hepatitis (SED-12, 132) (51–53), cholestatic hepatitis (SEDA-16, 71), and cholangitis ascribed to carbamazepine. Most acute hepatotoxic reactions caused by carbamazepine are accompanied by fever, rash, eosinophilia, and other signs of hypersensitivity, although they have also occurred without rash and eosinophilia (SEDA-19, 66).

Urinary tract

Carbamazepine-induced renal insufficiency has been described, but has not been firmly documented (SEDA-18, 63). Two diabetic patients who developed urinary retention on low doses (400–600 mg/day) were confirmed by rechallenge; there have been earlier reports, and pre-existing autonomic dysfunction may be a predisposing factor (54).

Skin

A skin rash occurs in 5–20% of patients started on carbamazepine, and is a common cause of early drug withdrawal. The rash is usually erythematous or maculopapular and may accompany systemic manifestations of hypersensitivity. Exfoliative dermatitis, Stevens–Johnson syndrome, and toxic epidermal necrolysis are relatively rare (SED-13, 148) (55,56).

There has been one case of toxic pustuloderma and two cases of lichenoid eruption attributed to carbamazepine (SEDA-16, 71) (SED-13, 148) (57–59). Patch testing for carbamazepine allergy tends to be positive only in some cases (60,61). A desensitization procedure, using gradually increasing dosages of carbamazepine over 6 weeks, has been described (SEDA-18, 64).

- A 58-year-old man developed stomatitis and widespread edematous erythema with papules and pustules after taking a combination of carbamazepine and paracetamol for 2 days, a most unusual treatment for headache and fever (62). The stomatitis improved but the eruption persisted for 2 months and was diagnosed as eosinophilic pustular folliculitis, a disorder that is rarely drug-induced. Recovery was achieved with glucocorticoid therapy.

A role of carbamazepine was suggested by reoccurrence of eosinophilic folliculitis after patch testing and low-dose (2 mg) oral rechallenge.

- A 17-year-old girl developed Stevens–Johnson syndrome after using carbamazepine 400 mg/day for 2 weeks (63). She was treated with intravenous immunoglobulin and intravenous methylprednisolone and recovered completely.

Immunologic

Hypersensitivity reactions are relatively common with carbamazepine. Most affect the skin, but systemic reactions with fever, lymphadenopathy, and/or involvement of the bone-marrow, the liver, the heart, the gastrointestinal system, the lungs, and other organs have been described. Severe serum sickness associated with immunoblastic lymphadenopathy has been reported in one case (SED-13, 148) (64). Occasional cases of systemic lupus erythematosus have occurred within the first few months, although an unusual case with onset after 8 years has been described (SEDA-22, 83).

- A 44-year-old woman, who was allergic to phenytoin, developed fever, lymphadenopathy, pneumonitis, hepatitis, and a morbilliform eruption after taking carbamazepine for 1 month (65). A skin biopsy of the dermis showed atypical lymphocytes that were CD3+, CD30+, and L26–. She improved quickly after carbamazepine was withdrawn.

This seems to have been the first report of carbamazepine-induced histological features of cutaneous pseudolymphoma, including CD30+ cells.

Cervical lymphadenopathy, fever, and a maculopapular skin rash developed in a 17-year-old boy after he had taken carbamazepine for 3 weeks (up to 600 mg/day) (66). Lymph node biopsies showed features typical of Kikuchi disease, a rare and self-limited immune-mediated lymphadenopathy that affects mostly the cervical region. The condition cleared rapidly after withdrawal.

- A 40-year-old man who had taken carbamazepine since childhood suffered for over 10 years from a lupus-like illness with hypocomplementemia, pancytopenia, and splenomegaly (67). He later developed cryoglobulinemia with membranoproliferative glomerulonephritis and raised ANA and pANCA titers. A causative role of carbamazepine in the latter syndrome was suggested by the observation that after withdrawal the antibodies fell and cryoglobulinemia resolved.

The carbamazepine hypersensitivity syndrome has been reviewed (68). Some of the following cases are examples of the different manifestations of this syndrome.

- A 12-year-old boy developed a maculopapular rash on two occasions after taking carbamazepine (69). A patch test was positive, but an in vitro lymphocyte transformation test was negative. However, T cells incubated with carbamazepine produced an excess of interferon-gamma.

The author proposed that this had been a delayed hypersensitivity response, perhaps mediated by a reactive metabolite.

- A 45-year-old man developed acute cardiac tamponade due to systemic lupus erythematosus associated with carbamazepine, which he had taken for 8 months (70).
- An 11-year-old girl developed a skin rash, fever, lymphadenopathy, and arthralgia after taking carbamazepine (plasma concentration 21 μmol/l) for 3 weeks (71). She had a lymphocytosis, mild thrombocytopenia, marked eosinophilia, and high transaminases. She was given betamethasone, and carbamazepine was gradually withdrawn. The fever and rash gradually abated and all the laboratory tests normalized by 2 weeks after the disappearance of the skin rash.

Long-Term Effects

Tumorigenicity

Carbamazepine and phenytoin have previously been associated with lymphoproliferative disorders, including dermatopathic lymphadenitis, atypical lymphoid proliferation, and cutaneous pseudolymphoma. In most reported cases, regression follows withdrawal of treatment with the causative drug. However, rarely true lymphoma can develop.

- A 13-year-old girl who had taken carbamazepine for about 8 months developed multiple painless reddish skin nodules, which grew and quickly ulcerated (72). The nodules were on the neck, trunk, and arms and varied in size. Neither lymphadenopathy nor splenomegaly was detected. Histology showed a CD30, primary, cutaneous, anaplastic, large-cell lymphoma. Carbamazepine was withdrawn, she received radiotherapy, and the lesions regressed. At 3 years after diagnosis she was still in complete remission.

Second-Generation Effects

Teratogenicity

Data from various studies in 1255 patients exposed to carbamazepine have been analysed to evaluate its potential teratogenicity (73). There was an increased rate of congenital anomalies, mainly neural tube defects, cardiovascular and urinary tract anomalies, and cleft palate. The combination of carbamazepine with other antiepileptic drugs was more teratogenic than carbamazepine monotherapy. Because this study was retrospective, the conclusions should not be seen as definitive.

There is an association of carbamazepine with cardiac malformations.

The Israeli Teratogen Information Service has prospectively followed 210 pregnancies with exposure to carbamazepine in the first trimester (74). The outcomes were compared with those in two overlapping groups of matched controls ($n = 629$) who had been exposed to non-teratogens. There was a two-fold increase in the rate of major congenital anomalies in the women who had used carbamazepine (12/160 on carbamazepine versus 18/560 controls; RR = 2.24; 95% CI = 1.10, 4.56) and a reduction in birth weight of about 250 g after in utero exposure to carbamazepine. There were no neural tube defects. These results are to be interpreted with caution, as they were obtained from a questionnaire in 87% of cases.

Fetotoxicity

Increased concentrations of PIVKA-II (prothrombin-induced by vitamin K absence for factor II) were found in four of six samples of cord blood collected at parturition from the placenta in 12 mothers exposed to carbamazepine during pregnancy (46). Prothrombin concentrations were also reduced in the whole group. High PIVKA-II concentrations were also recorded in cord blood from a newborn exposed prenatally to phenytoin and vigabatrin, but not in two exposed to phenytoin alone and one exposed to valproate alone. These results are consistent with evidence that enzyme-inducing anticonvulsants, particularly carbamazepine, interfere with vitamin K metabolism during pregnancy and can cause bleeding disorders in the newborn. Administration of vitamin K is recommended in these newborns at time of birth or in the mother toward the end of pregnancy. The authors also discussed the possibility that vitamin K supplementation in early pregnancy might reduce the risk of fetal facial dysmorphisms caused by enzyme-inducing anticonvulsants.

Lactation

In seven lactating women the mean concentrations of carbamazepine in milk and plasma samples were 15 and 26 μmol/l respectively; the concentrations of carbamazepine 10,11-epoxide were 5 and 8 μmol/l respectively (75). The mean milk/plasma ratios were 0.64 and 0.79 respectively. The amounts of carbamazepine and carbamazepine 10,11-epoxide that a breast-feeding child is likely to consume are thus very small.

Susceptibility Factors

Age

The elderly appear to be at increased risk of blood dyscrasias and liver reactions (39). Age above 55 years was associated with a greater risk of toxicity after rapid switch-over to a carbamazepine dosage designed to yield a plasma concentration of 10 μg/ml (76). Moderately severe to severe adverse effects in the 11 patients in either subgroup included sedation, ataxia, and confusion.

Hepatic disease

Because of the reactions described above, and because carbamazepine is mostly metabolized in the liver, it should be used with caution in patients with hepatic disorders.

Other features of the patient

Because of the reactions described above, carbamazepine should be used with caution in patients with cardiac disorders.

Alcohol abusers may represent a high-risk group for serious skin reactions (SED-13, 145) (39).

Carbamazepine is porphyrogenic (SED-12, 131) (77), (SED-13, 147) (78), and should not be used in patients with acute intermittent porphyria.

The presence of a static encephalopathy (defined as focal or diffuse structural brain lesions associated with mild to moderately severe cognitive dysfunction) was associated with a greater risk of toxicity after rapid switch-over to a carbamazepine dosage designed to yield a plasma concentration of 10 μg/ml (76). Moderately severe to severe adverse effects in the 11 patients in either subgroup included sedation, ataxia, and confusion.

Drug Administration

Drug formulations

When 14 patients taking a brand-named modified-release formulation of carbamazepine were switched to a generic modified-release formulation, nine developed adverse effects such as dizziness, nausea, ataxia, diplopia, and nystagmus, despite the fact that the two formulations met pharmacokinetic criteria for bioequivalence (79). Mean AUC and C_{max} values were about 10% higher with the generic formulation. The authors suggested that standard bioequivalence criteria (90% confidence limits of 80–125% for AUC and 70–143% for C_{max}) may be too broad for carbamazepine, which has a relatively narrow therapeutic ratio. While this may be correct, the findings could have been biased by the lack of a control group, lack of randomization in the sequence of the two treatments, and the use of a non-blinded design.

The suitability of a modified-release formulation of carbamazepine (Carbatrol) for administration through feeding tubes in six children has been assessed (80). Carbatrol was administered as follows: first, the tube was flushed with 10 ml of water, then the granular contents of a capsule of Carbatrol were added to 15 ml of water and administered via the tube; this was followed by an additional flush with 10 ml of water. Two of the six children had to be withdrawn from the study because of frequent tube occlusions, attributed to the Carbatrol granules.

Drug dosage regimens

The relations between plasma concentrations of carbamazepine and its two major metabolites, carbamazepine-10, 11-epoxide and carbamazepine-10,11-diol, and antimanic efficacy and adverse effects in patients with schizoaffective disorder have been studied in 10 patients (81). There were positive relations between plasma concentrations of the epoxide and the degree of clinical improvement and adverse effects, but not with plasma concentrations of carbamazepine or its diol.

Drug overdose

Acute interstitial pneumonia or diffuse alveolar damage in the context of other manifestations of overdose has been described (SEDA-22, 84).

There was impaired neuromuscular transmission at high frequency repetitive nerve stimulation in two children who presented in coma with diffuse hypotonia and areflexia after carbamazepine overdose (82). Both recovered with supportive care.

Acute massive carbamazepine intoxication has been reported in a 27-year-old man (83). The plasma concentration was 147 μmol/l. He had a sinus tachycardia and a leukocytosis.

In 14 children under the age of 5 years with peak serum carbamazepine concentrations of 76–134 μmol/l after acute accidental overdose there was nystagmus in 12, drowsiness in 10, ataxia in four, and mild tachycardia in two (84). None died.

Three drug dispensing errors causing carbamazepine overdose have been reported (85). In each case carbamazepine was given instead of another drug with a similar name—Tegretol instead of Trental (pentoxifylline, two cases) and carbamazepine–Neuroxpharm instead of piracetam–Neuraxpharm. All three developed mild cerebellar symptoms and all had high carbamazepine concentrations (50–55 μmol/l).

The postmortem blood concentration of carbamazepine has been reported in a case of suicide attributed to "mixed drug toxicity" with carbamazepine, lamotrigine, paroxetine, and thioridazine (86). It was 76 μmol/l.

Drug–Drug Interactions

General

Carbamazepine is an enzyme inducer, and its own metabolism can be induced or inhibited by other drugs, particularly those affecting cytochrome CYP3A4.

Antiretroviral protease inhibitors

Some antiretroviral protease inhibitors inhibit CYP3A4, which is mostly responsible for the metabolism of carbamazepine.

- Failure of antiretroviral drug therapy has been attributed to an interaction of carbamazepine with indinavir in a 48-year-old man taking indinavir, zidovudine, and lamivudine; his HIV-RNA viral load became undetectable after less than 2 months and he developed a Herpes zoster infection (87). Lower doses of carbamazepine are also required during co-administration of ritonavir, as has been shown in two recent cases.
- Within 4 days of the introduction of ritonavir in a 49-year-old woman taking carbamazepine 600 mg/day the serum carbamazepine concentration rose from 29 to 84 μmol/l and ataxia occurred (88). The dosage of carbamazepine was reduced to 300 mg/day and the serum concentration fell but then rose again. Finally, a serum carbamazepine concentration in the target range was achieved with a dosage of 100 mg/day.

- The serum carbamazepine concentration rose from 27 to 76 μmol/l after ritonavir was introduced in a 36-year-old man (89). Dizziness and a gait disorder resolved when carbamazepine was withdrawn. The serum phenytoin concentration was unaffected by ritonavir.

Clobazam

Negative myoclonus and more typical signs of carbamazepine intoxication (fatigue, ataxia, clumsiness) occurred in a 66-year-old man after he took add-on clobazam (10 mg/day) for 4 weeks (90). Plasma concentrations of carbamazepine (58 μmol/l) and carbamazepine-10, 11-epoxide (19 μmol/l) were higher than before clobazam therapy, and his symptoms resolved quickly when carbamazepine dosage was reduced and clobazam was withdrawn. The interaction was confirmed on rechallenge; however, it does not occur in most patients.

Coumarin anticoagulants

Carbamazepine reduces the effects of coumarin anticoagulants (SED-14, 1185) (91,92), including phenprocoumon (SEDA-22, 86), by inducing cytochrome P450 enzymes, and another case has been reported (93).

- A 53-year-old woman taking phenprocoumon had a large reduction in prothrombin time when carbamazepine was added. After withdrawal of carbamazepine, the prothrombin time returned to target values. Valproate had no effect on phenprocoumon.

Dextropropoxyphene

Dextropropoxyphene inhibits the oxidative metabolism of carbamazepine, leading to clinically significant rises in carbamazepine concentrations (94).

Fluconazole

In a 33-year-old man stabilized on carbamazepine, the addition of fluconazole (150 mg/day) led to severe carbamazepine toxicity associated with high carbamazepine concentrations (104 μmol/l) (95). The condition cleared after withdrawal of both drugs, and carbamazepine was then readministered without recurrence of toxicity. This interaction is likely to be mediated by inhibition of the CYP3A4-mediated metabolism of carbamazepine by fluconazole.

Grapefruit juice

In 10 patients grapefruit juice 300 ml taken with the morning dose of carbamazepine resulted in an approximate 50% increase of plasma carbamazepine concentrations (96). The interaction was ascribed to inhibition of cytochrome CYP3A4 by components of the juice.

Inhibitors of epoxide hydrolase

Clinically significant interactions can be caused by inhibitors of epoxide hydrolase, such as valpromide and valnoctamide, which increase the serum concentrations of the active metabolite carbamazepine-10,11-epoxide.

Lamotrigine

In dogs concurrent administration of lamotrigine had no significant effect on the pharmacokinetics of carbamazepine or the plasma concentration ratio of carbamazepine epoxide to carbamazepine (97).

In a retrospective study, in which 376 samples from 222 patients were analysed, carbamazepine reduced lamotrigine concentrations by 54% (98).

Lithium

A 42-year-old woman developed sinus node dysfunction during lithium toxicity (serum concentration 3.4 mmol/l) (99). The authors suggested that concomitant carbamazepine therapy (serum concentration 22 μmol/l) had exacerbated the effect of lithium on the sinus node.

Mianserin

In 12 patients, carbamazepine (400 mg/day for 4 weeks) markedly reduced the plasma concentrations of concomitantly administered mianserin, probably through enzyme induction (100). The concentration of *S*-mianserin, the more potent of the enantiomers of mianserin, fell by 45%, while the plasma concentrations of desmethylmianserin changed only slightly. These data suggest that patients co-medicated with carbamazepine may require higher dosages of mianserin.

Monoamine oxidase inhibitors

Carbamazepine is contraindicated in patients taking monoamine oxidase inhibitors (101,102). The combination can cause sudden high body temperature, extremely high blood pressure, and severe convulsions; at least 14 days should be allowed between stopping treatment with one medicine and starting the other.

Nefazodone

The pharmacokinetic interaction of nefazodone 200 mg bd with steady-state carbamazepine has been investigated in 12 healthy men (103). Nefazodone increased the steady-state plasma AUC of carbamazepine by 23% and reduced the AUC of active carbamazepine-10,11-epoxide by 20%. The steady-state AUC of nefazodone fell 14-fold and the AUCs of its metabolites (hydroxynefazodone, metachlorophenylpiperazine, and triazoledione) also fell significantly. Thus nefazodone had a small inhibitory effect on carbamazepine metabolism, while carbamazepine greatly increased the metabolism of nefazodone.

Olanzapine

In 11 healthy volunteers carbamazepine (400 mg/day for 2 weeks) reduces by about 30% the AUC of olanzapine, presumably by induction of olanzapine metabolism (104). Although the interaction was considered of little relevance, it cannot be excluded that some patients on carbamazepine may require higher olanzapine dosages than usual.

Rifampicin

Serum carbamazepine concentrations were reduced in a 44-year-old woman who also took rifampicin (105), presumably through induction of metabolism.

Risperidone

Risperidone significantly increases serum carbamazepine concentrations (106) and carbamazepine significantly reduces serum risperidone concentrations (107). The clinical relevance of these changes is uncertain.

Steady-state plasma concentrations of risperidone and 9-hydroxyrisperidone have been measured in 23 patients taking risperidone alone and in 11 patients co-medicated with carbamazepine (108). Carbamazepine markedly reduced the concentrations of both compounds, although the difference was significant only for the metabolite.

Sertraline

Loss of antidepressant activity of sertraline can occur at usual therapeutic doses when depressed patients have also taken drugs that induce CYP3A4, including carbamazepine, as has been reported in two cases, a 33-year-old woman and a 25-year-old man (109).

St. John's wort

St. John's wort contains an enzyme inducer that can reduce the plasma concentrations of drugs that are substrates of CYP3A4, such as indinavir and ciclosporin. However, in eight healthy volunteers aged 24–43 years, St. John's wort 300 mg/day (0.3% hypericin standardized tablet) for 14 days had no effect on the pharmacokinetics of carbamazepine (110).

Trazodone

In one case trazodone increased serum carbamazepine concentrations by about 30% (111). However, only one sample was taken after adding trazodone, and the rise in carbamazepine concentration might have been caused by random fluctuation.

Ziprasidone

In 25 healthy subjects, carbamazepine (up to 400 mg/day for 25 days) reduced the steady-state AUC of ziprasidone (40 mg/day) by about 35%, presumably through induction of the CYP3A4-mediated metabolism of the neuroleptic drug (112). Although the interaction was considered clinically insignificant, the dosage of carbamazepine was relatively low and a greater effect might occur at higher dosages.

The effect of steady-state carbamazepine administration on the steady-state pharmacokinetics of ziprasidone has been studied in 25 healthy young adults, in a randomized, placebo-controlled study (112). Carbamazepine caused small reductions in ziprasidone $AUC_{0 \rightarrow 12}$ and C_{max} (36% and 27% respectively). The authors concluded that carbamazepine had increased ziprasidone clearance by induction of CYP3A4.

Diagnosis of Adverse Drug Reactions

The usual target range for plasma carbamazepine concentrations is 17–42 μmol/l (4–10 μg/ml).

References

1. Harel L, Zecharia A, Straussberg R, Volovitz B, Amir J. Successful treatment of rheumatic chorea with carbamazepine. Pediatr Neurol 2000;23(2):147–51.
2. Gary NE, Byra WM, Eisinger RP. Carbamazepine poisoning: treatment by hemoperfusion. Nephron 1981;27(4–5):202–3.
3. Schwartau M, Wahl G, Bucking J. Intramyokardialer Block bei Carbamazepin-Intoxication. [Intramyocardial block in carbamazepine poisoning.] Dtsch Med Wochenschr 1983;108(48):1841–3.
4. Macnab AJ, Robinson JL, Adderly RJ, D'Orsogna L. Heart block secondary to erythromycin-induced carbamazepine toxicity. Pediatrics 1987;80(6):951–3.
5. Boesen F, Andersen EB, Jensen EK, Ladefoged SD. Cardiac conduction disturbances during carbamazepine therapy. Acta Neurol Scand 1983;68(1):49–52.
6. Jette N, Veregin T, Guberman A. Carbamazepine-induced hypertension. Neurology 2002;59(2):275–6.
7. Terrence CF, Fromm G. Congestive heart failure during carbamazepine therapy. Ann Neurol 1980;8(2):200–1.
8. Takayanagi K, Hisauchi I, Watanabe J, Maekawa Y, Fujito T, Sakai Y, Hoshi K, Kase M, Nishimura N, Inoue T, Hayashi T, Morooka S. Carbamazepine-induced sinus node dysfunction and atrioventricular block in elderly women. Jpn Heart J 1998;39(4):469–79.
9. Hennessy MJ, Tighe MG, Binnie CD, Nashef L. Sudden withdrawal of carbamazepine increases cardiac sympathetic activity in sleep. Neurology 2001;57(9):1650–4.
10. Perucca E, Gram L, Avanzini G, Dulac O. Antiepileptic drugs as a cause of worsening seizures. Epilepsia 1998;39(1):5–17.
11. Talwar D, Arora MS, Sher PK. EEG changes and seizure exacerbation in young children treated with carbamazepine. Epilepsia 1994;35(6):1154–9.
12. Traccis S, Monaco F, Sechi GP, Moglia A, Mutani R. Long-term therapy with carbamazepine: effects on nerve conduction velocity. Eur Neurol 1983;22(6):410–16.
13. Tridon P, Vidailhet C, Stehlin S. Dyskinésie linguale induite par la carbamazépine. Ann Med Nancy 1980;19:745.
14. Berchou RC, Rodin EA. Carbamazepine-induced oculogyric crisis. Arch Neurol 1979;36(8):522–3.
15. Crosley CJ, Swender PT. Dystonia associated with carbamazepine administration: experience in brain-damaged children. Pediatrics 1979;63(4):612–15.
16. Nisijima K, Kusakabe Y, Ohtuka K, Ishiguro T. Addition of carbamazepine to long-term treatment with neuroleptics may induce neuroleptic malignant syndrome. Biol Psychiatry 1998;44(9):930–1.
17. Hemet C, Chassagne P, Levade M. La carbamazepine, une cause rare de méningite aseptique. Rev Med Interne 1993;14:607.
18. Bogliun G, Di Viesti P, Monticelli LM, Beghi E, Zarrelli M, Simone P, Airoldi L, Frattola L. Anticonvulsants and peripheral nerve function results of prospective monitoring in patients with newly diagnosed epilepsy. Clin Drug Invest 2000;20:173–80.
19. Holtmann M, Korn-Merker E, Boenigk HE. Carbamazepine-induced combined phonic and motor tic in a boy with Down's syndrome. Epileptic Disord 2000;2(1):39–40.
20. Zgorzalewicz M, Galas-Zgorzalewicz B. Visual and auditory evoked potentials during long-term vigabatrin

treatment in children and adolescents with epilepsy. Clin Neurophysiol 2000;111(12):2150–4.
21. Ramsaransing G, Zwanikken C, De Keyser J. Worsening of symptoms of multiple sclerosis associated with carbamazepine. BMJ 2000;320(7242):1113.
22. Nousiainen I, Kalviainen R, Mantyjarvi M. Color vision in epilepsy patients treated with vigabatrin or carbamazepine monotherapy. Ophthalmology 2000;107(5):884–8.
23. Nousiainen I, Kalviainen R, Mantyjarvi M. Contrast and glare sensitivity in epilepsy patients treated with vigabatrin or carbamazepine monotherapy compared with healthy volunteers. Br J Ophthalmol 2000;84(6):622–5.
24. Miyaoka T, Seno H, Itoga M, Horiguchi J. Reversible pitch perception deficit caused by carbamazepine. Clin Neuropharmacol 2000;23(4):219–21.
25. Benatar MG, Sahin M, Davis RG. Antiepileptic drug-induced visual hallucinations in a child. Pediatr Neurol 2000;23(5):439–41.
26. Seidel WT, Mitchell WG. Cognitive and behavioral effects of carbamazepine in children: data from benign rolandic epilepsy. J Child Neurol 1999;14(11):716–23.
27. Martin R, Meador K, Turrentine L, Faught E, Sinclair K, Kuzniecky R, Gilliam F. Comparative cognitive effects of carbamazepine and gabapentin in healthy senior adults. Epilepsia 2001;42(6):764–71.
28. Isojarvi JI, Laatikainen TJ, Pakarinen AJ, Juntunen KT, Myllyla VV. Menstrual disorders in women with epilepsy receiving carbamazepine. Epilepsia 1995;36(7):676–81.
29. Stoffel-Wagner B, Bauer J, Flugel D, Brennemann W, Klingmuller D, Elger CE. Serum sex hormones are altered in patients with chronic temporal lobe epilepsy receiving anticonvulsant medication. Epilepsia 1998;39(11):1164–73.
30. Smith DB, Mattson RH, Cramer JA, Collins JF, Novelly RA, Craft B. Results of a nationwide Veterans Administration Cooperative Study comparing the efficacy and toxicity of carbamazepine, phenobarbital, phenytoin, and primidone. Epilepsia 1987;28(Suppl 3):S50–8.
31. Hogan RE, Bertrand ME, Deaton RL, Sommerville KW. Total percentage body weight changes during add-on therapy with tiagabine, carbamazepine and phenytoin. Epilepsy Res 2000;41(1):23–8.
32. Apeland T, Mansoor MA, Strandjord RE, Vefring H, Kristensen O. Folate, homocysteine and methionine loading in patients on carbamazepine. Acta Neurol Scand 2001;103(5):294–9.
33. Verrotti A, Pascarella R, Trotta D, Giuva T, Morgese G, Chiarelli F. Hyperhomocysteinemia in children treated with sodium valproate and carbamazepine. Epilepsy Res 2000;41(3):253–7.
34. Vilaseca MA, Monros E, Artuch R, Colome C, Farre C, Valls C, Cardo E, Pineda M. Anti-epileptic drug treatment in children: hyperhomocysteinaemia, B-vitamins and the 677C->T mutation of the methylenetetrahydrofolate reductase gene. Eur J Paediatr Neurol 2000; 4(6):269–77.
35. Huuskonen UEJ, Isojarvi JIT. Antiepileptic drugs and serum sodium. Epilepsia 1997;38(Suppl 8):89–90.
36. Van Amelsvoort T, Bakshi R, Devaux CB, Schwabe S. Hyponatremia associated with carbamazepine and oxcarbazepine therapy: a review. Epilepsia 1994;35(1):181–8.
37. Vogt H. Non-convulsive status epileptics or metabolic encephalopathy due to carbamazepine induced hyponatremia? Epilepsia 1999;40(Suppl 2):254.
38. Kelly BD, Hillery J. Hyponatremia during carbamazepine therapy in patients with intellectual disability. J Intellect Disabil Res 2001;45(Pt 2):152–6.
39. Askmark H, Wiholm BE. Epidemiology of adverse reactions to carbamazepine as seen in a spontaneous reporting system. Acta Neurol Scand 1990;81(2):131–40.
40. Sobotka JL, Alexander B, Cook BL. A review of carbamazepine's hematologic reactions and monitoring recommendations. DICP 1990;24(12):1214–19.
41. Tohen M, Castillo J, Cole JO, Miller MG, de los Heros R, Farrer RJ. Thrombocytopenia associated with carbamazepine: a case series. J Clin Psychiatry 1991;52(12):496–8.
42. Bradley JM, Sagraves R, Kimbrough AC. Carbamazepine-induced thrombocytopenia in a young child. Clin Pharm 1985;4(2):221–3.
43. Warren JA, Steinbook RM. Case report of carbamazepine-induced reticulocytes. Am J Psychiatry 1983;140(2):247–9.
44. Buitendag DJ. Pure red-cell aplasia associated with carbamazepine. A case report. S Afr Med J 1990; 78(4):214–15.
45. Cates M, Powers R. Concomitant rash and blood dyscrasias in geriatric psychiatry patients treated with carbamazepine. Ann Pharmacother 1998;32(9):884–7.
46. Howe AM, Oakes DJ, Woodman PD, Webster WS. Prothrombin and PIVKA-II levels in cord blood from newborn exposed to anticonvulsants during pregnancy. Epilepsia 1999;40(7):980–4.
47. Anttila VJ, Valtonen M. Carbamazepine-induced eosinophilic colitis. Epilepsia 1992;33(1):119–21.
48. Eland IA, Dofferhoff AS, Vink R, Zondervan PE, Stricker BH. Colitis may be part of the antiepileptic drug hypersensitivity syndrome. Epilepsia 1999;40(12):1780–3.
49. Linares Torres P, Fidalgo Lopez I, Castanon Lopez A, Martinez Pinto Y. Colitis linfocítica como causa de diarrea crónica: posible relación con carbamazepina. [Lymphocytic colitis as a cause of chronic diarrhea: possible association with carbamazepine.] Aten Primaria 2000;25(5):366–7.
50. Zucker P, Daum F, Cohen MI. Fatal carbamazepine hepatitis. J Pediatr 1977;91(4):667–8.
51. Levander HG. Granulomatous hepatitis in a patient receiving carbamazepine. Acta Med Scand 1980;208(4):333–5.
52. Levy M, Goodman MW, Van Dyne BJ, Sumner HW. Granulomatous hepatitis secondary to carbamazepine. Ann Intern Med 1981;95(1):64–5.
53. Mitchell MC, Boitnott JK, Arregui A, Maddrey WC. Granulomatous hepatitis associated with carbamazepine therapy. Am J Med 1981;71(4):733–5.
54. Steiner I, Birmanns B. Carbamazepine-induced urinary retention in long-standing diabetes mellitus. Neurology 1993;43(9):1855–6.
55. Breathnach SM, McGibbon DH, Ive FA, Black MM. Carbamazepine ('Tegretol') and toxic epidermal necrolysis: report of three cases with histopathological observations. Clin Exp Dermatol 1982;7(6):585–91.
56. Reed MD, Bertino JS Jr, Blumer JL. Carbamazepine-associated exfoliative dermatitis. Clin Pharm 1982;1(1):78–9.
57. Staughton RC, Payne CM, Harper JI, McMichen H. Toxic pustuloderma–a new entity? J R Soc Med 1984;77(Suppl 4):6–8.
58. Atkin SL, McKenzie TM, Stevenson CJ. Carbamazepine-induced lichenoid eruption. Clin Exp Dermatol 1990;15(5):382–3.
59. Ohtsuyama M, Maruyama T, Haruki T, Takahashi S, Morohashi M. Two cases of lichenoid drug eruption localised in the nails. Acta Dermatol 1990;85:221–6.
60. Alanko K. Patch testing in cutaneous reactions caused by carbamazepine. Contact Dermatitis 1993;29(5):254–7.
61. Tomson T, Kenneback G. Arrhythmia, heart rate variability, and antiepileptic drugs. Epilepsia 1997;38(Suppl 11):S48–51.
62. Mizoguchi S, Setoyama M, Higashi Y, Hozumi H, Kanzaki T. Eosinophilic pustular folliculitis induced by carbamazepine. J Am Acad Dermatol 1998;38(4):641–3.
63. Straussberg R, Harel L, Ben-Amitai D, Cohen D, Amir J. Carbamazepine-induced Stevens–Johnson syndrome

treated with IV steroids and IVIG. Pediatr Neurol 2000; 22(3):231–3.
64. Igarashi M, Bando Y, Shimanuki K, Hosoda N, Sunaoshi W, Shirai H, Miura H. Immunosuppressive factors detected during convalescence in a patient with severe serum sickness induced by carbamazepine. Int Arch Allergy Immunol 1993;100(4):378–81.
65. Nathan DL, Belsito DV. Carbamazepine-induced pseudolymphoma with CD-30 positive cells. J Am Acad Dermatol 1998;38(5 Pt 2):806–9.
66. Ganga A, Corda D, Gallo Carrabba G, Cossu S, Massarelli G, Rosati G. A case of carbamazepine-induced lymphadenopathy resembling Kikuchi disease. Eur Neurol 1998;39(4):247–8.
67. Lhotta K, Konig P. Cryoglobulinaemia, membranoproliferative glomerulonephritis and pANCA in a patient treated with carbamazepine. Nephrol Dial Transplant 1998;13(7):1890–1.
68. Elstner S, Sperling W. Das Carbamazepin-Hypersensitivitäts-Syndrome. Differentialdiagnostische Erwagungen an einer exemplarischen Fallvorstellungo. [The carbamazepine hypersensitivity syndrome. Differential diagnosis and a representative case history.] Fortschr Neurol Psychiatr 2000;68(4):188–92.
69. Koga T, Kubota Y, Nakayama J. Interferon-gamma production in the peripheral lymphocytes of a patient with carbamazepine hypersensitivity syndrome. Acta Dermatol Venereol 2000;80(1):73.
70. Verma SP, Yunis N, Lekos A, Crausman RS. Carbamazepine-induced systemic lupus erythematosus presenting as cardiac tamponade. Chest 2000;117(2):597–8.
71. Verrotti A, Feliciani C, Morresi S, Coscione G, Morgese G, Toto P, Chiarelli F. Carbamazepine-induced hypersensitivity syndrome in a child with epilepsy. Int J Immunopathol Pharmacol 2000;13(1):49–53.
72. Di Lernia V, Viglio A, Cattania M, Paulli M. Carbamazepine-induced, CD30+, primary, cutaneous, anaplastic large-cell lymphoma. Arch Dermatol 2001;137(5):675–6.
73. Matalon S, Schechtman S, Goldzweig G, Ornoy A. The teratogenic effect of carbamazepine: a meta-analysis of 1255 exposures. Reprod Toxicol 2002;16(1):9–17.
74. Diav-Citrin O, Shechtman S, Arnon J, Ornoy A. Is carbamazepine teratogenic? A prospective controlled study of 210 pregnancies. Neurology 2001;57(2):321–4.
75. Shimoyama R, Ohkubo T, Sugawara K. Monitoring of carbamazepine and carbamazepine 10,11-epoxide in breast milk and plasma by high-performance liquid chromatography. Ann Clin Biochem 2000;37(Pt 2):210–15.
76. Kanner AM, Bourgeois BF, Hasegawa H, Hutson P. Rapid switchover to carbamazepine using pharmacokinetic parameters. Epilepsia 1998;39(2):194–200.
77. Reynolds NC Jr, Miska RM. Safety of anticonvulsants in hepatic porphyrias. Neurology 1981;31(4):480–4.
78. Laiwah AC, Brodie MJ, Goldberg A. Carbamazepine-induced non-hereditary acute porphyria. Lancet 1983;1(8339):1442.
79. Mayer Th, May TW, Altenmuller DM, Sandmann M, Wolf P. Clinical problems with generic antiepileptic drugs. Comparison of sustained release formulations of carbamazepine. Clin Drug Invest 1999;18:17–26.
80. Riss JR, Kriel RL, Kammer NM, Judge MK, Montgomery MJ. Administration of Carbatrol to children with feeding tubes. Pediatr Neurol 2002;27(3):193–5.
81. Yoshimura R, Nakamura J, Eto S, Ueda N. Possible relationships between plasma carbamazepine-10,11-epoxide levels and antimanic efficacy and side effects in patients with schizoaffective disorde. Hum Psychopharmacol 2000;15(4):237–40.
82. Zaidat OO, Kaminski HJ, Berenson F, Katirji B. Neuromuscular transmission defect caused by carbamazepine. Muscle Nerve 1999;22(9):1293–6.
83. Campany Herrero D, Mateu De Antonio J, Del Villar Ruiz De La Torre JA, Grau Cerrato S, Salas Sanchez E, Ortiz Sagrista P. Intoxicación aguda por carbamazepina. Farm Hosp 2000;24:43–6.
84. Lifshitz M, Gavrilov V, Sofer S. Signs and symptoms of carbamazepine overdose in young children. Pediatr Emerg Care 2000;16(1):26–7.
85. Rosel T, Schneider J, Fischer JT, Druschky KF. "Carbamazepin Intoxikation" durch Verwechslung von Medikamenten. [Carbamazepine poisoning caused by confusing the drugs.] Dtsch Med Wochenschr 2000; 125(12):352–6.
86. Pricone MG, King CV, Drummer OH, Opeskin K, McIntyre IM. Postmortem investigation of lamotrigine concentrations. J Forensic Sci 2000;45(1):11–15.
87. Hugen PW, Burger DM, Brinkman K, ter Hofstede HJ, Schuurman R, Koopmans PP, Hekster YA. Carbamazepine–indinavir interaction causes antiretroviral therapy failure. Ann Pharmacother 2000;34(4):465–70.
88. Burman W, Orr L. Carbamazepine toxicity after starting combination antiretroviral therapy including ritonavir and efavirenz. AIDS 2000;14(17):2793–4.
89. Berbel Garcia A, Latorre Ibarra A, Porta Etessam J, Martinez Salio A, Perez Martinez D, Siaz Diaz R, Toledo Heras M. Protease inhibitor-induced carbamazepine toxicity. Clin Neuropharmacol 2000;23(4):216–18.
90. Genton P, Nguyen VH, Mesdjian E. Carbamazepine intoxication with negative myoclonus after the addition of clobazam. Epilepsia 1998;39(10):1115–18.
91. Denbow CE, Fraser HS. Clinically significant hemorrhage due to warfarin–carbamazepine interaction. South Med J 1990;83(8):981.
92. Hansen JM, Siersboek-Nielsen K, Skovsted L. Carbamazepine-induced acceleration of diphenylhydantoin and warfarin metabolism in man. Clin Pharmacol Ther 1971;12(3):539–43.
93. Schlienger R, Kurmann M, Drewe J, Muller-Spahn F, Seifritz E. Inhibition of phenprocoumon anticoagulation by carbamazepine. Eur Neuropsychopharmacol 2000; 10(3):219–21.
94. Hansen BS, Dam M, Brandt J, Hvidberg EF, Angelo H, Christensen JM, Lous P. Influence of dextropropoxyphene on steady state serum levels and protein binding of three anti-epileptic drugs in man. Acta Neurol Scand 1980;61(6):357–67.
95. Nair DR, Morris HH. Potential fluconazole-induced carbamazepine toxicity. Ann Pharmacother 1999;33(7–8): 790–2.
96. Garg SK, Kumar N, Bhargava VK, Prabhakar SK. Effect of grapefruit juice on carbamazepine bioavailability in patients with epilepsy. Clin Pharmacol Ther 1998; 64(3):286–8.
97. Matar KM, Nicholls PJ, Bawazir SA, Al-Khamis KI, Al-Hassan MI. Effect of lamotrigine on the pharmacokinetics of carbamazepine and its active metabolite in dogs. Eur J Drug Metab Pharmacokinet 2001;26(3):149–53.
98. May TW, Rambeck B, Jurgens U. Influence of oxcarbazepine and methsuximide on lamotrigine concentrations in epileptic patients with and without valproic acid comedication: results of a retrospective study. Ther Drug Monit 1999;21(2):175–81.
99. Lai CL, Chen WJ, Huang CH, Lin FY, Lee YT. Sinus node dysfunction in a patient with lithium intoxication. J Formos Med Assoc 2000;99(1):66–8.
100. Eap CB, Yasui N, Kaneko S, Baumann P, Powell K, Otani K. Effects of carbamazepine coadministration

on plasma concentrations of the enantiomers of mianserin and of its metabolites. Ther Drug Monit 1999;21(2): 166–70.
101. Thweatt RE. Carbamazepine/MAOI interaction. Psychosomatics 1986;27(7):538.
102. Barklage NE, Jefferson JW, Margolis D. Do monoamine oxidase inhibitors alter carbamazepine blood levels? J Clin Psychiatry 1992;53(7):258.
103. Laroudie C, Salazar DE, Cosson JP, Cheuvart B, Istin B, Girault J, Ingrand I, Decourt JP. Carbamazepine-nefazodone interaction in healthy subjects. J Clin Psychopharmacol 2000;20(1):46–53.
104. Lucas RA, Gilfillan DJ, Bergstrom RF. A pharmacokinetic interaction between carbamazepine and olanzapine: observations on possible mechanism. Eur J Clin Pharmacol 1998;54(8):639–43.
105. Zolezzi M. Antituberculosis agents and carbamazepine. Am J Psychiatry 2002;159(5):874.
106. Mula M, Monaco F. Carbamazepine-risperidone interactions in patients with epilepsy. Clin Neuropharmacol 2002;25(2):97–100.
107. Ono S, Mihara K, Suzuki A, Kondo T, Yasui-Furukori N, Furukori H, de Vries R, Kaneko S. Significant pharmacokinetic interaction between risperidone and carbamazepine: its relationship with CYP2D6 genotypes. Psychopharmacology (Berl) 2002;162(1): 50–4.
108. Spina E, Avenoso A, Facciola G, Salemi M, Scordo MG, Giacobello T, Madia AG, Perucca E. Plasma concentrations of risperidone and 9-hydroxyrisperidone: effect of comedication with carbamazepine or valproate. Ther Drug Monit 2000;22(4):481–5.
109. Khan A, Shad MU, Preskorn SH. Lack of sertraline efficacy probably due to an interaction with carbamazepine. J Clin Psychiatry 2000;61(7):526–7.
110. Burstein AH, Horton RL, Dunn T, Alfaro RM, Piscitelli SC, Theodore W. Lack of effect of St. John's wort on carbamazepine pharmacokinetics in healthy volunteers. Clin Pharmacol Ther 2000;68(6):605–12.
111. Romero AS, Delgado RG, Pena MF. Interaction between trazodone and carbamazepine. Ann Pharmacother 1999;33(12):1370.
112. Miceli JJ, Anziano RJ, Robarge L, Hansen RA, Laurent A. The effect of carbamazepine on the steady-state pharmacokinetics of ziprasidone in healthy volunteers. Br J Clin Pharmacol 2000;49(Suppl 1):S65–70.

Carbapenems

See also Beta-lactam antibiotics

General Information

Carbapenems differ from penicillins and cephalosporins by a methylene substitution for sulfur in the five-membered beta-ring structure. Imipenem and meropenem belong to this class of compounds.

In the last 25 years, various natural carbapenems have been discovered (1). However, their potential is limited by chemical instability. Imipenem (*N*-formimidoylthienamycin), the first carbapenem in use, is therefore a stabilized synthetic compound. To overcome a second difficulty, namely inactivation by a kidney dehydropeptidase, imipenem has to be combined with cilastatin, a competitive inhibitor of that enzyme. Meropenem has better stability in the presence of renal dehydropeptidase I (2). The antibacterial spectrum of carbapenems is among the broadest of all beta-lactam antibiotics, and they have good stability against many beta-lactamases.

General adverse reactions

The safety profile of the carbapenems is comparable to that of other beta-lactam antibiotics, in particular with regard to laboratory abnormalities, the most common ones being those related to liver function (3,4). In patients with pre-existing nervous system disease or who take dosages above the recommended limits (for example in renal impairment) seizures appear to be more common with imipenem + cilastatin.

Organs and Systems

Nervous system

Seizures associated with imipenem + cilastatin have repeatedly been reported (5–7). As with other beta-lactam antibiotics, it is difficult to assess clearly the cause of a seizure in patients with a cluster of other predisposing factors for neurotoxicity (8) and hence to reach clear estimates of frequency. In a review of 1754 patients there was a similar incidence of seizures with imipenem + cilastatin as with other antibiotic regimens usually containing another beta-lactam (9). In rabbits imipenem + cilastatin and another carbapenems were more neurotoxic than benzylpenicillin (10). In mice, ataxia and seizures were seen, with much lower blood concentrations of imipenem than cefotaxime or benzylpenicillin (1900 μg/ml versus 3400 μg/ml and 5800 μg/ml) (11). In mice imipenem also lowered the convulsive threshold of pentetrazol (pentylenetetrazole) more than cefazolin or two other carbapenems (12). Cilastatin alone was not proconvulsant, but it increased the effects of co-administered imipenem.

Imipenem is a more common cause of seizures than other beta-lactam antibiotics, particularly when high doses are given (13–15). In one study, seven of 21 children developed seizure activity while receiving imipenem + cilastatin for bacterial meningitis, a recognized risk factor (13). However, computer-assisted monitoring of imipenem + cilastatin dosages in relation to renal function resulted in a reduced incidence of seizures (16).

In animals, meropenem (17) and other carbapenems (18,19) were less epileptogenic than imipenem. In 403 children there was no meropenem-associated neurotoxicity (20) and meropenem was well tolerated in children with bacterial meningitis (21). In summary, a larger dose range of meropenem than imipenem appears to be tolerated, but when strictly observing known risk factors for seizure propensity the difference between the two compounds is very small (22,23).

Sensory systems

Taste alterations were seen in some early patients who were treated with carbapenems (24); these observations have not subsequently been confirmed.

Hematologic

As with some cephalosporins and clavulanic acid, the Coombs' test was positive in a number of patients taking carbapenems, but without hemolysis (25).

Mouth and teeth

Yellowish-brown staining of the teeth was related to imipenem in several cases (26,27). Staining was mostly removable with dental assistance.

Urinary tract

In animals, the tubular toxicity of imipenem was completely prevented by cilastatin. Accordingly, definite nephrotoxicity of this combination has not been documented in patients (25) or in healthy volunteers (28). The cilastatin component may even reduce the nephrotoxic effects of ciclosporin after kidney transplantation (29) or bone marrow transplantation (30).

Skin

Of all the drugs that have been implicated in drug-induced toxic epidermal necrolysis, antimicrobial drugs account for 29–42% (now more than 100 in number) (31,32), and almost all antimicrobial drugs have been implicated, including meropenem (33).

- A 75-year-old woman developed acute pneumonia. She was first given oral co-amoxiclav, fluconazole, and ciprofloxacin for 10 days, followed by cefotaxime and amikacin, both intravenously. Six days later, she developed a progressive erythematous rash, soon involving 40% of her body surface. The antibiotics were withdrawn and she was rehydrated and given intravenous immunoglobulins 0.75 g/kg for 5 days, but not systemic glucocorticoids. She then developed severe septic shock because of a combination of two very resistant bacterial strains and was given meropenem 1 g and teicoplanin 800 mg bd. However, within 2 days her skin lesions recurred, extending to previously uninvolved skin areas and including over 60% of her body. A biopsy showed typical features of toxic epidermal necrolysis. Meropenem was withdrawn and replaced by aztreonam. However, she died 5 days later.

Imipenem, which is related to meropenem, has also been reported to cause toxic epidermal necrolysis (34). The authors stated that to the best of their knowledge, this was the first report of a possible cross-reaction between two classes of antibiotics in causing toxic epidermal necrolysis. The time between first administration and the occurrence of epidermal necrolysis is considerably shorter in recurrence or provocation testing (35,36). They also claimed that it is likely that the beta-lactam ring is responsible for this hypersensitivity reaction, citing the evidence that the patient had been given amoxicillin 15 days before the cephalosporin, and that could have served as the sensitizing event. They did not discuss whether aztreonam, a monobactam, also could have caused a cross-reaction; however, it has been involved in two cases of fatal toxic epidermal necrolysis (37).

A pustular rash, as repeatedly observed with cephalosporins, has been described in one case (38). The frequencies of rash, urticaria, and pruritus were similar to those seen with other beta-lactam antibiotics (25).

Meropenem can cause occupational allergic contact dermatitis (39).

- A 45-year-old nurse presented with a 6-month history of recurrent periorbital erythema with itching and runny eyes. Each episode lasted about 5–6 days and settled on withdrawal from her place at work, where she handled a large number of drugs, including meropenem. She was patch-tested with the European standard series, and was negative to all except meropenem. She had complete remission after quitting her workplace.

The authors assumed that the localization to the periorbital region was due to involuntary contact with her hands or airborne contact.

Immunologic

There was a high degree of cross-reactivity between imipenem determinants, analogous to the penicillin determinants in penicillin-allergic patients. Nine of twenty patients with positive penicillin skin tests had positive skin reactions to analogous imipenem determinants (40). In view of this appreciable cross-reactivity, imipenem should not be given to patients with penicillin allergy.

Immediate hypersensitivity related to imipenem has been reported in a patient allergic to penicillin and aztreonam (41).

Drug–Drug Interactions

Ciclosporin

The addition of imipenem + cilastatin to long-term ciclosporin provoked seizures in patients without a corresponding history (42). In general, nervous system toxicity occurred shortly after the start of the antibiotic therapy and drug concentrations were stable, suggesting a synergistic effect.

Ciclosporin-induced acute nephrotoxicity was reduced by cilastatin, an inhibitor of active tubular resorption (30,43). Reduced renal parenchymal accumulation of the drug may account for this effect. Serum ciclosporin concentrations were unchanged or insignificantly reduced. A similar protective effect against tacrolimus is possible, but unproven (44).

GABA receptor antagonists

Carbapenems (imipenem more than meropenem) are believed to increase central nervous system excitation by inhibition of GABA binding to receptors. Combinations with other GABA inhibiting drugs such as theophylline or quinolones have been reported to provoke seizures (45,46).

Valproic acid

Two carbapenems, meropenem and panipenem + betamipron, reduced serum valproic acid concentrations, and increased the risk of seizures (47,48). The mechanism of the interaction was unclear. Accelerated renal elimination of valproic acid is probable, since the almost immediate fall in serum drug concentrations and low protein binding of carbapenems argue against enzyme induction or protein binding displacement (49).

Interference with Diagnostic Tests

Leukocyte urine dipstick test

Imipenem caused positive dipstick tests for leukocytes in patients with agranulocytosis and normal urinary sediments. This phenomenon was reproducible in vitro with imipenem, meropenem, and clavulanic acid. Sulbactam, tazobactam, three penicillins, three cephalosporins, and the basic structures of penicillins, cephalosporins, and monobactams tested negative (50).

References

1. Birnbaum J, Kahan FM, Kropp H, MacDonald JS. Carbapenems, a new class of beta-lactam antibiotics. Discovery and development of imipenem/cilastatin. Am J Med 1985;78(6A):3–21.
2. Fukasawa M, Sumita Y, Harabe ET, Tanio T, Nouda H, Kohzuki T, Okuda T, Matsumura H, Sunagawa M. Stability of meropenem and effect of 1 beta-methyl substitution on its stability in the presence of renal dehydropeptidase I. Antimicrob Agents Chemother 1992;36(7):1577–9.
3. Calandra GB, Brown KR, Grad LC, Ahonkhai VI, Wang C, Aziz MA. Review of adverse experiences and tolerability in the first 2,516 patients treated with imipenem/cilastatin. Am J Med 1985;78(6A):73–8.
4. Ahonkhai VI, Cyhan GM, Wilson SE, Brown KR. Imipenem–cilastatin in pediatric patients: an overview of safety and efficacy in studies conducted in the United States. Pediatr Infect Dis J 1989;8(11):740–4.
5. Brotherton TJ, Kelber RL. Seizure-like activity associated with imipenem. Clin Pharm 1984;3(5):536–40.
6. Job ML, Dretler RH. Seizure activity with imipenem therapy: incidence and risk factors. DICP 1990;24(5):467–9.
7. Tse CS, Hernandez Vera F, Desai DV. Seizure-like activity associated with imipenem–cilastatin. Drug Intell Clin Pharm 1987;21(7–8):659–60.
8. Schliamser SE, Cars O, Norrby SR. Neurotoxicity of beta-lactam antibiotics: predisposing factors and pathogenesis. J Antimicrob Chemother 1991;27(4):405–25.
9. Calandra G, Lydick E, Carrigan J, Weiss L, Guess H. Factors predisposing to seizures in seriously ill infected patients receiving antibiotics: experience with imipenem/cilastatin. Am J Med 1988;84(5):911–18.
10. Schliamser SE, Broholm KA, Liljedahl AL, Norrby SR. Comparative neurotoxicity of benzylpenicillin, imipenem/cilastatin and FCE 22101, a new injectible penem. J Antimicrob Chemother 1988;22(5):687–95.
11. Eng RH, Munsif AN, Yangco BG, Smith SM, Chmel H. Seizure propensity with imipenem. Arch Intern Med 1989;149(8):1881–3.
12. Williams PD, Bennett DB, Comereski CR. Animal model for evaluating the convulsive liability of beta-lactam antibiotics. Antimicrob Agents Chemother 1988;32(5):758–60.
13. Wong VK, Wright HT Jr, Ross LA, Mason WH, Inderlied CB, Kim KS. Imipenem/cilastatin treatment of bacterial meningitis in children. Pediatr Infect Dis J 1991;10(2):122–5.
14. Winston DJ, Ho WG, Bruckner DA, Champlin RE. Beta-lactam antibiotic therapy in febrile granulocytopenic patients. A randomized trial comparing cefoperazone plus piperacillin, ceftazidime plus piperacillin, and imipenem alone. Ann Intern Med 1991;115(11):849–59.
15. Leo RJ, Ballow CH. Seizure activity associated with imipenem use: clinical case reports and review of the literature. DICP 1991;25(4):351–4.
16. Pestotnik SL, Classen DC, Evans RS, Stevens LE, Burke JP. Prospective surveillance of imipenem/cilastatin use and associated seizures using a hospital information system. Ann Pharmacother 1993;27(4):497–501.
17. Patel JB, Giles RE. Meropenem: evidence of lack of proconvulsive tendency in mice. J Antimicrob Chemother 1989;24(Suppl A):307–9.
18. Kurihara A, Hisaoka M, Mikuni N, Kamoshida K. Neurotoxicity of panipenem/betamipron, a new carbapenem, in rabbits: correlation to concentration in central nervous system. J Pharmacobiodyn 1992;15(7):325–32.
19. Sunagawa M, Matsumura H, Fukasawa M. Structure-activity relationships of carbapenem and penem compounds for the convulsive property. J Antibiot (Tokyo) 1992; 45(12):1983–5.
20. Fujii R, Yoshioka H, Fujita K, Maruyama S, Sakata H, Inyaku F, Chiba S, Tsutsumi H, Wagatsuma Y, Fukushima N, et al. [Pharmacokinetic and clinical studies with meropenem in the pediatric field. Pediatric Study Group of Meropenem.] Jpn J Antibiot 1992; 45(6):697–717.
21. Klugman KP, Dagan R. Randomized comparison of meropenem with cefotaxime for treatment of bacterial meningitis. Meropenem Meningitis Study Group. Antimicrob Agents Chemother 1995;39(5):1140–6.
22. Norrby SR, Faulkner KL, Newell PA. Differentiating meropenem and imipenem/cilastatin. Inf Dis in Clin Pract 1997;6:291.
23. Norrby SR, Gildon KM. Safety profile of meropenem: a review of nearly 5,000 patients treated with meropenem. Scand J Infect Dis 1999;31(1):3–10.
24. Freimer EH, Donabedian H, Raeder R, Ribner BS. Empirical use of imipenem as the sole antibiotic in the treatment of serious infections. J Antimicrob Chemother 1985;16(4):499–507.
25. Calandra GB, Wang C, Aziz M, Brown KR. The safety profile of imipenem/cilastatin: worldwide clinical experience based on 3470 patients. J Antimicrob Chemother 1986;18(Suppl E):193–202.
26. Ku C, O'Neill D. Imipenem induced dental stains. Can J Hosp Pharm 1994;47:288.
27. Scanlon N, Wilsher M, Kolbe J. Imipenem induced dental staining. Aust NZ J Med 1997;27(2):190.
28. Drusano GL, Standiford HC, Bustamante CI, Rivera G, Forrest A, Leslie J, Tatem B, Delaportas D, Schimpff SC. Safety and tolerability of multiple doses of imipenem/cilastatin. Clin Pharmacol Ther 1985; 37(5):539–43.
29. Hammer C, Thies JC, Mraz W, Mihatsch M. Reduction of cyclosporin (CSA) nephrotoxicity by imipenem/cilastatin after kidney transplantation in rats. Transplant Proc 1989;21(1 Pt 1):931.
30. Gruss E, Tomas JF, Bernis C, Rodriguez F, Traver JA, Fernandez-Ranada JM. Nephroprotective effect of cilastatin in allogeneic bone marrow transplantation. Results from a retrospective analysis. Bone Marrow Transplant 1996;18(4):761–5.
31. Roujeau JC, Guillaume JC, Fabre JP, Penso D, Flechet ML, Girre JP. Toxic epidermal necrolysis (Lyell syndrome). Incidence and drug etiology in France, 1981–1985. Arch Dermatol 1990;126(1):37–42.
32. Schopf E, Stuhmer A, Rzany B, Victor N, Zentgraf R, Kapp JF. Toxic epidermal necrolysis and Stevens–Johnson

syndrome. An epidemiologic study from West Germany. Arch Dermatol 1991;127(6):839–42.
33. Paquet P, Jacob E, Damas P, Pierard GE. Recurrent fatal drug-induced toxic epidermal necrolysis (Lyell's syndrome) after putative beta-lactam cross-reactivity: case report and scrutiny of antibiotic imputability. Crit Care Med 2002; 30(11):2580–3.
34. Brand R, Rohr JB. Toxic epidermal necrolysis in Western Australia. Australas J Dermatol 2000;41(1):31–3.
35. Dreyfuss DA, Gottlieb LJ, Wilkerson DK, Parsons RW, Krizek TJ. Survival after a second episode of toxic epidermal necrolysis. Ann Plast Surg 1988;20(2):146–7.
36. Roujeau JC, Chosidow O, Saiag P, Guillaume JC. Toxic epidermal necrolysis (Lyell syndrome). J Am Acad Dermatol 1990;23(6 Pt 1):1039–58.
37. McDonald BJ, Singer JW, Bianco JA. Toxic epidermal necrolysis possibly linked to aztreonam in bone marrow transplant patients. Ann Pharmacother 1992;26(1):34–5.
38. Escallier F, Dalac S, Foucher JL, Lorcerie B, Lucet A, Lambert D. Pustulose exanthématique aiguë généralisée: imputabilité à l'imipénème (Tienam). [Acute generalized exanthematic pustulosis. Imputability of imipenem (Tienam).] Ann Dermatol Venereol 1989;116(5):407–9.
39. Yesudian PD, King CM. Occupational allergic contact dermatitis from meropenem. Contact Dermatitis 2001; 45(1):53.
40. Saxon A, Adelman DC, Patel A, Hajdu R, Calandra GB. Imipenem cross-reactivity with penicillin in humans. J Allergy Clin Immunol 1988;82(2):213–17.
41. Hantson P, de Coninck B, Horn JL, Mahieu P. Immediate hypersensitivity to aztreonam and imipenem. BMJ 1991;302(6771):294–5.
42. Bosmuller C, Steurer W, Konigsrainer A, Willeit J, Margreiter R. Increased risk of central nervous system toxicity in patients treated with ciclosporin and imipenem/cilastatin. Nephron 1991;58(3):362–4.
43. Carmellini M, Frosini F, Filipponi F, Boggi U, Mosca F. Effect of cilastatin on cyclosporine-induced acute nephrotoxicity in kidney transplant recipients. Transplantation 1997;64(1):164–6.
44. Paterson DL, Singh N. Interactions between tacrolimus and antimicrobial agents. Clin Infect Dis 1997; 25(6):1430–40.
45. De Sarro A, Ammendola D, De Sarro G. Effects of some quinolones on imipenem-induced seizures in DBA/2 mice. Gen Pharmacol 1994;25(2):369–79.
46. Semel JD, Allen N. Seizures in patients simultaneously receiving theophylline and imipenem or ciprofloxacin or metronidazole. South Med J 1991;84(4):465–8.
47. De Turck BJ, Diltoer MW, Cornelis PJ, Maes V, Spapen HD, Camu F, Huyghens LP. Lowering of plasma valproic acid concentrations during concomitant therapy with meropenem and amikacin. J Antimicrob Chemother 1998;42(4):563–4.
48. Yamagata T, Momoi MY, Murai K, Ikematsu K, Suwa K, Sakamoto K, Fujimura A. Panipenem–betamipron and decreases in serum valproic acid concentration. Ther Drug Monit 1998;20(4):396–400.
49. Nagai K, Shimizu T, Togo A, Takeya M, Yokomizo Y, Sakata Y, Matsuishi T, Kato H. Decrease in serum levels of valproic acid during treatment with a new carbapenem, panipenem/betamipron. J Antimicrob Chemother 1997;39(2):295–6.
50. Beer JH, Vogt A, Neftel K, Cottagnoud P. False positive results for leucocytes in urine dipstick test with common antibiotics. BMJ 1996;313(7048):25.

Carbenoxolone

General Information

Liquorice owes its ulcer-healing properties to glycyrrhizin and glycyrrhizic acid; carbenoxolone is related to the latter. All these substances have unwanted mineralocorticoid-like effects. Deglycyrrhizinated liquorice and lauryl glycyrrhetinic acid, which are also used in some countries for their ulcer-healing effects, do not have mineralocorticoid-like effects. It should be noted that liquorice is sometimes present in laxatives, for example those prepared by herbalists, and that hyperaldosteronism can occur unexpectedly in such cases when liquorice consumption has gone unrecognized (SEDA-16, 425). For example, hypokalemia and hypertension has been associated with the use of liquorice flavored chewing gum (1).

Organs and Systems

Endocrine

- Hyperprolactinemia occurred in a woman with secondary amenorrhea and hypertension who was taking large amounts of liquorice; all the abnormalities reversed on withdrawal (2).

This effect could have reflected involvement of prolactin in adrenal steroidogenesis or salt and water homeostasis.

Electrolyte balance

The mineralocorticoid properties of carbenoxolone are probably exerted by displacement of aldosterone from non-specific receptor sites in cells, thus making it more available to affect mineral metabolism. What this means in practice is that in normal doses carbenoxolone can cause salt and water retention, with occasional hypokalemia. These effects are common but usually mild; they are detected more often during treatment if patients are weighed, their blood pressure measured, and serum potassium concentrations checked. Those who take prolonged courses, elderly patients, and those with hepatic, cardiac, or renal impairment are at special risk; severe effects, with serious hypertension, heart failure, and hypokalemia of sufficient degree to induce myopathy and tubular necrosis, can usually be ascribed to ill-advised treatment of people in whom carbenoxolone is contraindicated, to its use in elderly patients, or to prolonged intake without supervision.

Liquorice-induced pseudohyperaldosteronism can cause hypokalemic myopathy (3).

- A 65-year-old man, diabetic and alcoholic, developed pseudohyperaldosteronism with hypokalemia, myopathy, and a reversible dilated cardiomyopathy associated with a small dose of liquorice-containing stomachics (0.06 of liquorice extract in total granules of 3 g/day) over a few years for gastritis and a total of 800 mg of glycyrrhizin intravenously over 2 months for worsening liver dysfunction.

Drug–Drug Interactions

Amiloride

Amiloride inhibits the ulcer-healing action of carbenoxolone (SEDA-6, 317).

Antihypertensive drugs

Because of its mineralocorticoid fluid-retaining properties, carbenoxolone opposes the therapeutic effects of diuretics and other drugs used to treat hypertension.

Spironolactone

Spironolactone inhibits the ulcer-healing action of carbenoxolone (SEDA-6, 317).

References

1. de Klerk GJ, Nieuwenhuis MG, Beutler JJ. Hypokalaemia and hypertension associated with use of liquorice flavoured chewing gum. BMJ 1997;314(7082):731–2.
2. Werner S, Brismar K, Olsson S. Hyperprolactinaemia and liquorice. Lancet 1979;1(8111):319.
3. Hasegawa J, Suyama Y, Kinugawa T, Morisawa T, Kishimoto Y. Echocardiographic findings of the heart resembling dilated cardiomyopathy during hypokalemic myopathy due to licorice-induced pseudoaldosteronism. Cardiovasc Drugs Ther 1998;12(6):599–600.

Carbocisteine

General Information

Carbocisteine is a mucolytic that is administered orally or from a metered dose inhaler. Its adverse effects include headache, nausea, vomiting, gastric discomfort and bleeding, diarrhea, and skin rash. It has, however, been shown to be an effective mucolytic which is generally well tolerated with few adverse effects (SEDA-17, 208).

The place of mucolytic drugs in respiratory disease has recently been reviewed (1). The authors suggested that they have been inappropriately used in the past. As mucolytic agents do not improve lung function tests in COPD, the European Respiratory Society and the American Thoracic Society guidelines discourage their use in the treatment of COPD. Future trials should evaluate clinical symptoms and quality of life as well as lung function tests. Mucolytic agents should be evaluated earlier in the natural history of COPD, when mucus hypersecretion is the major feature and before lung function has deteriorated.

Reference

1. Del Donno M, Olivieri D. Mucoactive drugs in the management of chronic obstructive pulmonary disease. Monaldi Arch Chest Dis 1998;53(6):714–19.

Carbon dioxide

General Information

Alternatives to iodinated X-ray contrast agents have been sought for cases in which they are contraindicated. One such agent is carbon dioxide (CO_2), a highly soluble gas, which is therefore relatively safe to inject into the circulation, where it displaces blood and reduces X-ray absorption, acting as a negative contrast agent (SEDA-20, 423) (1). No complication of any kind was reported with the use carbon dioxide in aortography or peripheral angiography (SEDA-20, 423).

In a UK study the safety and diagnostic efficacy of carbon dioxide as an arterial contrast agent have been investigated in 63 patients (36 men and 27 women, aged 46–86 years) who underwent angiographic examinations with carbon dioxide via an automated injector and iodinated contrast medium (2). There were adverse effects in 15 patients, including nausea ($n = 4$), abdominal pain ($n = 8$), and leg and groin pain ($n = 8$). All the symptoms were directly related to the injection of carbon dioxide and resolved within 1–2 minutes of injection. No arteriogram had to be abandoned because of adverse effects, and the incidence of adverse reactions was less with selective studies. Although it has been reported that carbon dioxide is well tolerated, with minimal discomfort, in this study there was a variety of mild to severe unpleasant symptoms, but no serious complications. The abdominal symptoms were related to the passage of a large volume of carbon dioxide into the mesenteric vessels. The catheter was above the mesenteric vessels in most of the patients with abdominal symptoms. These symptoms can be reduced by placing the tip of the catheter in non-selective studies at the aortic bifurcation to reduce the amount of carbon dioxide that passes into the superior or inferior mesenteric arteries. The symptoms are also reduced by injecting smaller volumes. The authors concluded that when iodinated contrast media are contraindicated carbon dioxide provides a diagnostic alternative.

The safety of carbon dioxide in vena cavography has been investigated in 119 patients (aged 17–89 years, 65 men). Patients with intracardiac shunts, severe pulmonary compromise, or non-dialysis-dependent renal insufficiency were excluded. Two patients developed mild adverse effects: one had nausea that resolved spontaneously and the other vomited several minutes after the administration of carbon dioxide but needed no treatment. The diagnostic quality of the venography was comparable to that with iodinated contrast media. The authors concluded that carbon dioxide cavography is well tolerated and is especially valuable in patients with a history of a reaction to iodinated contrast material or renal insufficiency.

References

1. Dewald CL, Jensen CC, Park YH, Hanks SE, Harrell DS, Peters GL, Katz MD. Vena cavography with CO(2) versus with iodinated contrast material for inferior vena cava filter placement: a prospective evaluation. Radiology 2000;216(3): 752–7.

2. Bees NR, Beese RC, Belli AM, Buckenham TM. Carbon dioxide angiography of the lower limbs: initial experience with an automated carbon dioxide injector. Clin Radiol 1999;54(12):833–8.

Carbonic anhydrase inhibitors

General Information

The carbonic anhydrase inhibitors, of which acetazolamide (rINN), a non-competitive inhibitor, is the prototype, are not suitable for normal diuretic use, because tolerance soon develops. However, they are well suited to brief intermittent use, particularly in the relief of glaucoma and in the prevention of acute mountain sickness. Acetazolamide and methazolamide (rINN) should be used with caution in the long-term control of glaucoma because of its serious systemic adverse effects. However, brinzolamide (rINN) and dorzolamide (rINN) are available for long-term topical administration.

The safety profile and efficacy of 2% dorzolamide hydrochloride (Trusopt) eye-drops have been evaluated. It was as effective as pilocarpine 2% and its ocular hypotensive efficacy was comparable with that of betaxolol 0.5%. The patients reported less interference with quality of life with dorzolamide than pilocarpine, particularly in regard to limitations in their ability to drive, read, and perform moderate activities. Long-term use was not associated with important electrolyte disturbances or the systemic effects commonly observed with oral carbonic anhydrase inhibitors (1–3).

In a 3-month prospective study of the adverse effects and efficacy of topical dorzolamide in 39 patients intolerant of systemic carbonic anhydrase inhibitors, the effect on mean intraocular pressure was similar to that of acetazolamide, and health assessment scores improved significantly in seven of the eight categories of the SF-36 health assessment questionnaire used to evaluate changes in well-being and quality of life (4). There were no adverse effects with the switch in medication.

General adverse effects

The incidence and severity of many adverse reactions to carbonic anhydrase inhibitors are dose-related and the problems usually abate when the dose is reduced or the drug is withdrawn. Symptoms of depression, confusion, fatigue, impotence, irritability, malaise, nervousness, and weight loss are often present to some extent in patients on long-term acetazolamide or methazolamide therapy. These symptoms may be related to systemic metabolic acidosis (due to renal excretion of bicarbonate), which is often accompanied by a reduction in serum potassium concentration (5). Gastrointestinal intolerance, manifested as abdominal cramping, dyspepsia, and nausea, with or without diarrhea, is another common problem. Carbonic anhydrase inhibitors reduce the urinary excretion of citrate and uric acid, which may lead to renal calculi and gouty arthritis. Pulmonary edema, taste disorders, and alopecia have also been reported. The most serious adverse effect of carbonic anhydrase inhibitors is bone-marrow depression.

Organs and Systems

Cardiovascular

Anaphylactic shock has been reported after a single oral dose of acetazolamide (6).

- A 70-year-old man was given acetazolamide 250 mg to control postoperative intravascular pressure 5 hours after cataract removal under local anesthetic. Thirty minutes later he complained of nausea, became cyanotic, and had an acute respiratory arrest. His systolic blood pressure was 70 mmHg, his heart rate was 180/minute, and there was tachypnea (40 breaths/minute). Arterial gases confirmed hypoxemia (PaO_2 6.34 kPa, 47 mmHg). Pulmonary embolism and high-pressure pulmonary edema were excluded by perfusion lung scanning and right-sided heart catheterization. Management was with ventilatory support, vasopressors, intravenous hydrocortisone, and diphenhydramine. Clinical improvement occurred over 12 hours. After stabilization, sulfonamide hypersensitivity was confirmed by skin testing, suggesting cross-sensitivity with a sulfonamide derivative (acetazolamide).

Physicians should be aware of the risk of anaphylaxis to acetazolamide, particularly in patients with a history of allergy to sulfonamides.

Nervous system

A case of possible Gerstmann syndrome has been attributed to acetazolamide (7).

- A 60-year-old woman became acutely confused 2 days after the removal of a cataract. She had long-standing diabetes mellitus, hypertension, and ischemic heart disease. There had been a minor stroke with complete recovery 2 years before. Her medication included aspirin, indapamide, enalapril, and oral hypoglycaemic agents. Acetazolamide 500 mg bd was added shortly after her eye operation. Neurological examination showed finger agnosia, nominal and receptive dysphasia, acalculia, astereognosis, and left–right disorientation. Other systems were normal. Withdrawal of acetazolamide resulted in rapid improvement with no residual neurological signs two days after admission.

Acetazolamide toxicity was suspected, because of the temporal association between drug treatment and the onset of the neurological symptoms, together with metabolic acidosis. Gerstmann syndrome is usually due to an acute stroke. Although a brain CT scan was negative, such an event was likely in this patient, who had a history of cerebrovascular disease and multiple risk factors, and a causal relation to acetazolamide must be considered tenuous.

Sensory systems

Eyes

In a multicenter, double-blind, prospective, parallel-group comparison of brinzolamide 1.0% bd or tds, dorzolamide 2.0% tds, and timolol 0.5% bd in 572 patients with primary open-angle glaucoma or ocular hypertension, the three drugs were equally effective (8). Brinzolamide 1.0% caused less ocular discomfort (burning and stinging) (bd 1.8%; tds 3.0%) than dorzolamide (16%).

- A 68-year-old woman developed bilateral marginal keratitis 2 weeks after starting to use dorzolamide eye-drops (9). One week after withdrawal she was asymptomatic, with complete resolution of her corneal infiltrates.

In this case the allergic reaction was caused by dorzolamide hydrochloride and not the preservative, benzalkonium chloride, since therapy was uneventfully continued with timolol maleate, which also contains benzalkonium chloride as a preservative. This is the first report of this phenomenon with a carbonic anhydrase inhibitor.

Taste

Acetazolamide can cause altered taste perception of carbonated drinks. The mechanism is unknown, but carbonic drinks may be a source of high concentrations of carbonic acid, which are reduced by carbonic anhydrase activity (SEDA-15, 219).

Endocrine

Thyrotoxic periodic paralysis occurs only occasionally in Caucasians, but for unknown reasons it can be worsened by acetazolamide (SEDA-15, 219).

Electrolyte balance

The carbonic anhydrase inhibitors are the most kaliuretic of all diuretics and can cause severe hypokalemia during the first few days of administration. However, hypokalemia is not a problem during long-term administration, because of compensatory potassium retention secondary to acidosis (10).

- A 46-year-old man with hypokalemic periodic paralysis and diabetes mellitus had worse muscle weakness after taking acetazolamide, possibly because of reduced muscle uptake of potassium (11).

Acid–base balance

Acetazolamide can produce severe lactic acidosis, with an increased lactate:pyruvate ratio, ketosis with a low beta-hydroxybutyrate:acetoacetate ratio, and a urinary organic acid profile consistent with pyruvate carboxylase deficiency. The acquired enzymatic injury that results from inhibition of mitochondrial carbonic anhydrase V, which provides bicarbonate to pyruvate carboxylase, can damage the tricarboxylic acid cycle.

Four preterm neonates with posthemorrhagic ventricular dilatation developed severe metabolic acidosis after being given acetazolamide (12). The acidosis suddenly disappeared after a transfusion of packed erythrocytes, which was attributed to the citrate contained in the blood.

Acetazolamide can cause a metabolic acidosis in 50% of elderly patients (SEDA-11, 199); occasionally (particularly if salicylates are being given or renal function is poor) the acidosis can be severe. It does this by inhibiting renal bicarbonate reabsorption. This effect is of particular use in treating patients with chronic respiratory acidosis with superimposed metabolic alkalosis. Life-threatening metabolic acidosis is rarely observed in the absence of renal insufficiency and/or diabetes mellitus. In three patients with central nervous system pathology alone conventional doses of acetazolamide resulted in severe metabolic acidosis (13). After withdrawal it took up to 48 hours for the metabolic acidosis and accompanying hyperventilation to resolve.

Metabolic acidosis has also been described with the topical carbonic anhydrase inhibitor dorzolamide.

- A 5-day-old boy, weighing 2.3 kg, developed a metabolic acidosis after receiving topical dorzolamide for 1 week for bilateral Peter's anomaly (a congenital corneal disorder characterized by a central leukoma and adhesions at the periphery of the corneal opacity) (14). The maximum base deficit was 20.2 mmol/l. On withdrawal of topical dorzolamide his acidosis resolved within 1 day.

Factors that may have contributed to this metabolic acidosis included low birth weight, renal tubular immaturity, and impaired renal function, which may have resulted in systemic accumulation with repetitive dosing. This case stresses the fact that topical medications can cause systemic effects if a sufficient amount of drug is absorbed in a susceptible subject.

Hematologic

Aplastic anemia occurs in about one in 18 000 patient-years of exposure to oral carbonic anhydrase inhibitors. Most cases occur within the first 6 months, and peak at 2–3 months.

Eleven cases of acetazolamide-associated aplastic anemia were reported in Sweden during a 17-year period (15). The median dose was 500 mg/day and the median duration of therapy was 3 (2–71) months. Ten of the eleven patients died within 8 weeks of diagnosis. The relative risk of aplastic anemia with acetazolamide was 13.3 (95% CI = 6.8, 25) and the estimated frequency was 1 in 18 000. These findings suggest that acetazolamide is associated with a substantially increased risk of aplastic anemia.

However, the National Registry of Drug-Induced Ocular Side Effects has not received a report of blood dyscrasias in patients who have taken oral carbonic anhydrase inhibitors for less than 2 weeks (16). Since there is generally some time before abnormal blood counts progress to bone-marrow failure, seeking a symptomless "early window" is precisely the point of routine hematological screening; thus, patients taking long-term oral carbonic anhydrase inhibitors should have erythrocyte, leukocyte, and platelet counts bimonthly during the first 6 months of therapy and then every 6 months thereafter. Routine hematological surveillance should always be accompanied by patient education about warning signs and symptoms of progressive marrow failure.

Urinary tract

In a French analysis of 22 510 urinary calculi performed by infrared spectroscopy, drug-induced urolithiasis was divided into two categories: first, stones with drugs physically embedded ($n = 238$; 1.0%), notably indinavir monohydrate ($n = 126$; 53%), followed by triamterene ($n = 43$; 18%), sulfonamides ($n = 29$; 12%), and amorphous silica ($n = 24$; 10%); secondly, metabolic nephrolithiasis induced by drugs ($n = 140$; 0.6%), involving mainly calcium/vitamin D supplementation ($n = 56$; 40%) and carbonic anhydrase inhibitors ($n = 33$; 24%) (17). Drug-induced stones are responsible for about 1.6% of all calculi in France. Physical analysis and a thorough drug history are important elements in the diagnosis.

Skin

Two Japanese-American women developed clinical features that satisfied the criteria for Stevens–Johnson syndrome during methazolamide treatment (18). Methazolamide is a sulfonamide, the most common group of drugs associated with Stevens–Johnson syndrome.

Topical dorzolamide caused severe periorbital dermatitis after an average exposure time of 20 weeks in 14 patients (19). Although dermatitis due to dorzolamide can resolve when it is withdrawn, this does not always occur, and in some patients all topical medications containing benzalkonium chloride must be withdrawn. Allergic contact blepharoconjunctivitis has also been reported with dorzolamide in a 72-year-old man (20).

Musculoskeletal

Chronic acetazolamide therapy is associated with greater spinal bone mineral density. This is probably the result of metabolic acidosis; urine calcium is increased and serum phosphate reduced. Osteomalacia has been reported during long-term therapy in combination with barbiturates in two patients.

Immunologic

Fatal anaphylactic shock with massive pulmonary edema has been reported in a 66-year-old woman who was taking acetazolamide for glaucoma (21). She had a history of sulfonamide allergy, and acetazolamide is a sulfonamide derivative. Sulfonamide allergy should be regarded as a contraindication to acetazolamide.

- Non-fatal anaphylactic shock with acute pulmonary edema has been reported in a 79-year-old woman after a first dose of acetazolamide (22). There was no history of sulfonamide allergy and she had been taking hydrochlorothiazide for some time.

Anaphylactic shock with acetazolamide should be recognized to occur as a first-dose phenomenon with no prior demonstrable sulfonamide allergy.

Long-Term Effects

Drug tolerance

Acetazolamide alkalinizes the urine and increases its volume. Urinary sodium, potassium, and bicarbonate concentrations rise, and chloride concentration falls. These effects are due to inhibition of carbonic anhydrase in the nephron, mainly in the proximal convoluted tubule, which reduces the number of protons available for Na/H antiporter exchange. Consequently, the concentration of bicarbonate in extracellular fluids falls, causing a metabolic acidosis, which itself limits the diuretic response to acetazolamide. Thus, the initial kaliuretic effect is lost within a few weeks.

Second-Generation Effects

Teratogenicity

Possible teratogenicity due to acetazolamide resulted in one case of congenital glaucoma, microphthalmia, and patent ductus arteriosus and one case of sacrococcygeal teratoma. One child was born with acidosis, hypercalcemia, and hypomagnesemia; these features resolved rapidly, but at 8 months there was mild hypotonicity of the legs. It has been suggested that acetazolamide should be avoided in the first trimester of pregnancy (SEDA-21, 228).

Fetotoxicity

The use of acetazolamide in pregnancy is ill-advised.

- Renal tubular acidosis occurred in a preterm boy shortly after birth (23). His mother had taken oral acetazolamide during pregnancy for glaucoma. When renal tubular acidosis developed, acetazolamide was detected in his serum, demonstrating transplacental passage of acetazolamide.

Susceptibility Factors

Carbonic anhydrase inhibitors should be used with caution in patients with respiratory acidosis or those with severe loss of respiratory capacity, and in patients with diabetes mellitus. They are contraindicated in patients with hepatic disease or insufficiency, reduced serum concentrations of sodium or potassium, adrenocortical insufficiency, hyperchloremic acidosis, or severe renal disease or dysfunction. They should also be avoided in patients taking salicylates.

Drug Administration

Drug administration route

Brinzolamide eye-drops can cause transient blurred vision (24).

Dorzolamide eye-drops can cause irreversible corneal edema in glaucoma patients with endothelial compromise (25).

Drug overdose

Overdosage with acetazolamide can destroy the gastric mucosal barrier, by interfering with prostaglandin and bicarbonate release, and can cause thrombocytopenia by bone marrow suppression, eventually leading to hemorrhagic gastritis. Although acetazolamide binds strongly to plasma proteins, and clearance by hemodialysis is generally poor, this approach and hemoperfusion (without heparin) appears to be effective (SEDA-22, 236).

Acetazolamide overdose has been reported in a child.

- A 12-month-old girl, weighing 10 kg, developed metabolic acidosis after taking 500–1250 mg of acetazolamide (26). The maximum base deficit recorded was 11.6. She was treated with sodium bicarbonate and recovered completely.

Accidental poisoning with acetazolamide should be included in the differential diagnosis of metabolic acidosis.

Drug–Drug Interactions

Furosemide

Acetazolamide inhibits cerebrospinal fluid production, and its effects are augmented by furosemide, suggesting a role for this combination in infants with ventricular dilatation resulting from severe periventricular hemorrhage. The International Posthaemorrhagic Ventricular Drug Trial Group has reported the results of a randomized, controlled trial of standard therapy alone or with the addition of acetazolamide plus furosemide in the first 151 of 177 randomized patients (27). The addition of acetazolamide plus furosemide was not only ineffective but also worsened the already poor outcome in these infants. At 1 year, death and the need for shunt placement were substantially commoner in the diuretic-treated group. There were adverse events (for example acidosis, nausea, anorexia, and diarrhea) in 37% of those given acetazolamide plus furosemide; in addition, 27% developed nephrocalcinosis (SEDA-21, 228). Altered cerebral blood flow due to acetazolamide may have caused additional brain injury.

In a commentary on this trial (28) it was pointed out that the use of acetazolamide alone or with furosemide in the treatment of posthemorrhagic hydrocephalus is another example of the use of untried therapy in neonatal care. The safety and efficacy of acetazolamide in children has never been established.

Salicylate

Two elderly patients developed lethargy, confusion, and incontinence, attributed to an interaction between acetazolamide and salicylate (29). Salicylate may reduce acetazolamide clearance by inhibiting its renal tubular secretion. Analgesic doses of salicylates should probably be avoided in elderly patients taking acetazolamide.

- A 50-year-old woman with chronic renal insufficiency treated with acetazolamide for simple glaucoma developed confusion, cerebellar ataxia, and metabolic acidosis 2 weeks after starting to take aspirin for acute pericarditis (30). A diagnosis of salicylism was made despite low serum salicylate concentrations.

The authors suggested that acetazolamide-induced acidosis increases the concentration of the unionized form of salicylate, which crosses membranes more rapidly, and hence explains the cerebral toxicity associated with low serum concentrations of salicylate. However, an increase in the plasma or erythrocyte concentrations of acetazolamide (not measured) is a much more convincing explanation for this patient's symptoms.

Other Environmental Interactions

Ketogenic diet

A ketogenic diet is sometimes used to control intractable seizures. Acetazolamide should be discontinued before starting the diet, because of the potential risk of severe secondary metabolic acidosis (31). Acetazolamide can be reintroduced once the acid–base status of the patient has stabilized.

Interference with Diagnostic Tests

HPLC assays for theophyline

Acetazolamide interferes with certain HPLC assays for theophylline, leading to spuriously increased theophylline concentrations (SEDA-21, 228).

References

1. Palmberg P. A topical carbonic anhydrase inhibitor finally arrives. Arch Ophthalmol 1995;113(8):985–6.
2. Strahlman E, Tipping R, Vogel R. A double-masked, randomized 1-year study comparing dorzolamide (Trusopt), timolol, and betaxolol. International Dorzolamide Study Group. Arch Ophthalmol 1995;113(8):1009–16.
3. Laibovitz R, Strahlman ER, Barber BL, Strohmaier KM. Comparison of quality of life and patient preference of dorzolamide and pilocarpine as adjunctive therapy to timolol in the treatment of glaucoma. J Glaucoma 1995; 4:306–13.
4. Nesher R, Ticho U. Switching from systemic to the topical carbonic anhydrase inhibitor dorzolamide: effect on the quality of life of glaucoma patients with drug-related side effects. Isr Med Assoc J 2003;5(4):260–3.
5. Fraunfelder FT, Meyer SM. Systemic adverse reactions to glaucoma medications. Int Ophthalmol Clin 1989;29(3):143–6.
6. Tzanakis N, Metzidaki G, Thermos K, Spyraki CH, Bouros D. Anaphylactic shock after a single oral intake of acetazolamide. Br J Ophthalmol 1998;82(5):588.
7. Lee YT, Wu JC, Chan FK. Acetazolamide-induced Gerstmann syndrome. Int J Clin Pract 1999;53(7):560–1.
8. Silver LH. Clinical efficacy and safety of brinzolamide (Azopt), a new topical carbonic anhydrase inhibitor for primary open-angle glaucoma and ocular hypertension. Brinzolamide Primary Therapy Study Group. Am J Ophthalmol 1998;126(3):400–8.
9. Taguri AH, Khan MA, Sanders R. Marginal keratitis: an uncommon form of topical dorzolamide allergy. Am J Ophthalmol 2000;130(1):120–2.
10. Critchlow AS, Freeborn SN, Roddie RA. Potassium supplements during treatment of glaucoma with acetazolamide. BMJ (Clin Res Ed) 1984;289(6436):21.
11. Ikeda K, Iwasaki Y, Kinoshita M, Yabuki D, Igarashi O, Ichikawa Y, Satoyoshi E. Acetazolamide-induced muscle weakness in hypokalemic periodic paralysis. Intern Med 2002;41(9):743–5.
12. Filippi L, Bagnoli F, Margollicci M, Zammarchi E, Tronchin M, Rubaltelli FF. Pathogenic mechanism, prophylaxis, and therapy of symptomatic acidosis induced by acetazolamide. J Investig Med 2002;50(2):125–32.

13. Venkatesha SL, Umamaheswara Rao GS. Metabolic acidosis and hyperventilation induced by acetazolamide in patients with central nervous system pathology. Anesthesiology 2000;93(6):1546–8.
14. Morris S, Geh V, Nischal KK, Sahi S, Ahmed MA. Topical dorzolamide and metabolic acidosis in a neonate. Br J Ophthalmol 2003;87(8):1052–3.
15. Keisu M, Wiholm BE, Ost A, Mortimer O. Acetazolamide-associated aplastic anaemia. J Intern Med 1990;228(6):627–32.
16. Fraunfelder FT, Bagby GC. Monitoring patients taking oral carbonic anhydrase inhibitors. Am J Ophthalmol 2000; 130(2):221–3.
17. Cohen-Solal F, Abdelmoula J, Hoarau MP, Jungers P, Lacour B, Daudon M. Les lithiases urinaires d'origine medicamenteuse. [Urinary lithiasis of medical origin.] Therapie 2001;56(6):743–50.
18. Flach AJ, Smith RE, Fraunfelder FT. Stevens–Johnson syndrome associated with methazolamide treatment reported in two Japanese–American women. Ophthalmology 1995;102(11):1677–80.
19. Delaney YM, Salmon JF, Mossa F, Gee B, Beehne K, Powell S. Periorbital dermatitis as a side effect of topical dorzolamide. Br J Ophthalmol 2002;86(4):378–80.
20. Mancuso G, Berdondini RM. Allergic contact blepharoconjunctivitis from dorzolamide. Contact Dermatitis 2001; 45(4):243.
21. Gerhards LJ, van Arnhem AC, Holman ND, Nossent GD. Fatale anafylactische reactie na inname van acetazolamide (Diamox) wegens glaucoom. [Fatal anaphylactic reaction after oral acetazolamide (Diamox) for glaucoma.] Ned Tijdschr Geneeskd 2000;144(25):1228–30.
22. Gallerani M, Manzoli N, Fellin R, Simonato M, Orzincolo C. Anaphylactic shock and acute pulmonary edema after a single oral dose of acetazolamide. Am J Emerg Med 2002;20(4):371–2.
23. Ozawa H, Azuma E, Shindo K, Higashigawa M, Mukouhara R, Komada Y. Transient renal tubular acidosis in a neonate following transplacental acetazolamide. Eur J Pediatr 2001;160(5):321–2.
24. Doyle JW, Smith MF. New aqueous inflow inhibitors. Semin Ophthalmol 1999;14(3):159–63.
25. Konowal A, Morrison JC, Brown SV, Cooke DL, Maguire LJ, Verdier DV, Fraunfelder FT, Dennis RF, Epstein RJ. Irreversible corneal decompensation in patients treated with topical dorzolamide. Am J Ophthalmol 1999;127(4):403–6.
26. Baer E, Reith DM. Acetazolamide poisoning in a toddler. J Paediatr Child Health 2001;37(4):411–12.
27. International PHVD Drug Trial Group. International randomised controlled trial of acetazolamide and furosemide in posthaemorrhagic ventricular dilatation in infancy. Lancet 1998;352(9126):433–40.
28. Hack M, Cohen AR. Acetazolamide plus furosemide for periventricular dilatation: lessons for drug therapy in children. Lancet 1998;352(9126):418–19.
29. Sweeney KR, Chapron DJ, Brandt JL, Gomolin IH, Feig PU, Kramer PA. Toxic interaction between acetazolamide and salicylate: case reports and a pharmacokinetic explanation. Clin Pharmacol Ther 1986;40(5):518–24.
30. Hazouard E, Grimbert M, Jonville-Berra AP, De Toffol MC, Legras A. Salicylisme et glaucome: augmentation reciproque de la toxicité de l'acétazolamide et de l'acide acetyl salicylique. [Salicylism and glaucoma: reciprocal augmentation of the toxicity of acetazolamide and acetylsalicylic acid.] J Fr Ophtalmol 1999;22(1):73–5.
31. Tallian KB, Nahata MC, Tsao CY. Role of the ketogenic diet in children with intractable seizures. Ann Pharmacother 1998;32(3):349–61.

Carboprost

See also Prostaglandins

General Information

Carboprost is a 15-methylated analogue of $PGF_{2\alpha}$. It is used in termination of pregnancy, in the management of labor, and to treat postpartum hemorrhage and uterine atony.

Organs and Systems

Respiratory

Pulmonary edema has been attributed to carboprost (1).

- An 18-year-old woman at 37 weeks gestation was given prostaglandin E_2 gel for cervical ripening followed by oxytocin. After delivery by cesarean section uterine atony, which did not respond to oxytocin and methylergometrine maleate, was treated with intramyometrial 15-methyl-prostaglandin $F_{2\alpha}$ 0.25 mg. After 5 minutes, her SpO_2 fell to 89 and she had dyspnea and sinus tachycardia due to acute pulmonary edema.

Gastrointestinal

Vomiting is a common adverse effect of $PGF_{2\alpha}$ (2).

Reproductive system

Uterine rupture has been reported after intramuscular injection of carboprost to terminate a mid-trimester pregnancy (3).

Drug Administration

Drug overdose

A neonate was accidentally given a large dose of carboprost and recovered (4).

- A full-term neonate was accidentally given carboprost 250 μg intramuscularly in an error for hepatitis vaccine. Within 15 minutes, he became tachypneic and hypertensive and then developed bronchospasm and dystonic movements and/or seizure activity in the arms. He was hyperthermic and had diarrhea. He recovered within 18 hours.

References

1. Rodriguez de la Torre MR, Gallego Alonso JI, Gil Fernandez M. Edema pulmonar en una cesarea relacionado con la administracion de 15-metil prostaglandina F2 alpha. [Pulmonary edema related to administration of 15-methyl-prostaglandin F2 alpha during a cesarean section.] Rev Esp Anestesiol Reanim 2004;51(2):104–7.
2. Biswas A, Roy S. A comparative study of the efficacy and safety of synthetic prostaglandin E2 derivative and 15-methyl prostaglandin F2 alpha in the termination of midtrimester pregnancy. J Indian Med Assoc 1996; 94(8):292–3.

3. Tripathy SN. Uterine rupture following intramuscular injection of carboprost in midtrimester pregnancy termination. J Indian Med Assoc 1985;83(9):328.
4. Mrvos R, Kerr FJ, Krenzelok EP. Carboprost exposure in a newborn with recovery. J Toxicol Clin Toxicol 1999; 37(7):865–7.

Cardiac glycosides

General Information

Many aspects of the pharmacology, clinical pharmacology, and adverse effects and interactions of cardiac glycosides have been reviewed (1–12).

Note on nomenclature

The most commonly used cardiac glycosides, digoxin and digitoxin, are derived from foxgloves, respectively *Digitalis lanata* and *Digitalis purpurea*. For this reason they are generally known as "digitalis." Most other cardiac glycosides, such as ouabain and proscillaridin, do not come from foxgloves but are nevertheless also commonly called "digitalis." Thus, the terms "cardiac glycoside" and "digitalis" are used interchangeably.

The cardiac glycosides that have been used therapeutically are listed in Table 1.

Mechanisms of digitalis toxicity

There is a large amount of evidence that the mechanisms of action of cardiac glycosides are mediated directly or indirectly by inhibition of the sodium/potassium pump enzyme, Na/K-ATPase (13). Their toxic effects on the myocardium may be due to excessive inhibition of cardiac Na/K-ATPase, although there is also evidence that effects on the nervous input to the heart may be involved (14), and it is not clear to what extent such an effect is mediated by inhibition of Na/K-ATPase. However, color vision disturbances associated with cardiac glycosides are due to inhibition of Na/K-ATPase (15).

Table 1 Cardiac glycosides that have been used therapeutically

Drug	Source	Main route of elimination
Acetyldigoxin	Semisynthetic derivative of digoxin	Renal
Digitoxin	*Digitalis purpurea*	Hepatic
Digoxin	*Digitalis lanata*	Renal
Gitoformate	*Digitalis purpurea*	Hepatic
Gitoxin	*Digitalis purpurea*	Hepatic
Lanatoside C	*Digitalis lanata*	Renal
Metildigoxin (betamethyldigoxin)	Semisynthetic derivative of digoxin	Hepatic/ renal
Ouabain (strophanthin-g)	*Strophanthus gratus, Acokanthera schimperi, Acokanthera ouabaio*	Renal
Peruvoside	*Nerium peruviana*	Hepatic
Proscillaridin	*Drimia maritima*	Hepatic
Strophanthin-k	*Strophanthus kombe*	Renal

Epidemiology of digitalis toxicity

Digitalis toxicity is common, since all cardiac glycosides have a low therapeutic index. Estimates vary widely from study to study, but in large prospective studies of hospital inpatients the frequency of digitalis toxicity has been as high as 29% (16). In outpatients the figure may be as high as 16% (7). The lower frequency in outpatients may be due partly to poor compliance and partly to digitalis toxicity being a reason for admission to hospital, thus increasing the numbers of toxic inpatients. The risk of toxicity may be lower with digitoxin than with digoxin (4), but when toxicity occurs it lasts longer, because of the very long half-life of digitoxin.

The overall mortality from digitalis toxicity also varies widely, having been reported as low as 4% and as high as 36% (7). However, it varies with dysrhythmias, and for paroxysmal supraventricular tachycardia with block may be as high as 50% (7).

In a study of serum digoxin concentrations in 1433 patients admitted to hospital, 115 had a raised concentration (17). Of the 82 in whom the blood sample had been taken at an appropriate time, 59 had electrocardiographic or clinical features of digoxin toxicity. The patients whose serum digoxin concentrations were over 3.2 nmol/l (2.5 ng/ml) were slightly older (78 versus 73 years) and had higher serum creatinine concentrations (273 versus 123 μmol/l) than those whose plasma concentrations were below 3.1 nmol/l. Of 47 patients with raised digoxin concentrations on admission, 21 were admitted because of digoxin toxicity, and impaired or worsening renal function contributed to high concentrations in 37 patients. A drug interaction was a contributory factor in 10 cases. These results suggest that digoxin toxicity is still very common and confirms the increased risk in elderly patients, patients with renal impairment, and patients taking drugs that may interact with digoxin. Serum potassium concentrations were not reported in this study.

In another study of this sort, serum digoxin concentrations were measured in 2009 patients (18). The concentration was over 2.6 nmol/l in 320 cases (9.3%) but in 51 of those the sample had been drawn too soon after the dose. When other results were omitted in cases in which the sampling time was not known, there were 138 evaluable patients, of whom 83 had clinical evidence of digoxin toxicity, an overall incidence of 4.1%. The authors concluded that digoxin toxicity was less common in their series than has previously been reported. There were no differences between the groups in serum potassium, calcium, or magnesium concentrations, but the serum creatinine concentration was significantly higher in those who had definite and possible toxicity. The mean age of the patients was 69 years. It is likely that the differences across studies of this sort are largely due to differences in renal function and age in the population being studied.

In a multicenter survey, conducted between 1988 and 1997, of 28 411 patients aged 70 (s.d. 16) years admitted to

81 hospitals throughout Italy, 1704 had adverse drug reactions (19). In 964 cases (3.4% of all admissions), adverse reactions were considered to be the cause of admission. Of these, 187 were regarded as severe. Gastrointestinal complaints (19%) were the most common, followed by metabolic and hemorrhagic complications (9%). The drugs most often responsible were diuretics, calcium channel blockers, non-steroidal anti-inflammatory drugs, and digoxin. Female sex (OR = 1.30; 95% CI = 1.10, 1.54), alcohol use (OR = 1.39; 95% CI = 1.20, 1.60), and number of drugs (OR = 1.24; 95% CI = 1.20, 1.27) were independent predictors of admission for adverse reactions. For severe adverse reactions, age (for age 65–79, OR = 1.50; 95% CI = 1.01, 2.23; for age 80 and over, OR = 1.53; 95% CI = 1.00, 2.33), co-morbidity (OR = 1.12; 95% CI = 1.05, 1.20 for each point on the Charlson Comorbidity Index), and number of drugs (OR = 1.18; 95% CI = 1.11, 1.25) were predisposing factors. Of the 28 411 patients, about 6700 were taking digoxin, and they suffered 82 adverse effects, either gastrointestinal ($n = 28$) or unspecified dysrhythmias ($n = 44$), or presumably both (data not given); of those, 11 were graded as severe (two gastrointestinal and nine dysrhythmias).

Of 603 adults aged 79 years, of whom 59% were women and 18% African-American, 376 patients (62%) were discharged taking digoxin, and 223 (37%) had no indication for its use, based on the absence of left ventricular systolic dysfunction or atrial fibrillation (20). After adjustment for various factors, prior digoxin use (OR = 11; 95% CI = 5.7, 23) and pulse over 100/minute (OR = 2.33; 95% CI = 1.1, 4.9) were associated with inappropriate digoxin use. Unfortunately, the authors did not report the frequency of adverse effects, and it is not therefore clear whether patients in whom digoxin is used inappropriately are more or less likely to suffer adverse reactions.

General adverse effects

The adverse effects of cardiac glycosides can be cardiac or non-cardiac. They mostly occur through toxicity and are time-independent (DoTS classification); susceptibility factors include electrolyte abnormalities (particularly hypokalemia), renal insufficiency, and age.

Frequent non-cardiac reactions include gastrointestinal effects (anorexia, nausea, vomiting, and diarrhea), central nervous system effects (drowsiness, dizziness, confusion, delirium), and less commonly visual effects (color vision abnormalities, photophobia, and blurred vision). Hypersensitivity reactions are rare and include thrombocytopenia and skin rashes. Tumor-inducing effects have not been reported.

Frequent cardiac adverse effects include heart block and ectopic dysrhythmias (ventricular extra beats, other ventricular tachydysrhythmias, and paroxysmal supraventricular tachycardia). The combination of heart block with an ectopic dysrhythmia, for example paroxysmal supraventricular tachycardia with block, is particularly suggestive of toxicity due to cardiac glycosides. Any other dysrhythmia can occasionally be caused by cardiac glycosides.

Of 332 residents of a nursing home, 52 had to be admitted to hospital because of adverse drug reactions (21). The drugs most commonly associated with adverse effects were non-steroidal anti-inflammatory drugs ($n = 30$), psychotropic drugs ($n = 14$), and digoxin ($n = 5$).

Individual cardiac glycosides

There are major pharmacokinetic differences among the different cardiac glycosides, the principal difference being between those that are mainly excreted via the kidneys (for example digoxin, metildigoxin, beta-acetyldigoxin, ouabain, and k-strophanthin) and those that are mainly excreted via hepatic metabolism (including digitoxin, gitoxin, pengitoxin (16-acetyldigoxin), and gitoformate).

It has also been suggested that there may be some pharmacodynamic differences among different cardiac glycosides (22), but these may at least partly be determined by differences in tissue distribution.

It is debatable whether any of these differences makes any particular cardiac glycoside preferable to another. The most strongly argued case is that digitoxin is preferable to digoxin in patients with renal insufficiency, since digitoxin is metabolized and digoxin is excreted by the kidneys. However, digitoxin has a much longer duration of action, and if toxicity occurs it will take longer to resolve. Furthermore, determining the effective dose of digitoxin is much more difficult, since there is great inter-individual variability in the extent to which digitoxin is metabolized, and hepatic metabolic function cannot be directly measured. Although digoxin excretion also varies from patient to patient, it can at least be gauged by measurement of creatinine clearance. The arguments for and against these preferences have been outlined (4,23) and it is probably best to choose a particular drug according to individual patient requirements.

Herbal formulations

Numerous plants worldwide contain cardiac glycosides that have been used both therapeutically as herbal formulations and for the purposes of self-poisoning. Details are given in Table 2.

- A 59-year-old man developed third-degree atrioventricular block after using an extract of *Nerium oleander* transdermally to treat psoriasis (24). A fatality due to drinking a herbal tea prepared from *N. oleander* leaves, erroneously believed to be eucalyptus leaves, has been reported (25).

Poisoning from ingestion of the seeds of *Thevetia peruviana* (yellow oleander) can be treated with oral multiple-dose activated charcoal (26).

In a Turkish case, the ingestion of two bulbs or *Urginea maritima* as a folk remedy for arthritic pains was sufficient to result in fatal poisoning (27).

Organs and Systems

Cardiovascular

Cardiac dysrhythmias and heart block

Percentage incidence figures for digitalis-induced dysrhythmias were given by Chung in his review of 726 patients (5). The commonest dysrhythmias are ventricular extra beats (54% of all dysrhythmias), coupled ventricular

Table 2 Some plants that contain cardiac glycosides

Plant	Common name(s)	Cardiac glycoside(s)	Comments
Adonis vernalis	False hellebore, pheasant's eye	Adonitoxin, strophanthidin	
Antiaris toxicaria	Upas tree	Antiarin	A Javanese tree of the mulberry family, used as an arrow poison
Convallaria majalis	Lily of the valley	Convallamarin	
Erysimum helveticum	Wallflower	Helveticoside	
Helleborus niger	Black hellebore, Christmas rose	Helleborcin	Also called melampodium after the Greek physician Melampus, who used it as a purgative
Nerium oleander	Pink oleander	Neriifolin	
Periploca graeca	Silk vine	Periplocin	
Tanghinia venenifera	Ordeal tree	Tanghinin	At one time used in Madagascar to test the guilt of someone suspected of a crime
Thevetia peruviana	Yellow oleander	Peruvoside, thevetins	Seeds widely used for self-poisoning in Southern India and Sri Lanka
Urginea (Scilla) maritima	Squill	Proscillaridin	Squill was a common remedy for dropsy in ancient times and up to the 19th century

extra beats (25%), and supraventricular tachycardia (33%). Sinus tachycardia was not common (3.4%). Atrial fibrillation (1.7%) or atrial flutter (1.8%) can cause difficulty in diagnosis, since digitalis is often used to treat those dysrhythmias.

Atrioventricular block was common (42%): first-degree, 14%; second-degree, 17%; and complete, 11%). However, first-degree heart block (that is prolongation of the PR interval) without higher degrees of atrioventricular nodal block can occur in the absence of digitalis intoxication.

Digitalis-induced dysrhythmias can be classified according to their sites of origin in the sinus node, the atria and atrioventricular node, and the ventricles.

Sinoatrial node

Digitalis can cause sinus bradycardia as a toxic effect, although patients with sinus bradycardia at rest often have no other evidence of digitalis toxicity, and this effect may simply represent increased vagal tone (28). Digitalis inhibits conduction through the sinoatrial node and has been reported to cause a syndrome mimicking that of the sick sinus syndrome (29–31); however, it is not clear whether or not it can impair sinus node function in patients who have previously normal sinoatrial nodes (32,33). Digitalis can certainly worsen sinus node function that has been otherwise impaired, for example by hyperthyroidism (34) or endotracheal suction (35).

Atria and atrioventricular node

Digitalis can cause supraventricular extra beats or tachycardia. The combination of such dysrhythmias with atrioventricular block is particularly suggestive of digitalis toxicity and carries a high mortality rate (3,36). Rarely atrial fibrillation (37) and atrial flutter (38) may be attributed to digitalis toxicity. The frequency of atrioventricular nodal block is mentioned above.

Paroxysmal atrial tachycardia with Wenckebach (Mobitz type I) atrioventricular block has been reported in a patient with a serum digoxin concentration of 3.2 ng/ml (39) and in a patient who in error took three times the recommended dose (40).

Ventricles

Ventricular extra beats, including coupled beats (that is ventricular bigeminy), are the most common cardiac effects of digitalis toxicity, although they are not specific. In more severe cases ventricular tachycardia, bidirectional tachycardia, and ventricular fibrillation can occur. There have also been reports of accelerated idioventricular rhythm (41,42).

Digoxin can cause ventricular fibrillation in children with Wolff–Parkinson–White syndrome (43,44).

- A male infant, whose narrow-complex tachycardia at birth had responded to adenosine, was treated with digoxin and 1 week later, during transesophageal electrophysiology with isoprenaline, developed coarse ventricular fibrillation after the induction of a supraventricular tachycardia (45). The serum digoxin concentration was not measured. The isoprenaline was withdrawn and the dysrhythmia resolved spontaneously at 160 seconds.

The effects of digoxin, isoprenaline, and transesophageal stimulation may have combined in this case to cause ventricular fibrillation.

Effects of digitalis on the electrocardiogram

Digitalis can prolong the PR interval and cause shortening of the QT interval, depression of the ST segment, and asymmetrical T wave inversion. These effects are non-specific and can occur in the absence of toxicity. However, there is evidence that the effects on the ST segment and T wave may be more common in patients with co-existing ischemic heart disease (46). Digitalis can also rarely cause both left (47) and right (48) bundle branch block.

The electrocardiographic effects of cardiac glycoside toxicity in 688 patients have been reviewed in the context of three cases of digoxin toxicity (49). The three cases featured bidirectional tachycardia in a 50-year-old man with a plasma digoxin concentration of 3.7 ng/ml, junctional tachycardia in a 59-year-old man with a plasma digoxin concentration of 4.3 ng/ml, and complete heart block in a 90-year-old woman whose postmortem digoxin concentration was 5.0 ng/ml.

Heart failure

In toxic doses digitalis impairs myocardial contractility and can cause or worsen heart failure. In one series of 148 patients with digitalis intoxication, worsening heart failure was diagnosed in 7.5% (50). In some cases worsening heart failure may be attributable to a cardiac dysrhythmia (51).

Vasoconstrictor and hypertensive effects

Giving a cardiac glycoside rapidly intravenously causes a transient increase in blood pressure, which has been attributed to an increase in peripheral resistance (52). However, digitalis does not seem to increase blood pressure during long-term treatment.

Myocardial ischemia

Subacute digitalis intoxication in dogs causes myocardial damage (53), and after intravenous administration there is increased creatine kinase activity in the plasma in man (54), suggesting ischemic damage.

There has been a report of coronary vasoconstriction in patients who were given acetyldigoxin 0.8 mg intravenously at angiography (55). Pretreatment with nisoldipine 10 mg, 2 hours before angiography, prevented the digoxin-induced vasoconstriction. These patients all had pre-existing coronary artery disease, but the vasoconstrictor effect occurred in both normal and abnormal coronary segments. However, the effect on high-grade stenoses was more pronounced. There is other evidence that ischemic damage can occur in patients who have been given digoxin intravenously, including an increase in the activity of serum creatinine kinase (54) and impaired left ventricular function after acute myocardial infarction (56).

- A 26-year-old woman who had taken a herbal supplement for stress relief which contained *Scutellaria lateriflora*, *Pedicularis canadensis*, *Cimifuga racemosa*, *Humulus lupulus*, *Valeriana officinalis*, and *Capsicum annuum* developed chest pain of 7 hours duration (57). Her medical history was otherwise unremarkable. Examination of her heart showed no abnormality, but during monitoring her heart rate fell to 39/minute and her blood pressure to 59/36 mmHg. Her serum digoxin concentration was 0.9 ng/ml. The authors therefore concluded that the herbal remedy contained digoxin-like factors that had caused digitalis toxicity.

Long-term use and cardiovascular adverse effects of cardiac glycosides

There have been many studies of the long-term efficacy of digitalis in patients in heart failure in sinus rhythm and also in patients with atrial fibrillation. These have been reviewed (SEDA-4, 123) (SEDA-14, 145) (SEDA-18, 196). The following is a brief resumé.

Atrial fibrillation is not necessarily an indication for long-term therapy with digitalis. In patients with controlled atrial fibrillation whose plasma digitalis concentration is below the lower limit of the target range (0.8 ng/ml for digoxin and 10 ng/ml for digitoxin) withdrawal rarely if ever results in deterioration. However, in those who have plasma digitalis concentrations within the target range withdrawal should not be attempted, since the risk of worsening atrial fibrillation outweighs the risk of toxicity, if there is careful monitoring of the plasma concentration.

In patients with heart failure in sinus rhythm there is no way of predicting which patients will benefit from long-term therapy, but the following recommendations can be made:

1. If the plasma digitalis concentration is below the therapeutic range (0.8 ng/ml for digoxin and 10 ng/ml for digitoxin) withdrawal is very unlikely to produce deterioration.
2. If a patient's condition is stable, and the plasma digitalis concentration is in the therapeutic range, with little risk of toxicity, withdrawal is probably not worthwhile because of the risk of deterioration.
3. If there is an increased risk of toxicity (for example because of renal impairment or if potassium balance is difficult to maintain) careful withdrawal of digitalis may be worth attempting.
4. In patients who have evidence of poor left ventricular function it may be better to continue therapy, even if there is an increased risk of toxicity, since these patients are very likely to deteriorate following withdrawal. In these cases careful monitoring of therapy will help to reduce the risk of toxicity.

The long-term adverse cardiovascular effects of digitalis have been reviewed (SEDA-10, 142) (SEDA-11, 153) (SEDA-15, 165). Briefly, in a number of retrospective studies, although mortality in the digitalis-treated patients was generally higher than in those not treated with digitalis, the difference was reduced when allowance was made for other confounding factors, such as the degree of heart failure, a history of dysrhythmias, and the use of other drugs. There may also be a higher mortality rate in patients who take long-term digitalis therapy after coronary artery bypass graft surgery (58), in patients who have had a cardiac arrest (59), and in those without evidence of heart failure or atrial fibrillation (60). In the first two studies the risk was increased further among those who were taking digitalis with diuretics, and it may be that these effects are due to digitalis toxicity secondary to potassium depletion, although it may simply indicate a greater prevalence of hypertension or heart failure among those treated with digitalis and diuretics.

Despite these earlier results, in the Digitalis Investigation Group (DIG) study (61) digoxin had no overall impact on mortality in patients with heart failure in sinus rhythm and with left ventricular ejection fractions equal to or less than 0.45.

It produced a small reduction in hospitalizations due to heart failure (nine per 1000 patients-years) balanced by a significant increase in deaths from presumed dysrhythmias. Digitalis is therefore indicated for a small number of patients who have severe heart failure associated with sinus rhythm after treatment with diuretics, vasodilators, beta-blockers, and spironolactone. It remains the drug of first choice in patients with heart failure accompanied by fast atrial fibrillation, especially if due to myocardial or mitral valve disease. A trial of withdrawal of digitalis therapy can be considered in some cases (as noted in point 3 above).

Of course, there are alternatives to digitalis in the long-term treatment of heart failure in sinus rhythm. It is not clear that any of these offers any particular advantage over digitalis in terms of therapeutic efficacy, although there may be fewer problems with toxicity. The comparative studies have been reviewed (SEDA-14, 141).

Sinus rhythm

The question of whether digoxin should be used to treat patients with mild to moderate heart failure in sinus rhythm, in the wake of randomized, controlled trials of its efficacy, including PROVED, RADIANCE, and DIG (SEDA-18, 196) (SEDA-20, 173), has been reviewed (62). The authors concluded that digoxin is effective in producing symptomatic improvement in patients with mild or moderate heart failure, but that because of concerns about its safety careful consideration must be taken in each case before using it.

Other positive inotropic drugs carry no extra benefit, and can increase mortality during long-term administration. There is no evidence that the combination of two drugs with positive inotropic actions is beneficial in chronic congestive heart failure. Vasodilators are as efficacious as digitalis, but there is a rationale for combining digitalis and a vasodilator, since by doing so it is possible to affect simultaneously the three important factors determining cardiac output (contractility, pre-load, and afterload). Furthermore, a vasodilator will oppose the small effect that digitalis has in increasing peripheral resistance, and which may reduce the beneficial effect of digitalis on cardiac output.

Of 2254 elderly patients, 724 were being treated with digoxin, of whom 187 had congestive heart failure, 90 had atrial fibrillation, and 447 were both free from heart failure and in sinus rhythm (60). Among those who did not have heart failure or atrial fibrillation, cardiovascular and total mortality were significantly higher among those taking digoxin. Digoxin was a predictor of mortality in those subjects. In addition, the incidence of non-fatal heart failure was higher among those taking digoxin. This is yet another non-randomized study purporting to show deleterious effects of digoxin during long-term use, in this case in patients in whom it was not indicated in the first place. Since similar non-randomized studies in patients with heart failure, which also showed deleterious effects (SEDA-20, 173), have since been contradicted by proper prospective randomized studies, this result should be ignored.

Atrial fibrillation

In uncomplicated atrial fibrillation a cardiac glycoside such as digoxin remains the drug of first choice. However, in those in whom digitalis is not completely effective or in whom symptoms (for example bouts of palpitation) persist despite adequate digitalization, a calcium antagonist, such as verapamil or diltiazem, can be added, or amiodarone used as an alternative. In patients with atrial fibrillation due to hyperthyroidism, a beta-adrenoceptor antagonist should be used in preference to digitalis, but digitalis can be added if there is an incomplete effect. In patients with atrial fibrillation secondary to an anomalous conduction pathway (for example Wolff–Parkinson–White syndrome), in most of whom digitalis is contraindicated, a calcium antagonist would be the treatment of choice. Paroxysmal atrial fibrillation generally does not respond to digitalis, and digitalis may in fact prolong the duration of a paroxysmal attack when it occurs. The treatment of paroxysmal atrial fibrillation is problematic, but many use amiodarone. Sotalol, propafenone, and flecainide are options, but there are doubts about the long-term safety of flecainide and sotalol, particularly in those who have had an acute myocardial infarction.

There has been a multicenter, randomized, placebo-controlled, double-blind comparison of aprindine and digoxin in the prevention of atrial fibrillation and its recurrence in 141 patients with symptomatic paroxysmal or persistent atrial fibrillation who had converted to sinus rhythm (63). They were randomized in equal numbers to aprindine 40 mg/day, digoxin 0.25 mg/day, or placebo, and were followed every 2 weeks for 6 months. After 6 months the Kaplan-Meier estimates of the numbers of patients who had no recurrences while taking aprindine, digoxin, and placebo were 33%, 29%, and 22% respectively. The rates of adverse events were similar in the three groups. This confirms that digoxin does not prevent relapse of symptomatic atrial fibrillation after conversion to sinus rhythm.

Cardioversion and digitalis

The presence of digitalis increases the risk of serious dysrhythmias after electrical cardioversion, even in the absence of frank toxicity (64). In order to minimize the risk of dysrhythmias in these circumstances digitalis should be withdrawn if possible a day or two before cardioversion and potassium depletion should be corrected. If cardioversion is required acutely, it has been recommended that low energies (for example 10 J) should be used initially (65).

Nervous system

Toxic effects of digitalis on the nervous system occur relatively often. Although in severe toxicity the incidence may be as high as 65% (66), in most series it has been below 25% (67).

Anorexia, nausea, and vomiting are mediated by the central nervous system. Other common nervous system effects of digitalis include confusion, dizziness, drowsiness, bad dreams, restlessness, nervousness, agitation, and amnesia.

Epilepsy occurs rarely and can be accompanied by electroencephalographic changes (68–70).

Other reported effects include transient global amnesia (71), trigeminal neuralgia (72,73), nightmares (74), organic brain syndrome (including impairment of long-term and short-term memory) (75), impairment of learning and memory (23), and a clinical syndrome resembling herpes encephalitis (76).

- Progressive stupor has been reported in an 85-year-old woman with mild renal insufficiency who was given digoxin 0.25 mg/day (77). The plasma digoxin concentration was 7.8 nmol/l. She recovered within 2 weeks after digoxin withdrawal, consistent with the likely half-life of digoxin. A 24-hour electrocardiogram showed one period of asystole for 4 seconds, but that is unlikely to have explained her symptoms.

Chorea has occasionally been reported in adults taking digitalis (SEDA-13, 138) (78), and also in a child (79).

- A 7-year-old girl with severe congenital heart disease who was given digoxin 0.125 mg bd developed chorea and had a serum digoxin concentration of 3.8 ng/ml. When digoxin was withheld and the serum concentration fell to 1.5 ng/ml her symptoms resolved. They recurred 4 days after rechallenge when her digoxin concentration was 2.5 mg/ml and again resolved after it had fallen to 1.3 mg/ml.

The authors hypothesized that digoxin caused chorea by virtue of an estrogenic effect in the basal ganglia, similar to the effect that is occasionally produced by oral contraceptives.

Sensory systems

Color vision abnormality is a well-known adverse effect of digitalis (SEDA-20, 173), and particularly occurs in patients with digitalis toxicity.

There have been two cases of digoxin-related visual disturbances in patients whose blood concentrations were in the usual target range (319).

- A 68-year-old woman had shimmering lights in her field of vision in both eyes when in sunlight, and a 63-year-old woman complained of blurring of vision in both eyes. The serum digoxin concentrations were 2.2 and 1.3 nmol/l (1.7 and 1.0 ng/ml) respectively. Withdrawal of digoxin caused resolution of their symptoms within 1–2 weeks.

Unfortunately the authors did not report serum electrolyte concentrations, and it is not clear in these cases whether the effect of digoxin was potentiated by potassium depletion.

In 30 patients (mean age 81 years) taking digoxin and an age-matched control group there was no correlation between color vision impairment and serum digoxin concentration (80). There was slight to moderate red-green impairment in 20–30% of those taking digoxin, depending on the test used; about 20% had a severe tritan defect. The authors suggested that color vision testing in elderly patients would have limited value in the detection of digitalis toxicity. However, this conclusion was based on using the digoxin concentration as a standard, while the point of pharmacodynamic tests, such as color vision measurement, is that they are supposed to reflect the effect of the drug better than the serum concentration.

Psychological, psychiatric

Acute psychosis and delirium can occur in digitalis toxicity, particularly in elderly people (81–83), and can be accompanied by visual or auditory hallucinations (84,85).

- Acute delirium occurred in a 61-year-old man whose serum digitoxin concentration was 44 ng/ml (86).

Digitalis toxicity can occasionally cause depression (87).

- A 77-year-old woman developed extreme fatigue, anorexia, psychomotor retardation, and social withdrawal 1 month after starting to take digoxin 0.5 mg/day for congestive heart failure (88). She did not respond to intravenous clomipramine 25 mg/day for 7 months. Her serum digoxin concentration was 3.2 ng/ml. Digoxin was withdrawn, and 12 days later, when her serum digoxin concentration was 0.5 ng/ml, she had improved, but was left with a memory disturbance, which was attributed to background dementia.

Endocrine

Digitalis has effects on sex hormones. It causes increased serum concentrations of follicle-stimulating hormone (FSH) and estrogen and reduced concentrations of luteinizing hormone (LH) and testosterone (89–92). These effects are probably not related to any direct estrogen-like structure of digitalis (despite structural similarities), but rather to an effect involving the synthesis or release of sex hormones. There are three possible clinical outcomes of these effects.

Gynecomastia in men and breast enlargement in women

Effects of cardiac glycosides in the breasts can be associated with demonstrable histological changes (93,94).

Stratification of the vaginal squamous epithelium in postmenopausal women

This can cause difficulty in the pathological interpretation of vaginal smears for cancer diagnosis (95).

A possible modifying effect on breast cancer

Digitalis can reduce the heterogeneity of breast cancer cell populations and reduce the rate of distant metastases (96). There is also evidence that the 5-year recurrence rate after mastectomy is lower in women who have been treated with digitalis (97). Early studies suggested that when breast tumors occurred in women with congestive heart failure taking cardiac glycosides, tumor size was significantly smaller and the tumor cells more homogeneous (SEDA-7, 194). It was originally thought that this action was due to an estrogen-like effect of cardiac glycosides, but more recent evidence suggests that it occurs because inhibition of the Na/K pump is involved in inhibiting proliferation and inducing apoptosis in various cell lines (98–101). Cardiac glycosides have different potencies in their effects on cell lines such as those of ovarian carcinoma and breast carcinoma (order of potency: proscillaridin A > digitoxin > digoxin > ouabain > lanatoside C) (102).

Metabolism

In three patients with diabetes mellitus, withdrawal of digoxin improved blood glucose control, implying that digoxin had impaired glucose tolerance (103). The authors conceded that the effect might have occurred coincidentally, but in one case glucose tolerance deteriorated again after rechallenge. Insulin increases the cellular uptake of glucose and stimulates the sodium/potassium pump, and it may be that inhibition of the sodium/potassium pump by digoxin has the opposite effect.

In 14 patients with morbid obesity, who were being given digoxin in the hope that reduced production of cerebrospinal fluid, with the consequent reduction in pressure, might be associated with weight reduction, the dosage of digoxin (Lanacrist 0.13 mg, equivalent to 0.065 mg of digoxin) was titrated to produce a minimum serum digoxin concentration of 1.0 nmol/l (104). One patient was already diabetic, and five developed fasting blood glucose concentrations greater than 5.0 mmol/l on three consecutive occasions, with accompanying glycosuria. Another had fasting blood glucose concentrations of 6.0–8.5 mmol/l. There was a significant relation between the dose of digoxin and the risk of impaired glucose tolerance. However, the diabetes mellitus did not abate after digoxin withdrawal, and since all these patients were obese, the occurrence of diabetes was probably coincidental.

Hematologic

Thrombocytopenia has been reported in patients taking digitoxin, acetyldigoxin, and digoxin (105–108).

There have been rare reports of eosinophilia in patients taking cardiac glycosides (109).

Gastrointestinal

Gastrointestinal symptoms are common in digitalis toxicity. These include anorexia, nausea, and vomiting (110), probably as a result of stimulation of the chemoreceptor trigger zone in the brain.

Diarrhea occurs occasionally (111).

Dysphagia has been rarely reported (112,113).

Other rare events include intestinal ischemia (SEDA-17, 215) (114), and hemorrhagic intestinal necrosis (115).

- A 79-year old woman with a serum digoxin concentration of 4.9 ng/ml had a mesenteric infarction (116). At postmortem no other causes were discovered.

Intestinal ischemia responds to verapamil and to anti-digoxin antibody (115).

Death

In a retrospective, non-randomized study of 484 patients, 90 of whom were taking digoxin, there was an increased death rate (RR = 2.12, CI = 1.21, 3.74) in those taking digoxin (117). In another non-randomized, retrospective analysis of the effects of digoxin in patients with acute myocardial infarction there was a higher rate of mortality in the 243 patients taking digoxin compared with the 1743 patients who were not (118). The results of these studies are reminiscent of the results of previous similar retrospective analyses. However, the prospective DIG study clearly showed no increase in mortality (SEDA-20, 173), and the results of these more recent non-randomized retrospective studies should be ignored.

In 345 patients with heart failure randomized to either digoxin ($n = 175$) or captopril ($n = 170$) and followed for a median of 4.5 years the death rate at 48 months was lower with captopril (21%) than with digoxin (32%), although this did not reach conventional significance (119). Since there was no placebo group for comparison it is not clear whether digoxin altered mortality in this study. Of the numerous adverse effects that were reported, the only one that differed between the two treatments was cough, which was significantly more frequent with captopril. In the absence of a placebo comparison it is impossible to say whether any of the other adverse effects were drug-related.

Despite the fact that the prospective study called DIG clearly showed that there was no increase in mortality in patients in taking long-term digoxin therapy (SEDA-20, 173), retrospective, non-randomized studies continue to be reported (SEDA-24, 201). In 180 patients with idiopathic dilated cardiomyopathy the overall mortality was 19% in those taking digoxin and 10% in those not taking digoxin (120). However, when the use of digoxin was adjusted for several predictive variables it no longer predicted cardiac death. This finding is reassuring, but results of studies like this, whatever their results, should be ignored, in view of the evidence that is currently available from the one large prospective, randomized study.

When interpreting the evidence presented in other accounts of the association between drug therapy and death it is important to remember that the current evidence suggests that digoxin does not cause excess mortality. For example, digoxin was the second most commonly encountered medication in an investigation of 2233 deaths reported to an American County Medical Examiner's office, with a medication history available in 775 cases (121). Furosemide was mentioned 181 times, digoxin 131 times, and glyceryl trinitrate 103 times. All other drugs were mentioned less than 100 times each. The authors suggested that the presence of digoxin at a death scene should suggest heart failure or a cardiac dysrhythmia, but they did not go further and stress that in such a case digoxin need not necessarily be implicated in the death. Postmortem diagnosis of digoxin toxicity is exceptionally difficult, but measurement of digoxin in the vitreous fluid can be helpful.

In a survey of 2 312 203 deaths in the USA in 1995, 206 (0.009%) were attributed to adverse drug reactions on death certificates (122). At the same time in the MedWatch program, 6894 deaths were reportedly attributed to adverse drug reactions, representing 6.3% of the 108 735 reports of adverse drug reactions. In the death certificate study 18 deaths were attributed to cardiac glycosides and in the MedWatch survey 15 deaths. This compares with figures of 289 and 782 from antimicrobial drugs, 449 and 280 from hormones, and 947 and 477 from drugs that affect the constituents of the blood (for example anticoagulants).

Sex-based differences in the effect of digoxin have been explored in a post-hoc analysis of the data from the DIG) study (SEDA-20, 173) (123). There was an absolute difference of 5.8% (95 CI = 0.5, 11) between men and women in the effect of digoxin on the case fatality rate from any cause. Women who were randomly assigned to digoxin had a significantly higher fatality rate than women who were randomly assigned to placebo (33 versus 29%), while the fatality rate was similar among men randomly assigned to digoxin or placebo (35% versus 37%). However, serum digoxin concentrations were higher in the women at 1 month, and this may have contributed to the increased risk of death (124).

In another post-hoc analysis of the data from the DIG study the patients who had been randomized to digoxin were divided into three groups, according to serum digoxin concentration, 0.5–0.8 ng/ml, 0.9–1.1 ng/ml, and 1.2 ng/ml and over (125). Higher concentrations were associated with higher all-cause fatality rates: 30%, 39%, and 48% respectively.

Both of these studies suggest that lower serum concentrations of digoxin (0.5–1.0 ng/ml) may be beneficial for routine therapy of heart failure than have traditionally been recommended (0.8–2.0 ng/ml), and this has been discussed in a brief review (126).

Second-Generation Effects

Pregnancy

Digoxin has been used to cause fetal death before termination of pregnancy (127). However, in a double-blind study in 126 women who had terminations by dilatation and evacuation at 20–23 weeks gestation intra-amniotic injection of digoxin 1 mg did not alter blood loss or pain; nor did it reduce difficulties with or the complications of the procedure (128). Significantly more women vomited after intra-amniotic digoxin. Digoxin given by this route is slowly absorbed into the systemic circulation, with a peak plasma concentration of 0.8 ng/ml at 11 hours (129).

Fetotoxicity

Digoxin crosses the placenta and enters the neonatal circulation (130). It has therefore been used, for example, to improve fetal cardiac function (131). In normal circumstances there seem to be no adverse effects on the neonate, and neonatal plasma concentrations are below those generally considered to be therapeutic. There has been one report of fatal toxicity in the fetus of a woman who took an overdose of digitoxin (132).

Susceptibility Factors

Age

Elderly people

The risk of digoxin toxicity is increased in old people, partly because they have poor renal function and lower body weight, factors that tend to increase the concentration of drug at the active site during steady-state therapy, and partly because they are liable to electrolyte imbalances, such as hypokalemia, which tend to increase the response of the tissues to a given concentration. Other factors, such as altered Na/K pump activity, may also contribute to increased tissue sensitivity. This means that the serum digoxin concentration that is associated with an increased risk of toxicity is slightly lower in elderly people than in younger people, and this has been confirmed in a recent study of 899 patients taking digoxin for heart failure or atrial fibrillation (133). No patients with serum digoxin concentrations below 1.4 ng/ml had evidence of digoxin toxicity. All patients who had a concentration of 3.0 ng/ml or more had severe toxicity. However in the range 1.4–2.9 ng/ml there were patients with and without evidence of toxicity, and the overlap was age-dependent. In patients aged 51–60 there was more evidence of toxicity with concentrations of 2.4–2.9 ng/ml; in patients aged 61–70 the range was 1.8–2.9 ng/ml, in patients aged 71–80 it was 1.4–2.7 ng/ml, and in those aged over 80 it was 1.4–2.6 ng/ml. The authors therefore suggested that serum digoxin concentrations should be no greater than 1.4 ng/ml during routine steady-state therapy. The incidences of toxicity were 16% in patients over 70 years of age and 7.3% in the whole group. The risk of toxicity was increased in the presence of renal insufficiency.

Because digitoxin is metabolized rather than being renally eliminated, the effects of renal impairment in elderly patients may not be so important in precipitating digitoxin toxicity. In 80 patients hospitalized 147 times, toxicity with digitoxin occurred in 7.6% of 92 admissions and digoxin toxicity occurred in 18.3% of 55 admissions (134). On the basis of these results the authors suggested that digitoxin is safer than digoxin in elderly patients. This is an old debate, and there are arguments in favor of both digoxin and digitoxin (135). However, there is currently no information on the long-term toxicity of digitoxin, and in particular its effects on mortality in patients with heart failure. Neither the severity of toxicity nor its duration was reported in this study.

A retrospective Bayesian analysis in 60 patients confirmed that age is a major factor in digoxin toxicity (136). However, an analysis of the data from the DIG study (SEDA-20, 173) has shown that while mortality in heart failure increases with age, the actions of digoxin are independent of age (137).

Children

Matters are also more complicated in young people. The pharmacokinetics of cardiac glycosides are different (138): the apparent volume of distribution of digoxin is higher in neonates, infants, and older children than in adults, and renal digoxin clearance is lower in children under 4–6 months. However, there may also be increased resistance to the effects of digoxin in infants because of changes in digitalis tissue receptors (139). Seriously ill children of low birth weight may be particularly at risk, even when low dosages of digitalis are used (140).

The risk of digitalis toxicity during the therapeutic use of cardiac glycosides is similar in children to that in adults, ranging in 12 separate published series from 12 to 50% (median 21%) (141). The most common non-cardiac effects are vomiting and feeding problems, and the most common cardiac effects are conduction defects, particularly atrioventricular block and ectopic rhythms, although (as in adults) any dysrhythmia can occur.

The pharmacokinetics of digoxin have been studied in 181 neonates and children with and without congestive heart failure (142). The clearance rate was lower in premature neonates than in neonates born at full term. Children with congestive heart failure also had lower digoxin clearance.

A population pharmacokinetic study in 172 neonates and infants showed that the clearance of digoxin is affected significantly by total body weight, age, renal function, and congestive heart failure (143).

Other features of the patient

Several factors increase patient susceptibility to digitalis intoxication. They can be considered in two groups (144).

Factors that alter the amount of digitalis that accumulates in the body or the plasma concentration at a fixed dose (pharmacokinetic factors)

Pharmacokinetic factors affect different cardiac glycosides differently.

Altered tissue distribution
The apparent volume of distribution of digoxin is reduced in hypothyroidism (145) and in renal insufficiency (146). This leads to increased plasma concentrations after a loading dose and hence an increased risk of toxicity, but does not affect the plasma concentration at steady state. The opposite occurs in hyperthyroidism.

Altered renal elimination
The effects of renal insufficiency on the pharmacokinetics of cardiac glycosides have been reviewed (146). The most important effect of renal failure is a reduced rate of elimination of digoxin, leading to increased accumulation during steady-state treatment. The same applies to some other glycosides, including beta-methyldigoxin, beta-acetyldigoxin, ouabain, and k-strophanthin, but not to glycosides that are mostly metabolized, such as digitoxin, the proscillaridins, and peruvoside (4). Drug interactions can also lead to reduced digoxin renal elimination.

A retrospective Bayesian analysis in 60 patients confirmed that renal impairment is a major factor in digoxin toxicity (136).

A population pharmacokinetic study in 172 neonates and infants showed that the clearance of digoxin is affected significantly by renal function (143).

Altered non-renal elimination
See Drug–Drug Interactions.

Factors that alter the clinical response to digitalis at a fixed amount of digitalis in the body and a fixed plasma concentration (pharmacodynamic factors)
Pharmacodynamic factors affect all cardiac glycosides in the same way.

Electrolyte disturbances
Of electrolyte disturbances that alter the response to a cardiac glycoside, hypokalemia is the most important. It has been estimated that a fall in plasma potassium concentration from 3.5 to 3.0 mmol/l is associated with a 50% increase in sensitivity to digoxin (144). Total body potassium depletion, even in the absence of hypokalemia, has a similar effect (147).

There is evidence that hypomagnesemia has the same effect as hypokalemia (148).

Hypercalcemia has the same effect as hypokalemia; hypocalcemia has the opposite effect, that is it causes resistance to the effects of digitalis.

Hypoxia and acidosis increase the risk of digitalis intoxication.

Renal insufficiency
In addition to its effect in reducing the elimination of digoxin, renal insufficiency may be associated with an increased sensitivity to the actions of digitalis (149).

Thyroid disease
Apart from the pharmacokinetic differences in thyroid disease (mentioned above), there may also be changes in tissue responsiveness, with reduced sensitivity in hyperthyroidism and the reverse in hypothyroidism (145). The reasons for these changes are not known, but they may be related to differences in tissue Na/K-ATPase activity.

Cardiac disease
All cardiac glycosides are best avoided in patients with acute myocardial infarction, since they increase oxygen demand in ischemic tissue, increase peripheral vascular resistance, and carry an increased risk of dysrhythmias, especially in the presence of tissue hypoxia and acidosis. Furthermore, there is evidence that digitalis is of little value in patients with acute myocardial infarction and either left ventricular failure or cardiogenic shock (150). The evidence that mortality in patients who take digitalis after an acute myocardial infarction is increased is discussed in the section Death in this monograph.

Cardiac glycosides are contraindicated in conditions in which there is obstruction to ventricular outflow, for example hypertrophic obstructive cardiomyopathy, constrictive pericarditis, and cardiac tamponade. Acute myocarditis may also increase the risk of toxicity.

Direct current cardioversion increases the risk of digitalis-induced dysrhythmias, but digitalis treatment is not a contraindication to cardioversion (151).

Hypercalcemia
The effects of digitalis are enhanced in the presence of hypercalcemia.

- An 81-year-old woman with congestive heart failure and hypercalcemia secondary to squamous cell carcinoma of the bronchus developed first-degree heart block and symptomatic sinus pauses when her serum digoxin concentration was only 1.5 mg/ml (152).

Drug Administration

Drug contamination

Digoxin toxicity has been reported in two patients who took herbal remedies (153). *D. lanata* was found as a contaminant.

Drug administration route

Intramuscular injection of digitalis can be painful and can cause local muscle necrosis, sometimes with pyrexia (154). The systemic availability of digitalis after intramuscular injection is poor (155), and this route of administration should be avoided if possible.

Digoxin has a rapid onset of action after oral administration, and there is rarely any justification for giving digoxin intravenously. This route of administration should be restricted to those who have severe atrial fibrillation that requires rapid treatment and in whom cardioversion or other drug therapy is not possible or indicated. If digoxin is given intravenously it should be infused over at least half-an-hour, since there is a risk of hypertension if it is infused faster.

There has been a randomized, double-blind comparison of intravenous diltiazem and digoxin in 40 patients with atrial fibrillation and a ventricular rate of over 100/minute (156). One patient given intravenous digoxin had a burning sensation at the site of injection.

Drug overdose

The most important complication of overdosage of digitalis in all age groups is disturbance of cardiac conduction, but in addition any dysrhythmia can occur. Death can result from asystole or ventricular fibrillation. Hyperkalemia is common, and the higher the plasma potassium concentration the poorer the prognosis (157).

Other common effects of overdosage are nausea, vomiting, and central nervous system and visual disturbances (66).

- Accidental overdose of digoxin in a 22-month-old boy caused vomiting, lethargy, and dehydration. The plasma digoxin concentration was 12 mg/ml. There was a relative bradycardia of 90/minute and Mobitz type 1 second-degree heart block on the electrocardiogram (158).

The pharmacokinetics of digoxin are altered after overdosage, the half-life being reportedly rapid, but there is too little information to define the kinetics precisely (157).

- Plasma glycoside concentrations have been documented after an overdose with purple foxglove in a 36-year-old woman (159). Apart from gitaloxin, which peaked on the fifth day at 113 ng/ml, all the glycosides detected peaked on the first day (gitoxin 13 ng/ml, digitoxin 113 ng/ml, digitoxigenin 3.3 ng/ml, and digitoxigenin monodigitoxoside 8.9 ng/ml). There was a second peak of digitoxin at about 70 hours, and this is consistent with the known enterohepatic recirculation of digitoxin.

Treatment of toxicity and overdosage

The treatment of digitalis toxicity and overdose have been reviewed (SEDA-5, 172) (SEDA-12, 149). In summary, the following measures should be taken.

Remove digitalis from the stomach

If the patient is seen within 1 hour of overdosage try to remove whatever drug still remains in the stomach by gastric lavage, although the risk of dysrhythmias may be increased. There is no evidence that emesis is beneficial.

Give activated charcoal

The use of activated charcoal in the treatment of digitalis overdose has been reviewed (160). The rationale for its use is that after absorption into the systemic circulation digitoxin is secreted into the bile and digoxin (161) (and probably other cardiac glycosides) is secreted into the gut lumen by the action of the P glycoprotein. Activated charcoal in the gut binds this secreted digoxin and encourages further secretion. To be fully effective charcoal should be given at regular intervals (for example 50 g 4-hourly).

In pigs, repeated doses of activated charcoal reduced the half-life of intravenous digoxin significantly from 65 to 17 hours and increased the clearance from 2.3 to 7.1 ml/minute/kg (162).

There is evidence of the efficacy of charcoal in healthy volunteers. In six adult volunteers repeated doses of activated charcoal significantly reduced the half-life of digoxin from 23 to 17 hours without a significant increase in clearance; the half-life of digitoxin was also reduced from 110 to 51 hours, and this was accompanied by a significant increase in clearance from 0.24 to 0.47 l/hour (163). In a volunteer with chronic renal insufficiency charcoal reduced the digoxin half-life from 93 to 29 hours and increased the clearance from 3.6 to 10 l/hour (163). Similarly, during maintenance therapy in six individuals, daily activated charcoal significantly reduced the mean plasma digoxin concentration by 31% and serum digitoxin concentration by 18% (164). In 10 healthy volunteers given intravenous digoxin 10 μg/kg repeated doses of activated charcoal significantly increased the total body clearance from 12 to 18 l/hour and reduced the half-life from 37 to 22 hours (161).

There have also been reports of the value of multiple doses of activated charcoal in patients with digoxin and digitoxin poisoning. In 23 patients with plasma digoxin concentrations over 2.5 ng/ml multiple doses of activated charcoal increased the mean clearance of digoxin to 98 ml/minute compared with 55 ml/minute in 16 patients who were not treated, and reduced the half-life from 68 to 36 hours (165). Anecdotal reports have also appeared.

- In a 69-year-old man the plasma digoxin concentration of 8.3 ng/ml fell with a half-life of 14 hours (166).
- In a 71-year-old woman with chronic renal insufficiency and a plasma digoxin concentration of 9 ng/ml charcoal shortened the half-life from 7.3 to 1.4 days (167).
- In a 66-year-old man with chronic renal insufficiency whose serum digoxin concentration did not respond to daily hemodialysis, multiple doses of activated charcoal caused a rapid reduction in the serum concentration (168).
- In a patient with a peak plasma digoxin concentration of 264 ng/ml multiple doses of activated charcoal reduced the half-life of digitoxin from 162 hours to 18 hours (169).
- In a patient on hemodialysis, activated charcoal caused a fall in the plasma digoxin concentration with a half-life of 29 hours (170).
- In another patient there was convincing evidence of a change in the digoxin half-life after repeated doses of activated charcoal (166).
- In a 73-year-old woman who took 12.5 mg of digoxin, gastric lavage and activated charcoal tided the patient over until antibodies became available (171).

However, the best evidence of the usefulness of repeated oral doses of activated charcoal in cardiac glycoside poisoning comes from the results of a randomized, placebo-controlled study in 402 individuals who took overdoses of the seeds of the yellow oleander tree in Sri Lanka. Repeated doses of activated charcoal reduced mortality from 8.0% to 2.5% (26).

Thus, the use of repeated doses of activated charcoal in patients with digitalis toxicity is a cheap way of increasing the rate of cardiac glycoside clearance.

Colestyramine has been used for the same purpose. In two elderly patients with congestive heart failure and raised serum digoxin concentrations it enhanced the elimination of digoxin (172). In one case the half-life of digoxin was 20 hours and in the other 24 hours.

Correct electrolyte disturbances

Hypokalemia should be treated with potassium chloride.

Hyperkalemia carries a poor prognosis and is usually an indication for antidigoxin antibody. The suggestion that intravenous calcium should be used to treat the hyperkalemia that can occur in digitalis intoxication (173) has been challenged, on the grounds that it can increase the risk of cardiac dysrhythmias in such cases (174).

Give antidigoxin antibody

Antidigoxin antibody (Fab fragments) is the treatment of choice in patients with severe digitalis toxicity due to any cardiac glycoside. It is effective after self-poisoning with digitoxin, lanatoside C, and acylated forms of digoxin, as well as digoxin itself (175). It should be used when there are life-threatening dysrhythmias or heart block, and when the plasma potassium concentration is above 5.0 mmol/l or is rising, since hyperkalemia is evidence of serious toxicity and carries a poor prognosis. Evidence of the efficacy of antidigoxin Fab antibody fragments in reducing the risk of cardiac dysrhythmias in the treatment of intoxication due to oleander poisoning, previously only anecdotally reported (176,177), has come from a prospective study (178), although the study was too small to assess the effect on mortality. The role of antidigoxin antibody fragments in treating milder forms of digitalis toxicity has not been fully assessed.

In a systematic review of 250 publications no controlled, randomized trials were found, and the authors concluded that there was little or no scientific evidence of efficacy, because there are no randomized, controlled trials (179). However, this is one case in which the cumulative anecdotal evidence is overwhelmingly convincing, and there can be no doubt that antidigoxin antibodies are highly effective in the treatment of digoxin intoxication and of intoxication with other cardiac glycosides. The important question is whether there are cases in which the antibodies need not be used, and guidelines have yet to be developed.

- Overdose of digoxin in a neonate caused complete atrioventricular block and cardiogenic shock, which were completely reversed within 4 hours after administration of the first dose of antidigoxin antibody; a second dose was given 48 hours later, when first-degree atrioventricular block occurred (180).

However, it is not known whether antidigoxin antibody reduces mortality after digitalis poisoning; one randomized, controlled study (178) was too small to detect an effect on mortality after self-poisoning with seeds of the yellow oleander, which contains cardiac glycosides such as peruvoside. Another study that suggested reduced mortality (181) was confounded by being retrospective and inferential, based on changes in death rates as antibody was introduced and reintroduced; furthermore, the change in mortality that was attributed to the use of antibody occurred at the same time as multiple-dose activated charcoal was introduced, and that has definitively been shown to reduce mortality.

The dose of antidigoxin antibody should be based on the dose of digitalis taken and, when possible, the plasma digitalis concentration. The recommended doses for cases of poisoning with digoxin and digitoxin are given in Table 3. Although the clearance of the fragments is reduced in patients who also have severe renal impairment (182,183), there is no need to reduce the dose of antibody in such patients (184–187).

Different formulations of antidigoxin antibody are available. Digibind is an ovine antibody to digoxin, whose production is stimulated by the administration of digoxin conjugated to human albumin. In contrast, DigiFab, also ovine, is stimulated by injecting a conjugate of digoxin to keyhole-limpet hemocyanin (188). In 15 adults with digoxin toxicity who were given DigiFab, electrocardiographic abnormalities resolved within 4 hours in 10 patients and the signs of toxicity completely resolved within 4 hours in seven patients and within 20 hours in 14 patients. In one patient loss of the effect of digoxin resulted in pulmonary edema, pleural effusions, and renal insufficiency. The half-life of DigiFab is slightly shorter than that of Digibind (15 versus 23 hours), but their pharmacodynamic properties are similar. It is said that DigiFab may be preferred in patients who are allergic to sheep proteins, papain, chymopapain, or bromelains.

Antidigoxin antibody fragments cause adverse events in about 7% of cases. These include allergic responses, possible recurrence of digitalis toxicity after treatment, and some effects attributable to the withdrawal of digitalis, such as worsening of heart failure. In one series allergic reactions occurred in only six of 717 patients reviewed, and consisted of pruritic rash and flushing or facial swelling (189). The risk of an allergic reaction was increased in patients who had a history of previous allergy or asthma. Recurrence of digitalis toxicity after treatment was usually due to inadequate treatment with the antibody.

Plasma exchange has been used to enhance the rate of removal of antidigoxin antibody Fab fragments in a

Table 3 Methods for calculating the required dose of antidigoxin antibody fragments in cases of digoxin or digitoxin intoxication

Digoxin

(1) When the ingested dose is known:

(a) Tablets	dose in mg x 40
(b) Elixir	dose in mg x 48
(c) Capsules	dose in mg x 55
(d) Intravenous	dose in mg x 60

(2) When the plasma or serum concentration is known:
ng/ml x lean body weight x 0.34
or
nmol/l x lean body weight x 0.26

Example: Plasma digoxin concentration = 24 ng/ml in a 75 kg patient
Dose of antibody = 24 x 75 x 0.34 = 612 mg
Give 640 mg (for example 16 ampoules of Digibind)

Digitoxin

(1) When the ingested dose is known (all formulations):
Dose in mg x 60

(2) When the plasma or serum concentration is known:
ng/ml x lean body weight x 0.034
or
nmol/l x lean body weight x 0.026

Example: Plasma digitoxin concentration = 280 ng/ml in a 70 kg patient
Dose of antibody = 280 x 70 x 0.034 = 666 mg
Give 680 mg (for example 17 ampoules of Digibind)

46-year-old man with renal insufficiency (190). Removal of the digoxin-Fab complexes in this case prevented their subsequent dissociation and a further increase in the unbound concentration of digoxin. The authors proposed that plasma exchange is best used in these cases within the first 3 hours after the administration of antidigoxin antibodies.

Treat dysrhythmias
Cardiac dysrhythmias in digitalis overdose should be treated only if they are life-threatening. Phenytoin is probably the treatment of choice for ventricular tachydysrhythmias, but lidocaine or a beta-adrenoceptor antagonist, such as propranolol, are options. After an overdose of 300 tablets of digoxin (plasma digoxin concentration 50 ng/ml), recurrent ventricular fibrillation was successfully treated with bretylium tosylate (191). Sinus bradycardia may respond to atropine.

Treat or anticipate heart block
Heart block is the most serious consequence of digitalis poisoning and should be anticipated by the insertion of a temporary pacemaker. If this is postponed until heart block or dysrhythmias occur, there may be difficulty in inserting the pacemaker (because of ventricular excitability), and delay in treatment can be deleterious.

Other measures
Because digoxin has a large apparent volume of distribution, plasma exchange, hemodialysis, and hemoperfusion are not effective methods of removing digoxin from the body.

Hemoperfusion
Hemoperfusion has been used to treat digitalis overdose (SEDA-5, 174) but once a cardiac glycoside has been distributed to the body tissues hemoperfusion is unlikely to be of benefit. For digitoxin, which has a lower apparent volume of distribution than digoxin, charcoal hemoperfusion may be more valuable.

- In an 88-year-old woman whose serum digoxin concentration was 6.4 ng/ml, hemoperfusion with an adsorption column containing beta$_2$-microglobulin caused a fall in serum concentration from 6 ng/ml to 2.3 ng/ml, with improvement in gastrointestinal symptoms (192). The serum digoxin concentration then rose again to 3.5 ng/ml over the next 3 days, and a further hemoperfusion treatment reduced it to 1.7 ng/ml, after which the serum concentration gradually fell and the patient improved. Because of chronic renal insufficiency, she also had repeated hemodialyses on alternate days, which also contributed to the reduction in serum digoxin concentrations.

The clearance of digoxin was measured in eight patients receiving hemodialysis during the use of a beta$_2$-microglobulin column (193). After 240 minutes of hemoperfusion the serum digoxin concentration fell from 1.11 to 0.57 ng/ml and digoxin clearance was about 145 ml/minute. However, this clearance rate cannot have been the true total body clearance, since it merely reflected the change in plasma concentration during hemoperfusion, which would have been almost entirely due to removal of digoxin from the plasma only and not from the tissues. This method cannot be recommended as a substitute for the use of antidigoxin antibodies in the treatment of digitalis toxicity.

Hemofiltration
Hemofiltration has been used to treat digitalis poisoning (SEDA-12, 149), but there is no convincing evidence of its efficacy.

Exchange transfusion
There have been reports of the use of exchange transfusion to remove Fab antibody fragment-digoxin complexes in patients with acute anuric renal insufficiency (194).

- Plasma exchange was used to enhance the rate of removal of antidigoxin antibody Fab fragments in a 46-year-old man with renal insufficiency (190). Removal of the digoxin-Fab complexes in this case prevented their subsequent dissociation and a further increase in the unbound concentration of digoxin.

The authors proposed that plasma exchange is best used in these cases within the first 3 hours after the administration of antidigoxin antibodies.

- A 70-year-old man with alcoholic cirrhosis was given amiodarone and digoxin for atrial fibrillation after a hemicolectomy for adenocarcinoma (195). He developed acute renal insufficiency and digoxin toxicity, with a serum concentration of 4.4 ng/ml. A dose of Fab antidigoxin antibody fragments was followed 16 hours later by exchange transfusion and another dose was followed by two exchanges. He recovered slowly over the next few days. The total digoxin concentration (antibody bound and unbound) rose after the first dose of Fab fragments but did not fall until after the second plasma exchange (after the second dose of Fab fragments).

In this case digoxin was recovered from the plasma collection bags, but the total amount recovered seems to have been less than 100 μg, so the efficacy of plasma exchange was not clear.

Drug–Drug Interactions

General

Drug interactions with cardiac glycosides can be subdivided into six types, according to mechanism. Interactions with digoxin have been reviewed (SEDA-6, 173) (196–198). Drug interactions with digitoxin have been briefly reviewed in the context of its use in the treatment of congestive heart failure (199).

Absorption
Absorption interactions with digitalis are probably not of great clinical importance, since (a) the dosages of drugs that reduce the absorption of digitalis are usually larger than those used clinically, and (b) the major effect on absorption probably occurs only if the two drugs are taken together.

The effect of activated charcoal in reducing digitalis absorption is mentioned under the treatment of poisoning, and binding resins such as colestyramine and colestipol have similar actions (200,201).

Certain combinations of cytotoxic drugs (cyclophosphamide, vincristine, and prednisone, with and without procarbazine) reduced plasma digoxin concentrations by about 50% during treatment with beta-acetyldigoxin, perhaps through impaired absorption of beta-acetyldigoxin (202); digitoxin was not affected (203).

Absorption interactions involving altered gastrointestinal motility have been described. These include interactions of digoxin with propantheline (204), metoclopramide (204), and cisapride (205). However, the clinical relevance of these interactions is unclear and they are probably unimportant.

Some antacids, such as magnesium trisilicate, reduce the absorption of digoxin slightly, but these interactions are probably of no clinical importance (206).

Protein-binding displacement

Interactions of this kind are of no importance for digoxin, which is only about 20% bound and has a high apparent volume of distribution.

An interaction of heparin with digitoxin has been described and ascribed to altered protein binding, secondary to changes in fatty acid concentrations, but the clinical relevance, for example in patients undergoing hemodialysis, is unclear (207).

Renal clearance

Digoxin is cleared by the kidneys by glomerular filtration and active secretion, and retained by passive reabsorption, the last two roughly balancing each other, so that clearance is usually proportional to creatinine clearance. A major mechanism for drug interactions with digoxin is inhibition of its renal tubular secretion by inhibition of P glycoprotein. This mechanism has been reviewed in relation to an in vitro tissue culture model, consisting of confluent polarized renal tubular cell monolayers (208). This model has confirmed the action of several drugs that can inhibit the renal tubular secretion of digoxin in this way, including amiodarone, ciclosporin, itraconazole and ketoconazole, mifepristone, propafenone, quinidine, spironolactone, verapamil, and vinblastine and vincristine.

In three large studies using either population pharmacokinetic analysis or Bayesian techniques, drugs that inhibit the transport of digoxin by inhibiting P glycoprotein significantly increased the serum digoxin concentration (143,209,210). These drugs included quinidine, spironolactone, and the calcium channel blockers diltiazem, nicardipine, nifedipine, and verapamil. The effects varied from about 22% to about 36%.

Vasodilators may increase the active secretion of digoxin, which is a high clearance process and is therefore affected by renal blood flow.

Uptake by the end-organ

The interaction of quinidine with digoxin involves displacement of digoxin from tissues.

Hyperkalemia, due to potassium chloride, potassium-retaining diuretics, ACE inhibitors, or angiotensin-receptor antagonists, reduces the apparent affinity of digitalis for Na/K-ATPase and thereby reduces its tissue binding.

Response of the end-organ

Interactions involving changes in the response of the end-organ to digitalis are the most common of all interactions with cardiac glycosides.

Potassium depletion, for example due to diuretics or corticosteroids, potentiates the effects of cardiac glycosides on the myocardium and may also have a small effect in reducing the renal tubular secretion of digoxin (211,212).

Magnesium depletion may have a similar effect (213), but the data are not as clear-cut as those for potassium.

Anecdotal reports suggest that intravenous infusion of calcium salts in patients taking digitalis can result in dangerous cardiac dysrhythmias. This may also be the basis of reports that edrophonium and suxamethonium enhance the actions of digitalis, since both of these drugs might cause altered disposition of calcium. Conversely, there is good anecdotal evidence that hypocalcemia causes reduced plasma responsiveness to digoxin (214).

Alpha-glucosidase inhibitors

Acarbose

In patients taking steady-state digoxin therapy the addition of acarbose reduced the plasma digoxin concentration (215,216). The association was confirmed in both cases by withdrawal of acarbose. The likely mechanism of this interaction is inhibition of the absorption of digoxin by acarbose, although the authors also suggested that acarbose might interfere with the hydrolysis of digoxin before absorption, thus altering the pattern of metabolites in the blood; however, this is a much less likely mechanism. The authors recommended that if acarbose be used in conjunction with digoxin, the doses should be separated by about 6 hours. This absorption interaction has previously been highlighted (217,218).

However, in a formal study of the pharmacokinetics of a single dose of digoxin 0.75 mg before and after the administration of acarbose 50 mg tds for 12 days in healthy volunteers, apart from a small increase in C_{max}, the pharmacokinetics of digoxin were unaffected by acarbose (219). It is not uncommon for anecdotal reports of a possible interaction to be unconfirmed by formal kinetic studies, and it is possible in such cases that there is a subset of patients who are susceptible to the interaction who have not been included in the formal study. In this case, for example, it may be that the interaction occurs in people with diabetes and not in healthy subjects. There may also be a difference in the effect of acarbose on a single dose of digoxin, compared with steady-state therapy. Advice that acarbose and digoxin should be administered 6 hours apart is still reasonable.

Voglibose

In eight healthy men voglibose, another inhibitor of alpha-glucosidase, had no effect on the pharmacokinetics of digoxin (220). This result suggests that inhibition of alpha-glucosidase is not the mechanism whereby acarbose alters the absorption of digoxin; however, acarbose also inhibits alpha-amylase and such inhibition cannot be ruled out as a mechanism of the interaction with acarbose, perhaps by altered gastrointestinal motility.

Amiodarone

Amiodarone inhibits the renal tubular secretion of digoxin (SEDA-22, 201) and it has also been suggested that it increases its absorption (SEDA-10, 144) (SEDA-12, 150). This interaction has also been reported with acetyldigoxin (SEDA-18, 198) (221).

Amiodarone also interacts with digitoxin (222). In two cases the half-life of digitoxin was prolonged, but there was no other information that suggested a mechanism. The author suggested that amiodarone might displace digitoxin from tissue sites, but that would have led to a shortening of the half-life rather than a prolongation. It seems more likely that amiodarone inhibits the clearance of digitoxin by inhibiting renal and gut P glycoprotein and perhaps by inhibiting its metabolism.

Antacids

Although digoxin is not extensively metabolized in most patients, it is metabolized before its absorption from the gut by two mechanisms, hydrolysis by gastric acid and hydrogenation by intestinal bacteria. In patients who have hypochlorhydria presystemic metabolism is reduced and increasing concentrations of digoxin are achieved systemically. This means that drugs that reduce gastric acid secretion, such as cimetidine, ranitidine, other histamine H_2 receptor antagonists, and omeprazole would be expected to increase the systemic availability of digoxin, and there is some supporting evidence (223,224), although this is not conclusive (SEDA-17, 216).

Antidysrhythmic drugs

Digoxin does not interact with a variety of antidysrhythmic drugs, including ajmaline, aprindine, lidocaine, lidoflazine (225), and moracizine (226). Other drugs that may have minor and clinically unimportant interactions include captopril, carvedilol, disopyramide, and flosequinan.

Antifungal imidazoles

Itraconazole increases steady-state serum digoxin concentrations, perhaps by inhibiting the renal tubular secretion of digoxin (SEDA-22, 202) (227–229). An alternative proposed mechanism is inhibition of CYP3A (SEDA-21, 196), and this has been reported in rats with ketoconazole (230), although an effect on P glycoprotein was also possible. Whatever the mechanism, ketoconazole increased the systemic availability of digoxin from 0.68 to 0.84 and reduced the mean absorption time from 1.1 hours to 0.3 hours. The increased systemic availability could have been explained by inhibition of CYP3A or P glycoprotein in the gut, but the increased rate of absorption could only be explained by inhibition of the P glycoprotein. Since the t_{max} was unaffected, the authors hypothesized that inhibition of P glycoprotein increased the absorption rate, which would have tended to reduce the t_{max}, while inhibition of CYP3A, which would have reduced the elimination rate of digoxin, would have tended to increase the t_{max}. Thus a combination of these two effects would have had no effect on t_{max}. It should be noted that CYP3A is an important route of metabolism of digoxin in rats, but not in man.

Digoxin toxicity sometimes accompanies this interaction.

- A 62-year-old woman who was taking digoxin took itraconazole 400 mg/day for 3 days developed nausea, anorexia, and lethargy; the symptoms improved within 48 hours after withdrawal of itraconazole (231). The serum digoxin concentrations were not reported.
- In a 75-year-old man who took itraconazole in a low dose (200 mg/day) the steady-state serum digoxin concentration only rose from 0.8 to 1.1 ng/ml after 8 days (232).
- Two renal transplant patients developed digoxin toxicity when they also took itraconazole (233).

Itraconazole increases the digoxin AUC_{0-72} by about 50%, and reduces its renal clearance by about 20% (234). Apart from inhibition of the renal secretion of digoxin, which is probably mediated by inhibition of P glycoprotein, a study in guinea pigs also showed significantly reduced biliary excretion of digoxin by itraconazole, suggesting that the interaction between itraconazole and digoxin may be due not only to a reduction in renal clearance, but also to a reduction in the metabolic clearance of digoxin by itraconazole (235).

Argatroban

The thrombin inhibitor argatroban had no effect on the steady-state pharmacokinetics of oral digoxin 0.375 mg/day in 12 healthy volunteers; the argatroban was given as an intravenous infusion of 2 micrograms/kg/minute on days 11–15 (236).

Bosentan

In a randomized study in 18 young men, bosentan caused a small (12%) reduction in the AUC of digoxin, without changing either the C_{max} or the C_{min} (237). This was a steady-state study, with plasma concentration measurements for only 24 hours, and so the half-life of digoxin was not measured. Bosentan is an antagonist at endothelin type 1 receptors and could therefore have increased renal blood flow by pre- and postglomerular vasoconstriction, increasing the elimination of digoxin. Furthermore, bosentan is a substrate for P glycoprotein, which mediates the renal tubular secretion of digoxin, and may induce its expression, increasing digoxin renal clearance. However, whatever the mechanism of this putative interaction, it is clearly unlikely to be of clinical significance.

Calcium channel blockers

Calcium channel blockers have varying effects on the disposition of digoxin. The calcium channel blockers for which varying amounts of information are available include cinnarizine, diltiazem, felodipine, fendiline, gallopamil, isradipine, lidoflazine, mibefradil, nicardipine, nifedipine, nitrendipine, tiapamil, and verapamil (238).

Diltiazem

Studies of the effects of diltiazem on the pharmacokinetics of digoxin have yielded variable results. In one study, diltiazem reduced the steady-state total body clearance of beta-acetyldigoxin in 12 healthy men, perhaps because of reduced renal and non-renal clearances (SEDA-10, 145). In some studies diltiazem 120–240 mg/day increased steady-state plasma digoxin concentrations by about 20–40% (SEDA-14, 146) (239), although not in other studies (SEDA-14, 146), and reduced the total body clearance of digoxin, with changes in both renal and non-renal clearances (SEDA-11, 154), although others did not find this (240). In at least one case digoxin toxicity was attributed to this interaction (SEDA-17, 216). In eight patients with chronic heart failure taking digoxin 0.25 mg/day, diltiazem 180 mg/day increased the AUC and mean steady-state serum concentrations of digoxin by 50% and reduced its total clearance (241).

Mibefradil

In 40 healthy subjects mibefradil 50 or 100 mg/day for 6 days had no significant effects on the steady-state pharmacokinetics of digoxin, apart from a very small increase in the C_{max} (242).

Tiapamil

Tiapamil reversed digoxin-induced splanchnic vasoconstriction in healthy men (243), but this has no direct effect on systemic hemodynamics.

Verapamil

Verapamil increases plasma digoxin concentrations at steady state by inhibiting the active tubular secretion and non-renal clearance of digoxin (244,245). There is only anecdotal evidence that this can result in digitalis toxicity (245,246).

Verapamil reversed digoxin-induced splanchnic vasoconstriction in healthy men (243), but this has no direct effect on systemic hemodynamics.

Captopril

There have been contradictory results in studies of the effects of captopril on digoxin pharmacokinetics. In some cases, captopril increased steady-state plasma digoxin concentrations (247), while in others there was no evidence of an interaction (248–251). In eight patients with NHYA Class IV congestive heart failure, captopril 12.5 mg tds for 1 week increased the peak digoxin concentration, reduced the time to peak, and increased the AUC during a single dosage interval at steady state; trough digoxin concentrations did not change (252). There are two possible explanations for these findings: that captopril reduced the clearance of digoxin or that it increased both the rate and extent of absorption of digoxin; unfortunately, the authors did not measure either the mean steady-state concentration or the half-life, which would have clarified this. On the whole, however, it is unlikely that this interaction is of any clinical significance, since in no study has there been evidence of digoxin toxicity during concomitant captopril therapy, and in one formal study (251) there was evidence of no pharmacodynamic interaction.

Cilomilast

In 12 healthy young adults the phosphodiesterase inhibitor cilomilast 15 mg bd for 5 days had no effect on the steady-state pharmacokinetics of digoxin, apart from a small reduction in the maximal concentration and a small increase in the time to peak (253). This was consistent with a small effect on the rate of digoxin absorption, which is unlikely to be of clinical significance. Digoxin had no effect on the disposition of cilomilast.

Cisapride

- In a 90-year-old woman the addition of cisapride 5 mg bd reduced the mean steady-state digoxin concentration from 0.9 ng/ml to 0.6 ng/ml and 5 mg tds reduced it to 0.4 ng/ml, with recurrence of her severe biventricular failure (254). When the doses of digoxin and cisapride were separated, the serum digoxin concentration rose again. The mechanism of this effect is thought to be increased gastrointestinal motility, although in this case the effect of separating the doses suggests that there might be a direct chemical interaction between the two drugs.

Citalopram

In 11 healthy adults citalopram 40 mg/day had no effect on the pharmacokinetics of a single oral dose of digoxin 1 mg (255). Digoxin did not affect citalopram pharmacokinetics.

Clopidogrel

In 12 healthy men steady-state clopidogrel 75 mg/day had no effect on the steady-state plasma concentrations of digoxin (256).

Dihydroergocriptine

The effect of dihydroergocriptine on the pharmacokinetics of a single oral dose of digoxin has been studied in 12 healthy men aged 23–39 years (257). There was no interaction.

Dofetilide

In 14 healthy men dofetilide 250 μg bd for 5 days had no effect on the pharmacokinetics of digoxin at a steady-state trough concentration of 1.0 ng/ml (258). However, in a placebo-controlled study in patients with atrial fibrillation or atrial flutter, conversion to sinus rhythm in patients given dofetilide was more likely if they were also given digoxin (259), so there may be a pharmacodynamic interaction.

Fondaparinux

Fondaparinux sodium, a selective inhibitor of coagulation factor Xa, is eliminated by the kidneys. In a randomized, crossover study in 24 healthy volunteers the pharmacokinetics and pharmacodynamics of digoxin 0.25 mg/day orally for 7 days were unaffected by fondaparinux sodium 10 mg/day subcutaneously for 7 days (260).

Hydralazine

The vasodilator hydralazine increases the renal clearance of digoxin, perhaps by increasing renal blood flow and therefore renal tubular secretion (261). This causes a small fall in plasma digoxin concentration the clinical significance of which is unclear.

Indometacin

Indometacin increased plasma digoxin concentrations in premature neonates with a patent ductus arteriosus (262), but a formal study in healthy adults showed no interaction (263). It may be that pre-existing impairment of renal function is required for this interaction, but this remains to be elucidated.

Levetiracetam

In 11 healthy adults in a double-blind, placebo-controlled study levetiracetam had no effect on the steady-state pharmacokinetics of digoxin or the actions of digoxin on the electrocardiogram (264).

Macrogol

Macrogol 20 g/day for 8 days caused a 30% reduction in the AUC and a 40% reduction in the C_{max} of a single dose of digoxin in 18 healthy volunteers; the t_{max} and half-life were not affected (265). This interaction was probably due to reduced absorption of digoxin, perhaps by a physicochemical interaction between the two compounds.

Macrolide antibiotics

Although digoxin is not extensively metabolized in the majority of patients, in some it is metabolized before its absorption from the gut, by two mechanisms: hydrolysis by gastric acid and hydrogenation by intestinal bacteria, mainly *Eubacterium lentum*. The macrolide antibiotics and tetracycline increase the systemic availability of digoxin, by inhibiting its breakdown by intestinal bacteria (266,267).

Macrolides have also been suggested to interact with digoxin by inhibiting P glycoprotein (SEDA-26, 200). However, in a study of this mechanism in nine healthy Japanese men, clarithromycin 200 mg bd and erythromycin 200 mg qds did not alter the plasma concentration versus time curve of a single intravenous dose of digoxin 0.5 mg, but increased its renal clearance (268). This contrasts with an observation of reduced renal clearance of digoxin in two patients taking clarithromycin (SEDA-23, 194). That inhibition of renal P glycoprotein may not reduce the renal clearance of digoxin has also been suggested by studies with talinolol (SEDA-25, 172) and atorvastatin (269). Other transport mechanisms for digoxin, including the organic anion-transporting polypeptides, have not been well studied and may play a role in digoxin disposition and hence drug interactions.

Azithromycin

- In a 31-month-old boy with Down's syndrome and Fallot's tetralogy during a 5-day course of azithromycin 5 mg/kg/day the serum digoxin concentration rose and the child had anorexia, diarrhea, and second-degree atrioventricular block with junctional extra beats (270).

The mechanism was not investigated.

Clarithromycin

- In a 72-year-old woman taking digoxin 0.25 mg/day, the addition of clarithromycin caused a rise in the serum digoxin concentration to 4.6 ng/ml (271).

In two other cases in which clarithromycin increased serum digoxin concentrations there was an associated reduction in the rate of renal digoxin clearance, which may be another mechanism for this interaction (272). The authors hypothesized that clarithromycin inhibited P glycoprotein. This was supported by the observation of a concentration-dependent effect of clarithromycin on in vitro transcellular transport of digoxin.

There is anecdotal evidence that this interaction may be clinically important. Digoxin toxicity occurred in a patient taking clarithromycin (273).

Erythromycin

- Digoxin toxicity occurred in a neonate who was also given erythromycin (274). She had bradycardia and coupled extra beats. Digoxin and erythromycin were withdrawn and she was given antidigoxin antibodies. Her plasma digoxin concentration, which had previously been 1.8 ng/ml, had risen to 8.0 ng/ml.

Meglitinides

In 12 healthy volunteers aged 19–36 years nateglinide had no effects on the pharmacokinetics of a single dose of digoxin (275). Similarly, in 14 healthy adults, repaglinide 2 mg three times had no effect on the steady-state pharmacokinetics of digoxin (276). These results suggest that the meglitinides do not affect P glycoprotein.

Nitrates

The effects of nitrates on the pharmacokinetics of digoxin are probably small.

In eight patients with chronic heart failure taking digoxin 0.25 mg/day, isosorbide dinitrate 10 mg tds caused only a small increase in C_{max} (15%) and had no effect on the mean steady-state serum concentration or AUC (241).

Nitroprusside increased the renal clearance of digoxin, perhaps by increasing renal blood flow and therefore renal tubular secretion (261). This caused a small fall in plasma digoxin concentration, the clinical significance of which is unclear.

Phenobarbital

The metabolism of digitoxin can be increased, with resulting increasing dosage requirements, by enzyme-inducing drugs (200). For example, phenobarbital 100 mg daily reduces steady-state serum digitoxin concentrations by 50%.

Propafenone

Propafenone causes a small increase in plasma digoxin concentrations by an unknown mechanism (277,278). Although this effect is perhaps not clinically significant, in patients with dysrhythmias it was accompanied by an increase in PR interval (214).

Quinidine

Digoxin

The quinidine–digoxin interaction has been reviewed (SEDA-6, 173) (SEDA-7, 195) (SEDA-9, 159) (SEDA-10, 145) (SEDA-15, 166) (SEDA-18, 198).

Although the major mechanism of the interaction is probably inhibition of the active tubular secretion of digoxin by quinidine, other mechanisms are involved, including reduced non-renal clearance and displacement of digoxin from the tissues. The reduction in non-renal clearance is at least partly due to a reduction in biliary clearance. This interaction affects most patients and on average causes a two-fold increase in steady-state plasma digoxin concentrations. Because both clearance and apparent volume of distribution are reduced, the half-life of digoxin is either unaffected or perhaps slightly prolonged.

In addition to the pharmacokinetic interaction, there may be a pharmacodynamic interaction, since there is some evidence that quinidine reduces the positive inotropic effect of digoxin on the heart, in addition to having a negative inotropic effect of its own. Thus, the outcome of the interaction is a 24-fold increased risk of digoxin toxicity and a reduction in its beneficial effect on the heart, at least in sinus rhythm. If the two drugs are used together, the initial digoxin dosage should be halved and adjusted subsequently on the basis of the patient's clinical condition and the plasma digoxin concentration.

Lanatoside C and metildigoxin are theoretically likely to be similarly affected by quinidine, and there is anecdotal evidence of this (279).

The pharmacokinetic interaction of quinidine with digoxin also occurs with quinine (280,281) and hydroxychloroquine (282). However, the effects of these drugs are smaller than those with quinidine. Quinine reduces the extrarenal clearance of digoxin, perhaps by altering its biliary secretion (283).

Digitoxin

In five healthy adults quinidine prolonged the half-life of a single dose of digitoxin from 174 to 261 hours and reduced its total body clearance from 1.54 to 1.09 ml/hour/kg and renal clearance from 0.65 to 0.46 ml/hour/kg. Digitoxin volume of distribution and protein binding were unaffected. Quinidine caused a rise in serum digitoxin concentrations (284).

In eight healthy subjects steady-state digitoxin plasma concentrations and renal excretion increased from 13.6 ng/ml and 16.1 μg/day before dosing to 19.7 ng/ml and 23.4 μg/day respectively during quinidine dosing for 32 days (285). Renal digitoxin clearance was not noticeably changed by quinidine, but total and extrarenal digitoxin clearances fell by 32% and 41% respectively. The half-life of digitoxin was prolonged from 150 to 203 hours. There were corresponding pharmacodynamic effects, as assessed by electrocardiography and systolic time intervals.

Quinolone antibiotics

The quinolone antimicrobial drugs gemifloxacin, levofloxacin, and sparfloxacin do not interact with digoxin.

In a crossover study in 14 healthy elderly individuals gemifloxacin 320 mg/day had no effect on the steady-state pharmacokinetics of digoxin (286).

Levofloxacin 500 mg bd for 6 days in 12 healthy volunteers did not interact with digoxin (287).

The interaction of sparfloxacin with digoxin, both at steady state, has been studied in a double-blind, placebo-controlled, crossover study in 24 healthy men aged 20–49 years. Sparfloxacin had no effect on the steady-state mean plasma concentration, C_{min}, t_{max}, or AUC of digoxin (288). Conversely digoxin did not alter the steady-state pharmacokinetics of sparfloxacin.

Rifampicin

The metabolism of digitoxin can be increased, with resulting increasing dosage requirements, by rifampicin (289).

Rifampicin also induces P glycoprotein and should therefore increase the clearance of digoxin by that mechanism. Some reports (290,291) have suggested that rifampicin reduces the steady-state concentration of digoxin. Another study in eight healthy men has shown that steady-state rifampicin significantly reduced the AUC of oral digoxin but had less of an effect on intravenous digoxin (292). The authors attributed this to induction of P glycoprotein in the intestine, with increased secretion of the drug into the gut lumen. Rifampicin has previously been reported to reduce steady-state plasma digitoxin concentrations, an effect that was attributed to induction of the metabolism of digitoxin to digoxin (289); however, in that study plasma digoxin concentrations were not measured separately, and it may be that rifampicin also increases the secretion of digitoxin into the gut lumen.

Ropinirole

In 10 patients with Parkinson's disease steady-state ropinirole treatment caused small reductions in the AUC and C_{max} of digoxin at steady state (10% and 25% respectively) (293). However, the C_{min} was unaffected and overall there was probably no significant effect of ropinirole on digoxin disposition.

Sevelamer

Sevelamer, a non-absorbed phosphate-binding polymer, in a dose of 2.4 g, had no effect on the pharmacokinetics of single doses of digoxin in 19 healthy volunteers (294).

Spironolactone

Spironolactone inhibits the active tubular secretion of digoxin by about 25% and in some cases digoxin dosages may have to be reduced (295).

St. John's wort (*Hypericum perforatum*)

St. John's wort (*Hypericum perforatum*) had no effect on the pharmacokinetics of digoxin after a single dose in 25 healthy volunteers, but during steady-state therapy it reduced the AUC of digoxin by 25% (296). There were also significant reductions in C_{max} and C_{min} (26% and 33% respectively). This effect was attributed to induction of P glycoprotein.

In Japan enough patients take St. John's wort with a cardiac glycoside to make this interaction potentially important; of 741 outpatients taking St. John's wort, 171 had been given a prescription for either digoxin or metildigoxin (297).

Statins

The effects of statins on the pharmacokinetics of digoxin have been variable. There is no simple explanation that reconciles the disparate findings.

- A 52-year-old man developed rhabdomyolysis while taking simvastatin, digoxin, ciclosporin, and verapamil (298). The authors proposed that this had been due in part to inhibition of the biliary secretion of simvastatin by digoxin; however, it is likely that the major mechanism of the interaction was inhibition of CYP3A4 by ciclosporin.

Atorvastatin

Atorvastatin 80 mg/day increased the AUC and C_{max} of digoxin 0.25 mg/day by 15% and 20% respectively during steady-state therapy, without affecting renal digoxin clearance (269).

Cerivastatin

In 20 healthy men, cerivastatin had no effect on the steady-state pharmacokinetics of digoxin (299). Digoxin had no significant effect on the pharmacokinetics of cerivastatin.

Fluvastatin

A single dose of fluvastatin increased the steady-state C_{max} of digoxin 0.125–0.5 mg/day by 11% and renal clearance by 15%, without changing AUC or t_{max} (300).

Rosuvastatin

Rosuvastatin 40 mg/day had no effect on the pharmacokinetics of a single oral dose of digoxin 0.5 mg in 18 healthy men (301).

Talinolol

The effects of talinolol on the pharmacokinetics of digoxin have been studied in 10 healthy volunteers aged 23–30 years in a crossover study (302). Oral talinolol 100 mg increased the AUC of digoxin significantly, but the renal clearance and half-life of digoxin were unchanged. Intravenous talinolol 30 mg had no effect on the pharmacokinetics of oral digoxin. The authors concluded that the change in AUC after oral talinolol was due to increased systemic availability of digoxin, through inhibition of intestinal P glycoprotein. They did not discuss the possibility that talinolol had also reduced the non-renal clearance of digoxin by inhibiting its biliary secretion, and indeed there was a small, albeit non-significant reduction in non-renal clearance of digoxin after both oral and intravenous talinolol. In contrast, digoxin did not affect the kinetics of talinolol.

Tamsulosin

The alpha$_1$-adrenoceptor antagonist tamsulosin 0.4 and 0.8 mg/day had no effect on the pharmacokinetics of a single intravenous dose of digoxin 0.5 mg in 10 healthy men (303).

Tegaserod

In 12 healthy subjects the 5-HT$_4$ receptor partial agonist tegaserod 6 mg bd for 3 days had a small effect on the pharmacokinetics of a single oral dose of digoxin 1 mg, reducing the mean AUC by 12% and the C_{max} by 15% (304). There was a small delay in the time to peak, which was not significant. These results suggest that tegaserod slightly reduces the systemic availability of digoxin, perhaps because it increases gastrointestinal motility, but that the effect is of no clinical significance.

Telmisartan

Multiple-dose telmisartan 120 mg/day administered with digoxin 0.25 mg/day resulted in higher serum digoxin concentrations (305). Digoxin AUC rose by 22% and C_{max} by 50%; the rise in C_{min} (13%) was not significant. These results suggest that telmisartan reduces the clearance of digoxin. The magnitude of this effect is comparable to that observed with calcium channel blockers, carvedilol, captopril, amiodarone, quinidine, and propafenone. Monitoring serum digoxin concentrations should be considered when patients first use telmisartan and when the dosage of telmisartan is changed.

Tetracycline

Although digoxin is not extensively metabolized in the majority of patients, in some it is metabolized before its absorption from the gut, by two mechanisms: hydrolysis by gastric acid and hydrogenation by intestinal bacteria, mainly *E. lentum*. Tetracycline increases the systemic availability of digoxin, by inhibiting its breakdown by intestinal bacteria (252).

Tiagabine

Tiagabine, which is principally metabolized by CYP3A, had no effect on the steady-state pharmacokinetics of digoxin in 13 healthy volunteers (306). This is evidence that CYP3A is not important in the metabolism of digoxin.

Warfarin

It has been claimed that digoxin potentiated the effects of warfarin in a 66-year-old man (307). However, the discussion of the possible mechanisms of this observation was flawed, and there is no reason to expect such an interaction, which probably does not occur (308).

Zaleplon

The effects of zaleplon on the pharmacokinetics and pharmacodynamics of steady-state digoxin have been studied in 20 healthy men aged 18–45 years (309). There was no interaction.

Interference with Diagnostic Tests

Digoxin radioimmunoassays

Spironolactone interferes with some digoxin radioimmunoassays, because it and its metabolites, such as canrenone and 7-alpha-thiomethylspironolactone, are immunoreactive with some forms of antidigoxin antibody (310–312). However, in contrast to this there has been a recent report that canrenoate, the main metabolite of spironolactone, interfered with the immunoassay of digoxin (313). The effect was largest with the AxSym MEIA II assay, and there was also some interference with the EMIT assay. However, the TDx assay did not show any interference. Spironolactone also caused some interference in the AxSym assay but less than canrenoate. In this case the failure to measure high digoxin concentrations resulted in clinical toxicity in a 71-year-old man who was given 3.8 mg over 11 days.

In a study of the use of the TDx II assay in 80 children and adults, there was apparent digoxin immunoreactivity in 3.7% of healthy subjects ($n = 80$), 3.6% of pregnant women ($n = 28$), 10% of patients with renal transplants ($n = 31$), and 23% of immature infants ($n = 40$) (314).

In nine assays (AxSYM, IMx, TDx, Emit, Dimension, aca, TinaQuant, Elecsys, and Vitros) interference by spironolactone, canrenone, and three metabolites was sought in vitro, and all routine digoxin measurements using the AxSYM system over 16.5 months ($n = 3089$) were reviewed (315). There was a reduction in the expected concentrations by canrenone (3125 ng/ml) in the following assays: AxSYM (42% of expected), IMx (51%), and Dimension (78%). There was positive bias in aca (0.7 ng/ml), TDx (0.62 ng/ml), and Elecsys (>0.58 ng/ml). Of 669 routinely monitored patients, 25 had falsely low results and 19 of them actually had potentially toxic digoxin concentrations; this was attributable to concurrent therapy with spironolactone, canrenone, hydrocortisone, or prednisolone. However, standard doses of spironolactone (up to 50 mg/day) in patients with heart failure produced less than 11% inhibition.

Monitoring Therapy

The use of plasma digitalis concentrations in monitoring therapy has been reviewed (133,316).

In a retrospective analysis of 210 randomly selected digoxin plasma concentration determinations in inpatients, the indications were considered to have been inappropriate in 67, appropriate in 81, and unevaluable in 4 (317). Timing of the blood sample was wrong in 17 cases (samples should be taken at least 6 hours and preferably about 11 hours after the dose). Of the measurements whose indications were considered to have been inappropriate, most (52) were performed as part of "routine" monitoring.

The following are the main uses of plasma digitalis concentration measurements.

Individualizing therapy

In the absence of factors that alter the response to digitalis it may be worth measuring the plasma concentration during the initial stages of therapy to ensure that a reasonable concentration has been achieved (1.0–1.5 ng/ml for digoxin, 10–15 ng/ml for digitoxin). In cases where there is still a poor response to treatment it is justifiable to increase digitalis dosages cautiously, but the risk of toxicity starts to rise markedly at plasma concentrations above 2.0 and 20 ng/ml respectively. If there are subsequent changes in the patient's condition, for example renal impairment, then plasma concentration measurement may help in readjusting dosages.

Monitoring adherence

The commonest cause of a low plasma digitalis concentration in a patient taking a cardiac glycoside is poor adherence to therapy.

Making decisions about long-term therapy

If the plasma digitalis concentration is below the target range in a patient whose condition is stable (for example atrial fibrillation with a ventricular rate of 80/minute) digitalis can usually be withdrawn safely.

Diagnosis of toxicity

The underlying principles in using plasma digitalis concentrations to diagnose toxicity are as follows:

1. The plasma digitalis concentration must be considered in conjunction with other clinical information, that is symptoms, the signs of possible intoxication, the stability of the underlying condition, age, renal function, the dosage, and biochemical measurements such as the plasma potassium concentration.
2. At plasma digitalis concentrations above 3.0 ng/ml (digoxin) or 30 ng/ml (digitoxin) toxicity is highly likely. At concentrations below 1.5 or 15 ng/ml, respectively, toxicity is unlikely. However, toxicity can occur even with low concentrations and should be suspected particularly if there is hypokalemia.
3. Certain factors increase the risk of digitalis toxicity at a given plasma concentration (see Susceptibility Factors). These factors will alter the interpretation of the plasma digitalis concentration and should lower the threshold for suspicion.
4. When in doubt it is far better to withhold digitalis and monitor progress than to continue treatment, thereby running the risk of perpetuating toxicity.

In patients whose condition is satisfactory and stable and whose plasma digoxin concentration is low (below 0.8 ng/ml), withdrawal of digoxin is recommended and is highly unlikely to affect the patient's condition (discussed in the section Making decisions about long-term therapy). Probably the same applies for digitoxin at concentrations below 8.0 ng/ml, although that has not been demonstrated.

It has yet again been confirmed that the serum digoxin concentration distinguishes between patients with and without digoxin toxicity, but with considerable overlap (318). Of 99 patients, 41 with toxicity had mean serum digoxin concentrations of 3.1 ng/ml compared with 1.6 ng/ml in 58 non-toxic patients. However the digoxin concentration was below 2 ng/ml in 10 patients with toxicity and higher than 2 ng/ml in 16 patients without. There were no significant differences in serum electrolyte concentrations between the toxic and non-toxic patients, and the authors therefore concluded that such abnormalities are less important than they have usually been considered to be. However, this study does not demonstrate that at all; rather it shows that even if serum electrolyte concentrations are well controlled it may not be possible to avoid digitalis toxicity for other reasons. Indeed, in this study the patients with toxicity had significantly worse renal function, which would have explained their increased risk.

References

1. Various authors. Digoxin symposium. Br Heart J 1985;54:227.
2. Fisch, C editor. William Withering: An account of the foxglove and some of its medical uses 1785–1985. J Am Coll Cardiol 1985;5(Suppl A).
3. Erdman E, Greeff K, Shou JC, editor. Cardiac Glycosides 1785–1984. Biochemistry, Pharmacology, Clinical Relevance. Darmstadt: Steinkopff Verlag, 1985.
4. Rietbrock N, Woodcock BG. Handbook of Renal-Independent Cardiac Glycosides: Pharmacology and Clinical Pharmacology. Chichester: Ellis Horwood, 1989.
5. Chung EK. Digitalis Intoxication. Amsterdam: Excerpta Medica, 1969.
6. Smith TW, Antman EM, Friedman PL, Blatt CM, Marsh JD. Digitalis glycosides: mechanisms and manifestations of toxicity. Prog Cardiovasc Dis 1984;26(6):495–540; 1984;27(1):21–56.
7. Aronson JK. Digitalis intoxication. Clin Sci (Lond) 1983;64(3):253–8.
8. Buchanan JF, Olson KR. Current management of digitalis toxicity. Part I: Clinical manifestations. Pract Cardiol 1988;14:75–9.
9. Buchanan JF, Olson KR. Current management of digitalis toxicity. Part II: Treatment of digitalis intoxication. Pract Cardiol 1988;14:92–5.
10. Hauptman PJ, Kelly RA. Digitalis. Circulation 1999;99(9):1265–70.
11. Haji SA, Movahed A. Update on digoxin therapy in congestive heart failure. Am Fam Physician 2000;62(2):409–16.
12. Gibbs CR, Davies MK, Lip GY. ABC of heart failure. Management: digoxin and other inotropes, beta blockers, and antiarrhythmic and antithrombotic treatment. BMJ 2000;320(7233):495–8.
13. Schwartz A, Lindenmayer GE, Allen JC. The sodium-potassium adenosine triphosphatase: pharmacological, physiological and biochemical aspects. Pharmacol Rev 1975;27(01):3–134.
14. Levitt B, Cagin N, Kleid J, Somberg J, Gillis R. Role of the nervous system in the genesis of cardiac rhythm disorders. Am J Cardiol 1976;37(7):1111–13.
15. Aronson JK, Ford AR. The use of colour vision measurement in the diagnosis of digoxin toxicity. Q J Med 1980;49(195):273–82.
16. Beller GA, Smith TW, Abelmann WH, Haber E, Hood WB Jr. Digitalis intoxication. A prospective clinical study with serum level correlations. N Engl J Med 1971;284(18):989–97.
17. Marik PE, Fromm L. A case series of hospitalized patients with elevated digoxin levels. Am J Med 1998;105(2):110–15.
18. Williamson KM, Thrasher KA, Fulton KB, LaPointe NM, Dunham GD, Cooper AA, Barrett PS, Patterson JH. Digoxin toxicity: an evaluation in current clinical practice. Arch Intern Med 1998;158(22):2444–9.
19. Onder G, Pedone C, Landi F, Cesari M, Della Vedova C, Bernabei R, Gambassi G. Adverse drug reactions as cause of hospital admissions: results from the Italian Group of Pharmacoepidemiology in the Elderly (GIFA). J Am Geriatr Soc 2002;50(12):1962–8.
20. Ahmed A, Allman RM, DeLong JF. Inappropriate use of digoxin in older hospitalized heart failure patients. J Gerontol A Biol Sci Med Sci 2002;57(2):M138–43.
21. Cooper JW. Adverse drug reaction-related hospitalizations of nursing facility patients: a 4-year study. South Med J 1999;92(5):485–90.
22. Joubert PH. Are all cardiac glycosides pharmacodynamically similar? Eur J Clin Pharmacol 1990;39(4):317–20.
23. Tucker AR, Ng KT. Digoxin-related impairment of learning and memory in cardiac patients. Psychopharmacology (Berl) 1983;81(1):86–8.
24. Wojtyna W, Enseleit F. A rare cause of complete heart block after transdermal botanical treatment for psoriasis. Pacing Clin Electrophysiol 2004;27(12):1686–8.
25. Haynes BE, Bessen HA, Wightman WD. Oleander tea: herbal draught of death. Ann Emerg Med 1985;14(4):350–3.
26. de Silva HA, Fonseka MM, Pathmeswaran A, Alahakone DG, Ratnatilake GA, Gunatilake SB, Ranasinha CD, Lalloo DG, Aronson JK, de Silva HJ. Multiple-dose activated charcoal for treatment of yellow oleander poisoning: a single-blind, randomised, placebo-controlled trial. Lancet 2003;361(9373):1935–8.
27. Tuncok Y, Kozan O, Cavdar C, Guven H, Fowler J. *Urginea maritima* (squill) toxicity. J Toxicol Clin Toxicol 1995;33(1):83–6.
28. Williams P, Aronson J, Sleight P. Is a slow pulse-rate a reliable sign of digitalis toxicity? Lancet 1978;2(8104–5):1340–2.
29. Hamer SS, Lemberg L. Digitalis excess mimicking the sick sinus syndrome. Heart Lung 1976;5(4):652–6.
30. Di Giacomo V, Carmenini G, Sciacca A. Su un caso di malattia del nodo del seno insorto in corso di trattamento digilatico. Progr Med 1977;33:775.
31. Margolis JR, Strauss HC, Miller HC, Gilbert M, Wallace AG. Digitalis and the sick sinus syndrome. Clinical and electrophysiologic documentation of severe toxic effect on sinus node function. Circulation 1975;52(1):162–9.
32. Engel TR, Schaal SF. Digitalis in the sick sinus syndrome. The effects of digitalis on sinoatrial automaticity and atrioventricular conduction. Circulation 1973;48(6):1201–7.
33. Vera Z, Miller RR, McMillin D, Mason DT. Effects of digitalis on sinus nodal function in patients with sick sinus syndrome. Am J Cardiol 1978;41(2):318–23.
34. Talley JD, Wathen MS, Hurst JW. Hyperthyroid-induced atrial flutter-fibrillation with profound sinoatrial nodal pauses due to small doses of digoxin, verapamil, and propranolol. Clin Cardiol 1989;12(1):45–7.
35. McCauley CS, Boller LR. Bradycardic responses to endotracheal suctioning. Crit Care Med 1988;16(11):1165–6.
36. Lown B, Wyatt NF, Levine HD. Paroxysmal atrial tachycardia with block. Circulation 1960;21:129–43.
37. Tawakkol AA, Nutter DO, Massumi RA. A prospective study of digitalis toxicity in a large city hospital. Med Ann Dist Columbia 1967;36(7):402–9.
38. Agarwal BL, Agrawal BV, Agarwal RK, Kansal SC. Atrial flutter. A rare manifestation of digitalis intoxication. Br Heart J 1972;34(4):392–5.
39. Spodick DH. Well concealed atrial tachycardia with Wenckebach (Mobitz I) atrioventricular block: digitalis toxicity. Am J Geriatr Cardiol 2001;10(1):59.
40. Barold SS, Hayes DL. Non-paroxysmal junctional tachycardia with type I exit block. Heart 2002;88(3):288.
41. Pellegrino L. Ritmo idioventriculare accelerato da intoxicazione digitalica. Studio clinico ed elettrocardiografico su due casi. [Accelerated idioventricular rhythm in patients with digitalic intoxication. Clinical and electrocardiographic study of two cases.] G Ital Cardiol 1976;6(3):527–31.
42. Castellanos A, Shin EK, Luceri RM, Myerburg RJ. Parasystolic accelerated idioventricular rhythms producing bidirectional tachycardia patterns. J Electrophysiol 1988;2:296.
43. Deal BJ, Keane JF, Gillette PC, Garson A Jr. Wolff-Parkinson–White syndrome and supraventricular tachycardia during infancy: management and follow-up. J Am Coll Cardiol 1985;5(1):130–5.

44. Pfammatter JP, Stocker FP. Re-entrant supraventricular tachycardia in infancy: current role of prophylactic digoxin treatment. Eur J Pediatr 1998;157(2):101–6.
45. Sanatani S, Saul JP, Walsh EP, Gross GJ. Spontaneously terminating apparent ventricular fibrillation during trans-esophageal electrophysiological testing in infants with Wolff-Parkinson-White syndrome. Pacing Clin Electrophysiol 2001;24(12):1816–18.
46. Lehmann HU, Witt E, Hochrein H. Zunahme von Angina pectoris und ST-Strecken-Senkung im EKG durch Digitalis (Koronare Funktionsuntersuchungen bei Gesunden und Koranarkranken ohne Herzinsuffizienz mittels rechtsatrialer Frequenzstimulation). [Digitalis-induced increase in angina pectoris and segment depression on electrocardiograms (Investigations of coronary function of healthy subjects and of coronary patients without cardiac insufficiency by means of atrial pacing).] Z Kardiol 1978;67(1):57–66.
47. Singh RB, Agrawal BV, Somani PN. Left bundle branch block: a rare manifestation of digitalis intoxication. Acta Cardiol 1976;31(2):175–9.
48. Gould L, Patel C, Betzu R, Judge D, Lee J. Right bundle branch block: a rare manifestation of digitalis toxicity—case report. Angiology 1986;37(7):543–6.
49. Ma G, Brady WJ, Pollack M, Chan TC. Electrocardiographic manifestations: digitalis toxicity. J Emerg Med 2001;20(2):145–52.
50. Von Capeller D, Copeland GD, Stern TN. Digitalis intoxication: a clinical report of 148 cases. Ann Intern Med 1959;50(4):869–78.
51. Somlyo AP. The toxicology of digitalis. Am J Cardiol 1960;5:523–33.
52. Braunwald E, Bloodwell RD, Goldberg LI, Morrow AG. Studies on digitalis. IV. Observations in man on the effects of digitalis preparations on the contractility of the non-failing heart and on total vascular resistance. J Clin Invest 1961;40:52–9.
53. Teske RH, Bishop SP, Righter HF, Detweiler DK. Subacute digoxin toxicosis in the beagle dog. Toxicol Appl Pharmacol 1976;35(2):283–301.
54. Varonkov Y, Shell WE, Smirnov V, Gukovsky D, Chazov EI. Augmentation of serum CPK activity by digitalis in patients with acute myocardial infarction. Circulation 1977;55(5):719–27.
55. Nolte CW, Jost S, Mugge A, Daniel WG. Protection from digoxin-induced coronary vasoconstriction in patients with coronary artery disease by calcium antagonists. Am J Cardiol 1999;83(3):440–2.
56. Balcon R, Hoy J, Sowton E. Haemodynamic effects of rapid digitalization following acute myocardial infarction. Br Heart J 1968;30(3):373–6.
57. Scheinost ME. Digoxin toxicity in a 26-year-old woman taking a herbal dietary supplement. J Am Osteopath Assoc 2001;101(8):444–6.
58. Eaker ED, Kronmal R, Kennedy JW, Davis K. Comparison of the long-term, postsurgical survival of women and men in the Coronary Artery Surgery Study (CASS). Am Heart J 1989;117(1):71–81.
59. Ross DL, Davis KB, Pettinger MB, Alderman EL, Killip T, Mason JW. Features of cardiac arrest episodes with and without acute myocardial infarction in the Coronary Artery Surgery Study (CASS). Am J Cardiol 1987;60(16):1219–24.
60. Casiglia E, Tikhonoff V, Pizziol A, Onesto C, Ginocchio G, Mazza A, Pessina AC. Should digoxin be proscribed in elderly subjects in sinus rhythm free from heart failure? A population-based study. Jpn Heart J 1998;39(5):639–51.
61. The Digitalis Investigation Group. The effect of digoxin on mortality and morbidity in patients with heart failure. N Engl J Med 1997;336(8):525–33.
62. Soler-Soler J, Permanyer-Miralda G. Should we still prescribe digoxin in mild-to-moderate heart failure? Is quality of life the issue rather than quantity? Eur Heart J 1998;19(Suppl P):P26–31.
63. Atarashi H, Inoue H, Fukunami M, Sugi K, Hamada C, Origasa H; Sinus Rhythm Maintenance in Atrial Fibrillation Randomized Trial (SMART) Investigators. Double-blind placebo-controlled trial of aprindine and digoxin for the prevention of symptomatic atrial fibrillation. Circ J 2002;66(6):553–6.
64. Deglin S, Deglin J, Chung EK. Direct current shock and digitalis therapy. Drug Intell Clin Pharm 1977;11:76.
65. Ali N, Dais K, Banks T, Sheikh M. Titrated electrical cardioversion in patients on digoxin. Clin Cardiol 1982;5(7):417–19.
66. Lely AH, van Enter CH. Large-scale digitoxin intoxication. BMJ 1970;3(725):737–40.
67. Lely AH, van Enter CH. Non-cardiac symptoms of digitalis intoxication. Am Heart J 1972;83(2):149–52.
68. Miller S, Forker AD. Digitalis toxicity. Neurologic manifestations. J Kans Med Soc 1974;75(8):263–4.
69. Kerr DJ, Elliott HL, Hillis WS. Epileptiform seizures and electroencephalographic abnormalities as manifestations of digoxin toxicity. BMJ (Clin Res Ed) 1982;284(6310):162–3.
70. Douglas EF, White PT, Nelson JW. Three per second spike-wave in digitalis toxicity. Report of a case. Arch Neurol 1971;25(4):373–5.
71. Greenlee JE, Crampton RS, Miller JQ. Transient global amnesia associated with cardiac arrhythmia and digitalis intoxication. Stroke 1975;6(5):513–16.
72. Bernat JL, Sullivan JK. Trigeminal neuralgia from digitalis intoxication. JAMA 1979;241(2):164.
73. Batterman RC, Guter LB. Hitherto undescribed neurological manifestations of digitalis toxicity. Am Heart J 1984;36:582–6.
74. Brezis M, Michaeli J, Hamburger R. Nightmares from digoxin. Ann Intern Med 1980;93(4):639–40.
75. Eisendrath SJ, Gershengorn KN, Unger R. Digoxin-induced organic brain syndrome. Am Heart J 1983;106(2):419–20.
76. Greenaway JR, Abuaisha B, Bramble MG. Digoxin toxicity presenting as encephalopathy. Postgrad Med J 1996;72(848):367–8.
77. Eberhard SM, Woolley S, Zellweger U. Adynamie und Apathie bei Digitalisintoxikation. [Powerlessness and apathy in digitalis intoxication.] Schweiz Rundsch Med Prax 1999;88(17):772–4.
78. Mulder LJ, van der Mast RC, Meerwaldt JD. Generalised chorea due to digoxin toxicity. BMJ (Clin Res Ed) 1988;296(6631):1262. Erratum in: BMJ (Clin Res Ed) 1988;297(6647):562.
79. Sekul EA, Kaminer S, Sethi KD. Digoxin-induced chorea in a child. Mov Disord 1999;14(5):877–9.
80. Lawrenson JG, Kelly C, Lawrenson AL, Birch J. Acquired colour vision deficiency in patients receiving digoxin maintenance therapy. Br J Ophthalmol 2002; 86(11):1259–61.
81. Singh RB, Singh VP, Somani PN. Psychosis: a rare manifestation of digoxin intoxication. J Indian Med Assoc 1977;69(3):62–3.
82. Shear MK, Sacks MH. Digitalis delirium: report of two cases. Am J Psychiatry 1978;135(1):109–10; Digitalis delirium: psychiatric considerations Int J Psychiatry Med 1977–78;8(4):371–81.
83. Portnoi VA. Digitalis delirium in elderly patients. J Clin Pharmacol 1979;19(11–12):747–50.
84. Gorelick DA, Kussin SZ, Kahn I. Paranoid delusions and auditory hallucinations associated with digoxin intoxication. J Nerv Ment Dis 1978;166(11):817–19.

85. Volpe BT, Soave R. Formed visual hallucinations as digitalis toxicity. Ann Intern Med 1979;91(6):865–6.
86. Kardels B, Beine KH. Acute delirium as a result of digitalis intoxication. Notf Med 2001;27:542–5.
87. Wamboldt FS, Jefferson JW, Wamboldt MZ. Digitalis intoxication misdiagnosed as depression by primary care physicians. Am J Psychiatry 1986;143(2):219–21.
88. Song YH, Terao T, Shiraishi Y, Nakamura J. Digitalis intoxication misdiagnosed as depression—revisited. Psychosomatics 2001;42(4):369–70.
89. Donat J, Jirkalova V, Havel V, Mikulecka D. Kotazce estrogenniho ucinku digitalisu u zen po menopauze. [On the question of the estrogenic effect of digitalis in women after menopause.] Cesk Gynekol 1980;45(1):19–23.
90. Burckhardt D, Vera CA, LaDue JS. Effect of digitalis on urinary pituitary gonadotrophine excretion. A study in postmenopausal women. Ann Intern Med 1968;68(5):1069–71.
91. Stoffer SS, Hynes KM, Jiang NS, Ryan RJ. Digoxin and abnormal serum hormone levels. JAMA 1973;225(13):1643–4.
92. Neri A, Aygen M, Zukerman Z, Bahary C. Subjective assessment of sexual dysfunction of patients on long-term administration of digoxin. Arch Sex Behav 1980;9(4):343–7.
93. LeWinn EB. Gynecomastia during digitalis therapy; report of eight additional cases with liver-function studies. N Engl J Med 1953;248(8):316–20.
94. Calov WL, Whyte MH. Oedema and mammary hypertrophy: a toxic effect of digitalis leaf. Med J Aust 1954;41(1:15):556–7.
95. Navab A, Koss LG, LaDue JS. Estrogen-like activity of digitalis: its effect on the squamous epithelium of the female genital tract. JAMA 1965;194(1):30–2.
96. Stenkvist B, Bengtsson E, Eklund G, Eriksson O, Holmquist J, Nordin B, Westman-Naeser S. Evidence of a modifying influence of heart glucosides on the development of breast cancer. Anal Quant Cytol 1980;2(1):49–54.
97. Stenkvist B, Pengtsson E, Dahlqvist B, Eriksson O, Jarkrans T, Nordin B. Cardiac glycosides and breast cancer, revisited. N Engl J Med 1982;306(8):484.
98. Haux J, Lam M, Marthinsen ABL, Strickert T, Lundgren S. Digitoxin, in non toxic concentrations, induces apoptotic cell death in Jurkat cells in vitro. Z Onkol 1999;31:14–20.
99. Haux J. Digitoxin is a potential anticancer agent for several types of cancer. Med Hypotheses 1999;53(6):543–8.
100. Haux J, Solheim O, Isaksen T, Anglesen A. Digitoxin, in non toxic concentrations, inhibits proliferation and induces cell death in prostate cancer cell line. Z Onkol 2000;32:11–16.
101. Nobel CS, Aronson JK, van den Dobbelsteen DJ, Slater AF. Inhibition of Na+/K(+)-ATPase may be one mechanism contributing to potassium efflux and cell shrinkage in CD95-induced apoptosis. Apoptosis 2000;5(2):153–63.
102. Johansson S, Lindholm P, Gullbo J, Larsson R, Bohlin L, Claeson P. Cytotoxicity of digitoxin and related cardiac glycosides in human tumor cells. Anticancer Drugs 2001;12(5):475–83.
103. Spigset O, Mjorndal T. Increased glucose intolerance related to digoxin treatment in patients with type 2 diabetes mellitus. J Intern Med 1999;246(4):419–22.
104. Hannerz J. Decrease of intracranial pressure and weight with digoxin in obesity. J Clin Pharmacol 2001;41(4):465–8.
105. Karpatkin S. Drug-induced thrombocytopenia. Am J Med Sci 1971;262(2):68–78.
106. Schneider AW, Gilfrich HJ, Fechler L. Thrombozytopenie bei Digitoxin-Intoxikation. [Thrombocytopenia in digitoxin poisoning.] Dtsch Med Wochenschr 1992;117(9):337–40.
107. Pirovino M, Ohnhaus EE, von Felten A. Digoxin-associated thrombocytopaenia. Eur J Clin Pharmacol 1981;19(3):205–7.
108. Forzy P, Joram F. Thrombopénie sévère en rapport avec une intoxication a l'acétyl digitoxine. Sem Hop Paris 1989;65:235–6.
109. Almeyda J, Levantine A. Cutaneous reactions to cardiovascular drugs. Br J Dermatol 1973;88(3):313–19.
110. Holt DW, Volans GN. Gastrointestinal symptoms of digoxin toxicity. BMJ 1977;2(6088):704.
111. Willems J, De Geest H. Digitalis intoxicatie. Ned Tijdschr Geneeskd 1968;24:617.
112. Kelton JG, Scullin DC. Digitalis toxicity manifested by dysphagia. JAMA 1978;239(7):613–14.
113. Cordeiro MF, Arnold KG. Digoxin toxicity presenting as dysphagia and dysphonia. BMJ 1991;302(6783):1025.
114. Adar R, Salzman EW. Letter: Intestinal ischemia and digitalis. JAMA 1974;229(12):1577.
115. Bourhis F, Riard P, Danel V, Hostein J, Fournet J. Intoxication digitalique avec ischémie colique grave: évolution favorable après traitement par anticorps spécifiques. [Digitalis poisoning with severe ischemic colitis: a favorable course after treatment with specific antibodies.] Gastroenterol Clin Biol 1990;14(1):95.
116. Guglielminotti J, Tremey B, Maury E, Alzieu M, Offenstadt G. Fatal non-occlusive mesenteric infarction following digoxin intoxication. Intensive Care Med 2000;26(6):829.
117. Lindsay SJ, Kearney MT, Prescott RJ, Fox KA, Nolan J. Digoxin and mortality in chronic heart failure. UK Heart Investigation. Lancet 1999;354(9183):1003.
118. Spargias KS, Hall AS, Ball SG. Safety concerns about digoxin after acute myocardial infarction. Lancet 1999;354(9176):391–2.
119. Cosin-Aguilar J, Marrugat J, Sanz G, Masso J, Gil M, Vargas R, Perez-Casar F, Simarro E, De Armas D, Garcia-Garcia J, Azpitarte J, Diago JL, Rodrigo-Trallero G, Lekuona I, Domingo E, Marin-Huerta E. Long-term results of the Spanish trial on treatment and survival of patients with predominantly mild heart failure. J Cardiovasc Pharmacol 1999;33(5):733–40.
120. Fauchier L, Babuty D, Cosnay P, Fauchier JP. Digoxin and mortality in idiopathic dilated cardiomyopathy. Eur Heart J 2000;21(10):858–9.
121. Heninger MM. Commonly encountered prescription medications in medical-legal death investigation: a guide for death investigators and medical examiners. Am J Forensic Med Pathol 2000;21(3):287–99.
122. Chyka PA. How many deaths occur annually from adverse drug reactions in the United States? Am J Med 2000;109(2):122–30.
123. Rathore SS, Wang Y, Krumholz HM. Sex-based differences in the effect of digoxin for the treatment of heart failure. N Engl J Med 2002;347(18):1403–11.
124. Eichhorn EJ, Gheorghiade M. Digoxin—new perspective on an old drug. N Engl J Med 2002;347(18):1394–5.
125. Rathore SS, Curtis JP, Wang Y, Bristow MR, Krumholz HM. Association of serum digoxin concentration and outcomes in patients with heart failure. JAMA 2003;289(7):871–8.
126. Sameri RM, Soberman JE, Finch CK, Self TH. Lower serum digoxin concentrations in heart failure and reassessment of laboratory report forms. Am J Med Sci 2002; 324(1):10–13.
127. Hern WM, Zen C, Ferguson KA, Hart V, Haseman MV. Outpatient abortion for fetal anomaly and fetal death from 15–34 menstrual weeks' gestation: techniques and clinical management. Obstet Gynecol 1993;81(2):301–6.
128. Jackson RA, Teplin VL, Drey EA, Thomas LJ, Darney PD. Digoxin to facilitate late second-trimester abortion: a randomized, masked, placebo-controlled trial. Obstet Gynecol 2001;97(3):471–6.
129. Drey EA, Thomas LJ, Benowitz NL, Goldschlager N, Darney PD. Safety of intra-amniotic digoxin administration before late second-trimester abortion by dilation and evacuation. Am J Obstet Gynecol 2000;182(5):1063–6.

130. Aronson JK. Clinical pharmacokinetics of digoxin. Clin Pharmacokinet 1980;5(2):137–49.
131. Rotmensch HH, Rotmensch S, Elkayam U. Management of cardiac arrhythmias during pregnancy. Current concepts. Drugs 1987;33(6):623–33.
132. Nishimura H, Tanimura T. Clinical Aspects of the Teratogenicity of Drugs. Amsterdam: Excerpta Medica, 1976.
133. Miura T, Kojima R, Sugiura Y, Mizutani M, Takatsu F, Suzuki Y. Effect of aging on the incidence of digoxin toxicity. Ann Pharmacother 2000;34(4):427–32.
134. Roever C, Ferrante J, Gonzalez EC, Pal N, Roetzheim RG. Comparing the toxicity of digoxin and digitoxin in a geriatric population: should an old drug be rediscovered? South Med J 2000;93(2):199–202.
135. Aronson JK. Book review: Handbook of renal-independent cardiac glycosides: pharmacology and clinical pharmacology, by N Rietbrock and BG Woodcock. Lancet 1989;2:1130–1.
136. Lecointre K, Pisante L, Fauvelle F, Mazouz S. Digoxin toxicity evaluation in clinical practice with pharmacokinetic correlations. Clin Drug Invest 2001;21:225–32.
137. Rich MW, McSherry F, Williford WO, Yusuf S; Digitalis Investigation Group. Effect of age on mortality, hospitalizations and response to digoxin in patients with heart failure: the DIG study. J Am Coll Cardiol 2001; 38(3):806–13.
138. Steinberg C, Notterman DA. Pharmacokinetics of cardiovascular drugs in children. Inotropes and vasopressors. Clin Pharmacokinet 1994;27(5):345–67.
139. Kearin M, Kelly JG, O'Malley K. Digoxin "receptors" in neonates: an explanation of less sensitivity to digoxin than in adults. Clin Pharmacol Ther 1980;28(3):346–9.
140. Johnson GL, Desai NS, Pauly TH, Cunningham MD. Complications associated with digoxin therapy in low-birth weight infants. Pediatrics 1982;69(4):463–5.
141. Hastreiter AR, van der Horst RL, Chow-Tung E. Digitalis toxicity in infants and children. Pediatr Cardiol 1984; 5(2):131–48.
142. Suematsu F, Minemoto M, Yukawa E, Higuchi S. Population analysis for the optimization of digoxin treatment in Japanese paediatric patients. J Clin Pharm Ther 1999;24(3):203–8.
143. Suematsu F, Yukawa E, Yukawa M, Minemoto M, Ohdo S, Higuchi S, Goto Y. Population-based investigation of relative clearance of digoxin in Japanese neonates and infants by multiple-trough screen analysis. Eur J Clin Pharmacol 2001;57(1):19–24.
144. Aronson JK. Digoxin: clinical aspects. In: Richens A, Marks V, editors. Therapeutic Drug Monitoring. London, Edinburgh: Churchill-Livingstone, 1981:404.
145. Shenfield GM. Influence of thyroid dysfunction on drug pharmacokinetics. Clin Pharmacokinet 1981;6(4):275–97.
146. Aronson JK. Clinical pharmacokinetics of cardiac glycosides in patients with renal dysfunction. Clin Pharmacokinet 1983;8(2):155–78.
147. Brater DC, Morrelli HF. Digoxin toxicity in patients with normokalemic potassium depletion. Clin Pharmacol Ther 1977;22(1):21–33.
148. Young IS, Goh EM, McKillop UH, Stanford CF, Nicholls DP, Trimble ER. Magnesium status and digoxin toxicity. Br J Clin Pharmacol 1991;32(6):717–21.
149. Piergies AA, Worwag EM, Atkinson AJ Jr. A concurrent audit of high digoxin plasma levels. Clin Pharmacol Ther 1994;55(3):353–8.
150. Hamer J. The paradox of the lack of the efficacy of digitalis in congestive heart failure with sinus rhythm. Br J Clin Pharmacol 1979;8(2):109–13.
151. Hagemeijer F, Van Houwe E. Titrated energy cardioversion of patients on digitalis. Br Heart J 1975; 37(12):1303–7.
152. Vella A, Gerber TC, Hayes DL, Reeder GS. Digoxin, hypercalcaemia, and cardiac conduction. Postgrad Med J 1999;75(887):554–6.
153. Slifman NR, Obermeyer WR, Aloi BK, Musser SM, Correll WA Jr, Cichowicz SM, Betz JM, Love LA. Contamination of botanical dietary supplements by *Digitalis lanata.* N Engl J Med 1998;339(12):806–11.
154. Andersen KE, Damsgaard T. The effect on serum enzymes of intramuscular injections of digoxin, bumetanide, pentazocine and isotonic sodium chloride. Acta Med Scand 1976;199(4):317–19.
155. Lewis WS, Doherty JE. Another disadvantage of intramuscular digoxin. N Engl J Med 1973;288(20):1077.
156. Tisdale JE, Padhi ID, Goldberg AD, Silverman NA, Webb CR, Higgins RS, Paone G, Frank DM, Borzak S. A randomized, double-blind comparison of intravenous diltiazem and digoxin for atrial fibrillation after coronary artery bypass surgery. Am Heart J 1998;135(5 Pt 1):739–47.
157. Bismuth C, Gaultier M, Conso F, Efthymiou ML. Hyperkalemia in acute digitalis poisoning: prognostic significance and therapeutic implications. Clin Toxicol 1973;6(2):153–62.
158. Gittelman MA, Stephan M, Perry H. Acute pediatric digoxin ingestion. Pediatr Emerg Care 1999;15(5):359–62.
159. Lacassie E, Marquet P, Martin-Dupont S, Gaulier JM, Lachatre G. A non-fatal case of intoxication with foxglove, documented by means of liquid chromatography–electrospray-mass spectrometry. J Forensic Sci 2000;45(5):1154–8.
160. American Academy of Clinical Toxicology; European Association of Poisons Centres and Clinical Toxicologists. Position statement and practice guidelines on the use of multi-dose activated charcoal in the treatment of acute poisoning. J Toxicol Clin Toxicol 1999;37(6):731–51.
161. Lalonde RL, Deshpande R, Hamilton PP, McLean WM, Greenway DC. Acceleration of digoxin clearance by activated charcoal. Clin Pharmacol Ther 1985;37(4):367–71.
162. Chyka PA, Holley JE, Mandrell TD, Sugathan P. Correlation of drug pharmacokinetics and effectiveness of multiple-dose activated charcoal therapy. Ann Emerg Med 1995;25(3):356–62.
163. Park GD, Goldberg MJ, Spector R, Johnson GF, Feldman RD, Quee CK, Roberts P. The effects of activated charcoal on digoxin and digitoxin clearance. Drug Intell Clin Pharm 1985;19(12):937–41.
164. Reissell P, Manninen V. Effect of administration of activated charcoal and fibre on absorption, excretion and steady state blood levels of digoxin and digitoxin. Evidence for intestinal secretion of the glycosides. Acta Med Scand Suppl 1982;668:88–90.
165. Ibanez C, Carcas AJ, Frias J, Abad F. Activated charcoal increases digoxin elimination in patients. Int J Cardiol 1995;48(1):27–30.
166. Boldy DA, Smart V, Vale JA. Multiple doses of charcoal in digoxin poisoning. Lancet 1985;2(8463):1076–7.
167. Lake KD, Brown DC, Peterson CD. Digoxin toxicity: enhanced systemic elimination during oral activated charcoal therapy. Pharmacotherapy 1984;4(3):161–3.
168. Critchley JA, Critchley LA. Digoxin toxicity in chronic renal failure: treatment by multiple dose activated charcoal intestinal dialysis. Hum Exp Toxicol 1997;16(12):733–5.
169. Pond S, Jacobs M, Marks J, Garner J, Goldschlager N, Hansen D. Treatment of digitoxin overdose with oral activated charcoal. Lancet 1981;2(8256):1177–8.
170. Papadakis MA, Wexman MP, Fraser C, Sedlacek SM. Hyperkalemia complicating digoxin toxicity in a patient with renal failure. Am J Kidney Dis 1985;5(1):64–6.
171. Lopez-Gomez D, Valdovinos P, Comin-Colet J, Esteve F, Sabate X, Esplugas E. Intoxicación grave por digoxina. Utilización exitosa del tratamiento clásico. [Severe digoxin

poisoning. The successful use of the classic treatment.] Rev Esp Cardiol 2000;53(3):471–2.
172. Roberge RJ, Sorensen T. Congestive heart failure and toxic digoxin levels: role of cholestyramine. Vet Hum Toxicol 2000;42(3):172–3.
173. Ahee P, Crowe AV. The management of hyperkalaemia in the emergency department. J Accid Emerg Med 2000;17(3):188–91.
174. Davey M. Calcium for hyperkalaemia in digoxin toxicity. Emerg Med J 2002;19(2):183.
175. Lapostolle F, Adnet F, Baud F, Lapandry C. Intoxications digitaliques: l'antidote existe. Rev Prat Med Gen 2000;14:345–7.
176. Safadi R, Levy I, Amitai Y, Caraco Y. Beneficial effect of digoxin-specific Fab antibody fragments in oleander intoxication. Arch Intern Med 1995;155(19):2121–5.
177. Shumaik GM, Wu AW, Ping AC. Oleander poisoning: treatment with digoxin-specific Fab antibody fragments. Ann Emerg Med 1988;17(7):732–5.
178. Eddleston M, Rajapakse S, Rajakanthan, Jayalath S, Sjostrom L, Santharaj W, Thenabadu PN, Sheriff MH, Warrell DA. Anti-digoxin Fab fragments in cardiotoxicity induced by ingestion of yellow oleander: a randomised controlled trial. Lancet 2000;355(9208):967–72.
179. Gonzalez Andres VL. Revisión sistemática sobre la efectividad e indicaciones de los anticuerpos antidigoxina en la intoxicación digitálica. [Systematic review of the effectiveness and indications of antidigoxin antibodies in the treatment of digitalis intoxication.] Rev Esp Cardiol 2000;53(1):49–58.
180. Laurent G, Poulet B, Falcon-Eicher S, Petit A, Ballout J, Iovescu D, Gouyon JB, Louis P. Anticorps antidigoxine au cours d'une intoxication digitalique sévère chez un nouveau-né de 11 jours. Revue de la litterature. [Anti-digoxin antibodies in severe digitalis poisoning in an 11-day old infant. Review of the literature.] Ann Cardiol Angeiol (Paris) 2001;50(5):274–84.
181. Eddleston M, Senarathna L, Mohamed F, Buckley N, Juszczak E, Sheriff MH, Ariaratnam A, Rajapakse S, Warrell D, Rajakanthan K. Deaths due to absence of an affordable antitoxin for plant poisoning. Lancet 2003;362(9389):1041–4.
182. Erdmann E, Mair W, Knedel M, Schaumann W. Digitalis intoxication and treatment with digoxin antibody fragments in renal failure. Klin Wochenschr 1989;67(1):16–19.
183. Clifton GD, McIntyre WJ, Zannikos PN, Harrison MR, Chandler MH. Free and total serum digoxin concentrations in a renal failure patient after treatment with digoxin immune Fab. Clin Pharm 1989;8(6):441–5.
184. Proudfoot AT. A star treatment for digoxin overdose? BMJ (Clin Res Ed) 1986;293(6548):642–3.
185. Butler VP Jr, Smith TW. Immunologic treatment of digitalis toxicity: a tale of two prophecies. Ann Intern Med 1986;105(4):613–14.
186. Robinson CP. Digoxin immune Fab (ovine). Drugs Future 1986;11:922–6.
187. Aronson J. Digitalis intoxication and its treatment. Top Circ 1987;2:9–12.
188. Thompson CA. FDA approves digoxin-toxicity remedy. Am J Health Syst Pharm 2001;58(21):2021.
189. Kelly RA, Smith TW. Recognition and management of digitalis toxicity. Am J Cardiol 1992;69(18):G108–18.
190. Zdunek M, Mitra A, Mokrzycki MH. Plasma exchange for the removal of digoxin-specific antibody fragments in renal failure: timing is important for maximizing clearance. Am J Kidney Dis 2000;36(1):177–83.
191. Krynicki R, Szumski B, Perkowska J, Dyduszynski A. Digitalis intoxication complicated by recurrent ventricular fibrillation and successfully treated with bretylium tosylate—a case report. Kardiol Pol 1999;50:230–4.
192. Kaneko T, Kudo M, Okumura T, Kasiwagi T, Turuoka S, Simizu M, Iino Y, Katayama Y. Successful treatment of digoxin intoxication by haemoperfusion with specific columns for beta$_2$-microgloblin-adsorption (Lixelle) in a maintenance haemodialysis patient. Nephrol Dial Transplant 2001;16(1):195–6.
193. Tsuruoka S, Osono E, Nishiki K, Kawaguchi A, Arai T, Furuyoshi S, Saito T, Takata S, Sugimoto K, Kurihara S, Fujimura A. Removal of digoxin by column for specific adsorption of beta(2)-microglobulin: a potential use for digoxin intoxication. Clin Pharmacol Ther 2001; 69(6):422–30.
194. Rabetoy GM, Price CA, Findlay JW, Sailstad JM. Treatment of digoxin intoxication in a renal failure patient with digoxin-specific antibody fragments and plasmapheresis. Am J Nephrol 1990;10(6):518–21.
195. Chillet P, Korach JM, Petitpas D, Vincent N, Poiron L, Barbier B, Boazis M, Berger PH. Digoxin poisoning and anuric acute renal failure: efficiency of the treatment associating digoxin-specific antibodies (Fab) and plasma exchanges. Int J Artif Organs 2002;25(6):538–41.
196. Binnion PF. Drug interactions with digitalis glycosides. Drugs 1978;15(5):369–80.
197. Brown DD, Spector R, Juhl RP. Drug interactions with digoxin. Drugs 1980;20(3):198–206.
198. Lampe D, Lampe H, Banaschak H. Arzneimittelwechselwirkungen mit Herzglykosiden. Dtsch Gesundheitsw 1980;35:1081–7.
199. Belz GG, Breithaupt-Grogler K, Osowski U. Treatment of congestive heart failure—current status of use of digitoxin. Eur J Clin Invest 2001;31(Suppl 2):10–17.
200. Bazzano G, Bazzano GS. Digitalis intoxication. Treatment with a new steroid-binding resin. JAMA 1972;220(6):828–30.
201. Fresard F, Balant L, Noble J, Garcia B, Muller AF. Choléstyramine et intoxication a la digoxine: éfficacité therapeutique? [Cholestyramine and digoxin intoxication: therapeutic efficacy?] Schweiz Med Wochenschr 1979;109(12):431–6.
202. Kuhlmann J, Zilly W, Wilke J. Effects of cytostatic drugs on plasma level and renal excretion of beta-acetyldigoxin. Clin Pharmacol Ther 1981;30(4):518–27.
203. Kuhlmann J, Wilke J, Rietbrock N. Cytostatic drugs are without significant effect on digitoxin plasma level and renal excretion. Clin Pharmacol Ther 1982;32(5): 646–51.
204. Manninen V, Apajalahti A, Melin J, Karesoja M. Altered absorption of digoxin in patients given propantheline and metoclopramide. Lancet 1973;1(7800):398–400.
205. Kirch W, Janisch HD, Santos SR, Duhrsen U, Dylewicz P, Ohnhaus EE. Effect of cisapride and metoclopramide on digoxin bioavailability. Eur J Drug Metab Pharmacokinet 1986;11(4):249–50.
206. D'Arcy PF, McElnay JC. Drug–antacid interactions: assessment of clinical importance. Drug Intell Clin Pharm 1987;21(7–8):607–17.
207. Lohman JJ, Merkus FW. Plasma protein binding of digitoxin and some other drugs in renal disease. Pharm Weekbl Sci 1987;9(2): 75–8.
208. Woodland C, Ito S, Koren G. A model for the prediction of digoxin-drug interactions at the renal tubular cell level. Ther Drug Monit 1998;20(2):134–8.
209. Yukawa E, Suematu F, Yukawa M, Minemoto M, Ohdo S, Higuchi S, Goto Y, Aoyama T. Population pharmacokinetics of digoxin in Japanese patients: a 2-compartment pharmacokinetic model. Clin Pharmacokinet 2001;40(10):773–81.
210. Nakamura T, Kakumoto M, Yamashita K, Takara K, Tanigawara Y, Sakaeda T, Okumura K. Factors influencing the prediction of steady state concentrations of digoxin. Biol Pharm Bull 2001;24(4):403–8.

211. Shapiro W. Correlative studies of serum digitalis levels and the arrhythmias of digitalis intoxication. Am J Cardiol 1978;41(5):852–9.
212. Steiness E. Suppression of renal excretion of digoxin in hypokalemic patients. Clin Pharmacol Ther 1978;23(5):511–14.
213. Storstein O, Hansteen V, Hatle L, Hillestad L, Storstein L. Studies on digitalis. XIII. A prospective study of 649 patients on maintenance treatment with digitoxin. Am Heart J 1977;93(4):434–43.
214. Chopra D, Janson P, Sawin CT. Insensitivity to digoxin associated with hypocalcemia. N Engl J Med 1977;296(16):917–18.
215. Ben-Ami H, Krivoy N, Nagachandran P, Roguin A, Edoute Y. An interaction between digoxin and acarbose. Diabetes Care 1999;22(5):860–1.
216. Nagai Y, Hayakawa T, Abe T, Nomura G. Are there different effects of acarbose and voglibose on serum levels of digoxin in a diabetic patient with congestive heart failure? Diabetes Care 2000;23(11):1703.
217. Serrano JS, Jimenez CM, Serrano MI, Balboa B. A possible interaction of potential clinical interest between digoxin and acarbose. Clin Pharmacol Ther 1996;60(5):589–92.
218. Miura T, Ueno K, Tanaka K, Sugiura Y, Mizutani M, Takatsu F, Takano Y, Shibakawa M. Impairment of absorption of digoxin by acarbose. J Clin Pharmacol 1998;38(7):654–7.
219. Cohen E, Almog S, Staruvin D, Garty M. Do therapeutic doses of acarbose alter the pharmacokinetics of digoxin? Isr Med Assoc J 2002;4(10):772–5.
220. Kusumoto M, Ueno K, Fujimura Y, Kameda T, Mashimo K, Takeda K, Tatami R, Shibakawa M. Lack of kinetic interaction between digoxin and voglibose. Eur J Clin Pharmacol 1999;55(1):79–80.
221. Lelarge P, Bauer P, Royer-Morrot MJ, Meregnani JL, Larcan A, Lambert H. Intoxication digitalique après administration conjointe d'acétyl digitoxine et d'amiodarone. Ann Med Nancy Est 1993;32:307.
222. Laer S, Scholz H, Buschmann I, Thoenes M, Meinertz T. Digitoxin intoxication during concomitant use of amiodarone. Eur J Clin Pharmacol 1998;54(1):95–6.
223. Fraley DS, Britton HL, Schwinghammer TL, Kalla R. Effect of cimetidine on steady-state serum digoxin concentrations. Clin Pharm 1983;2(2):163–5.
224. Oosterhuis B, Jonkman JH, Andersson T, Zuiderwijk PB, Jedema JN. Minor effect of multiple dose omeprazole on the pharmacokinetics of digoxin after a single oral dose. Br J Clin Pharmacol 1991;32(5):569–72.
225. Doering W. Quinidine-digoxin interaction: Pharmacokinetics, underlying mechanism and clinical implications. N Engl J Med 1979;301(8):400–4.
226. Antman EM, Arnold M, Friedman PL, White H, Bosak M, Smith TW. Drug interactions with cardiac glycosides: evaluation of a possible digoxin–ethmozine pharmacokinetic interaction. J Cardiovasc Pharmacol 1987;9(5):622–7.
227. Alderman CP, Jersmann HP. Digoxin–itraconazole interaction. Med J Aust 1993;159(11–12):838–9.
228. Sachs MK, Blanchard LM, Green PJ. Interaction of itraconazole and digoxin. Clin Infect Dis 1993;16(3):400–3.
229. Lomaestro BM, Piatek MA. Update on drug interactions with azole antifungal agents. Ann Pharmacother 1998;32(9):915–28.
230. Salphati L, Benet LZ. Effects of ketoconazole on digoxin absorption and disposition in rat. Pharmacology 1998;56(6):308–13.
231. Brodell RT, Elewski B. Antifungal drug interactions. Avoidance requires more than memorization. Postgrad Med 2000;107(1):41–3.
232. Mochizuki M, Murase S, Takahashi K, Shimada S, Kume H, Iizuka T, Fukuda M. Serum itraconazole and hydroxyitraconazole concentrations and interaction with digoxin in a case of chronic hypertrophic pachymenigitis caused by *Aspergillus flavus*. Nippon Ishinkin Gakkai Zasshi 2000;41(1):33–9.
233. Mathis AS, Friedman GS. Coadministration of digoxin with itraconazole in renal transplant recipients. Am J Kidney Dis 2001;37(2):E18.
234. Jalava KM, Partanen J, Neuvonen PJ. Itraconazole decreases renal clearance of digoxin. Ther Drug Monit 1997;19(6):609–13.
235. Nishihara K, Hibino J, Kotaki H, Sawada Y, Iga T. Effect of itraconazole on the pharmacokinetics of digoxin in guinea pigs. Biopharm Drug Dispos 1999;20(3):145–9.
236. Inglis AM, Sheth SB, Hursting MJ, Tenero DM, Graham AM, DiCicco RA. Investigation of the interaction between argatroban and acetaminophen, lidocaine, or digoxin. Am J Health Syst Pharm 2002;59(13):1258–66.
237. Weber C, Banken L, Birnboeck H, Nave S, Schulz R. The effect of bosentan on the pharmacokinetics of digoxin in healthy male subjects. Br J Clin Pharmacol 1999;47(6):701–6.
238. Pliakos ChC, Papadopoulos K, Parcharidis G, Styliadis J, Tourkantonis A. Effects of calcium channel blockers on serum concentrations of digoxin. Epitheorese Klin Farmakol Farmakokinetikes 1991;9:118–25.
239. North DS, Mattern AL, Hiser WW. The influence of diltiazem hydrochloride on trough serum digoxin concentrations. Drug Intell Clin Pharm 1986;20(6):500–3.
240. Halawa B, Mazurek W. Interakcje digoksyny z nifedypina i diltiazemem. [Interactions of digoxin with nifedipine and diltiazem.] Pol Tyg Lek 1990;45(23–24):467–9.
241. Mahgoub AA, El-Medany AH, Abdulatif AS. A comparison between the effects of diltiazem and isosorbide dinitrate on digoxin pharmacodynamics and kinetics in the treatment of patients with chronic ischemic heart failure. Saudi Med J 2002;23(6):725–31.
242. Peters J, Welker HA, Bullingham R. Pharmacokinetic and pharmacodynamic aspects of concomitant mibefradil–digoxin therapy at therapeutic doses. Eur J Drug Metab Pharmacokinet 1999;24(2):133–40.
243. Gasic S, Eichler HG, Korn A. Effect of calcium antagonists on basal and digitalis-dependent changes in splanchnic and systemic hemodynamics. Clin Pharmacol Ther 1987;41(4):460–6.
244. Pedersen KE, Dorph-Pedersen A, Hvidt S, Klitgaard NA, Nielsen-Kudsk F. Digoxin–verapamil interaction. Clin Pharmacol Ther 1981;30(3):311–16.
245. Klein HO, Lang R, Weiss E, Di Segni E, Libhaber C, Guerrero J, Kaplinsky E. The influence of verapamil on serum digoxin concentration. Circulation 1982; 65(5):998–1003.
246. Zatuchni J. Verapamil–digoxin interaction. Am Heart J 1984;108(2):412–13.
247. Cleland JG, Dargie HJ, Pettigrew A, Gillen G, Robertson JI. The effects of captopril on serum digoxin and urinary urea and digoxin clearances in patients with congestive heart failure. Am Heart J 1986;112(1):130–5.
248. Douste-Blazy P, Blanc M, Montastruc JL, Conte D, Cotonat J, Galinier F. Is there any interaction between digoxin and enalapril? Br J Clin Pharmacol 1986;22(6):752–3.
249. Magelli C, Bassein L, Ribani MA, Liberatore S, Ambrosioni E, Magnani B. Lack of effect of captopril on serum digoxin in congestive heart failure. Eur J Clin Pharmacol 1989;36(1):99–100.
250. Miyakawa T, Shionoiri H, Takasaki I, Kobayashi K, Ishii M. The effect of captopril on pharmacokinetics of digoxin in patients with mild congestive heart failure. J Cardiovasc Pharmacol 1991;17(4):576–80.
251. de Mey C, Elich D, Schroeter V, Butzer R, Belz GG. Captopril does not interact with the pharmacodynamics

and pharmacokinetics of digitoxin in healthy man. Eur J Clin Pharmacol 1992;43(4):445–7.
252. Kirimli O, Kalkan S, Guneri S, Tuncok Y, Akdeniz B, Ozdamar M, Guven H. The effects of captopril on serum digoxin levels in patients with severe congestive heart failure. Int J Clin Pharmacol Ther 2001;39(7):311–14.
253. Zussman BD, Kelly J, Murdoch RD, Clark DJ, Schubert C, Collie H. Cilomilast: pharmacokinetic and pharmacodynamic interactions with digoxin. Clin Ther 2001;23(6):921–31.
254. Kubler PA, Pillans PI, McKay JR. Possible interaction between cisapride and digoxin. Ann Pharmacother 2001;35(1):127–8.
255. Larsen F, Priskorn M, Overo KF. Lack of citalopram effect on oral digoxin pharmacokinetics. J Clin Pharmacol 2001;41(3):340–6.
256. Peeters PA, Crijns HJ, Tamminga WJ, Jonkman JH, Dickinson JP, Necciari J. Clopidogrel, a novel antiplatelet agent, and digoxin: absence of pharmacodynamic and pharmacokinetic interaction. Semin Thromb Hemost 1999;25(Suppl 2):51–4.
257. Retzow A, Althaus M, de Mey C, Mazur D, Vens-Cappell B. Study on the interaction of the dopamine agonist alpha-dihydroergocryptine with the pharmacokinetics of digoxin. Arzneimittelforschung 2000;50(7):591–6.
258. Kleinermans D, Nichols DJ, Dalrymple I. Effect of dofetillide on the pharmacokinetics of digoxin. Am J Cardiol 2001;87(2):248–50.
259. Norgaard BL, Wachtell K, Christensen PD, Madsen B, Johansen JB, Christiansen EH, Graff O, Simonsen EH. Efficacy and safety of intravenously administered dofetilide in acute termination of atrial fibrillation and flutter: a multicenter, randomized, double-blind, placebo-controlled trial. Danish Dofetilide in Atrial Fibrillation and Flutter Study Group. Am Heart J 1999;137(6):1062–9.
260. Mant T, Fournie P, Ollier C, Donat F, Necciari J. Absence of interaction of fondaparinux sodium with digoxin in healthy volunteers. Clin Pharmacokinet 2002;41(Suppl 2):39–45.
261. Cogan JJ, Humphreys MH, Carlson CJ, Benowitz NL, Rapaport E. Acute vasodilator therapy increases renal clearance of digoxin in patients with congestive heart failure. Circulation 1981;64(5):973–6.
262. Schimmel MS, Inwood RJ, Eidelman AI, Eylath U. Toxic digitalis levels associated with indomethacin therapy in a neonate. Clin Pediatr (Phila) 1980;19(11):768–9.
263. Finch MB, Kelly JG, Johnston GD, McDevitt DG. Evidence against a digoxin–indomethacin interaction. Br J Clin Pharmacol 1983;16:P212–13.
264. Levy RH, Ragueneau-Majlessi I, Baltes E. Repeated administration of the novel antiepileptic agent levetiracetam does not alter digoxin pharmacokinetics and pharmacodynamics in healthy volunteers. Epilepsy Res 2001;46(2):93–9.
265. Ragueneau I, Poirier JM, Radembino N, Sao AB, Funck-Brentano C, Jaillon P. Pharmacokinetic and pharmacodynamic drug interactions between digoxin and macrogol 4000, a laxative polymer, in healthy volunteers. Br J Clin Pharmacol 1999;48(3):453–6.
266. Lindenbaum J, Rund DG, Butler VP Jr, Tse-Eng D, Saha JR. Inactivation of digoxin by the gut flora: reversal by antibiotic therapy. N Engl J Med 1981; 305(14):789–94.
267. Ford A, Smith LC, Baltch AL, Smith RP. Clarithromycin-induced digoxin toxicity in a patient with AIDS. Clin Infect Dis 1995;21(4):1051–2.
268. Tsutsumi K, Kotegawa T, Kuranari M, Otani Y, Morimoto T, Matsuki S, Nakano S. The effect of erythromycin and clarithromycin on the pharmacokinetics of intravenous digoxin in healthy volunteers. J Clin Pharmacol 2002;42(10):1159–64.
269. Boyd RA, Stern RH, Stewart BH, Wu X, Reyner EL, Zegarac EA, Randinitis EJ, Whitfield L. Atorvastatin coadministration may increase digoxin concentrations by inhibition of intestinal P-glycoprotein-mediated secretion. J Clin Pharmacol 2000;40(1):91–8.
270. Ten Eick AP, Sallee D, Preminger T, Weiss A, Reed MD. Possible drug interaction between digoxin and azithromycin in a young child. Clin Drug Invest 2000;20:61–4.
271. Gooderham MJ, Bolli P, Fernandez PG. Concomitant digoxin toxicity and warfarin interaction in a patient receiving clarithromycin. Ann Pharmacother 1999; 33(7–8):796–9.
272. Wakasugi H, Yano I, Ito T, Hashida T, Futami T, Nohara R, Sasayama S, Inui K. Effect of clarithromycin on renal excretion of digoxin: interaction with P-glycoprotein. Clin Pharmacol Ther 1998;64(1):123–8.
273. Trivedi S, Hyman J, Lichstein E. Clarithromycin and digoxin toxicity. Ann Intern Med 1998;128(7):604.
274. Coudray S, Janoly A, Belkacem-Kahlouli A, Bourhis Y, Bleyzac N, Bourgeois J, Putet G, Aulagner G. Erythromycin-induced digoxin toxicity in a neonatal intensive care unit. J Pharm Clin 2001;20:129–31.
275. Zhou H, Walter YH, Smith H, Devineni D, McLeod JF. Nateglinide, a new mealtime glucose regulator. Lack of pharmacokinetic interaction with digoxin in healthy volunteers. Clin Drug Invest 2000;19:465–71.
276. Hatorp V, Thomsen MS. Drug interaction studies with repaglinide: repaglinide on digoxin or theophylline pharmacokinetics and cimetidine on repaglinide pharmacokinetics. J Clin Pharmacol 2000;40(2):184–92.
277. Cardaioli P, Compostella L, De Domenico R, Papalia D, Zeppellini R, Libardoni M, Pulido E, Cucchini F. Influenza del propafenone sulla farmacocinetica della digossina somministrata per via orale: studio su volontari sani. [Effect of propafenone on the pharmacokinetics of digoxin administered orally: a study in healthy volunteers.] G Ital Cardiol 1986;16(3):237–40.
278. Palumbo E, Svetoni N, Casini M, Spargi T, Biagi G, Martelli F, Lanzetta T. Interazione digoxina–propafenone: valori e limiti del dosaggio plasmatico dei due farmaci. Efficacia antiaritmica del propafenone. [Digoxin–propafenone interaction: values and limitations of plasma determination of the 2 drugs. Anti-arrhythmia effectiveness of propafenone.] G Ital Cardiol 1986;16(10):855–62.
279. Malek I, Gebauerova M, Stanek V. Riziko soucasného podávání chinidinu a digitalisu. [Risk of simultaneous administration of quinidine and digitalis.] Vnitr Lek 1980;26(3):358–61.
280. Pedersen KE, Lysgaard Madsen J, Klitgaard NA, Kjaer K, Hvidt S. Effect of quinine on plasma digoxin concentration and renal digoxin clearance. Acta Med Scand 1985; 218(2):229–32.
281. Aronson JK, Carver JG. Interaction of digoxin with quinine. Lancet 1981;1(8235):1418.
282. Leden I. Digoxin–hydroxychloroquine interaction? Acta Med Scand 1982;211(5):411–12.
283. Hedman A. Inhibition by basic drugs of digoxin secretion into human bile. Eur J Clin Pharmacol 1992; 42(4):457–9.
284. Fenster PE, Powell JR, Graves PE, Conrad KA, Hager WD, Goldman S, Marcus FI. Digitoxin–quinidine interaction: pharmacokinetic evaluation. Ann Intern Med 1980;93(5):698–701.
285. Kuhlmann J, Dohrmann M, Marcin S. Effects of quinidine on pharmacokinetics and pharmacodynamics of digitoxin achieving steady-state conditions. Clin Pharmacol Ther 1986;39(3):288–94.
286. Vousden M, Allen A, Lewis A, Ehren N. Lack of pharmacokinetic interaction between gemifloxacin and digoxin in healthy elderly volunteers. Chemotherapy 1999;45(6):485–90.

287. Chien SC, Rogge MC, Williams RR, Natarajan J, Wong F, Chow AT. Absence of a pharmacokinetic interaction between digoxin and levofloxacin. J Clin Pharm Ther 2002;27(1):7–12.
288. Johnson RD, Dorr MB, Hunt TL, Conway S, Talbot GH. Pharmacokinetic interaction of sparfloxacin and digoxin. Clin Ther 1999;21(2):368–79.
289. Boman G, Eliasson K, Odar-Cederlof I. Acute cardiac failure during treatment with digitoxin—an interaction with rifampicin. Br J Clin Pharmacol 1980;10(1):89–90.
290. Gault H, Longerich L, Dawe M, Fine A. Digoxin–rifampin interaction. Clin Pharmacol Ther 1984;35(6):750–4.
291. Novi C, Bissoli F, Simonati V, Volpini T, Baroli A, Vignati G. Rifampin and digoxin: possible drug interaction in a dialysis patient. JAMA 1980;244(22):2521–2.
292. Greiner B, Eichelbaum M, Fritz P, Kreichgauer HP, von Richter O, Zundler J, Kroemer HK. The role of intestinal P-glycoprotein in the interaction of digoxin and rifampin. J Clin Invest 1999;104(2):147–53.
293. Taylor A, Beerahee A, Citerone D, Davy M, Fitzpatrick K, Lopez-Gil A, Stocchi F. The effect of steady-state ropinirole on plasma concentrations of digoxin in patients with Parkinson's disease. Br J Clin Pharmacol 1999;47(2):219–22.
294. Burke S, Amin N, Incerti C, Plone M, Watson N. Sevelamer hydrochloride (Renagel), a nonabsorbed phosphate-binding polymer, does not interfere with digoxin or warfarin pharmacokinetics. J Clin Pharmacol 2001;41(2):193–8.
295. Waldorff S, Andersen JD, Heeboll-Nielsen N, Nielsen OG, Moltke E, Sorensen U, Steiness E. Spironolactone-induced changes in digoxin kinetics. Clin Pharmacol Ther 1978;24(2):162–7.
296. Johne A, Brockmoller J, Bauer S, Maurer A, Langheinrich M, Roots I. Pharmacokinetic interaction of digoxin with an herbal extract from St. John's wort (*Hypericum perforatum*). Clin Pharmacol Ther 1999; 66(4):338–45.
297. Homma M, Takeda M, Yamamoto Y, Suga H, Horiuchi M, Satoh S, Kohda Y. [Consultation and survey for drug interaction in outpatients taking the medicines potentially interact with St. John's Wort.] Yakugaku Zasshi 2000; 120(12):1435–40.
298. Kusus M, Stapleton DD, Lertora JJ, Simon EE, Dreisbach AW. Rhabdomyolysis and acute renal failure in a cardiac transplant recipient due to multiple drug interactions. Am J Med Sci 2000;320(6):394–7.
299. Weber P, Lettieri JT, Kaiser L, Mazzu AL. Lack of mutual pharmacokinetic interaction between cerivastatin, a new HMG-CoA reductase inhibitor, and digoxin in healthy normocholesterolemic volunteers. Clin Ther 1999;21(9):1563–75.
300. Garnett WR, Venitz J, Wilkens RC, Dimenna G. Pharmacokinetic effects of fluvastatin in patients chronically receiving digoxin. Am J Med 1994;96(6A):S84–6.
301. Martin PD, Kemp J, Dane AL, Warwick MJ, Schneck DW. No effect of rosuvastatin on the pharmacokinetics of digoxin in healthy volunteers. J Clin Pharmacol 2002;42(12):1352–7.
302. Westphal K, Weinbrenner A, Giessmann T, Stuhr M, Franke G, Zschiesche M, Oertel R, Terhaag B, Kroemer HK, Siegmund W. Oral bioavailability of digoxin is enhanced by talinolol: evidence for involvement of intestinal P-glycoprotein. Clin Pharmacol Ther 2000; 68(1):6–12.
303. Miyazawa Y, Paul Starkey L, Forrest A, Schentag JJ, Kamimura H, Swarz H, Ito Y. Effects of the concomitant administration of tamsulosin (0.8 mg) on the pharmacokinetic and safety profile of intravenous digoxin (Lanoxin) in normal healthy subjects: a placebo-controlled evaluation. J Clin Pharm Ther 2002;27(1):13–19.
304. Zhou H, Horowitz A, Ledford PC, Hubert M, Appel-Dingemanse S, Osborne S, McLeod JF. The effects of tegaserod (HTF 919) on the pharmacokinetics and pharmacodynamics of digoxin in healthy subjects. J Clin Pharmacol 2001;41(10):113.
305. Stangier J, Su CA, Hendriks MG, van Lier JJ, Sollie FA, Oosterhuis B, Jonkman JH. The effect of telmisartan on the steady-state pharmacokinetics of digoxin in healthy male volunteers. J Clin Pharmacol 2000;40(12 Pt 1):1373–9.
306. Snel S, Jansen JA, Pedersen PC, Jonkman JH, van Heiningen PN. Tiagabine, a novel antiepileptic agent: lack of pharmacokinetic interaction with digoxin. Eur J Clin Pharmacol 1998;54(4):355–7.
307. Bhattacharyya A, Bhavnani M, Tymms DJ. Serious interaction between digoxin and warfarin. Br J Cardiol 2002;9:356–7.
308. Richards D, Aronson JK. Serious interaction between digoxin and warfarin. Br J Cardiol 2002;9:446.
309. Sanchez Garcia P, Paty I, Leister CA, Guerra P, Frias J, Garcia Perez LE, Darwish M. Effect of zaleplon on digoxin pharmacokinetics and pharmacodynamics. Am J Health Syst Pharm 2000;57(24):2267–70.
310. Huffman DH. The effect of spironolactone and canrenone on the digoxin radioimmunoassay. Res Commun Chem Pathol Pharmacol 1974;9(4):787–90.
311. Pleasants RA, Williams DM, Porter RS, Gadsden RH Sr. Reassessment of cross-reactivity of spironolactone metabolites with four digoxin immunoassays. Ther Drug Monit 1989;11(2):200–4.
312. Valdes R Jr, Jortani SA. Unexpected suppression of immunoassay results by cross-reactivity: now a demonstrated cause for concern. Clin Chem 2002;48(3):405–6.
313. Steimer W, Muller C, Eber B, Emmanuilidis K. Intoxication due to negative canrenone interference in digoxin drug monitoring. Lancet 1999;354(9185):1176–7.
314. Capone D, Gentile A, Basile V. Possible interference of digoxin-like immunoreactive substances using the digoxin fluorescence polarization immunoassay. J Appl Ther Res 1999;2:305–8.
315. Steimer W, Muller C, Eber B. Digoxin assays: frequent, substantial, and potentially dangerous interference by spironolactone, canrenone, and other steroids. Clin Chem 2002;48(3):507–16.
316. Aronson JK. Digoxin. In: Widdop B, editor. Contemporary Issues in Biochemistry. Edinburgh: Churchill Livingstone, 1985:3.
317. Mordasini MR, Krahenbuhl S, Schlienger RG. Appropriateness of digoxin level monitoring. Swiss Med Wkly 2002;132(35–36):506–12.
318. Abad-Santos F, Carcas AJ, Ibanez C, Frias J. Digoxin level and clinical manifestations as determinants in the diagnosis of digoxin toxicity. Ther Drug Monit 2000;22(2):163–8.
319. Wolin MJ. Digoxin visual toxicity with therapeutic blood levels of digoxin. Am J Ophthalmol 1998;125(3):406–7.

Carisoprodol

General Information

Carisoprodol is a precursor of meprobamate, an oral anxiolytic with similarities to benzodiazepines. The spasmolytic effect of carisoprodol is thought to be due to interruption of neuronal communication within the reticular formation and spinal cord. Major adverse effects are sedation and drowsiness.

Organs and Systems

Nervous system

In 104 cases carisoprodol and its metabolite meprobamate were detected in the blood of car drivers who were either involved in accidents or arrested for impaired driving (1). In many of these cases, either alcohol or other nervous system depressants were also found. In 21 cases carisoprodol/meprobamate were the only drugs detected. Symptoms and reported driving behavior were similar in all cases. Impairment of driving ability appeared to be possible at any concentration of these two drugs. However, the most severe driving impairment and most overt symptoms of intoxication were noted when the combined concentration of carisoprodol and meprobamate exceeded 10 mg/l.

Long-Term Effects

Drug dependence

Because of its relation to benzodiazepines, dependence on carisoprodol can be a problem. Among patients who had taken carisoprodol for 3 months or more, up to 40% had used it in amounts larger than prescribed, and up to 30% had used it for an effect other than that for which it was prescribed (2). A significant percentage of physicians were unaware of the potential of carisoprodol for abuse and of its metabolism to meprobamate. Patients with carisoprodol withdrawal can present with agitation, restlessness, hallucinations, seizures, anorexia, and vomiting.

Drug Administration

Drug overdose

Carisoprodol overdose is reportedly rarely fatal. However, a review of the deaths examined at the Jefferson County Medical Examiner Office from 1986 to 1997 revealed 24 cases of carisoprodol overdosage (3). In all 24 cases other co-intoxicants were involved. Since the mechanism of death was respiratory depression in 82% of the cases, the authors suggested that carisoprodol had contributed to the fatal outcome. Carisoprodol overdosage should be regarded as potentially fatal if other respiratory depressants add to its effect.

Carisoprodol intoxication can also be associated with symptoms of nervous system overactivity rather than depression. Agitation and myoclonic movement disorders have been observed (4).

As carisoprodol and its metabolite meprobamate are GABA receptor agonists, the use of the benzodiazepine receptor antagonist flumazenil might be considered in some cases of carisoprodol toxicity (5).

- A 51-year-old woman took 87 tablets of carisoprodol (350 mg each) over 13 days and developed lethargy and abnormal speech. She was confused and her Glasgow Coma Score was 9/15. Her pupils were small and reactive. Two boluses of naloxone 2 mg were administered with no effect. After flumazenil 0.2 mg she became more alert but was still mildly somnolent. After a second dose of flumazenil 0.2 mg all signs of intoxication were reversed within 2 minutes. Her blood concentrations at admission were 7.4 μg/ml for carisoprodol and 30.7 μg/ml for meprobamate.

This suggests that flumazenil may be an effective therapeutic option if carisoprodol intoxication results in nervous system depression. However, carisoprodol overdose can also produce myoclonic movements or agitation (4), in which case it is questionable if flumazenil should be used.

References

1. Logan BK, Case GA, Gordon AM. Carisoprodol, meprobamate, and driving impairment. J Forensic Sci 2000;45(3):619–23.
2. Reeves RR, Carter OS, Pinkofsky HB, Struve FA, Bennett DM. Carisoprodol (Soma): abuse potential and physician unawareness. J Addict Dis 1999;18(2):51–6.
3. Davis GG, Alexander CB. A review of carisoprodol deaths in Jefferson County, Alabama. South Med J 1998; 91(8):726–30.
4. Roth BA, Vinson DR, Kim S. Carisoprodol-induced myoclonic encephalopathy. J Toxicol Clin Toxicol 1998;36(6):609–12.
5. Roberge RJ, Lin E, Krenzelok EP. Flumazenil reversal of carisoprodol (Soma) intoxication. J Emerg Med 2000; 18(1):61–4.

Carnidazole

General Information

Carnidazole is an imidazole derivative, less potent than most other similar compounds (1). In early studies, its adverse effects were mild; nausea and vomiting, abdominal discomfort, dry mouth, dizziness, headache, and tiredness were reported (SEDA-6, 264). Metronidazole-like adverse effects should be anticipated.

Reference

1. Jokipii L, Jokipii AM. Comparative evaluation of the 2-methyl-5-nitroimidazole compounds dimetridazole, metronidazole, secnidazole, ornidazole, tinidazole, carnidazole, and panidazole against *Bacteroides fragilis* and other bacteria of the *Bacteroids fragilis* group. Antimicrob Agents chemother 1985;28(4):561–4.

Carprofen

See also Non-steroidal anti-inflammatory drugs

General Information

The main adverse effects of the NSAID carprofen are cutaneous and hepatic. Photoreactions are being increasingly reported and its chemical similarity to benoxaprofen is worth noting (SEDA-12, 84). The photosensitivity mechanism is either toxic or allergic. Other cutaneous symptoms, such as burning, pruritus, dermatitis, and skin redness, have also been reported (1). In trials in the USA, 14% of 1500 patients had slight transient rises in liver function tests, the significance of which is unclear (SEDA-13, 79). Headache, dizziness, gastrointestinal discomfort, and dysuria have also been described (1). Asthma can be precipitated in aspirin-sensitive patients.

Susceptibility Factors

Other features of the patient

Although carprofen is reported to be well tolerated by patients with peptic ulcers taking ranitidine (2), it cannot be presumed to be without risk in patients with ulcer disease.

References

1. Jensen EM, Fossgren J, Kirchheiner B, et al. Treatment of rheumatoid arthritis with carprofen (Imadyl) or indometacin: a randomized multicentre trial. Curr Ther Res 1980;28:882.
2. Czarnobilski Z, Bem S, Czarnobilski K, Konturek SJ. Carprofen and the therapy of gastroduodenal ulcerations by ranitidine. Hepatogastroenterology 1985;32(1):20–3.

Carvedilol

See also Beta-adrenoceptor antagonists

General Information

Carvedilol is a highly lipophilic non-selective beta-adrenoceptor antagonist with $alpha_1$-blocking action, promoting peripheral vasodilatation. It also has free radical scavenging and antimitogenic effects.

The safety and tolerability profile of carvedilol in heart failure appears to be reassuring (1). In trials in patients with congestive heart failure, carvedilol was withdrawn in only about 5% (2). The most common adverse reactions were edema, dizziness, bradycardia, hypotension, nausea, diarrhea, and blurred vision. The rate of drug withdrawal was not different among patients under 65 years and among older ones.

The largest trial of carvedilol in patients with heart failure documented only a 5% withdrawal rate in 1197 patients during the open phase that preceded randomization. The major reasons for withdrawal were worsening heart failure (2%), dizziness (1.1%), bradycardia (0.2%), and death (0.5%). Overall, 78% of the patients who entered the trial and were randomized to carvedilol achieved the target dose of 50 mg/day, and withdrawal rates were comparable with carvedilol and placebo (11–14% over 6.5 months of treatment).

The issue of tolerability is particularly important in patients with severe heart failure (NYHA class IV). Unfortunately, so far all trials with carvedilol have failed to recruit a large number of such patients. A retrospective analysis of the tolerability profile of carvedilol in 63 patients with NYHA class IV heart failure showed that non-fatal adverse events while taking carvedilol were more frequent than in patients with class II-III heart failure (43 versus 24%) and more often resulted in permanent withdrawal of the drug (25 versus 13%) (3). However, 59% of the patients with class IV heart failure improved by one or more functional class after 3 months of treatment. The conclusion was that carvedilol is a useful adjunctive therapy for patients with NYHA class IV heart failure, but these patients require close observation during the start of treatment and titration of the dose.

In patients with heart failure, amiodarone is often required for the treatment of serious ventricular dysrhythmias. The beneficial effects of carvedilol on left ventricular remodeling, systolic function, and symptomatic status were not altered by amiodarone in 80 patients with heart failure. Adverse effects that necessitated withdrawal of carvedilol were no more frequent in patients taking amiodarone than in those taking carvedilol alone (26 versus 25%) (4).

In 10 patients with gastroesophageal varices, none having bled, treated with oral carvedilol 12.5 mg/day for 4 weeks, hemodynamic measurements were performed before the first administration and at 1 hour and 4 weeks after (5). After acute administration, the hepatic venous pressure gradient was significantly reduced by 23% (from 16.4 to 12.6 mmHg), with a significant reduction in heart rate. After 4 weeks, the hepatic venous pressure gradient was further significantly reduced to 9.3 mmHg. Carvedilol was well tolerated, and only one patient had asymptomatic hypotension. The results of this study suggest that low-dose carvedilol significantly reduces portal pressure without significantly systemic hemodynamic effects. The reduction in portal pressure with carvedilol was larger than that obtained with propranolol, encouraging specific trials of carvedilol for the primary prevention of variceal hemorrhage.

Organs and Systems

Cardiovascular

Since the adrenergic system is activated to support reduced contractility of the failing heart, the administration of a beta-blocker in a patient with heart failure can cause myocardial depression. This effect is more marked with non-selective first-generation beta-blockers, such as propranolol. Carvedilol has an acceptable tolerability profile, reducing after-load and thus counteracting the negative inotropic properties of adrenoceptor blockade. While these vasodilatory properties can play a favorable role at the start of treatment, it is less likely that vasodilatation can make a substantial contribution to the long-term effects of third-generation beta-blockers.

As with other alpha-blockers, postural hypotension is quite common with carvedilol, especially in elderly people (6). In a comparison of carvedilol with pindolol in elderly patients, postural hypotension occurred even with small doses of carvedilol (12.5 mg) (7). The authors concluded that lower starting doses should be used in elderly people, in patients taking diuretics, and in patients with heart failure.

Liver

Liver function abnormalities in trials of carvedilol occurred in 1.1% of patients taking carvedilol compared with 0.9% in patients taking placebo (2). However, in all trials the patients with pre-existing liver disease were excluded, and so information on the effects of carvedilol in these patients is not available.

Urinary tract

Renal insufficiency can occur in patients with heart failure treated with carvedilol, usually when pre-existing renal insufficiency, low blood pressure, or diffuse vascular disease are present (2). Patients at high risk of renal dysfunction should be carefully monitored, particularly at the beginning of treatment, and the drug should be withdrawn in case renal function worsens.

Skin

- Stevens–Johnson syndrome occurred in a 71-year-old man with stable ischemic cardiomyopathy taking carvedilol (8).

Sexual function

In a comparison of carvedilol with valsartan in 160 patients with hypertension (mean age 46 years) each treatment was continued for 16 weeks, with crossover after 4 weeks of placebo (9). Blood pressure was significantly lowered by both drugs (48% normalization with valsartan and 45% with carvedilol). In the first month of treatment, sexual activity (assessed as the number of episodes of sexual intercourse per month) fell with both treatments compared with baseline, although the change was statistically significant only with carvedilol. After the first month of treatment, sexual activity further worsened with carvedilol, but it improved or recovered fully with valsartan. The results were confirmed by the crossover. This confirms that beta-blockers can cause chronic worsening of sexual function.

Drug Administration

Drug overdose

Overdosage of carvedilol results mainly in hypotension and bradycardia (2). For excessive bradycardia, atropine has been used successfully, while to support ventricular function intravenous glucagon, dobutamine, or isoprenaline have been recommended. For severe hypotension, adrenaline or noradrenaline can be given.

References

1. Tang WHW, Fowler MB. Clinical trials of carvedilol in heart failure. Heart Fail Rev 1999;4:79–88.
2. Frishman WH. Carvedilol. N Engl J Med 1998;339(24):1759–65.
3. Macdonald PS, Keogh AM, Aboyoun CL, Lund M, Amor R, McCaffrey DJ. Tolerability and efficacy of carvedilol in patients with New York Heart Association class IV heart failure. J Am Coll Cardiol 1999;33(4):924–31.
4. Macdonald PS, Keogh AM, Aboyoun C, Lund M, Amor R, McCaffrey D. Impact of concurrent amiodarone treatment on the tolerability and efficacy of carvedilol in patients with chronic heart failure. Heart 1999;82(5):589–93.
5. Tripathi D, Therapondos G, Lui HF, Stanley AJ, Hayes PC. Haemodynamic effects of acute and chronic administration of low-dose carvedilol, a vasodilating beta-blocker, in patients with cirrhosis and portal hypertension. Aliment Pharmacol Ther 2002;16(3):373–80.
6. Louis WJ, Krum H, Conway EL. A risk-benefit assessment of carvedilol in the treatment of cardiovascular disorders. Drug Saf 1994;11(2):86–93.
7. Krum H, Conway EL, Broadbear JH, Howes LG, Louis WJ. Postural hypotension in elderly patients given carvedilol. BMJ 1994;309(6957):775–6.
8. Kowalski BJ, Cody RJ. Stevens–Johnson syndrome associated with carvedilol therapy. Am J Cardiol 1997; 80(5):669–70.
9. Fogari R, Zoppi A, Poletti L, Marasi G, Mugellini A, Corradi L. Sexual activity in hypertensive men treated with valsartan or carvedilol: a crossover study. Am J Hypertens 2001;14(1):27–31.

Catheters

General Information

Adverse effects can arise from physical effects of catheters used for intravenous, intra-arterial, urinary, or spinal access. Adverse reactions can also occur from the latex that some catheters contain or from the antiseptics with which they are sometimes combined.

Central venous catheters are reluctantly used as blood access for hemodialysis because of safety concerns and frequent complications, for example sepsis, thrombosis, and vessel stenosis. Nevertheless, 20% or more of all patients rely on atrial catheters for chronic dialysis because of lack of other access. Potentially fatal risks related to central venous catheters include air embolism (1), severe blood loss (2), and electric shock (3). These specific risks have been substantially eliminated by the inherent design and implantation of Dialock (Biolink Corporation, USA). Dialock is a subcutaneous device consisting of a titanium housing with two passages with integrated valves connected to two silicone catheters. The system is implanted subcutaneously below the clavicle. The tips of the catheters are placed in the right atrium. The port is accessed percutaneously with needle cannulas.

The results of a study of Dialock/CLS have been reported in 70 patients (29 men, 41 women; mean age at implantation 63 (range 30–88) years), of whom 42 had no infection (45 when infections occurring within 30 days after implantation were omitted) (4). Excluding these early events, 25 patients had a total of 30 infections. The majority (22 events in 20 patients) were pocket infections. The first seven of these pocket infections caused loss of the Dialock. After local treatment with gentamicin no further devices were lost through pocket infection. No infections were recorded during the last 3 months, although the expected rate calculated on the basis of previous occurrences would have been about four. This may have been related to increased nursing care.

Fracture of a central venous catheter due to compression between the clavicle and the adjacent first rib has been reported (5). A "pinched-off sign" on X-ray indicates the need to remove the catheter, because of a significant risk of subsequent fracture, which has an incidence of 0.9%. Catheters lying anterior to the subclavian vein between the clavicle and the first rib are liable to be compressed and to fracture subsequently. This is a potentially life-threatening complication that can be averted by correct placing of the central venous catheter and by immediate chest radiography to search for evidence of catheter kinking or compression.

Totally implantable venous devices are being increasingly used in patients who require long-term continuous parenteral drug therapy, especially in cancer chemotherapy. Inevitably there have been complications, including catheter fracture, as a consequence of "pinched-off" syndrome (6).

- A 67-year-old woman was provided with a totally implantable venous device in the right subclavian vein by the Seldinger technique with a peel-away sheath. The device was used for a course of chemotherapy. After about 1 month there was subcutaneous extravasation of the drug. A chest X-ray showed that the silicone catheter had fractured below the clavicle and the distal portion of the catheter had embolized into the right atrium. The fragments were removed.

This "pinched-off" effect appears to be due to narrowing of the catheter as it passes over the first rib and beneath the clavicle, when using the Seldinger technique, but it is usually only observed after long-term use. The authors recommended that the cephalic cut-down (Seldinger) technique is best avoided.

Continuous venous access for extended periods is commonly required in patients with cancer for chemotherapy delivery. Transcutaneously tunnelled central venous lines provide one means for the administration of such therapy, although they account for significant costs and morbidity (7). In a prospective study, 923 central venous tunnelled catheters in 791 patients were evaluated for devise-specific events. The most important adverse events included 11 insertion complications. Subsequent to placement, a proven or suspected devise-specific complication occurred in 540 lines. For every 10 000 catheter days there were 17.6 episodes of infection, 8.1 thrombotic complications, 6.9 instances of catheter breakage, 3.5 accidental or inadvertent cases of catheter displacement, and 0.6 device leaks. The devices were in position for a median of 365 days, but the median duration of device-specific complications was 167 days, reflecting a highly significant device salvage rate after complications. The authors concluded that central lines can be placed safely for use in long-term administration of cancer chemotherapy. Factors determining outcome are related to where the device is placed as well as the patient's disease.

Migration of a catheter caused failure of parenteral nutrition in a baby (8).

- A premature small-for-dates girl (34 weeks gestation, birth weight 1000 g) received parenteral nutrition for necrotizing enterocolitis. On day 7, among several septic spots that developed on the skin, an abscess developed on the left shoulder and ruptured spontaneously, leaving a superficial ulcer with purulent discharge. This was cleaned daily with isotonic saline and covered with gauze. On day 11, the blood glucose fell to 1.3 mmol/l and 10% glucose was given. Four further episodes of hypoglycemia during the next 12 hours were similarly treated. Over the next 12 hours the baby became lethargic, hypothermic, and apneic. Her blood glucose remained low (0.9–1.6 mmol/l). Several hours later she became bradycardic and hypotensive. It was then noticed that her bed linen was wet, and some fluid was seen trickling from the ulcer on her shoulder. A chest X-ray showed that the catheter tip had migrated to the left cephalic vein adjacent to the site of the ulcer. Despite rigorous resuscitation she died.

The authors speculated that the catheter tip had spontaneously migrated because the ulcer on the left shoulder had eroded deeply to form a venocutaneous fistula with the left cephalic vein. Continuous leakage of parenteral nutrition fluid through the fistula was soaked up by the gauze pads used to cover the ulcer, preventing early recognition of the problem.

In a systematic review of randomized studies of the use of different catheter materials for umbilical catheterization in newborn infants of any birth weight or gestation, there were no significant differences between heparin-bonded polyurethane catheters and polyvinyl chloride (PVC) catheters (9).

Organs and Systems

Cardiovascular

A major complication of intravenous infusion is thrombophlebitis, which is a principle limitation of peripheral parenteral nutrition. Its precise pathogenesis is unclear, but venospasm has been proposed as the most likely cause. However, in a study with ultrasound techniques to monitor vein caliber, there was no evidence to support this hypothesis, although thrombophlebitis was observed (10). The author suggested that the initiating event may be venous endothelial trauma, caused by the venepuncture itself, abrasion at the catheter tip, or the delivery of the feeding solution.

Venous reactions could also theoretically be influenced by the composition of the fat emulsion, because long-chain triglycerides, in particular, generate prostaglandin synthesis which can in turn effect vein tolerance. This potentially important issue has been assessed in a randomized, comparative trial of peripheral parenteral nutrition regimens with fat emulsions containing either long-chain triglycerides alone or in equal proportions with medium-chain triglycerides (11). All other factors were standardized. Long-chain triglyceride-based fat emulsions significantly prolonged the life of the peripheral vein, compared with mixtures of medium-chain and long-chain triglycerides. The authors hypothesized that this effect was due to a reduced reaction of the venous epithelium to the irritating nutritional mixture.

Superior vena cava thrombosis has been described after frequent central venous catheterization and total parenteral nutrition, with eventual partial recovery (12).

The possible etiological factors included the catheter material, catheter-related sepsis, endothelial trauma, osmotic injury, and hypercoagulability. Although thrombosis of the great veins of the thorax is rare, it is life-threatening, characterized by swelling of the head, upper limbs, and torso, and on chest X-ray by mediastinal widening. Confirmation of thrombosis is best achieved by contrast venography or contrast-enhanced CT scan.

Cardiac tamponade is a serious complication of central venous catheterization. A classical case history has been described with detailed discussion of prevention and management (13). Most serious complications, including air embolism, pneumothorax, hemothorax, chylothorax, chylopericardium, rupture of the right atrium, ventricular dysrhythmias, and cardiac tamponade, are essentially mechanical injuries relating to catheter insertion. Cardiac tamponade can be caused by acute perforation of the superior vena cava during insertion. Alternatively, a delayed event may be due to catheter-related erosion of the vascular wall, either in the vena cava or in the ventricular wall. The consequences are impairment of diastolic filling and a dramatic decrease in cardiac output, with a very high death rate (about 70%).

- A 63-year-old man with cancer of the esophagus developed severe dysphagia. A central venous catheter was introduced for presurgical parenteral nutrition and 3 hours later he reported severe epigastric and retrosternal pain. His condition deteriorated rapidly, with loss of consciousness, a weak pulse, hypotension, distant heart sounds, and jugular venous distension. A chest X-ray showed an enlarged mediastinal shadow and an electrocardiogram showed reduced voltage. The catheter was promptly removed. An emergency laparotomy showed only hepatic engorgement and about 100 ml of ascites, but at thoracotomy the pericardial sac was distended by about 500 ml of clear fluid. There was no apparent injury to the right subclavian artery or evidence of pleural hemorrhage.

The authors concluded that the right ventricle had been perforated by the catheter and they pointed out that these events can be insidious, and can take several months before symptoms suddenly start, requiring quick diagnosis and immediate intervention. This includes immediate removal of the catheter and often also emergency surgical intervention.

Respiratory

Lung transplant patients appear to be at increased risk of air embolism from catheters perhaps because of the considerable negative intrathoracic pressure that can develop when the diseased lung is replaced with a normal lung. Lung transplant patients are often also emaciated and have little subcutaneous tissue, allowing for a short tract from the central venous line insertion site to the opening of the central vein.

- A 53-year-old woman developed a serious air embolism from the central venous catheter tract after lung transplantation, at the time of removal of the catheter (14).

The authors referred in their report to four other cases of air embolism in lung transplant patients.

Nervous system

Complications have been described after the insertion of 157 intrathecal catheters in 142 patients (15). In most cases problems were related to the placement procedure, with subsequent neurological complications. Clinically unsuspected degeneration of the posterior columns, perhaps related to intraspinal infusion of morphine or to a paraneoplastic effect, has been observed postmortem in two patients with implanted pumps (16).

Paraplegia has been reported 2 months after morphine infusion by intrathecal catheter (17). Another case of paraplegia was reported in a 73-year-old man with an intrathecal catheter and a spinal cord stimulator (18).

Fluid balance

Umbilical venous catheters are commonly used in neonatal care for drug administration and parenteral nutrition. However, many risks are associated with their use. Ascites associated with parenteral nutrition have been reported (19).

- A girl weighing 1488 g was born by emergency cesarean section at 28 weeks gestation. An umbilical venous catheter was inserted as sole venous access. An abdominal X-ray showed that the catheter was at the level of T11/T12 in the midline. Owing to complications with oral feeding, parenteral nutrition was begun on day 2. The baby developed necrotizing enterocolitis and had to be ventilated. An abdominal X-ray suggested abdominal ascites. A diagnostic paracentesis produced 90 ml of bloodstained opalescent fluid, which settled to show a white layer on the surface (presumed to be fat emulsion). Following this procedure, respiratory status improved. Ultrasound and aerated saline tests on the umbilical venous catheter suggested that it had not migrated to the peritoneal cavity. However, it was removed and the abdominal distension resolved. The baby was extubated 3 days later and subsequently thrived with no further abdominal problems.

Hematologic

Heparinization of the fluid infused through an umbilical arterial catheter with heparin 0.25 units/ml reduces the likelihood of catheter occlusion; heparinization of flushes without heparinizing the infusate is ineffective (20).

Immunologic

Anaphylaxis to a central venous catheter (ARROWg+ard Blue Catheter) coated with chlorhexidine and sulfadiazine has been reported in a 50-year-old man (21).

Infection risk

Systemic catheter-related infections and local infections at catheter exit sites have been studied in relation to 479 central venous catheters in a prospective study in 311 patients in a general hospital in Australia (22). Local infections developed in association with 54 catheters (11%) and systemic infections with 32 (6.7%). Local infections predicted systemic infections, but the absence of a local infection did not exclude the possibility of systemic infection. Local complications included entry-site abscesses, cellulitis, and septic thrombophlebitis. Hemodialysis catheters were responsible for a higher rate of systemic infections than other types. Of all cases of bacteremia (33/160) detected in the hospital, 20% occurred in patients with a central venous catheter, and 24 of these (73%) were definitely or probably due to the catheter. The most common organism responsible was methicillin-resistant *Staphylococcus aureus*, and 40% of cases were due to catheter-related infection. Infection complications were few: three patients developed local abscesses, one developed endocarditis, and two died. In other surveys infective endocarditis has complicated 20% of systemic catheter-related infections, but it occurred only once in this study. It is possible that the short duration of this study (5 months) resulted in an underestimate of the real incidence of late complications of catheter-related infections. Innocuous in situ catheters can apparently be responsible for systemic infections. In other studies the risk of infection depended mainly on the duration of catheter therapy (23,24).

Catheter-related bacteremia due to *Pseudomonas paucimobilis* has been reported in two patients with cancer-associated neutropenia (25). This organism has rarely been implicated in community-acquired and nosocomial infections. Both patients had been undergoing intensive chemotherapy, and both required removal of the catheter to eradicate the infection.

There is some disagreement as to whether infectious complications differ with the use of different types of chronic central venous access devices in patients with cancer. In one study there was no significant difference in the risk of infection between subcutaneous ports and external catheters (26). However, this has been disputed by other workers, who found that in children with cancer there was a lower infection rate when subcutaneous ports were used compared with external catheters (27). The differences between the studies and the conclusions reached may be the result of their size and design, rather than real differences.

In 55 patients, continuous lumbar sympathetic blockade with local anesthetics administered via a catheter to treat sympathetic pain caused a psoas abscess in two patients, both of whom were treated with a continuous infusion of 0.25% bupivacaine (28). It was assumed that the catheter had been dislodged and that the drug had been injected into the psoas muscle or the psoas sheath. Another reason for this complication could have been local trauma due to a hematoma around the vertebrae during the insertion of the needle. The main drawbacks of the technique were the high incidences of infections and displacement of the catheters.

Infective endocarditis is a serious complication of centrally placed venous access devices. The successful treatment in situ of a large thrombus associated with the tip of the catheter has been described (29). The antibiotic regimen was gentamicin and vancomycin, both delivered via the venous access device; vancomycin was allowed to remain in situ between each 8-hourly dosing. This regimen successfully eradicated the thrombus within 3 weeks, without removal of the line.

In a prospective, double-blind study, the use of either vancomycin + heparin + ciprofloxacin or vancomycin + heparin flush solution, compared with heparin alone, significantly reduced the infective complications associated with tunnelled central venous lines in immunocompromised children. Neither antibiotic could be detected after flushing and there were no adverse events (30).

The incidence and types of complications related to central venous catheters in 71 patients with AIDS have been studied and compared with two control groups of patients without AIDS (65 immunocompromised patients and 14 immunocompetent patients receiving home total parenteral nutrition) (31). Three groups of patients requiring permanent venous access for administration of virustatics and/or total parenteral nutrition were investigated retrospectively. The Port-A-Cath system of implantation was used in all cases. Catheter-related mortality was low in all the groups (0–1%). Infectious complications could not be related to the degree of immunosuppression (CD4+ lymphocyte counts or white blood cell count). The incidence of both infectious and non-infectious complications was significantly higher in the immunocompetent subjects than in the others, probably because of the type of medium used and/or differences in handling of the catheter. The overall conclusions were that central venous catheters are safe and well tolerated by patients with AIDS and that they present no greater risk to them than they do to other categories of patients, regardless of degrees of immune competence. This conclusion should be regarded with some caution, given the retrospective nature of the study and the imbalance in the number of subjects studied in each category. However, it appears that totally implantable central venous catheters are safe and well tolerated by patients with AIDS, no differently to other immunocompromised patients and immunocompetent patients.

Total parenteral nutrition

Catheter sepsis rates in total parenteral nutrition are variable, depending on several patient factors. These include immunosuppression or associated critical illness, multiple intravascular catheters, and bacterial transfer from another source in the body. Catheter-related sepsis can present as fever, chills, change in mental status, hypotension, and leukocytosis. In patients with suspected catheter-related infection whose peripheral blood cultures do not grow the same organism as a culture drawn directly from the catheter, a guide wire exchange of the catheter may be effective. However, this is a surgical procedure which can become complicated by catheter malposition, air embolism, dislodgement of a septic thrombus, or cardiac dysrhythmias (32).

In a study of catheter infection in patients treated with total parenteral nutrition a distant septic focus was present in 165 of 244 patients (188 of 269 catheters: 70%). There was a colonization rate of 19% of the catheters of the patients with a distant septic focus, compared with 7.4% in patients without a distant septic focus. There was a high mortality rate in patients with a distant septic focus and a colonized catheter; sepsis was responsible for 33 of the 48 deaths (69%) in this group (33).

If a centrally placed venous catheter is required, tunnelling of the catheter under the skin from the entry point to the appropriate vein minimizes the risk of infection, and the inclusion of an internal cuff on the catheter provides a more reliable subcutaneous anchor point. The purpose of the cuff is to fibrose to the wall of subcutaneous tissue, helping to prevent dislodgement of the catheter and reduce the risk that infection will migrate from the entrance site in the skin. Cuffed catheters can be composed of polyurethane or silicone. It has been suggested that the former is better, because they are theoretically less thrombogenic. However, in a prospective study there was no difference between the two types (34). Mean catheter lifespans were similar, as were complication rates (including sepsis, obstruction, dislodgement, and thrombosis). However, fractures were entirely associated with the detachable flow-control devise. The authors therefore concluded that there was little evidence to support the hypothesis that polyurethane catheters offer more security in long-term parenteral nutrition.

Catheter infections in recipients of parenteral nutrition are of particular concern in children and can result in line removal, deep vein thrombosis, or an increased risk of liver disease. The incidence of catheter-related infections in 47 children receiving long-term parenteral nutrition has been studied retrospectively, one goal being to identify potential risk factors (35). The children had 125 catheters and 207 catheter-years. The average infection rate was 2.1/1000 parenteral nutrition days. The only factor identified was that early onset of infection after starting parenteral nutrition appeared to predict a poor prognosis.

HIV-positive subjects are expected to be at even greater risk of line-related infection. A prospective study of 212 subjects with HIV infection with 327 central venous catheters has provided evidence of this enhanced risk (36). Over the period 1994–97, 33% were suspected as being infected, although only 61 episodes were diagnosed as catheter-related sepsis. Three variables affected the rate of sepsis: parenteral nutrition, low numbers of circulating CD+ cells, and a high Apache score.

References

1. Orebaugh SL. Venous air embolism: clinical and experimental considerations. Crit Care Med 1992;20(8):1169–77.
2. Lau G. Iatrogenically-related, fatal haemorrhage occurring in end-stage renal failure: a series of three cases. Forensic Sci Int 1995;73(2):117–24.
3. Jonsson P, Stegmayr BG. Current leakage in haemodialysis machines varies. Int J Artif Organs 1999;22:425.
4. Sodemann K, Polaschegg HD, Feldmer B. Two years' experience with Dialock and CLS (a new antimicrobial lock solution). Blood Purif 2001;19(2):251–4.
5. Ramsden WH, Cohen AT, Blanshard KS. Case report: central venous catheter fracture due to compression between the clavicle and first rib. Clin Radiol 1995;50(1):59–60.
6. di Carlo I, Fisichella P, Russello D, Puleo S, Latteri F. Catheter fracture and cardiac migration: a rare complication of totally implantable venous devices. J Surg Oncol 2000;73(3):172–3.
7. Schwarz RE, Coit DG, Groeger JS. Transcutaneously tunneled central venous lines in cancer patients: an analysis of device-related morbidity factors based on prospective data collection. Ann Surg Oncol 2000;7(6):441–9.
8. Cheah FC, Boo NY, Latif JY. An unusual case of refractory hypoglycaemia in a neonate receiving total parenteral nutrition. Acta Paediatr 2000;89(4):497–8.
9. Barrington KJ. Umbilical artery catheters in the newborn: effects of catheter materials (Cochrane Review). In: The Cochrane Library. 1st ed. Oxford: Update Software, 1999.
10. Everitt NJ. Effect of prolonged infusion on vein calibre: a prospective study. Ann R Coll Surg Engl 1999;81(2):109–12.
11. Smirniotis V, Kotsis TE, Antoniou S, Kostopanagiotou G, Labrou A, Kourias E, Papadimitriou J. Incidence of vein thrombosis in peripheral intravenous nutrition: effect of fat emulsions. Clin Nutr 1999;18(2):79–81.
12. Muckart DJ, Neijenhuis PA, Madiba TE. Superior vena caval thrombosis complicating central venous catheterisation and total parenteral nutrition. S Afr J Surg 1998; 36(2):48–51.
13. Gluszek S, Kot M, Matykiewicz J. Cardiac tamponade as a complication of catheterization of the subclavian vein—prevention and principles of management. Nutrition 1999; 15(7–8):580–2.
14. McCarthy PM, Wang N, Birchfield F, Mehta AC. Air embolism in single-lung transplant patients after central venous catheter removal. Chest 1995;107(4):1178–9.
15. Nitescu P, Appelgren L, Hultman E, Linder LE, Sjoberg M, Curelaru I. Long-term, open catheterization of the spinal subarachnoid space for continuous infusion of narcotic and bupivacaine in patients with "refractory" cancer pain. A technique of catheterization and its problems and complications. Clin J Pain 1991;7(2):143–61.
16. Coombs DW, Fratkin JD, Meier FA, Nierenberg DW, Saunders RL. Neuropathologic lesions and CSF morphine concentrations during chronic continuous intraspinal morphine infusion. A clinical and post-mortem study. Pain 1985;22(4):337–51.
17. North RB, Cutchis PN, Epstein JA, Long DM. Spinal cord compression complicating subarachnoid infusion of morphine: case report and laboratory experience. Neurosurgery 1991;29(5):778–84.
18. Aldrete JA, Vascello LA, Ghaly R, Tomlin D. Paraplegia in a patient with an intrathecal catheter and a spinal cord stimulator. Anesthesiology 1994;81(6):1542–5.
19. Panetta J, Morley C, Betheras R. Ascites in a premature baby due to parenteral nutrition from an umbilical venous catheter. J Paediatr Child Health 2000;36(2):197–8.
20. Barrington KJ. Umbilical artery catheters in the newborn: effects of heparin (Cochrane Review). In: The Cochrane Library. 4th ed. Oxford: Update Software, 2001.
21. Stephens R, Mythen M, Kallis P, Davies DW, Egner W, Rickards A. Two episodes of life-threatening anaphylaxis in the same patient to a chlorhexidine–sulphadiazine-coated central venous catheter. Br J Anaesth 2001;87(2):306–8.
22. Gosbell IB, Duggan D, Breust M, Mulholland K, Gottlieb T, Bradbury R. Infection associated with central venous catheters: a prospective survey. Med J Aust 1995; 162(4):210–13.
23. Du Pen SL, Peterson DG, Williams A, Bogosian AJ. Infection during chronic epidural catheterization: diagnosis and treatment. Anesthesiology 1990;73(5):905–9.
24. Ericsson M, Algers G, Schliamser SE. Spinal epidural abscesses in adults: review and report of iatrogenic cases. Scand J Infect Dis 1990;22(3):249–57.
25. Salazar R, Martino R, Sureda A, Brunet S, Subira M, Domingo-Albos A. Catheter-related bacteremia due to Pseudomonas paucimobilis in neutropenic cancer patients: report of two cases. Clin Infect Dis 1995;20(6):1573–4.
26. Keung YK, Watkins K, Chen SC, Groshen S, Silberman H, Douer D. Comparative study of infectious complications of different types of chronic central venous access devices. Cancer 1994;73(11):2832–7.
27. Hidalgo M. Comparative study of infectious complications of different types of chronic central venous access devices. Cancer 1995;75(1):132–3.
28. Strumpf M, Zenz M, Donner B, Tryba M. Continuous block of the lumbar sympathetic trunk via catheter. Pain Digest 1994;1:21–8.

29. Venugopalan P, Louon A, Akinbami FO, Elnour IB. Endocarditis with a large thrombus complicating a central venous access device. Ann Trop Paediatr 1999; 19(1):101–3.
30. Henrickson KJ, Axtell RA, Hoover SM, Kuhn SM, Pritchett J, Kehl SC, Klein JP. Prevention of central venous catheter-related infections and thrombotic events in immunocompromised children by the use of vancomycin/ciprofloxacin/heparin flush solution: A randomized, multicenter, double-blind trial. J Clin Oncol 2000; 18(6):1269–78.
31. Consten ECJ, Van Lanschot JJB, Movig FM, Rijsman L, Oosting J, Danner SA. Safety and complications of central venous catheters in AIDS patients. Clin Microbiol Infect 1998;4:508–13.
32. Cahill SL, Benotti PN. Catheter infection control in parenteral nutrition. Nutr Clin Pract 1991;6(2):65–7.
33. Chuang JH, Chuang SF. Implication of a distant septic focus in parenteral nutrition catheter colonization. J Parenter Enteral Nutr 1991;15(2):173–5.
34. Beau P, Matrat S. A comparative study of polyurethane and silicone cuffed-catheters in long-term home total parenteral nutrition patients. Clin Nutr 1999;18(3):175–7.
35. Colomb V, Fabeiro M, Dabbas M, Goulet O, Merckx J, Ricour C. Central venous catheter-related infections in children on long-term home parenteral nutrition: incidence and risk factors. Clin Nutr 2000;19(5):355–9.
36. Tacconelli E, Tumbarello M, de Gaetano Donati K, Bertagnolio S, Pittiruti M, Leone F, Morace G, Cauda R. Morbidity associated with central venous catheter-use in a cohort of 212 hospitalized subjects with HIV infection. J Hosp Infect 2000;44(3):186–92.

Celastraceae

See also Herbal medicines

General Information

The genera in the family of Celastraceae (Table 1) include bittersweet and khat.

Table 1 The genera of Celastraceae

Canotia (canotia)
Cassine (cassine)
Catha (khat)
Celastrus (bittersweet)
Crossopetalum (crossopetalum)
Euonymus (spindle tree)
Gyminda (false box)
Lophopyxis
Maytenus (mayten)
Mortonia (saddlebush)
Pachystima (pachystima)
Paxistima (paxistima)
Perrottetia (perrottetia)
Pristimera (pristimera)
Salacia
Schaefferia (schaefferia)
Torralbasia (torralbasia)
Tripterygium

Catha edulis

Chewing the leaves of *Catha edulis* (khat, qat) results in subjective mental stimulation, increased physical endurance, and increased self-esteem and social interaction. Until recently, this habit was confined to Arabian and East African countries, because only fresh leaves are active, but because of increased air transportation, khat is now also chewed in other parts of the world. Although cathine (norpseudoephedrine) is quantitatively the main alkaloid, the amphetamine-like euphorigenic and sympathomimetic cardiovascular effects of khat are primarily attributed to cathinone (1). In Yemen chewers of khat produced in fields where chemical pesticides are used regularly have more symptoms than chewers of khat produced in fields where chemical pesticides are rarely or never used (2).

The toxicologist Louis Lewin described the effects of chewing khat in his monograph *Phantastica* (1924): "The khat eater is happy when he hears everyone talk in turn and tries to contribute to this social entertainment. In this way the hours pass in a rapid and agreeable manner. Khat produces joyous excitation and gaiety. Desire for sleep is banished, energy is revived during the hot hours of the day, and the feeling of hunger on long marches is dispersed. Messengers and warriors use khat because it makes the ingestion of food unnecessary for several days."

Adverse effects

Tachycardia and increased blood pressure, irritability, psychosis, and psychic dependence have been described as acute adverse effects of khat.

The long term adverse effects were well described by Louis Lewin: "Those organs functions which are incessantly subjected to the influence of the drug finally flag or are diverted into another channel of activity ... The khat eater is seized with a restlessness which robs him of sleep. The excited cerebral hemispheres do not return to their normal state of repose, and in consequence the functions of the peripheral organs, especially those of the heart, suffer to such a degree that serious cardiac affectations have been ascertained in a great number of khat eaters. The disorders of the nervous system in many cases also give rise to troubles of general metabolism partly due to the chronic loss of appetite from the consumption of khat ... In Yemen it was openly stated that inveterate eaters of khat were indifferent to sexual excitation and desire, and did not marry at all, or for economic reasons waited until they had saved enough money. The lost of libido sexualis has been also observed in other inhabitants of these countries."

Cardiovascular

When 80 healthy volunteers chewed fresh khat leaves for 3 hours there were significant progressive rises in systolic and diastolic blood pressures and heart rate, without return to baseline 1 hour after chewing had ceased (3).

Of 247 chronic khat chewers 169 (62%) had hemorrhoids and 124 (45%) underwent hemorrhoidectomy; by comparison, of 200 non-khat chewers 8 (4%) had hemorrhoids and one underwent hemorrhoidectomy (4).

Nervous system
Of 19 khat users suspected of driving under the influence of drugs, three had impaired driving and 10 had marked impairment of psychophysical functions with effects on the nervous system (slow pupil reaction to light, dry mouth, increased heart rate), trembling, restlessness/nervousness, daze/apathy/dullness, and impaired attention, walking, and standing on one leg; however, the concentrations of the khat alkaloids assayed in blood did not correlate with the symptoms of impairment (5).

A leukoencephalopathy has been associated with khat (6).

Psychiatric
Khat has amphetamine-like effects and can cause psychoses (7–13), including mania (14) and hypnagogic hallucinations (15). Two men developed relapsing short-lasting psychotic episodes after chewing khat leaves; the psychotic symptoms disappeared without any treatment within 1 week (16).

In 800 Yemeni adults (aged 15–76 years) symptoms that might have been caused by the use of khat were elicited by face-to-face interviews; 90 items covered nine scales of the following domains: somatization, depression, anxiety, phobia, hostility, interpersonal sensitivity, obsessive-compulsive, hostility, interpersonal sensitivity, paranoia, and psychoticism (17). At least one life-time episode of khat use was reported in 82% of men and 43% of women. The incidence of adverse psychological symptoms was not greater in khat users, and there was a negative association between the use of khat and the incidence of phobic symptoms.

Psychological
In 25 daily khat-chewing flight attendants, 39 occasional khat-chewing flight attendants, and 24 non-khat-chewing aircrew members, memory function test scores were significantly lower in khat chewers than non-chewers and in regular chewers than occasional chewers (18).

Sensory systems
Bilateral optic atrophy occurred in two patients who were long-standing users of khat leaves and had chewed larger quantities than usual (19).

Metabolism
Chronic khat chewing increased plasma glucose and C-peptide concentrations in people with type 2 diabetes mellitus (20).

Mouth
In 20 volunteers who chewed khat regularly (10–160 g/day), there was an eight-fold increase in micronucleated buccal mucosa cells compared with 10 controls (21). Among heavy khat chewers, 81% of nuclei had a centromere signal, suggesting that khat is aneuploidogenic. The effects of khat, tobacco, and alcohol were additive. The highest frequency of abnormality occurred during the fourth week after consumption.

Of 2500 Yemeni citizens (mean age 27 years) 1528 (61%) were khat chewers; of them, 342 cases (22%) had oral keratotic white lesions at the site of khat chewing, while only 6 (0.6%) non-chewers had such lesions; the prevalence and severity of these lesions increased as duration and frequency of use increased (22).

However, in a case-control study in 85 khat-chewing Kenyans and 141 matched controls, smoking unprocessed tobacco (Kiraiku) and smoking cigarettes were the most significant factors for oral leukoplakia; traditional beer, khat, and chili peppers were not significantly associated with oral leukoplakia (23).

A 30-year-old immigrant from Somalia developed a plasma-cell gingivitis in the mandibular gums, probably caused by chewing khat (24).

Chewing khat can cause a generalized mousy brown pigmentation of the gums (25).

Gastrointestinal
In 12 healthy volunteers who chewed Khat leaves or lettuce for 2 hours gastric emptying was significantly prolonged by khat (26).

Chewing khat is said to be a risk factor of duodenal ulceration. (27).

Urinary tract
In 11 healthy men khat chewing produced a fall in average and maximum urine flow rate; this effect was inhibited by the alpha$_1$-adrenoceptor antagonist indoramin (28).

Sexual function
Chewing khat lowers libido and can also lead to erectile impotence after long-term use (29).

Fertility
In 65 Yemeni khat addicts (mean duration of addiction 25 years; mean age 40 years), semen volume, sperm count, sperm motility and motility index, and percentage of normal spermatozoa were lower than in 50 controls (30). There were significant negative correlations between the duration of khat consumption and all semen parameters. On electron microscopy, about 65% of the spermatozoa were deformed, with different patterns of deformation, including both the head and flagella in complete spermatozoa, aflagellate heads, headless flagella, and multiple heads and flagella. Deformed heads had aberrant nuclei with immature nuclear chromatin and polymorphic intranuclear inclusions; these were associated with acrosomal defects.

Fetotoxicity
In pregnant women, consumption of khat affects fetal growth by inhibiting placental blood flow (29), and birth weights are reduced (31). In 1141 consecutive deliveries in Yemen, non-users of khat ($n = 427$) had significantly fewer low birth-weight babies (less than 2500 g) than occasional users ($n = 223$) and regular users ($n = 391$) (32). Khat-chewing mothers were older, of greater parity, and had more surviving children than the non-chewers. Significantly more khat-chewers had concomitant diseases. There was no difference in rates of stillbirth or congenital malformations.

Lactation
Khat chewing by a breastfeeding mother can lead to the presence of cathine in the urine of the suckling child.

Drug interactions
The speed and extent of ampicillin systemic availability were reduced significantly by khat chewing in eight healthy adult Yemeni men, except when they took it 2 hours after the khat (33).

***Euonymus* species**

The fruit of *Euonymus europaeus* (the European spindle tree) and the bark of *Euonymus atropurpureus* (Wahoo bark) have cathartic and emetic activity, due to sesquiterpenoids and cardiac glycosides that they contain.

Adverse effects
IgE-mediated type I allergy to *E. europaeus* wood has been described in a 44-year-old goldsmith who developed rhinitis and conjunctivitis after having worked with dust from the wood for 15 years (34).

Tripterygium wilfordii

Extracts from the root of *Tripterygium wilfordii* (Lei gong teng) are used in China for the treatment of various disorders, such as rheumatoid arthritis, ankylosing spondylitis, systemic lupus erythematosus, and glomerulonephritis. The potential benefits in such serious diseases should be carefully weighed against a substantial risk of adverse reactions, including gastrointestinal disturbances, skin rashes, amenorrhea, leukopenia, and thrombocytopenia (35).

Adverse effects
Cardiovascular

- A previously healthy young man developed profuse vomiting and diarrhea, leukopenia, renal insufficiency, profound hypotension, and shock after taking an extract of *T. wilfordii* (36). Serial electrocardiograms, cardiac enzymes, and echocardiography showed evidence of coexisting cardiac damage. He died of intractable shock 3 days later.

Gastrointestinal
In a double-blind, placebo-controlled study in 35 patients with long-standing rheumatoid arthritis in whom conventional therapy had failed, an extract of *T. wilfordii* was used in either a low-dose (180 mg/day) or a high-dose (360 mg/day) for 20 weeks, followed by an open extension period (37). Only 21 patients completed the study, of whom one in each group withdrew because of adverse events. The most common adverse effect of *T. wilfordii* was diarrhea, which caused one patient in the high-dose group to withdraw.

Reproductive system
In men, prolonged use of *T. wilfordii* can cause oligospermia and azoospermia, and a reduction in testicular size (38–40).

In 14 women with rheumatoid arthritis *T. wilfordii* caused amenorrhea associated with increased FSH and LH concentrations, which began to rise after 2–3 months and reached menopausal values after 4–5 months; estradiol concentrations began to fall after 3–4 months and reached very low concentrations at 5 months, suggesting an effect on the ovary (41).

Immunologic
The immunosuppressive properties of Lei gong teng can promote the development of infectious diseases (42).

Teratogenicity
A boy whose mother had taken *T. wilfordii* for rheumatoid arthritis early in her pregnancy was born with an occipital meningoencephalocele and cerebellar agenesis, which the authors attributed to the herb (43).

References

1. Widler P, Mathys K, Brenneisen R, Kalix P, Fisch HU. Pharmacodynamics and pharmacokinetics of khat: a controlled study. Clin Pharmacol Ther 1994;55(5):556–62.
2. Date J, Tanida N, Hobara T. Qat chewing and pesticides: a study of adverse health effects in people of the mountainous areas of Yemen. Int J Environ Health Res 2004;14(6):405–14.
3. Hassan NA, Gunaid AA, Abdo-Rabbo AA, Abdel-Kader ZY, al-Mansoob MA, Awad AY, Murray-Lyon IM. The effect of qat chewing on blood pressure and heart rate in healthy volunteers. Trop Doct 2000;30(2):107–8.
4. Al-Hadrani AM. Khat induced hemorrhoidal disease in Yemen. Saudi Med J 2000;21(5):475–7.
5. Toennes SW, Kauert GF. Driving under the influence of khat—alkaloid concentrations and observations in forensic cases. Forensic Sci Int 2004;140(1):85–90.
6. Morrish PK, Nicolaou N, Brakkenberg P, Smith PE. Leukoencephalopathy associated with khat misuse. J Neurol Neurosurg Psychiatry 1999;67(4):556.
7. Alem A, Shibre T. Khat induced psychosis and its medico-legal implication: a case report. Ethiop Med J 1997;35(2): 137–9.
8. Jager AD, Sireling L. Natural history of khat psychosis. Aust NZ J Psychiatry 1994;28(2):331–2.
9. Pantelis C, Hindler CG, Taylor JC. Use and abuse of khat (*Catha edulis*): a review of the distribution, pharmacology, side effects and a description of psychosis attributed to khat chewing. Psychol Med 1989;19(3):657–68.
10. Maitai CK, Dhadphale M. khat-induced paranoid psychosis. Br J Psychiatry 1988;152:294.
11. McLaren P. Khat psychosis. Br J Psychiatry 1987;150:712–13.
12. Kalix P. Amphetamine psychosis due to khat leaves. Lancet 1984;1(8367):46.
13. Dhadphale M, Mengech A, Chege SW. Miraa (*Catha edulis*) as a cause of psychosis. East Afr Med J 1981;58(2):130–5.
14. Giannini AJ, Castellani S. A manic-like psychosis due to khat (*Catha edulis* Forsk.). J Toxicol Clin Toxicol 1982;19(5):455–9.
15. Granek M, Shalev A, Weingarten AM. Khat-induced hypnagogic hallucinations. Acta Psychiatr Scand 1988;78(4):458–61.
16. Nielen RJ, van der Heijden FM, Tuinier S, Verhoeven WM. Khat and mushrooms associated with psychosis. World J Biol Psychiatry 2004;5(1):49–53.
17. Numan N. Exploration of adverse psychological symptoms in Yemeni khat users by the Symptoms Checklist-90 (SCL-90). Addiction 2004;99(1):61–5.
18. Khattab NY, Amer G. Undetected neuropsychophysiological sequelae of khat chewing in standard aviation medical examination. Aviat Space Environ Med 1995;66(8):739–44.

19. Roper JP. The presumed neurotoxic effects of *Catha edulis*—an exotic plant now available in the United Kingdom. Br J Ophthalmol 1986;70(10):779–81.
20. Saif-Ali R, Al-Qirbi A, Al-Geiry A, AL-Habori M. Effect of *Catha edulis* on plasma glucose and C-peptide in both type 2 diabetics and non-diabetics. J Ethnopharmacol 2003;86(1):45–9.
21. Kassie F, Darroudi F, Kundi M, Schulte-Hermann R, Knasmuller S. Khat (*Catha edulis*) consumption causes genotoxic effects in humans. Int J Cancer 2001;92(3):329–32.
22. Ali AA, Al-Sharabi AK, Aguirre JM, Nahas R. A study of 342 oral keratotic white lesions induced by qat chewing among 2500 Yemeni. J Oral Pathol Med 2004; 33(6):368–72.
23. Macigo FG, Mwaniki DL, Guthua SW. The association between oral leukoplakia and use of tobacco, alcohol and khat based on relative risks assessment in Kenya. Eur J Oral Sci 1995;103(5):268–73.
24. Marker P, Krogdahl A. Plasma cell gingivitis apparently related to the use of khat: report of a case. Br Dent J 2002;192(6):311–13.
25. Ashri N, Gazi M. More unusual pigmentations of the gingiva. Oral Surg Oral Med Oral Pathol 1990;70(4):445–9.
26. Heymann TD, Bhupulan A, Zureikat NE, Bomanji J, Drinkwater C, Giles P, Murray-Lyon IM. Khat chewing delays gastric emptying of a semi-solid meal. Aliment Pharmacol Ther 1995;9(1):81–3.
27. Raja'a YA, Noman TA, al Warafi AK, al Mashraki NA, al Yosofi AM. Khat chewing is a risk factor of duodenal ulcer. East Mediterr Health J 2001;7(3):568–70.
28. Nasher AA, Qirbi AA, Ghafoor MA, Catterall A, Thompson A, Ramsay JW, Murray-Lyon IM. Khat chewing and bladder neck dysfunction. A randomized controlled trial of alpha 1-adrenergic blockade. Br J Urol 1995;75(5):597–8.
29. Mwenda JM, Arimi MM, Kyama MC, Langat DK. Effects of khat (*Catha edulis*) consumption on reproductive functions: a review. East Afr Med J 2003;80(6):318–23.
30. el-Shoura SM, Abdel Aziz M, Ali ME, el-Said MM, Ali KZ, Kemeir MA, Raoof AM, Allam M, Elmalik EM. Deleterious effects of khat addiction on semen parameters and sperm ultrastructure. Hum Reprod 1995;10(9):2295–300.
31. Abdul Ghani N, Eriksson M, Kristiansson B, Qirbi A. The influence of khat-chewing on birth-weight in full-term infants. Soc Sci Med 1987;24(7):625–7.
32. Eriksson M, Ghani NA, Kristiansson B. Khat-chewing during pregnancy-effect upon the off-spring and some characteristics of the chewers. East Afr Med J 1991;68(2):106–11.
33. Attef OA, Ali AA, Ali HM. Effect of khat chewing on the bioavailability of ampicillin and amoxycillin. J Antimicrob Chemother 1997;39(4):523–5.
34. Herold DA, Wahl R, Maasch HJ, Hausen BM, Kunkel G. Occupational wood-dust sensitivity from *Euonymus europaeus* (spindle tree) and investigation of cross reactivity between E.e. wood and *Artemisia vulgaris* pollen (mugwort). Allergy 1991;46(3):186–90.
35. Pyatt DW, Yang Y, Mehos B, Le A, Stillman W, Irons RD. Hematotoxicity of the chinese herbal medicine *Tripterygium wilfordii* Hook F in CD34-positive human bone marrow cells. Mol Pharmacol 2000;57(3):512–18.
36. Chou WC, Wu CC, Yang PC, Lee YT. Hypovolemic shock and mortality after ingestion of *Tripterygium wilfordii* Hook F.: a case report. Int J Cardiol 1995;49(2):173–7.
37. Tao X, Younger J, Fan FZ, Wang B, Lipsky PE. Benefit of an extract of *Tripterygium wilfordii* Hook F in patients with rheumatoid arthritis: a double-blind, placebo-controlled study. Arthritis Rheum 2002;46(7):1735–43.
38. Yu DY. Clinical observation of 144 cases of rheumatoid arthritis treated with glycoside of radix *Tripterygium wilfordii*. J Tradit Chin Med 1983;3(2):125–9.
39. Tao XL, Sun Y, Dong Y, Xiao YL, Hu DW, Shi YP, Zhu QL, Dai H, Zhang NZ. A prospective, controlled, double-blind, cross-over study of *Tripterygium wilfodii* Hook F in treatment of rheumatoid arthritis. Chin Med J (Engl) 1989;102(5):327–32.
40. Qian SZ. *Tripterygium wilfordii*, a Chinese herb effective in male fertility regulation. Contraception 1987; 36(3):335–45.
41. Gu CX. [Cause of amenorrhea after treatment with *Tripterygium wilfordii* F.] Zhongguo Yi Xue Ke Xue Yuan Xue Bao 1989;11(2):151–3.
42. Guo JL, Yuan SX, Wang XC, Xu SX, Li DD. *Tripterygium wilfordii* Hook F in rheumatoid arthritis and ankylosing spondylitis. Preliminary report. Chin Med J (Engl) 1981;94(7):405–12.
43. Takei A, Nagashima G, Suzuki R, Hokaku H, Takahashi M, Miyo T, Asai J, Sanada Y, Fujimoto T. Meningoencephalocele associated with *Tripterygium wilfordii* treatment. Pediatr Neurosurg 1997;27(1):45–8.

Celecoxib

See also COX-2 inhibitors

General Information

Celecoxib is a selective COX-2 inhibitor.

Organs and Systems

Psychological, psychiatric

A 78-year-old woman had auditory hallucinations while taking celecoxib for osteoarthritis (1). Her symptoms occurred after she had taken celecoxib 200 mg bd for 48 hours and progressed over the next 8 days. Celecoxib was withdrawn and her hallucinations gradually disappeared over the next 4 days. Rechallenge with a lower dose (100 mg bd) caused recurrence.

There have been two reports of visual hallucinations in patients taking celecoxib.

- A 79-year-old woman presented to her optometrist with a 2-day history of seeing orange spots in both visual fields 2 months after starting to take celecoxib 100 mg/day (2). Physical examination and a CT scan were normal. Celecoxib was withdrawn and her symptoms resolved within 3 days.
- An 81-year-old woman took celecoxib 100 mg/day, and over the next 2 weeks developed delirium and auditory and visual hallucinations (3). Celecoxib was withdrawn and her symptoms resolved over several days. She took a few doses of rofecoxib 12.5 mg/day 6 months later without any problem. She began to take rofecoxib regularly again 2 months later, and after 1 month developed agitation, confusion, and hallucinations. Physical examination suggested no cause of the delirium other than rofecoxib. A CT scan was negative. The rofecoxib was withdrawn, and over the next 2 days her symptoms resolved

Auditory hallucinations have been previously reported in a patient taking celecoxib (SEDA-25, 134) but are probably uncommon.

Hematologic

A report has raised the possibility that patients with a known prothrombotic state and raised platelet thromboxane A_2 production may be at high risk of thrombosis when selective COX-2 inhibitors are used (4).

Thrombosis occurred during celecoxib therapy (400 mg/day) in four women (aged 37–56 years) with connective tissue diseases and conditions that predisposed them to thrombosis, including Raynaud's phenomenon, raised anticardiolipin antibody titers, and a previous history of thrombosis. Peripheral artery thrombosis (three patients) and pulmonary embolism (one patient) were documented after starting celecoxib. Symptoms of thrombosis began to appear within 1 week of starting celecoxib in three patients and 2 months after starting celecoxib in the fourth patient.

A causal relation between celecoxib and these thrombotic events cannot be established with certainty on the basis of the available evidence. However, the temporal relation between the start of treatment and the thrombotic event was impressive, at least in three patients, and the findings were consistent with the hypothesis that thrombosis is an adverse consequence of reduced production of systemic prostaglandin I_2 brought about by COX-2 inhibition. Reduced synthesis of prostaglandin I_2 may act in concert with other thrombotic risk factors (such as those occurring in this series of patients) to precipitate acute vascular occlusion.

Gastrointestinal

Celecoxib reportedly exacerbated inflammatory bowel disease in two patients (5).

- An 80-year-old woman with ulcerative colitis started taking celecoxib for arthritic pain, and 3 days later developed abdominal pain and diarrhea. Celecoxib was withdrawn and her symptoms improved.
- A 35-year-old woman with ileal and perianal Crohn's disease took four doses of celecoxib for an orthopedic injury, and had rectal bleeding, severe abdominal pain, and worse diarrhea. Celecoxib was withdrawn and her symptoms returned to baseline within 5 days.

The possible association of NSAIDs with inflammatory bowel disease is a matter of controversy (SEDA-25, 131), and there is little clinical experience with the selective COX-2 inhibitors. Coxibs should not be prescribed for patients with chronic inflammatory bowel disease until more experience has accumulated.

Liver

A 67-year-old woman developed acute hepatocellular and cholestatic liver damage after taking celecoxib 100 mg/day for 1 week (6). Celecoxib was withdrawn and the liver function tests normalized within 2 weeks.

There have been three case reports of acute cholestatic hepatitis in patients taking celecoxib.

- A 55-year-old non-alcoholic obese woman, who was allergic to sulfa drugs, presented with a 5-day history of jaundice, malaise, and a pruritic rash that began 3 weeks after she started to take celecoxib 200 mg/day for radicular pain (7). There were marked increases in liver enzymes and bilirubin and a peripheral eosinophilia. Liver biopsy showed marked intrahepatocyte cholestasis with eosinophil-rich inflammation, consistent with a drug reaction. Her symptoms and laboratory abnormalities completely resolved after withdrawal of celecoxib but took a long time (4 months) to normalize.
- A 54-year-old woman took celecoxib 200 mg/day for sacroiliac pain (8). After 4 days her pain resolved, but she developed generalized pruritus, which resolved when celecoxib was withdrawn. A week later, the pain recurred and celecoxib was restarted; 2 days later she again developed pruritus associated with dark urine, and 5 days later jaundice and raised bilirubin and liver enzymes. Her eosinophil count was raised. On withdrawal of celecoxib her liver function tests improved and her symptoms resolved.
- A 49-year-old man with alcoholic cirrhosis developed jaundice, fatigue, and choluria after he started to take celecoxib 200 mg/day for musculoskeletal pain (9). There were increases in transaminases, alkaline phosphatase, and bilirubin (to 547 μmol/l). Liver biopsy showed cirrhosis and marked hepatocellular cholestasis. On withdrawal of celecoxib the bilirubin began to fall very slowly; 1 year later he was well, with a total bilirubin concentration of 44 μmol/l.

The histories, clinical findings, and laboratory tests in these cases all suggested celecoxib-induced acute cholestatic hepatitis. The first case suggested that a sulfonamide-like allergic reaction was the pathogenic mechanism, and the same mechanism cannot be excluded in the other two patients, as sulfonamide allergy is often ignored and is discovered only when an adverse reaction occurs. Celecoxib should not be given to patients who are allergic to sulfa drugs.

Urinary tract

As more experience accumulates it appears clear that COX-2 inhibitors have a nephrotoxic potential similar to that of the non-selective NSAIDs. Sixteen cases of tubulointerstitial nephritis were reported to the manufacturers of celecoxib between the time when it was launched in 1999 and July 2001, but the diagnosis was not confirmed in 12 of these cases (10). Most of these renal adverse reactions occur in patients with susceptibility factors associated with prostaglandin-dependent renal function (11–13).

Skin

Skin reactions, including rashes, urticaria, and other allergic reactions, are not uncommon, according to data reported to the Australian Adverse Reactions Advisory Committee (14) and other reports (15–17).

Stevens–Johnson syndrome occurred in a 58-year-old man taking celecoxib (18). He recovered promptly after withdrawal. The reaction recurred 1 month later, after one dose of celecoxib.

Sweet's syndrome can be associated with several drugs. A case involving celecoxib has been reported (19).

- A 57-year-old man developed the typical cutaneous erosions and plaques of Sweet's syndrome after taking celecoxib 100 mg bd for 1 week for bursitis. Celecoxib was withdrawn and the mucocutaneous lesions began to clear. However, the bursitis recurred and he restarted celecoxib. The cutaneous lesions worsened dramatically. After withdrawal of celecoxib for the second time the lesions cleared completely.

Drug–Drug Interactions

Clopidogrel

Co-administration of celecoxib and clopidogrel can increase the hemorrhagic potential of clopidogrel, possibly by a pharmacokinetic interaction involving CYP2C9 (20). However, this possibility requires confirmation, as serious, sometimes fatal, hemorrhage has been reported during the postmarketing use of clopidogrel alone (21).

Warfarin

Celecoxib can potentiate the anticoagulant effects of warfarin. Although concomitant administration of celecoxib and warfarin had no significant effect on prothrombin time or the steady-state pharmacokinetics of *S*-warfarin or *R*-warfarin in 24 healthy volunteers (22), serious bleeding complications have been reported to adverse drug reactions monitoring systems (23) and in journals (24–26). These data suggest that celecoxib potentiates the anticoagulant effects of warfarin in some patients. Patients taking warfarin must be fully monitored when celecoxib is adding, changed, or withdrawn.

References

1. Lantz MS, Giambanco V. Acute onset of auditory hallucinations after initiation of celecoxib therapy. Am J Psychiatry 2000;157(6):1022–3.
2. Lund BC, Neiman RF. Visual disturbance associated with celecoxib. Pharmacotherapy 2001;21(1):114–15.
3. Macknight C, Rojas-Fernandez CH. Celecoxib- and rofecoxib-induced delirium. J Neuropsychiatry Clin Neurosci 2001;13(2):305–6.
4. Crofford LJ, Oates JC, McCune WJ, Gupta S, Kaplan MJ, Catella-Lawson F, Morrow JD, McDonagh KT, Schmaier AH. Thrombosis in patients with connective tissue diseases treated with specific cyclooxygenase 2 inhibitors. A report of four cases. Arthritis Rheum 2000;43(8):1891–6.
5. Bonner GF. Exacerbation of inflammatory bowel disease associated with use of celecoxib. Am J Gastroenterol 2001;96(4):1306–8.
6. Nachimuthu S, Volfinoz L, Gopal LN. Acute liver injury induced by celecoxib. Gastroenterology 2000;118:1471.
7. Galan MV, Gordon SC, Silverman AL. Celecoxib-induced cholestatic hepatitis. Ann Intern Med 2001;134(3):254.
8. O'Beirne JP, Cairns SR. Drug Points: Cholestatic hepatitis in association with celecoxib. BMJ 2001;323(7303):23.
9. Alegria P, Lebre L, Chagas C. Celecoxib-induced cholestatic hepatotoxicity in a patient with cirrhosis. Ann Intern Med 2002;137(1):75.
10. Demke D, Zhao S, Arellano FM. Interstitial nephritis associated with celecoxib. Lancet 2001;358(9294):1726–7.
11. Graham MG. Acute renal failure related to high-dose celecoxib. Ann Intern Med 2001;135(1):69–70.
12. Pfister AK, Crisalli RJ, Carter WH. Cyclooxygenase-2 inhibition and renal function. Ann Intern Med 2001;134(11):1077author reply 1078.
13. Alkhuja S, Menkel RA, Alwarshetty M, Ibrahimbacha AM. Celecoxib-induced nonoliguric acute renal failure. Ann Pharmacother 2002;36(1):52–4.
14. Anonymous. Celecoxib: early Australian reposting experience. Aust Adv Drug React Bull 2000;19:6.
15. Grob M, Scheidegger P, Wuthrich B. Allergic skin reaction to celecoxib. Dermatology 2000;201(4):383.
16. Crouch TE, Stafford CT. Urticaria associated with COX-2 inhibitors. Ann Allergy Asthma Immunol 2000; 84:140.
17. Cummins R, Wagner-Weiner L, Paller A. Pseudoporphyria induced by celecoxib in a patient with juvenile rheumatoid arthritis. J Rheumatol 2000;27(12):2938–40.
18. Gill S, Hermolin RH. Case report of a Stevens–Johnson type reaction to celecoxib. Can J Hosp Pharm 2001; 54:146.
19. Fye KH, Crowley E, Berger TG, LeBoit PE, Connolly MK. Celecoxib-induced Sweet's syndrome. J Am Acad Dermatol 2001;45(2):300–2.
20. Fisher AA, Le Couteur DG. Intracerebral hemorrhage following possible interaction between celecoxib and clopidogrel. Ann Pharmacother 2001;35(12):1567–9.
21. Irish Medicines Board. Clopidogrel (Plavix). Newsletter National Pharmacovigilance Center 2001;2–3.
22. Karim A, Tolbert D, Piergies A, Hubbard RC, Harper K, Wallemark CB, Slater M, Geis GS. Celecoxib does not significantly alter the pharmacokinetics or hypoprothrombinemic effect of warfarin in healthy subjects. J Clin Pharmacol 2000;40(6):655–63.
23. McMorran M, Morawiecka I. Celecoxib (Celebrex): 1 year later. CMAJ 2000;162(7):1044–61048–50.
24. Linder JD, Monkemuller KE, Davis JV, Wilcox CM. Cyclooxygenase-2 inhibitor celecoxib: a possible cause of gastropathy and hypoprothrombinemia. South Med J 2000;93(9):930–2.
25. Mersfelder TL, Stewart LR. Warfarin and celecoxib interaction. Ann Pharmacother 2000;34(3):325–7.
26. Haase KK, Rojas-Fernandez CH, Lane L, Frank DA. Potential interaction between celecoxib and warfarin. Ann Pharmacother 2000;34(5):666–7.

Celiprolol

See also Beta-adrenoceptor antagonists

General Information

Celiprolol is a $beta_1$-selective antagonist with partial $beta_2$-agonist activity. In healthy volunteers it caused "particularly unpleasant" subjective adverse effects, including headache, sleepiness, and feeling cold and generally unwell (1). However, it has beneficial effects on lipids, reducing total cholesterol by 6% and low-density lipoproteins by 10% (SEDA-17, 235). Whether this translates into clinical benefit is not known, and celiprolol has no convincing advantages over other beta-blockers (2).

Organs and Systems

Respiratory

There has been a report of hypersensitivity pneumonitis secondary to celiprolol (3).

References

1. Busst CM, Bush A. Comparison of the cardiovascular and pulmonary effects of oral celiprolol, propranolol and placebo in normal volunteers. Br J Clin Pharmacol 1989;27(4):405–10.
2. Anonymous. Celiprolol—a better beta blocker? Drug Ther Bull 1992;30(9):35–6.
3. Lombard JN, Bonnotte B, Maynadie M, Foucher P, Reybet Degat O, Jeannin L, Camus P. Celiprolol pneumonitis. Eur Respir J 1993;6(4):588–91.

Cephalosporins

See also Beta-lactam antibiotics

General Information

The cephalosporins represent a family of beta-lactam antibiotics originally derived from the naturally occurring cephalosporin C. Isolation of the cephalosporin C nucleus, 7-aminocephalosporanic acid, made it possible to introduce new groups into this molecule to obtain the current variety of compounds (1). Cephalosporins vary widely in their antibacterial properties, beta-lactamase stability, and pharmacokinetic behavior, but there is as yet no unequivocal classification (2). For reasons more practical than pharmacological, cephalosporins are often classified into first-, second-, third- and fourth-generation compounds, as shown in Table 1.

General adverse effects

Reactions that parallel those observed with penicillins include local reactions to parenteral administration, epileptogenicity, effects on sodium and potassium balance, autoimmune hemolytic anemia, neutropenia, thrombocytopenia, and altered platelet function.

More specifically associated with cephalosporins are false-positive Coombs' tests (also seen with clavulanic acid and imipenem + cilastatin), impaired vitamin K-dependent clotting factor synthesis with cephalosporins that contain the *N*-methylthiotetrazole side chain, biliary sludge formation with ceftriaxone, tubular nephrotoxicity of some older compounds (cefaloridine, cefaloglycin, and cefalotin), and disulfiram-like interactions with alcohol. Anaphylactic shock and other IgE antibody-mediated reactions are rare, but analogous to those experienced with the penicillins. Sufficiently reliable tests to predict or prove these reactions are still lacking for the cephalosporins. Other hypersensitivity reactions include acute interstitial nephritis, the majority of drug-inducible mucocutaneous manifestations, and various combinations of symptoms often referred to as "serum sickness-like reactions."

Table 1 Some cephalosporins and cephamycins (all rINNs except where stated)

Orally active cephalosporins	Injectable cephalosporins
Cefaclor[2] (pINN)	Cefamandole[2] (pINN)
Cefadroxil[3] (pINN)	Cefazolin[3] (pINN)
Cefalexin[2] (pINN)	Cefotaxime[3]
Cefetamet[3]	Cefoxitin[2]
Cefixime[3]	Ceftazidime[3]
*Cefradine[1]	Ceftizoxime[3]
*Cefuroxime[2]	Ceftriaxone[3]
	Cefuroxime[2]
	Latamoxef[3] (pINN)

[1]First-generation drugs
[2]Second-generation drugs
[3]Third-generation drugs
*Can also be given by injection

Organs and Systems

Cardiovascular

In isolated cases, cefalotin (3) and cefaclor (4) have been suspected to cause hypersensitivity myocarditis.

Respiratory

Diffuse pulmonary inflammation, as documented by gallium scanning in one case, was possibly caused by ceftriaxone (5). Cefotiam and in another case cefotiam followed by ceftazidime have been suspected to have caused pulmonary hypersensitivity (6,7).

Cefotetan-induced hiccup recurred after each cefotetan infusion and disappeared immediately after withdrawal; it did not recur after administration of another antibiotic (8). Intractable hiccups in a boy were attributed to ceftriaxone-induced pseudolithiasis (9).

Nervous system

In rats, intracerebroventricular injection of various cephalosporins produced markedly different responses in epileptogenic potential (10), later confirmed with a total of 15 compounds (11). Compounds with two heterocyclic rings at both position 3 and position 7 of the cephalosporin molecule, for example ceftriaxone, cefoperazone, and ceftazidime, were even more epileptogenic than benzylpenicillin, while others, with only one heterocyclic ring at position 7, for example cefotaxime and cefonicid, were less potent. Cefazolin, a tetrazole derivative, similar to the convulsant phenyltetrazole, was most potent.

Neurotoxicity has been reported with intracerebroventricular cefazolin (12) and with systemic cefazolin (13–15), cefepime (16), cefotaxime (17–19), ceftazidime (20,21), and cefuroxime (22). Ceftazidime also caused truncal asterixis (23) and absence status and toxic hallucinations (24). Even the least epileptogenic of 15 cephalosporins, namely cefonicid (11), caused seizures (25), although this effect was disputed (26). As expected, seizures after systemic treatment were predominant in uremic patients, and neurotoxicity has been associated with intraperitoneal ceftazidime therapy in a patient undergoing CAPD (27). Of practical interest was a patient treated with intravenous cefmetazole in whom the CSF concentration was twice as high as the corresponding blood concentration (236 versus 103 μg/ml) (28). Uremia may have contributed to this unusual distribution pattern.

- A 66-year-old woman had several episodes of recurrent aseptic meningitis associated with cefalexin, cefazolin, and ceftazidime (29). Intrathecal ceftazidime-specific IgG antibodies were isolated and a skin test with cefazolin provoked recurrence of the aseptic meningitis.

Two patients developed status epilepticus during treatment with cefepime for *Pseudomonas aeruginosa* sepsis (30).

- A 44-year-old man, who had previously had bilateral lung transplantation and who was on hemodialysis for chronic renal insufficiency, was given cefepime 2 g/day. Within 24 hours he started to become confused and developed diffuse hyper-reflexia. Two days later an electroencephalogram showed nearly continuous, generalized sharp-wave/slow-wave activity. After lorazepam 2 mg the status epilepticus resolved, but he remained confused. A follow-up electroencephalogram showed recurrence of generalized sharp-wave activity. Cefepime was withdrawn, and within hours he rapidly recovered his mental status. An electroencephalogram showed absence of epileptiform discharges.
- A 28-year-old woman with a thoracic spina bifida was given cefepime 1 g bd for an infection with *P. aeruginosa*. After a time (not stated) an electroencephalogram showed a continuous generalized spike and wave pattern. She was given lorazepam 2 mg, which resulted in resolution. Cefepime was withdrawn and she promptly recovered.

In the first case the dose was inappropriate for the degree of renal impairment and in the second case the dose was inappropriate for the patient's body weight. The authors underlined the importance of giving cefepime with great care, especially to patients with renal impairment and low body weight.

Five patients developed severe symptoms after receiving cefepime (31). The patients, three men and two women, aged 16–75 years, received 2 g/day ($n = 3$) 4 g/day ($n = 1$) or 9 g/day ($n = 1$). The symptoms started 12–16 days after the start of therapy. In all cases, the initial neurological symptoms (disorientation, confusion, and reduced consciousness) were progressive and were attributed to the infection. Facial or multifocal myoclonic movements occurred subsequently and were rapidly followed by convulsive or non-convulsive status epilepticus. The dose of cefipime had not been adjusted for renal function in any of the patients. Cefepime serum concentrations were measured in three cases, and were 72, 73, and 134 μg/ml. All the patients underwent hemodialysis, and the serum concentrations of cefepime fell to 4.3, 21, and 25 μg/ml respectively. In the other two patients, the serum concentrations after dialysis were 14 and 54 μg/ml, suggesting high concentrations before dialysis. There was complete recovery in four of the patients. One, a 73-year-old woman, died of multiorgan failure with refractory status epilepticus and coma. The authors referred to four other reports of cefepime-induced generalized seizures. They seriously questioned whether the actual frequency of this complication might not be underestimated, owing to insufficient knowledge, underreporting, and/or lack of specificity of clinical features.

- An 82-year-old man on chronic hemodialysis had pneumonia, for which he was given intravenous cefepime 1 g/day (32). After 4 days he developed a seizure and cefepime was withdrawn. Hemodialysis was started and his conscious level improved. On the next day, after a second hemodialysis, he recovered completely.

The authors recommended that in elderly patients with severe renal impairment, other agents than cefepime should be considered.

Psychological, psychiatric

It has long been known that intramuscular procaine penicillin can cause some peculiar psychological adverse reactions, and that other penicillin derivatives, such as amoxicillin, can cause psychiatric reactions, such as hallucinations (SEDA-21, 259). In a report from the Netherlands, neuropsychiatric symptoms occurred in six patients who received cefepime for febrile neutropenia (33). The patients, two men and four women, aged 32–75 years, received 6 g/day ($n = 5$) or 3 g/day ($n = 1$). The symptoms started 1–5 days after the first dose and varied from nightmares, anxiety, agitation, and visual and auditory hallucinations to coma and seizures. After withdrawal of cefepime, they recovered within 1–5 days. The causality between their neuropsychiatric symptoms and cefepime was considered as probable (WHO criteria) because of the temporal relation, lack of other causal neurological explanations, and positive rechallenge in five patients.

The mechanisms of these adverse effects are unknown, although it might be of value to take a closer look at the theory that drug-induced limbic kindling may be the principal pathogenic factor (SEDA-21, 259).

Hematologic

Since the days when chloramphenicol was more commonly used, it has been recognized that many antimicrobial drug are associated with severe blood dyscrasias, such as aplastic anemia, neutropenia, agranulocytosis, thrombocytopenia, and hemolytic anemia. Information on this association has come predominantly from case series and hospital surveys (34–36). Some evidence can be extracted from population-based studies that have focused on aplastic anemia and agranulocytosis and their association with many drugs, including antimicrobial drugs (37,38). The incidence rates of blood dyscrasias in the general population have been estimated in a cohort study with a nested case-control analysis, using data from a General Practice Research Database in Spain (39). The study population consisted of 822 048 patients aged 5–69 years who received at least one prescription (in all 1 507 307 prescriptions) for an antimicrobial drug during January 1994 to September 1998. The main outcome measure was a diagnosis of neutropenia, agranulocytosis, hemolytic anemia, thrombocytopenia, pancytopenia, or aplastic anemia. The incidence was 3.3 per 100 000 person-years in the general population. Users of antimicrobial drugs had a relative risk (RR), adjusted for age and sex, of 4.4, and patients who took more than one class of antimicrobial drug had a relative risk of 29. Among individual antimicrobial drugs, the greatest risk was with cephalosporins (RR = 14), followed by the sulfonamides (RR = 7.6) and penicillins (RR = 3.1).

Hemolytic anemia

Autoimmune hemolytic anemia has rarely been reported with the older cephalosporins, including cefalexin (40), cefalotin (41,42), cefazolin (43), and cefaloridine (44). The main laboratory findings correspond to the "drug adsorption" mechanism classically found in benzylpenicillin-induced immune hemolysis. Antibodies cross-reacting with cefalotin and benzylpenicillin were found in both benzylpenicillin-induced and cefalotin-induced hemolysis (43,45) Cases have also been reported with cefamandole (46), cefalexin (47), ceftriaxone (48), cefotaxime (49,50), cefotetan (51,52) and ceftazidime (53).

Cefotetan-induced hemolytic anemia has been discussed in a review of 35 cases, eight of which were discussed in greater detail (54). All eight cases were associated with the prophylactic use of cefotetan in gynecological or obstetric procedures. The patients had received 1–4 doses of cefotetan, and they left hospital in good shape, but all were re-admitted with hemolytic anemia within 2 weeks after the last dose. All needed several blood transfusions and two underwent plasmapheresis twice. They all survived, but the authors underlined the seriousness of this adverse effect. Of 43 cases of drug-induced hemolytic anemia that had been referred to their laboratory in the previous 8 years, 35 had been caused by cefotetan and three by ceftriaxone; 11 had a fatal outcome, eight and three caused by cefotetan and ceftriaxone respectively.

Hemolytic anemia has also been attributed to ceftizoxime (55).

- A 76-year-old Japanese man, who had been given 23 courses of intravenous antibiotic therapy over 2 years for chronic bronchitis, was given intravenous ceftizoxime 1 g/day. He developed anaphylactic shock and hemolysis. Despite very extensive therapy he died 2 weeks later.

The patient's serum was tested for antibodies against five penicillins and 30 different cephems (that is all types of cephalosporins), using protocols to detect drug adsorption as well as immune-complex mechanisms. His serum contained an IgM antibody that formed immune complexes with 10 of the 30 cephems. The 10 drugs were classified as oxime-type cephalosporins, that is they had a common structural formula at the C7 position on 7-aminocephalosporinic acid. This antibody did not show any cross-reactivity with five kinds of penicillins (ampicillin, aspoxicillin, carbenicillin, piperacillin, sulbenicillin). The authors asked a difficult question: Why did anaphylactic shock accompany acute hemolysis? Their answer was that the complex of ceftizoxime with IgM anti-ceftizoxime might act like anti-A or anti-B. This hypothesis will surely be further tested. In the meantime, it would be wise not to use the newer cephalosporins too freely.

Ceftriaxone has been associated with autoimmune hemolytic anemia, erythroblastocytopenia, and acute hepatitis (56). The ceftriaxone in this case was given intravenously and not orally, as erroneously published (written communication from the authors). Other cases of hemolysis have been reported after ceftriaxone (57).

- A 38-year-old man with no known disease rapidly developed disturbed consciousness 4 days after having taken co-amoxiclav for sinusitis (58). On admission, he was given intravenous ceftriaxone 2 g bd for purulent meningitis. On the 10th day of therapy, he developed icterus and hemolytic anemia. Despite vigorous resuscitative efforts, he died with evidence of multiple organ failure on day 5.
- A 48-year-old woman who had been given ceftriaxone 2 g/day intravenously for 7 days for Lyme disease developed severe hemolytic anemia (59). She had previously been given ceftriaxone twice without any adverse effects. An immune complex mechanism was suggested.
- A 14-year-old girl, perinatally infected with HIV, had a medical history of recurrent infections that had been treated with several antibiotics, including ceftriaxone. She was given ceftriaxone (60 mg/kg intravenously) for pneumonia and 30 minutes later complained of severe back pain, became nauseated, vomited, and collapsed. Despite intensive medical care she died within a few hours with massive intravascular hemolysis and disseminated intravascular coagulopathy. Autopsy was refused.

Of 10 patients with hemolysis due to ceftriaxone, seven died, six of them children (48,57,60–62).

- A 5-year-old girl, who had taken co-trimoxazole prophylaxis for recurrent urinary tract infections since the age of 1 year, received ceftriaxone intramuscularly for 7 days at the age of 5 years, uneventfully (63). Six months later she was given intramuscular ceftriaxone 50 mg/kg/day and amikacin 20 mg/kg for a new urinary tract infection. After 3 days she became unexpectedly ill and had a generalized seizure 30 minutes after the administration of both drugs. A day later, her seizures recurred, she rapidly became worse, and she was referred to an ICU for ventilatory support. There, she had two cardiac arrests and was resuscitated successfully. Her hematocrit and reticulocyte count were eight and 0.2% respectively. A direct antiglobulin test was strongly positive. She was given methylprednisone 5 mg/kg/day and three units of red blood cells. The direct antiglobulin test became negative on day 3, and the dose of methylprednisone was reduced to 3 mg/kg/day but then had to be increased again to 5 mg/kg/day because of recurring hemolysis. The steroid was withdrawn uneventfully after 8 weeks. She remained well and had no neurological deficit.

The authors stated that in children, hemolysis usually starts within minutes to some few hours after the administration of the drug, whereas in adults it starts after a period of days.

Mechanism

In addition to the "drug-adsorption" mechanism, the findings in some instances of anemia associated with cephalosporins were consistent with concomitant formation of auto-antibodies (51) or the so-called "innocent bystander" mechanism, leading to acute intravascular hemolysis, one with ceftriaxone being fatal (48). After this, another six cases were reported, of which five were fatal (57,60,61,64–66). All were due to ceftriaxone and all were in children aged 2–14 years, who were immunocompromised and/or had a hematological disease. All had been previously exposed to ceftriaxone and in some instances also to other cephalosporins. The hemolysis occurred abruptly within 5–54 minutes. However, it is not settled whether the risk reflected by those observations is specific to ceftriaxone or occurs with all cephalosporins. Ceftriaxone has a large share of the cephalosporin market, and three of the reports (61,65,66) were stimulated by a foregoing one (60), which may point to publication bias. Cross-reactivity of ceftriaxone antibodies with other cephalosporins was not studied. The significance of the underlying immunological or hematological diseases and the youth of the patients is also uncertain. Cefalotin and other cephalosporins can cause a positive direct antiglobulin test (67,68). This phenomenon is due to non-specific serum protein adsorption on to the erythrocyte membrane and is not related to immune hemolytic processes. Detection of non-immunologically bound serum proteins improves if reagents used in the direct antiglobulin test include additional antialbumin activity (69). The phenomenon is a known source of difficulties in evaluating suspected immune hemolysis or in routine cross-matching of blood products (70). The true frequency with many individual cephalosporins is unclear, since it has not been positively sought. However, it may depend on daily doses and in particular on the duration of treatment. For example, in a study with cefepime there were positive direct antiglobulin tests in 43% (71). The mean duration of treatment was 19 days and positive direct antiglobulin tests were principally seen in patients taking long-term treatment for osteomyelitis (mean duration of treatment 32 days). On the other hand, ceftazidime given for 9 days induced positive direct antiglobulin tests in 12% of patients (72). Positive direct antiglobulin tests can turn negative again while treatment with cephalosporins continues (71).

In a case of hemolysis associated with ceftriaxone the causative antibodies appeared to be stimulated solely by a degradation product of ceftriaxone (62).

- A 16-year-old girl with craniofacial dysplasia was given ceftriaxone 4 g/day for pneumococcal meningitis. On the seventh day of therapy she developed neck muscle spasms, dizziness, and tachypnea immediately after the administration of ceftriaxone. On the next day, the same symptoms occurred about 30 minutes after the end of the infusion of ceftriaxone. Her plasma was red and her hemoglobin had fallen to 2.4 g/dl. A direct antiglobulin test was positive only for C3d and no ceftriaxone-dependent antibodies were detected. Her serum reacted strongly with erythrocytes in the presence of ex vivo antigen related to ceftriaxone (urine samples from patients receiving ceftriaxone). All therapeutic attempts were unsuccessful and she developed renal insufficiency and died.

The authors concluded that this was the first reported case in which the causative antibodies appeared to be stimulated solely by a degradation product of ceftriaxone. Unfortunately, they were not able to characterize the degradation products. They ended their report by advising that degradation products should be taken into account in all suspected cases of drug-dependent hemocytopenia in which the antibody remains undetectable.

Neutropenia

Virtually all cephalosporins can cause neutropenia and agranulocytosis (73). This has been associated with cefapirin (74), cefepime (75), cefmenoxime (76), cefmetazole (77), ceftriaxone (78–81), moxalactam (82), and others. All of these cases were seen after high cumulative doses given in one treatment course. In one series, cefapirin-induced neutropenia occurred in five of 19 patients who took a total of 90 g or more, but not in 113 patients who took smaller cumulative doses (74). It has not been settled whether toxic mechanisms, immunological mechanisms, or both are involved.

Thrombocytopenia

Thrombocytopenia has rarely been reported, always associated with cefalotin (83–85). In one case there were drug-dependent antibodies. In two other cases the role of drug-dependent antibodies was further evaluated. In one case the antibodies only reacted with platelets in the presence of exogenous cefotetan, but not with cefotetan-coated platelets (86). In another case associated with cefamandole, antibodies cross-reacted with two cephalosporins that had a thiomethyltetrazole group at position 3 but not with other cephalosporins (87). In an additional case, cefuroxime has been implicated (88). In about one-third of cases with cephalosporin-induced neutropenia, slight concomitant thrombocytopenia has been found (73).

Impaired hemostasis

As with other beta-lactam antibiotics, cephalosporins can cause impaired hemostasis and bleeding by altering coagulation and platelet function.

Pseudolymphoma

Pseudolymphoma leukemia (Sézary syndrome) has been reported to occur mainly after the use of phenytoin and other anticonvulsant drugs (89,90), but cefixime has also been implicated (91).

- A 48-year-old woman developed fever and cough, for which she was given oral cefixime. After 48 hours she developed an itchy diffuse erythematous maculopapular rash all over her body. Her white blood cell count was 20×10^9/l, with 8% eosinophils; 5 days later it was 12.5×10^9/l, with atypical, so-called Sézary-like, cells and 64% eosinophils. A bone marrow aspirate showed 20% atypical lymphocytes with a Sézary-like appearance, having large cerebriform nuclei. An increase in eosinophil precursors was also noted. Cefixime was withdrawn, and as she continued to be febrile with a rash and her eosinophil count increased to 72% she was given corticosteroids. Her fever fell to 37.5°C, the rash improved, and her white cell count fell. At follow-up 12 months later her leukocytosis and eosinophilia had completely resolved and she did not have any other problems.

The authors stressed that, like patients with phenytoin-induced pseudolymphoma, this patient will need long-term follow-up to differentiate true prelymphoma. This case can be taken as a reminder that every new beta-lactam coming on the market may have an adverse effects profile of its own.

Mouth and teeth

Three children receiving cefaclor developed intraoral ulcers covered with a thick pseudomembrane together with various skin lesions, suggesting a viral disease at first sight (92).

Gastrointestinal

Acute hemorrhagic colitis without pseudomembranes has been reported after oral cefuroxime (SEDA 21, 261). In mice, some cephalosporins accelerated gastric emptying, in some instances even more effectively than erythromycin or metoclopramide (93). The relevance of this to the gastrointestinal adverse effects of cephalosporins, such as nausea and vomiting, is uncertain.

Liver

As with all beta-lactam antibiotics, slight increases in serum transaminases and alkaline phosphatase have been reported with cephalosporins. However, in contrast to the isoxazolylpenicillins and co-amoxiclav, only very sporadic cases with more severe liver disease have occurred (94–98). Very prolonged cholestasis was reported in isolated cases with cefmenoxime (99) and ceftibuten (98).

Biliary tract

Ceftriaxone has been associated with mostly asymptomatic and reversible biliary sludge. The condition is defined by the presence of low amplitude echoes with absent postacoustic shadows in the gallbladder on ultrasonography and has also been called "biliary pseudolithiasis" (100). Findings consistent with the presence of cholelithiasis (high amplitude echoes with acoustic shadowing) have also been reported (101).

The frequency of biliary sludge in 37 children treated for serious infections was 40% and was lower in adults (about 20%) (100,102,103). The condition usually runs a benign course and ultrasound becomes normal after withdrawal of ceftriaxone within a mean of 15 days (100). However, clinical evidence of cholecystitis has been reported (104). Gallstones containing mostly ceftriaxone have been described (105). In a case-control study of patients treated with ceftriaxone for Lyme disease, more serious biliary complications (cholecystitis and cholelithiasis) were observed in 2%. Age over 18 years and female sex were risk factors (106).

Ceftriaxone does not seem to predispose to subsequent gallbladder stone formation, as assessed 6 and 12 months later (107). The pathogenesis relates to ceftriaxone's high rate of biliary excretion and the subsequent formation of calcium-containing precipitates (108). Thus, apart from the risk factors mentioned above, the risk of biliary sludge may increase with the use of high doses, rapid bolus injection, gall bladder stasis, and renal insufficiency associated with enhanced biliary excretion. Routine ultrasound scans are not required in patients taking ceftriaxone. In the presence of symptoms possibly due to ceftriaxone-associated sludge or cholelithiasis, confirmed by ultrasonography, the drug should be withdrawn. Surgery is mostly unnecessary.

Pancreas

Ceftriaxone has been reported to have caused pancreatitis (109).

- A 13-year-old boy received long-term intravenous ceftriaxone after surgical drainage of a right frontal subdural empyema secondary to sinusitis. After about 5 weeks he developed abdominal pain with profuse emesis; his serum amylase was 1133 U/l and lipase 3528 U/l. Abdominal ultrasound showed cholelithiasis, and he had an uncomplicated cholecystectomy. The material in the gallbladder was 100% ceftriaxone.

The authors ended by stating that patients taking long-term ceftriaxone may be at risk of cholelithiasis and pancreatitis. Ultrasound screening might be useful for monitoring such patients.

Urinary tract

Two of the older cephalosporins, cefaloridine and cefalotin, are nephrotoxic and have often caused renal dysfunction (110,111). The nephrotoxicity of cefaloridine is related to its unusual renal transport, resulting in higher intracellular concentrations in the proximal tubular cells than with other cephalosporins (112). Since less toxic cephalosporins are available, the clinical use of cefaloridine is no longer justified.

Cefalotin can cause two types of renal disease in man (111): acute tubular necrosis, similar to that seen with cefaloridine, although less often; and acute interstitial nephritis, often accompanied by a rash, fever, or eosinophilia, resembling the same disorder as that caused by methicillin.

Beta-lactam nephrotoxicity has been reviewed, particularly considering structure-activity relations (112). Acute proximal tubular necrosis as a consequence of beta-lactam toxicity develops in proportion to:

- uptake by the cupular cell
- acylation inactivation of mitochondrial substrate transporters
- in the case of cefaloridine, lipid peroxidation.

For example, cefaloglycin, which is no longer used, is highly nephrotoxic because of its reactivity, while cefalexin, being comparably sequestered in the tubular cells, is not (112).

Broad clinical use of second- and third-generation cephalosporins has not produced clear evidence of significant nephrotoxicity. In two groups of 10 and 17 patients treated with ceftazidime 3 or 4 g/day, falls in glomerular filtration rate of about 10 ml/minute were seen after treatment courses of 4–9 days or 7–31 days respectively (113,114). For many other cephalosporins comparable data are lacking. Furthermore, an increase in aminoglycoside nephrotoxicity have only been documented with cefalotin and cefaloridine when used in combination (110,115). Nevertheless, adjustment of cephalosporin dosages in renal insufficiency is justified, and acute tubular necrosis can occur with very high doses of cephalosporins other than cefaloridine and cefalotin (116). Isolated cases of acute interstitial nephritis with newer compounds have been related to cefaclor (117), cefamandole (118), cefotaxime (119,120), cefotetan (121), cefoxitin (122), ceftazidime (123), ceftriaxone (124), and cefuroxime (125). Ceftriaxone, on the other hand, protects against tobramycin nephrotoxicity in rats (126). In addition to biliary sludge and stone formation with ceftriaxone, occasional patients developing urinary stones have been described (127,128).

In a report of acute tubulointerstitial nephritis in a patient receiving cefdinir, it was stated that among 41 kinds of cephalosporins available in Japan, this complication has been reported with 12 (129).

- A 58-year-old woman developed acute renal insufficiency soon after a 7-day course of cefdinir 300 mg/day for acute bronchitis. Renal histology showed tubular atrophy and interstitial fibrosis accompanied by moderate lymphocyte infiltration. A lymphocyte stimulation test with cefdinir was positive. Serum creatinine concentrations continued to rise even after withdrawal of cefdinir, but steroid therapy normalized renal function.

The outcome of drug-induced acute tubulointerstitial nephritis can be life-long dialysis or renal transplantation if it is not adequately treated in time. The authors therefore concluded that it is important to look out for this complication when using any cephalosporin.

Skin

Generalized pustular eruptions, histologically presenting as leukocytoclastic vasculitis with neutrophils forming subcorneal pustules, have been reported with different cephalosporins, such as cefaclor (130), cefazolin (131,132), cefalexin (133), and cefradine (134).

Isolated cases of the following syndromes have been reported more recently in connection with cephalosporins:

- pseudolymphoma leukemia syndrome after cefixime presenting with itchy rash, atypical Sézary-like cells, and lymphadenopathy (91);
- pemphigus vulgaris with cefadroxil (135) and cefalexin (136);
- erythema multiforme with cefotaxime (137) and cefalotin (138);
- adult linear IgA disease associated with an erythema multiforme-like reaction with cefamandole (139);
- Stevens–Johnson syndrome with cefalexin (140);
- toxic epidermal necrolysis with cefsulodin (141) and cefazolin (142);
- photosensitivity due to intravenous ceftazidime in a patient with cystic fibrosis (143);
- fixed drug eruption with cefalexin (144);
- occupational contact allergy with ceftiofur (145).

The frequencies of rashes have been retrospectively investigated in 5923 children (146). All the children who developed a rash after treatment with one or more of the commonly used oral antibiotics were identified, 472 in all. Significantly more rashes were documented with cefaclor (4.79%) compared with sulfonamides (3.46%), penicillins (2.72%), and other cephalosporins (1.04%). Based on the numbers of patients for whom the antibiotics were prescribed, the frequencies of rashes were 12.3% for cefaclor, 8.5% for sulfonamides, 7.4% for penicillins, and 2.6% for other cephalosporins.

Telangiectasiae in a light-exposed distribution have rarely been reported with cephalosporins.

- An otherwise healthy 57-year-old man developed telangiectatic skin lesions after receiving intramuscular cefotaxime 1 g bd for 7 days for a urinary tract infection (147). He had used no other medications, and there was no history of photosensitivity or rosacea. He had several asymptomatic telangiectasiae widely distributed on the forehead and on the backs of both hands. Antinuclear antibodies and antineutrophil cytoplasmic antibodies were negative. Skin biopsy showed dilated capillaries without signs of vasculitis. A light provocation test produced telangiectatic lesions at 36 hours. Because of the relation between the administration of cefotaxime and the onset of the telangiectasiae, confirmed by light testing, cefotaxime was withdrawn, with progressive improvement and complete resolution after 2 months; rechallenge was not performed.

Iatrogenic telangiectasis is a poorly understood dermatological adverse effect of several drugs, including cephalosporins (143,148). Telangiectasiae localized to light-exposed areas, as in this case, have been described with some calcium channel blockers (149,150).

Immunologic

Type I reactions

Immediate hypersensitivity reactions, mediated through IgE antibodies to cephalosporin determinants, are a major factor limiting their use. Early cases of anaphylaxis to cephalosporins were probably due to contamination with trace amounts of penicillin (151). These studies may therefore have over-reported cross-sensitivity.

In a retrospective study the frequency of systemic anaphylaxis to cefaloridine, cefalotin, or cefalexin was two out of 9388 patients (0.02%) without a history of penicillin allergy, and two out of 450 patients (0.4%) with a history of penicillin allergy (152). In the first group, two of the 1983 patients treated with cefalotin accounted for the adverse event.

Two of 178 prospective patients, of whom 151 had a history of penicillin allergy but were negative on penicillin skin testing, had reactions to a cephalosporin (153). There were 27 who had a positive penicillin skin test but did not react to a cephalosporin. Similar results were found by others (154).

However, a history of penicillin allergy is often vague, and many studies have suggested that it is an unreliable indicator, which has been confirmed (155). In 62 penicillin skin-test-positive patients, cephalosporins produced only one reaction of mild urticaria and bronchospasm (156).

Primary cephalosporin allergy in patients not allergic to penicillin has been reported, but the exact frequency is not known (157,158). The true incidence of allergic reactions may differ among the cephalosporins. Several reports implicating particular compounds have been published (159–163).

An accurate molecular definition of cephalosporin allergy is not currently available. Relevant determinants of cephalosporin-induced anaphylaxis may not reside in the bicyclic core, but rather in the side chain (164,165).

Neither in vitro tests nor skin tests reliably predict cephalosporin allergy (166). The true frequency of allergic reactions in penicillin-allergic patients exposed to cephalosporins has been estimated to be 1 or 2% (167). Nevertheless, when there is a history of penicillin anaphylaxis or other severe IgE-mediated reactions, it is wise to avoid cephalosporins.

An acute, life-threatening, anaphylactic reaction has been described in a child who received his first intravenous injection of ceftriaxone (168).

- A 3-year-old boy developed a high fever and a petechial rash. In the past he had been treated four times with amoxicillin for upper respiratory tract infections without allergic reactions. At presentation he had multiple petechiae over the trunk and limbs. There were no signs of meningeal irritation. He was given intravenous ceftriaxone 100 mg/kg and after 1 minute developed excitation and a generalized papular urticarial rash. His heart rate increased to 160/minute and the blood pressure was not measurable. He was given subcutaneous adrenaline 0.15 mg plus intravenous clemastine fumarate 2 mg, dexamethasone 3 mg, and fluids. Within 15 minutes his circulation was restored and the urticarial rash abated. Instead of ceftriaxone, he was given chloramphenicol for 7 days, and no further allergic reaction was observed. *Neisseria meningitidis*, sensitive to chloramphenicol and ceftriaxone, was cultured from his blood and spinal fluid. He was discharged well 12 days after admission. One month later, skin tests for ceftriaxone and benzylpenicillin were negative, as was a test for ceftriaxone-specific IgE. Because hypersensitivity could not be demonstrated, a controlled intravenous challenge with ceftriaxone 100 mg/kg was performed, and 20 seconds later there was again excitation and a generalized papular urticarial rash. He was treated as before and recovered within 15 minutes.

According to the authors, anaphylaxis after a single injection of ceftriaxone without previous exposure to the drug is very rare, and they referred to only one previous report (169). However, despite the fact that hypersensitivity could not be demonstrated by skin testing or the presence of ceftriaxone-specific IgE, the outcome of the challenge to ceftriaxone very clearly pointed to an anaphylactic reaction.

An anaphylactic reaction to a subconjunctival injection of cefazolin has been described.

- A 70-year-old white woman with a history of penicillin allergy underwent an uncomplicated eye operation, at the end of which she received a subconjunctival injection of cefazolin 50 mg (170). About 90 minutes postoperatively she developed acute respiratory distress and an erythematous macular rash over the face, neck, chest, forearms, and lateral thighs. The rash became urticarial without pruritus. She was given bronchodilators and intravenous glucocorticoids, with little improvement, but repeated subcutaneous injections of adrenaline gave some improvement in breathing. However, she had to be intubated, and was weaned from the ventilator only after some hours.

The main lesson from this case is that a small amount of a beta-lactam antibiotic anywhere in the body can cause life-threatening anaphylaxis.

Type III reactions

Serum sickness was first described by von Pirquet and Schick in 1905 and was regarded as a syndrome resulting from the administration of heterologous serum or other foreign proteins. The immunopathology of classic serum sickness results from antigen-antibody complex formation with a foreign protein as the antigen. Characteristic symptoms include fever, cutaneous eruptions, edema, arthralgias, and lymphadenopathy. The incidence of classical serum sickness has fallen secondary to the refinement of foreign proteins. However, a serum sickness-like reaction that is clinically similar to classical serum sickness can result from the administration of a number of non-protein drugs, such as tetracyclines, penicillins, cephalosporins (171). The reaction typically occurs within 1 month of the start of therapy and resolves after withdrawal.

Most cephalosporins have sporadically been reported to cause reactions closely resembling classical serum sickness (172,173), and intriguingly comparable syndromes were seen in the majority of a series of volunteers treated for up to 4 weeks with high doses of cefalotin and cefapirin (174). There is so far no clear evidence of drug-specific antibodies. The outcome has always been benign. Earlier suspicions that cefaclor increases the risk of serum sickness-like syndromes (175) have subsequently been confirmed (176–181). The true incidence is still a matter of debate. Data suggest that it is several-fold higher than with other cephalosporins or comparator antimicrobials, such as amoxicillin-containing products, penicillin, flucloxacillin, trimethoprim, and others (182,183). More children are affected, which might at least in part reflect preferential use of cefaclor in this age group (184,185).

Serum sickness has been attributed to cefaclor (186).

- A 2-year-old girl was given cefaclor for an infection, having been given it on one previous occasion without any adverse effects. However, on this occasion, after 6 days she developed a rash, edema, and joint swelling. Her symptoms were thought to be due to serum sickness caused by cefaclor, which was withdrawn. The rash resolved within 2 days and the arthralgia settled within 1 week.

It is still uncertain whether cefaclor-associated serum sickness-like reactions correspond to true hypersensitivity. It has indeed been suggested that they may result from inherited defects in the metabolism of reactive intermediates and may be a unique adverse reaction requiring biotransformation of the parent drug (187). A lymphocyte-based cytotoxicity assay has shown that cefaclor metabolites, as generated by murine hepatic microsomes, mediated cytotoxicity among patients with cefaclor-induced serum sickness-like disease, but not with other immediate or delayed hypersensitivity reactions (188). The positive tests were not shared with loracarbef, a carbacephem with a methylene (instead of a sulfur) substituent at position 5, but otherwise structurally identical to cefaclor. It is not known whether the chemical degradation of cefaclor in vivo (189) contributes to the pathophysiology of serum sickness-like reactions.

Second-Generation Effects

Teratogenicity

Sporadic reports of findings in cell cultures (190) and animals (191) have suggested potential second-generation effects of cephalosporins; however, no such effects are known in man.

Drug Administration

Drug administration route

Thrombophlebitis is a common reaction to the administration of cephalosporins into peripheral veins. The use of buffered solutions mitigated the reaction with cefalotin (192). Published trials have mainly compared older cephalosporins, but the overall results are still contradictory (193,194). Pain and inflammatory reactions after intramuscular injection are also common. Ceftriaxone is probably given more often intramuscularly now than any other cephalosporin. Its local tolerability does not differ from that of other compounds (195).

Drug–Drug Interactions

ACE inhibitors

Intestinal absorption of beta-lactams occurs at least in part by an active mechanism involving a dipeptide carrier, and this pathway can result in interactions with dipeptides and tripeptides (196,197), which reduce the rate of absorption of the beta-lactams. In particular, angiotensin-converting enzyme (ACE) inhibitors, which have an oligopeptide structure, are absorbed by the same carrier (198) and interact with beta-lactams in isolated rat intestine (199). However, there might be a second site of interaction between ACE inhibitors and beta-lactams. Both groups of substances are excreted by the renal anionic transport system, and concomitant administration of both drugs sometimes results in pronounced inhibition of the elimination of beta-lactams (200). In the case of cefalexin, it may not lead to toxic effects. However, when more toxic beta-lactams are used, the possibility of this interaction has to be kept in mind.

In rats, ACE inhibitors reduced renal cefdinir excretion, probably by competition at the tubular anionic carrier (201).

Alcohol

Cephalosporins that contain a methyltetrazole-thiol side chain (as in cefamandole, cefmenoxime, cefmetazole, cefonizid, cefoperazone, ceforanide, cefotetan, cefotiam, latamoxef, and moxalactam) and chemically similar structures (cefepime, ceftriaxone) co-administered with alcohol can produce a disulfiram-like syndrome by inhibiting aldehyde dehydrogenase (195,202,203).

Transient toxic reactions to cefepime and alcohol in the inner ear have been reported (204). Alcohol intolerance needs some time to build up and has been described for up to 5 days after the ingestion of the antibiotic (205,206). It has to be kept in mind that many pharmacological formulations contain alcohol.

Sudden but reversible bilateral labyrinthine hearing loss occurred after cefepime therapy for one-sided otitis and simultaneous intake of alcohol (204). An abortive form of the acetaldehyde syndrome was assumed.

Ciclosporin

Ceftriaxone reportedly increases ciclosporin blood concentrations (207).

Iron

There was a more than 10-fold reduction in AUC when cefdinir was given concomitantly with iron (208). Since the formation of a chelation complex is believed to account for this effect, similar interactions with aluminium- and magnesium-containing antacids are likely.

Vancomycin

Ceftazidime formed microprecipitates when it was mixed with vancomycin (209).

Verapamil

Competitive albumin binding of drugs with high serum protein affinity can increase pharmacologically active unbound concentrations and enhance the metabolism of low clearance drugs. Acute verapamil toxicity with ceftriaxone and clindamycin may be explained by this mechanism (210).

Interference with Diagnostic Tests

Galactose absorption

Some cephalosporins non-competitively inhibited the active absorption of D-galactose by reducing the activity of Na/K-ATPase (211). Theoretically, this effect might interfere with galactose tolerance testing.

Jaffee Test

Certain cephalosporins (cefoxitin, cefpirome, cefacetrile, cefaloglycin, cefaloridine, cefalotin) react with alkaline picrate solution, forming a chromogen with the same spectrum of absorbance as that formed by creatinine and alkaline picrate, producing falsely high serum creatinine values (212,213). This reaction occurs at therapeutic concentrations. Other cephalosporins (cefamandole, cefazolin, cefoperazone, cefotaxime, ceftazidime, ceftriaxone, cefuroxime, latamoxef) do not interfere with this assay (214).

References

1. Abraham EP. Cephalosporins 1945–1986. Drugs 1987;34(Suppl 2):1–14.
2. Williams JD. Classification of cephalosporins. Drugs 1987;34(Suppl 2):15–22.
3. Burke AP, Saenger J, Mullick F, Virmani R. Hypersensitivity myocarditis. Arch Pathol Lab Med 1991;115(8):764–9.
4. Beghetti M, Wilson GJ, Bohn D, Benson L. Hypersensitivity myocarditis caused by an allergic reaction to cefaclor. J Pediatr 1998;132(1):172–3.
5. Krasnow AZ, McNamara M, Akhtar R, Holanders E, Collier BD, Isitman AT. Cephalosporin-induced diffuse pulmonary inflammation depicted by Ga-67 scintigraphy. Clin Nucl Med 1989;14(5):379–80.
6. Irie M, Teshima H, Matsuura T, Sogawa H, Kihara H, Kubo C, Nakagawa T. [Pulmonary infiltration with eosinophilia possibly induced by cefotiam in a case of steroid-dependent asthma.] Nihon Kyobu Shikkan Gakkai Zasshi 1990;28(10):1353–8.
7. Suzuki K, Inagaki T, Adachi S, Matsuura T, Yamamoto T. [A case of ceftazidime-induced pneumonitis.] Nihon Kyobu Shikkan Gakkai Zasshi 1993;31(4):512–16.
8. Morris JT, McAllister CK. Cefotetan-induced singultus. Ann Intern Med 1992;116(6):522–3.
9. Bonioli E, Bellini C, Toma P. Pseudolithiasis and intractable hiccups in a boy receiving ceftriaxone. N Engl J Med 1994;331(22):1532.
10. De Sarro A, De Sarro GB, Ascioti C, Nistico G. Epileptogenic activity of some beta-lactam derivatives: structure–activity relationship. Neuropharmacology 1989;28(4):359–65.
11. De Sarro A, Ammendola D, Zappala M, Grasso S, De Sarro GB. Relationship between structure and convulsant properties of some beta-lactam antibiotics following intracerebroventricular microinjection in rats. Antimicrob Agents Chemother 1995;39(1):232–7.
12. Manzella JP, Paul RL, Butler IL. CNS toxicity associated with intraventricular injection of cefazolin. Report of three cases. J Neurosurg 1988;68(6):970–1.
13. Herd AM, Ross CA, Bhattacharya SK. Acute confusional state with postoperative intravenous cefazolin. BMJ 1989;299(6695):393–4.
14. Josse S, Godin M, Fillastre JP. Cefazolin-induced encephalopathy in a uraemic patient. Nephron 1987;45(1):72.
15. Geyer J, Hoffler D, Demers HG, Niemeyer R. Cephalosporin-induced encephalopathy in uremic patients. Nephron 1988;48(3):237.
16. Chetaille E, Hary L, de Cagny B, Gras-Champel V, Decocq G, Andrejak M. Crises convulsives associées à un surdosage en céfépime. [Convulsive crisis associated with an overdose of cefepime.] Therapie 1998;53(2):167–8.
17. Vincent JP, Dervanian P, Bodak A. Encéphalopathie sous céfotaxime. Une observation chez un sujet âgé insuffisant rénal. [Encephalopathy caused by cefotaxime. A case in an aged patient with renal failure.] Ann Med Interne (Paris) 1989;140(4):322.
18. Pascual J, Liano F, Ortuno J. Cefotaxime-induced encephalopathy in an uremic patient. Nephron 1990; 54(1):92.
19. Wroe SJ, Ellershaw JE, Whittaker JA, Richens A. Focal motor status epilepticus following treatment with azlocillin and cefotaxime. Med Toxicol 1987;2(3):233–4.
20. Douglas MA, Quandt CM, Stanley DA. Ceftazidime-induced encephalopathy in a patient with renal impairment. Arch Neurol 1988;45(9):936–7.
21. Hoffler D, Demers HG, Niemeyer R. Neurotoxizität moderner Cefalosporine. [Neurotoxicity of modern cephalosporins.] Dtsch Med Wochenschr 1986; 111(5):197–8.
22. Herishanu YO, Zlotnik M, Mostoslavsky M, Podgaietski M, Frisher S, Wirguin I. Cefuroxime-induced encephalopathy. Neurology 1998;50(6):1873–5.
23. Hillsley RE, Massey EW. Truncal asterixis associated with ceftazidime, a third-generation cephalosporin. Neurology 1991;41(12):2008.
24. Jackson GD, Berkovic SF. Ceftazidime encephalopathy: absence status and toxic hallucinations. J Neurol Neurosurg Psychiatry 1992;55(4):333–4.
25. Tse CS, Madura AJ, Vera FH. Suspected cefonicid-induced seizure. Clin Pharm 1986;5(8):629.
26. Higbee M, Ramsey R, Swenson E. Cefonicid-induced seizure. Clin Pharm 1987;6(4):271–2.
27. Lye WC, Leong SO. Neurotoxicity associated with intraperitoneal ceftazidime therapy in a CAPD patient. Perit Dial Int 1994;14(4):408–9.
28. Uchihara T, Tsukagoshi H. Myoclonic activity associated with cefmetazole, with a review of neurotoxicity of cephalosporins. Clin Neurol Neurosurg 1988;90(4): 369–71.
29. Creel GB, Hurtt M. Cephalosporin-induced recurrent aseptic meningitis. Ann Neurol 1995;37(6):815–17.
30. Dixit S, Kurle P, Buyan-Dent L, Sheth RD. Status epilepticus associated with cefepime. Neurology 2000; 54(11):2153–5.
31. Chatellier D, Jourdain M, Mangalaboyi J, Ader F, Chopin C, Derambure P, Fourrier F. Cefepime-induced neurotoxicity: an underestimated complication of antibiotherapy in patients with acute renal failure. Intensive Care Med 2002;28(2):214–17.
32. Ferrara N, Abete P, Giordano M, Ferrara P, Carnovale V, Leosco D, Beneduce F, Ciarambino T, Varricchio M, Rengo F. Neurotoxicity induced by cefepime in a very old hemodialysis patient. Clin Nephrol 2003;59(5):388–90.
33. Diemont W, MacKenzie M, Schaap N, Goverde G, Van Heereveld H, Hekster Y, Van Grootheest K. Neuropsychiatric symptoms during cefepime treatment. Pharm World Sci 2001;23:36.
34. George JN, Raskob GE, Shah SR, Rizvi MA, Hamilton SA, Osborne S, Vondracek T. Drug-induced thrombocytopenia: a systematic review of published case reports. Ann Intern Med 1998;129(11):886–90.
35. Wright MS. Drug-induced hemolytic anemias: increasing complications to therapeutic interventions. Clin Lab Sci 1999;12(2):115–18.
36. Arneborn P, Palmblad J. Drug-induced neutropenia—a survey for Stockholm 1973–1978. Acta Med Scand 1982;212(5):289–92.
37. Baumelou E, Guiguet M, Mary JY. Epidemiology of aplastic anemia in France: a case-control study. I. Medical history and medication use. The French Cooperative Group for Epidemiological Study of Aplastic Anemia. Blood 1993;81(6):1471–8.
38. International Agranulocytosis and Aplastic Anemia Study Group. Anti-infective drug use in relation to the risk of agranulocytosis and aplastic anemia. Arch Intern Med 1989;149(5):1036–40.
39. Huerta C, Garcia Rodriguez LA. Risk of clinical blood dyscrasia in a cohort of antibiotic users. Pharmacotherapy 2002;22(5):630–6.

40. Forbes CD, Craig JA, Mitchell R, McNicol GP. Acute intravascular haemolysis associated with cephalexin therapy. Postgrad Med J 1972;48(557):186–8.
41. Gralnick HR, McGinniss M, Elton W, McCurdy P. Hemolytic anemia associated with cephalothin. JAMA 1971;217(9):1193–7.
42. Jeannet M, Bloch A, Dayer JM, Farquet JJ, Girard JP, Cruchaud A. Cephalothin-induced immune hemolytic anemia. Acta Haematol 1976;55(2):109–117.
43. Moake JL, Butler CF, Hewell GM, Cheek J, Spruell MA. Hemolysis induced by cefazolin and cephalothin in a patient with penicillin sensitivity. Transfusion 1978; 18(3):369–73.
44. Kaplan K, Reisberg B, Weinstein L. Cephaloridine. Studies of therapeutic activity and untoward effects. Arch Intern Med 1968;121(1):17–23.
45. Nesmith LW, Davis JW. Hemolytic anemia caused by penicillin. Report of a case in which antipenicillin antibodies cross-reacted with cephalothin sodium. JAMA 1968;203(1):27–30.
46. Branch DR, Berkowitz LR, Becker RL, Robinson J, Martin M, Gallagher MT, Petz LD. Extravascular hemolysis following the administration of cefamandole. Am J Hematol 1985;18(2):213–19.
47. Manoharan A, Kot T. Cephalexin-induced haemolytic anaemia. Med J Aust 1987;147(4):202.
48. Garratty G, Postoway N, Schwellenbach J, McMahill PC. A fatal case of ceftriaxone (Rocephin)-induced hemolytic anemia associated with intravascular immune hemolysis. Transfusion 1991;31(2):176–9.
49. Shulman IA, Arndt PA, McGehee W, Garratty G. Cefotaxime-induced immune hemolytic anemia due to antibodies reacting in vitro by more than one mechanism. Transfusion 1990;30(3):263–6.
50. Salama A, Gottsche B, Schleiffer T, Mueller-Eckhardt C. 'Immune complex' mediated intravascular hemolysis due to IgM cephalosporin-dependent antibody. Transfusion 1987;27(6):460–3.
51. Chenoweth CE, Judd WJ, Steiner EA, Kauffman CA. Cefotetan-induced immune hemolytic anemia. Clin Infect Dis 1992;15(5):863–5.
52. Eckrich RJ, Fox S, Mallory D. Cefotetan-induced immune hemolytic anemia due to the drug-adsorption mechanism. Immunohematol 1994;10(2):51–4.
53. Chambers LA, Donovan LM, Kruskall MS. Ceftazidime-induced hemolysis in a patient with drug-dependent antibodies reactive by immune complex and drug adsorption mechanisms. Am J Clin Pathol 1991; 95(3):393–6.
54. Garratty G, Leger RM, Arndt PA. Severe immune hemolytic anemia associated with prophylactic use of cefotetan in obstetric and gynecologic procedures. Am J Obstet Gynecol 1999;181(1):103–4.
55. Endoh T, Yagihashi A, Sasaki M, Watanabe N. Ceftizoxime-induced hemolysis due to immune complexes: case report and determination of the epitope responsible for immune complex-mediated hemolysis. Transfusion 1999;39(3):306–9.
56. Longo F, Hastier P, Buckley MJ, Chichmanian RM, Delmont JP. Acute hepatitis, autoimmune hemolytic anemia, and erythroblastocytopenia induced by ceftriaxone. Am J Gastroenterol 1998;93(5):836–7.
57. Moallem HJ, Garratty G, Wakeham M, Dial S, Oligario A, Gondi A, Rao SP, Fikrig S. Ceftriaxone-related fatal hemolysis in an adolescent with perinatally acquired human immunodeficiency virus infection. J Pediatr 1998; 133(2):279–81.
58. Punar M, Ozsut H, Eraksoy H, Calangu S, Dilmener M. An adult case of fatal hemolysis induced by ceftriaxone. Clin Microbiol Infect 1999;5(9):585–6.
59. Maraspin V, Lotric-Furlan S, Strle F. Ceftriaxone associated hemolysis. Wien Klin Wochenschr 1999; 111(9):368–70.
60. Bernini JC, Mustafa MM, Sutor LJ, Buchanan GR. Fatal hemolysis induced by ceftriaxone in a child with sickle cell anemia. J Pediatr 1995;126(5 Pt 1):813–15.
61. Scimeca PG, Weinblatt ME, Boxer R. Hemolysis after treatment with ceftriaxone. J Pediatr 1996;128(1):163.
62. Meyer O, Hackstein H, Hoppe B, Gobel FJ, Bein G, Salama A. Fatal immune haemolysis due to a degradation product of ceftriaxone. Br J Haematol 1999; 105(4): 1084–5.
63. Citak A, Garratty G, Ucsel R, Karabocuoglu M, Uzel N. Ceftriaxone-induced haemolytic anaemia in a child with no immune deficiency or haematological disease. J Paediatr Child Health 2002;38(2):209–10.
64. Lo G, Higginbottom P. Ceftriaxone induced hemolytic anemia. Transfusion 1993;33(Suppl):25S.
65. Lascari AD, Amyot K. Fatal hemolysis caused by ceftriaxone. J Pediatr 1995;126(5 Pt 1):816–17.
66. Borgna-Pignatti C, Bezzi TM, Reverberi R. Fatal ceftriaxone-induced hemolysis in a child with acquired immunodeficiency syndrome. Pediatr Infect Dis J 1995; 14(12):1116–17.
67. Molthan L, Reidenberg MM, Eichman MF. Positive direct Coombs tests due to cephalothin. N Engl J Med 1967;277(3):123–5.
68. Garratty G. Review: Immune hemolytic anemia and/or positive direct antiglobulin tests caused by drugs. Immunohematol 1994;10(2):41–50.
69. Petz LD, Garratty G. Acquired Immune Hemolytic Anemias. New York: Churchill Livingstone, 1980.
70. Williams ME, Thomas D, Harman CP, Mintz PD, Donowitz GR. Positive direct antiglobulin tests due to clavulanic acid. Antimicrob Agents Chemother 1985; 27(1):125–7.
71. Jauregui L, Matzke D, Scott M, Minns P, Hageage G. Cefepime as treatment for osteomyelitis and other severe bacterial infections. J Antimicrob Chemother 1993; 32(Suppl B):141–9.
72. Joshi M, Bernstein J, Solomkin J, Wester BA, Kuye O. Piperacillin/tazobactam plus tobramycin versus ceftazidime plus tobramycin for the treatment of patients with nosocomial lower respiratory tract infection. Piperacillin/Tazobactam Nosocomial Pneumonia Study Group. J Antimicrob Chemother 1999;43(3):389–97.
73. Neftel KA, Hauser SP, Muller MR. Inhibition of granulopoiesis in vivo and in vitro by beta-lactam antibiotics. J Infect Dis 1985;152(1):90–8.
74. Vidal Pan C, Gonzalez Quintela A, Roman Garcia J, Millan I, Martin Martin F, Moya Mir M. Cephapirin-induced neutropenia. Chemotherapy 1989;35(6):449–53.
75. Dahlgren AF. Two cases of possible cefepime-induced neutropenia. Am J Health Syst Pharm 1997;54(22):2621–2.
76. Lucht F, Guy C, Perrot JL, et al. Agranulocytose à la cefménoxime. Therapie 1988;43:506.
77. Sugimoto M, Saito K, Hashimoto M, Horie S, Wakabayashi Y, Hirose S, Murata Y, Kobayashi M. [Antibiotics-induced agranulocytosis. Patient's IgG inhibits a GM colony formation.] Rinsho Ketsueki 1989; 30(5):768–73.
78. Rey D, Martin T, Albert A, Pasquali JL. Ceftriaxone-induced granulopenia related to a peculiar mechanism of granulopoiesis inhibition. Am J Med 1989;87(5):591–2.
79. Baciewicz AM, Skiest DJ, Weinshel EL. Ceftriaxone-associated neutropenia. Drug Intell Clin Pharm 1988; 22(10):826–7.
80. Becq-Giraudon B, Cazenave F, Breux JP. Agranulocytose aiguë réversible au cours d'un traitement

par la ceftriaxone. [Acute reversible agranulocytosis during ceftriaxone treatment.] Pathol Biol (Paris) 1986; 34(5):534–5.

81. Osterwalder P, Stocker D. Agranulozytose. [Agranulocytosis.] Schweiz Rundsch Med Prax 1998;87(33):1030–3.
82. Miyano T, Kawauchi K, Suto Y, Yokoyama M, Sato Y. [Latamoxef-induced agranulocytosis—direct inhibition of CFU-C by in vitro colony assay.] Rinsho Ketsueki 1988; 29(2):174–9.
83. Gralnick HR, McGinniss M, Halterman R. Thrombocytopenia with sodium cephalothin therapy. Ann Intern Med 1972;77(3):401–4.
84. Sheiman L, Spielvogel AR, Horowitz HI. Thrombocytopenia caused by cephalothin sodium. Occurrence in a penicillin-sensitive individual. JAMA 1968;203(8):601–3.
85. Naraqi S, Raiser M. Nonrecurrence of cephalothin-associated granulocytopenia and thrombocytopenia. J Infect Dis 1982;145(2):281.
86. Christie DJ, Lennon SS, Drew RL, Swinehart CD. Cefotetan-induced immunologic thrombocytopenia. Br J Haematol 1988;70(4):423–6.
87. Lown JA, Barr AL. Immune thrombocytopenia induced by cephalosporins specific for thiomethyltetrazole side chain. J Clin Pathol 1987;40(6):700–1.
88. Aitken P, Zaidi SM. Cefuroxime-induced thrombocytopenia? Postgrad Med J 1996;72(854):757–8.
89. Rosenthal CJ, Noguera CA, Coppola A, Kapelner SN. Pseudolymphoma with mycosis fungoides manifestations, hyperresponsiveness to diphenylhydantoin, and lymphocyte disregulation. Cancer 1982;49(11):2305–14.
90. D'Incan M, Souteyrand P, Bignon YJ, Fonck Y, Roger H. Hydantoin-induced cutaneous pseudolymphoma with clinical, pathologic, and immunologic aspects of Sézary syndrome. Arch Dermatol 1992;128(10):1371–4.
91. Jabbar A, Siddique T. A case of pseudolymphoma leukaemia syndrome following cefixime. Br J Haematol 1998;101(1):209.
92. Blignaut E. Cefaclor associated with intra-oral ulceration. S Afr Med J 1990;77(8):426–7.
93. Kuo WH, Wadwa KS, Ferris CD. Cephalosporin antibiotics accelerate gastric emptying in mice. Dig Dis Sci 1998;43(8):1690–4.
94. Horsmans Y, Larrey D, Pessayre D, Benhamou JP. Hépatotoxicité des médicaments anti-infectieux. [Hepatotoxicity of antimicrobial agents.] Gastroenterol Clin Biol 1990;14(12):911–24.
95. Vial T, Biour M, Descotes J, Trepo C. Antibiotic-associated hepatitis: update from 1990. Ann Pharmacother 1997;31(2):204–20.
96. Ammann R, Neftel K, Hardmeier T, Reinhardt M. Cephalosporin-induced cholestatic jaundice. Lancet 1982;2(8293):336–7.
97. Kojima N, Kumamoto I, Masumoto T, Onji M. A case report of drug-induced allergic hepatitis probably due to the N-methyltetrazolethiol group cephalosporin. Arerugi 1994;43(3):511–14.
98. Combe C, Banas B, Zoller WG, Manns MP, Schlondorff D. Antibiotikumreduzierte prolongierte Cholestase: Verdacht der Auslösung durch Ceftibuten. [Antibiotic-induced prolonged cholestasis: suspected induction by ceftibuten.] Z Gastroenterol 1996;34(7): 434–7.
99. Kajii N, Matsuda S, Okazaki M, Nishizaki Y, Ohmura R , Fukumoto Y, Harada T. [A case of granulomatous hepatitis caused by administration of antibiotics.] Nippon Shokakibyo Gakkai Zasshi 1993; 90(3): 710–14.
100. Schaad UB, Wedgwood-Krucko J, Tschaeppeler H. Reversible ceftriaxone-associated biliary pseudolithiasis in children. Lancet 1988;2(8625):1411–13.
101. Sahni PS, Patel PJ, Kolawole TM, Malabarey T, Chowdhury D, el-Rashed Gorish M. Ultrasound of ceftriaxone-associated reversible cholelithiasis. Eur J Radiol 1994;18(2):142–5.
102. Heim-Duthoy KL, Caperton EM, Pollock R, Matzke GR, Enthoven D, Peterson PK. Apparent biliary pseudolithiasis during ceftriaxone therapy. Antimicrob Agents Chemother 1990;34(6):1146–9.
103. Pigrau C, Pahissa A, Gropper S, Sureda D, Martinez Vazquez JM. Ceftriaxone-associated biliary pseudolithiasis in adults. Lancet 1989;2(8655):165.
104. Jacobs RF. Ceftriaxone-associated cholecystitis. Pediatr Infect Dis J 1988;7(6):434–6.
105. Lopez AJ, O'Keefe P, Morrissey M, Pickleman J. Ceftriaxone-induced cholelithiasis. Ann Intern Med 1991;115(9):712–14.
106. Genese C, Finelli L, Parkin W, Spitalny KC. From the Centers for Disease Control and Prevention. Ceftriaxone-associated biliary complications of treatment of suspected disseminated Lyme disease—New Jersey, 1990–1992. JAMA 1993;269(8):979–80.
107. Cometta A, Gallot-Lavallee-Villars S, Iten A, Cantoni L, Anderegg A, Gonvers JJ, Glauser MP. Incidence of gallbladder lithiasis after ceftriaxone treatment. J Antimicrob Chemother 1990;25(4):689–95.
108. Shiffman ML, Keith FB, Moore EW. Pathogenesis of ceftriaxone-associated biliary sludge. In vitro studies of calcium-ceftriaxone binding and solubility. Gastroenterology 1990;99(6):1772–8.
109. Maranan MC, Gerber SI, Miller GG. Gallstone pancreatitis caused by ceftriaxone. Pediatr Infect Dis J 1998;17(7):662–3.
110. Zhanel GG. Cephalosporin-induced nephrotoxicity: does it exist? DICP 1990;24(3):262–5.
111. Foord RD. Cephaloridine, cephalothin and the kidney. J Antimicrob Chemother 1975;1(Suppl 3):119–33.
112. Tune BM. Nephrotoxicity of beta-lactam antibiotics: mechanisms and strategies for prevention. Pediatr Nephrol 1997;11(6):768–72.
113. Norrby SR, Burman LA, Linderholm H, Trollfors B. Ceftazidime: pharmacokinetics in patients and effects on the renal function. J Antimicrob Chemother 1982;10(3):199–206.
114. Alestig K, Trollfors B, Andersson R, Olaison L, Suurkula M, Norrby SR. Ceftazidime and renal function. J Antimicrob Chemother 1984;13(2):177–81.
115. Rankin GO, Sutherland CH. Nephrotoxicity of aminoglycosides and cephalosporins in combination. Adverse Drug React Acute Poisoning Rev 1989; 8(2):73–88.
116. Lentnek AL, Rosenworcel E, Kidd L. Acute tubular necrosis following high-dose cefamandole therapy for *Hemophilus parainfluenzae* endocarditis. Am J Med Sci 1981;281(3):164–8.
117. Pommer W, Krause PH, Berg PA, Neumayer HH, Mihatsch MJ, Molzahn M. Acute interstitial nephritis and non-oliguric renal failure after cefaclor treatment. Klin Wochenschr 1986;64(6):290–3.
118. Csanyi P, Rado JP, Hormay M. Acute renal failure due to cephamandole. BMJ (Clin Res Ed) 1988; 296(6619):433.
119. Grcevska L, Polenakovic M. Second attack of acute tubulointerstitionephritis induced by cefataxim and pregnancy. Nephron 1996;72(2):354–5.
120. al Shohaib S, Satti MS, Abunijem Z. Acute interstitial nephritis due to cefotaxime. Nephron 1996;73(4):725.

121. Nguyen VD, Nagelberg H, Agarwal BN. Acute interstitial nephritis associated with cefotetan therapy. Am J Kidney Dis 1990;16(3):259–61.
122. Toll LL, Lee M, Sharifi R. Cefoxitin-induced interstitial nephritis. South Med J 1987;80(2):274–5.
123. Ladagnous JF, Rousseau JM, Gaucher A, Saissy JM, Pitti R. Néphrite interstitielle aiguë: rôle de la ceftazidime. [Acute interstitial nephritis. Role of ceftazidime.] Ann Fr Anesth Reanim 1996;15(5):677–80.
124. Mancini S, Iacovoni R, Fierimonte V, Spaini A, Parisi MC, Pichi A. Nefrite interstiziale da farmaci. Descrizione di un caso clinico. [Drug-induced interstitial nephritis. A case report.] Minerva Pediatr 1994;46(12):557–60.
125. Goddard JK, Janning SW, Gass JS, Wilson RF. Cefuroxime-induced acute renal failure. Pharmacotherapy 1994; 14(4):488–91.
126. Beauchamp D, Theriault G, Grenier L, Gourde P, Perron S, Bergeron Y, Fontaine L, Bergeron MG. Ceftriaxone protects against tobramycin nephrotoxicity. Antimicrob Agents Chemother 1994;38(4):750–6.
127. Schaad UB, Suter S, Gianella-Borradori A, Pfenninger J, Auckenthaler R, Bernath O, Cheseaux JJ, Wedgwood J. A comparison of ceftriaxone and cefuroxime for the treatment of bacterial meningitis in children. N Engl J Med 1990;322(3):141–7.
128. Cochat P, Cochat N, Jouvenet M, Floret D, Wright C, Martin X, Vallon JJ, David L. Ceftriaxone-associated nephrolithiasis. Nephrol Dial Transplant 1990; 5(11):974–6.
129. Diemont W, MacKenzie M, Schaap N, Goverde G, van Heereveld H, Hekster Y, van Grootheest K. Neuropsychiatric symptoms during cefepime treatment. Pharm World Sci 2001;23(1):36.
130. Ogoshi M, Yamada Y, Tani M. Acute generalized exanthematic pustulosis induced by cefaclor and acetazolamide. Dermatology 1992;184(2):142–4.
131. Stough D, Guin JD, Baker GF, Haynie L. Pustular eruptions following administration of cefazolin: a possible interaction with methyldopa. J Am Acad Dermatol 1987;16(5 Pt 1):1051–2.
132. Fayol J, Bernard P, Bonnetblanc JM. Pustular eruption following administration of cefazolin: a second case report. J Am Acad Dermatol 1988;19(3):571.
133. Jackson H, Vion B, Levy PM. Generalized eruptive pustular drug rash due to cephalexin. Dermatologica 1988;177(5):292–4.
134. Kalb RE, Grossman ME. Pustular eruption following administration of cephradine. Cutis 1986;38(1):58–60.
135. Wilson JP, Koren JF, Daniel RC 3rd, Chapman SW. Cefadroxil-induced ampicillin-exacerbated pemphigus vulgaris: case report and review of the literature. Drug Intell Clin Pharm 1986;20(3):219–23.
136. Wolf R, Dechner E, Ophir J, Brenner S. Cephalexin. A nonthiol drug that may induce pemphigus vulgaris. Int J Dermatol 1991;30(3):213–15.
137. Green ST, Natarajan S, Campbell JC. Erythema multiforme following cefotaxime therapy. Postgrad Med J 1986;62(727):415.
138. Munoz D, Del Pozo MD, Audicana M, Fernandez E, Fernandez De Corres LF. Erythema-multiforme-like eruption from antibiotics of 3 different groups. Contact Dermatitis 1996;34(3):227–8.
139. Argenyi ZB, Bergfeld WF, Valenzuela R, McMahon JT, Taylor JS. Adult linear IgA disease associated with an erythema multiforme-like drug reaction. Cleve Clin J Med 1987;54(5):445–50.
140. Murray KM, Camp MS. Cephalexin-induced Stevens–Johnson syndrome. Ann Pharmacother 1992; 26(10):1230–3.
141. Okano M, Kitano Y, Ohzono K. Toxic epidermal necrolysis due to cephem. Int J Dermatol 1988;27(3):183–4.
142. Julsrud ME. Toxic epidermal necrolysis. J Foot Ankle Surg 1994;33(3):255–9.
143. Vinks SA, Heijerman HG, de Jonge P, Bakker W. Photosensitivity due to ambulatory intravenous ceftazidime in cystic fibrosis patient. Lancet 1993; 341(8854): 1221–2.
144. Baran R, Perrin C. Fixed-drug eruption presenting as an acute paronychia. Br J Dermatol 1991;125(6):592–5.
145. Garcia F, Juste S, Garces MM, Carretero P, Blanco J, Herrero D, Perez R. Occupational allergic contact dermatitis from ceftiofur without cross-sensitivity. Contact Dermatitis 1998;39(5):260.
146. Ibia EO, Schwartz RH, Wiedermann BL. Antibiotic rashes in children: a survey in a private practice setting. Arch Dermatol 2000;136(7):849–54.
147. Borgia F, Vaccaro M, Guarneri F, Cannavo SP. Photodistributed telangiectasia following use of cefotaxime. Br J Dermatol 2000;143(3):674–5.
148. Flax SH, Uhle P. Photo recall-like phenomenon following the use of cefazolin and gentamicin sulfate. Cutis 1990;46(1):59–61.
149. Collins P, Ferguson J. Photodistributed nifedipine-induced facial telangiectasia. Br J Dermatol 1993; 129(5):630–3.
150. Basarab T, Yu R, Jones RR. Calcium antagonist-induced photo-exposed telangiectasia. Br J Dermatol 1997; 136(6):974–5.
151. Pedersen-Bjergaard J. Cephalotin in the treatment of penicillin-sensitive patients. Acta Allergol 1967;22:299.
152. Petz LD. Immunologic reactions of humans to cephalosporins. Postgrad Med J 1971;47(Suppl):64–9.
153. Solley GO, Gleich GJ, Van Dellen RG. Penicillin allergy: clinical experience with a battery of skin-test reagents. J Allergy Clin Immunol 1982;69(2):238–44.
154. Van Arsdel PP Jr, Miller S. Antimicrobial treatment of patients with a penicillin allergy history. J Allergy Clin Immunol 1990;85:188.
155. Surtees SJ, Stockton MG, Gietzen TW. Allergy to penicillin: fable or fact? BMJ 1991;302(6784):1051–2.
156. Saxon A, Beall GN, Rohr AS, Adelman DC. Immediate hypersensitivity reactions to beta-lactam antibiotics. Ann Intern Med 1987;107(2):204–15.
157. Abraham GN, Petz LD, Fudenberg HH. Cephalothin hypersensitivity associated with anti-cephalothin antibodies. Int Arch Allergy Appl Immunol 1968; 34(1):65–74.
158. Ong R, Sullivan T. Detection and characterization of human IgE to cephalosporin determinants. J Allergy Clin Immunol 1988;81:222.
159. Nishioka K, Katayama I, Kobayashi Y, Takijiri C. Anaphylaxis due to cefaclor hypersensitivity. J Dermatol 1986;13(3):226–7.
160. Hama R, Mori K. High incidence of anaphylactic reactions to cefaclor. Lancet 1988;1(8598):1331.
161. Levine LR. Quantitative comparison of adverse reactions to cefaclor vs. amoxicillin in a surveillance study. Pediatr Infect Dis 1985;4(4):358–61.
162. Bloomberg RJ. Cefotetan-induced anaphylaxis. Am J Obstet Gynecol 1988;159(1):125–6.
163. Hashimoto Y, Soeda A, Takarada M, Tanioka H. Anaphylaxis to moxalactam: report of a case. J Oral Maxillofac Surg 1990;48(9):1004–6.
164. Blanca M, Fernandez J, Miranda A, Terrados S, Torres MJ, Vega JM, Avila MJ, Perez E, Garcia JJ, Suau R. Cross-reactivity between penicillins and cephalosporins: clinical and immunologic studies. J Allergy Clin Immunol 1989;83(2 Pt 1):381–5.

165. Anderson JA. Cross-sensitivity to cephalosporins in patients allergic to penicillin. Pediatr Infect Dis 1986;5(5):557–61.
166. Saxon A, Beall GN, Rohr AS, et al. Immediate hypersensitivity reactions to beta-lactam antibiotics. Urology 1988;31(Suppl):14.
167. Saxon A. Antibiotic choices for the penicillin-allergic patient. Postgrad Med 1988;83(4):135–8, 141–2, 147–8.
168. Ernst MR, van Dijken PJ, Kabel PJ, Draaisma JM. Anaphylaxis after first exposure to ceftriaxone. Acta Paediatr 2002;91(3):355–6.
169. Romano A, Piunti E, Di Fonso M, Viola M, Venuti A, Venemalm L. Selective immediate hypersensitivity to ceftriaxone. Allergy 2000;55(4):415–16.
170. Berrocal AM, Schuman JS. Subconjunctival cephalosporin anaphylaxis. Ophthalmic Surg Lasers 2001;32(1):79–80.
171. Mannik M. Serum sickness and pathophysiology of immune complexes. In: Rich RR, Fleisher TA, Schwartz BD, editors. Clinical Immunology, Principles and Practice. St Louis: Mosby Year Book Inc, 1996:1062–71.
172. Lowery N, Kearns GL, Young RA, Wheeler JG. Serum sickness-like reactions associated with cefprozil therapy. J Pediatr 1994;125(2):325–8.
173. Plantin P, Milochau P, Dubois D. Nefrite interstiziale da farmaci. Descrizione di un caso clinico. [Drug-induced serum sickness after ingestion of cefatrizine. First reported case.] Presse Méd 1992;21(40):1915.
174. Sanders WE Jr, Johnson JE 3rd, Taggart JG. Adverse reactions to cephalothin and cephapirin. Uniform occurrence on prolonged intravenous administration of high doses. N Engl J Med 1974;290(8):424–9.
175. Murray DL, Singer DA, Singer AB, Veldman JP. Cefaclor—a cluster of adverse reactions. N Engl J Med 1980;303(17):1003.
176. Platt R, Dreis MW, Kennedy DL, Kuritsky JN. Serum sickness-like reactions to amoxicillin, cefaclor, cephalexin, and trimethoprim–sulfamethoxazole. J Infect Dis 1988;158(2):474–7.
177. Heckbert SR, Stryker WS, Coltin KL, Manson JE, Platt R. Serum sickness in children after antibiotic exposure: estimates of occurrence and morbidity in a health maintenance organization population. Am J Epidemiol 1990;132(2):336–42.
178. Stricker BH, Tijssen JG. Serum sickness-like reactions to cefaclor. J Clin Epidemiol 1992;45(10):1177–84.
179. Vial T, Pont J, Pham E, Rabilloud M, Descotes J. Cefaclor-associated serum sickness-like disease: eight cases and review of the literature. Ann Pharmacother 1992;26(7–8):910–14.
180. Hebert AA, Sigman ES, Levy ML. Serum sickness-like reactions from cefaclor in children. J Am Acad Dermatol 1991;25(5 Pt 1):805–8.
181. Parra FM, Igea JM, Martin JA, Alonso MD, Lezaun A, Sainz T. Serum sickness-like syndrome associated with cefaclor therapy. Allergy 1992;47(4 Pt 2):439–40.
182. Parshuram CS, Phillips RJ. Retrospective review of antibiotic-associated serum sickness in children presenting to a paediatric emergency department. Med J Aust 1998;169(2):116.
183. Martin J, Abbott G. Serum sickness like illness and antimicrobials in children. NZ Med J 1995;108(997):123–4.
184. Boyd IW. Cefaclor-associated serum sickness. Med J Aust 1998;169(8):443–4.
185. Anonymous. Canadian Adverse Drug Reaction Newsletter. Can Med Assoc J 1996;155:913.
186. Isaacs D. Serum sickness-like reaction to cefaclor. J Paediatr Child Health 2001;37(3):298–9.
187. Kearns GL, Wheeler JG, Childress SH, Letzig LG. Serum sickness-like reactions to cefaclor: role of hepatic metabolism and individual susceptibility. J Pediatr 1994;125(5 Pt 1):805–11.
188. Kearns GL, Wheeler JG, Rieder MJ, Reid J. Serum sickness-like reaction to cefaclor: lack of in vitro cross-reactivity with loracarbef. Clin Pharmacol Ther 1998;63(6):686–93.
189. Sourgens H, Derendorf H, Schifferer H. Pharmacokinetic profile of cefaclor. Int J Clin Pharmacol Ther 1997;35(9):374–80.
190. Jaju M, Jaju M, Ahuja YR. Effect of cephaloridine on human chromosomes in vitro in lymphocyte cultures. Mutat Res 1982;101(1):57–66.
191. Hoover DM, Buening MK, Tamura RN, Steinberger E. Effects of cefamandole on spermatogenic development of young CD rats. Fundam Appl Toxicol 1989;13(4):737–46.
192. Berger S, Ernst EC, Barza M. Comparative incidence of phlebitis due to buffered cephalothin, cephapirin, and cefamandole. Antimicrob Agents Chemother 1976;9(4):575–9.
193. Cole DR. Double-blind comparison of phlebitis associated with cefazolin and cephalothin. Int J Clin Pharmacol Biopharm 1976;14(1):75–7.
194. Browning MC, Tune BM. Toxicology of Betalactam Antibiotics. In: Demain AL, Solomon NA, editors. Antibiotics Containing the Betalactam Structure, Part II. Berlin: Springer-Verlag, 1983:371.
195. Moskovitz BL. Clinical adverse effects during ceftriaxone therapy. Am J Med 1984;77(4C):84–8.
196. Sugawara M, Toda T, Iseki K, Miyazaki K, Shiroto H, Kondo Y, Uchino J. Transport characteristics of cephalosporin antibiotics across intestinal brush-border membrane in man, rat and rabbit. J Pharm Pharmacol 1992;44(12):968–72.
197. Dantzig AH, Bergin L. Uptake of the cephalosporin, cephalexin, by a dipeptide transport carrier in the human intestinal cell line, Caco-2. Biochim Biophys Acta 1990;1027(3):211–17.
198. Friedman DI, Amidon GL. Intestinal absorption mechanism of dipeptide angiotensin converting enzyme inhibitors of the lysyl-proline type: lisinopril and SQ 29,852. J Pharm Sci 1989;78(12):995–8.
199. Hu M, Amidon GL. Passive and carrier-mediated intestinal absorption components of captopril. J Pharm Sci 1988;77(12):1007–11.
200. Padoin C, Tod M, Perret G, Petitjean O. Analysis of the pharmacokinetic interaction between cephalexin and quinapril by a nonlinear mixed-effect model. Antimicrob Agents Chemother 1998;42(6):1463–9.
201. Jacolot A, Tod M, Petitjean O. Pharmacokinetic interaction between cefdinir and two angiotensin-converting enzyme inhibitors in rats. Antimicrob Agents Chemother 1996;40(4):979–82.
202. Kitson TM. The effect of cephalosporin antibiotics on alcohol metabolism: a review. Alcohol 1987;4(3):143–8.
203. Norrby SR. Side effects of cephalosporins. Drugs 1987;34(Suppl 2):105–20.
204. Klemm E, Mross C. Akute beidseitige Innenohrschwerhörigkeit durch Cefepim und Alkohol. [Sudden bilateral labyrinthine hearing loss due to cefepime and alcohol.] Otorhinolaryngol Nova 1997;7/1:45.
205. Buening MK, Wold JS. Ethanol–moxalactam interactions in vivo. Rev Infect Dis 1982;4(Suppl):S555–63.
206. Heizmann WR, Trautmann M, Marre R. Antiinfektiöse Chemotherapie. Stuttgart: Wissenschaftliche Verlags gesellschaft, 1996:176.
207. Soto Alvarez J, Sacristan Del Castillo JA, Alsar Ortiz MJ. Interaction between ciclosporin and ceftriaxone. Nephron 1991;59(4):681–2.
208. Stoeckel K, Hayton WL, Edwards DJ. Clinical pharmacokinetics of oral cephalosporins. Antibiot Chemother 1995;47:34–71.

209. Fiscella RG. Physical incompatibility of vancomycin and ceftazidime for intravitreal injection. Arch Ophthalmol 1993;111(6):730.
210. Kishore K, Raina A, Misra V, Jonas E. Acute verapamil toxicity in a patient with chronic toxicity: possible interaction with ceftriaxone and clindamycin. Ann Pharmacother 1993;27(7–8):877–80.
211. Idoate I, Mendizabal MV, Urdaneta E, Larralde J. Interactions of cephradine and cefaclor with the intestinal absorption of D-galactose. J Pharm Pharmacol 1996;48(6):645–50.
212. Swain RR, Briggs SL. Positive interference with the Jaffe reaction by cephalosporin antibiotics. Clin Chem 1977;23(7):1340–2.
213. Grotsch H, Hajdu P. Interference by the new antibiotic cefpirome and other cephalosporins in clinical laboratory tests, with special regard to the "Jaffe" reaction. J Clin Chem Clin Biochem 1987;25(1):49–52.
214. Kroll MH, Elin RJ. Mechanism of cefoxitin and cephalothin interference with the Jaffe method for creatinine. Clin Chem 1983;29(12):2044–8.

Cerivastatin

See also HMG Co-A reductase inhibitors

General Information

Weight for weight, cerivastatin is the most potent statin. Like other statins, the chance of rhabdomyolysis increases when cerivastatin is taken together with certain other drugs (1). Although cerivastatin is degraded by two different isoforms of P_{450} in the liver, and therefore should be less likely to take part in drug interactions than most of the other statins, clinically important interactions do occur, and reports of drug interactions in 2001 triggered its withdrawal, after 31 people in the USA taking cerivastatin, 12 of whom had also taken gemfibrozil, died of severe rhabdomyolysis (2).

In other respects, the adverse effects of cerivastatin are similar to those of other statins (3), and a pooled analysis of studies of cerivastatin 100–400 micrograms/day taken for at least 8 weeks showed no differences in drug-related adverse events between cerivastatin and placebo (4). There was no association between plasma transaminase or creatine kinase activities and cerivastatin dosages. Cerivastatin 800 micrograms/day for 4 weeks had only mild transient adverse effects (5).

Organs and Systems

Liver

There were increases in serum transaminase activities to more than three times the top end of the reference range in under 1% of patients taking cerivastatin, which is similar to findings with other statins (6).

Musculoskeletal

There were no cases of myalgia in 94 patients taking cerivastatin 50–300 micrograms/day for 72 weeks, whereas in the same study, two of 59 patients taking simvastatin had myalgia (7). At dosages of 300–400 micrograms/day for 8 weeks in 349 patients there were no rises in creatine kinase activity above 10 times the upper limit of the reference range, and asymptomatic increases (to over three times the upper limit of the reference range) occurred more often with placebo (2.8%) than with cerivastatin (1.4% with 0.4 mg; none with 0.3 mg) (8).

Drug–Drug Interactions

Ciclosporin

Cerivastatin 0.2 mg/day was well tolerated when given together with ciclosporin, although there were 3- to 5-fold increases in the plasma concentrations of cerivastatin and its metabolites when single-dose cerivastatin was given to 12 kidney transplant recipients taking ciclosporin 200 mg bd and to 12 healthy controls (9). Ciclosporin may have affected both the distribution of cerivastatin and its biotransformation in the liver.

Gemfibrozil

Cerivastatin was withdrawn in 2001 after 31 people in the USA taking cerivastatin, 12 of whom had also taken gemfibrozil, died of severe rhabdomyolysis (2).

- Myalgia and a marked increase in creatine kinase was precipitated in a 74-year-old woman with normal renal function who took gemfibrozil 1200 mg/day 3 weeks after she had started to take cerivastatin 300 μg/day (10).

References

1. Horsmans Y. Differential metabolism of statins: importance in drug–drug interactions. Eur Heart J Suppl 1999;1(Suppl T):T7–12.
2. Thompson CA. Cerivastatin withdrawn from market. Am J Health Syst Pharm 2001;58(18):1685.
3. McClellan KJ, Wiseman LR, McTavish D. Cerivastatin. Drugs 1998;55(3):415–20.
4. Stein E, Schopen U, Catagay M. A pooled efficacy analysis of cerivastatin in the treatment of primary hyperlipidaemia. Clin Drug Invest 1999;18:433–44.
5. Stein E, Isaacsohn J, Stoltz R, Mazzu A, Liu MC, Lane C, Heller AH. Pharmacodynamics, safety, tolerability, and pharmacokinetics of the 0.8-mg dose of cerivastatin in patients with primary hypercholesterolemia. Am J Cardiol 1999;83(10):1433–6.
6. Anonymous. Cerivastatin for hypercholesterolemia. Med Lett Drugs Ther 1998;40(1018):13–14.
7. Leiter LA, Hanna K. Efficacy and safety of cerivastatin in primary hypercholesterolemia: a long term comparative titration study with simvastatin. Can J Cardiol 1999;15(5):545–55.
8. Davignon J, Hanefeld M, Nakaya N, Hunninghake DB, Insull W Jr, Ose L. Clinical efficacy and safety of cerivastatin: summary of pivotal phase IIb/III studies. Am J Cardiol 1998;82(4B):J32–9.
9. Muck W, Mai I, Fritsche L, Ochmann K, Rohde G, Unger S, Johne A, Bauer S, Budde K, Roots I, Neumayer HH, Kuhlmann J. Increase in cerivastatin systemic exposure after single and multiple dosing in cyclosporine-treated

kidney transplant recipients. Clin Pharmacol Ther 1999; 65(3):251–61.
10. Pogson GW, Kindred LH, Carper BG. Rhabdomyolysis and renal failure associated with cerivastatin–gemfibrozil combination therapy. Am J Cardiol 1999;83(7):1146.

Ceruletide

General Information

Ceruletide is a synthetic decapeptide that resembles cholecystokinin and causes contraction of the gallbladder. It has sometimes been used instead of the traditional "fatty meal" in cholecystography. After intramuscular injection, nausea, vomiting, diarrhea, and cramps have been reported.

Intravenous injection can cause spasm of the gall-bladder neck and severe pain with tingling sensations, sweating, and mild hypotension (1).

Reference

1. Sargent EN, Boswell W, Hubsher J. Cholecystokinetic cholecystography: efficacy and tolerance studies of ceruletide. Am J Roentgenol 1978;130(6):1051–5.

Cetirizine

See also Antihistamines

General Information

Cetirizine is a non-sedating metabolite of hydroxyzine (SEDA-18, 181) (SEDA-19, 172) (SEDA-21, 172) (SEDA-22, 178). There is only minor hepatic metabolism of cetirizine (1), which is excreted unchanged in the urine. It has not been associated with dysrhythmias. Skin reactions have been reported, and the anticoagulant activity of acenocoumarol may be potentiated (SEDA-22, 178).

Seasonal allergic rhinitis affects about 10% of school-age children, and there is evidence of a significant impact of the disease on health-related quality of life. The effect on health-related quality of life of once-daily of cetirizine syrup 10 mg/day for 4 weeks has been studied in 544 children with seasonal allergic rhinitis in a multicenter, open, non-comparative study (2). In addition to improvements in symptom scores the authors also reported significant improvements in health-related quality of life, with good tolerability of the drug. Treatment-related adverse effects were reported in 22 subjects, of which somnolence was the most frequent problem, reported by six of the subjects. Only 12 of subjects discontinued treatment owing to an adverse effect.

Health-related quality of life and clinical outcomes in 865 adult patients with seasonal allergic rhinitis treated with cetirizine or placebo for 2 weeks have been evaluated in a double-blind, randomized, parallel-group study (3). Cetirizine significantly improved both symptoms and health-related quality of life, while treatment-related adverse effects were comparable with those in the placebo group.

Organs and Systems

Cardiovascular

In a prospective, double-blind, parallel-group study for 18 months in 817 children with atopic dermatitis aged 12–24 months, cetirizine 0.25 mg/kg bd had no effect on the QT_c interval (4).

In a double-blind, randomized, placebo-controlled study in 85 infants aged 6–11 months there were no differences in the frequencies of adverse events between those who were given cetirizine or placebo, and no electrocardiographic changes, particularly in the QT interval (5).

Nervous system

Oculogyric crisis has been described in nine patients treated with cetirizine; eight cases occurred in children (6).

The effects of cetirizine (5, 10, and 15 mg) on sleep latency, subjective sleepiness, and performance from 0.5 to 7.5 hours after ingestion have been studied (7). Cetirizine produced shortened sleep latencies, increased subjective sleepiness, and impaired tracking. The authors considered that cetirizine should not be used by personnel involved in critical occupations.

Psychological, psychiatric

In a double-blind, crossover study levocetirizine 5 mg once daily for 4 days was compared with cetirizine 10 mg, loratadine 10 mg, promethazine 30 mg, and placebo in terms of nervous system inhibitory effects in 20 healthy volunteers (8). With the exception of promethazine, none of the drugs had disruptive or sedative effects on objective measurements in a comprehensive battery of psychomotor and cognitive tests.

The Early Treatment of the Atopic Child (ETAC) Study has provided evidence that cetirizine may be able to halt the progression to asthma in high-risk groups of young children and infants with atopic dermatitis (9). However, the study involved giving relatively high doses of cetirizine to very young children (aged 1–2 years at study entry) over a long period of time. Therefore, the impact of prolonged use of high-dose cetirizine (0.25 mg/kg bd over 18 months) on behavior and cognitive ability in young children and infants has been assessed in a double-blind, randomized, placebo-controlled study (10). Well-validated and standardized assessments of behavior or cognition were used, and the ages at which psychomotor milestones were attained were established. The authors concluded that, compared with placebo, cetirizine had no significant effects on behavior, cognition, or psychomotor milestones in young children with atopic dermatitis.

Liver

Severe hepatitis has been reported in a 23-year-old man taking cetirizine (11) and cholestasis in a 28-year-old man who had taken cetirizine for 2 years (12). However, a causal relation between these uncommon events and cetirizine was difficult to confirm.

Skin

Cutaneous reactions have been reported with cetirizine (13).

- A man taking cetirizine developed a multifocal fixed drug eruption (14).
- In a 45-year-old man cetirizine caused multiple fixed erythematous lesions on the trunk (15). Cetirizine was withdrawn for 15 days and an oral challenge test was performed. The same skin lesions developed in the previously affected skin sites when cetirizine was taken.
- A 14-year-old girl with house dust mite allergy had generalized skin eruptions after taking cetirizine. She also had symptoms of acute hepatitis, which also resolved after withdrawal of cetirizine (16).
- A 73-year-old man had skin eruptions associated with cetirizine and hydroxyzine therapy, which healed after drug withdrawal (17).

There have been several case reports of urticaria due to cetirizine.

- Generalized urticaria developed in a woman 2 hours after she took cetirizine (18).
- Acute generalized urticaria occurred in a 42-year-old woman taking cetirizine for seasonal allergic rhinitis and conjunctivitis, which had previously been treated with loratadine (19).
- A 32-year-old woman with recurrent idiopathic urticaria, asthma, and metal-induced contact dermatitis had 5–10 episodes of urticaria a year, with pruritic wheals of less than 24 hours duration (20). Cetirizine 10 mg/day was associated with the appearance of pruritic wheals on her neck, forehead, and arms. The symptoms resolved on drug withdrawal and reappeared on rechallenge. Double-blind challenge tests with mizolastine, loratadine, fexofenadine, dexchlorphenamine, ebastine, ketotifen, and placebo were negative, whereas hydroxyzine and its active metabolite, cetirizine, reproduced the urticaria.
- A 36-year-old woman noted intense exacerbation of urticarial wheals and facial edema 3–4 hours after taking cetirizine 10 mg (21). Skin tests with cetirizine produced an urticarial reaction 5 hours after challenge. Placebo-controlled oral challenge resulted in generalized urticaria, edema of the hands, and intense pruritus 90 minutes after administration of cetirizine, with symptoms lasting up to 12 hours. Skin biopsies showed inflammation typical of urticaria.

Susceptibility Factors

Age

The long-term safety of cetirizine (0.25 mg/kg bd) has been studied in children with atopic dermatitis (22). The mean duration of exposure to cetirizine in 399 children was 17 months. The frequency of dropouts and serious events did not differ between cetirizine and placebo. There were no clinically important differences in neurological or cardiovascular events, growth, or behavioral or cardiovascular assessments between the groups. No child taking cetirizine had prolongation of the QT_c interval.

The effects of cetirizine 0.25 mg/kg bd for 18 months have been investigated in a prospective, double-blind, parallel-group study in 817 children with atopic dermatitis aged 12–24 months (4). Dropouts and serious events, including hospitalization, were infrequent and were less common in the children who took cetirizine, although the differences were not statistically significant. Most of the adverse events were mild and were not related to medication.

Drug–Drug Interactions

Alcohol

Cetirizine did not potentiate the effects of ethanol on psychomotor and driving performance (SEDA-20, 163), but did affect tracking speed and performance in divided attention tests.

References

1. Gillard M, Van Der Perren C, Moguilevsky N, Massingham R, Chatelain P. Binding characteristics of cetirizine and levocetirizine to human H(1) histamine receptors: contribution of Lys(191) and Thr(194). Mol Pharmacol 2002;61(2):391–9.
2. Gillman SA, Blatter M, Condemi JJ, Collins M, Olufade AO, Leidy NK, Chapman D, Kramer B. The health-related quality of life effects of once-daily cetirizine HCl syrup in children with seasonal allergic rhinitis. Clin Pediatr (Phila) 2002;41(9):687–96.
3. Murray JJ, Nathan RA, Bronsky EA, Olufade AO, Chapman D, Kramer B. Comprehensive evaluation of cetirizine in the management of seasonal allergic rhinitis: impact on symptoms, quality of life, productivity, and activity impairment. Allergy Asthma Proc 2002;23(6):391–8.
4. Estelle F, Simons R. Prospective, long-term safety evaluation of the H_1-receptor antagonist cetirizine in very young children with atopic dermatitis. Allergologie 2000;23:244–55.
5. Simons FE, Silas P, Portnoy JM, Catuogno J, Chapman D, Olufade AO. Safety of cetirizine in infants 6 to 11 months of age: a randomized, double-blind, placebo-controlled study. J Allergy Clin Immunol 2003;111(6):1244–8.
6. Fraunfelder FW, Fraunfelder FT. Oculogyric crisis in patients taking cetirizine. Am J Ophthalmol 2004;137(2):355–7.
7. Nicholson AN, Turner C. Central effects of the H1-antihistamine, cetirizine. Aviat Space Environ Med 1998;69(2):166–71.
8. Hindmarch I, Johnson S, Meadows R, Kirkpatrick T, Shamsi Z. The acute and sub-chronic effects of levocetirizine, cetirizine, loratadine, promethazine and placebo on cognitive function, psychomotor performance, and weal and flare. Curr Med Res Opin 2001;17(4):241–55.
9. Early Treatment of the Atopic Child. Allergic factors associated with the development of asthma and the influence of

cetirizine in a double-blind, randomised, placebo-controlled trial: first results of ETAC. Pediatr Allergy Immunol 1998;9(3):116–24.
10. Stevenson J, Cornah D, Evrard P, Vanderheyden V, Billard C, Bax M, Van Hout A; ETAC Study Group. Long-term evaluation of the impact of the H_1-receptor antagonist cetirizine on the behavioral, cognitive, and psychomotor development of very young children with atopic dermatitis. Pediatr Res 2002;52(2):251–7.
11. Watanabe M, Kohge N, Kaji T. Severe hepatitis in a patient taking cetirizine. Ann Intern Med 2001;135(2):142–3.
12. Fong DG, Angulo P, Burgart LJ, Lindor KD. Cetirizine-induce cholestasis. J Clin Gastroenterol 2000;31(3):250–3.
13. Karamfilov T, Wilmer A, Hipler UC, Wollina U. Cetirizine-induced urticarial reaction. Br J Dermatol 1999;140(5):979–80.
14. Kranke B, Kern T. Multilocalized fixed drug eruption to the antihistamine cetirizine. J Allergy Clin Immunol 2000;106(5):988.
15. Inamadar AC, Palit A, Athanikar SB, Sampagavi VV, Deshmukh NS. Multiple fixed drug eruptions due to cetirizine. Br J Dermatol 2002;147(5):1025–6.
16. Sanchez-Lombrana JL, Alvarez RP, Saez LR, Oliva NP, Martinez RM. Acute hepatitis associated with cetirizine intake. J Clin Gastroenterol 2002;34(4):493–5.
17. Assouere MN, Mazereeuw-Hautier J, Bonafe JL. Toxidernie à deux histaminiques ayant une parente chimique: la cétirizine et l'hydroxyzine. [Cutaneous drug eruption with two antihistaminic drugs of a same chemical family: cetirizine and hydroxyzine.] Ann Dermatol Venereol 2002;129(11):1295–8.
18. Demoly P, Messaad D, Benahmed S, Sahla H, Bousquet J. Hypersensitivity to H_1-antihistamines. Allergy 2000;55(7):679–80.
19. Calista D, Schianchi S, Morri M. Urticaria induced by cetirizine. Br J Dermatol 2001;144(1):196.
20. Tella R, Gaig P, Bartra J, Garcia-Ortega P. Urticaria to cetirizine. J Investig Allergol Clin Immunol 2002; 12(2):136–7.
21. Schroter S, Damveld B, Marsch WC. Urticarial intolerance reaction to cetirizine. Clin Exp Dermatol 2002; 27(3):185–7.
22. Simons FE. Prospective, long-term safety evaluation of the H_1-receptor antagonist cetirizine in very young children with atopic dermatitis. ETAC Study Group. Early Treatment of the Atopic Child. J Allergy Clin Immunol 1999;104(2 Pt 1):433–40.

Cetrimonium bromide and cetrimide

See also Disinfectants and antiseptics

General Information

Cetrimonium bromide and cetrimide are quaternary ammonium antiseptics, trimethylammonium derivatives, with similar structures. Cetrimonium bromide is hexadecyltrimethylammonium. Cetrimide is a mixture of tetradecyltrimethylammonium (mostly), dodecyltrimethylammonium, and hexadecyltrimethylammonium. They dissociate in aqueous solution, forming a relatively large and complex cation, which is responsible for their surface activity, and a smaller inactive anion. They are emulsifiers and detergents and have bactericidal activity against Gram-positive and, at higher concentrations, some Gram-negative bacteria.

In three hospitals, 378 patients with hydatid cysts were treated surgically, including irrigation with cetrimide solutions in concentrations between 0.05 and 1% (1). No adverse effects were observed.

Organs and Systems

Sensory systems

Accidental use of cetrimide solution 0.1% as an irrigation solution during cataract surgery in two cases resulted in immediate corneal edema, which in turn resulted in a severe bullous keratopathy (2).

Acid–base balance

Severe metabolic acidosis without signs of peritonitis occurred after more than 1 liter of 1% cetrimide was instilled into hydatid cysts (SEDA-11, 490) (3).

Hematologic

Severe methemoglobinemia has been reported after excision of hydatid cysts and liberal irrigation of the cysts in the liver with a 0.1% solution of cetrimide (4).

Skin

Eighteen cases of an ichthyosiform contact dermatitis caused by antiseptic solutions containing 3% cetrimide and 0.3% chlorhexidine have been reported (5,6). Biopsies showed hyperkeratosis with striking vesiculation of lamellar bodies in the granular cells and upper spinous cells, premature secretion of lamellar bodies, and abundant remnants of lamellar bodies and retention of desmosomes between corneocytes. Cetrimide, and not chlorhexidine, was said to be the cause of the dermatitis.

References

1. Frayha GJ, Bikhazi KJ, Kachachi TA. Treatment of hydatid cysts (*Echinococcus granulosus*) by Cetrimide®. Trans R Soc Trop Med Hyg 1981;75(3):447–50.
2. van Rij G, Beekhuis WH, Eggink CA, Geerards AJ, Remeijer L, Pels EL. Toxic keratopathy due to the accidental use of chlorhexidine, cetrimide and cialit. Doc Ophthalmol 1995;90(1):7–14.
3. Momblano P, Pradere B, Jarrige N, Concina D, Bloom E. Metabolic acidosis induced by cetrimonium bromide. Lancet 1984;2(8410):1045.
4. Baraka A, Yamut F, Wakid N. Cetrimide-induced methaemoglobinaemia after surgical excision of hydatid cyst. Lancet 1980;2(8185):88–9.
5. Lee JY, Wang BJ. Contact dermatitis caused by cetrimide in antiseptics. Contact Dermatitis 1995;33(3):168–71.
6. Lee JY. Pathogenesis of abnormal keratinization in ichthyosiform cetrimide dermatitis: an ultrastructural study. Am J Dermatopathol 1997;19(2):162–7.

Chenopodiaceae

See also Herbal medicines

General Information

The genera in the family of Chenopodiaceae (Table 1) include beet and spinach.

Table 1 The genera of Chenopodiaceae

Allenrolfea (allenrolfea)
Aphanisma (coastalcreeper)
Arthrocnemum (arthrocnemum)
Atriplex (saltbush)
Axyris (Russian pigweed)
Bassia (smotherweed)
Beta (beet)
Ceratoides (winterfat)
Chenopodium (goosefoot)
Corispermum (bugseed)
Cycloloma (cycloloma)
Dysphania (dysphania)
Endolepis (endolepis)
Grayia (hopsage)
Halogeton (saltlover)
Kochia (molly)
Krascheninnikovia (winterfat)
Microtea (jumby pepper)
Monolepis (povertyweed)
Nitrophila (niterwort)
Polycnemum (polycnemum)
Proatriplex (proatriplex)
Salicornia (pickleweed)
Salsola (Russian thistle)
Sarcobatus (greasewood)
Sarcocornia (swampfire)
Spinacia (spinach)
Suaeda (seepweed)
Suckleya (suckleya)
Zuckia (zuckia)

Chenopodium ambrosioides

Chenopodium ambrosioides (American wormseed) contains the diterpenoid aritasone and the toxic principle ascaridole, which was formerly used as an antihelminthic drug, but has now been superseded.

Chloral hydrate

General Information

Chloral hydrate, which was synthesized by Justus Liebig in 1832, continues to be used for sleep disorders and for sedation before surgery or radiology, especially in children (1). As an alternative to the benzodiazepines, it has essentially similar properties and problems, but is associated with perhaps rather more frequent gastrointestinal disturbances, up to 7% in one large sample of children. Chloral hydrate had a reputation for safety, which has been challenged by data that suggest that it and short-acting barbiturates are particularly lethal when taken in overdose (2). Liver damage and cardiac toxicity, consistent with the chemical similarities between trichloroethanol, chloroform, and alcohol, can occur.

Organs and Systems

Cardiovascular

A single dose (1.2 g) in a 4-year-old girl gave rise to a reversible ventricular dysrhythmia (SEDA-21, 39).

Nervous system

Two generalized seizures occurred in a 2-year-old boy after he was sedated before echocardiography (SEDA-22, 42).

Gastrointestinal

A 78-year-old woman and a 45-year-old man developed pneumatosis cystoides coli. Both were taking chloral hydrate (3). It was speculated that chloral hydrate had caused the abdominal symptoms in these patients.

- A 69-year-old man had daily loose stools with mucous discharge. Repeated stool cultures were negative. Histology confirmed the appearances of pneumatosis cystoides coli. Various treatments had little effect on his symptoms. He had taken chloral hydrate for insomnia for 10 years. Subjectively, his symptoms were worse while taking the drug and resolved after withdrawal. With his consent, an unblinded controlled challenge with chloral hydrate was performed. The results, recorded meticulously in a symptoms diary, were dramatic. Before chloral hydrate, his bowels opened 18 times per week and only two motions contained mucus. After one tablet of chloral hydrate on days 1, 2, 5, and 7 he passed 49 stools in one week, 35 containing mucus. Two weeks later his bowel habit had returned to normal, with 15 movements per week, and only one stool contained mucus. Subsequently his bowel frequency fell to 8–10 times per week with considerable colonoscopic improvement.

Liver

Hyperbilirubinemia in neonates associated with chloral hydrate (4) may be due to the more prolonged half-life of trichloroethanol in newborns compared with adults (37 versus 14 hours).

Skin

Allergic skin reactions continue to be reported (5).

Immunologic

Several reports have highlighted the importance of gelatin allergy in young children, with some deaths due to anaphylaxis.

- A 2-year-old boy and a 4-year-old boy developed anaphylactic symptoms after being given a chloral hydrate suppository, which contained gelatin, for sedation before electroencephalography (6).

Chloral hydrate suppositories are often used to sedate children during various examinations and the authors suggested using gelatin-free formulations.

Long-Term Effects

Drug dependence

Chloral hydrate dependence can occur (7), the most famous case being that of Anna O. (Bertha Pappenheim), who was treated by Breuer from 1880 to 1882, and whose pathology was discussed by him and Freud in 1895 (8).

Tumorigenicity

Concerns about carcinogenicity are not supported by its persisting and generally successful therapeutic use.

Drug Administration

Drug formulations

Several reports have highlighted the importance of gelatin allergy in young children, with some deaths due to anaphylaxis. Some formulations of chloral hydrate contain gelatin.

- A 2-year-old boy and a 4-year-old boy developed anaphylactic symptoms after being given a chloral hydrate suppository, which contained gelatin, for sedation before electroencephalography (6).

Chloral hydrate suppositories are often used to sedate children during various examinations and the authors suggested using gelatin-free formulations.

Drug overdose

Chloral hydrate toxicity can cause a number of dysrhythmias, including supraventricular tachycardia, ventricular tachycardia, ventricular fibrillation, and torsade de pointes.

- A 27-year-old man with a history of psychiatric illness became unconscious after taking about 20 g of chloral hydrate, 1000 mg of loxapine, and 180 mg of fluoxetine (9). He became unresponsive and hypotensive and had intermittent episodes of ventricular tachycardia, which was successfully treated with intravenous propranolol.

References

1. Fox BE, O'Brien CO, Kangas KJ, Murphree AL, Wright KW. Use of high dose chloral hydrate for ophthalmic exams in children: a retrospective review of 302 cases. J Pediatr Ophthalmol Strabismus 1990;27(5):242–4.
2. Buckley NA, Whyte IM, Dawson AH, McManus PR, Ferguson NW. Correlations between prescriptions and drugs taken in self-poisoning. Implications for prescribers and drug regulation. Med J Aust 1995;162(4):194–7.
3. Marigold JH. Pneumatosis cystoides coli and chloral hydrate. Gut 1998;42(6):899–900.
4. Lambert GH, Muraskas J, Anderson CL, Myers TF. Direct hyperbilirubinemia associated with chloral hydrate administration in the newborn. Pediatrics 1990;86(2):277–81.
5. Lindner K, Prater E, Schubert H, Siegmund S. Arzneimittel exanthem auf chlorhydrat. [Drug exanthema due to chloral hydrate.] Dermatol Monatsschr 1990;176(8):483–5.
6. Yamada A, Ohshima Y, Tsukahara H, Hiraoka M, Kimura I, Kawamitsu T, Kimura K, Mayumi M. Two cases of anaphylactic reaction to gelatin induced by a chloral hydrate suppository. Pediatr Int 2002;44(1):87–9.
7. Stone CB, Okun R. Chloral hydrate dependence: report of a case. Clin Toxicol 1978;12(3):377–80.
8. de Paula Ramos S. Revisiting Anna O: a case of chemical dependence. Hist Psychol 2003;6(3):239–50.
9. Zahedi A, Grant MH, Wong DT. Successful treatment of chloral hydrate cardiac toxicity with propranolol. Am J Emerg Med 1999;17(5):490–1.

Chloramphenicol

General Information

Chloramphenicol is one of the older broad-spectrum antibiotics. It was introduced in 1948 and grew in popularity because of its high antimicrobial activity against a wide range of Gram-positive and Gram-negative bacteria, *Rickettsiae*, *Chlamydia*, and *Mycoplasma* species. It is particularly useful in infections caused by *Salmonella typhi* and *Haemophilus influenzae*. It is mainly bacteriostatic. It readily crosses tissue barriers and diffuses rapidly into nearly all tissues and body fluids.

The main route of elimination of chloramphenicol is metabolic transformation by glucuronidation. The microbiologically inactive metabolites are excreted rapidly and only a small proportion of unchanged drug is excreted in the urine. The usual daily dose is 50 mg/kg for adults and children over 2 months. The total dose should not exceed 3.0–3.5 g/70 kg. The statement that neither the dose nor the interval of chloramphenicol administration needs to be adjusted in patients with significant renal dysfunction (1) probably has to be modified in view of recent findings (2).

By 1950 it became evident that chloramphenicol could cause serious and fatal blood dyscrasias. Its use has therefore steadily fallen during the past 50 years. Since the risk of serious chloramphenicol toxicity is so small (1:18 000 or probably less) it is of more than historical interest. There are still many areas in which its benefits outweigh its risks. These include:

- typhoid and paratyphoid fever;
- other septic forms of *Salmonella* infections;
- meningitis due to *H. influenzae*, *Streptococcus pneumoniae*, and *Neisseria meningitidis* when the patient is allergic to beta-lactam antibiotics or when the strains (*H. influenzae*, Enterobacteriaceae) are resistant to aminopenicillins and cephalosporins;
- brain abscess;
- serious infections caused by *Bacteroides fragilis* (as an alternative to clindamycin or metronidazole).

Since chloramphenicol is still one of the cheapest antibiotics, this list of indications is longer in developing countries, where chloramphenicol may be more readily available than newer expensive antibiotics. However, most infections can be readily, safely, and effectively treated with alternative drugs. Therefore, the role of chloramphenicol in the treatment of infectious diseases is likely to diminish further.

Chloramphenicol and its metabolites act primarily on the 50S ribosomal subunit, with suppression of the activity of the enzyme peptidyltransferase. It inhibits mitochondrial membrane protein synthesis, leading to suppression of mitochondrial respiration and ultimately to cessation of cell proliferation (3). Analogous mechanisms may operate in the production of the reversible type of bone marrow depression, which is the most prominent toxic effect in patients taking chloramphenicol. Its potency to induce toxic effects on mitochondria in maturing or rapidly proliferating eukaryotic cells is very close to that for inhibiting prokaryotic cells (bacteria and blue-green algae). However, little progress has been made in elucidating the pathogenesis of irreversible bone marrow aplasia (3–5).

Observational studies

The response to chloramphenicol has been assessed in cases of bacteremia due to vancomycin-resistant enterococci, of whom 65% received chloramphenicol (6). Among those in whom a response could be assessed, 61% had a clinical response and 79% had a microbiological response. Mortality was non-significantly lower in patients treated with chloramphenicol. In cases with central line-related bacteremia, there was no difference in mortality among those treated with chloramphenicol, line removal, or both. No adverse effect could be definitely attributed to chloramphenicol.

General adverse effects

Chloramphenicol has been associated with two serious but rare toxic effects, each with a high mortality. One is the "gray syndrome," vasomotor collapse in neonates caused by excessive parenteral doses. The second is bone marrow aplasia, which is a hypersusceptibility reaction. Prolonged use can result in neuropathies. Mild gastrointestinal disturbances are common. Chloramphenicol can cause a Jarisch–Herxheimer reaction, for example in patients with louse-borne relapsing fever (7). Hypersensitivity reactions are commonly mild and more frequent with topical use (allergic contact dermatitis, rashes, glossitis). The late, severe type of bone marrow reaction may be of allergic origin. Tumor-inducing effects have not been described; a statement that chloramphenicol might cause cancer in the fetus appears to have been purely speculative.

Organs and Systems

Cardiovascular

The "gray syndrome" is the term given to the vasomotor collapse that occurs in neonates who are given excessive parenteral doses of chloramphenicol. The syndrome is characterized by an ashen gray, cyanotic color of the skin, a fall in body temperature, vomiting, a protuberant abdomen, refusal to suck, irregular and rapid respiration, and lethargy. It is mainly seen in newborn infants, particularly when premature. It usually begins 2–9 days after the start of treatment.

Inadequate glucuronyl transferase activity combined with reduced glomerular filtration in the neonatal period is responsible for a longer half-life and accumulation of the drug. In addition, the potency of chloramphenicol to inhibit protein synthesis is higher in proliferating cells and tissues. The most important abnormality seems to be respiratory deficiency of mitochondria, due, for example to suppressed synthesis of cytochrome oxidase. The dosage should be adjusted according to the age of the neonate, and blood concentrations should be monitored. In most cases of gray syndrome, the daily dose of chloramphenicol has been higher than 25 mg/kg (8,9). Occasionally, treatment of older children and teenagers with large doses of chloramphenicol (about 100 mg/kg) has resulted in a similar form of vasomotor collapse (10).

Nervous system

Peripheral neuropathy has been seen after prolonged courses of chloramphenicol (11).

Retrobulbar optic neuritis and polyneuritis have been attributed to prolonged chloramphenicol therapy (12).

Sensory systems

Eyes

Optic neuropathy has been seen after prolonged courses of chloramphenicol (13). Alterations in color perception and optic neuropathy, in some cases resulting in optic atrophy and blindness, have been observed, especially in children with cystic fibrosis receiving relatively high doses for many months (12,14). Most of these complications were reversible and were attributed to a deficiency of B vitamins.

Ears

Local application of chloramphenicol can cause hearing defects. Asymmetrical hearing loss with lowered perception of high tones has been documented after treatment of chronic bilateral otitis media with chloramphenicol powder (15). Propylene glycol is often used as a vehicle for chloramphenicol ear-drops, and ototoxicity may be due to chloramphenicol and/or propylene glycol, which is itself strongly ototoxic. Ototoxic effects can also occur after systemic drug administration (16).

Hematologic

The first death resulting from bone marrow aplasia induced by chloramphenicol eye-drops was described in 1955 (17). Chloramphenicol causes two types of bone marrow damage (18).

- A frequent, early, dose-related, reversible suppression of the formation of erythrocytes, thrombocytes, and granulocytes (early toxicity).
- A rare, late type of bone marrow aplasia, a hypersusceptibility reaction, which is generally irreversible, and has a high mortality rate (aplastic anemia) (19–21).

Chloramphenicol inhibits mRNA translation by the 70S ribosomes of prokaryotes, but does not affect 80S eukaryotic ribosomes. Most mitochondrial proteins are encoded by nuclear DNA and are imported into the organelles from the cytosol where they are synthesized. Mitochondria retain the capacity to translate, on their own ribosomes, a few proteins encoded by the mitochondrial genome. True to its prokaryotic heritage, mitochondrial ribosomes are similar to those of bacteria, meaning that chloramphenicol inhibits protein synthesis by these ribosomes. Chloramphenicol-induced anemia is believed to result from this inhibition (22). Chloramphenicol can also cause apoptosis in purified human bone marrow CD34+ cells (23).

Dose-related bone marrow suppression

The early, dose-related type of chloramphenicol toxicity is usually seen after the second week of treatment, and is characterized by inhibited proliferation of erythroid cells and reduced incorporation of iron into heme. The clinical correlates in the peripheral blood are anemia, reticulocytopenia, normoblastosis, and a shift to early erythrocyte forms. The plasma iron concentration is increased. Early erythroid forms and granulocyte precursors show cytoplasmic vacuolation. After withdrawal, complete recovery is the rule. Leukopenia and thrombocytopenia are less frequent.

Although there is no evidence that these abnormalities progress to frank bone marrow aplasia, continuation of chloramphenicol after the appearance of early toxicity is thought to be hazardous. Pre-existing liver damage (for example due to infectious hepatitis or alcoholism) and impaired kidney function can lead to reduced elimination of chloramphenicol and its metabolites, thereby aggravating marrow toxicity. As a rule, this is not the irreversible type.

Aplastic anemia

Although bone marrow aplasia has not been related with certainty to either the daily or the total dose of chloramphenicol or to the sex or age of the patients, it has occurred almost exclusively in individuals who were taking prolonged therapy, particularly if they were exposed to the drug on more than one occasion (24). The condition is rare, occurring about once in every 18 000–50 000 subjects in various countries. These variations may in part depend on ethnic factors (25,26). For example, there have been very few cases reported in blacks (27). Bone marrow aplasia due to chloramphenicol has usually resulted in aplastic anemia with pancytopenia; other forms, such as red cell hypoplasia, selective leukopenia, or thrombocytopenia, are less common.

When bone marrow aplasia was complete, the fatality rate approached 100%. As a rule, it has been found that the longer the interval between the last dose of chloramphenicol and the appearance of the first sign of a blood dyscrasia, the more severe the resulting aplasia. Nearly all patients in whom the interval was longer than 2 months died as a result of this complication. However, fatal aplastic anemia can also occur shortly after normal doses of chloramphenicol (28).

The pathogenesis of bone marrow aplasia after chloramphenicol is still uncertain. Compared with normal cells, bone marrow aspirates from patients with bone marrow aplasia are relatively resistant to the toxic effects of chloramphenicol in vitro. This has been explained by the hypothesis that during treatment with chloramphenicol, chloramphenicol-sensitive cells were eliminated, leaving behind only a chloramphenicol-insensitive population of blood cell precursors with poor proliferative capacity (29). Chloramphenicol can induce apoptosis in purified human bone marrow CD34+ cells; however, there was no protection from a variety of antioxidants on chloramphenicol-induced suppression of burst-forming unit erythroid and colony-forming unit granulocyte/monocyte in vitro (30). In contrast, a caspase inhibitor ameliorated the apoptotic-inducing effects of chloramphenicol.

Since thiamphenicol, which causes very few cases of aplastic anemia, differs from chloramphenicol by substitution of the para-nitro group by a methylsulfonyl group, interest has been focused on the para-nitro group and metabolites of that part of the molecule, nitrosochloramphenicol and chloramphenicol hydroxylamine. In human bone marrow, nitrosochloramphenicol inhibited DNA synthesis at 10% of the concentration of chloramphenicol required for the same effect, and proliferation of myeloid progenitors was irreversibly inhibited. The covalent binding of nitrosochloramphenicol to marrow cells was 15 times greater than that of chloramphenicol (31). This has lent support to the hypothesis that abnormal metabolism may contribute to the susceptibility to bone marrow aplasia. The production of reduced derivatives by intestinal microbes may contribute to toxicity, but oral administration of chloramphenicol is not essential for the development of aplastic anemia (32). There is evidence that genetic predisposition may play a role (33,34). The wide geographical variations in the incidence of aplastic anemia may also reflect environmental factors.

For many years it had been said that there were no cases of aplastic anemia after parenteral administration of chloramphenicol; however, a few cases of aplastic anemia have been reported (35). There have also been reports of bone marrow hypoplasia after the use of chloramphenicol eye-drops (36,37).

There is controversy about the risk of aplastic anemia with topical chloramphenicol. In a prospective case-control surveillance of aplastic anemia in a population of patients who had taken chloramphenicol for a total of 67.2 million person-years, 145 patients with aplastic anemia and 1226 controls were analysed. Three patients and five controls had been exposed to topical chloramphenicol, but two had also been exposed to other known causes of aplastic anemia. Based on these findings, an association between ocular chloramphenicol and aplastic anemia could not be excluded, but the risk was less than one per million treatment courses (38). In another study, a review of the literature identified seven cases of idiosyncratic hemopoietic reactions associated with topical chloramphenicol. However, the authors failed to find an association between the epidemiology of acquired aplastic anemia and topical chloramphenicol. Furthermore, after topical therapy they failed to detect serum accumulation of chloramphenicol by high performance liquid chromatography. They concluded that these findings support the view that topical chloramphenicol was not a risk factor for dose-related bone marrow toxicity and that calls for abolition of treatment with topical chloramphenicol based on current data are not supported (39).

In a study using general practitioner-based computerized data, 442 543 patients were identified who received 674 148 prescriptions for chloramphenicol eye-drops. Among these patients, there were three with severe hematological toxicity and one with mild transient leukopenia. The causal link between topical chloramphenicol and hematological toxicity was not further evaluated in detail (40).

Leukemia

In a small fraction of patients who survive the chronic type of bone marrow damage, myeloblastic leukemia develops (41,42). In most instances this complication has appeared within a few months of the diagnosis of aplasia and was considered to be a sequel of chloramphenicol treatment. Sometimes the delay was shorter. The majority were either children or adults aged 50–70 years.

The occurrence of acute leukemia has been studied in relation to preceding use of drugs (before the 12 months preceding the diagnosis) in a case-control study of 202 patients aged over 15 years with a diagnosis of acute leukemia and age- and sex-matched controls (43). Among users of chloramphenicol or thiamphenicol the odds ratio for any use was 1.1 (0.6–2.2) whereas the odds ratio for high doses was 1.8 (0.6–5.3). Other systemic antibiotics showed no substantial relation with the occurrence of leukemia.

Gastrointestinal

Mild gastrointestinal disturbances are common in patients taking chloramphenicol. In 51 children with Mediterranean spotted fever randomized for 7 days to either clarithromycin, 15 mg/kg/day orally in two divided doses, or chloramphenicol, 50 mg/kg/day orally in four divided doses, the two drugs were equally well tolerated and there were no major adverse effects; there was vomiting in two patients treated with clarithromycin and in one treated with chloramphenicol (44). None of the patients required drug withdrawal.

Skin

Hypersensitivity occurs about four times more often after topical than after oral use (45). In fact, there has been a continuous increase in chloramphenicol hypersensitivity, owing to the use of dermatological formulations (46). Allergic contact dermatitis and macular or vesicular skin rashes are usually limited to skin areas previously exposed to the drug. Contact conjunctivitis has also been reported.

A case of a facial contact dermatitis due to chloramphenicol with cross-sensitivity to thiamphenicol has been reported (47).

Immunologic

Systemic reactions with collapse, bronchospasm, angioedema, and urticaria occur rarely (48,49).

Infection risk

The number and types of microorganisms that constitute the normal microflora of the alimentary, respiratory, and genital tracts change during therapy with chloramphenicol. Superinfections can then develop with *Staphylococcus aureus*, *Pseudomonas*, *Proteus*, and fungi. The changes in intestinal flora may be partly responsible for a reduction in the synthesis of vitamin K-dependent clotting factors, especially in patients with severe illnesses and malnutrition or during the administration of oral anticoagulants.

Long-Term Effects

Drug tolerance

There have been reports of chloramphenicol-resistant *H. influenzae* from various countries, but there have been few cases (50). Outbreaks of chloramphenicol-resistant *S. typhi* have been observed in several countries (51,52).

High-level chloramphenicol-resistant strains of *N. meningitidis* serogroup B were isolated from 11 patients in Vietnam and one patient in France. Resistance was due to the presence of the catP gene on a truncated transposon that has lost mobility because of internal deletions (53).

Salmonella typhimurium DT104 is usually resistant to ampicillin, chloramphenicol, streptomycin, sulfonamides, and tetracycline. An outbreak of 25 culture-confirmed cases of multidrug-resistant *S. typhimurium* DT104 has been identified in Denmark (54). The strain was resistant to the above-mentioned antibiotics and nalidixic acid and had reduced susceptibility to fluoroquinolones. A swineherd was identified as the primary source (54). The DT104 strain was also found in cases of salmonellosis in Washington State, and soft cheese made with unpasteurized milk was identified as an important vehicle of its transmission (55).

A high rate of resistance of non-typhoid *Salmonella* to commonly used antimicrobial agents was found in Taiwan; 67% of the isolated strains were resistant to chloramphenicol (56).

Streptococcus pneumoniae was isolated in 30% of 40 HIV-infected and 50% of 162 HIV-negative children living in a Romanian orphanage (57). Multidrug-resistant streptococci were highly prevalent, and 21% of the isolates were resistant to chloramphenicol.

Esterases in serum from rabbits and to a lesser extent humans can convert diacetyl chloramphenicol back to an active antibiotic. Therefore, in vitro findings may not accurately reflect the level of chloramphenicol resistance by chloramphenicol acetyltransferase-bearing bacteria in vivo, when growth media supplemented with serum are used (58).

The flo gene that confers resistance to chloramphenicol and the veterinary antibiotic florfenicol have previously been identified in *Photobacterium piscicida* and *Salmonella enterica serovar typhimurium* DT104 (59). Florfenicol-resistant isolates of *Escherichia coli* were tested and found to contain large flo-positive plasmids, suggesting that several of these isolates may have a chromosomal flo gene. The *E. coli* flo gene also specifies non-enzymatic cross-resistance to both florfenicol and chloramphenicol (60). Florfenicol resistance has emerged among veterinary isolates of *E. coli* incriminated in bovine diarrhea.

Second-Generation Effects

Teratogenicity

In the large population-based dataset of the Hungarian Case Control Surveillance of Congenital Abnormalities, of 38 151 pregnant women who had babies without any defects and 22 865 pregnant women who had neonates or fetuses with congenital abnormalities, 51 and 52 had been treated with oral chloramphenicol respectively. Treatment during early pregnancy presented little, if any, teratogenic risk to the fetus (61).

Fetotoxicity

Chloramphenicol penetrates the fetal circulation and should therefore be avoided during the last phase of pregnancy (62,63). The gray syndrome has been observed in babies born to mothers who had received chloramphenicol in the final stage of pregnancy.

Lactation

Chloramphenicol has been found in relatively large amounts in breast milk. It should therefore be avoided during breast-feeding (62,63).

Susceptibility Factors

Age

In children, a high cumulative dose seems to be an important risk factor. As leukopenia can occur in the early phase of treatment, a complete blood count every third day is recommended (SEDA-15, 267).

Renal disease

Impaired kidney function, with reduced clearance of chloramphenicol, may be a risk factor for toxicity.

Hepatic disease

Liver damage, with reduced clearance of chloramphenicol, may be a risk factor for toxicity.

Other features of the patient

In a retrospective study of 30 consecutive children with sepsis treated with oral chloramphenicol, weight, albumin, and white blood cell count were the most important determinants for chloramphenicol distribution volume, whereas age, white blood cell count, and serum creatinine were most important for drug clearance (64). A pre-existing blood dyscrasia is generally considered to be an absolute contraindication to the use of chloramphenicol.

Drug Administration

Drug administration route

In 1993 the American National Register of Drug Induced Ocular Side Effects received reports of 23 patients with blood dyscrasias that could have been related to topical ocular administration of chloramphenicol (65).

Of the two types of bone marrow toxicity that chloramphenicol can cause, it may cause the late type only in genetically predisposed patients. The overall risk of aplastic anemia after oral administration of chloramphenicol is 1:30 000 to 1:50 000, which is 13 times greater than the risk of idiopathic aplastic anemia in the population as a whole. Since topical administration achieves systemic effects by absorption through the conjunctival membrane or through drainage down the lacrimal duct, with eventual absorption from the gastrointestinal tract, the risk may be similar to that after oral administration. However, based on two case-control studies and a cohort study, the incidence of blood dyscrasias due to chloramphenicol eye-drops was estimated to be somewhat lower, namely 1:100 000 treated patients (40,66).

It is difficult to justify subjecting patients to this small potential risk, in view of the availability of other antibiotics for use in the eye. In the USA the Physician's Desk Reference emphasizes with repeated warnings the importance of not using ocular chloramphenicol unless there is no alternative, and this warning should be respected on both sides of the Atlantic (67,68).

Allergic reactions to chloramphenicol eye-drops include conjunctivitis, keratitis, and palpebral and periocular eczema (47).

Erythema multiforme caused by local treatment with chloramphenicol eye-drops has been described (47). The possible role of an allergic mechanism in this reaction was suggested, based on a positive mast cell degranulation test (69).

Drug–Drug Interactions

Ciclosporin

A possible interaction between ciclosporin and chloramphenicol has been observed (70).

- A morbidly obese 17-year-old Hispanic girl, who had a cadaveric renal transplantation 5 years before, took ciclosporin and prednisone for stabilization. She was treated with chloramphenicol 875 mg qds and ceftazidime 2 g tds for vancomycin-resistant enterococcal sinusitis. There was a substantial and sustained increase in ciclosporin concentrations after chloramphenicol was added. Normalization was achieved after withdrawal of chloramphenicol.

Cyclophosphamide

Chloramphenicol inhibits the biotransformation of cyclophosphamide (71).

Cytochrome P450

Chloramphenicol can interfere with the elimination of drugs that are inactivated by hepatic metabolism, probably through a mechanism involving inhibition of microsomal enzymes. The mechanism has been claimed to be inactivation of microsomal enzymes via an intermediate reactive metabolite that binds covalently to the protein moiety of cytochrome P450 (71). Assuming such a mechanism, chloramphenicol would be expected to interact with the metabolism of other drugs dealt with by cytochrome P450.

Oral anticoagulants

Chloramphenicol inhibits the biotransformation of oral anticoagulants (71).

Paracetamol (acetaminophen)

Paracetamol altered the pharmacokinetics of chloramphenicol in some studies but not in others.

In six adults the half-life of chloramphenicol, 1 g intravenously was increased from 3.3 to 15 hours by paracetamol 100 mg intravenously (72).

In contrast, in five children aged 2.5–5 years paracetamol 50 mg/kg/day for several days significantly lowered the C_{max} of chloramphenicol, increased its apparent volume of distribution and clearance, and slightly shortened its half-life (73).

Other studies have failed to show any interaction in children (74) or adults (75).

Phenobarbital

Phenobarbital can increase the rate of chloramphenicol metabolism and so lead to abnormally low serum chloramphenicol concentrations. In 17 children receiving chloramphenicol succinate alone, mean peak and trough serum concentrations were 25 and 13 μg/ml respectively. In six patients phenobarbital reduced these concentrations to 17 and 7.5 μg/ml respectively (76).

Phenytoin

The ability of chloramphenicol to inhibit the biotransformation of phenytoin is well established and clinically relevant (77).

Conversely, phenytoin can increase the rate of chloramphenicol metabolism and so lead to abnormally low serum chloramphenicol concentrations, as has been anecdotally reported (78). However, contrary to expectation, in another study serum chloramphenicol concentrations rose during concomitant phenytoin therapy (76).

Rifampicin

Rifampicin can increase the rate of chloramphenicol metabolism and so lead to abnormally low serum chloramphenicol concentrations (79,80).

Tacrolimus

Inhibition of tacrolimus clearance has been observed in an adolescent renal transplant recipient who was treated with standard doses of chloramphenicol for vancomycin-resistant enterococci. Toxic concentrations of tacrolimus were observed on the second day of chloramphenicol treatment, requiring an 83% reduction in the dose of tacrolimus (81).

A significant interaction has also been reported in an adult (82).

- A 47-year-old white man with a cadaveric liver transplant took chloramphenicol for a urinary tract infection due to a vancomycin-resistant *Enterococcus* and inadvertently received 1850 mg qds (roughly twice the maximum recommended dose). On day 4 he had a 12-hour trough tacrolimus concentration of over 60 ng/ml, and complained of fatigue, lethargy, headache, and tremor, symptoms consistent with tacrolimus toxicity.

It was suggested that the underlying mechanism might be inhibition of CYP3A4 by chloramphenicol.

Tolbutamide

Chloramphenicol inhibits the biotransformation of tolbutamide (71).

Warfarin

An interaction of warfarin with ocular chloramphenicol (5 mg/ml; 1 drop qds in each eye), which led to an increase in INR, has been suspected in an 83-year-old white woman (83). The authors suggested that the effect may be due to chloramphenicol inhibition of hepatic microsomal CYP2C9, since the pharmacologically active enantiomer *S*-warfarin is metabolized by this enzyme).

References

1. Bennett WM, Aronoff GR, Morrison G, Golper TA, Pulliam J, Wolfson M, Singer I. Drug prescribing in renal failure: dosing guidelines for adults. Am J Kidney Dis 1983;3(3):155–93.
2. Phelps SJ, Tsiu W, Barrett FF, Nahata MC, Disessa TG, Stidham G, Roy S 3rd. Chloramphenicol-induced cardiovascular collapse in an anephric patient. Pediatr Infect Dis J 1987;6(3):285–8.
3. Yunis AA. Effects of chloramphenicol on erythropoiesis. In: Dimitrov NV, Nodine JH, editors. Drugs and Hematological Reactions. London, New York: Grune and Stratton, 1974:133.
4. Keiser G. Co-operative study of patients treated with thiamphenicol. Comparative study of patients treated with chloramphenicol and thiamphenicol. Postgrad Med J 1974;50(Suppl 5):143–5.
5. Polin HB, Plaut ME. Chloramphenicol. NY State J Med 1977;77(3):378–81.
6. Lautenbach E, Schuster MG, Bilker WB, Brennan PJ. The role of chloramphenicol in the treatment of bloodstream infection due to vancomycin-resistant enterococcus. Clin Infect Dis 1998;27(5):1259–65.
7. Perine PL, Teklu B. Antibiotic treatment of louse-borne relapsing fever in Ethiopia: a report of 377 cases. Am J Trop Med Hyg 1983;32(5):1096–100.
8. Lietman PS. Chloramphenicol and the neonate—1979 view. Clin Perinatol 1979;6(1):151–62.
9. Nahata MC. Lack of predictability of chloramphenicol toxicity in paediatric patients. J Clin Pharm Ther 1989;14(4):297–303.
10. Brown RT. Chloramphenicol toxicity in an adolescent. J Adolesc Health Care 1982;3(1):53–5.
11. Bomb BS, Bedi HK. Chloramphenicol-induced peripheral neuropathy (a case report). J Assoc Physicians India 1974;22(8):623–5.
12. Murayama E, Miyakawa T, Sumiyoshi S, Deshimaru M, Sugita K. [Retrobulbar optic neuritis and polyneuritis due to prolonged chloramphenicol therapy.] Rinsho Shinkeigaku 1973;13(4):213–20.
13. Venegas-Francke P, Fruns-Quintana M, Oporto-Caroca M. Neuritis optica bilateral por cloranfenicol. [Bilateral optic neuritis caused by chloramphenicol.] Rev Neurol 2000;31(7):699–700.
14. Beyer CR. Chloramphenicol-induced acute bilateral optic neuritis in cystic fibrosis. J Pediatr Ophthalmol Strabismus 1978;15:291.

15. Anonymous. Ear drops and iatrogenic deafness. Med J Aust 1975;2(16):626.
16. Iqbal SM, Srivatsav CB. Chloramphenicol ototoxicity. A case report. J Laryngol Otol 1984;98(5):523–5.
17. Rosenthal RL, Blackman A. Bone-marrow hypoplasia following the use of chloramphenicol eye drops. JAMA 1965;191:136–7.
18. Yunis AA. Chloramphenicol toxicity: 25 years of research. Am J Med 1989;87(3N):N44–8.
19. Turton JA, Andrews CM, Havard AC, Robinson S, York M, Williams TC, Gibson FM. Haemotoxicity of thiamphenicol in the BALB/c mouse and Wistar Hanover rat. Food Chem Toxicol 2002;40(12):1849–61.
20. Holdiness MR. Management of cutaneous erythrasma. Drugs 2002;62(8):1131–41.
21. Lam RF, Lai JS, Ng JS, Rao SK, Law RW, Lam DS. Topical chloramphenicol for eye infections. Hong Kong Med J 2002;8(1):44–7.
22. Alcindor T, Bridges KR. Sideroblastic anaemias. Br J Haematol 2002;116(4):733–43.
23. Ahmed SG, Ibrahim UA. Bone marrow morphological features in anaemic patients with acquired immune deficiency syndrome in Nigeria. Niger Postgrad Med J 2001;8(3):112–15.
24. Najean Y, Guerin MN, Chomienne C. Etiology of acquired aplastic anemia. In: Najean Y, Tognoni G, Yunis AA, editors. Safety Problems Related to Chloramphenicol and Thiamphenicol Therapy. New York: Raven Press, 1981:61.
25. Wallerstein RO, Condit PK, Kasper CK, Brown JW, Morrison FR. Statewide study of chloramphenicol therapy and fatal aplastic anemia. JAMA 1969;208(11): 2045–50.
26. Mary JY, Baumelou E, Guiguet M. Epidemiology of aplastic anemia in France: a prospective multicentric study. The French Cooperative Group for Epidemiological Study of Aplastic Anemia. Blood 1990;75(8):1646–53.
27. Froese EA. Chloramphenicol-associated aplastic anemia: its occurrence in Africans and with parenteral administration. Cent Afr J Med 1978;;24:58.
28. Daum RS, Cohen DL, Smith AL. Fatal aplastic anemia following apparent "dose-related" chloramphenicol toxicity. J Pediatr 1979;94(3):403–6.
29. Yunis AA, Mayan DR, Arimura GK. Comparative metabolic effects of chloramphenicol and thiamphenicol in mammalian cells. J Pediatr 1974;94:403.
30. Kong CT, Holt DE, Ma SK, Lie AK, Chan LC. Effects of antioxidants and a caspase inhibitor on chloramphenicol-induced toxicity of human bone marrow and HL-60 cells. Hum Exp Toxicol 2000;19(9):503–10.
31. Murray TR, Downey KM, Yunis AA. Chloramphenicol-mediated DNA damage and its possible role in the inhibitory effects of chloramphenicol on DNA synthesis. J Lab Clin Med 1983;102(6):926–32.
32. Chaplin S. Bone marrow depression due to mianserin, phenylbutazone, oxyphenbutazone, and chloramphenicol—Part II. Adverse Drug React Acute Poisoning Rev 1986;5(3):181–96.
33. Nagao T, Mauer AM. Concordance for drug-induced aplastic anemia in identical twins. N Engl J Med 1969;281(1):7–11.
34. Yunis AA. Differential in-vitro toxicity of chloramphenicol, nitroso-chloramphenicol, and thiamphenicol. Sex Transm Dis 1984;11(Suppl 4):340–2.
35. Fink TJ, Gump DW. Chloramphenicol: an impatient study of use and abuse. J Infect Dis 1978;138(5):690–4.
36. West BC, DeVault GA Jr, Clement JC, Williams DM. Aplastic anemia associated with parenteral chloramphenicol: review of 10 cases, including the second case of possible increased risk with cimetidine. Rev Infect Dis 1988;10(5):1048–51.
37. Brodsky E, Biger Y, Zeidan Z, Schneider M. Topical application of chloramphenicol eye ointment followed by fatal bone marrow aplasia. Isr J Med Sci 1989;25(1):54.
38. Laporte JR, Vidal X, Ballarin E, Ibanez L. Possible association between ocular chloramphenicol and aplastic anaemia—the absolute risk is very low. Br J Clin Pharmacol 1998;46(2):181–4.
39. Walker S, Diaper CJ, Bowman R, Sweeney G, Seal DV, Kirkness CM. Lack of evidence for systemic toxicity following topical chloramphenicol use. Eye 1998;12(Pt 5):875–9.
40. Lancaster T, Swart AM, Jick H. Risk of serious haematological toxicity with use of chloramphenicol eye drops in a British general practice database. BMJ 1998;316(7132):667.
41. Baumelou E, Najean Y. Why still prescribe chloramphenicol in 1983? Comparison of the clinical and biological hematologic effects of chloramphenicol and thiamphenicol. Blut 1983;47(6):317–20.
42. Shu XO, Gao YT, Linet MS, Brinton LA, Gao RN, Jin F, Fraumeni JF Jr. Chloramphenicol use and childhood leukaemia in Shanghai. Lancet 1987;2(8565):934–7.
43. Traversa G, Menniti-Ippolito F, Da Cas R, Mele A, Pulsoni A, Mandelli F. Drug use and acute leukemia. Pharmacoepidemiol Drug Saf 1998;7(2):113–23.
44. Cascio A, Colomba C, Di Rosa D, Salsa L, di Martino L, Titone L. Efficacy and safety of clarithromycin as treatment for Mediterranean spotted fever in children: a randomized controlled trial. Clin Infect Dis 2001;33(3):409–11.
45. Forck G. Häufigkeit und Bedeutung von Chloramphenicol-Allergien. [Incidence and significance of chloramphenicol hypersensitivities with respect to different ways of sensitization.] Dtsch Med Wochenschr 1971;96(4):161–5.
46. van Joost T, Dikland W, Stolz E, Prens E. Sensitization to chloramphenicol; a persistent problem. Contact Dermatitis 1986;14(3):176–8.
47. Le Coz CJ, Santinelli F. Facial contact dermatitis from chloramphenicol with cross-sensitivity to thiamphenicol. Contact Dermatitis 1998;38(2):108–9.
48. Palchick BA, Funk EA, McEntire JE, Hamory BH. Anaphylaxis due to chloramphenicol. Am J Med Sci 1984;288(1):43–5.
49. Liphshitz I, Loewenstein A. Anaphylactic reaction following application of chloramphenicol eye ointment. Br J Ophthalmol 1991;75(1):64.
50. Kinmonth AL, Storrs CN, Mitchell RG. Meningitis due to chloramphenicol-resistant *Haemophilus influenzae* type b. BMJ 1978;1(6114):694.
51. Butler T, Linh NN, Arnold K, Pollack M. Chloramphenicol-resistant typhoid fever in Vietnam associated with R factor. Lancet 1973;2(7836):983–5.
52. Cherubin CE, Neu HC, Rahal JJ, Sabath LD. Emergence of resistance to chloramphenicol in *Salmonella*. J Infect Dis 1977;135(5):807–12.
53. Galimand M, Gerbaud G, Guibourdenche M, Riou JY, Courvalin P. High-level chloramphenicol resistance in *Neisseria meningitidis*. N Engl J Med 1998;339(13): 868–74.
54. Villar RG, Macek MD, Simons S, Hayes PS, Goldoft MJ, Lewis JH, Rowan LL, Hursh D, Patnode M, Mead PS. Investigation of multidrug-resistant *Salmonella* serotype typhimurium DT104 infections linked to raw-milk cheese in Washington State. JAMA 1999;281(19):1811–16.
55. Molbak K, Baggesen DL, Aarestrup FM, Ebbesen JM, Engberg J, Frydendahl K, Gerner-Smidt P, Petersen AM, Wegener HC. An outbreak of multidrug-resistant, quinolone-resistant *Salmonella enterica* serotype typhimurium DT104. N Engl J Med 1999;341(19):1420–5.
56. Chen YH, Chen TP, Tsai JJ, Hwang KP, Lu PL, Cheng HH, Peng CF. Epidemiological study of human salmonellosis

during 1991–1996 in southern Taiwan. Kaohsiung J Med Sci 1999;15(3):127–36.
57. Leibovitz E, Dragomir C, Sfartz S, Porat N, Yagupsky P, Jica S, Florescu L, Dagan R. Nasopharyngeal carriage of multidrug-resistant *Streptococcus pneumoniae* in institutionalized HIV-infected and HIV-negative children in northeastern Romania. Int J Infect Dis 1999;3(4):211–15.
58. Sohaskey CD, Barbour AG. Esterases in serum-containing growth media counteract chloramphenicol acetyltransferase activity in vitro. Antimicrob Agents Chemother 1999;43(3):655–60.
59. Cloeckaert A, Sidi Boumedine K, Flaujac G, Imberechts H, D'Hooghe I, Chaslus-Dancla E. Occurrence of a *Salmonella enterica* serovar typhimurium DT104-like antibiotic resistance gene cluster including the floR gene in *S. enterica* serovar agona. Antimicrob Agents Chemother 2000;44(5):1359–61.
60. White DG, Hudson C, Maurer JJ, Ayers S, Zhao S, Lee MD, Bolton L, Foley T, Sherwood J. Characterization of chloramphenicol and florfenicol resistance in *Escherichia coli* associated with bovine diarrhea. J Clin Microbiol 2000;38(12):4593–8.
61. Czeizel AE, Rockenbauer M, Sorensen HT, Olsen J. A population-based case-control teratologic study of oral chloramphenicol treatment during pregnancy. Eur J Epidemiol 2000;16(4):323–7.
62. Havelka J, Frankova A. Prispevek K Vedlejsim ucinkum chloramfenikolu u nororozencu. [Adverse effects of chloramphenicol in newborn infants.] Cesk Pediatr 1972;27(1):31–3.
63. Kunz J, Schreiner WE. Breitspektrumantibiotika. In: Kunz J, Schreiner WE, editors. Pharmakotherapie während Schwangerschaft und Stillperiode. Stuttgart, New York: Thieme Verlag, 1982:28.
64. Lugo Goytia G, Lares-Asseff I, Perez Guille MG, Perez AG, Mejia CL. Relationship between clinical and biologic variables and chloramphenicol pharmacokinetic parameters in pediatric patients with sepsis. Ann Pharmacother 2000;34(3):393–7.
65. Fraunfelder FT, Morgan RL, Yunis AA. Blood dyscrasias and topical ophthalmic chloramphenicol. Am J Ophthalmol 1993;115(6):812–13.
66. Wiholm BE, Kelly JP, Kaufman D, Issaragrisil S, Levy M, Anderson T, Shapiro S. Relation of aplastic anaemia to use of chloramphenicol eye drops in two international case-control studies. BMJ 1998;316(7132):666.
67. Doona M, Walsh JB. Use of chloramphenicol as topical eye medication: time to cry halt? BMJ 1995; 310(6989):1217–18.
68. Fraunfelder FT. In: Drug-induced Ocular Side Effects. 4th ed. Baltimore, MD: Williams and Wilkins, 1996:23–6.
69. Amichai B, Grunwald MH, Halevy S. Erythema multiforme resulting from chloramphenicol in eye drops: confirmation by mast cell degranulation test. Ann Ophthalmol Glaucoma 1998;30:225–7.
70. Bui L, Huang DD. Possible interaction between cyclosporine and chloramphenicol. Ann Pharmacother 1999;33(2):252–3.
71. Halpert J, Naslund B, Betner I. Suicide inactivation of rat liver cytochrome P-450 by chloramphenicol in vivo and in vitro. Mol Pharmacol 1983;23(2):445–52.
72. Buchanan N, Moodley GP. Interaction between chloramphenicol and paracetamol. BMJ 1979;2(6185):307–8.
73. Spika JS, Davis DJ, Martin SR, Beharry K, Rex J, Aranda JV. Interaction between chloramphenicol and acetaminophen. Arch Dis Child 1986;61(11):1121–4.
74. Kearns GL, Bocchini JA Jr, Brown RD, Cotter DL, Wilson JT. Absence of a pharmacokinetic interaction between chloramphenicol and acetaminophen in children. J Pediatr 1985;107(1):134–9.
75. Stein CM, Thornhill DP, Neill P, Nyazema NZ. Lack of effect of paracetamol on the pharmacokinetics of chloramphenicol. Br J Clin Pharmacol 1989;27(2):262–4.
76. Krasinski K, Kusmiesz H, Nelson JD. Pharmacologic interactions among chloramphenicol, phenytoin and phenobarbital. Pediatr Infect Dis 1982;1(4):232–5.
77. Rose JQ, Choi HK, Schentag JJ, Kinkel WR, Jusko WJ. Intoxication caused by interaction of chloramphenicol and phenytoin. JAMA 1977;237(24):2630–1.
78. Powell DA, Nahata MC, Durrell DC, Glazer JP, Hilty MD. Interactions among chloramphenicol, phenytoin, and phenobarbital in a pediatric patient. J Pediatr 1981; 98(6):1001–3.
79. Prober CG. Effect of rifampin on chloramphenicol levels. N Engl J Med 1985;312(12):788–9.
80. Kelly HW, Couch RC, Davis RL, Cushing AH, Knott R. Interaction of chloramphenicol and rifampin. J Pediatr 1988;112(5):817–20.
81. Schulman SL, Shaw LM, Jabs K, Leonard MB, Brayman KL. Interaction between tacrolimus and chloramphenicol in a renal transplant recipient. Transplantation 1998;65(10):1397–8.
82. Taber DJ, Dupuis RE, Hollar KD, Strzalka AL, Johnson MW. Drug–drug interaction between chloramphenicol and tacrolimus in a liver transplant recipient. Transplant Proc 2000;32(3):660–2.
83. Leone R, Ghiotto E, Conforti A, Velo G. Potential interaction between warfarin and ocular chloramphenicol. Ann Pharmacother 1999;33(1):114.

Chlordiazepoxide

See also Benzodiazepines

General Information

Chlordiazepoxide, which has a long duration of action ($t_{1/2}$ = 10–25 hours), is useful for the management of alcohol withdrawal and is arguably better tolerated than other benzodiazepines when used for this indication. As with diazepam, loading doses are possible and simplify clinical management.

Organs and Systems

Metabolism

A San Francisco woman with a history of diabetes and high blood pressure was hospitalized in January 2001 with a life-threatening low blood sugar concentration after she consumed Anso Comfort capsules (1). The authors conjectured that hospitalization may have been necessitated by a drug interaction of chlordiazepoxide with medications that she was taking for other medical conditions.

Hematologic

- A 68-year-old man, who had been taking lorazepam, perphenazine, and amitriptyline for many years, developed acute thrombocytopenic purpura after combination therapy of chlordiazepoxide 5 mg and clidinium 2.5 mg tds for irritable bowel syndrome (2). His disease improved after withdrawal of chlordiazepoxide and clidinium and treatment with intravenous prednisolone.

In this case it was not clear which of the two compounds caused the purpura; it is possible that it was due to the combination.

Drug Administration

Drug formulations

The California State Health Director has warned consumers to stop using the herbal product Anso Comfort capsules immediately, because the product contains the undeclared prescription drug chlordiazepoxide (1). Anso Comfort capsules, available by mail or telephone order from the distributor in 60-capsule bottles, are clear with dark green powder inside. The label is yellow with green English printing and a picture of a plant. An investigation by the California Department of Health Services Food and Drug Branch and Food and Drug Laboratory showed that the product contains chlordiazepoxide. The ingredients for the product were imported from China and the capsules were manufactured in California. Advertising for the product claims that the capsules are useful for the treatment of a wide variety of illnesses, including high blood pressure and high cholesterol, in addition to claims that it is a natural herbal dietary supplement. The advertising also claims that the product contains only Chinese herbal ingredients and that consumers may reduce or stop their need for prescribed medicines. No clear medical evidence supports any of these claims. The distributor, NuMeridian (formerly known as Top Line Project), has voluntarily recalled the product.

Drug–Drug Interactions

Heparin

In normal non-fasting subjects, 100–1000 IU of heparin given intravenously caused a rapid increase in the free fractions of diazepam, chlordiazepoxide, and oxazepam (3,4), but no change in the case of lorazepam (3). The clinical implications of this finding are not known.

Oral contraceptives

In 7 healthy young women who had taken oral contraceptives for more than 6 months the protein binding of chlordiazepoxide was reduced and its volume of distribution increased (5). The clearance of chlordiazepoxide is also reportedly reduced by oral contraceptives (6).

Mid-cycle spotting occurred in a large proportion of 72 women taking oral contraceptives and chlordiazepoxide; however, there were no pregnancies (7).

References

1. Anonymous. Herbal medicine. Warning: found to contain chlordiazepoxide. WHO Pharm Newslett 2001;1:2–3.
2. Alexopoulou A, Michael A, Dourakis SP. Acute thrombocytopenic purpura in a patient treated with chlordiazepoxide and clidinium. Arch Intern Med 2001;161(14):1778.
3. Desmond PV, Roberts RK, Wood AJ, Dunn GD, Wilkinson GR, Schenker S. Effect of heparin administration on plasma binding of benzodiazepines. Br J Clin Pharmacol 1980;9(2):171–5.
4. Routledge PA, Kitchell BB, Bjornsson TD, Skinner T, Linnoila M, Shand DG. Diazepam and N-desmethyldiazepam redistribution after heparin. Clin Pharmacol Ther 1980; 27(4):528–32.
5. Roberts RK, Desmond PV, Wilkinson GR, Schenker S. Disposition of chlordiazepoxide: sex differences and effects of oral contraceptives. Clin Pharmacol Ther 1979;25(6):826–31.
6. Back DJ, Orme ML. Pharmacokinetic drug interactions with oral contraceptives. Clin Pharmacokinet 1990;18(6):472–84.
7. Somos P. Interaction between certain psychopharmaca and low-dose oral contraceptives. Ther Hung 1990;38(1):37–40.

Chlorhexidine

See also Disinfectants and antiseptics

General Information

Chlorhexidine (1,1′-hexamethylene-*bis*[5-(*p*-chlorophenyl) biguanide]) is a widely used antibacterial agent with activity against Gram-positive bacteria, Gram-negative bacteria (less against *Pseudomonas* species), and yeasts. It was introduced as an antiseptic in the early 1950s. It has been primarily used for topical antisepsis, for example in preoperative skin disinfection, and for disinfection of materials, mainly in combination with cetrimide. Long-term experience has shown a low incidence of sensitization and a low irritant potential (SEDA-11, 480).

Unwanted effects have resulted from undue reliance on the disinfecting properties of chlorhexidine. Hospital-acquired infections have been caused by infected chlorhexidine used for bladder irrigation and for storage or disinfection of catheter spigots and needles (SEDA-11, 480) (1,2). A microbiological analysis of chlorhexidine-cream tubes, repeatedly used by patients with indwelling urethral catheters, showed high contamination with potential pathogens in 32% of cream samples and in 35% of swabs taken from the outside of the tubes beneath the screw cap (SEDA-11, 480) (3).

Use of chlorhexidine in dentistry

Chlorhexidine has been used as an adjuvant for plaque control and in the treatment of gingival inflammation. It is generally considered to be effective in the control of plaque and can be helpful in the treatment of gingivitis. It can be applied in the form of a solution, used as a mouth rinse or with a toothbrush, in dentifrice or as a gel. The concentrations used are 0.05–2%.

It is very difficult to summarize the effect of chlorhexidine on oral hygiene, since studies differ markedly as regards the population studied, the occurrence of gingival lesions, the use of other oral hygiene regimens, previous scaling, and polishing of the teeth. The most frequently reported adverse effects of oral use are discoloration of the teeth, tongue, and buccal mucosa, taste disorders, and desquamation of the oral mucosa. A mild increase in gingival bleeding was reported after the use of chlorhexidine mouthwash compared with mechanical cleaning methods.

Use of chlorhexidine in neonatal skin care

The withdrawal of hexachlorophene-containing products for routine neonatal skin care stimulated investigations into the possible use of chlorhexidine in this field. Its activity range includes effectiveness of high dilutions against Gram-positive and Gram-negative bacteria, yeasts, and molds. In studies of nursery populations, chlorhexidine appears to be as effective as hexachlorophene in preventing staphylococcal colonization and infection. However, there is no evidence that chlorhexidine promotes Gram-negative colonization in neonates bathed in water-containing chlorhexidine (SEDA-11, 482).

Data presented in three studies have provided substantial evidence that there is very low percutaneous absorption in full-term infants and also in excessively exposed newborn rhesus monkeys. However, traces of chlorhexidine were found in adipose tissue (two of five monkeys), kidneys (five of five), and liver (one of five), suggesting some absorption percutaneously or by oral ingestion, following the rigorous bathing procedure in the above study. The grooming habits of the monkeys could have played a role (SEDA-12, 578) (4).

Use of chlorhexidine in routine neonatal cord care

About 0.2 ml of undiluted 4% chlorhexidine solution with a detergent was included in the daily routine of rubbing the dry cord stump and the surrounding skin, which were then rinsed and dried. No chlorhexidine was detectable in the blood samples of the neonates, taken on the fifth day (5).

Use of chlorhexidine in spermicides

The use of chlorhexidine in spermicides has been promoted as a strategy for protecting against sexually transmitted diseases, including HIV infection. However, both the claim of protection and the cytotoxicity of chlorhexidine, with a risk of damage to the epithelia of the vagina, cervix, and glans penis due to chronic exposure, have to be further validated (6).

Vaginal use of chlorhexidine

Five studies of the prophylactic intravaginal use of chlorhexidine vaginal suppositories before delivery and in obstetrics have been reviewed (7). No severe adverse reactions were reported.

Accidental ingestion

A newborn had cyanotic spells associated with sinus bradycardia but not with apnea on the third day of life(8). The mother had used a chlorhexidine spray on her breasts from the third feed onwards. Bradycardia became less frequent and less severe from day 4 after the spray was stopped, and had abated completely by day 6.

Five healthy newborn breast-fed babies were accidentally fed a dilute antiseptic solution containing chlorhexidine 0.05% with cetrimide 1% instead of sterile water (9). They developed caustic burns of the lips, mouth, and tongue within minutes. One baby became severely ill due to acute pulmonary edema, but all survived without sequelae.

Organs and Systems

Respiratory

Chlorhexidine gluconate when ingested usually causes relatively mild symptoms, with poor gastrointestinal absorption, and is considered relatively safe. However, a rare fatality, with acute respiratory distress syndrome, has been reported (10).

- An 80-year-old woman with dementia accidentally took about 200 ml of chlorhexidine gluconate 5%. She aspirated her gastric contents and despite intensive treatment died of acute respiratory distress syndrome 12 hours later. The serum concentration of chlorhexidine gluconate was markedly high (25 μg/ml).

It is possible that in this case, although chlorhexidine was poorly absorbed from the gastrointestinal tract, absorption occurred through the pulmonary alveoli.

Occupational asthma caused by chlorhexidine alcohol disinfectant spray was well documented in three nurses (11).

Ear, nose, throat

Reversible hyposmia occurred after Hardy's operation for pituitary adenomas following preoperative disinfection of the nasal cavity with chlorhexidine (12). The olfactory disturbance improved after 3–7 weeks. Degeneration of the olfactory epithelium was also seen in guinea pigs when the nasal cavities were irrigated 3 times with 5 ml 0.5% chlorhexidine solution; regeneration of the epithelium started after 14 days and the surfaces appeared normal after 1 month.

Nervous system

The middle ear should be carefully protected against chlorhexidine solutions in preoperative skin disinfection in otolaryngology. Severe sensorineural deafness occurred in 14 of 97 patients who underwent myringoplasty (13). The only common factor in all these patients was the preoperative skin disinfection of the ear with 0.5% chlorhexidine in a 70% alcoholic solution.

In extensive investigations of the ototoxicity caused by chlorhexidine after introducing it into the middle ear of guinea pigs, the extent of severe vestibular and cochlear damage was related to the concentration of chlorhexidine, to the duration of exposure, and to the time-lapse after exposure (14–16).

Sensory systems

Eyes

Accidental contamination of the eye with chlorhexidine can cause adverse effects. Care should be taken during preoperative skin preparation to keep chlorhexidine out of the eye and to flush copiously with sterile saline solution or sterile water if contact accidentally occurs.

- Accidental use of chlorhexidine solutions (1:666 and 1:1000) as irrigation during cataract surgery resulted in immediate corneal edema, which resulted in a bullous keratopathy (17).

- Chlorhexidine disinfectant was accidentally used to irrigate the eyes of four patients; despite immediate treatment, corneal burns occurred in all (18).
- In four patients, accidental corneal exposure to Hibiclens (4% chlorhexidine formulated with a detergent) resulted in keratitis, with severe and permanent corneal opacification (19).
- Epithelial and stromal edema of the cornea and a diffuse bullous keratopathy developed in a 39-year-old woman 2 weeks after a preoperative disinfection of the face with an alcoholic chlorhexidine solution. This led to penetrating keratoplasty 10 months later (20).

The histopathological findings in the cornea have been described in such cases; they include epithelial edema with bullous changes, marked loss of keratocytes, thickening of Descemet's membrane, and an attenuated disrupted cell layer (21).

Chlorhexidine has also been accidentally irrigated into the anterior chamber of the eye, instead of balanced salt solution, during cataract surgery (22). Later in the operation, a decrease in corneal clarity was noted and an epithelial abrasion had to be performed. The inadvertent use of chlorhexidine in this patient resulted in reduced endothelial function and loss of corneal clarity.

Progressive ulcerative keratitis related to the use of chlorhexidine gluconate 0.02% eye-drops has been reported (23).

- A 45-year-old woman was treated for presumed *Acanthamoeba* keratitis with chlorhexidine gluconate 0.02% and propamidine 0.1% eye-drops. After using the eye-drops for 8 weeks she developed a near total loss of the corneal epithelium and progressive ulcerative keratitis, which eventually required penetrating keratoplasty. Histopathological examination of the corneal button showed ulceration and loss of Bowman's membrane, massive loss of keratocytes with apparent apoptosis, and loss of endothelial cells, with inflammatory cells adherent to the remaining cells. These findings were similar to those seen in chlorhexidine 4% keratopathy. No organisms were seen in stained sections and immune histochemistry showed no significant findings.

Taste

Taste impairment and/or disturbance is especially seen with chlorhexidine mouthwashes (SEDA-11, 481) (SEDA-12, 577) (24). It occurs in about one-third of subjects and is perhaps the main complaint. Symptoms include a burning sensation, a feeling of soreness, a dry mouth, and a bitter aftertaste lasting from a few minutes up to several hours. However, these types of symptoms also occur, albeit to a lesser extent, in placebo or control groups.

Mouth and teeth

Desquamation and ulceration of the oral mucosa has been observed after the use of chlorhexidine mouthwashes. The frequency of this adverse effect must be very low. Histological and histochemical examination of mucosal biopsies taken after 18 months of daily exposure to chlorhexidine did not show any adverse effect on the oral mucosa. There was increased keratinization of human gingival cells in vitro in cell cultures if the chlorhexidine concentration exceeded 25 μg/ml, and the same acceleration of keratinization of human gingival cells in gingival swabs occurred after rinsing with 0.025, 0.05, and 0.1% chlorhexidine solutions (25). In one case there was excessive impairment of wound healing after daily rinses with a 0.1% chlorhexidine solution after oral surgery.

Staining of the teeth was the first and principal adverse effect observed with the dental use of chlorhexidine. In a 4-month study of soldiers who used chlorhexidine mouthwashes in concentrations of 0.1 and 0.2%, 15% of the interproximal surface and 62% of the fillings, especially the old and porous ones, were discoloured (26,27). The stain intensity seems to be directly correlated to the concentration of the chlorhexidine and to the frequency and duration of use. The type of administration (0.2% mouthwash, 0.2% spray, or 1% gel) does not seem to influence the amount of tooth-staining. The initial discoloration is yellow-brown, but prolonged use and stronger concentrations result in a dark-brown color. Extensive investigations have been performed to evaluate factors that influence tooth-staining and the possibility of avoiding it. The cause of extrinsic tooth discoloration is not fully understood. However, the available evidence suggests that browning and formation of pigmented metal sulfides are the most likely causes, while dietary factors (such as beverages or red wine) and smoking may play an aggravating role only (SEDA-10, 427).

A discoloration of the dorsum of the tongue occurs in up to one-third of subjects using chlorhexidine mouth rinses. It does not occur during the use of chlorhexidine-containing dentifrices or gels (SEDA-11, 481) (27,28).

Reversible swelling of the parotid glands has been reported occasionally after the use of chlorhexidine mouthwashes; this is probably due to mechanical obstruction of the parotid duct by over-rigorous rinsing (SEDA-11, 481) (29).

Gastrointestinal

- Atrophic gastritis was reported in a 72-year-old man with Parkinson's disease who had used a 4% chlorhexidine solution as a daily mouthwash but had also swallowed it. Gastroscopy showed multiple erosions in the lower part of his stomach and the first part of the duodenum (30).

Skin

Of 551 patients with venous or traumatic ulcers of the leg who were patch-tested with chlorhexidine, 10 developed severe dermatitis and 4 developed skin infections on the face and/or scalp (31).

Serosae

Sclerosing peritoneal disease occurred in peritoneal dialysis patients in whom the tubing connection had been disinfected with chlorhexidine (32–34); 214 cases were reported from 112 centers in European countries up to 1984 (SEDA-15, 250).

Musculoskeletal

Chlorhexidine is not normally used in arthroscopy, but it is a common irrigating fluid for surgical wounds. In three of five patients with pain, swelling, crepitus, and loss of range of movement following arthroscopy of the knee, there had been accidental irrigation with 1% aqueous chlorhexidine. Histological examination showed partial necrosis of the cartilage, with slight non-specific inflammation and fibrosis of synovial specimens (35). This shows that particular care is needed in checking irrigation fluids.

Even very dilute solutions of chlorhexidine can cause marked chondrolysis of articular cartilage, leading to severe permanent damage of the knee (36).

- A 20-year-old woman, a 30-year-old man, and a 62-year-old woman all had arthroscopic reconstruction of the anterior cruciate ligament performed by the same surgeon. The only difference in technique in these three cases, compared with the rest of his cases, was the use of chlorhexidine 0.02% for irrigation throughout the procedure. All had good immediate postoperative recovery with no sign of infection, and none had preceding rheumatoid or other inflammatory joint disease, systemic disease, or chronic use of drugs. However, they all developed pain, swelling, stiffness, and loud crepitus at 2–4 months after the procedure and had radiological evidence of loss of joint space, especially in the medial compartment. Arthroscopy in all three cases showed a large amount of loose chondral material, a "snowstorm" appearance, which could be washed out. Severe erosion of the articular cartilage and a mild synovitis were also demonstrated. The ligaments were all intact and culture of the synovial fluid was sterile. Histopathology of the fragments of cartilage showed non-viable chondrocytes, with an absence of acute inflammatory cells and very few chronic inflammatory cells. The synovial biopsies showed evidence of fibrosis. All three patients had severely damaged knees which required total knee replacement.

These cases of chondrolysis did not result from accidental use of relatively concentrated solutions of chlorhexidine, but from the use of a very low concentration, 0.02%, which is widely used as an irrigation solution during surgical procedures. Chlorhexidine has a damaging effect on the articular cartilage of the knee, and should not be used, even in low concentrations, to irrigate exposed articular cartilage.

Immunologic

Allergic reactions, including anaphylaxis, from chlorhexidine are reported with all types of use and are well documented. However, chlorhexidine may still not be suspected as a possible cause of anaphylaxis when several agents are used in the anesthetized surgical patient, and hypersensitivity to chlorhexidine may not be tested for (37). If a reaction occurs during anesthesia, there is often doubt about the exact agent responsible; patch-testing will help if there is doubt about causality.

Mechanism

The molecular basis of the recognition of chlorhexidine in a sensitive patient has been examined (38).

- A 75-year-old man had three anaphylactic events after the use of chlorhexidine. The first occurred in September 1995 during general anesthesia for coronary artery bypass grafts. Ten minutes after induction he developed a marked fall in blood pressure, bronchospasm, tachycardia, and increased pulmonary artery pressure. In July 1996, a transurethral resection of the prostate was performed under spinal anesthetic. At cystoscopy he developed a headache, a rash, and bronchospasm, which settled after treatment. He had a further cystoscopy in February 1998, during which he became flushed, wheezy, and hypotensive, and had a cardiac arrest. He was successfully resuscitated. He had raised serum tryptase activities (60.4 and 26.6 μg/l at 3.5 and 9.5 hours after the event), suggesting a true anaphylactic reaction. Since the only pharmacological agent common to all three procedures was urethral jelly containing lidocaine 2% and chlorhexidine 0.05%, he subsequently had skin prick tests, intradermal tests, and sequential subcutaneous challenges to lidocaine without any positive or adverse effects. Because he had developed profound anaphylaxis with cardiac arrest after the topical administration of chlorhexidine, skin tests were deemed unethical, and an in vitro method for detecting sensitivity to chlorhexidine was pursued. Detailed quantitative hapten inhibition studies were carried out with chlorhexidine-reactive IgE antibodies identified in the serum of the patient.

The authors concluded that unlike most drug allergic determinants the whole chlorhexidine molecule is complementary to the IgE antibody combining sites and that the 4-chlorophenol, biguanide, and hexamethylene structures together comprise the allergenic component.

Frequency and susceptibility factors

In a collaborative Danish study, 2061 patients were patch-tested with chlorhexidine gluconate 1% in water. There was a positive reaction in 2.3% of the patients. This was more common in patients with leg eczema (6.8%) or leg ulcer (10.6%) than in those with eczema of the hands (1.9%) or at other sites (1.6%). Of the 14 patients who were retested with chlorhexidine, only one was positive to the 1% solution and none to a solution of 0.01%. This apparent loss of sensitivity may be due to irritable skin at the initial testing, the so-called excited skin syndrome. This study suggests that the sensitizing potential of chlorhexidine is very low, but that it should be used with caution in dressings for leg ulcers.

In 1063 consecutive eczema patients tested with the ICDRG standard series, supplemented with chlorhexidine gluconate 1% in water and 1% in petrolatum, the frequency of positive reactions was similar to that in the collaborative study (39).

Application to the skin

In a report of generalized urticaria after skin cleansing with and urethral instillation of chlorhexidine-containing products, the authors suggest that there is under-reporting of such reactions and that alternative antiseptics should be considered in urological and gynecological procedures (40).

- Life-threatening anaphylactic reactions with generalized urticaria, dyspnea, and shock occurred in six patients after the use of 0.05, 0.5, or 1% chlorhexidine (41), and in one patient after topical use of an alcoholic 0.5% chlorhexidine digluconate solution (42). A severe systemic allergic response was observed in a patient in whom the large donor area of skin graft was dressed with Bactigras, which contains 0.5% chlorhexidine acetate (43).
- An acute anaphylactic reaction occurred in a 19-year-old man after cleaning of burns on the left arm (44). A scratch test with chlorhexidine acetate 0.05% was positive.
- Anaphylaxis occurred in four surgical patients after the use of chlorhexidine as a skin disinfectant. All four had a history of minor symptoms, such as rashes or faints, in connection with previous surgery or invasive procedures (45).
- Following disinfection of a drain insertion site with chlorhexidine digluconate 2% solution, a 43-year-old man had severe anaphylaxis, manifest as dyspnea, shock, and ST segment elevation (46). In the past he had had two episodes of contact dermatitis with chlorhexidine antiseptics.
- A 14-year-old girl had combined delayed and immediate types of allergy, with urticarial rash and syncope, after long-term use of an antiacne formulation containing chlorhexidine in an unknown concentration.
- When chlorhexidine was used as a skin disinfectant in a 53-year-old man undergoing lung resection for adenocarcinoma, anaphylaxis was complicated by coronary artery spasm (47). He had two anaphylactic reactions accompanied by severe myocardial ischemia. Immunological testing indicated chlorhexidine as the causative substance.

In the last two cases, epicutaneous tests with 1% chlorhexidine gluconate and acetate, and prick tests with 0.05 and 0.01% of the acetate solution were positive (48).

Local hypersensitivity reactions to chlorhexidine-impregnated patches occur in neonates (49). In a randomized comparison of povidone-iodine and a chlorhexidine gluconate impregnated dressing for the prevention of central venous catheter infections in neonates, the risk of local contact dermatitis limited the use of the chlorhexidine dressing (50).

Application to mucous membranes

Anaphylaxis has been reported after nasal application of chlorhexidine.

- Anaphylactic circulatory arrest occurred in a 53-year-old man with acromegaly when his nasal mucosa was cleaned with an aqueous solution of chlorhexidine gluconate 0.05% (51).

A report to the Japanese Ministry of Welfare about reactions observed between 1967 and 1984 included 22 cases with a fall in blood pressure, 13 with dyspnea, 9 with anaphylactic shock, 4 with cyanosis, 19 with erythema, 11 with urticaria, 9 with pruritus, and 7 with facial wheals; following this report, in 1984, the Japanese Ministry of Welfare recommended that the use of chlorhexidine on mucous membranes be prohibited because of the evidence of the risk of anaphylactic shock (41).

Application to wounds

Application of chlorhexidine to wounds is generally safe, but it should be used at the lowest bactericidal concentration of 0.05% (41).

Application to the urethra

Anaphylaxis after cystoscopy or urinary catheterization has been reported repeatedly (SEDA-18, 255) (SEDA-19, 235) (SEDA-20, 225) (52).

- A 64-year-old man had severe anaphylaxis induced by intraurethral chlorhexidine gel 0.05% (53). Previous hypersensitivity reactions during urethral dilatation had been thought to be due to lidocaine. Chlorhexidine-specific IgE antibodies were demonstrated, and the chlorhexidine gel had been used in all the preceding urological procedures the patient had undergone.

Severe allergic reactions occurred in five patients after the insertion of an intra-urethral lidocaine jelly containing chlorhexidine gluconate and instrumentation of the urethra (54). All had a positive response to chlorhexidine gluconate (0.0005%) and a negative response to lidocaine (0.2%).

Impregnated intravenous catheters

Chlorhexidine-coated catheters have been developed in the hope of reducing the incidence of central venous line sepsis. Package inserts warn that these should not be used in individuals who are thought to be sensitive to chlorhexidine.

It is possible that the potential benefit of reducing the incidence of central venous sepsis by using chlorhexidine-coated catheters is outweighed by the risk of sudden and profound anaphylaxis. Certainly a high degree of suspicion of chlorhexidine allergy should be exercised and skin tests performed.

In a randomized clinical study of the efficacy of catheters impregnated with antiseptics for the prevention of central venous catheter-related infections in intensive care units in 204 patients with 235 central venous catheters between November 1998 and June 1999, a standard triple-lumen polyurethane catheter and a catheter impregnated with chlorhexidine and silver sulfadiazine were indistinguishable from each other (55). Compared with standard polyurethane catheters, antiseptic catheters were less likely to be colonized by micro-organisms when they were cultured at removal (8 versus 20 colonized catheters per 100 catheters; relative risk 0.34 (95% CI = 0.15, 0.74). There were no significant differences between the groups in catheter-related infections (0.9 versus 4.9 infections per 100 catheters; relative risk 0.17 (95% CI = 0.03, 1.15)). Gram-positive cocci and fungi were more likely to colonize the standard polyurethane catheters than antiseptic catheters. Two of the cases in the control group died because of catheter-related candidemia. There were no adverse reactions such as hypersensitivity or leukopenia with the antiseptic catheters. The authors concluded that central venous catheters with antiseptic coating are safe and carry less risk of colonization of bacteria and fungi than standard catheters in critically ill patients.

However, although randomized studies have failed to show an association between hypersensitivity reactions and chlorhexidine-impregnated central venous catheters, there have been reports of anaphylaxis after insertion of these catheters (SEDA-22, 262) (56,57), and two life-threatening episodes of anaphylaxis in the same patient were attributed to a central venous catheter that had been impregnated with chlorhexidine and sulfadiazine (58).

- In a 51-year-old man, two episodes of pronounced, refractory cardiovascular collapse accompanied the insertion of a chlorhexidine-coated central venous catheter (59). Sensitivity to chlorhexidine was not at first suspected, but 5 months later, a skin prick test with chlorhexidine resulted in a characteristic sustained wheal and flare response, strongly suggesting IgE-mediated sensitivity. The patient subsequently underwent uneventful surgery following strict avoidance of chlorhexidine exposure.

Bronchospasm was not a feature in any of these cases.

The FDA has issued a public health notice to inform health-care professionals about the potential for serious hypersensitivity reactions to medical devices impregnated with chlorhexidine. The Agency is also seeking information and reports to better evaluate the potential health hazard these products might pose, and to decide on what action, if any, should be taken. Devices that incorporate chlorhexidine that the FDA has cleared for marketing include intravenous catheters, topical antimicrobial skin dressings, and implanted antimicrobial surgical mesh. The notice describes non-US reports of systemic reactions to chlorhexidine-impregnated gels or lubricants used during urological procedures and similarly impregnated central venous catheters. It also describes other types of reactions that have been reported in the USA, including localized reactions to impregnated patches in neonates and occupational asthma in nurses exposed to chlorhexidine and alcohol aerosols (49).

A meta-analysis of the clinical and economic effects of chlorhexidine and silver sulfadiazine antiseptic-impregnated catheters has been undertaken (60). The costs of hypersensitivity reactions were considered as part of the analysis, and the use of catheters impregnated with antiseptics resulted in reduced costs. The analysis used the higher estimated incidence of hypersensitivity reactions occurring in Japan, where the use of chlorhexidine-impregnated catheters is still banned (61).

Polyhexanide

Caution also seems to be warranted concerning polyhexanide, a chlorhexidine polymer, used in disinfectants for a relatively short time.

- Polyhexanide caused severe anaphylaxis in two young patients (62). Both were exposed to the disinfectant Lavasept®, containing polyhexanide, on surgical wounds during orthopedic interventions. They had never been exposed to polyhexanide before, but had been exposed to chlorhexidine. However, skin prick tests were positive for polyhexanide in both cases, while chlorhexidine was negative. Negative skin prick tests to polyhexanide were obtained from controls.

References

1. Mitchell RG, Hayward AC. Postoperative urinary-tract infections caused by contaminated irrigating fluid. Lancet 1966;1(7441):793–5.
2. Speller DC, Stephens ME, Viant AC. Hospital infection by *Pseudomonas cepacia*. Lancet 1971;1(7703):798–9.
3. Salveson A, Bergan T. Contamination of chlorhexidine cream used to prevent ascending urinary tract infections. J Hyg (Lond) 1981;86(3):295–301.
4. Gongwer LE, Hubben K, Lenkiewicz RS, Hart ER, Cockrell BY. The effects of daily bathing of neonatal rhesus monkeys with an antimicrobial skin cleanser containing chlorhexidine gluconate. Toxicol Appl Pharmacol 1980;52(2):255–61.
5. Johnsson J, Seeberg S, Kjellmer I. Blood concentrations of chlorhexidine in neonates undergoing routine cord care with 4% chlorhexidine gluconate solution. Acta Paediatr Scand 1987;76(4):675–6.
6. Salole EG, Shepherd AJ. Spermicides: anti-HIV activity and cytotoxicity in vitro. AIDS 1993;7(2):293–5.
7. Weidinger H, Passloer HJ, Kovacs L, Berle B. Nutzen der prophylaktischen Vaginalantiseptik mit Hexetidin in Geburtshilfe und Gynäkologie. [The advantage of preventive vaginal antisepsis with hexetidine in obstetrics and gynecology.] Geburtshilfe Frauenheilkd 1991; 51(11):929–35.
8. Quinn MW, Bini RM. Bradycardia associated with chlorhexidine spray. Arch Dis Child 1989;64(6):892–3.
9. Mucklow ES. Accidental feeding of a dilute antiseptic solution (chlorhexidine 0.05% with cetrimide 1%) to five babies. Hum Toxicol 1988;7(6):567–9.
10. Hirata K, Kurokawa A. Chlorhexidine gluconate ingestion resulting in fatal respiratory distress syndrome. Vet Hum Toxicol 2002;44(2):89–91.
11. Waclawski ER, McAlpine LG, Thomson NC. Occupational asthma in nurses caused by chlorhexidine and alcohol aerosols. BMJ 1989;298(6678):929–30.
12. Yamagishi M, Kawana M, Hasegawa S, et al. Impairment of olfactory epithelium treated with chlorhexidine digluconate (Hibitane): postoperative olfactory disturbances after Hardy's operation and results of experimental study. Pract Otol 1985;78:399.
13. Bicknell PG. Sensorineural deafness following myringoplasty operations. J Laryngol Otol 1971;85(9):957–61.
14. Parker FL, James GW. The effect of various topical antibiotic and antibacterial agents on the middle and inner ear of the guinea-pig. J Pharm Pharmacol 1978;30(4):236–9.
15. Aursnes J. Vestibular damage from chlorhexidine in guinea pigs. Acta Otolaryngol 1981;92(1–2):89–100.
16. Aursnes J. Cochlear damage from chlorhexidine in guinea pigs. Acta Otolaryngol 1981;92(3–4):259–71.
17. van Rij G, Beekhuis WH, Eggink CA, Geerards AJ, Remeijer L, Pels EL. Toxic keratopathy due to the accidental use of chlorhexidine, cetrimide and cialit. Doc Ophthalmol 1995;90(1):7–14.
18. Nakamura Y, Inatomi T, Nishida K, Sotozono C, Kinoshita S. Four cases of chemical corneal burns by misuse of disinfectant. Jpn J Clin Ophthalmol 1998;52:786–8.
19. Tabor E, Bostwick DC, Evans CC. Corneal damage due to eye contact with chlorhexidine gluconate. JAMA 1989;261(4):557–8.
20. Phinney RB, Mondino BJ, Hofbauer JD, Meisler DM, Langston RH, Forstot SL, Benes SC. Corneal edema related to accidental Hibiclens exposure. Am J Ophthalmol 1988;106(2):210–15.
21. Varley GA, Meisler DM, Benes SC, McMahon JT, Zakov ZN, Fryczkowski A. Hibiclens keratopathy. A clinicopathologic case report. Cornea 1990;9(4):341–6.

22. Klebe S, Anders N, Wollensak J. Inadvertent use of chlorhexidine as intraocular irrigation solution. J Cataract Refract Surg 1998;24(6):729–30.
23. Murthy S, Hawksworth NR, Cree I. Progressive ulcerative keratitis related to the use of topical chlorhexidine gluconate (0.02%). Cornea 2002;21(2):237–9.
24. Bain MJ. Chlorhexidine in dentistry—a review. NZ Dent J 1980;76(344):49–54.
25. Heidemann D. Wundheiliungsstörungen nach Chlorhexidin-Anwedung: ein Fallbericht. [Disturbances in the wound healing process after chlorhexidine use—a case report.] ZWR 1981;90(9):68–70.
26. Flotra L, Gjermo P, Rolla G, Waerhaug J. Side effects of chlorhexidine mouth washes. Scand J Dent Res 1971;79(2):119–25.
27. Flotra L. Different modes of chlorhexidine application and related local side effects. J Periodontal Res Suppl 1973;12:41–4.
28. Prayitno S, Taylor L, Cadogan S, Addy M. An in vivo study of dietary factors in the aetiology of tooth staining associated with the use of chlorhexidine. J Periodontal Res 1979;14(5):411–17.
29. Rushton A. Safety of Hibitane. II. Human experience. J Clin Periodontol 1977;4(5):73–9.
30. Roche S, Chinn R, Webb S. Chlorhexidine-induced gastritis. Postgrad Med J 1991;67(784):210–11.
31. Osmundsen PE. Contact dermatitis to chlorhexidine. Contact Dermatitis 1982;8(2):81–3.
32. Junor BJ, Briggs JD, Forwell MA, et al. Sclerosing peritonitis—the contribution of chlorhexidine in alcohol. Periton Dial Bull 1985;5:101.
33. Oules R, Challah S, Brunner FP. Case-control study to determine the cause of sclerosing peritoneal disease. Nephrol Dial Transplant 1988;3(1):66–9.
34. Lo WK, Chan KT, Leung AC, Pang SW, Tse CY. Sclerosing peritonitis complicating prolonged use of chlorhexidine in alcohol in the connection procedure for continuous ambulatory peritoneal dialysis. Perit Dial Int 1991;11(2):166–72.
35. Douw CM, Bulstra SK, Vandenbroucke J, Geesink RG, Vermeulen A. Clinical and pathological changes in the knee after accidental chlorhexidine irrigation during arthroscopy. Case reports and review of the literature. J Bone Joint Surg Br 1998;80(3):437–40.
36. Schroder CH, Severijnen RS, Monnens LA. Vergiftiging door desinfectans bij conservatieve behandeling van twee patiënten met omfalokele. [Poisoning by disinfectants in the conservative treatment of 2 patients with omphalocele.] Tijdschr Kindergeneeskd 1985;53(2):76–9.
37. Evans P, Foxell RM. Chlorhexidine as a cause of anaphylaxis. Int J Obstet Anaesth 2002;11:145–6.
38. Pham NH, Weiner JM, Reisner GS, Baldo BA. Anaphylaxis to chlorhexidine. Case report. Implication of immunoglobulin E antibodies and identification of an allergenic determinant. Clin Exp Allergy 2000;30(7):1001–7.
39. Lasthein Andersen B, Brandrup F. Contact dermatitis from chlorhexidine. Contact Dermatitis 1985;13(5):307–9.
40. Stables GI, Turner WH, Prescott S, Wilkinson SM. Generalized urticaria after skin cleansing and urethral instillation with chlorhexidine-containing products. Br J Urol 1998;82(5):756–7.
41. Okano M, Nomura M, Hata S, Okada N, Sato K, Kitano Y, Tashiro M, Yoshimoto Y, Hama R, Aoki T. Anaphylactic symptoms due to chlorhexidine gluconate. Arch Dermatol 1989;125(1):50–2.
42. Ohtoshi T, Yamauchi N, Tadokoro K, Miyachi S, Suzuki S, Miyamoto T, Muranaka M. IgE antibody-mediated shock reaction caused by topical application of chlorhexidine. Clin Allergy 1986;16(2):155–61.
43. Cheung J, O'Leary JJ. Allergic reaction to chlorhexidine in an anaesthetised patient. Anaesth Intensive Care 1985;13(4):429–30.
44. Evans RJ. Acute anaphylaxis due to topical chlorhexidine acetate. BMJ 1992;304(6828):686.
45. Garvey LH, Roed-Petersen J, Husum B. Anaphylactic reactions in anaesthetised patients — four cases of chlorhexidine allergy. Acta Anaesthesiol Scand 2001;45(10):1290–4.
46. Ebo DG, Stevens WJ, Bridts CH, Matthieu L. Contact allergic dermatitis and life-threatening anaphylaxis to chlorhexidine. J Allergy Clin Immunol 1998;101(1 Pt 1):128–9.
47. Conraads VM, Jorens PG, Ebo DG, Claeys MJ, Bosmans JM, Vrints CJ. Coronary artery spasm complicating anaphylaxis secondary to skin disinfectant. Chest 1998;113(5):1417–19.
48. Thune P. To pasienter med klorheksidinallergi–anafylaktiske reaksjoner og eksem. [Two patients with chlorhexidine allergy—anaphylactic reactions and eczema.] Tidsskr Nor Laegeforen 1998;118(21):3295–6.
49. Nightingale SL. Hypersensitivity to chlorhexidine-impregnated medical devices. JAMA 1998;279:1684.
50. Garland JS, Alex CP, Mueller CD, Otten D, Shivpuri C, Harris MC, Naples M, Pellegrini J, Buck RK, McAuliffe TL, Goldmann DA, Maki DG. A randomized trial comparing povidone-iodine to a chlorhexidine gluconate-impregnated dressing for prevention of central venous catheter infections in neonates. Pediatrics 2001;107(6):1431–6.
51. Chisholm DG, Calder I, Peterson D, Powell M, Moult P. Intranasal chlorhexidine resulting in anaphylactic circulatory arrest. BMJ 1997;315(7111):785.
52. Leuer J, Mayser P, Schill WB. Anaphylaktischer schock durch intraoperative Anwendung von Chlorhexidin. HGZ Hautkr 2001;76:160–3.
53. Wicki J, Deluze C, Cirafici L, Desmeules J. Anaphylactic shock induced by intraurethral use of chlorhexidine. Allergy 1999;54(7):768–9.
54. Yong D, Parker FC, Foran SM. Severe allergic reactions and intra-urethral chlorhexidine gluconate. Med J Aust 1995;162(5):257–8.
55. Sheng WH, Ko WJ, Wang JT, Chang SC, Hsueh PR, Luh KT. Evaluation of antiseptic-impregnated central venous catheters for prevention of catheter-related infection in intensive care unit patients. Diagn Microbiol Infect Dis 2000;38(1):1–5.
56. Nikaido S, Tanaka M, Yamoto M, Minami T, Akatsuka M, Mori H. [Anaphylactoid shock caused by chlorhexidine gluconate.] Masui 1998;47(3):330–4.
57. Terazawa E, Shimonaka H, Nagase K, Masue T, Dohi S. Severe anaphylactic reaction due to a chlorhexidine-impregnated central venous catheter. Anesthesiology 1998;89(5):1296–8.
58. Stephens R, Mythen M, Kallis P, Davies DW, Egner W, Rickards A. Two episodes of life-threatening anaphylaxis in the same patient to a chlorhexidine-sulphadiazine-coated central venous catheter. Br J Anaesth 2001;87(2):306–8.
59. Pittaway A, Ford S. Allergy to chlorhexidine-coated central venous catheters revisited. Br J Anaesth 2002;88(2):304–5.
60. Veenstra DL, Saint S, Sullivan SD. Cost-effectiveness of antiseptic-impregnated central venous catheters for the prevention of catheter-related bloodstream infection. JAMA 1999;282(6):554–60.
61. Raad I, Hanna H. Intravascular catheters impregnated with antimicrobial agents: a milestone in the prevention of bloodstream infections. Support Care Cancer 1999; 7(6):386–90.
62. Olivieri J, Eigenmann PA, Hauser C. Severe anaphylaxis to a new disinfectant: polyhexanide, a chlorhexidine polymer. Schweiz Med Wochenschr 1998;128(40):1508–11.

Chlormezanone

General Information

Chlormezanone is a tranquillizer with central muscle relaxant effects. In reaction to some case reports of serious, sometimes fatal, cutaneous toxicity and after intervention by drug regulatory authorities in some European countries, all major manufacturers have stopped production of chlormezanone. It may still be available in combination products in some Asian countries.

For the most part chlormezanone causes only minor adverse effects, such as sedation, dizziness, nausea, and headache, which clear on stopping the drug.

Organs and Systems

Hematologic

Rarely, thombocytopenia can occur in a patient taking chlormezanone (1).

Liver

Rarely, cholestatic hepatitis can occur with chlormezanone.

- A 46-year-old woman with rheumatoid arthritis developed cholestatic liver disease while taking chlormezanone and paracetamol (2).
- Fulminant liver necrosis requiring liver transplantation occurred in a young pregnant woman who had taken chlormezanone 600 mg/day for 3 weeks (SEDA-17, 157).

Skin

Toxic epidermal necrolysis and Stevens–Johnson syndrome have been attributed to chlormezanone (3).

Drug–Drug Interactions

Paracetamol

The concomitant use of paracetamol may increase the chance of adverse effects, especially erythema and urticaria (4).

References

1. Finney RD, Apps J. Unreviewed reports: Trancopal (chlormezanone) and thrombocytopenia. BMJ (Clin Res Ed) 1985;290:1112.
2. Pomiersky C, Blaich E. Arzneimittelbedingte Hepatitis mit Cholestase nach Therapie mit Chlormezanon.. [Drug-induced hepatitis with cholestasis following therapy with chlormezanone.] Z Gastroenterol 1985;23(12):684–6.
3. Roujeau JC, Kelly JP, Naldi L, Rzany B, Stern RS, Anderson T, Auquier A, Bastuji-Garin S, Correia O, Locati F, et al. Medication use and the risk of Stevens-Johnson syndrome or toxic epidermal necrolysis. N Engl J Med 1995;333(24):1600–7.
4. Verbov J. Fixed drug eruption due to a drug combination but not to its constituents. Dermatologica 1985;171(1):60–1.

Chloroform

See also General anesthetics

General Information

Chloroform (SED-8, 250) should no longer be used, because of its toxic effects on the heart, liver, and kidneys, although the exact nature and extent of these complications has been debated (1). The very serious adverse effects of chloroform anesthesia when poorly administered have been briefly reviewed (2).

References

1. Payne JP. Chloroform in clinical anaesthesia. Br J Anaesth 1981;53(Suppl 1):S11–15.
2. Defalque RJ, Wright AJ. An anesthetic curiosity in New York (1875–1900): a noted surgeon returns to "open drop" chloroform. Anesthesiology 1998;88(2):549–51.

Chloroprocaine

See also Local anesthetics

General Information

Chloroprocaine is a local anesthetic, an aminoester of para-aminobenzoic acid. Its systemic toxicity is low, owing to rapid hydrolysis by plasma pseudocholinesterases (1).

Organs and Systems

Cardiovascular

Of 25 patients who received epidural chloroprocaine for various day procedures, 23 had a fall in arterial blood pressure of 15%, and in two it fell by 25% (2).

Neuromuscular function

Prolonged neuromuscular blockade has been reported after epidural chloroprocaine (3).

- A 29-year-old woman in labor was given an epidural infusion of bupivacaine 0.04% plus fentanyl 1.66 micrograms/ml, running at 15 ml/hour for 7 hours. She then required an urgent cesarean section and 15 ml of chloroprocaine 3% was given, followed 20 minutes later by 12 ml of 2% lidocaine. Half an hour later she showed signs of high epidural blockade with dyspnea followed by unresponsiveness, and required immediate intubation with suxamethonium. She then developed prolonged neuromuscular blockade with a first-twitch response occurring after 1.75 hours. It took 3.75 hours before she could be extubated. Her plasma cholinesterase activity was low immediately postpartum, with a concentration of 1.3 U/ml (reference range 2.8–11), returning to normal within 7 weeks.

The authors believed that the high epidural blockade and the prolonged neuromuscular block had resulted from reduced pseudocholinesterase activity.

Second-Generation Effects

Pregnancy

Reduced pseudocholinesterase activity has been described both in pregnancy and with magnesium therapy. As most ester local anesthetics (with the exception of cocaine) are metabolized by this enzyme, caution should be exercised when using ester local anesthetics in pregnancy, especially with the increasing use of magnesium sulfate in this field.

Susceptibility Factors

Genetic factors

When there is an atypical pseudocholinesterase, complications can occur, notably convulsions (1).

Drug Administration

Drug formulations

Chloroprocaine does not itself appear to be neurotoxic at clinical concentrations. However, formulations that contain EDTA can cause burning back pain when used in epidurals (SEDA-22, 142).

Local neural irritation can occur when large doses of formulations containing sodium bisulfate as a preservative are used epidurally or intrathecally, probably because of the low pH and the sodium bisulfate content rather than the local anesthetic (SEDA-14, 111). Prolonged neural deficits have been described, the pathophysiology of which is controversial (SEDA-10, 105).

Drug–Drug Interactions

Suxamethonium

Because it is hydrolysed by plasma cholinesterase, chloroprocaine may competitively enhance the action of suxamethonium (4).

References

1. Smith AR, Hur D, Resano F. Grand mal seizures after 2-chloroprocaine epidural anesthesia in a patient with plasma cholinesterase deficiency. Anesth Analg 1987;66(7):677–8.
2. Allen RW, Fee JP, Moore J. A preliminary assessment of epidural chloroprocaine for day procedures. Anaesthesia 1993;48(9):773–5.
3. Monedero P, Hess P. High epidural block with chloroprocaine in a parturient with low pseudocholinesterase activity. Can J Anaesth 2001;48(3):318–19.
4. Matsuo S, Rao DB, Chaudry I, Foldes FF. Interaction of muscle relaxants and local anesthetics at the neuromuscular junction. Anesth Analg 1978;57(5):580–7.

Chloroquine and hydroxychloroquine

General Information

Chloroquine is rapidly and almost completely absorbed from the intestinal tract, peak serum concentrations being reached in 1–6 hours (average 3 hours). It is extensively distributed and redistribution follows. It is slowly metabolized by side-chain de-ethylation. The half-life is 30–60 days. Elimination is mainly via the kidney. Malnutrition can slow down the rate of metabolism.

Comparative studies

Amodiaquine and chloroquine have been compared in an open, randomized trial in uncomplicated falciparum malaria in Nigerian children (1). The doses were amodiaquine ($n = 104$) 10 mg/kg/day for 3 days and chloroquine ($n = 106$) 10 mg/kg/day for 3 days. After 28 days, the cure rate was significantly higher with amodiaquine than chloroquine (95% versus 58%). The rates of adverse events, most commonly pruritus (10%) and gastrointestinal disturbances (3%), were similar in the two groups. Cross-resistance between the two aminoquinolines is common, and there are concerns regarding toxicity of amodiaquine with repeated use.

General adverse effects

There are relatively few adverse effects at the doses of chloroquine that are used for malaria prophylaxis and standard treatment doses. However, the use of higher doses than those recommended, for example because of problems with resistance, can cause problems. Infants are very easily overdosed (SEDA-16, 302). In the treatment of rheumatoid arthritis and lupus erythematosus, larger doses are used, often for long periods of time, and with this use the incidence of adverse effects is high. Neuromyopathy, neuritis, myopathy, and cardiac myopathy can cause serious problems. Retinopathy can lead to blindness. Chloroquine has a long half-life and accumulates in the tissues, including the brain. Concentrations in the brain can have a bearing on mental status and psychotic syndromes. Chloroquine interferes with the action of several enzymes, including alcohol dehydrogenase, and blocks the sulfhydryl–disulfide interchange reaction. Allergic reactions are generally limited to rashes and pruritus.

Organs and Systems

Cardiovascular

Electrocardiographic changes, comprising altered T waves and prolongation of the QT interval, are not uncommon during high-dose treatment with chloroquine. The clinical significance of this is uncertain. With chronic intoxication, a varying degree of atrioventricular block can be seen; first-degree right bundle branch block and total atrioventricular block have been described. Symptoms depend on the severity of the effects: syncope, Stokes–Adams attacks, and signs of cardiac failure can occur. Acute intoxication can cause cardiovascular collapse and/or respiratory failure. Cardiac complications can prove fatal in both chronic and acute intoxication.

Third-degree atrioventricular conduction defects have been reported in two patients with rheumatoid arthritis after prolonged administration of chloroquine (2,3).

Intravenous administration can result in dysrhythmias and cardiac arrest; the speed of administration is relevant, but also the concentration reached: deaths have been recorded with blood concentrations of 1 μg/ml; concentrations after a 300 mg dose are usually 50–100 μg/ml (SEDA-13, 803).

Long-term chloroquine can cause cardiac complications, such as conduction disorders and cardiomyopathy (restrictive or hypertrophic), by structural alteration of the interventricular septum (4). Thirteen cases of cardiac toxicity associated with long-term chloroquine and hydroxychloroquine have been reported in patients with systemic autoimmune diseases. The cumulative doses were 600–2281 g for chloroquine and 292–4380 g for hydroxychloroquine.

- A 64-year-old woman with systemic lupus erythematosus took chloroquine for 7 years (cumulative dose 1000 g). She developed syncope, and the electrocardiogram showed complete heart block; a permanent pacemaker was inserted. The next year she presented with biventricular cardiac failure, skin hyperpigmentation, proximal muscle weakness, and chloroquine retinopathy. Coronary angiography was normal. An echocardiogram showed a restrictive cardiomyopathy. A skeletal muscle biopsy was characteristic of chloroquine myopathy. Chloroquine was withdrawn and she improved rapidly with diuretic therapy.
- Chloroquine cardiomyopathy occurred during long-term (7 years) treatment for rheumatoid polyarthritis in a 42-year-old woman, who had an isolated acute severe conduction defect, confirmed by histological study with electron microscopy (5).

Regular cardiac evaluation should be considered for those who have taken a cumulative chloroquine dose of 1000 g, particularly elderly patients.

More than one mechanism may underlie the cardiac adverse effects of chloroquine. Severe hypokalemia after a single large dose of chloroquine has been documented, and some studies show a correlation between plasma potassium concentrations and the severity of the cardiac effects (6).

Light and electron microscopic abnormalities were found on endomyocardial biopsy in two patients with cardiac failure. The first had taken hydroxychloroquine 200 mg/day for 10 years, then 400 mg/day for a further 6 years; the second had taken hydroxychloroquine 400 mg/day for 2 years (SEDA-13, 239). A similar case was reported after the use of 250 mg/day for 25 years (SEDA-18, 286).

Respiratory

Respiratory collapse can occur with acute overdosage.

Acute pneumonitis probably due to chloroquine has been described (7).

- A 41-year-old man with chronic discoid lupus erythematosus was given chloroquine 150 mg bd for 10 days followed by 150 mg/day. After 2 weeks he developed fever, a diffuse papular rash, dyspnea, and sputum. A chest X-ray showed peripheral pulmonary infiltrates. He improved on withdrawal of chloroquine and treatment with cefpiramide and roxithromycin. No organism was isolated. A subsequent oral challenge with chloroquine provoked a similar reaction.

Nervous system

The incidence of serious nervous system events among patients taking chloroquine for less than a year has been estimated as one in 13 600.

Chloroquine, especially in higher doses, can cause a marked neuromyopathy, characterized by slowly progressive weakness of insidious onset. In many cases this weakness first affects the proximal muscles of the legs. Reduction in nerve conduction time and electromyographic abnormalities typical of both neuropathic and myopathic changes can be found. Histologically there is a vacuolar myopathy. Neuromyopathy is a rare adverse effect and is usually limited to patients taking 250–750 mg/day for prolonged periods. The symptoms can be accompanied by other manifestations of chloroquine toxicity (SEDA-11, 583). An 80-year-old woman developed symptoms after taking chloroquine 300 mg/day for 6 months (8), once more demonstrating that a standard dosage can be too much for elderly people.

A spastic pyramidal tract syndrome of the legs has been reported. In young children the features of an extrapyramidal syndrome include abnormal eye movements, trismus, torticollis, and torsion dystonia.

Chloroquine can cause seizures in patients with epilepsy. The mechanism is uncertain, but it may include reductions in inhibitory neurotransmitters and pharmacokinetic interactions that alter anticonvulsant concentrations. Tonic–clonic convulsions were reported in four patients in whom chloroquine was part of a prophylactic regimen. Antiepileptic treatment was required to control the seizures. None had further seizures after withdrawal of the antimalarial drugs (9).

Chloroquine and desethylchloroquine concentrations have been studied in 109 Kenyan children during the first 24 hours of admission to hospital with cerebral malaria (10). Of the 109 children 100 had received chloroquine before admission. Blood chloroquine and desethylchloroquine concentrations were no higher in children who had seizures than in those who did not, suggesting that chloroquine does not play an important role in the development of seizures in malaria.

- A 59-year-old woman had a generalized convulsion 24 hours after returning from a trip to Vietnam (11). She had a history of partial complex seizures (controlled with carbamazepine) due to a previous ruptured cerebral aneurysm. For the preceding 3 weeks she had been taking chloroquine 100 mg/day and proguanil 200 mg/day. A blood film was negative for malaria. A CT scan of the brain showed changes compatible with the previous hemorrhage. She was successfully treated with clobazam (dose not stated) until withdrawal of chemoprophylaxis.

The interaction between chloroquine and carbamazepine was not examined. Chloroquine should not be given to adults with a history of epilepsy.

Neuromuscular function

Severe neuromyopathy has been reported in patients taking chloroquine (SEDA-21, 295).

Chloroquine-induced neuromyopathy is a complication of chloroquine treatment of autoimmune disorders or long-term use of chloroquine as a prophylactic antimalarial drug (12).

Sensory systems

Eyes

Chloroquine and its congeners can cause two typical effects in the eye, a keratopathy and a specific retinopathy. Both of these effects are associated with the administration of the drug over longer periods of time.

Keratopathy

Chloroquine-induced keratopathy is limited to the corneal epithelium, where high concentrations of the drug are readily demonstrable. Slit lamp examination shows a series of punctate opacities scattered diffusely over the cornea; these are sometimes seen as lines just below the center of the cornea, while thicker yellow lines may be seen in the stroma. The keratopathy is often asymptomatic, fewer than 50% of patients having complaints. The commonest symptoms are the appearance of halos around lights and photophobia. Keratopathy can appear after 1–2 months of treatment, but dosages of under 250 mg/day usually do not cause it. Dust exposure can lead to similar changes. The incidence of keratopathy is high, occurring in 30–70% of patients treated with higher dosages of chloroquine. The condition is usually reversible on withdrawal and does not seem to involve a threat to vision (SEDA-13, 805). There are differences in incidence between chloroquine and hydroxychloroquine. In a survey of 1500 patients, 95% of the patients taking chloroquine had corneal deposition of the drug, while less than 10% of patients taking hydroxychloroquine showed any corneal changes (SEDA-16, 303).

Retinopathy

The retinopathy encountered with the prolonged use of chloroquine or related drugs is a much more serious adverse effect and can lead to irreversible damage to the retina and loss of vision. However, it is not possible to predict in which patients and in what proportion of patients an early retinopathy will progress to blindness. The typical picture is that of the "bull's eye," an intact foveal area surrounded by a depigmented ring, the whole lesion being enclosed in a scattered hyperpigmented area. At this stage the retinal vessels are contracted, there are changes in the peripheral retinal pigment epithelium, and the optic disk is atrophic. In the early stages there are changes in the macular retinal pigment epithelium. However, the picture is not always clear, and peripheral retinal changes may appear as the first sign. Another sign may be unilateral paramacular retinal edema. The macular changes and the "bull's eye" are occasionally seen in patients who have never been treated with chloroquine or related drugs (SED-13, 805). Retinopathy can occur after chloroquine antimalarial chemoprophylaxis for less than 10 years: the lowest reported total dose was 110 g (13). A case of hydroxychloroquine-induced retinopathy in a 45-year-old woman with systemic lupus erythematosus has illustrated that maculopathy can be associated with other 4-aminoquinolines (14).

The resulting functional defects are varied: difficulty in reading, scotomas, defective color vision, photophobia, light flashes, and a reduction in visual acuity. Symptoms do not parallel the retinal changes. By the time that visual acuity has become impaired, irreversible changes will have taken place.

Testing of visual acuity, central fields (with or without the use of red targets), contrast sensitivity, dark adaptation, and color vision provides no early indication of chloroquine retinopathy. Careful ophthalmoscopic examination of the macula can be a sensitive index when visual acuity remains intact. More sophisticated tests, such as the measurement of the critical flicker fusion frequency and the Amsler grid test (detection of small peripheral scotoma), can be useful. It is important to trace, if at all possible, the results of a pretreatment ophthalmological examination after dilatation of the pupils, thus reducing the possibility of confusing senile degenerative changes with chloroquine-induced abnormalities.

Despite the fact that the retinopathy has been known for many years, it is still not clear why certain patients develop these changes while others do not. There is a clear relation to daily dosage: the retinopathy is rarely seen with daily doses below 250 mg of chloroquine or 400 mg of hydroxychloroquine; the daily dose seems to be more important than the total dose. Nevertheless, cases of retinopathy have been described after the use of small doses for relatively short periods of time, while prolonged treatment and total doses of a kilogram or more have been used in many other patients without any evidence of macular changes. In the published cases there is usually no information about other treatments given previously or concomitantly. More cases are seen in older people. Patients with lupus erythematosus are more susceptible than patients with rheumatoid arthritis. The presence of nephropathy increases the likelihood of retinopathy, as does the concomitant use of probenecid. Exposure to sunlight may be of importance, since light amplifies the risk of retinopathy. The retinopathic changes are probably connected with the concentrating capacity of the melanin-containing epithelium. Chloroquine inhibits the incorporation of amino acids into the retinal pigment epithelium.

Little is yet known about the development of the retinopathy after withdrawal of treatment. Retinal changes in the early stages are probably reversible if the drug is withdrawn, and progression of a severe maculopathy to blindness seems to be less frequent than feared. In 1650 patients with 6/6 vision and relative scotomas there was no further decline in visual acuity after drug withdrawal, but 63% of patients who presented with absolute scotomas lost further vision over a median period of 6 years.

This suggests that withdrawal of chloroquine at an early stage halts progression of the disease (SEDA-17, 327).

Three patients with chloroquine retinopathy have been studied with multifocal electroretinography (15). All three had been taking chloroquine for rheumatological diseases and all had electroretinographic changes that were more sensitive than full field electroretinography. It may be that multifocal electroretinography will be a useful technique in the assessment of suspected cases of subtle chloroquine retinopathy.

The need for routine ophthalmological testing of all patients who take chloroquine is under discussion, an obvious element being the cost/benefit ratio. The best current opinion seems to be that at doses not exceeding 6.5 mg/kg/day of hydroxychloroquine, given for not longer than 10 years and with periodic checking of renal and hepatic function, the likelihood of retinal damage is negligible and ophthalmological follow-up is not required (SEDA-16, 303) (SEDA-17, 327). However, patients taking chloroquine or higher doses of hydroxychloroquine should be checked.

Other adverse effects on the eyes

Rhegmatogenous retinal detachment and bitemporal hemianopsia have both been seen in association with chloroquine retinopathy. Bilateral edema of the optic nerve occurred in a woman who took chloroquine 200 mg/day for 2.5 months. Diplopia and impaired accommodation (characterized by difficulty in changing focus quickly from near to far vision and vice versa) also affect a minority of patients (SEDA-13, 806).

Ears

Ototoxicity has been mentioned occasionally over the years; tinnitus and deafness can occur in relation to high doses; symptoms described after injection of chloroquine phosphate include a case of cochlear vestibular dysfunction in a child (16). However, there is insufficient evidence to attribute ototoxicity to chloroquine in humans, except as a rare individualized phenomenon. In guinea pigs given chloroquine 25 mg/kg/day intraperitoneally, one of the first signs of intoxication was ototoxicity (SEDA-11, 586).

- Unilateral sensorineural hearing loss occurred in a 7-year-old girl with idiopathic pulmonary hemosiderosis after she had taken hydroxychloroquine 100 mg bd for 2 years (17).

Taste

Disturbances of taste and smell have been attributed to chloroquine (18).

Psychological, psychiatric

Many mental changes attributed to chloroquine have been described, notably agitation, aggressiveness, confusion, personality changes, psychotic symptoms, and depression. Acute mania has also been recognized (SEDA-18, 287). The mental changes can develop slowly and insidiously. Subtle symptoms, such as fluctuating impairment of thought, memory, and perception, can be early signs, but may also be the only signs. The symptoms may be connected with the long half-life of chloroquine and its accumulation, leading to high tissue concentrations (SEDA-11, 583). Chloroquine also inhibits glutamate dehydrogenase activity and can reduce concentrations of the inhibitory transmitter GABA.

In some cases with psychosis after the administration of recommended doses, symptoms developed after the patients had taken a total of 1.0–10.5 g of the drug, the time of onset of behavioral changes varying from 2 hours to 40 days. Most cases occurred during the first week and lasted from 2 days to 8 weeks (SEDA-11, 583).

Transient global amnesia occurred in a healthy 62-year-old man, 3 hours after he took 300 mg chloroquine. Recovery was spontaneous after some hours (SEDA-16, 302).

In one center, toxic psychosis was reported in four children over a period of 18 months (SEDA-16, 302). The children presented with acute delirium, marked restlessness, outbursts of increased motor activity, mental inaccessibility, and insomnia. One child seemed to have visual hallucinations. In each case, chloroquine had been administered intramuscularly because of fever. The dosages were not recorded. The children returned to normal within 2 weeks.

Metabolism

Hypoglycemia was reported in a fatal chloroquine intoxication in a 32-year-old black Zambian male (SEDA-13, 240). Hypoglycemia has also been seen in patients, especially children, with cerebral malaria (SEDA-13, 240). Further studies have shown that the hypoglycemia in these African children was usually present before the antimalarial drugs had been started; in a study in Gambia hypoglycemia occurred after treatment with the drug had been started, although it was not necessarily connected with the treatment (SEDA-13, 240). Convulsions were more common in hypoglycemic children. This commonly unrecognized complication contributes to morbidity and mortality in cerebral *Plasmodium falciparum* malaria. Hypoglycemia is amenable to treatment with intravenous dextrose or glucose, which may help to prevent brain damage (SEDA-13, 804).

Although hydroxychloroquine has been used to treat porphyria cutanea tarda (19), there are reports that it can also worsen porphyria (20,21).

Electrolyte balance

Severe hypokalemia after a single large dose of chloroquine has been documented, and some studies show a correlation between plasma potassium concentrations and the severity of the cardiac effects. In a retrospective study of 191 consecutive patients who had taken an overdose of chloroquine (mean blood chloroquine concentration 20 μmol/l; usual target concentration up to 6 μmol/l), the mean plasma potassium concentration was 3.0 mmol/l (0.8) and was significantly lower in those who died than in those who survived (6). Plasma potassium varied directly with the systolic blood pressure and inversely with the QRS and QT intervals. Plasma potassium varied inversely with the blood chloroquine.

Hematologic

Chloroquine inhibits myelopoiesis in vitro at therapeutic concentrations and higher. In a special test procedure, a short-lasting anti-aggregating effect could be seen with chloroquine concentrations of 3.2–32 μg/ml (SEDA-16, 303). These effects have clinical consequences. Chloroquine and related aminoquinolines have reportedly caused blood dyscrasias at antimalarial doses. Leukopenia, agranulocytosis, and the occasional case of thrombocytopenia have been reported (SEDA-13, 804) (22). There is some evidence that myelosuppression is dose-dependent. This is in line with the hypothesis that 4-aminoquinoline therapy merely accentuates the cytopenia linked to other forms of bone marrow damage (SEDA-11, 584) (SEDA-16, 302).

Some studies have pointed to inhibitory effects of chloroquine on platelet aggregability. In an investigation, this aspect of chloroquine was studied in vitro in a medium containing ADP, collagen, and ristocetin. There was a highly significant effect at chloroquine concentrations of 3.2–32 μg/ml. However, there were no significant differences in platelet responses to ADP or collagen 2 or 6 hours after adding chloroquine, compared with pre-drug values. The investigators believed that these data provided no cause for concern in using chloroquine for malaria prophylaxis in patients with impaired hemostasis (SEDA-16, 303).

Mouth and teeth

Pigmentation of the palate can occur as a part of a more generalized pigmentation in patients taking chloroquine (23).

Several patients seen with chloroquine retinopathy in Accra have been observed to present with depigmented patches in the skin of the face. This may be associated with a greyish pigmentation of the mucosa of the hard palate. Two such cases are reported here to illustrate the condition. Stomatitis with buccal ulceration has occasionally been mentioned (SEDA-11, 584).

Gastrointestinal

Gastrointestinal discomfort is not unusual in patients receiving chloroquine, and diarrhea can occur. Changes in intestinal motility may be to blame; intramuscular injection of chloroquine caused a shortened orofecal time in the five cases in which this was measured. Overdosage can cause vomiting.

Skin

Skin lesions and eruptions of different types have been attributed to chloroquine, including occasional cases of epidermal necrolysis (24).

The most common dermatological adverse event associated with chloroquine is skin discomfort (often called pruritus). It is much more common in people with darker skins and has been ascribed to chloroquine binding to increased melanin concentrations in the skin. In a pharmacokinetic study, the ratio of AUC_{0-48} for chloroquine and its major metabolite desethylchloroquine was significantly higher in the plasma and urine of 18 patients with chloroquine-induced pruritus than in that of 18 patients without (25). These results imply that differences in metabolism and higher chloroquine concentrations may be partly responsible for chloroquine-induced pruritus.

Pruritus begins about 10 hours after the start of treatment, with a maximum intensity at about 24 hours. These times correspond to maximum serum concentrations of chloroquine and its metabolites after oral ingestion. In many cases, the itch is confined to the palms of the hands and the soles of the feet. In a study in Nigeria, the incidence of pruritus was 60–75%; the itch was considered unbearable in 40%, and 30% refused further chloroquine (26). In a second study, there was an even higher incidence. In a study elsewhere, the incidence of pruritus was 27% (SEDA-16, 304). Not surprisingly, pruritus is a major cause of non-adherence to treatment, and it may contribute largely to the emergence and spread of resistant *P. falciparum* (SEDA-16, 304). Pruritus is more often seen in black-skinned than in white-skinned people in Africa, a difference that has been ascribed to the binding of chloroquine to melanin, and hence a racial predisposition. No such reports have come from America (SEDA-11, 584) (SEDA-16, 303) (SEDA-17, 327) (SEDA-18, 288). Antihistamine treatment can have a preventive effect on pruritus. Other treatments that have been mentioned include prednisone and niacin, but the results were not impressive (27).

A few cases of psoriasis, or severe exacerbation of psoriasis shortly after the start of treatment, have been reported (SEDA-13, 804) (SEDA-16, 304) (SEDA-17, 327).

Photosensitivity and photo-allergic dermatitis have been seen, particularly during prolonged therapy with high doses.

Blue–black pigmentation involving the palate and facial, pretibial, and subungual areas occurs rarely, but it has been associated with retinopathy (SEDA-11, 584). The nail bed can turn blue–brown and the nail itself may develop longitudinal stripes and show a blue–grey fluorescence (SEDA-11, 584).

Chloroquine can cause vitiligo (SEDA-17, 327).

Fatal toxic epidermal necrolysis has been associated with hydroxychloroquine (28).

- A 39-year-old woman with rheumatoid arthritis took hydroxychloroquine 200 mg bd for painful synovitis, in addition to meloxicam, co-dydramol, and Gaviscon. She inadvertently took twice the prescribed dose of hydroxychloroquine, but stopped it after 2 weeks because of nausea. The next day she developed a widespread blotchy erythema and 2 weeks later was admitted to hospital with clinical and histological toxic epidermal necrolysis and deteriorated rapidly with multiorgan failure; she died 1 week later.

There have been only a few isolated reports of Stevens–Johnson syndrome associated with hydroxychloroquine. Recently, a clear temporal relation to the start of treatment with hydroxychloroquine has been documented in a patient with rheumatoid arthritis (29).

An increased frequency of skin reactions to hydroxychloroquine was noted in 11 patients (seven of whom had systemic lupus erythematosus, two discoid lupus, and two a lupus-like syndrome) when a coloring agent (sunshine yellow E110) was removed from the formulation; the authors were unable to explain this unexpected finding (30).

There have been four case reports of photosensitivity associated with hydroxychloroquine (31) which has an estimated incidence of about 10 per 1000 patient-years (32).

Hydroxychloroquine causes skin reactions such as urticaria. There is some support for the contention that hydroxychloroquine causes skin reactions more often than chloroquine.

Nails

Chloroquine can turn the nail bed blue–brown and the nail itself can develop longitudinal stripes and show a blue–grey fluorescence (SEDA-11, 584).

Immunologic

- Allergic contact dermatitis, which progressed to generalized dermatitis and conjunctivitis, followed later by severe asthma, occurred in a 60-year-old worker in the pharmaceutical industry after exposure to hydroxychloroquine (33). Patch-testing showed delayed sensitivity to hydroxychloroquine. Equivalent tests in five healthy volunteers were negative. The patch test reactions were pustular, and a biopsy was interpreted as multiform contact dermatitis. Bronchial exposure to hydroxychloroquine dust produced delayed bronchial obstruction over the next 20 hours, progressing to fever and generalized erythema (hematogenous contact dermatitis).

Long-Term Effects

Drug tolerance

Chloroquine-resistant falciparum malaria was first reported in 1960. As of 1996, chloroquine resistance became widespread throughout the world and in many areas there is multidrug resistance. Preventive administration of drugs such as chloroquine, primaquine, and pyrimethamine, as well as the use of various sulfonamide mixtures and combinations of sulfonamides with trimethoprim, has progressively lost its usefulness. Currently, hardly half a century after the therapeutic breakthroughs occurred, quinine is once more one of the most valuable drugs in the treatment of malaria and there is a desperate need for other effective drugs.

Alongside the well-known development of resistance by *P. falciparum* to chloroquine, the emergence of chloroquine-resistant *Plasmodium vivax* is now clear (SEDA-13, 801). An increased frequency of cerebral malaria appears to coincide with the growing emergence of the chloroquine-resistant strains in Francophone Africa.

Second-Generation Effects

Pregnancy

Chloroquine inactivates DNA, and crosses the placenta in animals. Caution has generally been advised with respect to the use of chloroquine and related compounds during pregnancy, but except for one (perhaps coincidental) case, there have been no reports of complications to mother or child from treatment with chloroquine during pregnancy (SEDA-14, 239) (SEDA-17, 326).

An observational comparison in a rural Ghanaian hospital of 2083 pregnant women and 3084 historical controls showed no serious adverse events with chloroquine chemoprophylaxis (300 mg/week), but a high rate of pruritus (34). There was a decrease in anemia in pregnancy but no increase in perinatal mortality or birth weight in the chloroquine-treated mothers, although this was only in comparison with historical controls.

Susceptibility Factors

Genetic factors

Mutations in the ABCR gene (a photoreceptor-specific ATP-binding cassette transporter gene) have been associated with Stargardt disease, which has some features similar to chloroquine-induced retinopathy. In a case-control study of eight cases of chloroquine-induced retinopathy, five of the eight cases had mis-sense mutations in the ABCR gene, two of which have been associated with Stargardt disease (35). It may be that polymorphisms in the ABCR gene predispose to chloroquine-induced retinopathy.

Age

Small children have usually been considered as being relatively more sensitive to the effects of overdosage, but it has been calculated that on a mg/kg body weight basis, adults are in fact equally sensitive. Young children seem to be truly more susceptible to gastric irritation. Patients with a history of mania or epilepsy should be careful in taking chloroquine (9). The hypoxemic effects of chloroquine, reflecting cardiac and respiratory toxicity, pose a particular problem in the newborn, in whom existing malarial infection may not become clinically manifest until some months after birth (SEDA-16, 302).

Compared with adults, mortality in children after acute chloroquine poisoning is extremely high. Although the clinical presentation is mostly similar to that in adults (apnea, seizures, cardiac dysrhythmias), a single 300 mg chloroquine tablet was enough to kill a 12-month-old female infant (SEDA-16, 302).

Other features of the patient

Skin reactions to hydroxychloroquine occur more often in patients with dermatomyositis than in patients with systemic lupus erythematosus, as has been shown in a retrospective, age-, sex-, and race-matched case-control study in 78 patients (36). Twelve of 39 patients with dermatomyositis developed a skin reaction to hydroxychloroquine, compared with only one of 39 patients with lupus erythematosus.

Drug Administration

Drug formulations

Chloroquine has a bitter taste, which can deter children from taking it, so a sweet effervescent formulation of chloroquine phosphate has been compared with chloroquine tablets in a pharmacodynamic study (37). However, sweet-tasting medications carry a risk of accidental overdose in children.

Drug administration route

If given intravenously, chloroquine should be diluted and infused slowly, since rapid injection causes toxic concentrations. Toxicity and even death have been reported after intramuscular administration of larger doses; this is probably connected with rapid absorption in such cases (SEDA-17, 327).

Drug overdose

Acute intoxication, either accidental or in attempted suicide, can cause headache, drowsiness, vision disturbance, vomiting and diarrhea, cardiovascular collapse, and respiratory failure. Deaths have been recorded at blood concentrations of 1 μg/ml (SEDA-11, 586) (38,39). Compared with adults, mortality in children after acute chloroquine poisoning is extremely high. Although the clinical presentation is mostly similar to that in adults (apnea, seizures, cardiac dysrhythmias), a single 300 mg chloroquine tablet was enough to kill a 12-month-old female infant (SEDA-16, 302).

Deaths from chloroquine overdose have been reported with doses as low as 2–3 g in adults, and the death rate is as high as 25%. The effects of chloroquine overdose include cardiac effects (such as dysrhythmias, reduced myocardial contractility, and hypotension) and central nervous system complications (such as confusion, coma, and seizures).

There have been three reports of chloroquine overdose, two from Oman (40) and one from the Netherlands (41). The two reports from Oman were similar to previously published reports of chloroquine overdose associated with cardiac dysfunction, confusion, and coma; both patients had standard treatment with activated charcoal, diazepam infusions, and positive inotropic drugs, and both survived. The single case report from the Netherlands gave pharmacokinetic measurements performed before, during, and after hemoperfusion. This showed that hemoperfusion extracted very little chloroquine and was unlikely to be of any use in chloroquine overdose, as would be expected from the high protein binding and large volume of distribution of chloroquine.

In Zimbabwe, 544 cases of poisoning by a single agent were identified in a retrospective hospital record review (42). Antimalarial drugs accounted for the largest proportion of admissions (53%), and chloroquine accounted for 96% of these (279 cases). The median length of hospital stay in those who took chloroquine was significantly shorter (1 versus 2 days) and more patients took chloroquine deliberately (80% versus 69%). The mortality rate from chloroquine poisoning was significantly higher than from poisoning with other drugs (5.7% versus 0.7%).

Overdose with hydroxychloroquine is far less common than with chloroquine. Three of eight patients died (43). Life-threatening symptoms, such as hypotension, conduction disturbances, and hypokalemia can occur within 30 minutes of ingestion and are similar to those seen in chloroquine overdose. The lethal plasma concentration of hydroxychloroquine is not well established. Therapeutic drug concentrations are usually less than 1 μmol/l. Serious toxicity has been reported at plasma concentrations of 2.1–29 μmol/l.

Management of hydroxychloroquine overdose is similar to that of chloroquine overdose, including the use of charcoal for drug adsorption, diazepam for seizures and sedation, early intubation and mechanical ventilation, and potassium replacement for severe hypokalemia.

Drug–Drug Interactions

Amlodipine

Syncope occurred in a hypertensive 48-year-old man who took oral chloroquine sulfate (total 600 mg base) while also taking amlodipine 5 mg/day (44). Chloroquine and amlodipine both cause vasodilatation, perhaps by release of nitric oxide, and the syncope in this case was probably due to a synergistic mechanism. Malaria itself can also provoke orthostatic reactions, which may be why syncope is not a reported adverse effect of chloroquine. However, in this patient malaria had been excluded.

Antibiotics

Studies of chloroquine used in combination with antibiotics showed an antagonistic effect with penicillin but a synergistic effect with chlortetracycline. Urinary tests after single doses of ampicillin 1 g and chloroquine 1 g showed a significant reduction in the systemic availability of the ampicillin.

Chlorphenamine

Chlorphenamine enhances the efficacy of chloroquine in acute uncomplicated falciparum malaria, but the disposition of chloroquine in these circumstances is unpredictable. Chloroquine (25 mg/kg) was given orally over 3 days in combination with chlorphenamine to Nigerian children with parasitemia (45). The peak whole blood chloroquine concentration was increased and the time to peak concentration shortened. In small trials there seemed to be an increase in QT interval with this combination, but less than with halofantrine (46). However, in other studies, the addition of chlorphenamine to chloroquine did not amplify the cardiac effects of chloroquine (46).

Ciclosporin

Chloroquine can increase ciclosporin blood concentrations (47).

Cimetidine

Cimetidine enhanced the susceptibility of *P. falciparum* to chloroquine in vitro in 60% of isolates (48).

Digoxin

The pharmacokinetic interaction of quinidine with digoxin also occurs with quinine and hydroxychloroquine (49).

Fansidar (sulfadoxine + pyrimethamine)

The combined use of Fansidar (sulfadoxine + pyrimethamine) with chloroquine has been reported to result in more severe adverse reactions (50). However, an increased risk has not been reported in recent studies (51).

Halofantrine

There is an increased risk of dysrhythmias, including torsade de pointes, when halofantrine is combined with quinine/quinidine or chloroquine and any other drug that prolongs the QT interval (52).

Insulin

There may be an interaction of chloroquine with insulin. An oral glucose load given to healthy subjects and to patients with non-insulin-dependent diabetes mellitus, before and during a short course of chloroquine, showed a small but significant reduction in fasting blood glucose concentration in the control group and improvement in glucose tolerance in the patients (SEDA-12, 240). The response seems to reflect reduced degradation of insulin rather than increased pancreatic output.

Quinine

Chloroquine antagonizes the action of quinine against *P. falciparum* in vivo. However, no such evidence of antagonism was found in a study in which Malawian children with cerebral malaria were treated with quinine. There was no difference in survival and rate of recovery in patients who had also been given chloroquine compared with those who had not (SEDA-13, 816).

Thyroxine

A marked increase in serum TSH occurred in the same patient on two occasions after several weeks of antimalarial prophylaxis with chloroquine and proguanil, the likely mechanism being enzyme induction and increased thyroxine catabolism (SEDA-22, 469).

Vaccines

Chloroquine 300 mg/week adversely affected the antibody response to human diploid-cell rabies vaccine administered concurrently. The mean rabies-neutralizing antibody titer was significantly reduced on each day of testing (SEDA-13, 806) (8). In contrast, retrospective studies of the response to pneumococcal polysaccharide in patients with systemic lupus erythematosus taking chloroquine or hydroxychloroquine, and of the response to tetanus–measles–meningococcal vaccine in a region of Nigeria where malaria is endemic, did not show an effect on antibody production. However, it was pointed out that the altered immune status of patients with systemic lupus erythematosus makes it difficult to compare their response to that of young healthy adults receiving rabies vaccine. Illness and nutritional state could have influenced the findings in the Nigerian study (SEDA-13, 807) (53).

Verapamil

Verapamil completely reversed pre-existing in vitro resistance to chloroquine to below the cut-off point of 70 nmol/l (48).

Smoking

Antimalarial drugs (chloroquine, hydroxychloroquine, or quinacrine) were given to 36 patients with cutaneous lupus, of whom 17 were smokers and 19 non-smokers (8). The median number of cigarettes smoked was one pack/day, with a median duration of 12.5 years. There was a reduction in the efficacy of antimalarial therapy in the smokers. Patients with cutaneous lupus should therefore be encouraged to stop smoking and consideration may be given to increasing the doses of antimalarial drugs in smokers with refractory cutaneous lupus before starting a cytotoxic agent.

References

1. Sowunmi A, Ayede AI, Falade AG, Ndikum VN, Sowunmi CO, Adedeji AA, Falade CO, Happi TC, Oduola AM. Randomized comparison of chloroquine and amodiaquine in the treatment of acute, uncomplicated, *Plasmodium falciparum* malaria in children. Ann Trop Med Parasitol 2001;95(6):549–58.
2. Veinot JP, Mai KT, Zarychanski R. Chloroquine related cardiac toxicity. J Rheumatol 1998;25(6):1221–5.
3. Guedira N, Hajjaj-Hassouni N, Srairi JE, el Hassani S, Fellat R, Benomar M. Third-degree atrioventricular block in a patient under chloroquine therapy. Rev Rhum Engl Ed 1998;65(1):58–62.
4. Cervera A, Espinosa G, Font J, Ingelmo M. Cardiac toxicity secondary to long term treatment with chloroquine. Ann Rheum Dis 2001;60(3):301.
5. Charlier P, Cochand-Priollet B, Polivka M, Goldgran-Toledano D, Leenhardt A. Cardiomyopathie a la chloroquine revelée par un bloc auriculo-ventriculaire complete. A propos d'une observation. [Chloroquine cardiomyopathy revealed by complete atrio-ventricular block. A case report.] Arch Mal Coeur Vaiss 2002;95(9):833–7.
6. Clemessy JL, Favier C, Borron SW, Hantson PE, Vicaut E, Baud FJ. Hypokalaemia related to acute chloroquine ingestion. Lancet 1995;346(8979):877–80.
7. Mitja K, Izidor K, Music E. Chloroquin-induzierte arzneimitteltoxische Alveolitis. [Chloroquine-induced drug hypersensitivity alveolitis.] Pneumologie 2000;54(9):395–7.
8. Blaison G, Tranchant C, Mohr M, Roth T, Warter JM. Les complications neuromusculaires des traitements par la chloroquine. Sem Hop Paris 1990;66:2425–8.
9. Fish DR, Espir ML. Convulsions associated with prophylactic antimalarial drugs: implications for people with epilepsy. BMJ 1988;297(6647):526–7.
10. Crawley J, Kokwaro G, Ouma D, Watkins W, Marsh K. Chloroquine is not a risk factor for seizures in childhood cerebral malaria. Trop Med Int Health 2000;5(12):860–4.
11. Guilloton L, Burckard E, Fresse S, Drouet A, Felten D. Crise epileptique apres chimioprophylaxie antipalustre par chloroquine. [Epileptic crisis after antimalaria chemoprophylaxis with chloroquine.] Presse Méd 2001;30(35):1745.
12. Wasay M, Wolfe GI, Herrold JM, Burns DK, Barohn RJ. Chloroquine myopathy and neuropathy with elevated CSF protein. Neurology 1998;51(4):1226–7.

13. Bertagnolio S, Tacconelli E, Camilli G, Tumbarello M. Case report: retinopathy after malaria prophylaxis with chloroquine. Am J Trop Med Hyg 2001;65(5):637–8.
14. Warner AE. Early hydroxychloroquine macular toxicity. Arthritis Rheum 2001;44(8):1959–61.
15. Kellner U, Kraus H, Foerster MH. Multifocal ERG in chloroquine retinopathy: regional variance of retinal dysfunction. Graefes Arch Clin Exp Ophthalmol 2000; 238(1):94–7.
16. Mukherjee DK. Chloroquine ototoxicity—a reversible phenomenon? J Laryngol Otol 1979;93(8):809–15.
17. Coutinho MB, Duarte I. Hydroxychloroquine ototoxicity in a child with idiopathic pulmonary haemosiderosis. Int J Pediatr Otorhinolaryngol 2002;62(1):53–7.
18. Weber JC, Alt M, Blaison G, Welsch M, Martin T, Pasquali JL. Modifications du gout et de l'odorat imputables a l'hydroxychloroquine. [Changes in taste and smell caused by hydroxychloroquine.] Presse Méd 1996; 25(5):213.
19. Petersen CS, Thomsen K. High-dose hydroxychloroquine treatment of porphyria cutanea tarda. J Am Acad Dermatol 1992;26(4):614–19.
20. Kutz DC, Bridges AJ. Bullous rash and brown urine in a systemic lupus erythematosus patient treated with hydroxychloroquine. Arthritis Rheum 1995;38(3):440–3.
21. Baler GR. Porphyria precipitated by hydroxychloroquine treatment of systemic lupus erythematosus. Cutis 1976;17(1):96–8.
22. Don PC, Kahn TA, Bickers DR. Chloroquine-induced neutropenia in a patient with dermatomyositis. J Am Acad Dermatol 1987;16(3 Pt 1):629–30.
23. Bentsi-Enchill KO. Pigmentary skin changes associated with ocular chloroquine toxicity in Ghana. Trop Geogr Med 1980;32(3):216–20.
24. Boffa MJ, Chalmers RJ. Toxic epidermal necrolysis due to chloroquine phosphate. Br J Dermatol 1994; 131(3):444–5.
25. Onyeji CO, Ogunbona FA. Pharmacokinetic aspects of chloroquine-induced pruritus: influence of dose and evidence for varied extent of metabolism of the drug. Eur J Pharm Sci 2001;13(2):195–201.
26. Osifo NG. Chloroquine-induced pruritus among patients with malaria. Arch Dermatol 1984;120(1):80–2.
27. Ajayi AA, Akinleye AO, Udoh SJ, Ajayi OO, Oyelese O, Ijaware CO. The effects of prednisolone and niacin on chloroquine-induced pruritus in malaria. Eur J Clin Pharmacol 1991;41(4):383–5.
28. Murphy M, Carmichael AJ. Fatal toxic epidermal necrolysis associated with hydroxychloroquine. Clin Exp Dermatol 2001;26(5):457–8.
29. Leckie MJ, Rees RG. Stevens–Johnson syndrome in association with hydroxychloroquine treatment for rheumatoid arthritis. Rheumatology (Oxford) 2002;41(4):473–4.
30. Salido M, Joven B, D'Cruz DP, Khamashta MA, Hughes GR. Increased cutaneous reactions to hydroxychloroquine (Plaquenil) possibly associated with formulation change: comment on the letter by Alarcon. Arthritis Rheum 2002;46(12):3392–6.
31. Metayer I, Balguerie X, Courville P, Lauret P, Joly P. Toxidermies photo-induites parl'hydroxychloroquine: 4 cas. [Photodermatosis induced by hydroxychloroquine: 4 cases.] Ann Dermatol Venereol 2001;128(6–7):729–31.
32. Singh G, Fries JF, Williams CA, Zatarain E, Spitz P, Bloch DA. Toxicity profiles of disease modifying antirheumatic drugs in rheumatoid arthritis. J Rheumatol 1991; 18(2):188–94.
33. Meier H, Elsner P, Wuthrich B. Berufsbedingtes kontaktekzem und Asthma bronchiale bei ungewohnlicher allergischer Reaktion vona Spattyp auf Hydroxychloroquin. [Occupationally-induced contact dermatitis and bronchial asthma in a unusual delayed reaction to hydroxychloroquine.] Hautarzt 1999;50(9):665–9.
34. Geelhoed DW, Visser LE, Addae V, Asare K, Schagen van Leeuwen JH, van Roosmalen J. Malaria prophylaxis and the reduction of anemia at childbirth. Int J Gynaecol Obstet 2001;74(2):133–8.
35. Shroyer NF, Lewis RA, Lupski JR. Analysis of the ABCR (ABCA4) gene in 4-aminoquinoline retinopathy: is retinal toxicity by chloroquine and hydroxychloroquine related to Stargardt disease? Am J Ophthalmol 2001; 131(6):761–6.
36. Pelle MT, Callen JP. Adverse cutaneous reactions to hydroxychloroquine are more common in patients with dermatomyositis than in patients with cutaneous lupus erythematosus. Arch Dermatol 2002;138(9):1231–3.
37. Yanze MF, Duru C, Jacob M, Bastide JM, Lankeuh M. Rapid therapeutic response onset of a new pharmaceutical form of chloroquine phosphate 300 mg: effervescent tablets. Trop Med Int Health 2001;6(3):196–201.
38. Bochner F, Carruthers G, Kampmann J, Steiner J. Handbook of Clinical Pharmacology. Boston, MA: Little Brown, 1978.
39. Di Maio VJ, Henry LD. Chloroquine poisoning. South Med J 1974;67(9):1031–5.
40. Reddy VG, Sinna S. Chloroquine poisoning: report of two cases. Acta Anaesthesiol Scand 2000;44(8):1017–20.
41. Boereboom FT, Ververs FF, Meulenbelt J, van Dijk A. Hemoperfusion is ineffectual in severe chloroquine poisoning. Crit Care Med 2000;28(9):3346–50.
42. Ball DE, Tagwireyi D, Nhachi CF. Chloroquine poisoning in Zimbabwe: a toxicoepidemiological study. J Appl Toxicol 2002;22(5):311–15.
43. Marquardt K, Albertson TE. Treatment of hydroxychloroquine overdose. Am J Emerg Med 2001;19(5):420–4.
44. Ajayi AA, Adigun AQ. Syncope following oral chloroquine administration in a hypertensive patient controlled on amlodipine. Br J Clin Pharmacol 2002;53(4):404–5.
45. Okonkwo CA, Coker HA, Agomo PU, Ogunbanwo JA, Mafe AG, Agomo CO, Afolabi BM. Effect of chlorpheniramine on the pharmacokinetics of and response to chloroquine of Nigerian children with falciparum malaria. Trans R Soc Trop Med Hyg 1999; 93(3):306–11.
46. Sowunmi A, Fehintola FA, Ogundahunsi OA, Ofi AB, Happi TC, Oduola AM. Comparative cardiac effects of halofantrine and chloroquine plus chlorpheniramine in children with acute uncomplicated falciparum malaria. Trans R Soc Trop Med Hyg 1999;93(1):78–83.
47. Guiserix J, Aizel A. Interactions ciclosporine–chloroquine. [Cyclosporine–chloroquine interactions.] Presse Méd 1996;25(26):1214.
48. Ndifor AM, Howells RE, Bray PG, Ngu JL, Ward SA. Enhancement of drug susceptibility in *Plasmodium falciparum* in vitro and *Plasmodium berghei* in vivo by mixed-function oxidase inhibitors. Antimicrob Agents Chemother 1993;37(6):1318–23.
49. Leden I. Digoxin–hydroxychloroquine interaction? Acta Med Scand 1982;211(5):411–12.
50. Rombo L, Stenbeck J, Lobel HO, Campbell CC, Papaioanou M, Miller KD. Does chloroquine contribute to the risk of serious adverse reactions to Fansidar? Lancet 1985;2(8467):1298–9.
51. Rahman M, Rahman R, Bangali M, Das S, Talukder MR, Ringwald P. Efficacy of combined chloroquine and sulfadoxine–pyrimethamine in uncomplicated *Plasmodium falciparum* malaria in Bangladesh. Trans R Soc Trop Med Hyg 2004;98(7):438–41.
52. Simooya OO, Sijumbil G, Lennard MS, Tucker GT. Halofantrine and chloroquine inhibit CYP2D6 activity in healthy Zambians. Br J Clin Pharmacol 1998; 45(3):315–17.
53. Van der Straeten C, Klippel JH. Antimalarials and pneumococcal immunization. N Engl J Med 1986;315(11):712–13.

Chlorotrianisene

General Information

Chlorotrianisene is a non-steroidal triphenylethylene with estrogen and antiestrogen activity. Diethylstilbestrol and other non-steroidal estrogens came into vogue at a time when the cost of producing steroidal estrogens, whether synthetic or of natural origin, was still prohibitive. They have fallen out of favor, in view of the association between diethylstilbestrol in pregnancy and second-generation injury. There is no reason for believing that the short-term acute adverse reactions to these non-steroidal compounds differ from those of estrogenic steroids.

Chlorotrianisene does not bind in vitro to the uterine estrogen receptor but has potent estrogenic and antiestrogenic actions in vivo, suggesting that it is a prodrug. Its antiestrogenic activity has been proposed to be due to a reactive intermediate (1).

Organs and Systems

Hematologic

In 50 postpartum women who took chlorotrianisene for lactation suppression in a double-blind, randomized, placebo-controlled study, antithrombin III concentrations were significantly lower on the third day postpartum compared with placebo (2).

References

1. Kupfer D, Bulger WH. Inactivation of the uterine estrogen receptor binding of estradiol during P-450 catalyzed metabolism of chlorotrianisene (TACE). Speculation that TACE antiestrogenic activity involves covalent binding to the estrogen receptor. FEBS Lett 1990;261(1):59–62.
2. Niebyl JR, Bell WR, Schaaf ME, Blake DA, Dubin NH, King TM. The effect of chlorotrianisene as postpartum lactation suppression on blood coagulation factors. Am J Obstet Gynecol 1979;134(5):518–22.

Chloroxylenol

See also Disinfectants and antiseptics

General Information

Since the withdrawal of hexachlorophene from the non-prescription drug market in the USA, the antiseptic chloroxylenol, which is less antigenic, has been a substitute in a large number of products.

Organs and Systems

Skin

Topical exposure can cause rashes.

- A 10-day-old baby who was given a bath in a 25% solution of Dettol containing 1.2% chloroxylenol became dehydrated and developed diffuse erythema and vesicles, and afterwards exfoliative dermatitis (1). There was a good response to therapy with systemic glucocorticoids and supportive measures.

Immunologic

Allergic contact dermatitis can occur after sensitization to chloroxylenol, for example in medicated Vaseline or in electrocardiographic paste (2).

In a retrospective analysis of patch tests in 951 patients 1.8% had positive reactions to chloroxylenol (3). Most of the patients had been sensitized by popular proprietary formulations containing chloroxylenol (SEDA-11, 221).

Drug Administration

Drug overdose

There have been many cases of intoxication with oral Dettol liquid, a widespread household disinfectant that contains chloroxylenol 4.8%, pine oil, and isopropyl alcohol (4–8). Dettol was involved in 10% of hospital admissions related to self-poisoning in Hong Kong. In a retrospective study of 67 cases, serious complications were relatively common (8%) and these included aspiration of Dettol with gastric contents, resulting in pneumonia, cardiopulmonary arrest, bronchospasm, adult respiratory distress syndrome, and severe laryngeal edema with upper airway obstruction. Of 89 patients, five developed minor hematemesis, in the form of coffee-colored or blood-stained vomitus (6). One patient had a gastroscopy performed on the day after admission, which showed signs of chemical burns in the esophagus and stomach. Gastroscopy in another patient on day 11, done to rule out an esophageal stricture, showed no abnormality. All patients with hematemesis recovered completely. The authors suggest that upper gastrointestinal hemorrhage after Dettol ingestion tends to be mild and self-limiting. Gastroscopy, which may increase the risk of aspiration in patients with impaired consciousness, is not required unless other causes of gastrointestinal bleeding are suspected. Furthermore, Dettol poisoning can be associated with an increased risk of aspiration, possibly caused by the use of gastrointestinal lavage in 88% of the patients and vomiting in 62% (6,7).

Of 121 patients who ingested Dettol 200–500 ml, three developed renal impairment, as evidenced by raised plasma urea and creatinine (7). Two of these patients also had serious complications, including aspiration leading to pneumonia and adult respiratory distress syndrome; one died. Renal impairment only appears to be observed when relatively large amounts of Dettol are ingested (7).

References

1. Kumar B, Singh G, Roy SN. Dettol induced irritant dermatitis. Indian J Dermatol Venereol Leprol 1981;47:128.
2. Storrs FJ. Para-chloro-meta-xylenol allergic contact dermatitis in seven individuals. Contact Dermatitis 1975; 1(4):211–13.
3. Myatt AE, Beck MH. Contact sensitivity to parachlorometaxylenol (PCMX). Clin Exp Dermatol 1985; 10(5):491–4.
4. Chan TY, Lau MS, Critchley JA. Serious complications associated with Dettol poisoning. Q J Med 1993; 86(11):735–8.
5. Chan TY, Critchley JA. Is chloroxylenol nephrotoxic like phenol? A study of patients with DETTOL poisoning. Vet Hum Toxicol 1994;36(3):250–1.
6. Chan TY, Critchley JA, Lau JT. The risk of aspiration in Dettol poisoning: a retrospective cohort study. Hum Exp Toxicol 1995;14(2):190–1.
7. Chan TY, Sung JJ, Critchley JA. Chemical gastro-oesophagitis, upper gastrointestinal haemorrhage and gastroscopic findings following Dettol poisoning. Hum Exp Toxicol 1995;14(1):18–19.
8. Chan TY, Critchley JA. Pulmonary aspiration following Dettol poisoning: the scope for prevention. Hum Exp Toxicol 1996;15(10):843–6.

Chlorphenamine maleate

See also Antihistamines

General Information

Chlorphenamine (chlorpheniramine) is a first-generation antihistamine, an alkylamine derivative, with sedative and antimuscarinic activity.

Organs and Systems

Psychological, psychiatric

Functional neuroimaging of cognition was impaired by chlorphenamine (1).

Skin

Lichen-planus-like contact dermatitis after topical use of chlorphenamine has been described in one case report, with positive patch-testing (2).

Drug–Drug Interactions

Chloroquine

Chlorphenamine enhances the efficacy of chloroquine in acute uncomplicated falciparum malaria, but the disposition of chloroquine in these circumstances is unpredictable. Chloroquine (25 mg/kg) was given orally over 3 days in combination with chlorphenamine to Nigerian children with parasitemia (3). The peak whole blood chloroquine concentration was increased and the time to peak concentration shortened. However, in further studies the addition of chlorphenamine to chloroquine did not amplify the cardiac effects of chloroquine (4).

Ranitidine

In the same way that pharmacokinetic studies have been used to ascertain whether co-administration of an inhibitor of CYP3A4 can lead to cardiotoxicity, similar studies have been carried out to indicate whether the co-administration of an inhibitor can enhance a limited sedative effect. Healthy subjects took a single dose of racemic chlorphenamine 4 mg on two separate occasions; the second occasion coincided with the sixth day of dosing with ranitidine 75 mg bd for 8 days. Serum concentrations and urinary excretion of chlorphenamine were not altered, and so it was considered unlikely that co-administration with ranitidine would enhance the potential of chlorphenamine to cause drowsiness (5).

References

1. Okamura N, Yanai K, Higuchi M, Sakai J, Iwata R, Ido T, Sasaki H, Watanabe T, Itoh M. Functional neuroimaging of cognition impaired by a classical antihistamine, d-chlorpheniramine. Br J Pharmacol 2000; 129(1):115–23.
2. Kuroda K, Hisanaga Y. The diagnosis of lichen-planus-like contact dermatitis to chlorpheniramine maleate. Dermatology 2002;205(3):281–4.
3. Okonkwo CA, Coker HA, Agomo PU, Ogunbanwo JA, Mafe AG, Agomo CO, Afolabi BM. Effect of chlorpheniramine on the pharmacokinetics of and response to chloroquine of Nigerian children with falciparum malaria. Trans R Soc Trop Med Hyg 1999;93(3):306–11.
4. Sowunmi A, Fehintola FA, Ogundahunsi OA, Ofi AB, Happi TC, Oduola AM. Comparative cardiac effects of halofantrine and chloroquine plus chlorpheniramine in children with acute uncomplicated falciparum malaria. Trans R Soc Trop Med Hyg 1999;93(1):78–83.
5. Koch KM, O'Connor-Semmes RL, Davis IM, Yin Y. Stereoselective pharmacokinetics of chlorpheniramine and the effect of ranitidine. J Pharm Sci 1998;87(9):1097–100.

Chlorphenoxamine

General Information

Chlorphenoxamine is an antihistamine closely related to diphenhydramine with a similar metabolic pathway (1). It appears to have been developed in the hope of producing a greater effect in Parkinson's disease by combining both anticholinergic and antihistaminic effects in a single molecule (2).

In the doses commonly used well-recognized anticholinergic effects can occur (3). Some patients become drowsy, whilst others are stimulated; with increasing dosages, some patients go into coma; others have agitation, convulsions, and marked euphoria, perhaps with hallucinations and disorientation.

References

1. Koppel C, Tenczer J, Arndt I, Ibe K. Urinary metabolism of chlorphenoxamine in man. Arzneimittelforschung 1987;37(9):1062–4.
2. Strang RR. A clinical evaluation of chlorphenoxamine with caffeine in the treatment of Parkinson's disease, including a comparison with methixene. J Clin Pharmacol J New Drugs 1967;7(4):214–20.
3. Kerley TL, Newberne JW, Brinkman DC, Weaver LC. The acute and chronic toxicities of chlorphenoxamine. Toxicol Appl Pharmacol 1962;4:638–49.

Chlorphentermine

See also Anorectic drugs

General Information

Chlorphentermine is an anorectic sympathomimetic amine, with actions and adverse effects similar to those of amfepramone (diethylpropion).

Organs and Systems

Respiratory

Pathological changes in the lungs were produced with chlorphentermine in laboratory animals (SED-9, 14). Pulmonary complications might therefore occur in humans, which puts in doubt the wisdom of continuing to recommend chlorphentermine as an anorectic drug until more definitive information is available.

Nervous system

Much less stimulation of the central nervous system has been reported in patients taking chlorphentermine than in those taking dexamphetamine; less frequent too were complaints of light-headedness, tremors, restlessness, nervousness, and insomnia; patients taking chlorphentermine can paradoxically become drowsy (1).

Gastrointestinal

In 25 patients who had taken chlorphentermine, constipation and dryness of the mouth were more frequent than with other appetite depressants. In another comparative study with phenmetrazine in volunteers, constipation and dry mouth were again among the more frequent adverse reactions, along with sleepiness and increases in motor activity and urinary urgency (SED-8, 16).

Reference

1. Sletten IW, Sundland D, Pichardo J, Viamontes G. Chlorphentermine and phenmetrazine compared: weight reduction, side effects and psychological change. Mo Med 1967;64(11):927–9.

Chlorpromazine

See also Neuroleptic drugs

General Information

Chlorpromazine is a phenothiazine with a large range of pharmacological actions; it is a dopamine receptor antagonist, an alpha-adrenoceptor antagonist, a muscarinic antagonist, and an antihistamine.

Organs and Systems

Cardiovascular

The possibility that some of the cardiac effects of chlorpromazine may be related to metabolites as well as the parent compound has been explored (1,2).

Some cases of sudden death in apparently young healthy individuals may be directly attributable to cardiac dysrhythmias after treatment with thioridazine or chlorpromazine (3).

Nervous system

In 15 schizophrenic inpatients aged 16–55 years, there was a 50% probability that a patient would have a tremor when the plasma concentration of chlorpromazine was 46 ng/ml or more, corresponding to the minimum plasma concentration that has been associated with a good clinical response (4).

Skin

Chlorpromazine most often causes photosensitivity reactions (incidence around 3%), which may result from formation of a cytotoxic by-product after exposure to ultraviolet light. Patients should be advised to avoid prolonged exposure to strong indoor light, to wear protective clothing, and to use a combined para-aminobenzoic acid plus benzophenone sunscreen when exposure to strong sunlight is unavoidable.

Toxic epidermal necrolysis has been reported in association with chlorpromazine (5).

Chlorpromazine is thought to have caused an immunologically mediated contact urticaria (6–10).

Sexual function

Two cases of priapism have been attributed to chlorpromazine: a 65-year-old man who took a single dose of chlorpromazine 25 mg and a 27-year-old man who took chlorpromazine 200 mg for agitation after a suicide attempt (11).

Drug–Drug Interactions

Amfetamine

Chlorpromazine has sometimes been used to treat amfetamine psychosis, for example due to acute poisoning in children who did not respond to barbiturates (12).

Beta-adrenoceptor antagonists

Lipophilic beta-adrenoceptor antagonists are metabolized to varying degrees by oxidation by liver microsomal cytochrome P450 (for example propranolol by CYP1A2 and CYP2D6 and metoprolol by CYP2D6). They can therefore reduce the clearance and increase the steady-state plasma concentrations of other drugs that undergo similar metabolism, potentiating their effects. Drugs that interact in this way include chlorpromazine (13).

- A schizophrenic patient experienced delirium, tonic-clonic seizures, and photosensitivity after the addition of propranolol to chlorpromazine, suggesting that chlorpromazine concentrations are increased by propranolol (14).

Although high dosages of propranolol (up to 2 g) have been used in combination with chlorpromazine to treat schizophrenia, the combination of propranolol or pindolol with chlorpromazine should be avoided if possible (15).

Haloperidol

- A 40-year-old man with schizophrenia developed a raised plasma concentration of haloperidol in combination with chlorpromazine and during overlap treatment with clozapine (16).

Like haloperidol, chlorpromazine is a competitive inhibitor of CYP2D6; however, clozapine appears to be largely metabolized by CYP1A2.

Monoamine oxidase inhibitors

Hyperthermia and labile blood pressure occurred in a patient taking chlorpromazine, phenelzine, and clomipramine (17).

Smoking

Chlorpromazine concentrations were reduced by 36% in smokers (18). Of factors that can affect chlorpromazine concentrations, smoking may be second in importance only to dosage (19).

Interference with Diagnostic Tests

Cholesterol

Chlorpromazine can cause overestimation of cholesterol (Zlatkis–Zak reaction) (20).

CSF protein

Chlorpromazine can cause falsely increased CSF protein (Folin–Ciocalteau method) (20).

Haptoglobin

Chlorpromazine can cause falsely reduced serum haptoglobin concentrations (20).

References

1. Axelsson R, Aspenstrom G. Electrocardiographic changes and serum concentrations in thioridazine-treated patients. J Clin Psychiatry 1982;43(8):332–5.
2. Dahl SG. Active metabolites of neuroleptic drugs: possible contribution to therapeutic and toxic effects. Ther Drug Monit 1982;4(1):33–40.
3. Risch SC, Groom GP, Janowsky DS. The effects of psychotropic drugs on the cardiovascular system. J Clin Psychiatry 1982;43(5 Pt 2):16–31.
4. Chetty M, Gouws E, Miller R, Moodley SV. The use of a side effect as a qualitative indicator of plasma chlorpromazine levels. Eur Neuropsychopharmacol 1999;9(1–2): 77–82.
5. Purcell P, Valmana A. Toxic epidermal necrolysis following chlorpromazine ingestion complicated by SIADH. Postgrad Med J 1996;72(845):186.
6. Leliever WC. Topical gentamicin-induced positional vertigo. Otolaryngol Head Neck Surg 1985;93(4):553–5.
7. De Groot AC, Weyland JW, Nater JP. Unwanted Effects of Cosmetics and Drugs used in Dermatology. 3rd ed. Amsterdam: Elsevier, 1994.
8. Hannuksela M. Mechanisms in contact urticaria. Clin Dermatol 1997;15(4):619–22.
9. Wistedt B. Neuroleptics and depression. Arch Gen Psychiatry 1982;39(6):745.
10. Wilkins-Ho M, Hollander Y. Toxic delirium with low-dose clozapine. Can J Psychiatry 1997;42(4):429–30.
11. Mutlu N, Ozkurkcugil C, Culha M, Turkan S, Gokalp A. Priapism induced by chlorpromazine. Int J Clin Pract 1999;53(2):152–3.
12. Espelin DE, Done AK. Amphetamine poisoning. Effectiveness of chlorpromazine. N Engl J Med 1968;278(25):1361–5.
13. Peet M, Middlemiss DN, Yates RA. Pharmacokinetic interaction between propranolol and chlorpromazine in schizophrenic patients. Lancet 1980;2(8201):978.
14. Miller FA, Rampling D. Adverse effects of combined propranolol and chlorpromazine therapy. Am J Psychiatry 1982;139(9):1198–9.
15. Markowitz JS, Wells BG, Carson WH. Interactions between antipsychotic and antihypertensive drugs. Ann Pharmacother 1995;29(6):603–9.
16. Allen SA. Effect of chlorpromazine and clozapine on plasma concentrations of haloperidol in a patient with schizophrenia. J Clin Pharmacol 2000;40(11): 1296–7.
17. Stern TA, Schwartz JH, Shuster JL. Catastrophic illness associated with the combination of clomipramine, phenelzine and chlorpromazine. Ann Clin Psychiatry 1992;4:81–5.
18. Pantuck EJ, Pantuck CB, Anderson KE, Conney AH, Kappas A. Cigarette smoking and chlorpromazine disposition and actions. Clin Pharmacol Ther 1982;31(4):533–8.
19. Sramek J, Herrera J, Roy S, Parent M, Hudgins R, Costa J, Alatorre E. An analysis of steady state chlorpromazine plasma levels in the clinical setting. J Clin Psychopharmacol 1987;7(2):117–18.
20. Sher PP. Drug interferences with clinical laboratory tests. Drugs 1982;24(1):24–63.

Chlorprothixene

See also Neuroleptic drugs

General Information

Chlorprothixene is a thioxanthene neuroleptic drug.

Organs and Systems

Immunologic

Rare disorders of connective tissue resembling systemic lupus erythematosus have been reported with chlorpromazine, perphenazine, and chlorprothixene (1).

Reference

1. McNevin S, MacKay M. Chlorprothixene-induced systemic lupus erythematosus. J Clin Psychopharmacol 1982;2(6):411–12.

Chlortalidone

See also Diuretics

General Information

Chlortalidone (chlorthalidone) is chemically unrelated to the thiazide diuretics but shares many of their actions and adverse effects.

It is so closely similar to the thiazide diuretics in most respects that data have generally been regarded as interchangeable.

Comparative studies

In the Antihypertensive and Lipid-Lowering Treatment to Prevent Heart Attack Trial (ALLHAT), over 40 000 participants aged 55 years or older with hypertension and at least one other risk factor for coronary heart disease were randomized to chlortalidone, amlodipine, doxazosin, or lisinopril (1,2). Doxazosin was discontinued prematurely because chlortalidone was clearly superior in preventing cardiovascular events, particularly heart failure (2). Otherwise, mean follow-up was 4.9 years. There were no differences between chlortalidone, amlodipine, and lisinopril in the primary combined outcome or all-cause mortality. Compared with chlortalidone, heart failure was more common with amlodipine and lisinopril, and chlortalidone was better than lisinopril at preventing stroke.

Organs and Systems

Electrolyte balance

In the past chlortalidone was thought to carry a greater risk of hypokalemia and hyponatremia (SED-8, 488), but this probably reflected relative overdosage with accumulation, because of its long half-life. With the much lower dosages now in use there appears to be no clear difference from the thiazides.

Skin

Pseudoporphyria has been attributed to chlortalidone (3).

Body temperature

Drug fever has been attributed to chlortalidone (4).

- A 58-year-old woman presented with intermittent nocturnal fever (up to 39.5°C) for 4 weeks beginning 2 weeks after the introduction of chlortalidone for hypertension. Otherwise, physical examination was normal. Investigations showed a normochromic normocytic anemia and a raised erythrocyte sedimentation rate and C-reactive protein. Other biochemical tests, blood cultures, and serological and immunological tests were negative. Chest radiography, lung scintigraphy, and abdominal ultrasound were unremarkable. There was no further fever after chlortalidone was withdrawn, and all biochemical tests became normal. The lymphocyte transformation test showed stimulation by chlortalidone.

References

1. ALLHAT Collaborative Research Group. Major cardiovascular events in hypertensive patients randomized to doxazosin vs chlorthalidone: the antihypertensive and lipid-lowering treatment to prevent heart attack trial (ALLHAT). JAMA 2000;283(15):1967–75.
2. ALLHAT Officers and Coordinators for the ALLHAT Collaborative Research Group. The Antihypertensive and Lipid-Lowering Treatment to Prevent Heart Attack Trial. Major outcomes in high-risk hypertensive patients randomized to angiotensin-converting enzyme inhibitor or calcium channel blocker vs diuretic: The Antihypertensive and Lipid-Lowering Treatment to Prevent Heart Attack Trial (ALLHAT). JAMA 2002;288(23):2981–97.
3. Baker EJ, Reed KD, Dixon SL. Chlorthalidone-induced pseudoporphyria: clinical and microscopic findings of a case. J Am Acad Dermatol 1989;21(5 Pt 1):1026–9.
4. Osterwalder P, Koch J, Wuthrich B, Pichler WJ, Vetter W. Unklarer status febrilis. [Intermittent fever of unknown origin.] Dtsch Med Wochenschr 1998;123(24):761–5.

Chlorzoxazone

General Information

Chlorzoxazone is a centrally acting benzoxazole derivative with a weak muscle relaxing effect (1). It is usually used in combination with paracetamol for the treatment of painful muscle spasms. The usual dose is 500 mg tds. Drowsiness, weakness, dizziness, and gastrointestinal complaints are the most frequent unwanted effects.

Organs and Systems

Nervous system

A spasmodic torticollis-like syndrome, repeatedly evoked after the ingestion of chlorzoxazone, is an unusual adverse effect of the drug. Benzatropine mesilate 1 mg intravenously led to resolution of the symptoms within 10 minutes (2).

Liver

The most serious adverse effect of chlorzoxazone, which fortunately occurs only rarely, is hepatotoxicity.

In one case jaundice occurred and rechallenge with a single tablet of Parafon Forte (chlorzoxazone plus paracetamol) resulted in a dramatic reaction after 5 hours, with fever, chills, nausea, vomiting, and recurrence of icterus. Paracetamol on its own had no adverse effect in this case.

The authors reviewed some 23 other cases (SEDA-12, 119) (3).

References

1. Elenbaas JK. Centrally acting oral skeletal muscle relaxants. Am J Hosp Pharm 1980;37(10):1313–23.
2. Rosin MA. Chlorzoxazone-induced spasmotic torticollis. JAMA 1981;246(22):2575.
3. Powers BJ, Cattau EL Jr, Zimmerman HJ. Chlorzoxazone hepatotoxic reactions. An analysis of 21 identified or presumed cases. Arch Intern Med 1986;146(6):1183–6.

Cholera vaccine

See also Vaccines

General Information

Cholera vaccines consist of live attenuated or heat-killed *Vibrio cholerae* organisms. They can be given orally or parenterally.

Following the administration of live oral cholera vaccine (containing the attenuated strain *V. cholerae* CVD 103-HgR, prepared from *V. cholerae* 01 strain 569B), there were significant rises in serum antitoxin concentrations and only few mild adverse effects (SED-13, 925). There was protective efficacy in 82–100% of healthy adult volunteers and no difference in adverse effects between 25 recipients of the vaccine and 26 controls (1).

A randomized, double-blind, placebo-controlled trial using a live oral cholera vaccine (strain CVD 103, derived from the *V. cholerae* 01 classical Inaba strain 569B by deletion of the genes encoding the A subunit of cholera toxin) was conducted in 50 healthy Swiss adults. There was a significant rise in serum antitoxin titers in 76% of the volunteers. Two vaccinees reported watery stools after immunization (2).

When an oral single-dose cholera vaccine against *V. cholerae* 0139 was given to ten volunteers there was 83% protective efficacy and the only adverse effect, in one volunteer, was mild diarrhea (3).

The results with an oral cholera vaccine consisting of the immunogenic but completely non-toxic B subunit of cholera toxin in combination with heat- and formalin-killed *V. cholerae* represent an improvement compared with previous parenteral vaccines (4). The frequency of adverse effects (pain at the injection site, nausea, diarrhea) was low (5).

Severe complications connected with cholera (or combined) immunization are extremely rare and the causal relation is always doubtful. However, when they do occur they constitute a contraindication to further administration. There are occasional reports of neurological and psychiatric reactions (SED-8, 706) (SEDA-1, 246), Guillain–Barré syndrome (SEDA-1, 246), myocarditis (6,7), myocardial infarction (SEDA-3, 261), a syndrome similar to immune complex disease (8), acute renal insufficiency accompanied by hepatitis (9), and pancreatitis (10).

Drug Administration

Drug formulations

A parenteral cholera vaccine consisting of a heat-killed, phenol-preserved, mixed suspension of the Inaba and Ogawa subtypes of *V. cholerae*, Serovar 01, has been used subcutaneously or intramuscularly, or for booster doses intradermally. About 1% of vaccinees develop mild local skin lesions comprising transitory soreness at the injection site within 5-7 days after injection, characterized by erythema, swelling, pain, and induration, and rarely resulting in ulceration. More general reactions are allergic: as a rule, these amount at most to slight pyrexia, headache, and malaise. However, considering the low protective efficacy and high reactogenicity of this vaccine, the World Health Organization and many national health authorities do not recommend it anymore and most manufacturers have stopped producing it.

References

1. Davis R, Spencer CM. Live oral cholera vaccine. A preliminary review of its pharmacology and clinical potential in providing protective immunity against cholera. Clin Immunother 1998;4:235–47.
2. Cryz SJ Jr, Levine MM, Kaper JB, Furer E, Althaus B. Randomized double-blind placebo controlled trial to evaluate the safety and immunogenicity of the live oral cholera vaccine strain CVD 103-HgR in Swiss adults. Vaccine 1990;8(6):577–80.
3. Coster TS, Killeen KP, Waldor MK, Beattie DT, Spriggs DR, Kenner JR, Trofa A, Sadoff JC, Mekalanos JJ, Taylor DN. Safety, immunogenicity, and efficacy of live attenuated *Vibrio cholerae* O139 vaccine prototype. Lancet 1995;345(8955):949–52.
4. Holmgren J, Svennerholm AM. New vaccines against bacterial enteric infections. Scand J Infect Dis Suppl 1990;70:149–56.
5. Markman B. Symptoms of reactogenicity in field trial of oral cholera vaccine. Lancet 1990;336(8710):320.
6. Gavrilesco S, Streian C, Constantinesco L. Tachycardie ventriculaire et fibrillation auriculaire associées après vaccination anticholériques. [Associated ventricular

tachycardia and auricular fibrillation after anticholera vaccination.] Acta Cardiol 1973;28(1):89–94.
7. Driehorst J, Laubenthal F. Akute Myocarditis nach Choleraschutzimpfung. [Acute myocarditis after cholera vaccination.] Dtsch Med Wochenschr 1984;109(5):197–8.
8. Mall T, Gyr K. Episode resembling immune complex disease after cholera vaccination. Trans R Soc Trop Med Hyg 1984;78(1):106–7.
9. Eisinger AJ, Smith JG. Acute renal failure after TAB and cholera vaccination. BMJ 1979;1(6160):381–2.
10. Gatt DT. Pancreatitis following monovalent typhoid and cholera vaccinations. Br J Clin Pract 1986;40(7):300–1.

Choline

General Information

Choline has been given in the past as an acetylcholine precursor to raise acetylcholine concentrations in the brain and thus enhance cholinergic neurotransmission. There is evidence that the symptoms of tardive dyskinesia can be reduced by choline or lecithin (1).

Organs and Systems

Psychological, psychiatric

Occasionally, doses of choline up to 9 g/day have been found to produce severe depression, presumably by altering the adrenaline/acetylcholine balance (2).

References

1. Rosenberg GS, Davis KL. The use of cholinergic precursors in neuropsychiatric diseases. Am J Clin Nutr 1982;36(4):709–20.
2. Tamminga C, Smith RC, Chang S, Haraszti JS, Davis JM. Depression associated with oral choline. Lancet 1976;2(7991):905.

Choline alfoscerate

General Information

Choline alfoscerate increases cerebral acetylcholine synthesis and release (1). In the light of animal studies it has been investigated as a possible treatment for vascular dementia (2). Adverse effects have been few, notably headache and flushing.

References

1. Sigala S, Imperato A, Rizzonelli P, Casolini P, Missale C, Spano P. L-alpha-glycerylphosphorylcholine antagonizes scopolamine-induced amnesia and enhances hippocampal cholinergic transmission in the rat. Eur J Pharmacol 1992;211(3):351–8.
2. Parnetti L, Amenta F, Gallai V. Choline alphoscerate in cognitive decline and in acute cerebrovascular disease: an analysis of published clinical data. Mech Ageing Dev 2001;122(16):2041–55.

Chromium

General Information

Chromium is a metallic element (symbol Cr; atomic no. 24) that occurs naturally in minerals such as fuchsite and picotite.

Certain salts of radioactive chromium (1) are used as radiopharmaceutical tracers in various hematological procedures. Chromium compounds are also used in oral and parenteral nutrition and in artificial hip and knee joints. Chromium picolinate has been promoted as a nutritional supplement and has received a great deal of interest because of its possible beneficial effects on muscle strength and body composition.

Trivalent chromium is supposedly an essential trace element, but its essentiality continues to be discussed (2). The biochemistry of chromium has been reviewed (3), as have the mechanisms of its toxicity, carcinogenicity, and allergenicity (4) and its general toxicology (5).

Trivalent chromium compounds (chromium chloride, chromium nicotinate, and chromium picolinate) are used by patients to enhance weight loss, to increase lean body mass, or to improve glycemic control. Drug histories should include attention to the use of over-the-counter nutritional supplements often regarded as harmless by the public and lay media. The recommended daily allowance of chromium picolinate is 50–200 micrograms, but information about its toxicity is limited.

The quest for the molecular mechanisms of chromium in relation to diabetes continues (6,7). Chromium picolinate may aid muscle insulin sensitivity, and initial reports suggest that it is an effective therapy for type 2 diabetes (8). Chromium picolinate supplementation alone does not improve insulin sensitivity (9).

- In a 28-year-old woman with an 18-year history of type 1 diabetes mellitus the glycosylated hemoglobin fell from 11.3 to 7.9% and her blood glucose concentration was 1.7–3.3 mmol/l lower after she had taken chromium picolinate (200 micrograms tds for 3 months) (10). There were no adverse effects.

Chromium in metal implants and prostheses

Complications from the use of metal implants and prostheses can arise because of biochemical and histological reactions to some of the materials used (SEDA-22, 250). These include titanium, stainless steel (10–14% nickel, 17–20% chromium), and cobalt chrome alloys (27–30% chromium, 57–68% cobalt, and up to 2.5% nickel). All of these metals can produce sensitization or elicit toxic reactions when they are solubilized and come into contact with tissues; it can be difficult or even impossible to differentiate between hypersensitivity and toxic reactions.

Metals from prostheses can continue to be released into the system for many years. The development of hypersensitivity takes time, and allergic reactions are usually delayed for weeks, months, or 1–2 years. The symptoms can assume a variety of forms. Local reactions can cause loosening of the device or local pain. Dermatological reactions include eczema, bullous pemphigoid, urticaria, and "muscle tumors."

Attempts continue to predict metal sensitivity in the individual patient so that the choice of material can be made accordingly. In vitro tests for metal allergies have been developed on the basis of lymphokine (MIF) release from sensitized T lymphocytes exposed to metal-protein complexes (11). About 6% of patients without a previous metal implant had positive reactions to nickel, chromium, or cobalt. However, it is still not clear whether such a positive reaction is a reliable predictor of clinical problems. In practice few patients have either local or systemic reactions; when symptoms occur and other causes are ruled out, the implant should be removed. Some workers recommend removal of an implant whenever there is both a positive MIF test and a positive skin test, even in the current absence of a serious reaction. Allergic dermatitis will clear up as soon as the metal has begun to be cleared from the tissue. The type of metal and the amount released into the tissue will affect the time taken for the disappearance of toxic dermatological phenomena.

Organs and Systems

Psychological, psychiatric

There have been three reports of the efficacy of chromium in depression, with adverse effects that included dizzy spells and vivid dreams (12).

- A 50-year-old man developed bipolar II disorder with the onset of a major depressive episode in his late twenties. His mood stabilized with lithium, but he continued to have periods of irritability and breakthrough depression. He started to take chromium picolinate 400 micrograms/day and within 2 days felt more relaxed and stable than he had since the onset of his disorder. He stopped taking lithium. Several months later he forgot to take his chromium, and within a few days his symptoms returned. In order to catch up he took 800 micrograms/day and developed sweating each morning and a mild hand tremor. After reducing the dosage to 600 micrograms/day he again went into complete remission. After more than 1 year of chromium treatment he developed uric acid kidney stones. One year after switching to a different chromium salt (the polynicotinate), there was no recurrence of kidney stones.
- A 38-year-old man with bipolar II disorder took chromium polynicotinate 400 micrograms/day. Shortly after the first dose his mood started to improve, but he had unusually vivid intense dreams. The dose of chromium was increased to 600 micrograms/day. He then developed intermittent brief dizzy spells due to orthostatic hypotension. After switching to chromium picolinate his dizzy spells did not recur.
- A 47-year-old man with a dysthymic disorder and intermittent panic attacks and rage outbursts took chromium 400 micrograms/day, and after 1 day had strikingly vivid dreams. Over the next several days there was a dramatic improvement in his mood and behavior. The efficacy of chromium was later confirmed by a double-blind, placebo-controlled, *n*-of-1 trial.

Liver

Hepatic injury is a risk that is associated primarily with occupational exposure to chromium, in this case among chromium platers (13), an occupation that has an increased incidence of chronic hepatitis or liver cirrhosis. There also appears to be a trend toward a significantly increased risk of lung cancer.

- A 35-year-old woman complained of nausea, fatigue, pruritus, dark urine, pale stools, and jaundice after taking a supplement containing chromium picolinate for weight loss (14). Infectious hepatitis was excluded and a liver biopsy was consistent with toxic liver damage. Hepatic chromium concentrations were more than 10 times normal. The chromium supplement was withdrawn and she received supportive treatment with a suspension containing "natural products," colestyramine 1 g qds, and hydroxyzine 25 mg tds. She fully recovered in 3 months.

Skin

Allergic contact dermatitis has apparently been most commonly due to occupational exposure of building workers to a form of cement containing a water-soluble form of chromium (SEDA-20, 208) (15). Such reactions to medical exposure have not been described but could in principle occur.

Chromium has been reported to cause dermatitis when ingested (16).

- A 35-year-old man developed a subacute dermatitis with scattered patches of erythema and scaling on the lower legs, ankles, hands, and wrists. He had no history of atopy but a prior history of allergy to a leather watch-strap. He had taken various oral vitamin and mineral formulations for several weeks. Patch-testing showed reactions to potassium dichromate at 48 and 96 hours.

Chromium picolinate has caused acute generalized exanthematous pustulosis (17).

- A 32-year-old previously healthy man developed an extensive rash of sudden onset associated with a low-grade fever (37.4°C), a sore throat, and malaise after taking chromium picolinate 1 mg/day for 4 days. He had a confluent symmetrical erythematous eruption with numerous non-follicular 1–2 mm pustules on the trunk and proximal limbs. The eruption was most prominent in the antecubital and popliteal fossae bilaterally. There was mild pharyngeal erythema and bilateral tender cervical adenopathy, but no tonsillar enlargement or exudate. Chromium picolinate was withdrawn and he was treated with oral prednisone 60 mg/day tapered over 15 days. The acute eruption resolved within 1 week, followed by post-inflammatory desquamation. It did not recur during follow-up for 15 months.

Musculoskeletal

- Rhabdomyolysis has been attributed to chromium picolinate in a 24-year-old body builder who took 1200 micrograms over 48 hours (18).

Long-Term Effects

Tumorigenicity

Hexavalent chromium compounds have no medical uses and are known as mutagens and carcinogens (19). In an in vitro study the coordination of chromium by picolinate ligands made chromium picolinate more toxic to cultured cells, leading to enhanced apoptosis (20). These observations support the hypothesis that chromium picolinate is a human carcinogen.

A mortality study among workers engaged in producing chromium compounds from chromite, performed using retrospective data (21), showed a significantly increased risk of lung cancer, despite cessation of exposure. The risk of nasal cavity/sinus cancer was also significantly increased.

Drug Administration

Drug overdose

Toxicity secondary to chronic ingestion of 6–12 times the recommended daily allowance of over-the-counter chromium picolinate has been reported (22).

- A 33-year-old white woman presented with weight loss, anemia, thrombocytopenia, hemolysis, liver dysfunction (transaminase activities 15–20 times normal, total bilirubin three times normal), and renal insufficiency. She had taken chromium picolinate 1200–2400 micrograms/day for the previous 4–5 months to enhance weight loss. Her plasma chromium concentrations were 2–3 times normal. After withdrawal of chromium picolinate, she was managed with supportive measures, blood transfusions, and hemodialysis. The hemolysis stabilized and her liver and renal function eventually recovered.

Drug–Drug Interactions

Sertraline

Chromium can potentiate antidepressant pharmacotherapy for manic-depressive disorder. In five patients taking sertraline, supplementation with chromium picolinate and chromium polynicotinate led to enhanced remission of dysthymic symptoms (23).

References

1. Ruiz-Maldonado R, Contreras-Ruiz J, Sierra-Santoyo A, Lopez-Corella E, Guevara-Flores A. Black granules on the skin after bismuth subsalicylate ingestion. J Am Acad Dermatol 1997;37(3 Pt 1):489–90.
2. Stearns DM. Is chromium a trace essential metal? Biofactors 2000;11(3):149–62.
3. Vincent JB. The biochemistry of chromium. J Nutr 2000;130(4):715–18.
4. Dayan AD, Paine AJ. Mechanisms of chromium toxicity, carcinogenicity and allergenicity: review of the literature from 1985 to 2000. Hum Exp Toxicol 2001;20(9):439–51.
5. Barceloux DG. Chromium. J Toxicol Clin Toxicol 1999;37(2):173–94.
6. Vincent JB. Quest for the molecular mechanism of chromium action and its relationship to diabetes. Nutr Rev 2000;58(3 Pt 1):67–72.
7. Anderson RA. Chromium in the prevention and control of diabetes. Diabetes Metab 2000;26(1):22–7.
8. McCarty MF. Toward practical prevention of type 2 diabetes. Med Hypotheses 2000;54(5):786–93.
9. Amato P, Morales AJ, Yen SS. Effects of chromium picolinate supplementation on insulin sensitivity, serum lipids, and body composition in healthy, nonobese, older men and women. J Gerontol A Biol Sci Med Sci 2000;55(5):M260–3.
10. Fox GN, Sabovic Z. Chromium picolinate supplementation for diabetes mellitus. J Fam Pract 1998;46(1):83–6.
11. Hierholzer S, Hierholzer G. Untersuchungen zur Metalallergie nach Osteosynthesen. [Allergy to metal following osteosynthesis.] Unfallchirurgie 1982;8(6):347–52.
12. McLeod MN, Golden RN. Chromium treatment of depression. Int J Neuropsychopharmacol 2000;3(4):311–14.
13. Itoh T, Takahashi K, Okubo T. [Mortality of chromium plating workers in Japan—a 16-year follow-up study.] J UOEH 1996;18(1):7–18.
14. Lanca S, Alves A, Vieira AI, Barata J, de Freitas J, de Carvalho A. Chromium-induced toxic hepatitis. Eur J Intern Med 2002;13(8):518–20.
15. Roto P, Sainio H, Reunala T, Laippala P. Addition of ferrous sulfate to cement and risk of chromium dermatitis among construction workers. Contact Dermatitis 1996;34(1):43–50.
16. Fowler JF Jr. Systemic contact dermatitis caused by oral chromium picolinate. Cutis 2000;65(2):116.
17. Young PC, Turiansky GW, Bonner MW, Benson PM. Acute generalized exanthematous pustulosis induced by chromium picolinate. J Am Acad Dermatol 1999;41(5 Pt 2):820–3.
18. Martin WR, Fuller RE. Suspected chromium picolinate-induced rhabdomyolysis. Pharmacotherapy 1998;18(4):860–2.
19. Bagchi D, Stohs SJ, Downs BW, Bagchi M, Preuss HG. Cytotoxicity and oxidative mechanisms of different forms of chromium. Toxicology 2002;180(1):5–22.
20. Manygoats KR, Yazzie M, Stearns DM. Ultrastructural damage in chromium picolinate-treated cells: a TEM study. Transmission electron microscopy. J Biol Inorg Chem 2002;7(7-8):791–8.
21. Rosenman KD, Stanbury M. Risk of lung cancer among former chromium smelter workers. Am J Ind Med 1996;29(5):491–500.
22. Cerulli J, Grabe DW, Gauthier I, Malone M, McGoldrick MD. Chromium picolinate toxicity. Ann Pharmacother 1998;32(4):428–31.
23. McLeod MN, Gaynes BN, Golden RN. Chromium potentiation of antidepressant pharmacotherapy for dysthymic disorder in 5 patients. J Clin Psychiatry 1999;60(4):237–40.

Chymotrypsin

General Information

The enzyme chymotrypsin has been used for enzymatic zonulolysis during operations for cataract (1). Its possible role in precipitating postoperative intraocular hypertension has been studied, but the use of enzymatic zonulolysis does not seem to increase significantly the risk of glaucoma (2).

References

1. Packer AJ, Fraioli AJ, Epstein DL. The effect of timolol and acetazolamide on transient intraocular pressure elevation following cataract extraction with alpha-chymotrypsin. Ophthalmology 1981;88(3):239–43.
2. Havener WH. Ocular Pharmacology. 4th ed. Saint Louis: C.V. Mosby, 1978.

Cianidanol

General Information

Cianidanol is an antioxidant flavonoid that occurs especially in woody plants. It is one constituent of green tea. It has immunomodulatory properties, including effects on T lymphocytes and killer cells (1).

Of 40 patients with chronic active hepatitis, 22 took cianidanol 3 g/day and 18 took placebo (2). Adverse effects of cianidanol were fever ($n = 4$), hemolysis ($n = 1$), and urticaria ($n = 1$).

Serious adverse effects were not observed when cianidanol was used to treat HBe-antigen-positive chronic hepatitis in 338 patients (3). The only adverse effect of note that appeared to be drug-related was transient pyrexia in 13, necessitating withdrawal of therapy in eight. Four patients also had a skin eruption.

Organs and Systems

Hematologic

Nine cases of acute intravascular hemolysis, severe enough to cause death in one and to necessitate hemodialysis in two others, were attributed to cianidanol on the basis of a close temporal relation and serological tests (4).

References

1. Berg AU, Baron DP, Berg PA. Immunomodulating properties of cianidanol on responsiveness and function of human peripheral blood T cells and K-cells. Int J Immunopharmacol 1988;10(4):387–94.
2. Bar-Meir S, Halpern Z, Gutman M, Shpirer Z, Baratz M, Bass D. Effect of (+)-cyanidanol-3 on chronic active hepatitis: a double blind controlled trial. Gut 1985; 26(9):975–9.
3. Suzuki H, Yamamoto S, Hirayama C, Takino T, Fujisawa K, Oda T. Cianidanol therapy for HBe-antigen-positive chronic hepatitis: a multicentre, double-blind study. Liver 1986;6(1):35–44.
4. Rotoli B, Giglio F, Bile M, Formisano S. Immune-mediated acute intravascular hemolysis caused by cianidanol (catergen). Haematologica 1985;70(6):495–9.

Cibenzoline

See also Antidysrhythmic drugs

General Information

Cibenzoline is an antidysrhythmic drug of Class Ia, with some additional properties of drugs of Class III and Class IV. Its pharmacology, electrophysiological effects, therapeutic effects and indications, pharmacokinetics, and adverse effects have been reviewed (1,2). Prolongation of the QT interval, leading to cardiac dysrhythmias, is the major adverse effect. Other effects include gastrointestinal disturbances, effects on the central nervous system, and hypoglycemia, perhaps related to inhibition of ATP-dependent potassium channels in the pancreas.

Comparative studies

Cibenzoline and flecainide have been compared in the prevention of recurrence of atrial tachydysrhythmias in 139 patients (3). During the study, 27 patients withdrew, in 13 cases with adverse effects, seven of which were due to cibenzoline. Overall there were 26 adverse effects in 23% of the patients taking cibenzoline; these included one case of ventricular dysrhythmia, four minor cardiac events, four cases of nausea or epigastric pain, eight cases of weakness, four cases of depression or insomnia, one skin rash, and one case of hypoglycemia. The QRS complex was prolonged by more than 13% in 14 patients, but the QT interval was not prolonged. Although this was not a placebo-controlled study, the incidence of adverse effects with cibenzoline was probably as one would expect in such a population.

Organs and Systems

Cardiovascular

Cibenzoline prolongs the PR interval, the QRS interval, and the QT_c interval (4–7). It also prolongs the AH and HV intervals (5,8) and shortens the sinus cycle length (5–8). Because of these effects it can cause dysrhythmias (4,6,7,9).

- Cardiac dysrhythmias have been attributed to cibenzoline in a 60-year-old man with hypertrophic cardiomyopathy (10).
- In a 72-year-old woman cibenzoline was associated with left bundle branch block and heart failure (11). Excess cibenzoline accumulation was suspected, because of reduced renal function, but plasma cibenzoline concentrations were not reported.

Right bundle branch block has also been reported (6).

In three patients in whom cibenzoline had caused sinus node dysfunction, normal sinus node recovery time was restored by cilostazol (12).

Cibenzoline has a negative inotropic effect and can therefore cause hypotension (6,7,13,14) and worsening heart failure (4).

Nervous system

Various nervous system complaints have been reported in occasional patients, including headache (15), disturbances of visual accommodation (15), and tremulousness (16). Dizziness and light-headedness have more commonly been reported, sometimes in association with hypertension (7,17).

There have been frequent reports of anticholinergic adverse effects, including dry mouth (7,9,13), blurred vision (4,9), and difficulty in micturition (18).

- Choreiform movements associated with persistent orofacial dystonia have been attributed to cibenzoline in a 77-year-old woman who took 260 mg/day for 1 week (19). When cibenzoline was eventually withdrawn the effects resolved within 1 month.

The authors proposed that the effect was due to inhibition of potassium channels.

A myasthenia-like syndrome has occasionally been attributed to cibenzoline (SEDA-21, 199) (20).

- A 57-year-old man with chronic renal insufficiency treated by continuous and ambulatory peritoneal dialysis took cibenzoline 150 mg/day for a ventricular dysrhythmia. Four days later he developed proximal muscle weakness, progressing to generalized muscle weakness, with dysphagia and dysarthria. Hemodiafiltration on six occasions caused complete improvement and cibenzoline was withdrawn. There was no further recurrence, even when other drugs that he had been taking were restarted.

The authors suggested that cibenzoline may have inhibited ATP-dependent potassium channels in skeletal muscle. The plasma cibenzoline concentration at the height of this patient's symptoms was very high at 1890 μg/ml (usual target range 300–600) and the authors counselled caution in patients with renal insufficiency (SEDA-15, 174).

Metabolism

Several cases of hypoglycemia have been attributed to cibenzoline (21–23) (SEDA-18, 204). In a case-control study of 14 156 outpatients, 91 had hypoglycemia, and each was matched with five controls (24). Eight of those with hypoglycemia were taking cibenzoline and three were taking disopyramide. In contrast, only seven of the controls were taking cibenzoline, a significant difference. However, 20 of the controls were taking disopyramide, which was not significant from the patients with hypoglycemia, although disopyramide is known to cause hypoglycemia. Insulin was also associated with hypoglycemia, but sulfonylureas were not. Furthermore, there was a positive association with what were termed "thyroid agents." All of these features cast some doubt on the validity of these results in relation to cibenzoline.

- A 65-year-old woman developed hypoglycemia while taking cibenzoline and alacepril (25).

It is possible that hypoglycemia due to cibenzoline can be enhanced by ACE inhibitors, which can increase insulin sensitivity (SED-14, 640).

Gastrointestinal

Various gastrointestinal adverse effects have been reported not infrequently, including nausea (15), sometimes in association with abdominal pain (7,9,13), vomiting, and diarrhea (7,8,14,16).

Liver

Hepatotoxicity with cibenzoline has been rarely reported. There has been a report of slight rises in the activities of serum transaminases (16), and one of ischemic hepatitis (26).

- A 67-year-old woman, who also had mild thrombocytopenia developed markedly abnormal liver function tests, which normalized within 3 months of withdrawal (27).

Susceptibility Factors

Renal disease

Cibenzoline is 60% eliminated by the kidneys (14,28,29). Its renal clearance falls with age (28); this is attributable to renal impairment.

- Three patients with severe renal insufficiency (creatinine clearance 10–16 ml/minute) had increased plasma cibenzoline concentrations during treatment with 300 mg/day (30). They developed prolonged QTc intervals, widened QRS complexes, dysrhythmias, hypotension, and hypoglycemia. Their plasma cibenzoline concentrations were 1944–2580 μg/l, 5–10 times higher than the usual target range. The half-lives of cibenzoline immediately after withdrawal were 69, 116, and 198 hours, 3–10 times longer than reported in patients with end-stage renal insufficiency (about 20 hours).

Drug Administration

Drug overdose

Overdose of cibenzoline has been reported.

- An 80-year-old woman who took an unknown number of 300 mg tablets had impaired consciousness, a low blood pressure (58/30 mmHg), coarse crackles in the lung, and a prolonged QT_c interval (0.64 seconds) (31). There was mild left ventricular global hypokinesia with a 50% left ventricular ejection fraction, severe mitral regurgitation, and left atrial dilatation. There was a mild partially compensated metabolic acidosis and hypoglycemia (2.9 mmol/l). The plasma concentration of cibenzoline was 2580 ng/ml. She was treated with sodium bicarbonate, dopamine, and noradrenaline. A pre-existing right ventricular pacemaker was not functioning, and the amplitude was increased from 2.5 to 7.5 volts at a rate of 90 per minute. Charcoal perfusion for 5 hours caused a dramatic fall in the plasma cibenzoline concentration in association with a reduction in the QT_c interval to 0.48 seconds and improvement in the pacing threshold.
- Fatal intoxication with cibenzoline has been reported in an 83-year-old man (32).

Diagnosis of Adverse Drug Reactions

It has been suggested that plasma concentrations of 100–200 mg/ml are necessary for efficacy and that at concentrations over 400 mg/ml there is an increased risk of adverse reactions (7). In most studies plasma cibenzoline concentrations have been around 200–400 mg/ml (4,6,8,17). Plasma concentrations correlate well with electrophysiological effects (6), its hemodynamic effects (33), and reduction in ventricular extra beats (34). In one study, patients who had adverse effects had a mean concentration of 913 mg/ml compared with 312 mg/ml in those who did not (8).

References

1. Miura DS, Keren G, Torres V, Butler B, Aogaichi K, Somberg JC. Antiarrhythmic effects of cibenzoline. Am Heart J 1985;109(4):827–33.
2. Kodama I, Ogawa S, Inoue H, Kasanuki H, Kato T, Mitamura H, Hiraoka M, Sugimoto T. Profiles of aprindine, cibenzoline, pilsicainide and pirmenol in the framework of the Sicilian Gambit. The Guideline Committee for Clinical Use of Antiarrhythmic Drugs in Japan (Working Group of Arrhythmias of the Japanese Society of Electrocardiology). Jpn Circ J 1999;63(1):1–12.
3. Babuty D, Maison-Blanche P, Fauchier L, Brembilla-Perrot B, Medvedowsky JL, Bine-Scheck F. Double-blind comparison of cibenzoline versus flecainide in the prevention of recurrence of atrial tachyarrhythmias in 139 patients. Ann Noninvasive Electrocardiol 1999;4:53–9.
4. Miura DS, Keren G, Torres V, Butler B, Aogaichi K, Somberg JC. Antiarrhythmic effects of cibenzoline. Am Heart J 1985;109(4):827–33.
5. Thizy JF, Jandot V, Andre-Fouet X, Viallet M, Pout M. Etude électrophysiologique de l'UP 339–01 chez l'homme. Lyon Med 1981;245:119–22.
6. Hoffmann E, Mattke S, Haberl R, Steinbeck G. Randomized crossover comparison of the electrophysiologic and antiarrhythmic efficacy of oral cibenzoline and sotalol for sustained ventricular tachycardia. J Cardiovasc Pharmacol 1993;21(1):95–100.
7. Kostis JB, Davis D, Kluger J, Aogaichi K, Smith M. Cifenline in the short-term treatment of patients with ventricular premature complexes: a double-blind placebo-controlled study. J Cardiovasc Pharmacol 1989; 14(1):88–95.
8. Kushner M, Magiros E, Peters R, Carliner N, Plotnick G, Fisher M. The electrophysiologic effects of oral cibenzoline. J Electrocardiol 1984;17(1):15–23.
9. Browne KF, Prystowsky EN, Zipes DP, Chilson DA, Heger JJ. Clinical efficacy and electrophysiologic effects of cibenzoline therapy in patients with ventricular arrhythmias. J Am Coll Cardiol 1984;3(3):857–64.
10. Nishida K, Fujiki A, Mizumaki K, Nagasawa H, Sakabe M, Sakurai K, Inoue H. Exercise-induced ventricular fibrillation during treatment with cibenzoline in a patient with hypertrophic cardiomyopathy. Ther Res 2001;22:832–6.
11. Paelinck BP, De Raedt H, Conraads V. Blurred vision, left bundle-branch block and cardiac failure. Acta Cardiol 2001;56(1):39–40.
12. Yamaji S, Imai S, Watanabe T, Takahashi N, Uenishi T, Matsudaira K, Sugino K, Yagi H, Kanmatsuse K. Cilostazol improved sinus nodal dysfunction induced by cibenzoline which was used for hybrid therapy in patients with paroxysmal atrial fibrillation. Ther Res 2002;23:882–6.
13. Humen DP, Lesoway R, Kostuk WJ. Acute, single, intravenous doses of cibenzoline: an evaluation of safety, tolerance, and hemodynamic effects. Clin Pharmacol Ther 1987;41(5):537–45.
14. Katoh T, Ishihara S, Tanaka T, Kobagasi Y, Takada K, Shimai S, Seino Y, Tanaka K, Takano T, Hayakawa H. Hemodynamic effects of intravenous cibenzoline, a new antiarrhythmic agent. Jpn J Clin Pharmacol Ther 1988;19:707–16.
15. Cocco G, Strozzi C, Pansini R, Rochat N, Bulgarelli R, Padula A, Sfrisi C, Kamal Al Yassini A. Antiarrhythmic use of cibenzoline, a new class 1 antiarrhythmic agent with class 3 and 4 properties, in patients with recurrent ventricular tachycardia. Eur Heart J 1984;5(2):108–14.
16. Klein RC, House M, Rushforth N. Efficacy and safety of oral cibenzoline in treatment of ventricular ectopy. Clin Res 1984;32:9A.
17. Lee MA, Fenster PE, Garcia ZM, Kipps JE, Huang SK. Cibenzoline for symptomatic ventricular arrhythmias: a prospective, randomized, double-blind, placebo controlled trial and a long term open label study. Can J Cardiol 1989;5(6):295–8.
18. Miura D, Torres V, Butler B, Gottlieb S, Aogaicki K, Somberg J. Effects of cibenzoline in patients with ventricular tachycardia. J Clin Pharmacol 1984;24:413.
19. Devos D, Defebvre L, Destee A, Caron J. Choreic movements induced by cibenzoline: an Ic class antiarrhythmic effect? Mov Disord 2000;15(5):1030–1.
20. Wakutani Y, Matsushima E, Son A, Shimizu Y, Goto Y, Ishida H. Myasthenialike syndrome due to adverse effects of cibenzoline in a patient with chronic renal failure. Muscle Nerve 1998;21(3):416–17.
21. Lefort G, Haissaguerre M, Floro J, Beauffigeau P, Warin JF, Latapie JL. Hypoglycémies au cours de surdosages par un nouvel anti-arythmique: la cibenzoline; trois observations. [Hypoglycemia caused by overdose of a new anti-arrhythmia agent: cibenzoline. 3 cases.] Presse Méd 1988;17(14):687–91.
22. Jeandel C, Preiss MA, Pierson H, Penin F, Cuny G, Bannwarth B, Netter P. Hypoglycaemia induced by cibenzoline. Lancet 1988;1(8596):1232–3.
23. Gachot BA, Bezier M, Cherrier JF, Daubeze J. Cibenzoline and hypoglycaemia. Lancet 1988;2(8605):280.
24. Takada M, Fujita S, Katayama Y, Harano Y, Shibakawa M. The relationship between risk of hypoglycemia and use of cibenzoline and disopyramide. Eur J Clin Pharmacol 2000;56(4):335–42.
25. Ogimoto A, Hamada M, Saeki H, Hiasa G, Ohtsuka T, Hashida H, Hara Y, Okura T, Shigematsu Y, Hiwada K. Hypoglycemic syncope induced by a combination of cibenzoline and angiotensin converting enzyme inhibitor. Jpn Heart J 2001;42(2):255–9.
26. Gutknecht J, Larrey D, Ychou M, Fedkovic Y, Janbon C. Ischémie hépatique grave après prise de cibenzoline. [Severe ischemic hepatitis after taking cibenzoline.] Ann Gastroenterol Hepatol (Paris) 1991;27(6):269–70.
27. Binois F, Guiserix J, Kilian D. Hépatite aiguë au cours d'un traitement par la cibenzoline. [Acute hepatitis during cibenzoline therapy.] Presse Méd 2000;29(13):703.
28. Canal M, Flouvat B, Tremblay D, Dufour A. Pharmacokinetics in man of a new antiarrhythmic drug, cibenzoline. Eur J Clin Pharmacol 1983;24(4):509–15.
29. Brazzell RK, Rees MM, Khoo KC, Szuna AJ, Sandor D, Hannigan J. Age and cibenzoline disposition. Clin Pharmacol Ther 1984;36(5):613–19.
30. Takahashi M, Echizen H, Takahashi K, Shimada S, Aoyama N, Izumi T. Extremely prolonged elimination of cibenzoline at toxic plasma concentrations in patients with renal impairments. Ther Drug Monit 2002;24(4):492–6.

31. Aoyama N, Sasaki T, Yoshida M, Suzuki K, Matsuyama K, Aizaki T, Izumi T, Kondo R, Kamijo Y, Soma K, Ohwada T. Effect of charcoal hemoperfusion on clearance of cibenzoline succinate (cifenline) poisoning. J Toxicol Clin Toxicol 1999;37(4):505–8.
32. Sadeg N, Richecoeur J, Dumontet M. Intoxication mortelle a la cibenzoline. [Fatal poisoning by cibenzoline.] Therapie 2001;56(2):188–9.
33. van den Brand M, Serruys P, de Roon Y, Aymard MF, Dufour A. Haemodynamic effects of intravenous cibenzoline in patients with coronary heart disease. Eur J Clin Pharmacol 1984;26(3):297–302.
34. Khoo KC, Szuna AJ, Colburn WA, Aogaichi K, Morganroth J, Brazzell RK. Single-dose pharmacokinetics and dose proportionality of oral cibenzoline. J Clin Pharmacol 1984;24(7):283–8.

Ciclosporin

General Information

Ciclosporin is an immunosuppressant drug that primarily inhibits T cell activation, therefore down-regulating the T cell responses that mediate graft rejection. Myelotoxic effects are therefore not expected. Ciclosporin has also been used in a wide range of chronic inflammatory or autoimmune diseases.

Considerable efforts have been devoted to defining the optimal dose to ensure minimal toxicity while retaining efficacy. In transplant patients, the daily maintenance dose is 2–6 mg/kg/day. In non-transplant patients, daily doses of 2.5 mg/kg up to a maximum of 4 mg/kg are usually recommended.

In renal transplantation, ciclosporin maintenance monotherapy can be effectively achieved in a subset of patients with the aim of reducing adverse effects associated with glucocorticoids or azathioprine, but this should be carefully balanced against the risks of acute or chronic allograft rejection. This approach was again emphasized, based on data from 100 adults and a review of the most recent literature (1). According to the authors, clinical predictors of successful ciclosporin maintenance therapy included compliant patients over 25 years old with a donor age younger than 40 years, patients with later azathioprine withdrawal, patients with serum creatinine concentrations of 125 μmol/l or less, patients without a history of rejection (or one rejection episode responding favorably to glucocorticoids), and patients who have successfully discontinued glucocorticoids 6 months before.

Comparative studies

Although the pattern of long-term toxicity of ciclosporin and tacrolimus is remarkably similar for most serious adverse effects (particularly nephrotoxicity), a higher incidence of several minor adverse effects with ciclosporin, namely hirsutism, gingivitis or gum hyperplasia, has been thought to underlie a moderate but significant decrease in the quality of life with ciclosporin compared with tacrolimus (2).

General adverse effects

As regards long-term toxicity, particularly nephrotoxicity, and frequent drug interactions, the benefit-to-harm balance of ciclosporin is still debatable. Whereas the adverse effects have generally been deemed acceptable, although occasionally treatment-limiting in patients with rheumatoid arthritis given low-dose ciclosporin rather than conventional antirheumatic drugs, conflicting opinions have been expressed on the acceptability of the risks in patients with psoriasis (SEDA-20, 343).

Of 20 patients with chronic idiopathic thrombocytopenic purpura refractory to glucocorticoids or splenectomy treated with ciclosporin, six withdrew owing to toxicity (3). The target blood concentration range was identical to that aimed at in the first 3 months after kidney transplantation. The most common adverse effects were hypertension, headache, and severe myalgia.

The antileukemic effect of ciclosporin has been harnessed in the treatment of cytopenias associated with chronic lymphatic leukemia. In 31 patients the most common adverse effect was a raised serum creatinine concentration of grade 2 or worse in six patients (19%); three patients developed opportunistic infections (4).

Drug interactions with ciclosporin have been comprehensively reviewed (5).

Organs and Systems

Cardiovascular

Compared with azathioprine, hypertension has been considered one of the main long-term risks in patients taking ciclosporin, with major concerns about the post-transplantion increase in cardiovascular morbidity and mortality. However, there are many susceptibility factors for cardiovascular disease in transplant patients (6), and it is difficult to take into account their complex interplay. Ciclosporin-associated hypertension appears to be dose-related, and higher whole-blood ciclosporin concentrations were found during the preceding months in patients who had thromboembolic complications compared with patients who did not (7).

De novo or aggravated hypertension is very common in patients taking ciclosporin, with the highest incidence in cases of heart transplant (71–100%) and the lowest incidence in bone marrow transplant recipients (33–60%) (8). In addition, 30–45% of patients with psoriasis, rheumatoid arthritis, or uveitis had hypertension, suggesting that ciclosporin is a significant cause of hypertension in organ transplantation. Ciclosporin-associated hypertension can cause acute vascular injury, with microangiopathic hemolysis, encephalopathy, seizures, and intracranial hemorrhage.

The incidence, clinical features, consequences, and management of ciclosporin-induced hypertension have been reviewed (9). The prevalence was 29–54% in non-transplant patients and 65–100% in heart and liver transplant patients also taking glucocorticoids. Disturbed circadian rhythm with a loss of nocturnal blood pressure fall was the main characteristic, and patients therefore had higher risks of left ventricular hypertrophy, cerebrovascular damage, microalbuminuria, and other target organ damage.

The pathophysiology of ciclosporin-induced hypertension is complex and not yet fully elucidated. Increased systemic vascular resistance subsequent to altered vascular endothelium function, renal vasoconstriction with reduced glomerular filtration and sodium-water retention, and/or increased activity of the sympathetic nervous system were suggested, while only a minor role or none was attributed to the renin–angiotensin system (10). However, hypertension often occurs before changes in renal function or sodium balance can be demonstrated, and ciclosporin nephrotoxicity alone does not explain ciclosporin-associated hypertension (8,11).

The effects of antihypertensive agents have been evaluated in patients taking ciclosporin. Collectively, dihydropyridine calcium channel blockers that do not affect ciclosporin blood concentrations substantially or at all (felodipine, isradipine, and nifedipine) are usually considered to be the drugs of choice. However, the risk of gingival hyperplasia with nifedipine, which ciclosporin also causes, should be borne in mind. Combination therapy with angiotensin-converting enzyme inhibitors or beta-blockers, or the use of other calcium channel blockers (verapamil or diltiazem) should also be considered, but careful monitoring of ciclosporin blood concentrations is recommended with the latter because they inhibit ciclosporin metabolism.

A possible role of ciclosporin in the exacerbation or development of Raynaud's disease has been suggested on one occasion; such an effect could be linked to endothelial damage or changes in platelet function (12).

A capillary leak syndrome with subsequent pulmonary edema has also been reported after intravenous ciclosporin (SEDA-21, 383).

Infusion phlebitis has been attributed to intravenous ciclosporin (13).

Respiratory

Adult respiratory distress syndrome has been described after intravenous ciclosporin. It was thought that a high concentration of the drug in the pulmonary vasculature due to administration through a central vein was responsible for capillary leakage, but in one patient the pulmonary capillary leak resolved rapidly when the intravenous ciclosporin was changed to oral (14). This suggested that Cremophor (polyoxyethylated castor oil), the solvent for parenteral ciclosporin, was responsible. However, there has been a report of an adult who developed respiratory distress syndrome in association with oral ciclosporin given after renal transplantation (15).

Hypersensitivity pneumonitis has been attributed to ciclosporin (16).

- A 35-year-old woman taking glibenclamide and mesalazine for Crohn's colitis was given ciclosporin for severe disease exacerbation. Within 6 weeks, she developed arthralgia and moderate thrombocytopenia, and ciclosporin was discontinued. Acute fever (41°C) and dyspnea were noted several days later, and a chest X-ray showed diffuse bilateral infiltrates. Bronchoalveolar lavage showed neutrophil preponderance and plasma cells, and a lung biopsy strongly suggested an acute hypersensitivity pneumonitis. All her symptoms subsided after a short course of prednisolone and oxygen.

Both the absence of an infectious cause and the rapid improvement without withdrawal of other drugs suggested that ciclosporin was the likely cause.

Nervous system

Neurological adverse effects of ciclosporin have been reported in up to 39% of all transplant patients. Most are mild. The most frequent is a fine tremor, the mechanism of which is not known. From many case reports or studies in transplant patients, the pattern of ciclosporin neurotoxicity ranges from common and mild to moderate symptoms, such as headaches, tremors, paresthesia, restlessness, mood changes, sleep disturbances, confusion, agitation, and visual hallucinations, to rare but severe or life-threatening disorders, including acute psychotic episodes, cerebellar disorders, cortical blindness (permanent in one report), spasticity or paralysis of the limbs, catatonia, speech disorders or mutism, chorea, seizures, leukoencephalopathy, and coma (SED-13, 1124) (SEDA-16, 516) (SEDA-17, 520) (SEDA-20, 343) (SEDA-21, 383) (17–19).

A 19% incidence of central nervous system toxicity with ciclosporin has been reported in pediatric renal transplantation patients; the symptoms included seizures, drowsiness, confusion, hallucinations, visual disturbances, and mental changes (20).

Neurological symptoms were observed in 12–25% of liver-transplant patients and in 29% of bone marrow transplant patients, but severe neurotoxicity occurred only in about 1% (18,19,21). They usually appeared within the first month of treatment, but were sometimes delayed (19). Particular attention should be paid to prompt recognition of severe neurotoxicity, because abnormalities of the white matter can occur. Patients usually improved rapidly after temporary ciclosporin withdrawal or dosage reduction, and tacrolimus has sometimes been used successfully instead (SEDA-21, 383) (18). However, recurrence of seizures and persistent electroencephalographic abnormalities were found in 46 and 70% of pediatric transplant patients respectively who had had ciclosporin acute encephalopathy and seizure syndrome and who were followed-up for 49 months (22).

Although the role of many other factors should be considered when neurological symptoms occur in transplant recipients, isolated reports of neurotoxicity in non-transplanted patients are in keeping with a causal role of ciclosporin. There are many susceptibility factors in ciclosporin neurotoxicity. Blood ciclosporin concentrations are sometimes raised, but severe neurological symptoms have been observed in some patients with concentrations in the usual target range (18). Other possible susceptibility factors for ciclosporin neurotoxicity include hypocholesterolemia, hypomagnesemia, aluminium overload, concomitant high-dose glucocorticoid therapy, hypertension, and concomitant microangiopathic hemolytic anemia (SED-13, 1124) (SEDA-21, 383). Acute graft-versus-host disease or HLA-mismatched and unrelated donor transplants were also potential susceptibility factors in recipients of bone marrow transplants (SEDA-22, 383) (19).

Ciclosporin-induced vasculopathy, with endothelial injury and derangement of the blood–brain barrier, is the postulated mechanism of neurological damage. Transient cerebral perfusion abnormalities, demonstrable in SPECT scans of the brain, have been suggested as a reliable indicator of ciclosporin neurotoxicity (SEDA-20, 344). Clinical symptoms as well as CT and/or MRI scans were very similar to those observed in hypertensive encephalopathy, with predominant and reversible white-matter occipital lesions (23). There was complete neurological recovery in most patients after blood pressure was normalized, and deaths due to intracranial hemorrhage are reported only exceptionally.

A retrospective study identified a significantly higher incidence of central nervous system symptoms in patients with Behçet's disease (24). Headache, fever, paralysis, ataxia, dysarthria, or disturbed consciousness occurred in 12 of 47 ciclosporin-treated patients compared with nine of 270 patients not treated or taking other drugs. CT and/or MRI scans were abnormal in all 12. As the clinical findings were very similar to the neurological effects of Behçet's disease, it was suggested that ciclosporin can promote the development of neurological complications in this population.

Ciclosporin neurotoxicity is particularly frequent in liver and bone marrow transplant patients, who usually recover after temporary dosage reduction or withdrawal. However, a fatal outcome has been reported (25).

- A 54-year-old man was given ciclosporin and methotrexate after allogeneic bone marrow transplantation. He noted blurred vision during several days and became confused 11 weeks after transplantation. Generalized tonic-clonic seizures occurred the day after and he was given phenytoin and antibiotics. His neurological condition deteriorated during the next 5 days, despite ciclosporin withdrawal, and he died from respiratory failure. Postmortem examination showed white matter edema and astrocyte injury without demyelination.

Most studies have focused on the central nervous system adverse effects of ciclosporin, and there have been few reports of peripheral neuropathy.

- In two patients, ciclosporin was suggested as a possible cause of an entrapment neuropathy, and surgery was required in both (26).

However, the report did not provide sufficient evidence to assess the causal relation fully.

- Another patient developed a symmetric polyneuropathy with flaccid paraplegia while her ciclosporin serum concentrations were about twice normal (27). Electromyography showed features of axonal degeneration in the peripheral nerves and neurological symptoms improved on ciclosporin dosage reduction.

Migraine associated with ciclosporin is sometimes resistant to classical treatment and the consequences can be even more severe.

- Three young adult renal transplant patients, including two with a previous history of moderate migraine, had severe attacks of unilateral throbbing migraine associated with vomiting during ciclosporin treatment (28). In two patients, vomiting was severe enough to reduce compliance with the immunosuppressive regimen, and both subsequently lost their grafts. The same sequence of events was again observed after retransplantation.

Substitution by tacrolimus may be beneficial in such cases.

Severe ciclosporin neurotoxicity has mostly been reported in transplant patients, but should also be considered in non-transplanted patients.

- An 87-year-old patient with resistant nodular prurigo was successfully treated with ciclosporin (3 mg/kg/day) and prednisone (10 mg/day) (29). Bilateral numbness and distal limb weakness developed after 18 months. Clinical examination, electromyography, and nerve conduction studies confirmed a diffuse axonal neuropathy which rapidly progressed over the next 2 months. Ciclosporin alone was withdrawn and complete remission was observed within 3 months.

Unfortunately, ciclosporin blood concentrations and renal function at the time of diagnosis were not reported.

Very severe or fatal neurotoxicity has been reported in isolated patients only.

- Based on postmortem findings in a 32-year-old woman who died with an acute encephalopathy (30) and another report of two patients investigated with transcranial Doppler ultrasound and MRI for symptoms of ciclosporin neurotoxicity (31), vascular changes with vasospasm and dissection of the vascular intima strongly suggest that vasculopathy is a possible mechanism of ciclosporin-induced encephalopathy.

Prolonged confusion is a recognized complication of ciclosporin, and can be due to non-convulsive status epilepticus (32). Three patients who developed neurotoxicity following treatment with ciclosporin manifested with generalized tonic-clonic seizures and dysarthria. The plasma ciclosporin concentration in these patients increased as the neurological signs appeared, and the signs resolved quickly after dosage reduction (33). Tonic-clonic seizures have been reported in a child taking ciclosporin (34).

- A 13-year-old boy with severe Crohn's disease developed hematochezia and required blood transfusion. He was given ciclosporin on day 22 because of persistent rectal bleeding and diarrhea, despite high-dose intravenous glucocorticoids. After 6 days he developed multiple episodes of generalized tonic-clonic seizures, with MRI findings typical but not pathognomonic of ciclosporin: prominent meningeal enhancement, bifrontal, bitemporal, biparietal, and bioccipital cortical and subcortical white matter high-signal changes, and swelling of the gyri, which obliterated the sulci.

This case illustrates that severe ciclosporin neurotoxicity can develop in patients with predisposing factors, such as hypomagnesemia, hypocholesterolemia, hypertension, and glucocorticoid therapy.

There is still debate about whether ciclosporin crosses the blood–brain barrier and enters the cerebrospinal fluid. Ciclosporin could not be identified in cerebrospinal fluid from 14 patients with liver transplants who had various neurological complications (35). Ciclosporin metabolites were measurable in the cerebrospinal fluid in only four patients, who had evidence of acute renal insufficiency, cholestasis, and raised blood concentrations of ciclosporin metabolites but identical ciclosporin parent drug blood concentrations compared with 10 patients with undetectable concentrations of ciclosporin metabolites in the cerebrospinal fluid. Ciclosporin metabolites enter the cerebrospinal fluid, and direct neurotoxicity is therefore possible in at least some patients with renal or hepatic dysfunction.

Endogenous ligands for ciclosporin and tacrolimus, known as immunophilins, are found in very high concentrations in the basal ganglia, and ciclosporin can alter dopamine phosphorylation in the medium-sized neurons in the striatum. Changes in basal ganglia glucose metabolism have been studied in a patient with severe ciclosporin-related tremor (36).

- A 37-year-old man received ciclosporin after bone marrow transplantation for chronic myelogenous leukemia. Soon afterwards he developed a severe tremor, which persisted despite dosage reduction. A brain MRI scan was normal. After 22 months he developed a personality change. A high resolution PET scan showed symmetrical increases in ^{18}F-deoxyglucose uptake in both caudate and putamen.

These results confirm that ciclosporin can modulate dopaminergic transmission in the striatum, presumably by inhibition of calcineurin.

- A 16-year-old girl with end-stage renal insufficiency underwent successful renal transplantation and was given ciclosporin on day 1 (37). On day 10 she complained of tinnitus and tremor and had a right facial nerve palsy. An MRI scan showed areas of increased signal in the white matter of the periventricular region. The dose of ciclosporin was reduced, since no other cause could be determined. Her tremor and tinnitus resolved, but the facial nerve palsy persisted. She was given tacrolimus, but the tremor and tinnitus recurred. She was then given mycophenolate mofetil and prednisone, and the tremor and tinnitus disappeared, although the facial nerve palsy persisted. The MRI scan 3 months later was normal.

The serum magnesium concentration was below the reference range in this case, which may have favored the development of neurotoxicity.

Sensory systems

Controversial reports of ocular symptoms have been published in patients taking oral ciclosporin, with ptosis and diplopia attributed to unilateral or bilateral sixth nerve palsies in four patients (who had also taken ganciclovir), and nystagmus in one patient (SEDA-21, 383). Peripheral optic neuropathy, with visual loss, nystagmus, and ophthalmoplegia, has also been reported (38). Acute cerebral cortical blindness complicating ciclosporin therapy in a 5-year-old girl (39) and transient cortical blindness and occipital seizures with visual impairment (40,41) have also been reported in association with ciclosporin.

Bilateral optic disc edema is sometimes associated with ciclosporin given for bone marrow transplantation, but unilateral papilledema with otherwise asymptomatic raised intracranial pressure can occur (42). Eight cases of optic disc edema have been reported in bone marrow transplant patients taking ciclosporin. In two of the patients there were other possible explanations, but in all cases withdrawal of ciclosporin resulted in resolution of the papilledema (43).

Ciclosporin eye-drops have been used after keratoplasty, in high-risk cases, to prevent graft rejection and to treat severe vernal conjunctivitis, keratoconjunctivitis sicca, and various immune-related corneal disorders. Despite its severe adverse effects after systemic use, topical ciclosporin can generally be used without serious adverse reactions (44,45).

Ciclosporin oil-in-water emulsion has been used in the local treatment of moderate to severe dry eye disease. Chronic dry eye disease results from inflammation mediated by cytokines and receptors for autoimmune antibodies in the lacrimal glands. It affects the lacrimal gland acini and ducts, leading to abnormalities in the tear film, and ultimately disrupting the homeostasis of the ocular surface. Topical ciclosporin reduces the cell-mediated inflammatory response associated with inflammatory ocular surface diseases.

In two large, randomized controlled trials in 977 patients, the adverse effects associated with ciclosporin ophthalmic emulsion for the treatment of dry eye disease were minimal and consisted mostly of mild ocular burning and stinging (46). However, topical application of ciclosporin eye-drops was the suspected cause of severe visual loss with bilateral white corneal deposits in a 45-year-old patient with dry eye syndrome caused by graft-versus-host disease (47). Infrared spectroscopy and X-ray analysis suggested that the deposits contained ciclosporin. A reduction in tear clearance and compromised epithelial barrier function caused by the concomitant use of oxybuprocaine may have precipitated this adverse effect.

The efficacy, safety, tolerability, and optimal dose of ciclosporin eye-drops have been studied in a randomized, double-masked, vehicle-controlled multicenter trial in 162 patients with keratoconjunctivitis sicca with or without Sjögren's disease and refractory to conventional treatment (48). Ciclosporin ophthalmic emulsion 0.05, 0.1, 0.2, or 0.4%, or the vehicle alone was instilled twice daily into both eyes for 12 weeks, followed by a 4-week observation period. There was no clear dose–response relation; ciclosporin 0.1% emulsion produced the most consistent improvement in objective and subjective end-points and ciclosporin 0.05% gave the most consistent improvement in symptoms. The vehicle also performed well, perhaps because of its long residence time on the ocular surface. There were no significant adverse effects, no microbial overgrowth, and no residence time of the vehicle emulsion on the ocular surface. All treatments were well tolerated and the highest ciclosporin blood concentration detected was 0.16 ng/ml.

To study the efficacy and safety of ciclosporin 0.05 and 0.1% ophthalmic emulsions and their vehicle in patients with moderate to severe dry eye disease, two identical multicenter, randomized, double-masked, vehicle-controlled trials have been performed in 877 patients for

6 months (46). More than 76% completed the course. Ciclosporin 0.05 or 0.1% eye-drops gave significantly greater improvement than the vehicle in two objective signs of dry eye disease (corneal staining and Schirmer values). Ciclosporin 0.05% also gave significantly greater improvement in three subjective measures (blurred vision, need for concomitant artificial tears, and the physician's evaluation of global response to treatment). There was no dose–response effect and there were no topical or systemic adverse findings.

Corneal deposition of ciclosporin can occur (47).

- A 45-year-old woman with dry eye syndrome caused by graft-versus-host disease after bone marrow transplantation for acute leukemia was given systemic ciclosporin and topical 0.1% sodium hyaluronate, 0.3% ofloxacin, 0.1% fluorometholone, and isotonic saline. She was also given 0.4% oxybuprocaine for the relief of severe ocular pain. The bilateral corneal epithelial defects persisted even after the application of punctal plugs, and 2% ciclosporin in olive oil was added as eye-drops three times a day bilaterally. Five days later she complained of severe visual loss in association with bilateral corneal opacities, which covered the pupil and the punctal plugs bilaterally. As she did not agree to keratectomy, infrared spectroscopy and X-ray analysis were conducted on the deposits on the plugs. The spectroscopic pattern and X-ray analysis showed that the deposits had the properties of ciclosporin.

As the corneal deposits did not abate after withdrawal of the ciclosporin eye-drops, the systemic ciclosporin as well as its topical use may have contributed to the deposits. One should be aware that precipitation of ciclosporin on a compromised cornea can lead to severe visual impairment.

Metabolism

Diabetes mellitus

Diabetes mellitus after transplantation is recognized as an important adverse effect of immunosuppressants, and has been extensively reviewed (49). However, the use of ciclosporin in immunosuppressive regimens is not associated with diabetes mellitus after transplantation (10–20%) (50).

Hyperlipidemia

Ciclosporin is potentially more toxic in patients with altered LDL concentrations or a low total serum cholesterol (51). Ciclosporin therapy itself significantly raises plasma lipoprotein concentrations by increasing the total serum cholesterol; this is due to an increase in LDL cholesterol, demonstrated in a prospective, double-blind, randomized, placebo-controlled trial in 36 men with amyotrophic lateral sclerosis (52). In 22 patients there were significant increases in mean serum triglycerides and cholesterol 2 weeks after they started to take low-dose ciclosporin (53). Hypertriglyceridemia developed in seven patients taking ciclosporin 2.0–7.5 mg/kg/day for psoriasis during the first month of therapy; the values were greater than the upper limit in age- and sex-matched controls (54).

The pathology of hyperlipidemia after transplantation is multifactorial, but it is clearly dose-dependently related to immunosuppressive therapy (55). This results in cardiovascular disease, which is one of the most common causes of morbidity and mortality in long-term survivors of organ transplantation (56). Hyperlipidemia can also cause renal atheroma, resulting in graft rejection. The possible impact of ciclosporin on lipids includes an increase in total cholesterol, LDL cholesterol, and apolipoprotein B concentrations, and a reduction in HDL cholesterol (SED-13, 1124). The influence of ciclosporin on lipoprotein(a) concentrations has been debated (SEDA-21, 383) (57). Post-transplant hyperlipidemia is multifactorial and can be affected by impaired renal function, diuretics and beta-blockers, increased age, and female sex. A combination of lipid-lowering drugs and optimization of immunosuppressive regimens compatible with long-term allograft survival is probably required to reduce post-transplantation hyperlipidemia.

Whereas azathioprine is considered to play no role, glucocorticoid use correlates positively with increased serum cholesterol concentrations. It is uncertain whether these lipid changes reflect primarily an effect of ciclosporin alone or an additive/synergistic effect of the drug plus glucocorticoids. Ciclosporin has been considered as a possible independent susceptibility factor by several investigators, but others were unable to find an association between hyperlipidemia and ciclosporin (SEDA-20, 344). There was indirect evidence for a causal role of ciclosporin in several studies; hyperlipidemia developed in non-transplant patients taking ciclosporin alone; there was a transient reduction in hyperlipidemia after ciclosporin withdrawal; there was a significant correlation between ciclosporin blood concentrations and lipid abnormalities; and there was a higher incidence of lipid abnormalities in patients taking ciclosporin alone compared with patients taking azathioprine and prednisolone (SED-8, 1131) (SEDA-17, 524) (SEDA-21, 383) (55,58). Other studies have provided striking evidence that hyperlipidemia is more frequent in patients taking ciclosporin than in those taking tacrolimus, with more patients classified as having high cholesterol concentrations in the ciclosporin group or a significant fall in total cholesterol or LDL cholesterol in patients switched from ciclosporin to tacrolimus (59,60). Although the glucocorticoid-sparing effect of tacrolimus may account for these differences, the concept that the glucocorticoid dose is a confounding factor has been disputed (SEDA-22, 412). Whether these differences translate to a higher risk of cardiovascular complications in patients taking ciclosporin has not been carefully assessed. The treatment of hyperlipidemia in transplant patients may represent a major dilemma, because of several drug interactions, with an increased risk of myopathy and rhabdomyolysis after the combined use of ciclosporin and several lipid-lowering drugs.

Hyperuricemia

Significant hyperuricemia has been observed in as many as 80% of patients taking ciclosporin (61). In one series, hyperuricemia occurred in 72% of male and 82% of female patients taking ciclosporin after cardiac transplantation; there was also an increased incidence of gouty arthritis in these patients (62). Episodes of gout developed mostly in men taking diuretics, but the incidence was lower than in the hyperuricemic population. In renal transplant patients, the incidence of gout was 5–24% and tophi sometimes developed rapidly after the onset of gout (63). The potential mechanisms of hyperuricemia include reduced renal function and impaired tubular secretion of acid uric, with hypertension and diuretics as confounding factors (SEDA-21, 383).

Nutrition

Higher plasma homocysteine concentrations, which may contribute to atherosclerosis, have been found in patients taking ciclosporin, compared with both transplant patients not taking ciclosporin and non-transplant patients with renal insufficiency (SEDA-20, 344).

Electrolyte balance

Mild and uncomplicated hyperkalemia is commonly observed in patients taking ciclosporin and is generally prevented by a low potassium diet. A reduction in distal nephron potassium secretion and tubular flow rate, with insensitivity to exogenous mineralocorticoids, and leakage of cellular potassium into the extracellular fluid are possible mechanisms (SED-13, 1124) (64).

Mineral balance

Hypomagnesemia and hypercalcemia occur infrequently during ciclosporin treatment (SED-13, 1124).

- In a 43-year-old renal transplant patient, hypomagnesemia was associated with muscle weakness and a near four-fold increase in serum creatine kinase activity (65). Both disorders resolved after magnesium supplementation, and ciclosporin was continued.

Renal magnesium wasting occurred in 24% of a series of renal transplant patients taking ciclosporin; other indicators of renal function were normal (66,67).

Hypomagnesemia in the early post-transplant period has been cited as a possible risk factor for acute ciclosporin neurotoxicity. Ciclosporin-induced sustained magnesium depletion has been investigated in 109 ciclosporin-treated patients with renal transplants who had been stable for more than 6 months (68). Total and ionized plasma magnesium concentrations were significantly lower than in 21 healthy volunteers and in 15 patients with renal transplants who were not taking ciclosporin. Ciclosporin-treated patients who were also taking hypoglycemic drugs had lower plasma magnesium concentrations, but patients taking diuretics did not.

Hematologic

A very few cases of ciclosporin-induced immune hemolytic anemia have been reported (SED-13, 1125) (69,70), but a direct causal relation with ciclosporin is difficult to establish. Ciclosporin-induced hypercoagulability was suggested in patients with aplastic anemia (SEDA-20, 344). Higher whole-blood ciclosporin concentrations were found during the preceding months in patients who experienced thromboembolic complications compared with patients who had not.

Ciclosporin-associated thrombotic microangiopathy occurs in 3–14% of patients with a renal transplant and can cause allograft loss. Renal impairment, reflected by an increase in serum creatinine concentration, is often the only change found, and hemolysis is not always present. Plasmapheresis has been used to treat this complication (71).

- A 47-year-old multiparous Hispanic woman received a living-unrelated kidney transplant for end-stage renal disease secondary to polycystic kidney disease. On the day of transplantation she received intravenous daclizumab 1 mg/kg plus methylprednisolone 300 mg and mycophenolate mofetil 3 g/day, and on day 3 ciclosporin emulsion 4 mg/kg/day. On day 8 she developed thrombotic microangiopathy without evidence of rejection. Ciclosporin was withdrawn. Plasmapheresis with fresh frozen plasma was started. Daclizumab on day 14 was postponed for 24 hours and plasmapheresis was stopped to avoid clearance of daclizumab. Thereafter she was given tacrolimus, without recurrence of hemolysis.

Mouth and teeth

Ciclosporin-induced gingival hyperplasia was noted in the early 1980s, and subsequent studies investigated the prevalence and pathophysiology of this adverse effect (SED-13, 1127). The reported incidence was 7–70%, and clinically significant gingival overgrowth, that is to say requiring treatment or surgical excision, affected about 30% of patients within the first 6 months of treatment (72). Clinical and histological features are similar to those associated with phenytoin or nifedipine. Compared with control specimens, ultrastructural gingival examinations in patients taking ciclosporin showed many fibroblasts, abundant amorphous substance, and marked plasma cell infiltration (73). Although an imbalance between the production and removal of collagen is supposed to account for gingival hyperplasia, the mechanism of ciclosporin-induced gingival overgrowth has not yet been clearly established. Possible local lymphocyte resistance to ciclosporin resulting in an increasing number of several inflammatory cells in the gingival lamina propria and ciclosporin-induced inhibition of prostaglandin I_2 synthesis have also been suggested (74,75).

There are many susceptibility factors for ciclosporin-induced gingival hyperplasia. The duration of treatment and the cumulative dose during the first 6 months play a major role. Accordingly, reduction of the ciclosporin dose can lessen the risk, and the use of lower doses is thought to reduce the overall incidence (76,77). There is also a positive correlation between the degree of gingival hyperplasia and changes in renal function (78). There are conflicting findings regarding the effects of blood concentrations on the incidence of gingival hyperplasia, and no clear relation between saliva and blood ciclosporin concentrations has been found. Lower age correlated significantly with the presence of gingival hyperplasia and children under 6 years of age are more susceptible to the complication in severe form (76,79). Male sex is a predisposing factor, a finding supported by the report of an increased androgen metabolism in gingival hyperplasia induced by ciclosporin (80). There has been also speculation concerning genetic differences in the susceptibility to develop these changes (72) (SEDA-21, 384). Finally, the combination of ciclosporin and nifedipine is additive with an increased prevalence and/or severity of gingival hyperplasia (SED-13, 1127) (76,77,80–82). As several other calcium channel blockers can produce gingival overgrowth, more frequent gingival hyperplasia should be expected, at least theoretically, when these drugs are combined with ciclosporin.

It is not yet clearly established whether bacterial plaque, gingival bleeding index, or inflammation are the cause or result of gingival hyperplasia. Certainly, poor oral health with subsequent local inflammation appears to be a contributing factor. Consequently, careful dental hygiene with plaque control is often sufficient to improve or resolve hyperplasia, but surgical treatment is sometimes necessary. Preliminary case reports have suggested that azithromycin or metronidazole can improve ciclosporin-induced gingival hyperplasia (SEDA-19, 350). This has been confirmed for azithromycin, with no indication that ciclosporin blood concentrations are modified during a short course of azithromycin (SEDA-22, 414).

Gastrointestinal

Gastrointestinal symptoms due to ciclosporin are usually mild and transient. In rheumatoid arthritis, gastrointestinal intolerance has been reported in 50% of patients, being the main cause for withdrawal of ciclosporin in 8% (83). Whereas worsening colitis did not occur in patients with inflammatory bowel disease, ciclosporin was involved in the development of acute colitis in isolated reports (SED-13, 1125).

Liver

There was at least one episode of hepatotoxicity in 228 of 466 patients (49%) with renal transplants who took ciclosporin; 110 (48%) had hyperalbuminemia, 108 (47%) a raised aspartate transaminase, and 167 (59%) a raised alkaline phosphatase (84). Ciclosporin dosage reduction resulted in resolution of hepatotoxicity in 185 patients (81%), while 32 (14%) had recurrent or persistent liver function abnormalities. Eleven (2.4%) developed biliary calculous disease. The serum ciclosporin concentration was high among the patients with hepatotoxicity. Pharmacokinetic studies showed an increased AUC in the patients with hepatotoxicity, probably due to reduced drug clearance.

A causal association has been shown between the hepatotoxicity of ciclosporin and cold ischemic liver damage that can occur during preservation before liver transplantation (85). This presents a problem when ciclosporin is used after liver transplantation. In more than 1000 patients there was an incidence of mild reversible hepatotoxicity of 40% in patients taking 5-fluorouracil and levamisole as adjuvants for more than 1 year; the incidence of mild hepatotoxicity in those taking levamisole alone and amongst those receiving no treatment at all was the same, a little over 16% (86).

Experiments with isolated human hepatocytes have shown that ciclosporin competitively inhibits the uptake of cholate and glycocholate bile acids; the biological features of ciclosporin-associated hepatotoxicity are therefore mostly those of cholestasis, with reduced bile excretion (87). The presence of underlying chronic viral hepatitis can increase the severity of ciclosporin-induced cholestasis (88).

Ciclosporin can cause cholestasis and cellular necrosis by an inhibitory effect on hepatocyte membrane transport proteins at both sinusoidal and canalicular levels. It induces oxidative stress by accumulation of various free radicals. Ademetionine (*S*-adenosylmethionine) is a naturally occurring substance that is involved in liver detoxification processes. The efficacy of ademetionine in the treatment and prevention of ciclosporin-induced cholestasis has been studied in 72 men with psoriasis (89). The patients who were given ciclosporin plus ademetionine had low plasma and erythrocyte concentrations of oxidants and high concentrations of antioxidants. The authors concluded that ademetionine may protect the liver against hepatotoxic substances such as ciclosporin.

A possible consequence of bile acid abnormalities and cholestasis associated with ciclosporin is the development of cholelithiasis in liver transplant patients when the donor has pre-existing susceptibility for cholesterol gallstone formation or abnormalities of bile composition.

- A young patient who received a liver from a 78-year-old donor subsequently developed cholesterol gallstones (SEDA-21, 383).

In a retrospective study in 50 consecutive patients who received both parenteral nutrition and glucocorticoids, with or without the addition of ciclosporin, at some stage in their management, there was no evidence that ciclosporin caused more liver dysfunction than that associated with parenteral nutrition (90).

Urinary tract

The renal toxicity of ciclosporin has been described as being an adverse effect of the drug on the compensatory mechanisms of the kidney, without effects on proximal tubular function (urea and sodium reabsorption) (91). A rise in serum creatinine concentration may be adequate to identify acute-onset ciclosporin nephrotoxicity, but it is not suitable for identification of chronic, late-onset ciclosporin nephrotoxicity (92).

Presentation

Acute renal impairment

Acute ciclosporin-induced nephrotoxicity, causing reduced renal function, develops within the first month, and includes a dose-related rise in serum creatinine concentrations and hyperkalemia. Fatal acute tubular necrosis has also been noted after very high intravenous doses (SEDA-19, 345). Although it is clinically often difficult to differentiate from acute allograft rejection in renal transplant patients, the alteration in renal function promptly resolves on ciclosporin withdrawal or dosage reduction, and initial acute renal insufficiency is not clearly associated with the development of subsequent chronic renal dysfunction (93). Several conditions, such as pre-existing hypovolemia, concomitant diuretic treatment, or renal artery stenosis, are susceptibility factors.

Hypothyroidism was thought to be involved in one patient (94), and the transplanted kidney itself rather than interindividual differences between recipients was thought to play a role (SEDA-21, 384).

Hemolytic–uremic syndrome and thrombotic microangiopathy

Hemolytic–uremic syndrome, with histological findings of thrombotic microangiopathy and possible evolution to graft loss or death, is another instance of very severe acute nephrotoxicity (SED-13, 1125). It usually occurs at between the second and fourth weeks after transplant, with associated fever, thrombocytopenia, erythrocyte fragmentation, neurotoxicity, and renal impairment. Uncommon clinical features have been reported.

- In two women, hemolytic–uremic syndrome was apparently revealed by an episode of severe acute depression (95).
- In another patient, a single injection of ciclosporin may have induced the development of fibrin thrombi seen in the perioperative graft biopsy (96). Later on, she was confirmed to have clinical and biological features of hemolytic–uremic syndrome, which reversed after ciclosporin withdrawal.

Hemolyti–uremic syndrome has also been reported during ciclosporin treatment for Behçet's disease (SEDA-21, 384). Both early and delayed hemolytic–uremic syndrome can occur after transplantation, and its actual incidence may have been underestimated. Thrombotic microangiopathy with clinical features of hemolytic–uremic syndrome was found in 3.5–5% of renal transplant patients (97,98). Graft loss was mostly found in patients who developed hemolytic–uremic syndrome early after transplantation, and the clinical distinction from acute rejection can be very difficult. Hemolytic–uremic syndrome does not recur after initial withdrawal and further ciclosporin reintroduction, once renal function has normalized, or even despite ciclosporin maintenance with dosage reduction (SED-13, 1125) (SEDA-20, 345). In some cases, the patient was successfully switched to tacrolimus, and only one case of hemolytic–uremic syndrome with recurrence on ciclosporin rechallenge has been reported (SEDA-21, 384). In contrast, both ciclosporin and tacrolimus were significant susceptibility factors for recurrence of hemolytic–uremic syndrome in patients who had undergone renal transplantation for end-stage renal disease (99).

The factors that contribute to the development of thrombotic microangiopathy have been retrospectively investigated in 50 of 188 patients with kidney or kidney + pancreas allografts who underwent graft biopsies and in 19 control patients who had never had renal graft dysfunction or a biopsy (100). There were definite histological features of thrombotic microangiopathy 4 days to 6 years after transplantation in 26 patients, of whom 24 were taking ciclosporin and two were taking tacrolimus, showing that this complication can occur at any time after transplantation. Eight patients had graft loss, but only two had associated systemic evidence of microangiopathy, that is thrombocytopenia and intravascular hemolysis, suggesting that thrombotic microangiopathy should be considered in any patients with renal graft dysfunction, even if there are no suggestive systemic symptoms. Although the more frequent use of the microemulsion form of ciclosporin (Neoral) in patients with confirmed thrombotic microangiopathy than in controls suggested a possible role of this formulation, this issue remains to be further investigated, because the number of evaluable patients was small. None of the other investigated variables (age, sex, race, living-related or cadaveric donor status, the degree of HLA mismatch, the type of allograft, or the incidence of urinary tract infections after transplantation) was significantly associated with the occurrence of thrombotic microangiopathy compared with patients without thrombotic microangiopathy. Finally, the most successful strategy was a switch from ciclosporin to tacrolimus, which resulted in normalization of graft function in 81% of these patients.

Chronic renal insufficiency

Chronic renal impairment, as first reported in cardiac transplant patients (101), is of major concern, because of possible irreversible renal dysfunction. A considerable amount of work has subsequently accumulated on the development of progressive renal dysfunction in patients receiving long-term ciclosporin for organ transplantation or chronic inflammatory disease (SED-13, 1125) (SEDA-20, 345) (SEDA-21, 384) (SEDA-22, 413), and there have been several comprehensive reviews (102–105). About one-third of all patients have increased serum creatinine concentrations and reduced glomerular filtration rate during ciclosporin maintenance therapy. The histopathological features of chronic nephropathy consist mostly of non-specific tubular atrophy and interstitial fibrosis (106); arteriolar lesions are considered very suggestive of ciclosporin nephrotoxicity. The prevalence of renal damage due to ciclosporin has fallen considerably since the use of lower doses. Arteriolopathy sometimes improves after reducing or withdrawing ciclosporin. Morphological features in patients with autoimmune diseases are non-specific, and include a wide range of lesions, mostly characterized by tubulointerstitial changes and arteriolopathy. There is no significant correlation between histological findings and ciclosporin dose. Severe histological lesions can be identified in some patients with normal renal function (107); the severity of tubulointerstitial lesions has been deemed to be a better index than the glomerular filtration rate for predicting the occurrence of chronic nephropathy, but in one study there was no correlation between histological renal findings and various measures of renal function (108).

Because the possibility of irreversible renal dysfunction is a major problem in ciclosporin maintenance in both transplant and non-transplant patients, this issue continues to receive attention. Even though many studies have been performed, the long-term prognosis is a source of conflicting opinions, and the initial assumption that long-term use of ciclosporin will sooner or later cause irreversible chronic nephropathy is hotly debated. It is still unclear to what extent long-term ciclosporin contributes to progressive renal insufficiency and whether chronic ciclosporin nephropathy is irreversible or improves after dosage reduction. A retrospective analysis of more than 12 000 renal transplant patients showed that long-term maintenance with a glucocorticoid-free ciclosporin regimen (ciclosporin alone or with azathioprine) significantly increased renal graft and patient survival, compared with patients taking other immunosuppressive regimens (109). This allowed the use of higher doses of ciclosporin without increasing the frequency of nephrotoxicity. In contrast, several investigators have considered a change to a ciclosporin-free regimen in 40% of patients, because of progressive renal deterioration with histological signs of nephrotoxicity (110). The incidence of end-stage renal insufficiency requiring dialysis or renal transplantation ranges from 1% in renal transplant patients to 3–6% in heart-transplant patients (111–114). Nevertheless, several investigators have shown that despite an initial reduction in renal function, serum creatinine concentrations stabilized with no strong evidence of progressive nephropathy after several years of surveillance in various organ transplant patients (93,112,115–117).

The potential long-term consequences of ciclosporin nephrotoxicity constitute a major disadvantage in non-transplant patients. Renal function was assessed 7 years after the end of a 1-year ciclosporin treatment period in 36 young patients from a randomized, placebo-controlled trial of ciclosporin in diabetes mellitus, 19 taking ciclosporin, and 17 taking placebo (118). Blood pressure did not differ between the groups. Compared with baseline values, urinary albumin excretion rate was significantly higher and estimated glomerular filtration rate significantly lower with ciclosporin. The results in the placebo group showed no change or increases. In addition, there was progression to micro- or macro-albuminuria in four patients taking ciclosporin, and two of five patients who underwent renal biopsy had arteriolar hyalinosis. It is not known whether these changes will translate to an increased risk of nephropathy, but they suggest that ciclosporin might enhance it. Of 91 consecutive patients with renal transplants with a minimum graft survival of 1 year who were followed for 7–8 years, 65% had stable renal function despite ciclosporin serum concentrations of 200–250 ng/ml (119). In addition, none of the 26 patients with worsening renal function had features of ciclosporin nephrotoxicity on renal biopsy.

Frequency

In a meta-analysis of 18 trials involving ciclosporin doses below 10 mg/kg/day for at least 2 months in autoimmune diseases, the weighted percentage increase in serum creatinine concentrations was 17% in ciclosporin-treated patients and 1.7% in controls (120). The corrected risk difference for an increase of more than 50% of pretreatment serum creatinine concentrations between the two groups was 21% (95% CI = 12, 30) (120). This meta-analysis did not fully consider the long-term outcome, but clinical and histological evidence of sustained or progressive ciclosporin nephropathy in this population continues to accumulate. Unfortunately, some of the findings are discordant (107,121–130).

In a retrospective study of 106 patients following renal transplantation who had been treated with ciclosporin, 85% were hypertensive compared with 54% of patients taking azathioprine (131). Renal function was significantly better in hypertensive patients treated with nifedipine than with other antihypertensive medication (beta-blockers and vasodilators), and it was similar to that of normotensive patients treated with ciclosporin.

Pathophysiology

The pathogenesis of chronic ciclosporin nephrotoxicity is not fully understood (105). Intrarenal afferent arteriolar vasoconstriction may play an important part, particularly in acute nephrotoxicity (132), in which a marked reduction in renal blood flow associated with an increase in renal vascular resistance, probably due to postglomerular vasoconstriction, has been demonstrated (133,134). The supposed mechanism is primarily an imbalance between several regulatory mechanisms of renal vasodilatation and vasoconstriction, leading to increased renal vasoconstriction, and the explanations that have been proposed include activation of the renin–angiotensin system, prostaglandin inhibition, and sympathetic nervous system activation (135). However, it is unclear whether a continuous increase in renal vascular resistance can account for chronic renal dysfunction in patients taking long-term ciclosporin. There are many possible mediators of renal vasoconstriction, for example nitric oxide, the renin–angiotensin and kallikrein–kinin systems, endothelin-1 release, and stimulation of sympathetic nervous system activity. A major effect of ciclosporin is to promote calcium accumulation in the mitochondrial matrix, which in turn reduces ATP synthesis (136). The main morphological abnormality that has been demonstrated in the kidneys of patients taking long-term ciclosporin is interstitial fibrosis. Vascular lesions, predominantly arteriolar, with arterial intimal fibrosis have been noted in renal biopsies from patients with chronic ciclosporin nephrotoxicity (137).

Renal morphology has been studied in 17 patients who received ciclosporin for sight-threatening uveitis. Most had not received other potentially nephrotoxic drugs. Variable interstitial fibrosis, frequently associated with tubular atrophy, was noted in all 17. The extent of the pathological changes did not correlate with the age, treatment duration, or average cumulative dose (138). Ciclosporin nephrotoxicity mimics the histological features of acute allograft rejection and tubular necrosis. It is important to be able to distinguish clinically between ciclosporin toxicity on the one hand (necessitating a reduction in dose) and rejection (requiring an increase in dose) on the other.

The long-term effects of ciclosporin on renal function in 11 liver transplant recipients were evaluated over a follow-up period of 6–26 months (135). Immediately postoperatively, glomerular filtration rate (GFR) and effective renal plasma flow (ERPF) fell by 60%, subsequently settling at 45–60% of normal. There were additional toxic effects on renal tubular function. Histopathological findings were mild to moderate; notably, arterial and arteriolar nephrosclerosis. Renal function improved as the dose of ciclosporin was reduced, despite continued administration of the drug. This suggests a persistent, potentially reversible, functional component to chronic ciclosporin nephrotoxicity.

The respective roles of organ preservation and ciclosporin in the pathogenesis of post-transplant renal damage have been studied in an in vitro model that simulates the hypothermic kidney preserved before surgery in Collins' solution and exposed after transplantation to ciclosporin (139). The results showed that preservation sensitizes the kidney to ciclosporin injury, which is consistent with clinical experience (140). If the preserved kidney cells were given a period of repair before administration of ciclosporin, further injury did not happen. In animal experiments, prolonged cold preservation causes progressive deterioration in the renal cortical microcirculation; concentration of ciclosporin in the renal cortex of hypoperfused kidneys markedly potentiates the vascular damage caused by cold preservation (131).

Large-scale studies with long periods of follow-up have emphasized the major role of graft arteriopathy (chronic graft rejection) rather than chronic ciclosporin nephrotoxicity as the primary cause of graft failure (111,116,141). Severe ciclosporin nephropathy was the cause of renal transplant failure in less than 1% of patients.

Susceptibility factors and prediction

Many factors have been postulated as being relevant to ciclosporin nephrotoxicity. Whereas in several studies initial high doses of ciclosporin increased the risk of chronic nephrotoxicity (115,121), others suggested that patients maintained on relatively high ciclosporin concentrations had no more chance than others of developing toxic nephropathy (116). Neither the daily dose nor the duration of ciclosporin treatment reasonably predicts the risk of chronic renal insufficiency. Chronic renal dysfunction can be observed, despite the maintenance of ciclosporin blood concentrations below 400 ng/ml. However, age, sustained hypertension, hypertriglyceridemia, low HDL cholesterol concentrations, and recurrent episodes of severe acute nephrotoxicity increase susceptibility to chronic ciclosporin nephrotoxicity (122,142).

From a prospective study in 36 heart transplant patients with stable renal function for at least 6 months after transplantation, it was suggested that high urinary retinol-binding protein concentrations may indicate tubulointerstitial damage and therefore detect patients who are at risk of ciclosporin nephrotoxicity (143). At the start of the study, 13 patients had high urinary retinol-binding protein concentrations and 23 had normal concentrations. After 5 years of follow-up, five of the 13 patients developed end-stage renal insufficiency requiring dialysis, whereas none of the 23 other patients had terminal renal insufficiency. Although these data await confirmation, the authors suggested that ciclosporin dosage reduction should be considered in patients with high urinary retinol-binding protein concentrations, in order to limit renal damage.

Ciclosporin can cause tubulointerstitial lesions, the pathogenesis of which is unclear. In 37 patients, the duration of ciclosporin treatment and of heavy proteinuria were independent risk factors for ciclosporin-induced tubulointerstitial disease (144).

Management

The possible risk of precipitating end-stage renal insufficiency should not be regarded as a major limitation to ciclosporin treatment in organ-transplant patients, and no matter how defective our knowledge of the susceptibility factors is, attempts must be made to prevent or manage ciclosporin nephrotoxicity. Delaying the introduction of ciclosporin until post-transplant renal function has returned to normal and reducing the dose of ciclosporin when increases in serum creatinine concentrations are more than 30% above baseline values are measures that may well reduce the risk of acute nephrotoxicity. In the long term, switching patients from ciclosporin to azathioprine, reducing ciclosporin doses, or even electively withdrawing ciclosporin have been suggested as helpful measures, but they should be regarded cautiously and set against the risk of rejection (145–149). Once-daily dosing of ciclosporin in the morning improves glomerular filtration rate and renal blood flow compared with half the dose taken twice daily (150). Despite evidence for a very similar profile of nephrotoxicity, conversion from ciclosporin to tacrolimus has been used successfully (SEDA-20, 347).

Finally, several drugs have been investigated in experimental and clinical studies to prevent ciclosporin nephrotoxicity. Calcium channel blockers, such as nifedipine, diltiazem, or verapamil, have repeatedly been proposed as reliable adjunctive drugs to minimize the long-term nephrotoxic effects of ciclosporin in renal transplant patients. Among anti-ischemic drugs, trimetazidine might be a good choice, because it prevents the loss of ATP synthesis caused by ciclosporin in rat kidney cells. S-15176 and S-16950 are trimetazidine derivatives that antagonize the mitochondrial toxicity of ciclosporin without changing its immunosuppressive effects.

Viewing the evidence as a whole, it appears that the use of lower doses of ciclosporin is probably the most important factor accounting for the fact that the majority of patients on long-term ciclosporin do not today have evidence of progressive nephrotoxicity.

Skin

Mild flushing often occurs during ciclosporin treatment, but more severe extensive erythema is uncommon.

- Recurrent episodes of diffuse flushing of the arms, the face, and the trunk reportedly occurred about 2 hours after each dose of ciclosporin in a 24-year-old man who had received a renal transplant 6 years before (151). These episodes were noted from the beginning of treatment, but worsened after he changed to Neoral, the microemulsion form of ciclosporin, and completely resolved after ciclosporin was replaced by tacrolimus.

Ciclosporin sometimes causes chronic inflammatory dermatitis, and there have been two reports of four male transplant recipients who developed clinical and histopathological features of keloid acne of the posterior scalp or neck (152,153). *Staphylococcus aureus* infection was identified in three. Ciclosporin-induced hypertrichosis was suggested as a possible cause, with local bacterial infection and immunosuppression as trigger factors.

- Multiple, large epidermoid cysts have been described in a 23-year-old man taking ciclosporin (154).

Acute generalized pustular psoriasis occurred 1 week after ciclosporin withdrawal in a 32-year-old woman who had taken ciclosporin for 12 weeks for chronic plaque psoriasis (155). This is in keeping with a similar phenomenon sometimes observed after glucocorticoid withdrawal.

Coarsening of facial features and a possibly more frequent occurrence of acne vulgaris and keratosis pilaris have been described in children taking ciclosporin (SED-8, 1125) (156). In 19 children who took ciclosporin and prednisone after renal transplantion, there was coarsening of facial features with thickening of the nares, lips, and ears, puffiness of the cheeks, prominence of the supraorbital ridges, and mandibular prognathism; this was found in all the children who had been treated for 6 months (157). Although the concurrent use of glucocorticoids may play a role in the development of acne, resolution of severe acne was in one reported case attained only after ciclosporin withdrawal (SEDA-20, 345). Convincing but anecdotal evidence of the worsening of subcutaneous sarcoidosis has been reported (SEDA-22, 384).

Sebaceous glands

Juxtaclavicular beaded lines are unique malformation of sebaceous glands or a variant of sebaceous hyperplasia.

- A 63-year-old man developed small, asymptomatic, linear papules over the neck and clavicles. He had taken prednisone and ciclosporin for 30 months after kidney transplantation (158). A skin biopsy showed sebaceous hyperplasia.

The pathogenesis of juxtaclavicular beaded lines is unclear. Some authors have reported a prevalence of 16% in heart transplant patients, but only in men. Because ciclosporin is highly lipophilic, it has many adverse effects associated with alterations of pilosebaceous follicles, such as hypertrichosis and acne. In this case the authors postulated that the combined effect of prednisone and ciclosporin may have induced sebaceous gland hyperplasia.

Hair

Widespread hypertrichosis is one of the most common complications of ciclosporin, and distichiasis (accessory eyelashes) has been reported in one patient (SEDA-20, 345). Ciclosporin-associated soft tissue proliferation with an abnormal hyperplastic reaction has been suggested to account for the development of hyperplastic pseudofolliculitis barbae (159).

Alopecia areata or alopecia totalis has been noted in isolated cases (SEDA-21, 384).

A white-headed man noted progressive darkening of the hair while taking ciclosporin (160).

Nails

Several nail changes (excess granulation tissue or ingrowing toenails) have been attributed to ciclosporin (SED-13, 1127).

- Marked pitting with Mees' lines (homogeneous transverse white lines in the nail plates) in the fingernails, a disorder that has not been previously reported, was attributed to ciclosporin-associated kidney dysfunction in a 41-year-old man who inadvertently took ciclosporin 300 mg/day for psoriasis (161).

Musculoskeletal

Muscle disorders attributed to ciclosporin have been mostly described in anecdotal case reports (SED-14, 1291). In an analysis of published or spontaneous case reports, the manufacturers found 29 cases of muscle disorders in patients taking ciclosporin; the complications fell into two categories (162). Myopathic symptoms, that is myalgia and muscle weakness without rhabdomyolysis, were reported in 0.17% of patients and abated after dose reduction or treatment withdrawal. Rhabdomyolysis occurred in under 0.05% of patients and was mostly observed in patients taking other drugs, such as lovastatin or colchicine.

This topic has been re-analysed in a systematic review of published papers, in which relevant information from a total of 34 patients was identified (163). All but two patients were also taking concomitant drugs known to affect the muscles, among which glucocorticoids, simvastatin, lovastatin, colchicine, and pyrazinamide were the most frequently cited. Ciclosporin is therefore difficult to implicate in most patients, but at least one case with positive ciclosporin re-administration supported a causative role. The clinical picture was non-specific, with myalgia, cramps, and muscle weakness, sometimes associated with raised serum creatine kinase activity, and heterogeneous histopathology. Finally, skeletal muscle abnormalities have rarely been described in patients without muscle symptoms.

Ciclosporin is increasingly cited as a possible cause of severe bone and joint pain (164). Acute bilateral deep bone pain, mostly involving the legs, has been retrospectively identified in 19% of patients taking ciclosporin, with the highest prevalence in renal transplant recipients (165). In addition, about half of the patients with osteonecrosis had a history of episodic bone pains. Another study showed features of acute bone marrow edema on MRI in six patients who had bone pain, including one patient who further developed avascular necrosis (SEDA-21, 385). Calcium channel blockers dramatically improved bone pain in prospectively evaluated transplant patients, suggesting a possible vascular etiology (165).

Osteopenia is another potential adverse effect after renal transplantation, but the possible contribution of ciclosporin to bone loss and subsequent osteoporosis is controversial (SEDA-19, 350) (SEDA-20, 345). Moreover, ciclosporin did not appear to have a negative influence on post-transplantation growth in prepubertal children (166).

Both ciclosporin and tacrolimus cause increased bone turnover and significant reductions in bone mass, more marked with tacrolimus (FK506). As most transplantation regimens include glucocorticoids, the individual effects of ciclosporin and tacrolimus are uncertain. As tacrolimus is the more potent immunosuppressant, theoretically, its use after transplantation should allow reduction in glucocorticoid doses, which would be associated with higher bone mineral density. Preliminary data suggest that there is a lower rate of vertebral fractures in patients taking tacrolimus compared with those taking ciclosporin. In 18 men who underwent liver transplantation and took ciclosporin and seven patients who took tacrolimus, bone mineral density in the lumbar spine and proximal femur was prospectively measured before and at 6, 12, and 24 months after transplantation (167). Serum concentrations of parathyroid hormone and 25-hydroxycolecalciferol were determined at the same time. Although the two groups had the same pattern of rapid early bone loss, tacrolimus was associated with lower doses of glucocorticoids and a trend to faster lumbar bone mass recovery. This may have a favorable effect on long-term bone mass evolution, especially in the femoral neck.

Reproductive system

Benign mammary hyperplasia occurs in 0.7% of women taking ciclosporin (168). The mechanism is poorly understood, but it may be related to trophic effects in the breast through ciclosporin receptors on fibroblasts (169), to an effect of ciclosporin on the hypothalamic-pituitary axis (170), or to antagonism at prolactin receptor sites on B and T (171,172).

Immunologic

Anaphylactoid reactions can occur with intravenous ciclosporin, sometimes after the first dose. Reported symptoms included pruritic rash, respiratory symptoms, chest pain, and, rarely, cardiopulmonary arrest. The presence of Cremophor EL, polyoxyethylated castor oil used as a solvent, is likely to account for this life-threatening reaction. The mechanism is still unclear, and results of skin tests were available in only three of 22 previously published patients.

In a report of an anaphylactic reaction, positive intradermal tests suggested a possible IgE-mediated reaction, most probably directed against Cremophor EL, as the patient subsequently tolerated the corn-oil-based soft gelatin formulation (173).

During a Phase I/II trial of high-dose intravenous ciclosporin, there was a high incidence of anaphylactoid reactions associated with improper mixing during preparation of the infusions, perhaps due to large initial bolus infusions of the vehicle, Cremophor EL (174).

Infection risk

Infections, in particular bacterial and viral (cytomegalovirus, *Herpes simplex* virus, Epstein–Barr virus), and also protozoal and fungal infections, are major causes of morbidity and mortality after transplantation, whatever the immunosuppressive regimen used (175–177). Based on an analysis of medical and autopsy records, infections were found to be the cause of death in 70% of transplant patients, with bacteria (50%) or fungi (29%) the most common pathogens (178).

Body temperature

Recurrent episodes of fever, which disappeared after ciclosporin withdrawal, have only been reported in one patient (SEDA-22, 414).

Long-Term Effects

Mutagenicity

An increase in chromosomal abnormalities correlated with serum ciclosporin concentrations in one study (179).

Tumorigenicity

Because of the varied indications for azathioprine and mercaptopurine, it is difficult to determine whether there is an increased incidence of cancer specifically related to prolonged drug exposure. Data from the Cincinnati Transplant Tumor Registry, published in 1993, helped to define comprehensively the characteristics of neoplasms observed in organ transplant recipients (180). Skin and lip cancers were the most common, and non-Hodgkin's lymphomas represent the majority of lymphoproliferative disorders, with an incidence some 30- to 50-fold higher than in controls. There is also an excess of Kaposi's sarcomas (181), carcinomas of the vulva and perineum, hepatobiliary tumors, various sarcomas, and renal cell carcinomas (182–184). In one case, complete regression of Kaposi's sarcoma followed withdrawal of ciclosporin (185). In contrast, the incidence of common neoplasms encountered in the general population is not increased. In renal transplant patients, the actuarial cumulative risk of cancer was 14–18% at 10 years and 40–50% at 20 years (186,187). Skin cancers accounted for about half of the cases. Very similar figures were found in later studies (SEDA-20, 341).

In patients with transplanted organs ciclosporin is associated with a small but significant risk of Epstein–Barr virus-associated lymphoproliferative disorders.

- A 39-year-old man with atopic eczema was given ciclosporin for an exacerbation, which responded well (188). After 2 years he developed a large ulcerated erythematous nodule, a CD30+ lymphoma of the skin. Ciclosporin was withdrawn and the lesion resolved within 2 months.

Of all transplant-related lymphomas 15% are of T cell origin and are unrelated to Epstein–Barr virus infection. Cutaneous T cell lymphomas are rare and carry a good prognosis, with a 90%, 4-year survival rate. Regression is often observed when immunosuppression is withdrawn or reduced.

While there is no doubt that the incidence of malignancies is increased in the transplant population, there has been controversy as to which factors (namely duration of treatment, total dosage, the degree of immunosuppression, or the type of immunosuppressive regimens) are the most relevant in determining risk. Partial or complete regression of lymphoproliferative disorders and Kaposi's sarcomas after reduction of immunosuppressive therapy argues strongly for the role of the degree of immunosuppression (180). The incidence of cancer was also significantly higher in renal transplant patients taking triple therapy regimens compared with dual therapy (189). Similarly, aggressive immunosuppressive therapy may account for the higher incidence of lymphomas in patients with cardiac versus renal allografts.

In a large, multicenter study in more than 52 000 kidney or heart transplant patients between 1983 and 1991, the rate of non-Hodgkin's lymphomas in the first post-transplantation year was 0.2% in kidney and 1.2% in heart recipients, and fell substantially thereafter

(190). Initial immunosuppression with azathioprine and ciclosporin, and prophylactic treatment with antilymphocyte antibodies or muromonab was associated with a significantly increased incidence of non-Hodgkin's lymphomas compared with other immunosuppressive regimens, which confirmed the major role of the level of immunosuppression. Later studies confirmed that immunosuppression per se rather than a single agent is responsible for the increased risk of cancer (SEDA-20, 340). Finally, the most striking difference between conventional and modern immunosuppressive regimens, including ciclosporin, was the average time to the appearance of tumors, in particular skin cancers and lymphomas, which was shorter in ciclosporin-treated patients (191,192).

Multiple factors with complex interactions are involved in the observed pattern and increased incidence of neoplasms. They include severely depressed immunity with an impaired immune surveillance against various carcinogens, the activation of several oncogenic viruses, and a possible mutagenic effect of the drugs. Viruses, such as papillomavirus, cytomegalovirus, and Epstein–Barr virus, are believed to play an important role in the development of several post-transplant cancers. From a theoretical point of view, the use of antiviral drugs active against herpes viruses which are commonly implicated as co-factors can be expected to produce a reduction in the incidence of post-transplant lymphoproliferative disorders.

In an in vitro and in vivo experiment, ciclosporin promoted tumor growth by a direct cellular effect (193). This was suggested to be due to increased synthesis of transforming growth factor beta (TGF beta); anti-TGF beta antibodies blocked the increased spread of cancer cells. The clinical relevance of these data awaits further careful clinical confirmation. Continuing analysis of clinical experience has not provided clear evidence for a ciclosporin-specific effect and has instead supported an immunosuppressive effect (194).

Fibroadenomata are the most common solid breast masses in young women. Between 1997 and 2000, five women who had had transplant surgery and who were taking ciclosporin developed new breast masses, which were histologically confirmed to be fibroadenomata (195).

Ciclosporin-associated soft tissue proliferation with an abnormal hyperplastic reaction has been suggested to account for the development of eruptive angiomatosis (196).

Second-Generation Effects

Pregnancy

Pregnancies in women who took ciclosporin resulted in live neonates in 68%; half were premature while the other half were of low birth weights (197). Reduced renal graft function during pregnancy was associated with greater risks of neonates of lower birth weights and graft loss. In another study, a ciclosporin-based regimen was associated with more frequent miscarriage, preterm birth and intrauterine growth retardation, compared with previous experience (198).

It has been suggested that ciclosporin is more likely to induce maternal renal dysfunction or pre-eclampsia than tacrolimus, but this view was based on a comparison involving only a small number of patients (SEDA-22, 414).

Teratogenicity

Maternal azathioprine treatment during pregnancy is clearly teratogenic in animals, but the mechanisms are not known. A large number of reports have described the outcome of pregnancies following the use of immunosuppressant drugs, in particular in renal transplant patients, and hundreds of pregnancies have been analysed (199). The largest experience is that derived from the National Transplantation Pregnancy Registry which has been built up in the USA since 1991 (200). This registry has accumulated data on more than 900 pregnancies, of which 83% followed kidney transplantation and in this and other studies there was no difference in the rate of malformations when comparing ciclosporin with other immunosuppressive regimens (197,198,201). Ectopic pregnancies and miscarriages seemed to occur at a similar rate as in the general population. The most common complications were frequent prematurity and more frequent intrauterine growth retardation with low birthweight. Risk factors associated with adverse pregnancy outcomes included a short time interval between transplantation and pregnancy (that is less than 1–2 years), graft dysfunction before or during pregnancy, and hypertension (202).

There have been no reports that physical and mental development or renal function are altered. In one study, there were changes in T lymphocyte development in seven children born to mothers who had taken azathioprine or ciclosporin, but immune function assays were normal (203). Thus, development of the fetal immune system is not affected by ciclosporin (204).

Renal function in 14 children born to women with transplants treated throughout pregnancy with a ciclosporin-based regimen has been extensively investigated at a mean of 2.6 years after delivery (205). No renal function abnormalities were found. In particular, glomerular filtration rate was within the reference range. Renal function was found to be normal in 22 children evaluated after a mean of 39 months after birth (206), and no adverse effects on the immune function were identified in the few infants examined in this respect (203).

In a meta-analysis of the effects of exposure to ciclosporin during pregnancy, 15 studies (total 410 patients; 6 studies with control groups who were not given ciclosporin) met inclusion criteria for malformations, 10 for preterm delivery, and five for low birth weight (207). Ciclosporin did not appear to be a major human teratogen, but was associated with increased rates of prematurity.

Lactation

Ciclosporin is excreted into human breast milk and because of potential immunosuppression, breastfeeding is usually regarded as contraindicated. Reassuring reports are now however available (SEDA-21, 385). After follow-up for 12–36 months in seven breast-fed infants (duration 4–12 months) whose mothers were treated with ciclosporin, none of them experienced renal or other long-term adverse consequences (208). Although ciclosporin concentrations measured in breast milk from six mothers were close to those measured in blood samples, it was calculated that the infants ingested less than 300 μg/day, and ciclosporin was not detectable in random blood samples.

Drug Administration

Drug formulations

In an attempt to overcome the poor and unpredictable absorption of the standard oral formulation, a microemulsion-based formulation (Neoral) has been developed. The benefit-to-harm balance of conversion from the standard to the microemulsion formulation have been discussed at length and guidelines for conversion have been proposed (209).

From the results of a retrospective study of 227 liver transplant patients who took Neoral as the primary immunosuppressant, it was suggested that this formulation may reduce the risk of severe neurotoxicity (210). Mild-to-moderate symptoms, that is headache ($n = 24$), mild hand tremor ($n = 13$), and paresthesia ($n = 5$), were the most frequent, whereas generalized seizures were reported in only two patients.

In one large study in 1097 patients, there was a significantly higher incidence of neurological complications, gastrointestinal disturbances, and increased serum creatinine concentrations during the first month of treatment with Neoral, compared with conventional ciclosporin (211). However, a meta-analysis showed that the adverse events profile was similar with the two formulations, while primary immunosuppression with Neoral produced significant benefit in terms of a lower incidence of rejection (212). In particular, in liver transplant patients treated with Neoral from the start, the incidence of adverse events was halved. All the same, because dosage adjustments were often required and often hazardous, owing to the risk of adverse effects and transplant rejection, other investigators concluded that switching to Neoral may be of little benefit, at least in previously stable liver transplant patients (213).

As the data from this meta-analysis were subject to many potential biases, the same authors reanalysed their results, taking into account only randomized, prospective studies (214). The incidence of adverse effects was higher with Sandimmune in open-label studies (840 patients) and higher with Neoral in blinded studies (3006 patients). In accordance with other investigators, these authors concluded that de novo immunosuppression with Neoral is beneficial, without significant differences in the incidence of adverse effects, whereas conversion from Sandimmune to Neoral in previously stable patients is associated with significantly more adverse effects with Neoral.

Drug dosage regimens

Several authors were unable to find convincing evidence that ciclosporin specifically increases the risk of tumors in transplant patients compared with previously used immunosuppressive regimens, and some even suggested a possibly lower incidence in ciclosporin-treated patients (191,192,215). However, in analyses from Japan and France (3454 patients), the average time that elapsed until the occurrence of cancer was significantly shorter in patients treated with ciclosporin compared with those taking conventional immunosuppressive treatment, that is 43–452 months versus 92–96 months (216,217). In addition, French authors found a higher cumulative risk of cancer after 10 years in ciclosporin-treated patients (14 versus 8.4%), and this was mostly due to an increased incidence of skin carcinomas (216). Other significant risk factors included age, a shorter duration of pretransplant dialysis and the combination with azathioprine treatment. The occurrence of cancer in ciclosporin-treated patients is thought to be dose-related, and one study found a significantly higher frequency of cancer in the normal than in the low-dose group (218). These positive findings were limited by the more frequent occurrence of acute rejection in the low-dose group.

Long-term ciclosporin also carries the risk of malignancies in non-transplant patients, and the overall incidence of lymphoma was estimated to be 0.14% among 3700 patients treated for autoimmune disease (219). However, the available studies are again conflicting. They are mostly based on a limited number of patients or a short duration of follow-up. Patients with rheumatoid arthritis receiving ciclosporin had an increased relative risk of malignancies compared with those given glucocorticoids, but it was similar to the risk in patients treated with disease-modifying antirheumatic drugs (220). Another study showed no increased risk of malignancies in ciclosporin-treated patients compared with controls who had never received ciclosporin (221). The spontaneous occurrence of cancers unrelated to the treatment cannot be excluded, and an increased risk of lymphomas has been repeatedly found in patients with rheumatoid arthritis. In patients with psoriasis and as compared to the expected incidence rate of cancer in this population, the relative risk of malignancies was 5.6 (95% CI = 3.9, 8.0) in a cohort of 1223 ciclosporin-treated patients (222). This was comparable to the increased risk of cancer in patients treated with other immunosuppressants.

Drug overdose

Experience with ciclosporin overdose has been reviewed by the manufacturers using published data or cases spontaneously reported (223). Accidental overdose was the most common, with doses of 20–400 mg/kg. In adults, no serious clinical consequences were observed with doses up to 100 mg/kg, and there were only minor clinical or biological effects (transient hypertension, tachycardia, headache, gastrointestinal symptoms, or slight increases in serum creatinine concentrations). However, life-threatening reactions occurred in three neonates, of whom one died after severe metabolic acidosis and renal insufficiency. Subchronic ciclosporin overdose over 8 days did not appear to cause any additional risk (224).

Taken together, the available data suggest that the acute toxicity of ciclosporin is low in adults, but that more severe intoxication could be expected in neonates. However, two reports, including one fatal case, have shown that accidental intoxication sometimes produces severe complications in adults (225,226).

- A 29-year-old man received a double lung transplantation for end-stage cystic fibrosis. After uneventful surgery, he was accidentally given ten times the intended dose of ciclosporin (30 instead of 3 mg/kg) and 18 hours later became anuric. His blood ciclosporin concentration was 4100 ng/ml. Hemodialysis was required for 6 weeks. A renal biopsy 7 weeks later showed typical features of acute tubular necrosis and lesions that resembled chronic nephrotoxicity. Renal function was still abnormal when he died from another cause 14 weeks after the accidental overdose.
- A 51-year-old man underwent double lung transplantation for pulmonary fibrosis, accidentally received an infusion of ciclosporin 30 mg/hour instead of 3 mg/hour, and 3 hours later had bilateral reactive mydriasis and absence of tendon reflexes. A CT brain scan showed diffuse cerebral edema, and massive intracranial hypertension rapidly developed. He died 5 hours later from brainstem compression, and pathological examination showed diffuse cerebral edema with neuronal necrosis.

The first of these cases suggested that acute renal dysfunction secondary to acute overdose can lead to renal sequelae. In the second patient, an isolated neurotoxic effect of ciclosporin was suggested because no predisposing factor except overdose was identified.

Drug–Drug Interactions

Acetazolamide

The interaction of ciclosporin with acetazolamide was previously supported by a single case report only. In three further patients, the addition of acetazolamide produced a near seven-fold increase in ciclosporin blood concentrations within 3 days (227).

Aciclovir

In an analysis of changes in ciclosporin clearance and systemic availability obtained from the medical records of 100 transplant patients, aciclovir altered ciclosporin pharmacokinetics (228).

The coadministration of ciclosporin with drugs with nephrotoxic effects carries a risk of increased renal dysfunction. Although a possible enhancement of nephrotoxicity has been suggested in patients also taking aciclovir (229), there were no such findings in a retrospective analysis of a double-blind study (230).

Aminoglycoside antibiotics

Severe nephrotoxicity has been reported in three renal transplant patients who received ciclosporin and gentamicin, and in others receiving both drugs before surgical procedures, even though toxic serum concentrations of either drug were not reached (231).

Angiotensin receptor blockers

In an analysis of changes in ciclosporin clearance and systemic availability obtained from the medical records of 100 transplant patients, losartan and valsartan altered ciclosporin pharmacokinetics (228).

Bisphosphonates

In an analysis of changes in ciclosporin clearance and systemic availability obtained from the medical records of 100 transplant patients, alendronic acid altered ciclosporin pharmacokinetics (228).

Calcium channel blockers

A large amount of data has accumulated on the effects of various calcium channel blockers on ciclosporin metabolism or a possible renal protective effect. Diltiazem, nicardipine, or verapamil inhibit ciclosporin metabolism, and this has been investigated as a potential beneficial combination for ciclosporin-sparing effects, particularly for diltiazem or verapamil (232,233). Any change in the formulation of calcium channel blockers in patients previously stabilized should be undertaken cautiously because unpredictable changes in ciclosporin concentrations can occur (234). In contrast, nifedipine, isradipine, or felodipine do not significantly affect ciclosporin pharmacokinetics (SED-13, 1129). Results obtained with amlodipine are conflicting; some studies have shown no effect, while others indicate an increase of up to 40% in ciclosporin blood concentrations (SEDA-19, 351) (SEDA-20, 345). Co-administration of calcium channel blockers is also regarded as a valuable option in the treatment of ciclosporin-induced hypertension, or to prevent ciclosporin nephrotoxicity.

There are conflicting results from studies on the protective role of calcium channel blockers in patients taking ciclosporin in regard to blood pressure and preservation of renal graft function. In a multicenter, randomized, placebo-controlled study in 131 de novo recipients of cadaveric renal allografts, lacidipine improved graft function from 1 year onwards, but had no effect on acute rejection rate, trough blood ciclosporin concentrations, blood pressure, number of antihypertensive drugs, hospitalization rate, or rate of adverse events (235).

The combination of ciclosporin with nifedipine produces an additive on gingival hyperplasia, with an increased prevalence and/or severity (SED-13, 1127) in both children (77,81) and adults (76,80,82). In contrast, verapamil had no significant additional effects on the prevalence or severity of ciclosporin-induced gingival overgrowth (SEDA-21, 385).

Chloramphenicol

Chloramphenicol was suspected of causing a dramatic increase in ciclosporin blood concentrations in a single patient (236). However, multiple concomitant confounding factors made this interaction purely speculative.

Clindamycin

In two lung-transplant patients aged 39 and 48 years, blood ciclosporin concentrations fell after the addition of oral clindamycin (1.8 g/day), and both patients required temporary increases in daily ciclosporin dose until clindamycin withdrawal (237).

Colchicine

The combination of colchicine with ciclosporin increased the risk of myopathy. In a retrospective study of 221 renal transplant patients, five of 10 patients who took both drugs developed acute or chronic proximal myopathy, whereas none of the 30 controls matched for age, sex, transplant duration, ciclosporin use, and cumulative dose of glucocorticoids had similar symptoms (238).

Cytotoxic drugs

High-dose chemotherapy with cyclophosphamide, vincristine, prednisolone, and intrathecal methotrexate given for post-transplant lymphoproliferative disease was suggested to have favored the occurrence of acute ciclosporin neurotoxicity (headache, fever, seizures, and visual agnosia) in a 9-year-old cardiac transplant patient (239). Ciclosporin serum concentrations were normal and a further similar episode occurred on ciclosporin readministration.

In 27 patients, ciclosporin caused a marked increase in the AUC of idarubicin and its main metabolite idarubicinol, perhaps due to inhibition of the multidrug transporter P-glycoprotein (240).

There was a dramatic increase in the systemic availability of paclitaxel when ciclosporin was administered concomitantly (241) and in a phase I study of the pharmacokinetics of twice-daily oral paclitaxel 60–160 mg/m^2 in 15 patients in combination with ciclosporin (15 mg/kg) there was a seven-fold increase in the systemic exposure to paclitaxel; the plasma concentration increased from negligible to therapeutic concentrations (242). The inhibitory effect of ciclosporin on the gastrointestinal multidrug transporter P-glycoprotein was suggested to account for these interactions.

Several studies have shown that ciclosporin reduces the clearance or increases the AUC of dactinomycin, etoposide, mitoxantrone, and vincristine (5,243).

Digoxin

In an analysis of changes in ciclosporin clearance and systemic availability obtained from the medical records of 100 transplant patients, digoxin increased ciclosporin systemic availability (228).

Doxorubicin

High-dose ciclosporin increased the AUC of doxorubicin and doxorubicinol and produced greater doxorubicin-related myelotoxicity (244).

Fibrates

A possible synergistic risk of muscle disorders should be considered in patients taking ciclosporin with fibric acid derivatives (SEDA-19, 351).

Fluoroquinolones

Although ciprofloxacin was initially thought to increase ciclosporin blood concentrations and enhance ciclosporin nephrotoxicity, no definite evidence to support this interaction has been found (245). A norfloxacin-induced increase in ciclosporin blood concentrations has been reported in children (5,246), while ofloxacin did not appear to alter ciclosporin metabolism (247).

Foscarnet

Foscarnet (248), but not ganciclovir (249), has also been involved in reversible renal insufficiency after concomitant use with ciclosporin.

Grapefruit juice

Following the observation that grapefruit juice ingestion can increase the systemic bioavailability of ciclosporin, there was considerable interest in its possible use to reduce ciclosporin doses (SEDA-19, 351). However, this has been strongly criticized and considered hazardous because of large interindividual variability and the commercial availability of different formulations of grapefruit juice with potentially different effects on ciclosporin pharmacokinetics (250).

Histamine H_2 receptor antagonists

The available data on a possible interaction between histamine H_2 receptor antagonists and ciclosporin are inconclusive. Whereas neither cimetidine nor ranitidine significantly altered ciclosporin pharmacokinetics, there was an increase in serum creatinine concentration in patients taking both ciclosporin and cimetidine, but not ranitidine. The clinical significance of this interaction is probably limited, and it has been attributed to competition of cimetidine with creatinine for tubular secretion (251).

HMG-CoA reductase inhibitors

Dosages of statins should be reduced in patients taking ciclosporin, because of pharmacodynamic and pharmacokinetic interactions.

Pharmacodynamic interactions

Patients taking ciclosporin with conventional dosages of lovastatin or simvastatin can develop acute muscle toxicity (SED-14, 1296) (SEDA-19, 351). Among 110 ciclosporin-treated patients with heart transplants, four of 18 patients taking simvastatin 20 mg/day developed rhabdomyolysis, whereas none of the patients taking simvastatin 10 mg/day (26 patients) or pravastatin 20 mg/day (66 patients) had similar symptoms (252). Inhibition of CYP3A by ciclosporin was the most likely mechanism. In another study, there was a five-fold higher AUC of lovastatin (10 mg/day for 10 days) in 16 patients taking ciclosporin compared with 13 patients not taking ciclosporin (253).

- The addition of atorvastatin (10 mg/day) to a multidrug regimen including ciclosporin in a 40-year-old patient with a renal transplant resulted in rhabdomyolysis within 2 months (254).

Similar interactions are expected with other HMG-CoA reductase inhibitors such as cerivastatin and rosuvastatin.

Pharmacokinetic interactions

Plasma concentrations of lovastatin- or simvastatin-active metabolites were increased in several patients and in a pharmacokinetic study, suggesting that ciclosporin can inhibit their metabolism (255–257). Lower doses of lovastatin and simvastatin can be safely administered (258). Fluvastatin or pravastatin may offer some advantages, as no significant drug interactions have been documented with ciclosporin, at least for pravastatin (259).

From an analysis of changes in ciclosporin clearance and systemic availability obtained from the medical records of 100 transplant patients, atorvastatin, fluvastatin, pravastatin, and simvastatin were found to affect ciclosporin pharmacokinetics (228).

In a study of the safety and efficacy of simvastatin in hyperlipidemia after renal transplantation in 15 patients, the C_{max} and AUC of simvastatin were increased seven-fold by ciclosporin (260). In contrast, in 17 patients, tacrolimus had no effect. Although there were no complications, such as myopathy or rhabdomyolysis, creatine kinase activity must be monitored during co-administration of simvastatin and ciclosporin.

Ciclosporin produced a three- to five-fold increase in the plasma concentrations of cerivastatin and its metabolites in 12 patients with renal transplants who took cerivastatin 0.2 mg/day for 7 days compared with a single dose in 12 healthy controls (261).

Hypericum perforatum (St. John's wort)

Hypericum perforatum (St. John's wort), which is used for mild depression, is an inducer of cytochrome P-450. It caused a rapid dramatic fall in ciclosporin blood concentrations, resulting in acute heart transplant rejection in two patients aged 61 and 63 years (262). It produces an average 50% reduction in ciclosporin blood concentrations (263). At least three other case reports have clearly confirmed that St. John's wort is dangerous in transplant patients, because it produced a rapid and dramatic reduction in blood ciclosporin concentration and resulted in acute organ rejection in two patients (264–266). Induction of CYP3A4 and/or P-glycoprotein was the most likely mechanism.

- A 44-year-old black woman with a living-related renal transplant had an acute rejection within 3 months and was given muromonab but was from then on stable. She was later given oral ciclosporin (Neoral 2 mg/kg bd), mycophenolate mofetil 1000 mg bd, and prednisolone 7.5 mg/day. Over 6 months her ciclosporin blood concentrations were consistently below the target concentration of 200 ng/ml. It was then discovered that she had also been taking 2–3 tablets/day of St. John's wort (Your Life, Leiner Health Products, Carson CA, 300 mg standardized to 0.3% hypericin). The St. John's wort was withdrawn and her blood ciclosporin concentrations reached the target within 2 weeks.
- A 29-year-old white woman with cadaveric kidney and pancreas transplants had two early rejection episodes but then stabilized on ciclosporin 100 mg bd and prednisolone 5 mg/day. Her blood ciclosporin concentration was consistently 200–350 ng/ml. She then started to take St. John's wort and over the next 30 days her blood ciclosporin concentration fell to 155 ng/ml and 3 weeks later to 97 ng/ml. Her serum creatinine rose to 1.3 mg/dl (115 μmol/l) and her serum amylase rose from a baseline of 60–90 to 314 U/l; this was associated with abdominal pain. Renal biopsy confirmed acute rejection, which was treated. She subsequently developed chronic rejection, confirmed by renal biopsy.

Imidazoles

Among the imidazole derivatives, numerous case reports or studies have shown that ketoconazole, fluconazole, and itraconazole can inhibit ciclosporin metabolism and increase blood ciclosporin concentrations (267). Ketoconazole, which is undoubtedly the most potent inhibitor, has been used to reduce the dose, and therefore the cost or adverse effects, of ciclosporin (268–270). There was also a beneficial effect on the rate of rejection or infection. In contrast, interactions with metronidazole and miconazole have only been described in isolated case histories (SEDA-19, 351) (5).

In a double-blind, randomized, placebo-controlled study in renal transplant patients taking ciclosporin, voriconazole increased the mean ciclosporin AUC 1.7-fold (271). The authors therefore recommend halving the dose of ciclosporin in these patients and carefully monitoring ciclosporin blood concentrations.

Imipenem/cilastatin

In contrast to what has previously been stated, there was no significant increase in the frequency of seizures among 77 patients with bone marrow transplants who were taking ciclosporin alone (three seizures), 45 patients taking ciclosporin plus imipenem/cilastatin (two seizures), and 44 patients taking imipenem/cilastatin alone (no seizures) (272).

Inducers, inhibitors, or substrates of 3A

Ciclosporin is absorbed to a variable extent from the gastrointestinal tract and almost completely metabolized in both the liver and small intestine by CYP3A, which metabolizes a large number of drugs. Inducers, inhibitors, or substrates of CYP3A therefore have the potential to interact with ciclosporin. In addition, ciclosporin has wide pharmacokinetic variability and a narrow therapeutic index. Conversely, ciclosporin can inhibit the hepatic metabolism of other drugs that share the same CYP3A metabolic pathway.

Drugs that increase the systemic availability of ciclosporin do not always have negative effects, and several ciclosporin-sparing agents have indeed been used for the purpose of improving efficacy while reducing the cost of treatment. However, use of such combinations should be balanced against their potential risks (273).

Table 1 lists drugs that have proven or possible clinically relevant drug interactions with ciclosporin.

Macrolide antibiotics

Erythromycin increases ciclosporin blood concentrations, and increased serum creatinine concentrations have been consistently demonstrated; isolated reports have also suggested possible interactions with clarithromycin, josamycin, midecamycin, or pristinamycin (SEDA-21, 385) (274). A two-fold increase in ciclosporin concentrations has been

Table 1 A summary of major interactions with ciclosporin

Pharmacokinetic	Pharmacodynamic
Anticonvulsants	**Increased risk of nephrotoxicity**
Carbamazepine*	ACE inhibitors
Phenobarbital*	Aciclovir (see text)
Phenytoin*	Aminoglycosides
Primidone*	Amphotericin
Antidepressants	Co-trimoxazole
Fluoxetine (unproven; see text)	Diuretics
Fluvoxamine	Foscarnet (see text)
Nefazodone	Melphalan
St. John's wort	Nafcillin (see text)
Antimicrobial drugs	NSAIDs (unproven, see text)
Antifungal drugs	**Increased risk of muscle toxicity (see text)**
Ketoconazole, fluconazole, itraconazole, metronidazole	Colchicine
Chloramphenicol (unproven)	Fibric acid derivatives
Clindamycin*	HMG CoA reductase inhibitors (statins)
Fluoroquinolones	Pyrazinamide (SEDA-20, 346)
Griseofulvin*	**Increased risk of gingival hyperplasia**
Macrolides or related drugs (see text)	Nifedipine
Clarithromycin, erythromycin, josamycin, midecamycin, miocamycin, pristinamycin	**Increased risk of neurotoxicity**
Protease inhibitors	Imipenem/cilastatin
Ritonavir, saquinavir	**Increased risk of hepatotoxicity**
Pyrazinamide*	Androgens
Quinupristin/dalfopristin (SEDA-21, 386)	Norethandrolone, oxymetholone
Rifamycins*	Parenteral nutrition (see text)
Sulfadiazine*	**Increased risk of hyperkalemia**
Terbinafine* (SEDA-21, 386)	Potassium salts
Cardiovascular drugs	Potassium-sparing diuretics
Amiodarone	
Calcium channel blockers	
Amlodipine, diltiazem, nicardipine, verapamil	
Carvedilol (SEDA-22, 415)	
Clonidine	
Propafenone	
Hypoglycemic drugs	
Glibenclamide	
Glipizide	
Troglitazone*	
Miscellaneous drugs	
Acetazolamide	
Allopurinol	
Bezafibrate	
Bile acid resin*	
Chloroquine	
Danazol	
Glucocorticoids	
Grapefruit juice	
Modafinil*	
Muromonab (SEDA-21, 386)	
Octreotide*	
Oral contraceptives (unproven)	
Orlistat*	
Probucol*	
Sulfasalazine*	
Sulfinpyrazone*	
Tacrolimus	
Ticlopidine*	
Vitamin E (water-soluble) (SEDA-20, 346)	

*These drugs reportedly reduce ciclosporin blood concentrations; the rest increase them

reported in patients receiving miocamycin. In contrast, spiramycin or roxithromycin did not significantly affect ciclosporin concentrations, and a single report involving azithromycin (SEDA-19, 351) was not substantiated by several prospective studies.

Mycophenolate mofetil

The interaction of ciclosporin with mycophenolate mofetil was investigated in 52 renal transplant patients taking triple therapy (ciclosporin, mycophenolate mofetil, and prednisone), who continued taking the same treatment ($n = 19$) or underwent elective ciclosporin withdrawal ($n = 19$) or prednisolone withdrawal ($n = 14$) 6 months after transplantation (275). Median mycophenolate mofetil trough concentrations 3 months later were about two-fold higher in patients who had discontinued ciclosporin compared with patients who continued to take triple therapy and patients who had discontinued prednisone. No clear mechanism readily explains these changes.

Nefazodone

Nefazodone can alter blood ciclosporin concentrations (276,277). In one case there was nearly a 10-fold increase in whole-blood ciclosporin concentrations in a cardiac transplant patient shortly after the addition of nefazodone (278).

NSAIDs

Based on the theoretical possibility of additive nephrotoxic effects, the combined use of NSAIDs with ciclosporin is expected to reduce renal function and therefore to increase ciclosporin-induced nephrotoxicity.

- In an 8-year-old girl with rheumatoid arthritis, the combination of ciclosporin with NSAIDs (indometacin and diclofenac) was suggested to have caused biopsy-proven, non-specific colitis, because her symptoms occurred only when the combination was used (279).

From several studies performed in healthy volunteers, repeated doses of diclofenac, aspirin, indometacin, or piroxicam did not significantly alter ciclosporin single-dose pharmacokinetics, but the AUC of diclofenac was increased by ciclosporin (280). In a further study of 20 patients with rheumatoid arthritis who took ciclosporin for 4 weeks, there was a two-fold increase in diclofenac AUC, and a small but significant increase in serum creatinine concentrations (281). Changes in renal function were easily managed by dosage titration of both drugs. In another study of 32 patients who received a 4-week course of paracetamol, indometacin, ketoprofen, or sulindac, changes in the calculated creatinine clearance were minimal (282). There were no striking differences among different NSAIDs. Taken together, the results of these studies and previous findings suggested that the clinical relevance of this interaction is limited.

Orlistat

Orlistat reduces plasma ciclosporin concentrations.

- A 29-year-old woman with increased body weight after renal transplantation was unable to adhere to a low-fat

diet and took orlistat, which gave her severe diarrhea (283). Her plasma ciclosporin concentrations fell to subtherapeutic, even though she took the orlistat 2 hours before the ciclosporin and even though the daily dose of orlistat was reduced to 240 mg/day.
- There was a two-fold reduction in blood ciclosporin concentrations 2 weeks after orlistat was given to a 61-year-old patient with a heart transplant (284).

The FDA has received six reports of subtherapeutic blood ciclosporin concentrations soon after transplant recipients started to take orlistat (285). Reduced absorption of ciclosporin is the most likely mechanism (286,287) by reduction in fat absorption rather than by a direct drug–drug interaction.

Oxycodone

In an analysis of changes in ciclosporin clearance and systemic availability obtained from the medical records of 100 transplant patients, oxycodone reduced ciclosporin systemic availability (228).

Parenteral nutrition

Cholestasis from other causes can increase the accumulation of ciclosporin or its metabolites, which in turn worsens hepatic cholestasis. This mechanism has been suggested in patients with bowel diseases who experienced an aggravation of hyperbilirubinemia or an increased incidence of hepatotoxicity from the combination of total parenteral nutrition and ciclosporin (SEDA-19, 348) (288).

Protease inhibitors

Interactions of ciclosporin with protease inhibitors should be expected, particularly with ritonavir, a potent inhibitor of CYP3A.

- Despite a prophylactic reduction in the dose of ciclosporin (100 mg/day) before antiretroviral treatment, a 40-year-old woman had an acute increase in ciclosporin trough concentrations (over 1000 ng/ml) and serum creatinine concentration (from 84 to 228 μmol/l) after taking zidovudine (600 mg/day), saquinavir (800 mg/day), and ritonavir (800 mg/day) for 11 days (289). Despite ciclosporin withdrawal, ciclosporin and creatinine blood concentrations remained high for over 10 days until triple drug therapy was withdrawn. Ritonavir was the most likely suspect.

Proton pump inhibitors

Conflicting data have emerged on the interaction of omeprazole with ciclosporin, with isolated case reports suggesting that omeprazole can increase or reduce ciclosporin concentrations, whereas no effect of omeprazole was demonstrated in a controlled trial (290–292).

Quinidine

In an analysis of changes in ciclosporin clearance and systemic availability obtained from the medical records of 100 transplant patients, digoxin increased ciclosporin systemic availability (228).

Saquinavir

A reciprocal interaction between ciclosporin and saquinavir has been reported in an HIV-positive kidney transplant patient (293). Whereas ciclosporin concentrations were previously acceptable, there was a three-fold increase in ciclosporin trough concentrations after 3 days of saquinavir (3600 mg/day). In addition, the saquinavir AUC was four times higher than that usually observed in patients taking similar dosages.

Selective serotonin reuptake inhibitors

Fluvoxamine and fluoxetine have been involved in isolated cases of increased blood ciclosporin concentrations, but fluoxetine was not confirmed to affect ciclosporin concentrations significantly in 13 patients (SEDA-20, 345) (SEDA-22, 385–386). In an analysis of changes in ciclosporin clearance and systemic availability obtained from the medical records of 100 transplant patients, sertraline altered ciclosporin pharmacokinetics (228).

Sulfasalazine

In a 51-year-old woman with a renal transplant who had been stable for the past 13.5 months with ciclosporin (9.6 mg/kg) and sulfasalazine (1.5 g/day) for ulcerative colitis, sulfasalazine withdrawal resulted in an almost two-fold increase in ciclosporin blood concentrations over the next 10 days (294).

Sulfinpyrazone

In 120 heart transplant patients, sulfinpyrazone (200 mg/day) for ciclosporin-associated hyperuricemia was associated with lowered blood ciclosporin concentrations despite an increase in the daily dose (295). The authors cited evidence (296) that sulfinpyrazone induces ciclosporin metabolism.

Sulfonylureas

Both glipizide and glibenclamide increase ciclosporin concentrations significantly (297).

Ticlopidine

Although there was no interaction between ciclosporin and ticlopidine in a pharmacokinetic study, a 64-year-old patient with a renal transplant had a reduction in the concentration:dose ratio of ciclosporin after each of two successive courses of ticlopidine (298).

Troglitazone

Case reports and a retrospective evaluation of seven renal transplant patients showed that troglitazone can increase ciclosporin metabolism with a subsequent reduction of 15–45% in ciclosporin trough concentrations (299). The interaction of ciclosporin with troglitazone has been confirmed in four heart transplant patients with a 30–60% fall in ciclosporin concentrations within days of taking troglitazone 200 mg/day (300).

Monitoring Therapy

Ciclosporin pharmacokinetics vary considerably between patients, and even in an individual patient from time to time, with changes in the clinical condition and treatment, particularly with administration of other drugs (301). Inadequate exposure to ciclosporin is a key factor in acute rejection and contributes to the development of chronic rejection and graft failure. Monitoring of ciclosporin concentrations is widely adopted as an accurate and practical measure of drug exposure (302).

In an open, randomized, parallel-group study in 307 patients, ciclosporin blood concentrations measured 2 hours after a dose were compared with conventional trough ciclosporin blood concentrations (303). The traditional predose blood concentration did not correlate well with drug exposure, and the 2-hour concentration was superior in preventing acute rejection. This is important, because data derived from the database of the United Network for Organ Sharing Scientific Liver Transplant Registry has shown that moderate and more severe grades of rejection are associated with poor graft function and outcome in liver transplant recipients.

Of 53 bone marrow transplant recipients in whom ciclosporin was used to suppress graft-versus-host disease, 63% developed acute nephrotoxicity (304). These patients had significantly higher plasma ciclosporin concentrations during the first month after transplantation than those who did not develop acute nephrotoxicity, even though they received the same cumulative dose. Children received a higher cumulative dose, but their plasma concentrations did not differ significantly from the adults, and they suffered less nephrotoxicity.

Although a correlation between early post-transplantation whole-blood concentrations of ciclosporin and the occurrence of ciclosporin-induced toxicity has been suggested, blood concentrations in most patients are in the target range, and the identification of patients susceptible to adverse effects has yet to be achieved (305).

References

1. Touchard G, Verove C, Bridoux F, Bauwen F. Cyclosporin maintenance monotherapy after renal transplantation. What factors predict success? BioDrugs 1999;12:91–113.
2. Shield CF III, McGrath MM, Goss TF. Assessment of health-related quality of life in kidney transplant patients receiving tacrolimus (FK506)-based versus cyclosporine-based immunosuppression. FK506 Kidney Transplant Study Group. Transplantation 1997;64(12):1738–43.
3. Kappers-Klunne MC, van't Veer MB. Cyclosporin A for the treatment of patients with chronic idiopathic thrombocytopenic purpura refractory to corticosteroids or splenectomy. Br J Haematol 2001;114(1):121–5.
4. Cortes J, O'Brien S, Loscertales J, Kantarjian H, Giles F, Thomas D, Koller C, Keating M. Cyclosporin A for the treatment of cytopenia associated with chronic lymphocytic leukemia. Cancer 2001;92(8):2016–22.
5. Campana C, Regazzi MB, Buggia I, Molinaro M. Clinically significant drug interactions with cyclosporin. An update. Clin Pharmacokinet 1996;30(2):141–79.
6. Kasiske BL, Guijarro C, Massy ZA, Wiederkehr MR, Ma JZ. Cardiovascular disease after renal transplantation. J Am Soc Nephrol 1996;7(1):158–65.
7. Kronenberg F, Lhotta K, Konigsrainer A, Konig P. Renal artery thromboembolism and immunosuppressive therapy. Nephron 1996;72(1):101.
8. Textor SC, Canzanello VJ, Taler SJ, Wilson DJ, Schwartz LL, Augustine JE, Raymer JM, Romero JC, Wiesner RH, Krom RA, et al. Cyclosporine-induced hypertension after transplantation. Mayo Clin Proc 1994;69(12):1182–93.
9. Taler SJ, Textor SC, Canzanello VJ, Schwartz L. Cyclosporin-induced hypertension: incidence, pathogenesis and management. Drug Saf 1999;20(5):437–49.
10. Ventura HO, Mehra MR, Stapleton DD, Smart FW. Cyclosporine-induced hypertension in cardiac transplantation. Med Clin North Am 1997;81(6):1347–57.
11. Sturrock ND, Lang CC, Struthers AD. Cyclosporin-induced hypertension precedes renal dysfunction and sodium retention in man. J Hypertens 1993;11(11):1209–16.
12. Davenport A. The effect of renal transplantation and treatment with cyclosporin A on the prevalence of Raynaud's phenomenon. Clin Transplant 1993;7:4–8.
13. Rottenberg Y, Fridlender ZG. Recurrent infusion phlebitis induced by cyclosporine. Ann Pharmacother 2004;38(12):2071–3.
14. Blaauw AA, Leunissen KM, Cheriex EC, Wolters J, Kootstra G, Van Hooff JP. Disappearance of pulmonary capillary leak syndrome when intravenous cyclosporine is replaced by oral cyclosporine. Transplantation 1987;43(5):758–9.
15. Carbone L, Appel GB, Benvenisty AI, Cohen DJ, Kunis CL, Hardy MA. Adult respiratory distress syndrome associated with oral cyclosporine. Transplantation 1987;43(5):767–8.
16. Roelofs PM, Klinkhamer PJ, Gooszen HC. Hypersensitivity pneumonitis probably caused by cyclosporine. A case report. Respir Med 1998;92(12):1368–70.
17. Hauben M. Cyclosporine neurotoxicity. Pharmacotherapy 1996;16(4):576–83.
18. Wijdicks EF, Wiesner RH, Krom RA. Neurotoxicity in liver transplant recipients with cyclosporine immunosuppression. Neurology 1995;45(11):1962–4.
19. Erer B, Polchi P, Lucarelli G, Angelucci E, Baronciani D, Galimberti M, Giardini C, Gaziev D, Maiello A. CsA-associated neurotoxicity and ineffective prophylaxis with clonazepam in patients transplanted for thalassemia major: analysis of risk factors. Bone Marrow Transplant 1996;18(1):157–62.
20. Bohlin AB, Berg U, Englund M, Malm G, Persson A, Tibell A, Tyden G. Central nervous system complications in children treated with ciclosporin after renal transplantation. Child Nephrol Urol 1990;10(4):225–30.
21. de Groen PC, Aksamit AJ, Rakela J, Forbes GS, Krom RA. Central nervous system toxicity after liver transplantation. The role of cyclosporine and cholesterol. N Engl J Med 1987;317(14):861–6.
22. Gleeson JG, duPlessis AJ, Barnes PD, Riviello JJ Jr. Cyclosporin A acute encephalopathy and seizure syndrome in childhood: clinical features and risk of seizure recurrence. J Child Neurol 1998;13(7):336–44.
23. Schwartz RB, Bravo SM, Klufas RA, Hsu L, Barnes PD, Robson CD, Antin JH. Cyclosporine neurotoxicity and its relationship to hypertensive encephalopathy: CT and MR findings in 16 cases. Am J Roentgenol 1995;165(3):627–31.
24. Kotake S, Higashi K, Yoshikawa K, Sasamoto Y, Okamoto T, Matsuda H. Central nervous system

symptoms in patients with Behçet disease receiving cyclosporine therapy. Ophthalmology 1999;106(3):586–9.
25. Gopal AK, Thorning DR, Back AL. Fatal outcome due to cyclosporine neurotoxicity with associated pathological findings. Bone Marrow Transplant 1999;23(2): 191–3.
26. Kaito K, Kobayashi M, Otsubo H, Ogasawara Y, Sekita T, Shimada T, Hosoya T. Cyclosporine and entrapment neuropathy. Report of two cases. Acta Haematol 1998;100(3):159.
27. Terrovitis IV, Nanas SN, Rombos AK, Tolis G, Nanas JN. Reversible symmetric polyneuropathy with paraplegia after heart transplantation. Transplantation 1998;65(10): 1394–5.
28. Maghrabi K, Bohlega S. Cyclosporine-induced migraine with severe vomiting causing loss of renal graft. Clin Neurol Neurosurg 1998;100(3):224–7.
29. Braun R, Arechalde A, French LE. Reversible ascending motor neuropathy as a side effect of systemic treatment with ciclosporine for nodular prurigo. Dermatology 1999;199(4): 372–3.
30. Koide T, Yamada M, Takahashi T, Igarashi S, Masuko M, Furukawa T, Kuroha T, Koike T, Sato M, Tanaka R, Tsuji S, Takahashi H. Cyclosporine A-associated fatal central nervous system angiopathy in a bone marrow transplant recipient: an autopsy case. Acta Neuropathol (Berl) 2000;99(6):680–4.
31. Shbarou RM, Chao NJ, Morgenlander JC. Cyclosporin A-related cerebral vasculopathy. Bone Marrow Transplant 2000;26(7):801–4.
32. Delpont E, Thomas P, Gugenheim J, Chichmanian RM, Mahagne MH, Suisse G, Dolisi C. Syndrome confusionnel prolongé au cours d'un traitement par ciclosporine: etat de mal à expression confusionnelle? [Prolonged confusion syndrome in the course of cyclosporine treatment: a state of confusion?] Neurophysiol Clin 1990;20(3):207–15.
33. Labar B, Bogdanic V, Plavsic F, Francetic I, Dobric I, Kastelan A, Grgicevic D, Vrtar M, Grgic-Markulin L, Balabanic-Kamauf B, et al. Cyclosporin neurotoxicity in patients treated with allogeneic bone marrow transplantation. Biomed Pharmacother 1986;40(4):148–50.
34. Rosencrantz R, Moon A, Raynes H, Spivak W. Cyclosporine-Induced neurotoxicity during treatment of Crohn's disease: lack of correlation with previously reported risk factors. Am J Gastroenterol 2001;96(9):2778–82.
35. Bronster DJ, Chodoff L, Yonover P, Sheiner PA. Cyclosporine levels in cerebrospinal fluid after liver transplantation. Transplantation 1999;68(9):1410–13.
36. Meyer MA. Elevated basal ganglia glucose metabolism in cyclosporine neurotoxicity: a positron emission tomography imaging study. J Neuroimaging 2002;12(1):92–3.
37. Ozkaya O, Kalman S, Bakkaloglu S, Buyan N, Soylemezoglu O. Cyclosporine-associated facial paralysis in a child with renal transplant. Pediatr Nephrol 2002;17(7):544–6.
38. Porges Y, Blumen S, Fireman Z, Sternberg A, Zamir D. Cyclosporine-induced optic neuropathy, ophthalmoplegia, and nystagmus in a patient with Crohn disease. Am J Ophthalmol 1998;126(4):607–9.
39. Rubin AM, Kang H. Cerebral blindness and encephalopathy with cyclosporin A toxicity. Neurology 1987;37(6):1072–6.
40. Rubin AM. Transient cortical blindness and occipital seizures with cyclosporine toxicity. Transplantation 1989;47(3):572–3.
41. Wilson SE, de Groen PC, Aksamit AJ, Wiesner RH, Garrity JA, Krom RA. Cyclosporin A-induced reversible cortical blindness. J Clin Neuroophthalmol 1988;8(4): 215–20.
42. Saito J, Kami M, Taniguchi F, Kanda Y, Takeda N, Mitani K, Hirai H, Araie M, Fujino Y. Unilateral papilledema after bone marrow transplantation. Bone Marrow Transplant 1999;23(9):963–5.
43. Avery R, Jabs DA, Wingard JR, Vogelsang G, Saral R, Santos G. Optic disc edema after bone marrow transplantation. Possible role of cyclosporine toxicity. Ophthalmology 1991;98(8):1294–301.
44. BenEzra D, Pe'er J, Brodsky M, Cohen E. Cyclosporine eyedrops for the treatment of severe vernal keratoconjunctivitis. Am J Ophthalmol 1986;101(3):278–82.
45. Zierhut M, Thiel HJ, Weidle EG, Waetjen R, Pleyer U. Topical treatment of severe corneal ulcers with cyclosporin A. Graefes Arch Clin Exp Ophthalmol 1989;227(1):30–5.
46. Sall K, Stevenson OD, Mundorf TK, Reis BL. Two multicenter, randomized studies of the efficacy and safety of cyclosporine ophthalmic emulsion in moderate to severe dry eye disease. CsA Phase 3 Study Group. Ophthalmology 2000;107(4):631–9.
47. Kachi S, Hirano K, Takesue Y, Miura M. Unusual corneal deposit after the topical use of cyclosporine as eyedrops. Am J Ophthalmol 2000;130(5):667–9.
48. Stevenson D, Tauber J, Reis BL. Efficacy and safety of cyclosporin A ophthalmic emulsion in the treatment of moderate-to-severe dry eye disease: a dose-ranging, randomized trial. The Cyclosporin A Phase 2 Study Group. Ophthalmology 2000;107(5):967–74.
49. Jindal RM, Sidner RA, Milgrom ML. Post-transplant diabetes mellitus. The role of immunosuppression. Drug Saf 1997;16(4):242–57.
50. Copstein LA, Zelmanovitz T, Goncalves LF, Manfro RC. Posttransplant patients: diabetes mellitus in cyclosporine-treated renal allograft a case-control study. Transplant Proc 2004;36(4):882–3.
51. Raine AE, Carter R, Mann JI, Morris PJ. Adverse effect of cyclosporin on plasma cholesterol in renal transplant recipients. Nephrol Dial Transplant 1988;3(4):458–63.
52. Ballantyne CM, Podet EJ, Patsch WP, Harati Y, Appel V, Gotto AM Jr, Young JB. Effects of cyclosporine therapy on plasma lipoprotein levels. JAMA 1989;262(1):53–6.
53. Stiller MJ, Pak GH, Kenny C, Jondreau L, Davis I, Wachsman S, Shupack JL. Elevation of fasting serum lipids in patients treated with low-dose cyclosporine for severe plaque-type psoriasis. An assessment of clinical significance when viewed as a risk factor for cardiovascular disease. J Am Acad Dermatol 1992;27(3):434–8.
54. Grossman RM, Delaney RJ, Brinton EA, Carter DM, Gottlieb AB. Hypertriglyceridemia in patients with psoriasis treated with cyclosporine. J Am Acad Dermatol 1991;25(4):648–51.
55. Hricik DE. Posttransplant hyperlipidemia: the treatment dilemma. Am J Kidney Dis 1994;23(5):766–71.
56. Massy ZA. Hyperlipidemia and cardiovascular disease after organ transplantation. Transplantation 2001;72(Suppl 6):S13–15.
57. Webb AT, Reaveley DA, O'Donnell M, O'Connor B, Seed M, Brown EA. Does cyclosporin increase lipoprotein(a) concentrations in renal transplant recipients? Lancet 1993;341(8840):268–70. (See also) Hunt BJ, Parratt R, Rose M, Yacoub M. Does cyclosporin affect lipoprotein(a) concentrations? Lancet 1994;343(8889):119–20.
58. Kuster GM, Drexel H, Bleisch JA, Rentsch K, Pei P, Binswanger U, Amann FW. Relation of cyclosporine blood levels to adverse effects on lipoproteins. Transplantation 1994;57(10):1479–83.
59. Claesson K, Mayer AD, Squifflet JP, Grabensee B, Eigler FW, Behrend M, Vanrenterghem Y, van Hooff J, Morales JM, Johnson RW, Buchholz B, Land W, Forsythe JL, Neumayer HH, Ericzon BG, Muhlbacher F.

Lipoprotein patterns in renal transplant patients: a comparison between FK 506 and cyclosporine A patients. Transplant Proc 1998;30(4):1292–4.
60. McCune TR, Thacker LR II, Peters TG, Mulloy L, Rohr MS, Adams PA, Yium J, Light JA, Pruett T, Gaber AO, Selman SH, Jonsson J, Hayes JM, Wright FH Jr, Armata T, Blanton J, Burdick JF. Effects of tacrolimus on hyperlipidemia after successful renal transplantation: a Southeastern Organ Procurement Foundation multicenter clinical study. Transplantation 1998;65(1):87–92.
61. Lin HY, Rocher LL, McQuillan MA, Schmaltz S, Palella TD, Fox IH. Cyclosporine-induced hyperuricemia and gout. N Engl J Med 1989;321(5):287–92.
62. Burack DA, Griffith BP, Thompson ME, Kahl LE. Hyperuricemia and gout among heart transplant recipients receiving cyclosporine. Am J Med 1992;92(2):141–6.
63. Ben Hmida M, Hachicha J, Bahloul Z, Kaddour N, Kharrat M, Jarraya F, Jarraya A. Cyclosporine-induced hyperuricemia and gout in renal transplants. Transplant Proc 1995;27(5):2722–4.
64. Laine J, Holmberg C. Renal and adrenal mechanisms in cyclosporine-induced hyperkalaemia after renal transplantation. Eur J Clin Invest 1995;25(9):670–6.
65. Cavdar C, Sifil A, Sanli E, Gulay H, Camsari T. Hypomagnesemia and mild rhabdomyolysis in living related donor renal transplant recipient treated with cyclosporine A. Scand J Urol Nephrol 1998;32(6):415–17.
66. Scoble JE, Freestone A, Varghese Z, Fernando ON, Sweny P, Moorhead JF. Cyclosporin-induced renal magnesium leak in renal transplant patients. Nephrol Dial Transplant 1990;5(9):812–15.
67. Nozue T, Kobayashi A, Kodama T, Uemasu F, Endoh H, Sako A, Takagi Y. Pathogenesis of cyclosporine-induced hypomagnesemia. J Pediatr 1992;120(4 Pt 1):638–40.
68. Vannini SD, Mazzola BL, Rodoni L, Truttmann AC, Wermuth B, Bianchetti MG, Ferrari P. Permanently reduced plasma ionized magnesium among renal transplant recipients on cyclosporine. Transpl Int 1999;12(4):244–9.
69. Faure JL, Causse X, Bergeret A, Meyer F, Neidecker J, Paliard P. Cyclosporine induced hemolytic anemia in a liver transplant patient. Transplant Proc 1989;21(1 Pt 2): 2242–3.
70. Rougier JP, Viron B, Ronco P, Khayat R, Michel C, Mignon F. Autoimmune haemolytic anaemia after ABO-match, ABDR full match kidney transplantation. Nephrol Dial Transplant 1994;9(6):693–7.
71. Trimarchi H, Freixas E, Rabinovich O, Schropp J, Pereyra H, Bullorsky E. Cyclosporine-associated thrombotic microangiopathy during daclizumab induction: a suggested therapeutic approach. Nephron 2001;87(4):361–4.
72. Seymour RA. Drug-induced gingival overgrowth. Adverse Drug React Toxicol Rev 1993;12(4):215–32.
73. Mariani G, Calastrini C, Carinci F, Marzola R, Calura G. Ultrastructural features of cyclosporine A-induced gingival hyperplasia. J Periodontol 1993;64(11):1092–7.
74. O'Valle F, Mesa FL, Gomez-Morales M, Aguilar D, Caracuel MD, Medina-Cano MT, Andujar M, Lopez-Hidalgo J, Garcia del Moral R. Immunohistochemical study of 30 cases of cyclosporin A-induced gingival overgrowth. J Periodontol 1994;65(7):724–30.
75. Nell A, Matejka M, Solar P, Ulm C, Sinzinger H. Evidence that cyclosporine inhibits periodontal prostaglandin I2 synthesis. J Periodontal Res 1996;31(2):131–4.
76. Thomason JM, Seymour RA, Ellis JS, Kelly PJ, Parry G, Dark J, Idle JR. Iatrogenic gingival overgrowth in cardiac transplantation. J Periodontol 1995;66(8):742–6.
77. Wondimu B, Dahllof G, Berg U, Modeer T. Cyclosporin-A-induced gingival overgrowth in renal transplant children. Scand J Dent Res 1993;101(5):282–6.
78. Wondimu B, Berg U, Modeer T. Renal function in cyclosporine-treated pediatric renal transplant recipients in relation to gingival overgrowth. Transplantation 1997;64(1):92–6.
79. Kilpatrick NM, Weintraub RG, Lucas JO, Shipp A, Byrt T, Wilkinson JL. Gingival overgrowth in pediatric heart and heart-lung transplant recipients. J Heart Lung Transplant 1997;16(12):1231–7.
80. Sooriyamoorthy M, Gower DB, Eley BM. Androgen metabolism in gingival hyperplasia induced by nifedipine and cyclosporin. J Periodontal Res 1990;25(1):25–30.
81. Bokenkamp A, Bohnhorst B, Beier C, Albers N, Offner G, Brodehl J. Nifedipine aggravates cyclosporine A-induced gingival hyperplasia. Pediatr Nephrol 1994;8(2):181–5.
82. Thomason JM, Seymour RA, Rice N. The prevalence and severity of cyclosporin and nifedipine-induced gingival overgrowth. J Clin Periodontol 1993;20(1):37–40.
83. Landewe RB, Goei The HS, van Rijthoven AW, Rietveld JR, Breedveld FC, Dijkmans BA. Cyclosporine in common clinical practice: an estimation of the benefit/risk ratio in patients with rheumatoid arthritis. J Rheumatol 1994;21(9):1631–6.
84. Lorber MI, Van Buren CT, Flechner SM, Williams C, Kahan BD. Hepatobiliary and pancreatic complications of cyclosporine therapy in 466 renal transplant recipients. Transplantation 1987;43(1):35–40.
85. Harihara Y, Sanjo K, Idezuki Y. Cyclosporine hepatotoxicity and cold ischemia liver damage. Transplant Proc 1992;24(5):1984.
86. Moertel CG, Fleming TR, Macdonald JS, Haller DG, Laurie JA. Hepatic toxicity associated with fluorouracil plus levamisole adjuvant therapy. J Clin Oncol 1993;11(12):2386–90.
87. Kowdley KV, Keeffe EB. Hepatotoxicity of transplant immunosuppressive agents. Gastroenterol Clin North Am 1995;24(4):991–1001.
88. Myara A, Cadranel JF, Dorent R, Lunel F, Bouvier E, Gerhardt M, Bernard B, Ghoussoub JJ, Cabrol A, Gandjbakhch I, Opolon P, Trivin F. Cyclosporin A-mediated cholestasis in patients with chronic hepatitis after heart transplantation. Eur J Gastroenterol Hepatol 1996;8(3):267–71.
89. Neri S, Signorelli SS, Ierna D, Mauceri B, Abate G, Bordonaro F, Cilio D, Malaguarnera M. Role of admethionine (S-adenosylmethionine) in cyclosporin-induced cholestasis. Clin Drug Invest 2002;22:191–5.
90. Chicharro M, Guarner L, Vilaseca J, Planas M, Malagelada J. Does cyclosporin A worsen liver function in patients with inflammatory bowel disease and total parenteral nutrition? Rev Esp Enferm Dig 2000;92(2):68–77.
91. Laskow DA, Curtis JJ, Luke RG, Julian BA, Jones P, Deierhoi MH, Barber WH, Diethelm AG. Cyclosporine-induced changes in glomerular filtration rate and urea excretion. Am J Med 1990;88(5):497–502.
92. Mobb GE, Veitch PS, Bell PR. Are serum creatinine levels adequate to identify the onset of chronic cyclosporine A nephrotoxicity? Transplant Proc 1990;22(4):1708–10.
93. Greenberg A, Thompson ME, Griffith BJ, Hardesty RL, Kormos RL, el-Shahawy MA, Janosky JE, Puschett JB. Cyclosporine nephrotoxicity in cardiac allograft patients—a seven-year follow-up. Transplantation 1990;50(4):589–93.
94. Leong SO, Lye WC, Tan CC, Lee EJ. Acute cyclosporine A nephrotoxicity in a renal allograft recipient with hypothyroidism. Am J Kidney Dis 1995;25(3):503–5.
95. van der Molen LR, van Son WJ, Tegzess AM, Stegeman CA. Severe vital depression as the presenting

feature of cyclosporin-A-associated thrombotic microangiopathy. Nephrol Dial Transplant 1999;14(4):998–1000.
96. Kohli HS, Sud K, Jha V, Gupta KL, Minz M, Joshi K, Sakhuja V. Cyclosporin-induced haemolytic–uraemic syndrome presenting as primary graft dysfunction. Nephrol Dial Transplant 1998;13(11):2940–2.
97. Wiener Y, Nakhleh RE, Lee MW, Escobar FS, Venkat KK, Kupin WL, Mozes MF. Prognostic factors and early resumption of cyclosporin A in renal allograft recipients with thrombotic microangiopathy and hemolytic uremic syndrome. Clin Transplant 1997;11(3):157–62.
98. Bren AF, Kandus A, Buturovic J, Koselj M, Kaplan Pavlovcic S, Ponikvar R, Kovac D, Lindic J, Vizjak A, Ferluga D. Cyclosporine-related hemolytic–uremic syndrome in kidney graft recipients: clinical and histomorphologic evaluation. Transplant Proc 1998;30(4):1201–3.
99. Ducloux D, Rebibou JM, Semhoun-Ducloux S, Jamali M, Fournier V, Bresson-Vautrin C, Chalopin JM. Recurrence of hemolytic–uremic syndrome in renal transplant recipients: a meta-analysis. Transplantation 1998;65(10):1405–7.
100. Zarifian A, Meleg-Smith S, O'donovan R, Tesi RJ, Batuman V. Cyclosporine-associated thrombotic microangiopathy in renal allografts. Kidney Int 1999;55(6):2457–66.
101. Myers BD, Ross J, Newton L, Luetscher J, Perlroth M. Cyclosporine-associated chronic nephropathy. N Engl J Med 1984;311(11):699–705.
102. Bennett WM, DeMattos A, Meyer MM, Andoh T, Barry JM. Chronic cyclosporine nephropathy: the Achilles' heel of immunosuppressive therapy. Kidney Int 1996;50(4):1089–100.
103. Mihatsch MJ, Ryffel B, Gudat F. The differential diagnosis between rejection and cyclosporine toxicity. Kidney Int Suppl 1995;52:S63–9.
104. Shihab FS. Cyclosporine nephropathy: pathophysiology and clinical impact. Semin Nephrol 1996;16(6):536–47.
105. Ader JL, Rostaing L. Cyclosporin nephrotoxicity: pathophysiology and comparison with FK-506. Curr Opin Nephrol Hypertens 1998;7(5):539–45.
106. Mihatsch MJ, Antonovych T, Bohman SO, Habib R, Helmchen U, Noel LH, Olsen S, Sibley RK, Kemeny E, Feutren G. Cyclosporin A nephropathy: standardization of the evaluation of kidney biopsies. Clin Nephrol 1994;41(1):23–32.
107. Habib R, Niaudet P. Comparison between pre- and post-treatment renal biopsies in children receiving ciclosporine for idiopathic nephrosis. Clin Nephrol 1994; 42(3):141–6.
108. Jacobson SH, Jaremko G, Duraj FF, Wilczek HE. Renal fibrosis in cyclosporin A-treated renal allograft recipients: morphological findings in relation to renal hemodynamics. Transpl Int 1996;9(5):492–8.
109. Opelz G. Effect of the maintenance immunosuppressive drug regimen on kidney transplant outcome. Transplantation 1994;58(4):443–6.
110. Thiel G, Bock A, Spondlin M, Brunner FP, Mihatsch M, Rufli T, Landmann J. Long-term benefits and risks of cyclosporin A (Sandimmun)—an analysis at 10 years. Transplant Proc 1994;26(5):2493–8.
111. Mihatsch MJ, Morozumi K, Strom EH, Ryffel B, Gudat F, Thiel G. Renal transplant morphology after long-term therapy with cyclosporine. Transplant Proc 1995;27(1):39–42.
112. Gonwa TA, Klintmalm GB, Levy M, Jennings LS, Goldstein RM, Husberg BS. Impact of pretransplant renal function on survival after liver transplantation. Transplantation 1995;59(3):361–5.
113. Kuo PC, Luikart H, Busse-Henry S, Hunt SA, Valantine HA, Stinson EB, Oyer PE, Scandling JD, Alfrey EJ, Dafoe DC. Clinical outcome of interval cadaveric renal transplantation in cardiac allograft recipients. Clin Transplant 1995;9(2):92–7.
114. Goldstein DJ, Zuech N, Sehgal V, Weinberg AD, Drusin R, Cohen D. Cyclosporine-associated end-stage nephropathy after cardiac transplantation: incidence and progression. Transplantation 1997;63(5):664–8.
115. Almond PS, Gillingham KJ, Sibley R, Moss A, Melin M, Leventhal J, Manivel C, Kyriakides P, Payne WD, Dunn DL, et al. Renal transplant function after ten years of cyclosporine. Transplantation 1992;53(2):316–23.
116. Burke JF Jr, Pirsch JD, Ramos EL, Salomon DR, Stablein DM, Van Buren DH, West JC. Long-term efficacy and safety of cyclosporine in renal-transplant recipients. N Engl J Med 1994;331(6):358–63.
117. Ruggenenti P, Perico N, Amuchastegui CS, Ferrazzi P, Mamprin F, Remuzzi G. Following an initial decline, glomerular filtration rate stabilizes in heart transplant patients on chronic cyclosporine. Am J Kidney Dis 1994;24(4):549–53.
118. Parving HH, Tarnow L, Nielsen FS, Rossing P, Mandrup-Poulsen T, Osterby R, Nerup J. Cyclosporine nephrotoxicity in type 1 diabetic patients. A 7-year follow-up study. Diabetes Care 1999;22(3):478–83.
119. Lipkowitz GS, Madden RL, Mulhern J, Braden G, O'Shea M, O'Shaughnessy J, Nash S, Kurbanov A, Freeman J, Rennke H, Germain M. Long-term maintenance of therapeutic cyclosporine levels leads to optimal graft survival without evidence of chronic nephrotoxicity. Transpl Int 1999;12(3):202–7.
120. Vercauteren SB, Bosmans JL, Elseviers MM, Verpooten GA, De Broe ME. A meta-analysis and morphological review of cyclosporine-induced nephrotoxicity in auto-immune diseases. Kidney Int 1998; 54(2):536–45.
121. Feutren G, Mihatsch MJ. Risk factors for cyclosporine-induced nephropathy in patients with autoimmune diseases. International Kidney Biopsy Registry of Cyclosporine in Autoimmune Diseases. N Engl J Med 1992;326(25):1654–60.
122. Pei Y, Scholey JW, Katz A, Schachter R, Murphy GF, Cattran D. Chronic nephrotoxicity in psoriatic patients treated with low-dose cyclosporine. Am J Kidney Dis 1994;23(4):528–36.
123. Korstanje MJ, Bilo HJ, Stoof TJ. Sustained renal function loss in psoriasis patients after withdrawal of low-dose cyclosporin therapy. Br J Dermatol 1992;127(5):501–4.
124. Young EW, Ellis CN, Messana JM, Johnson KJ, Leichtman AB, Mihatsch MJ, Hamilton TA, Groisser DS, Fradin MS, Voorhees JJ. A prospective study of renal structure and function in psoriasis patients treated with cyclosporin. Kidney Int 1994;46(4):1216–22.
125. Shupack J, Abel E, Bauer E, Brown M, Drake L, Freinkel R, Guzzo C, Koo J, Levine N, Lowe N, McDonald C, Margolis D, Stiller M, Wintroub B, Bainbridge C, Evans S, Hilss S, Mietlowski W, Winslow C, Birnbaum JE. Cyclosporine as maintenance therapy in patients with severe psoriasis. J Am Acad Dermatol 1997;36(3 Pt 1):423–32.
126. van den Borne BE, Landewe RB, The HS, Breedveld FC, Dijkmans BA. Low dose cyclosporine in early rheumatoid arthritis: effective and safe after two years of therapy when compared with chloroquine. Scand J Rheumatol 1996;25(5):307–16.
127. Zachariae H, Kragballe K, Hansen HE, Marcussen N, Olsen S. Renal biopsy findings in long-term cyclosporin treatment of psoriasis. Br J Dermatol 1997;136(4):531–5.
128. Lowe NJ, Wieder JM, Rosenbach A, Johnson K, Kunkel R, Bainbridge C, Bourget T, Dimov I, Simpson K, Glass E, Grabie MT. Long-term low-dose cyclosporine therapy for

severe psoriasis: effects on renal function and structure. J Am Acad Dermatol 1996;35(5 Pt 1):710–19.
129. Rodriguez F, Krayenbuhl JC, Harrison WB, Forre O, Dijkmans BA, Tugwell P, Miescher PA, Mihatsch MJ. Renal biopsy findings and followup of renal function in rheumatoid arthritis patients treated with cyclosporin A. An update from the International Kidney Biopsy Registry. Arthritis Rheum 1996;39(9):1491–8.
130. Landewe RB, Dijkmans BA, van der Woude FJ, Breedveld FC, Mihatsch MJ, Bruijn JA. Longterm low dose cyclosporine in patients with rheumatoid arthritis: renal function loss without structural nephropathy. J Rheumatol 1996;23(1):61–4.
131. Feehally J, Walls J, Mistry N, Horsburgh T, Taylor J, Veitch PS, Bell PR. Does nifedipine ameliorate cyclosporin A nephrotoxicity? BMJ (Clin Res Ed) 1987;295(6593):310.
132. Tindall RS, Rollins JA, Phillips JT, Greenlee RG, Wells L, Belendiuk G. Preliminary results of a double-blind, randomized, placebo-controlled trial of cyclosporine in myasthenia gravis. N Engl J Med 1987;316(12):719–24.
133. Hadj-Aissa A, Labeeuw M, Lareal MC, et al. Effets de la cyclosporine (CyA) sur le rein isole: comparaison avec l'excipient (Exc). Nephrologie 1987;8:73.
134. Hoyer PF, Krohn HP, Offner G, Byrd DJ, Brodehl J, Wonigeit K, Pichlmayr R. Renal function after kidney transplantation in children. A comparison of conventional immunosuppression with cyclosporine. Transplantation 1987;43(4):489–93.
135. Wheatley HC, Datzman M, Williams JW, Miles DE, Hatch FE. Long-term effects of cyclosporine on renal function in liver transplant recipients. Transplantation 1987;43(5):641–7.
136. Albengres E, Le Louet H, d'Athis P, Tillement JP. S15176 and S16950 interaction with cyclosporin A antiproliferative effect on cultured human lymphocytes. Fundam Clin Pharmacol 2001;15(1):41–6.
137. Mihatsch MJ, Thiel G, Ryffel B. Brief review of the morphology of cyclosporin A nephropathy. Nephrologie 1987;8(3):143–5.
138. Palestine AG, Austin HA 3rd, Balow JE, Antonovych TT, Sabnis SG, Preuss HG, Nussenblatt RB. Renal histopathologic alterations in patients treated with cyclosporine for uveitis. N Engl J Med 1986;314(20):1293–8.
139. Raphael L, Fish JC. An in vitro model for analyzing the nephrotoxicity of cyclosporine and preservation injury. Transplantation 1987;43(5):703–8.
140. Anaise D, Waltzer WC, Arnold AN, Rapaport FT. Adverse effects of cyclosporine A on the microcirculation of the cold preserved kidney. NY State J Med 1987;87(3):141–2.
141. Lewis RM. Long-term use of cyclosporine A does not adversely impact on clinical outcomes following renal transplantation. Kidney Int Suppl 1995;52:S75–8.
142. Sehgal V, Radhakrishnan J, Appel GB, Valeri A, Cohen DJ. Progressive renal insufficiency following cardiac transplantation: cyclosporine, lipids, and hypertension. Am J Kidney Dis 1995;26(1):193–201.
143. Camara NO, Matos AC, Rodrigues DA, Pereira AB, Pacheco-Silva A. Early detection of heart transplant patients with increased risk of ciclosporin nephrotoxicity. Lancet 2001;357(9259):856–7.
144. Iijima K, Hamahira K, Tanaka R, Kobayashi A, Nozu K, Nakamura H, Yoshikawa N. Risk factors for cyclosporine-induced tubulointerstitial lesions in children with minimal change nephrotic syndrome. Kidney Int 2002;61(5):1801–5.
145. Hollander AAMJ, Van der Woude FJ. Efficacy and tolerability of conversion from cyclosporin to azathioprine after kidney transplantation. A review of the evidence. BioDrugs 1998;9:197–210.
146. Kasiske BL, Heim-Duthoy K, Ma JZ. Elective cyclosporine withdrawal after renal transplantation. A meta-analysis. JAMA 1993;269(3):395–400.
147. Heim-Duthoy KL, Chitwood KK, Tortorice KL, Massy ZA, Kasiske BL. Elective cyclosporine withdrawal 1 year after renal transplantation. Am J Kidney Dis 1994;24(5):846–53.
148. Smith SR, Minda SA, Samsa GP, Harrell FE Jr, Gunnells JC, Coffman TM, Butterly DW. Late withdrawal of cyclosporine in stable renal transplant recipients. Am J Kidney Dis 1995;26(3):487–94.
149. Mourad G, Vela C, Ribstein J, Mimran A. Long-term improvement in renal function after cyclosporine reduction in renal transplant recipients with histologically proven chronic cyclosporine nephropathy Transplantation 1998;65(5):661–7.
150. Bunke M, Sloan R, Brier M, Ganzel B. An improved glomerular filtration rate in cardiac transplant recipients with once-a-day cyclosporine dosing. Transplantation 1995;59(4):537–40.
151. Ramsay HM, Harden PN. Cyclosporin-induced flushing in a renal transplant recipient resolving after substitution with tacrolimus. Br J Dermatol 2000;142(4):832–3.
152. Azurdia RM, Graham RM, Weismann K, Guerin DM, Parslew R. Acne keloidalis in caucasian patients on cyclosporin following organ transplantation. Br J Dermatol 2000;143(2):465–7.
153. Carnero L, Silvestre JF, Guijarro J, Albares MP, Botella R. Nuchal acne keloidalis associated with cyclosporin. Br J Dermatol 2001;144(2):429–30.
154. Gupta S, Radotra BD, Kumar B, Pandhi R, Rai R. Multiple, large, polypoid infundibular (epidermoid) cysts in a cyclosporin-treated renal transplant recipient. Dermatology 2000;201(1):78.
155. Mahendran R, Grech C. Generalized pustular psoriasis following a short course of cyclosporin (Neoral). Br J Dermatol 1998;139(5):934.
156. Halpert E, Tunnessen WW Jr, Fivush B, Case B. Cutaneous lesions associated with cyclosporine therapy in pediatric renal transplant recipients. J Pediatr 1991;119(3):489–91.
157. Reznik VM, Jones KL, Durham BL, Mendoza SA. Changes in facial appearance during cyclosporin treatment. Lancet 1987;1(8547):1405–7.
158. Lee MO, Park SK, Choi JH, Sung KJ, Moon KC, Koh JK. Juxta-clavicular beaded lines in a kidney transplant patient receiving immunosuppressants. J Dermatol 2002; 29(4):235–7.
159. Lear J, Bourke JF, Burns DA. Hyperplastic pseudofolliculitis barbae associated with cyclosporin. Br J Dermatol 1997;136(1):132–3.
160. Rebora A, Delmonte S, Parodi A. Cyclosporin A-induced hair darkening. Int J Dermatol 1999;38(3):229–30.
161. Siragusa M, Alberti A, Schepis C. Mees' lines due to cyclosporin. Br J Dermatol 1999;140(6):1198–9.
162. Arellano F, Krupp P. Muscular disorders associated with cyclosporin. Lancet 1991;337(8746):915.
163. Breil M, Chariot P. Muscle disorders associated with cyclosporine treatment. Muscle Nerve 1999;22(12):1631–6.
164. Stevens JM, Hilson AJ, Sweny P. Post-renal transplant distal limb bone pain. An under-recognized complication of transplantation distinct from avascular necrosis of bone? Transplantation 1995;60(3):305–7.
165. Barbosa LM, Gauthier VJ, Davis CL. Bone pain that responds to calcium channel blockers. A retrospective and prospective study of transplant recipients. Transplantation 1995;59(4):541–4.

166. Hokken-Koelega AC, Van Zaal MA, de Ridder MA, Wolff ED, De Jong MC, Donckerwolcke RA, De Muinck Keizer-Schrama SM, Drop SL. Growth after renal transplantation in prepubertal children: impact of various treatment modalities. Pediatr Res 1994;35(3): 367–71.
167. Monegal A, Navasa M, Guanabens N, Peris P, Pons F, Martinez de Osaba MJ, Rimola A, Rodes J, Munoz-Gomez J. Bone mass and mineral metabolism in liver transplant patients treated with FK506 or cyclosporine A. Calcif Tissue Int 2001;68(2):83–6.
168. Baildam AD, Higgins RM, Hurley E, Furlong A, Walls J, Venning MC, Ackrill P, Mansel RE. Cyclosporin A and multiple fibroadenomas of the breast. Br J Surg 1996;83(12):1755–7.
169. Foxwell BM, Woerly G, Husi H, Mackie A, Quesniaux VF, Hiestand PC, Wenger RM, Ryffel B. Identification of several cyclosporine binding proteins in lymphoid and non-lymphoid cells in vivo. Biochim Biophys Acta 1992;1138(2):115–21.
170. Lopez-Calderon A, Soto L, Villanua MA, Vidarte L, Martin AI. The effect of cyclosporine administration on growth hormone release and serum concentrations of insulin-like growth factor-I in male rats. Life Sci 1999;64(17):1473–83.
171. Russell DH, Kibler R, Matrisian L, Larson DF, Poulos B, Magun BE. Prolactin receptors on human T and B lymphocytes: antagonism of prolactin binding by cyclosporine. J Immunol 1985;134(5):3027–31.
172. Larson DF. Cyclosporin. Mechanism of action: antagonism of the prolactin receptor. Prog Allergy 1986;38:222–38.
173. Volcheck GW, Van Dellen RG. Anaphylaxis to intravenous cyclosporine and tolerance to oral cyclosporine: case report and review. Ann Allergy Asthma Immunol 1998;80(2):159–63.
174. Liau-Chu M, Theis JG, Koren G. Mechanism of anaphylactoid reactions: improper preparation of high-dose intravenous cyclosporine leads to bolus infusion of Cremophor EL and cyclosporine Ann Pharmacother 1997; 31(11):1287–91.
175. Garcia VD, Keitel E, Almeida P, Santos AF, Becker M, Goldani JC. Morbidity after renal transplantation: role of bacterial infection. Transplant Proc 1995;27(2):1825–6.
176. Wade JJ, Rolando N, Hayllar K, Philpott-Howard J, Casewell MW, Williams R. Bacterial and fungal infections after liver transplantation: an analysis of 284 patients. Hepatology 1995;21(5):1328–36.
177. Singh N, Yu VL. Infections in organ transplant recipients. Curr Opin Infect Dis 1996;9:223–9.
178. Reis MA, Costa RS, Ferraz AS. Causes of death in renal transplant recipients: a study of 102 autopsies from 1968 to 1991. J R Soc Med 1995;88(1):24–7.
179. Fukuda M, Ohmori Y, Aikawa I, Yoshimura N, Oka T. Mutagenicity of cyclosporine in vivo. Transplant Proc 1988;20(3 Suppl 3):929–30.
180. Penn I. Tumors after renal and cardiac transplantation. Hematol Oncol Clin North Am 1993;7(2):431–45.
181. Qunibi WY, Akhtar M, Ginn E, Smith P. Kaposi's sarcoma in cyclosporine-induced gingival hyperplasia. Am J Kidney Dis 1988;11(4):349–52.
182. Penn I. Cancers after cyclosporine therapy. Transplant Proc 1988;20(1 Suppl 1):276–9.
183. Penn I. Posttransplant malignancies. World J Urol 1988;6:125.
184. Penn I, Brunson ME. Cancers after cyclosporine therapy. Transplant Proc 1988;20(3 Suppl 3):885–92.
185. Pilgrim M. Spontane Manifestation und Regression eines Kaposi-Sarkoms unter Cyclosporin A. [Spontaneous manifestation and regression of a Kaposi's sarcoma under cyclosporin A therapy.] Hautarzt 1988;39(6): 368–70.
186. Gaya SB, Rees AJ, Lechler RI, Williams G, Mason PD. Malignant disease in patients with long-term renal transplants. Transplantation 1995;59(12):1705–9.
187. London NJ, Farmery SM, Will EJ, Davison AM, Lodge JP. Risk of neoplasia in renal transplant patients. Lancet 1995;346(8972):403–6.
188. Kirby B, Owen CM, Blewitt RW, Yates VM. Cutaneous T cell lymphoma developing in a patient on cyclosporin therapy. J Am Acad Dermatol 2002; 47(Suppl 2):S165–7.
189. Kehinde EO, Petermann A, Morgan JD, Butt ZA, Donnelly PK, Veitch PS, Bell PR. Triple therapy and incidence of de novo cancer in renal transplant recipients. Br J Surg 1994;81(7):985–6.
190. Opelz G, Henderson R. Incidence of non-Hodgkin lymphoma in kidney and heart transplant recipients. Lancet 1993;342(8886–8887):1514–16.
191. Gruber SA, Gillingham K, Sothern RB, Stephanian E, Matas AJ, Dunn DL. De novo cancer in cyclosporine-treated and non-cyclosporine-treated adult primary renal allograft recipients. Clin Transplant 1994; 8(4):388–95.
192. Hiesse C, Kriaa F, Rieu P, Larue JR, Benoit G, Bellamy J, Blanchet P, Charpentier B. Incidence and type of malignancies occurring after renal transplantation in conventionally and cyclosporine-treated recipients: analysis of a 20-year period in 1600 patients. Transplant Proc 1995;27(1):972–4.
193. Hojo M, Morimoto T, Maluccio M, Asano T, Morimoto K, Lagman M, Shimbo T, Suthanthiran M. Cyclosporine induces cancer progression by a cell-autonomous mechanism. Nature 1999;397(6719):530–4.
194. Jensen P, Hansen S, Moller B, Leivestad T, Pfeffer P, Geiran O, Fauchald P, Simonsen S. Skin cancer in kidney and heart transplant recipients and different long-term immunosuppressive therapy regimens. J Am Acad Dermatol 1999;40(2 Pt 1):177–86.
195. Weinstein SP, Orel SG, Collazzo L, Conant EF, Lawton TJ, Czerniecki B. Cyclosporin A-induced fibroadenomas of the breast: report of five cases. Radiology 2001;220(2):465–8.
196. De Felipe I, Redondo P. Eruptive angiomas after treatment with cyclosporine in a patient with psoriasis. Arch Dermatol 1998;134(11):1487–8.
197. Armenti VT, Ahlswede KM, Ahlswede BA, Cater JR, Jarrell BE, Mortiz MJ, Burke JF Jr. Variables affecting birthweight and graft survival in 197 pregnancies in cyclosporine-treated female kidney transplant recipients. Transplantation 1995;59(4):476–9.
198. Cararach V, Carmona F, Monleon FJ, Andreu J. Pregnancy after renal transplantation: 25 years experience in Spain. Br J Obstet Gynaecol 1993;100(2):122–5.
199. Ramsey-Goldman R, Schilling E. Immunosuppressive drug use during pregnancy. Rheum Dis Clin North Am 1997;23(1):149–67.
200. Armenti VT, Moritz MJ, Davison JM. Drug safety issues in pregnancy following transplantation and immunosuppression: effects and outcomes. Drug Saf 1998;19(3):219–32.
201. Armenti VT, Ahlswede KM, Ahlswede BA, Jarrell BE, Moritz MJ, Burke JF. National Transplantation Pregnancy Registry—outcomes of 154 pregnancies in cyclosporine-treated female kidney transplant recipients. Transplantation 1994;57(4):502–6.
202. Armenti VT, Ahlswede BA, Moritz MJ, Jarrell BE. National Transplantation Pregnancy Registry: analysis of pregnancy outcomes of female kidney recipients with

relation to time interval from transplant to conception. Transplant Proc 1993;25(1 Pt 2):1036–7.
203. Pilarski LM, Yacyshyn BR, Lazarovits AI. Analysis of peripheral blood lymphocyte populations and immune function from children exposed to cyclosporine or to azathioprine in utero. Transplantation 1994;57(1):133–44.
204. Baarsma R, Kamps WA. Immunological responses in an infant after cyclosporine A exposure during pregnancy. Eur J Pediatr 1993;152(6):476–7.
205. Giudice PL, Dubourg L, Hadj-Aissa A, Said MH, Claris O, Audra P, Martin X, Cochat P. Renal function of children exposed to cyclosporin in utero. Nephrol Dial Transplant 2000;15(10):1575–9.
206. Shaheen FA, al-Sulaiman MH, al-Khader AA. Long-term nephrotoxicity after exposure to cyclosporine in utero. Transplantation 1993;56(1):224–5.
207. Bar Oz B, Hackman R, Einarson T, Koren G. Pregnancy outcome after cyclosporine therapy during pregnancy: a meta-analysis. Transplantation 2001;71(8):1051–5.
208. Nyberg G, Haljamae U, Frisenette-Fich C, Wennergren M, Kjellmer I. Breast-feeding during treatment with cyclosporine. Transplantation 1998;65(2):253–5.
209. Olyaei AJ, deMattos AM, Bennett WM. Switching between cyclosporin formulations. What are the risks? Drug Saf 1997;16(6):366–73.
210. Wijdicks EF, Dahlke LJ, Wiesner RH. Oral cyclosporine decreases severity of neurotoxicity in liver transplant recipients. Neurology 1999;52(8):1708–10.
211. Keown P, Landsberg D, Halloran P, Shoker A, Rush D, Jeffery J, Russell D, Stiller C, Muirhead N, Cole E, Paul L, Zaltzman J, Loertscher R, Daloze P, Dandavino R, Boucher A, Handa P, Lawen J, Belitsky P, Parfrey P. A randomized, prospective multicenter pharmacoepidemiologic study of cyclosporine microemulsion in stable renal graft recipients. Report of the Canadian Neoral Renal Transplantation Study Group. Transplantation 1996;62(12):1744–52.
212. Shah MB, Martin JE, Schroeder TJ, First MR. Evaluation of the safety and tolerability of Neoral and Sandimmune: a meta-analysis. Transplant Proc 1998; 30(5):1697–700.
213. Freise CE, Galbraith CA, Nikolai BJ, Ascher NL, Lake JR, Stock PG, Roberts JP. Risks associated with conversion of stable patients after liver transplantation to the microemulsion formulation of cyclosporine. Transplantation 1998;65(7):995–7.
214. Shah MB, Martin JE, Schroeder TJ, First MR. Validity of open labeled versus blinded trials: a meta-analysis comparing Neoral and Sandimmune. Transplant Proc 1999;31(1–2):217–19.
215. Sheil AG, Disney AP, Mathew TH, Amiss N, Excell L. Cancer development in cadaveric donor renal allograft recipients treated with azathioprine (AZA) or cyclosporine (CyA) or AZA/CyA. Transplant Proc 1991;23(1 Pt 2): 1111–12.
216. Hiesse C, Rieu P, Kriaa F, Larue JR, Goupy C, Neyrat N, Charpentier B. Malignancy after renal transplantation: analysis of incidence and risk factors in 1700 patients followed during a 25-year period. Transplant Proc 1997;29(1–2):831–3.
217. Hoshida Y, Tsukuma H, Yasunaga Y, Xu N, Fujita MQ, Satoh T, Ichikawa Y, Kurihara K, Imanishi M, Matsuno T, Aozasa K. Cancer risk after renal transplantation in Japan. Int J Cancer 1997;71(4):517–20.
218. Dantal J, Hourmant M, Cantarovich D, Giral M, Blancho G, Dreno B, Soulillou JP. Effect of long-term immunosuppression in kidney-graft recipients on cancer incidence: randomised comparison of two cyclosporin regimens. Lancet 1998;351(9103):623–8.
219. Feutren G. The optimal use of cyclosporin A in autoimmune diseases. J Autoimmun 1992;5(Suppl A):183–95.
220. Arellano F, Krupp P. Malignancies in rheumatoid arthritis patients treated with cyclosporin A. Br J Rheumatol 1993;32(Suppl 1):72–5.
221. van den Borne BE, Landewe RB, Houkes I, Schild F, van der Heyden PC, Hazes JM, Vandenbroucke JP, Zwinderman AH, Goei The HS, Breedveld FC, Bernelot Moens HJ, Kluin PM, Dijkmans BA. No increased risk of malignancies and mortality in cyclosporin A-treated patients with rheumatoid arthritis. Arthritis Rheum 1998;41(11):1930–7.
222. Arellano F. Risk of cancer with cyclosporine in psoriasis. Int J Dermatol 1997;36(Suppl 1):15–17.
223. Arellano F, Monka C, Krupp PF. Acute cyclosporin overdose. A review of present clinical experience. Drug Saf 1991;6(4):266–76.
224. Sketris IS, Onorato L, Yatscoff RW, Givner M, Nicol D, Abraham I. Eight days of cyclosporine overdose: a case report. Pharmacotherapy 1993;13(6):658–60.
225. Dussol B, Reynaud-Gaubert M, Saingra Y, Daniel L, Berland Y. Acute tubular necrosis induced by high level of cyclosporine A in a lung transplant. Transplantation 2000;70(8):1234–6.
226. de Perrot M, Spiliopoulos A, Cottini S, Nicod L, Ricou B. Massive cerebral edema after I.V. cyclosporin overdose. Transplantation 2000;70(8):1259–60.
227. Tabbara KF, Al-Faisal Z, Al-Rashed W. Interaction between acetazolamine and cyclosporine. Arch Ophthalmol 1998;116(6):832–3.
228. Lill J, Bauer LA, Horn JR, Hansten PD. Cyclosporine-drug interactions and the influence of patient age. Am J Health Syst Pharm 2000;57(17):1579–84.
229. Ahmed T, Fenton T, McGraw M. Reversible renal failure in renal transplant patients receiving acyclovir. Pediatr Nephrol 1993;7:C58.
230. Dugandzic RM, Sketris IS, Belitsky P, Schlech WF 3rd, Givner ML. Effect of coadministration of acyclovir and cyclosporine on kidney function and cyclosporine concentrations in renal transplant patients. DICP 1991; 25(3):316–17.
231. Termeer A, Hoitsma AJ, Koene RA. Severe nephrotoxicity caused by the combined use of gentamicin and cyclosporine in renal allograft recipients. Transplantation 1986;42(2):220–1.
232. Sketris IS, Methot ME, Nicol D, Belitsky P, Knox MG. Effect of calcium-channel blockers on cyclosporine clearance and use in renal transplant patients. Ann Pharmacother 1994;28(11):1227–31.
233. Smith CL, Hampton EM, Pederson JA, Pennington LR, Bourne DW. Clinical and medicoeconomic impact of the cyclosporine–diltiazem interaction in renal transplant recipients. Pharmacotherapy 1994;14(4):471–81.
234. Jones TE, Morris RG, Mathew TH. Formulation of diltiazem affects cyclosporin-sparing activity. Eur J Clin Pharmacol 1997;52(1):55–8.
235. Kuypers DR, Neumayer HH, Fritsche L, Budde K, Rodicio JL, Vanrenterghem Y; Lacidipine Study Group. Calcium channel blockade and preservation of renal graft function in cyclosporine-treated recipients: a prospective randomized placebo-controlled 2-year study. Transplantation 2004;78(8):1204–11.
236. Bui L, Huang DD. Possible interaction between cyclosporine and chloramphenicol. Ann Pharmacother 1999; 33(2):252–3.
237. Thurnheer R, Laube I, Speich R. Possible interaction between clindamycin and cyclosporin. BMJ 1999; 319(7203):163.

238. Ducloux D, Schuller V, Bresson-Vautrin C, Chalopin JM. Colchicine myopathy in renal transplant recipients on cyclosporin. Nephrol Dial Transplant 1997;12(11):2389–92.
239. Tweddle DA, Windebank KP, Hewson QC, Yule SM. Cyclosporin neurotoxicity after chemotherapy. BMJ 1999;318(7191):1113.
240. Pea F, Damiani D, Michieli M, Ermacora A, Baraldo M, Russo D, Fanin R, Baccarani M, Furlanut M. Multidrug resistance modulation in vivo: the effect of cyclosporin A alone or with dexverapamil on idarubicin pharmacokinetics in acute leukemia. Eur J Clin Pharmacol 1999; 55(5):361–8.
241. Meerum Terwogt JM, Beijnen JH, ten Bokkel Huinink WW, Rosing H, Schellens JH. Co-administration of cyclosporin enables oral therapy with paclitaxel. Lancet 1998;352(9124):285.
242. Malingre MM, Beijnen JH, Rosing H, Koopman FJ, van Tellingen O, Duchin K, Ten Bokkel Huinink WW, Swart M, Lieverst J, Schellens JH. A phase I and pharmacokinetic study of bi-daily dosing of oral paclitaxel in combination with cyclosporin A. Cancer Chemother Pharmacol 2001;47(4):347–54.
243. Bisogno G, Cowie F, Boddy A, Thomas HD, Dick G, Pinkerton CR. High-dose cyclosporin with etoposide—toxicity and pharmacokinetic interaction in children with solid tumours. Br J Cancer 1998;77(12):2304–9.
244. Rushing DA, Raber SR, Rodvold KA, Piscitelli SC, Plank GS, Tewksbury DA. The effects of cyclosporine on the pharmacokinetics of doxorubicin in patients with small cell lung cancer. Cancer 1994;74(3):834–41.
245. Hoey LL, Lake KD. Does ciprofloxacin interact with cyclosporine? Ann Pharmacother 1994;28(1):93–6.
246. McLellan RA, Drobitch RK, McLellan H, Acott PD, Crocker JF, Renton KW. Norfloxacin interferes with cyclosporine disposition in pediatric patients undergoing renal transplantation. Clin Pharmacol Ther 1995; 58(3):322–7.
247. Wynckel A, Toupance O, Melin JP, David C, Lavaud S, Wong T, Lamiable D, Chanard J. Traitement des légionelloses par ofloxacine chez le transplanté rénal. Absence d'interférence avec la ciclosporine A. [Treatment of legionellosis with ofloxacin in kidney transplanted patients. Lack of interaction with cyclosporin A.] Presse Méd 1991;20(7):291–3.
248. Morales JM, Munoz MA, Fernandez Zatarain G, Garcia Canton C, Garcia Rubiales MA, Andres A, Aguado JM, Gonzalez Pinto I. Reversible acute renal failure caused by the combined use of foscarnet and cyclosporin in organ transplanted patients. Nephrol Dial Transplant 1995; 10(6):882–3.
249. Cantarovich M, Latter D. Effect of prophylactic ganciclovir on renal function and cyclosporine levels after heart transplantation. Transplant Proc 1994;26(5):2747–8.
250. Johnston A, Holt DW. Effect of grapefruit juice on blood cyclosporin concentration. Lancet 1995; 346(8967):122–3.
251. Lewis SM, McCloskey WW. Potentiation of nephrotoxicity by H2-antagonists in patients receiving cyclosporine. Ann Pharmacother 1997;31(3):363–5.
252. Rodriguez JA, Crespo-Leiro MG, Paniagua MJ, Cuenca JJ, Hermida LF, Juffe A, Castro-Beiras A. Rhabdomyolysis in heart transplant patients on HMG-CoA reductase inhibitors and cyclosporine. Transplant Proc 1999;31(6):2522–3.
253. Gullestad L, Nordal KP, Berg KJ, Cheng H, Schwartz MS, Simonsen S. Interaction between lovastatin and cyclosporine A after heart and kidney transplantation. Transplant Proc 1999;31(5):2163–5.
254. Maltz HC, Balog DL, Cheigh JS. Rhabdomyolysis associated with concomitant use of atorvastatin and cyclosporine. Ann Pharmacother 1999;33(11):1176–9.
255. East C, Alivizatos PA, Grundy SM, Jones PH, Farmer JA. Rhabdomyolysis in patients receiving lovastatin after cardiac transplantation. N Engl J Med 1988;318(1):47–8.
256. Campana C, Iacona I, Regazzi MB, Gavazzi A, Perani G, Raddato V, Montemartini C, Vigano M. Efficacy and pharmacokinetics of simvastatin in heart transplant recipients. Ann Pharmacother 1995;29(3):235–9.
257. Cheung AK, DeVault GA Jr, Gregory MC. A prospective study on treatment of hypercholesterolemia with lovastatin in renal transplant patients receiving cyclosporine. J Am Soc Nephrol 1993;3(12):1884–91.
258. Wanner C, Kramer-Guth A, Galle J. Use of HMG-CoA reductase inhibitors after kidney and heart transplantation. BioDrugs 1997;8:387–93.
259. Olbricht C, Wanner C, Eisenhauer T, Kliem V, Doll R, Boddaert M, O'Grady P, Krekler M, Mangold B, Christians U. Accumulation of lovastatin, but not pravastatin, in the blood of cyclosporine-treated kidney graft patients after multiple doses. Clin Pharmacol Ther 1997;62(3):311–21.
260. Ichimaru N, Takahara S, Kokado Y, Wang JD, Hatori M, Kameoka H, Inoue T, Okuyama A. Changes in lipid metabolism and effect of simvastatin in renal transplant recipients induced by cyclosporine or tacrolimus. Atherosclerosis 2001;158(2):417–23.
261. Muck W, Mai I, Fritsche L, Ochmann K, Rohde G, Unger S, Johne A, Bauer S, Budde K, Roots I, Neumayer HH, Kuhlmann J. Increase in cerivastatin systemic exposure after single and multiple dosing in cyclosporine-treated kidney transplant recipients. Clin Pharmacol Ther 1999;65(3):251–61.
262. Ruschitzka F, Meier PJ, Turina M, Luscher TF, Noll G. Acute heart transplant rejection due to Saint John's wort. Lancet 2000;355(9203):548–9.
263. Breidenbach T, Hoffmann MW, Becker T, Schlitt H, Klempnauer J. Drug interaction of St. John's wort with cyclosporin. Lancet 2000;355(9218):1912.
264. Barone GW, Gurley BJ, Ketel BL, Lightfoot ML, Abul-Ezz SR. Drug interaction between St. John's wort and cyclosporine. Ann Pharmacother 2000;34(9):1013–16.
265. Karliova M, Treichel U, Malago M, Frilling A, Gerken G, Broelsch CE. Interaction of *Hypericum perforatum* (St. John's wort) with cyclosporin A metabolism in a patient after liver transplantation. J Hepatol 2000;33(5):853–5.
266. Mai I, Kruger H, Budde K, Johne A, Brockmoller J, Neumayer HH, Roots I. Hazardous pharmacokinetic interaction of Saint John's wort (*Hypericum perforatum*) with the immunosuppressant cyclosporin. Int J Clin Pharmacol Ther 2000;38(10):500–2.
267. Schroeder TJ, Melvin DB, Clardy CW, Wadhwa NK, Myre SA, Reising JM, Wolf RK, Collins JA, Pesce AJ, First MR. Use of cyclosporine and ketoconazole without nephrotoxicity in two heart transplant recipients. J Heart Transplant 1987;6(2):84–9.
268. First MR, Schroeder TJ, Michael A, Hariharan S, Weiskittel P, Alexander JW. Cyclosporine–ketoconazole interaction. Long-term follow-up and preliminary results of a randomized trial. Transplantation 1993;55(5):1000–4.
269. Keogh A, Spratt P, McCosker C, Macdonald P, Mundy J, Kaan A. Ketoconazole to reduce the need for cyclosporine after cardiac transplantation. N Engl J Med 1995; 333(10):628–33.
270. Sobh M, el-Agroudy A, Moustafa F, Harras F, el-Bedewy M, Ghoneim M. Coadministration of ketoconazole to cyclosporin-treated kidney transplant recipients: a

prospective randomized study. Am J Nephrol 1995; 15(6):493–9.
271. Romero AJ, Pogamp PL, Nilsson LG, Wood N. Effect of voriconazole on the pharmacokinetics of cyclosporine in renal transplant patients. Clin Pharmacol Ther 2002; 71(4):226–34.
272. Turhal NS. Cyclosporin A and imipenem associated seizure activity in allogeneic bone marrow transplantation patients. J Chemother 1999;11(5):410–13.
273. Jones TE. The use of other drugs to allow a lower dosage of cyclosporin to be used. Therapeutic and pharmacoeconomic considerations. Clin Pharmacokinet 1997;32(5):357–67.
274. Amsden GW. Macrolides versus azalides: a drug interaction update. Ann Pharmacother 1995;29(9):906–17.
275. Gregoor PJ, de Sevaux RG, Hene RJ, Hesse CJ, Hilbrands LB, Vos P, van Gelder T, Hoitsma AJ, Weimar W. Effect of cyclosporine on mycophenolic acid trough levels in kidney transplant recipients. Transplantation 1999;68(10):1603–6.
276. Helms-Smith KM, Curtis SL, Hatton RC. Apparent interaction between nefazodone and cyclosporine. Ann Intern Med 1996;125(5):424.
277. Garton T. Nefazodone and CYP450 3A4 interactions with cyclosporine and tacrolimus1. Transplantation 2002;74(5):745.
278. Wright DH, Lake KD, Bruhn PS, Emery RW Jr. Nefazodone and cyclosporine drug–drug interaction. J Heart Lung Transplant 1999;18(9):913–15.
279. Constantopoulos A. Colitis induced by interaction of cyclosporine A and non-steroidal anti-inflammatory drugs. Pediatr Int 1999;41(2):184–6.
280. Kovarik JM, Mueller EA, Gerbeau C, Tarral A, Francheteau P, Guerret M. Cyclosporine and nonsteroidal antiinflammatory drugs: exploring potential drug interactions and their implications for the treatment of rheumatoid arthritis. J Clin Pharmacol 1997;37(4):336–43.
281. Kovarik JM, Kurki P, Mueller E, Guerret M, Markert E, Alten R, Zeidler H, Genth-Stolzenburg S. Diclofenac combined with cyclosporine in treatment refractory rheumatoid arthritis: longitudinal safety assessment and evidence of a pharmacokinetic/dynamic interaction. J Rheumatol 1996;23(12):2033–8.
282. Tugwell P, Ludwin D, Gent M, Roberts R, Bensen W, Grace E, Baker P. Interaction between cyclosporin A and nonsteroidal antiinflammatory drugs. J Rheumatol 1997;24(6):1122–5.
283. Barbaro D, Orsini P, Pallini S, Piazza F, Pasquini C. Obesity in transplant patients: case report showing interference of orlistat with absorption of cyclosporine and review of literature. Endocr Pract 2002;8(2):124–6.
284. Nagele H, Petersen B, Bonacker U, Rodiger W. Effect of orlistat on blood cyclosporin concentration in an obese heart transplant patient. Eur J Clin Pharmacol 1999;55(9):667–9.
285. Colman E, Fossler M. Reduction in blood cyclosporine concentrations by orlistat. N Engl J Med 2000; 342(15):1141–2.
286. Le Beller C, Bezie Y, Chabatte C, Guillemain R, Amrein C, Billaud EM. Co-administration of orlistat and cyclosporine in a heart transplant recipient. Transplantation 2000;70(10):1541–2.
287. Schnetzler B, Kondo-Oestreicher M, Vala D, Khatchatourian G, Faidutti B. Orlistat decreases the plasma level of cyclosporine and may be responsible for the development of acute rejection episodes. Transplantation 2000;70(10):1540–1.
288. Actis GC, Debernardi-Venon W, Lagget M, Marzano A, Ottobrelli A, Ponzetto A, Rocca G, Boggio-Bertinet D, Balzola F, Bonino F, et al. Hepatotoxicity of intravenous cyclosporin A in patients with acute ulcerative colitis on total parenteral nutrition. Liver 1995;15(6):320–3.
289. Gregoor PJ, van Gelder T, van der Ende ME, Ijzermans JN, Weimar W. Cyclosporine and triple-drug treatment with human immunodeficiency virus protease inhibitors. Transplantation 1999;68(8):1210.
290. Schouler L, Dumas F, Couzigou P, Janvier G, Winnock S, Saric J. Omeprazole–cyclosporin interaction. Am J Gastroenterol 1991;86(8):1097.
291. Arranz R, Yanez E, Franceschi JL, Fernandez-Ranada JM. More about omeprazole–cyclosporine interaction. Am J Gastroenterol 1993;88(1):154–5.
292. Blohme I, Idstrom JP, Andersson T. A study of the interaction between omeprazole and cyclosporine in renal transplant patients. Br J Clin Pharmacol 1993;35(2):156–60.
293. Brinkman K, Huysmans F, Burger DM. Pharmacokinetic interaction between saquinavir and cyclosporine. Ann Intern Med 1998;129(11):914–15.
294. Du Cheyron D, Debruyne D, Lobbedez T, Richer C, Ryckelynck JP, Hurault de Ligny B. Effect of sulfasalazine on cyclosporin blood concentration. Eur J Clin Pharmacol 1999;55(3):227–8.
295. Caforio AL, Gambino A, Tona F, Feltrin G, Marchini F, Pompei E, Testolin L, Angelini A, Dalla Volta S, Casarotto D. Sulfinpyrazone reduces cyclosporine levels: a new drug interaction in heart transplant recipients. J Heart Lung Transplant 2000;19(12):1205–8.
296. Pichard L, Fabre I, Fabre G, Domergue J, Saint Aubert B, Mourad G, Maurel P. Cyclosporin A drug interactions. Screening for inducers and inhibitors of cytochrome P-450 (cyclosporin A oxidase) in primary cultures of human hepatocytes and in liver microsomes. Drug Metab Dispos 1990;18(5):595–606.
297. Islam SI, Masuda QN, Bolaji OO, Shaheen FM, Sheikh IA. Possible interaction between cyclosporine and glibenclamide in posttransplant diabetic patients. Ther Drug Monit 1996;18(5):624–6.
298. Verdejo A, de Cos MA, Zubimendi JA, Lopez-Lazaro L. Drug points. Probable interaction between cyclosporin A and low dose ticlopidine. BMJ 2000;320(7241):1037.
299. Kaplan B, Friedman G, Jacobs M, Viscuso R, Lyman N, DeFranco P, Bonomini L, Mulgaonkar SP. Potential interaction of troglitazone and cyclosporine. Transplantation 1998;65(10):1399–400.
300. Park MH, Pelegrin D, Haug MT 3rd, Young JB. Troglitazone, a new antidiabetic agent, decreases cyclosporine level. J Heart Lung Transplant 1998;17(11):1139–40.
301. Le Bigot JF, Lavene D, Kiechel JR. Pharmacocinétique et métabolisme di la cyclosporine: interaction médicamenteuse. [Pharmacokinetics and metabolism of cyclosporin; drug interactions.] Nephrologie 1987;8(3):135–41.
302. Keown PA. New concepts in cyclosporine monitoring. Curr Opin Nephrol Hypertens 2002;11(6):619–26.
303. Levy G, Burra P, Cavallari A, Duvoux C, Lake J, Mayer AD, Mies S, Pollard SG, Varo E, Villamil F, Johnston A. Improved clinical outcomes for liver transplant recipients using cyclosporine monitoring based on 2-hr post-dose levels (C2). Transplantation 2002;73(6):953–9.
304. Lindholm A, Ringden O, Lonnqvist B. The role of cyclosporine dosage and plasma levels in efficacy and toxicity in bone marrow transplant recipients. Transplantation 1987;43(5):680–4.
305. Azoulay D, Lemoine A, Dennison A, Gries JM, Dolizy I, Castaing D, Beaune P, Bismuth H. Incidence of adverse reactions to cyclosporine after liver transplantation is predicted by the first blood level. Hepatology 1993; 17(6):1123–6.

Cidofovir

General Information

Cidofovir (*S*-1-3-hydroxy-2-phosphonylmethoxypropyl-cytosine), also known as HPMPC, is a nucleotide analogue with potent activity against cytomegalovirus (CMV) in vitro and in vivo.

Observational studies

Cidofovir has been used to treat 14 patients with cytomegalovirus infection after stem-cell transplantation; no adverse effects were reported in this small study (1).

In an open study of the use of intralesional cidofovir in treating laryngeal papilloma, 14 adults received monthly injections of cidofovir (maximum dose 37.5 mg per injection in 6 ml of saline; mean 22.5 mg) (2). Remission was achieved in all cases with an average of six injections and without additional laryngeal scarring, vocal cord damage, or systemic adverse effects.

Organs and Systems

Sensory systems

In a placebo-controlled study of the efficacy of cidofovir 1% eye-drops with and without ciclosporin 1% eye-drops four or ten times a day for acute adenovirus keratoconjunctivitis in 34 patients, the frequency of severe corneal opacities was lower with cidofovir (3). However, cidofovir caused conjunctival pseudomembranes, conjunctivitis, and erythematous inflammation of the skin of the eyelids, and the trial was stopped as a result.

Two cases of iritis shortly after intravenous administration of cidofovir have been reported (4). Intravitreal administration of cidofovir delays the progression of CMV retinitis, but can be associated with reduced intraocular pressure or vitreitis (5). In two cases the drug association with the iritis was demonstrated by withdrawal and rechallenge (6). These patients had also taken probenecid, but it is not clear whether or not that was involved. The evidence is that in such cases the cidofovir should be withdrawn; treatment should be with a mydriatic and glucocorticoids.

In a study of compassionate use of intravenous cidofovir in AIDS patients with CMV retinitis, iritis developed in 21 of 51 individuals (7). The appearance of this inflammatory process did not fit the characteristics of the vitritis associated with immune reconstitution, or with HIV-induced vitritis. The high rate in this cohort (compared with a 5–7% incidence in randomized trials) was associated with severe CMV retinitis, and the authors suggested that breakdown of the blood–ocular barrier in these patients may promote higher intraocular concentrations of cidofovir and thus enhance local toxicity. Previous correlations of prior use of HIV protease inhibitors with iritis were not confirmed in this study, although patients with iritis had better immunological and virological status than those without the disease.

Uveitis (8) and cystoid macular edema (9) are recognized risks associated with cidofovir treatment for cytomegalovirus retinitis. The latter is almost certainly an immune recovery phenomenon, since it is apparently encountered only in eyes with inactive CMV retinitis; the unaffected contralateral side never develops cystoid macular edema. The time range of appearance (3–48 weeks after administration) also makes a direct toxic effect of cidofovir unlikely.

In a retrospective record review of 18 HIV-infected patients (30 eyes) who were being treated with intravenous cidofovir for complicated cytomegalovirus retinitis, eight patients developed anterior uveitis after a median of four (range 2–8) doses of cidofovir or a median of 55 (20–131) days after the start of therapy (10). While they were receiving treatment with cidofovir, none of the patients showed any evidence of progression of CMV retinitis. Five of the eight had symptoms of photophobia and blurred vision at the onset of uveitis, and the other three were asymptomatic. There was no difference in the use of HIV-1 protease inhibitors between the patients who did or did not develop anterior uveitis. Baseline intraocular pressure measurements were available for 11/18 patients. With the introduction of cidofovir there was a fall in mean intraocular pressure, and a trend for this fall to be more pronounced in those who developed anterior uveitis. Withdrawal of cidofovir was necessary in only one patient, after which all symptoms and signs disappeared and vision returned to baseline within 1 month. In two of the seven other patients, cidofovir had to be withdrawn because of nephrotoxicity. In the other five patients, cidofovir was continued and the uveitis was controlled with topical therapy, consisting of corticosteroids with or without a cycloplegic agent.

During long-term follow-up of patients with AIDS treated with parenteral cidofovir for CMV retinitis, the median time to discontinuation for intolerance was 6.6 months (11). Cidofovir-associated uveitis occurred in 10 of 58 patients and ocular hypotony (a 50% fall in intraocular pressure from baseline to below 5 mmHg) occurred at a rate of 0.16 per person-year. There were 51 episodes of proteinuria in 30 of the 58 patients and 82% of these episodes resolved on withdrawal (median time to resolution 20 days). No nephrotoxic events required dialysis.

Urinary tract

The main adverse effect associated with intravenous cidofovir is renal tubular damage (12), although it is usually mild. However, cases of acute renal insufficiency leading to end-stage disease have been reported (13,14). Acute renal insufficiency has also been attributed to topical cidofovir (15).

- A 28-year-old bone marrow transplant recipient with chronic renal insufficiency developed genital condylomata resistant to standard therapy. After application of topical cidofovir (1% daily for 5 days, then 4% for 12 days) the lesions improved but local erosions appeared. He developed acute renal insufficiency with features of tubular acidosis on day 19. He recovered after cidofovir withdrawal.

It was not clear whether this effect was due to the cidofovir or to its vehicle, propylene glycol. The authors suggested that topical cidofovir should be avoided on abraded skin and should be carefully monitored.

The risk of renal toxicity was higher in patients with established CMV infections than in those who were taking it prophylactically, and there was no relation between dosage and nephrotoxicity; toxicity occurred early in therapy, usually within the first 3 weeks (16). Proteinuria seems to be an early indicator of this adverse effect. Other laboratory abnormalities associated with nephrotoxicity are glycosuria, reduced serum phosphate, uric acid, and bicarbonate, and an increased serum creatinine. Serious and potentially irreversible nephrotoxicity can generally be prevented by the concomitant administration of intravenous saline and oral probenecid, monitoring the blood and urine immediately before each infusion of cidofovir, and withdrawing the drug for low-threshold increases in either urinary protein or serum creatinine concentrations (17). Concomitant use of other nephrotoxic drugs should be avoided.

In a rare cytomegalovirus comparison trial, a ganciclovir insert (an intraocular implant) plus oral ganciclovir was compared with intravenous cidofovir (18). Based on data from 61 patients (the trial was stopped early owing to low recruitment), cidofovir was associated with a raised serum creatinine concentration of 142 μmol/l (1.6 mg/dl) or greater (0.48 per person-year), 3+ or greater proteinuria (0.29 per person-year), uveitis (0.35 per person-year), and neutropenia (0.11 per person-year).

Prophylactic cidofovir treatment for CMV antigenemia has been investigated in a prospective study in patients with transplants (19). Renal toxicity, occasionally with proteinuria, was reported, as was nausea. The renal toxicity was mild and reversible.

Susceptibility Factors

Renal disease

The pharmacokinetics of cidofovir were studied in 24 subjects with varying degrees of renal insufficiency, who were given a single intravenous dose of cidofovir 0.5 mg/kg over 1 hour (20). Those who were not receiving dialysis were given intravenous hydration and concomitant oral probenecid. Mean cidofovir clearance in control subjects (normal renal function; $n = 5$) was 1.7 ml/minute/kg, and this fell markedly with falling renal function. The mean steady-state volume of distribution did not change significantly in those with kidney disease, but the half-life of cidofovir was significantly prolonged in those with severe renal insufficiency. Cidofovir was not significantly cleared during continuous ambulatory peritoneal dialysis, but high-flux hemodialysis resulted in the removal of 52% of the dose. The authors concluded that very considerable aggressive dosage reduction of cidofovir would be necessary in subjects with kidney disease to ensure comparable drug exposure in terms of serum concentrations.

References

1. Bosi A, Bartolozzi B, Vannucchi AM, Orsi A, Guidi S, Rossi Ferrini P. Polymerase chain reaction-based "pre-emptive" therapy with cidofovir for cytomegalovirus reactivation in allogeneic hematopoietic stem cells transplantation recipients: a prospective study. Haematologica 2002;87(4):446–7.
2. Bielamowicz S, Villagomez V, Stager SV, Wilson WR. Intralesional cidofovir therapy for laryngeal papilloma in an adult cohort. Laryngoscope 2002;112(4):696–9.
3. Hillenkamp J, Reinhard T, Ross RS, Bohringer D, Cartsburg O, Roggendorf M, De Clercq E, Godehardt E, Sundmacher R. The effects of cidofovir 1% with and without cyclosporin a 1% as a topical treatment of acute adenoviral keratoconjunctivitis: a controlled clinical pilot study. Ophthalmology 2002;109(5):845–50.
4. Tseng AL, Mortimer CB, Salit IE. Iritis associated with intravenous cidofovir. Ann Pharmacother 1999;33(2):167–71.
5. Kirsch LS, Arevalo JF, Chavez de la Paz E, Munguia D, de Clercq E, Freeman WR. Intravitreal cidofovir (HPMPC) treatment of cytomegalovirus retinitis in patients with acquired immune deficiency syndrome. Ophthalmology 1995; 102(4):533–42. Erratum in: Ophthalmology 1995;102(5):702.
6. Neau D, Renaud-Rougier MB, Viallard JE, Dutronc H, Cazorla C, Ragnaud JM, Dupon M, Lacut JY. Intravenous cidofovir-induced iritis. Clin Infect Dis 1999;28(1):156–7.
7. Berenguer J, Mallolas J, Padilla B, Colmenero M, Santos I. Intravenous cidofovir for compassionate use in AIDS patients with cytomegalovirus retinitis. Spanish Cidofovir Study Group. Clin Infect Dis 2000;30(1):182–4.
8. Ambati J, Wynne KB, Angerame MC, Robinson MR. Anterior uveitis associated with intravenous cidofovir use in patients with cytomegalovirus retinitis. Br J Ophthalmol 1999;83(10):1153–8.
9. Kersten AJ, Althaus C, Best J, Sundmacher R. Cystoid macular edema following immune recovery and treatment with cidofovir for cytomegalovirus retinitis. Graefes Arch Clin Exp Ophthalmol 1999;237(11):893–6.
10. Akler ME, Johnson DW, Burman WJ, Johnson SC. Anterior uveitis and hypotony after intravenous cidofovir for the treatment of cytomegalovirus retinitis. Ophthalmology 1998;105(4):651–7.
11. Jabs DA, Freeman WR, Jacobson M, Murphy R, Van Natta ML, Meinert CL. Long-term follow-up of patients with AIDS treated with parenteral cidofovir for cytomegalovirus retinitis: the HPMPC Peripheral Cytomegalovirus Retinitis Trial. The Studies of Ocular Complications of AIDS Research Group in collaboration with the AIDS Clinical Trials Group. AIDS 2000;14(11):1571–81.
12. Skiest DJ, Duong M, Park S, Wei L, Keiser P. Complications of therapy with intravenous cidofovir: severe nephrotoxicity and anterior uveitis. Infect Dis Clin Pract 1999;83:151–7.
13. Vandercam B, Moreau M, Goffin E, Marot JC, Cosyns JP, Jadoul M. Cidofovir-induced end-stage renal failure. Clin Infect Dis 1999;29(4):948–9.
14. Meier P, Dautheville-Guibal S, Ronco PM, Rossert J. Cidofovir-induced end-stage renal failure. Nephrol Dial Transplant 2002;17(1):148–9.
15. Bienvenu B, Martinez F, Devergie A, Rybojad M, Rivet J, Bellenger P, Morel P, Gluckman E, Lebbe C. Topical use of cidofovir induced acute renal failure. Transplantation 2002;73(4):661–2.
16. Ljungman P, Deliliers GL, Platzbecker U, Matthes-Martin S, Bacigalupo A, Einsele H, Ullmann J, Musso M, Trenschel R, Ribaud P, Bornhauser M, Cesaro S, Crooks B, Dekker A, Gratecos N, Klingebiel T, Tagliaferri E, Ullmann AJ, Wacker P, Cordonnier C. Cidofovir for cytomegalovirus infection and disease in allogeneic stem cell transplant recipients. The Infectious Diseases Working Party of the European Group for Blood and Marrow Transplantation. Blood 2001;97(2):388–92.
17. Lalezari JP, Holland GN, Kramer F, McKinley GF, Kemper CA, Ives DV, Nelson R, Hardy WD, Kuppermann BD, Northfelt DW, Youle M, Johnson M, Lewis RA, Weinberg DV, Simon GL, Wolitz RA, Ruby AE, Stagg RJ, Jaffe HS. Randomized, controlled

study of the safety and efficacy of intravenous cidofovir for the treatment of relapsing cytomegalovirus retinitis in patients with AIDS. J Acquir Immune Defic Syndr Hum Retrovirol 1998;17(4):339–44.
18. Jabs DA. Studies of Ocular Complications of AIDS Research Group. The AIDS Clinical Trials Group. The ganciclovir implant plus oral ganciclovir versus parenteral cidofovir for the treatment of cytomegalovirus retinitis in patients with acquired immunodeficiency syndrome: The Ganciclovir Cidofovir Cytomegalovirus Retinitis Trial. Am J Ophthalmol 2001;131(4):457–67.
19. Platzbecker U, Bandt D, Thiede C, Helwig A, Freiberg-Richter J, Schuler U, Plettig R, Geissler G, Rethwilm A, Ehninger G, Bornhauser M. Successful preemptive cidofovir treatment for CMV antigenemia after dose-reduced conditioning and allogeneic blood stem cell transplantation. Transplantation 2001;71(7):880–5.
20. Brody SR, Humphreys MH, Gambertoglio JG, Schoenfeld P, Cundy KC, Aweeka FT. Pharmacokinetics of cidofovir in renal insufficiency and in continuous ambulatory peritoneal dialysis or high-flux hemodialysis. Clin Pharmacol Ther 1999;65(1):21–8.

Cilazapril

See also Angiotensin converting enzyme inhibitors

General Information

Cilazapril is a non-sulfhydryl ACE inhibitor (1). Like enalapril and ramipril it is a prodrug and is hydrolysed after absorption to cilazaprilat, which has a long half-life allowing once-daily administration (2).

Organs and Systems

Skin

Many cases of pemphigus have been reported with ACE inhibitors, related to the amide group they contain. This is the case for cilazapril.

- A 69-year-old white woman developed skin lesions of pemphigus foliaceus after she had taken cilazapril for 3 months; they resolved on withdrawal and the addition of prednisone and azathioprine (3).
- Pemphigus vulgaris possibly triggered by cilazapril has been reported (4).

References

1. Szucs T. Cilazapril. A review. Drugs 1991;41(Suppl 1):18–24.
2. Deget F, Brogden RN. Cilazapril. A review of its pharmacodynamic and pharmacokinetic properties, and therapeutic potential in cardiovascular disease. Drugs 1991;41(5):799–820.
3. Buzon E, Perez-Bernal AM, de la Pena F, Rios JJ, Camacho F. Pemphigus foliaceus associated with cilazapril. Acta Derm Venereol 1998;78(3):227.
4. Orion E, Gazit E, Brenner S. Pemphigus vulgaris possibly triggered by cilazapril. Acta Dermatol Venereol 2000;80(3):220.

Cilostazol

General Information

Cilostazol is a phosphodiesterase inhibitor that suppresses platelet aggregation and also acts as a direct arterial vasodilator. Small studies in Japan suggested that it might be useful for treating chronic arterial disease and symptoms of intermittent claudication. A trial in 81 patients with claudication substantiated this claim: claudication distance was improved by 35% for initial and 41% for absolute claudication distance.

Placebo-controlled studies

The efficacy and safety data of cilostazol in placebo-controlled clinical trials have been repeatedly subjected to meta-analysis, with the same conclusion (1,2). Cilostazol is well tolerated; headache, bowel complaints, and palpitation are the most common but mild adverse effects.

Six multicenter placebo-controlled trials have been conducted in the USA (3,4). They involved more than 2000 patients with intermittent claudication and established the efficacy of cilostazol in improving walking distance in these patients.

Cilostazol was approved by the FDA in January 1999 for the treatment of symptoms of intermittent claudication; from 1984 to 1999 pentoxifylline was the only drug approved in the USA for this indication. The two drugs have been compared with placebo in a large, randomized, double-blind, placebo-controlled trial (5). After 24 weeks of treatment the mean increase in maximal walking distance was 54% with cilostazol and only 30% with pentoxifylline and 34% with placebo. Headache, diarrhea, abnormal stools, and bouts of palpitation were significantly more common with cilostazol. They were reported as generally mild to moderate and self-limiting and have been previously recognized as being related to cilostazol.

The efficacy of antithrombotic prophylaxis with cilostazol for the secondary prevention of cerebral infarction has been studied in a Japanese, placebo-controlled trial in 1095 patients (6). There was a 42% relative risk reduction compared with placebo. As in the trials in patients with peripheral arterial disease, mild to moderate headache and palpitation were the most commonly observed symptomatic adverse events attributed to cilostazol; they respectively occurred in 13 and 5.3%. Headache with cilostazol is attributed to cerebral vasodilatation induced by relaxation of vascular smooth muscle.

In another placebo-controlled trial, there were gastrointestinal complaints in 44% of the cilostazol-treated patients and in 15% of the placebo group. The most commonly reported adverse effects included diarrhea, loose stools, flatulence, and nausea; they were usually mild and transient but persisted in some patients. Headache occurred in 20% of cilostazol-treated patients but also in 15% of those given placebo (7).

Safety data relating to the use of cilostazol in 2702 patients who participated in eight USA–UK placebo-controlled trials have been re-analysed (8). The most frequently recorded adverse events were headache (32%), diarrhea (17%), and abnormal stools (14%).

Palpitation, tachycardia, and dizziness were additional events that occurred more often in cilostazol-treated patients and were considered to be probably related to treatment. Headache led to withdrawal of cilostazol in 3.5% of patients, and palpitation and diarrhea led to withdrawal in another 1%. All adverse events quickly resolved after withdrawal. Cardiovascular and all-cause mortality were similar with cilostazol and placebo.

Organs and Systems

Cardiovascular

Ventricular tachycardia has been reported during cilostazol therapy (9).

- A 92-year-old woman developed sudden runs of ventricular tachycardia, a few days after she started to take cilostazol because of subacute leg ischemia. She was known to have atrial fibrillation and intraventricular conduction delay. The runs did not respond to empirical magnesium therapy but subsided shortly after withdrawal of cilostazol.

The phosphodiesterase III inhibitors have no known direct dysrhythmogenic effects. However, the authors speculated that raised concentrations of cAMP may have contributed to the ventricular tachycardia, mainly because ventricular dysrhythmias have been mentioned with other agents of the same family in patients with heart failure. Whether some populations are particularly vulnerable is unknown.

References

1. Thompson PD, Zimet R, Forbes WP, Zhang P. Meta-analysis of results from eight randomized, placebo-controlled trials on the effect of cilostazol on patients with intermittent claudication. Am J Cardiol 2002;90(12):1314–19.
2. Regensteiner JG, Ware JE Jr, McCarthy WJ, Zhang P, Forbes WP, Heckman J, Hiatt WR. Effect of cilostazol on treadmill walking, community-based walking ability, and health-related quality of life in patients with intermittent claudication due to peripheral arterial disease: meta-analysis of six randomized controlled trials. J Am Geriatr Soc 2002;50(12):1939–46.
3. Comp PC. Treatment of intermittent claudication in peripheral arterial disease. Recent clinical experience with cilostazol. Today's Ther Trends 1999;17:99–112.
4. Sorkin EM, Markham A. Cilostazol. Drugs Aging 1999;14(1):63–71.
5. Dawson DL, Cutler BS, Hiatt WR, Hobson RW 2nd, Martin JD, Bortey EB, Forbes WP, Strandness DE Jr. A comparison of cilostazol and pentoxifylline for treating intermittent claudication. Am J Med 2000;109(7):523–30.
6. Gotoh F, Tohgi H, Hirai S, Terashi A, Fukuuchi Y, Otomo E, Shinohara Y, Itoh E, Matsuda T, Sawada T, Yamaguchi T, Nishimaru K, Ohashi Y. Cilostazol stroke prevention study: a placebo-controlled double-blind trial for secondary prevention of cerebral infarction. J Stroke Cerebrovasc Dis 2000;9:147–57.
7. Dawson DL, Cutler BS, Meissner MH, Strandness DE Jr. Cilostazol has beneficial effects in treatment of intermittent claudication: results from a multicenter, randomized, prospective, double-blind trial. Circulation 1998;98(7):678–86.
8. Cariski AT. Cilostazol: a novel treatment option in intermittent claudication. Int J Clin Pract Suppl 2001;(119):11–18.
9. Gamssari F, Mahmood H, Ho JS, Villareal RP, Liu B, Rasekh A, Garcia E, Massumi A. Rapid ventricular tachycardias associated with cilostazol use. Tex Heart Inst J 2002;29(2):140–2.

Cimetidine

See also Histamine H_2 receptor antagonists

General Information

Cimetidine is a histamine H_2 receptor antagonist.

General adverse effects

The main varieties of adverse effects attributed to cimetidine relate to its antiandrogenic properties and its actions in sufficient concentrations on the central nervous system. There is also a spectrum of drug interactions, mainly attributable to inhibition of hepatic CYP isoforms, but they only have clinical consequences under special circumstances. Occasional adverse effects, which are generally minor, include bradycardia and conduction defects, thrombocytopenia, neutropenia, interstitial nephritis, mild hepatic dysfunction, and headache. Intestinal infection due to loss of the gastric acid barrier also occurs, and myalgia, fever, monoamine oxidase-like interactions, and neuropathies have been well documented occasionally. Allergic reactions, such as bronchospasm, have rarely been described. Anaphylaxis with recurrence on rechallenge is on record, as are asthma and skin effects.

Organs and Systems

Cardiovascular

Rapid infusion of cimetidine causes an increase in plasma histamine concentration, and this could be one reason for its cardiac effects. A marked degree of bradycardia (for example a 30% reduction in heart rate) is uncommon although well recognized (SEDA-17, 417); sinoatrial and atrioventricular conduction effects and dysrhythmias of every possible type have occasionally been noted, particularly after infusion but also with oral therapy. It has been suggested that if a patient is particularly at risk (for example because of poor renal function) the electrocardiogram should be monitored (SEDA-15, 394).

Symptoms of vasodilatation have been attributed to cimetidine (1).

- A 31-year-old white man taking maintenance hemodialysis had frequent episodes of hot flushes, sweating, palpitation, and dizziness, which started after about 1 month of treatment with cimetidine 400 mg/day. When the drug was temporarily discontinued and later when it was totally withdrawn, he noted marked improvement in 2–5 days.

Respiratory

Bronchospasm is occasionally reported, reflecting the possibility of allergy to cimetidine, and the need for some caution with its initial use in any patient with asthma (SEDA-15, 394). In pre-existing atopic asthma, H_2 receptor antagonists can enhance bronchial reactivity (SEDA-16, 421). Central nervous system effects can lead to respiratory depression, although this is rare.

Loss of the gastric acid barrier can predispose to intestinal infection, and pulmonary aspiration of infected gastrointestinal secretions can very occasionally cause pneumonia after anesthesia or during intensive care (2). Interstitial lung disease can occur under these conditions.

Nervous system

Cimetidine crosses the blood–brain barrier and its adverse events include central respiratory depression and extrapyramidal and cerebellar disturbances. There have been convincing isolated reports of choreiform movements (3,4).

Severe central neurological problems are not common with cimetidine. In one intensive survey of nearly 10 000 patients followed for 3 months there were only five cases of confusion, though there were 34 with sensations of dizziness, 23 with headache, and 74 with other milder central nervous effects (5). The overall incidence of adverse neurological effects reported to the US public health authorities (which naturally represent only a small proportion of those that actually occur) was 8.6 per million prescriptions for cimetidine and virtually the same for ranitidine. Healthy elderly people are probably not at particular risk.

Occasionally, neuropathies have been documented (6). The fear that cimetidine or ranitidine might increase the incidence of motor neuron disease was raised in the light of case-control work, but seems to have been allayed by data from the Oxford Record Linkage Study published in 1993 (7).

A dystonic reaction has been attributed to cimetidine (8).

- A 39-year-old woman developed a dystonic reaction (masseter spasm, lip smacking, oculogyric crisis, and mild neck spasm) within 5 minutes of intravenous administration of cimetidine 300 mg for epigastric pain. She had epilepsy and had not taken her antiepileptic medication regularly. She had developed a similar dystonic reaction to prochlorperazine 1 week before. She recovered within 5 minutes of treatment with intravenous diphenhydramine and lorazepam.

Psychological, psychiatric

Cimetidine crosses the blood–brain barrier and can cause confusion, particularly in elderly or sick individuals with compromised hepatic or renal function, and especially after intravenous treatment. Very rarely an acute confusional psychosis has been seen in a younger person (9). Delirium has been thought to be a particular problem with intravenous use, but this is more likely to be a reflection of patient selection. Depression has occasionally been attributed to cimetidine (10,11).

Metabolism

In the earlier years of cimetidine use there were scattered (although well-documented) reports of the drug having destabilized severe diabetes, resulting in impaired control (12); however, most people with diabetes are unlikely to be affected.

Modest increases in serum high-density lipoproteins have occasionally been noted in patients taking cimetidine (SED-12, 942) (13).

Hematologic

There was concern during the first years of cimetidine therapy that it might produce severe blood dyscrasias, but most of those that have been described have occurred in patients who were already severely ill or exposed to other toxic influences (SED-12, 942) (SEDA-15, 394).

Thrombocytopenia has been attributed to cimetidine, with recurrence on rechallenge, and neutropenia has also been documented as an occasional adverse effect, possibly related to inhibition of granulocyte colony growth (SEDA-10, 325). These effects appear to occur with all H_2 receptor antagonists in an incidence roughly proportional to their sales. Exceptionally, thrombocytopenia and leukopenia have occurred together (SEDA-17, 417). In one case of pancytopenia there was cimetidine dose-related inhibition of normal human CFU-GM colon formation (SEDA-16, 422).

Mouth and teeth

Parotitis with positive rechallenge has been documented in one case (14).

Gastrointestinal

An early concern was the possibility that H_2 receptor antagonists could predispose to gastric carcinogenesis, but this seems to have been allayed, as was the fear once expressed that ulcers might be more liable to perforate after cimetidine had been given and withdrawn.

Liver

The rate of acute liver injury due to cimetidine 800 mg/day in the UK has been estimated at over 10 per 100 000 users. The increased risk was seen mainly in the first 2 months of use. The risks of liver injury due to ranitidine and omeprazole were much lower (SEDA-22, 391) (15).

Cimetidine has rarely been reported to cause hepatic encephalopathy.

- Cimetidine-induced hyperammoniacal encephalopathy has been reported in a previously healthy 44-year-old man who had taken cimetidine 400 mg/day for 4 days; he recovered completely after drug withdrawal (16).

Pancreas

Pancreatitis has several times been suggested as a complication of treatment (17), but this is unconfirmed.

Urinary tract

Minor rises in serum creatinine concentrations reflect interference with tubular function; this seems to be clinically unimportant and fully reversible. There were two early reports of reversible acute renal insufficiency, one of them with positive rechallenge and a biopsy finding of interstitial infiltrates of inflammatory cells (18).

Skin

Allergic skin reactions to cimetidine include urticaria (19), exfoliative dermatitis (20), and the various forms of erythema multiforme (21–23).

Several cases of psoriasis have been precipitated or aggravated by cimetidine, and ranitidine has the same rare effect (24).

Xerosis and asteatotic dermatitis are among the rare cutaneous effects that can occur with cimetidine; they may be of antiandrogenic origin (25).

Hair

A possibly unique case of alopecia affecting the entire body was described in 1981; in that case the temporal association was convincing and there was a correlation with an antiandrogenic effect on hormone concentrations (26).

Musculoskeletal

A small proportion of patients develop troublesome myalgia when taking cimetidine (27). There have been incidental reports of polymyositis and a form of myopathy probably of motor neuron origin. Myalgia can also be associated with arthritis and joint effusion, but this is extremely unusual (SED-12, 942) (28).

Sexual function

Mild antiandrogenic properties, which are dose-related, are associated with binding of cimetidine to androgen receptors. Reduced sperm counts have been reported, as have modestly raised serum prolactin levels after intravenous treatment (SEDA-9, 313). Some slight degree of male breast enlargement is not uncommon (for example in one series of 25 men, five had it) (29), but it can regress with continued treatment; it is very rarely massive and unilateral; there is no strict parallel between the effects on the breasts and the blood prolactin concentration. In 81 535 men aged 25–84 years, the relative risk of gynecomastia among users of cimetidine compared with non-users was 7.2. The period of maximum risk lay between the 7th and the 12th months of treatment (SEDA-19, 313).

Erectile impotence has been suggested in the light of some case experiences; this type of effect is always difficult to prove but it has been described repeatedly with various H_2 receptor antagonists.

One well-documented case suggested that in an infant girl reversible premature puberty was induced, but it must be noted that domperidone was also being given (SEDA-15, 394); in another instance an 18-month-old infant had marked enlargement of one breast (SEDA-16, 421–422), but this is probably similar to the effect sometimes seen in adult men rather than a true endocrine effect.

Body temperature

Fever is occasionally noted with cimetidine (30).

Long-Term Effects

Drug withdrawal

A complex neurobehavioral and gastroenteric withdrawal syndrome has been seen with both cimetidine and ranitidine. The characteristics included anxiety, sleeplessness, anorexia with weight loss, irritability, tachycardia, diarrhea, nausea and vomiting, abdominal pain, headache, and vertigo. The syndrome virtually disappeared when the drugs were given again, but reappeared when they were withdrawn once more. The syndrome may be related to a fall in prolactin concentrations; it responded well to domperidone (31).

Susceptibility Factors

Age

Neurological adverse effects are more likely to occur in elderly patients with impaired hepatic or renal function.

Sex

It has been suggested that women with spinal cord injuries may be at increased risk of galactorrhea due to H_2 receptor antagonists, since such injuries can themselves cause galactorrhea (SEDA-17, 417).

Drug–Drug Interactions

General

The many drug interactions described with cimetidine are largely attributable to inhibition of CYP isozymes or renal clearance of other drugs. Cimetidine also reduces hepatic blood flow and so can, for example, reduce the clearance of lidocaine. In the kidneys cimetidine interferes with the tubular excretion of procainamide and quinidine. Both effects are small, and the long list of drugs for which interference is demonstrable (Table 1) is out of all proportion to the number for which interference is of clinical significance.

Table 1 Groups of drugs interacting with cimetidine

Drug	Effect	References
Analgesics		
Methadone	Potentiation	(32)
Anticoagulants		
Acenocoumarol	Potentiation	(33,34)
Phenindione	Potentiation	(33)
Warfarin	Potentiation	(35,36)
Antiepileptic drugs		
Carbamazepine	Transient rise in concentrations	(37,38)
Phenytoin	Increased steady-state concentrations Small reduction in to clearance	(39)
Valproate		(40)
Antidepressants		
Tricyclics		
Amitriptyline	Reduced metabolism	(41)

Drug	Effect	References
Desipramine	Reduced metabolism in extensive hydroxylators	(42)
Doxepin	Reduced metabolism	(43)
Imipramine	Reduced metabolism	(44,45)
Nortriptyline	Reduced metabolism	(45)
SSRIs		
Fluoxetine	Parkinsonism	(46)
Paroxetine	Reduced metabolism	(47)
Antidysrhythmic drugs		
Cifenline	Increased serum concentrations	(48)
Encainide	Increased serum concentrations	(49)
Flecainide	Increased serum concentrations	(50)
Lidocaine	Toxic concentrations	(51)
Moracizine	Reduced metabolism	(52)
Procainamide	Increased plasma concentrations	(53)
Quinidine	Increased plasma concentrations	(54,55)
Tocainide	Reduced oral systemic availability	(56)
Anti-inflammatory to drugs		
Indometacin	Reduced serum concentrations	(57)
Benzodiazepines		
Adinazolam	Increased plasma concentrations	(58)
Alprazolam	Increased plasma concentrations	(59,60)
Chlordiazepoxide	Increased plasma concentrations	(61)
Clobazam	Increased plasma concentrations	(62)
Clorazepate	Prolonged elimination	(63)
Diazepam	Increased plasma concentrations	(64,65)
Flurazepam	Increased plasma concentrations	(66)
Nitrazepam	Increased plasma concentrations	(67)
Triazolam	Increased plasma concentrations	(59,60)
Beta-blockers		
Atenolol	Slightly prolonged half-life	(68)
Labetalol	Increased systemic availability; toxicity Increased plasma concentrations	(69,70)
Metoprolol	Increased plasma concentrations	(71)
Propranolol		(72)
Bronchodilators		
Theophylline	Increased plasma concentrations; toxicity	(73,74)
Calcium channel blockers		
Diltiazem	Increased plasma concentrations	(75)
Felodipine	Increased plasma concentrations	(76)
Nifedipine	Increased plasma concentrations	(77)
Nimodipine	Increased systemic availability	(78)
Nisoldipine	Increased systemic availability	(79)
Nitrendipine	Increased systemic availability	(80)
Verapamil	Increased systemic availability	(81)
	Reduced clearance	(82)
Cytotoxic drugs		
Fluorouracil	Increased plasma concentrations	(83)
	Increased antiproliferative effect	(84)
Diuretics		
Furosemide	Increased AUC	(85)
Hypoglycemic drugs		
Gliclazide	Hypoglycemia	(86)
Immunosuppressants		
Ciclosporin	Increased plasma concentrations; toxicity	(87)
Neuromuscular blockers		
Suxamethonium	Delayed recovery (not confirmed)	(88,89)
Vecuronium	Delayed recovery	(90,91)

In most cases the slowing of the metabolism of other drugs, by a third at most, is only likely to be troublesome for drugs with a narrow margin between the therapeutic and toxic dose, such as theophylline, phenytoin, and warfarin; the clearance of theophylline may be reduced by up to 22% and the half-life increased by 50% (SEDA-16, 421).

Alcohol

Cimetidine slightly reduces the rate of metabolism of alcohol and alters its absorption (92–94), but it is doubtful if these effects are clinically significant.

References

1. Bastani B, Galli D, Gellens ME. Cimetidine-induced climacteric symptoms in a young man maintained on chronic hemodialysis. Am J Nephrol 1998;18(6):538–40.
2. Holtmann BJ, Schott D, Ulmer WT. Diffuse interstitielle Lungerkrankung nach Anwendung von Cimetidin bei einem Patienten mit schwerer Refluxkrankheit der Speiseröhre. [Diffuse interstitial lung disease following the use of cimetidine in a patient with severe reflux disease of the esophagus.] Med Klin (Munich) 1989;84(8):405–10.
3. Kushner MJ. Chorea and cimetidine. Ann Intern Med 1982;96(1):126.
4. Lehmann AB. Reversible chorea due to ranitidine and cimetidine. Lancet 1988;2(8603):158.
5. Guckenbiehl W, Gilfrich HJ, Just H. Einfluss von Laxantien und Metoclopramid auf die Chinidin-Plasmakonzentration während Langzeittherapie bei Patienten mit Herzrhythmusstörungen. [Effect of laxatives and metoclopramide on plasma quinidine concentration during prolonged administration in patients with heart rhythm disorders.] Med Welt 1976;27(26):1273–6.

6. Pouget J, Pellissier JF, Jean P, Jouglard J, Toga M, Serratrice G. Neuropathie périphérique au cours d'un traitement par la cimétidine. [Peripheral neuropathy during treatment with cimetidine.] Rev Neurol (Paris) 1986;142(1):34–41.
7. Vessey MP, Goldacre MJ, Seagroatt V, Yeates D. Peptic ulcer, cimetidine, and motor neurone disease—a record linkage study. Gut 1993;34(12):1660–1.
8. Peiris RS, Peckler BF. Cimetidine-induced dystonic reaction. J Emerg Med 2001;21(1):27–9.
9. Bhatia MS, Agrawal P, Khastgir U, Malik SC. Cimetidine induced psychosis. Indian Pediatr 1989;26(10):1061–2.
10. Pierce JR Jr. Cimetidine-associated depression and loss of libido in a woman. Am J Med Sci 1983;286(3):31–4.
11. Billings RF, Tang SW, Rakoff VM. Depression associated with cimetidine. Can J Psychiatry 1981;26(4):260–1.
12. Pomare EW. Hyperosmolar non-ketotic diabetes and cimetidine. Lancet 1978;1(8075):1202.
13. Miller NE, Lewis B. Cimetidine and HDL cholesterol. Lancet 1983;1(8323):529–30.
14. Trechot PF, De Romemont E, De Romemont M, et al. Parotidite récidivante avec un antihistaminique H2. J Fr Oto-Rhino-Laryngol 1991;40:173–4.
15. Garcia Rodriguez LA, Wallander MA, Stricker BH. The risk of acute liver injury associated with cimetidine and other acid-suppressing anti-ulcer drugs. Br J Clin Pharmacol 1997;43(2):183–8.
16. Duval L, Hautecoeur P, Mahieu M. Encephalopathie hyperammoniémique après prise de cimétidine. [Cimetidine-induced hyperammonemic encephalopathy.] Presse Méd 1999;28(11):582–3.
17. Arnold F, Doyle PJ, Bell G. Acute pancreatitis in a patient treated with cimetidine. Lancet 1978;1(8060):382–3.
18. Payne CR, Ackrill P, Ralston AJ. Acute renal failure and rise in alkaline phosphatase activity caused by cimetidine. BMJ (Clin Res Ed) 1982;285(6335):100.
19. Mitchell GG, Magnusson AR, Weiler JM. Cimetidine-induced cutaneous vasculitis. Am J Med 1983;75(5):875–6.
20. Yantis PL, Bridges ME, Pittman FE. Cimetidine-induced exfoliative dermatitis. Dig Dis Sci 1980;25(1):73–4.
21. Bjaeldager PA. Erythema ultiforme som sandsynlig bivirkning til cimetidinbehandling. [Erythema multiforme as a possible side-effect of treatment with cimetidine.] Ugeskr Laeger 1981;143(22):1406–7.
22. Talvard O, Fischbein L, Robineau M, Kemeny JL, Rancourt A, Sachs RN, Lanfranchi J. Syndrome de Stevens–Johnson lie a la cimetidine. [Stevens–Johnson syndrome related to cimetidine.] Presse Méd 1987; 16(17):825.
23. Tidwell BH, Paterson TM, Burford B. Cimetidine-induced toxic epidermal necrolysis. Am J Health Syst Pharm 1998;55(2):163–4.
24. Andersen M. Forvμrring af psoriasis under behandling med H2-antagonister. [Exacerbation of psoriasis during treatment with H2 antagonists.] Ugeskr Laeger 1991; 153(2):132.
25. Greist MC, Epinette WW. Cimetidine-induced xerosis and asteatotic dermatitis. Arch Dermatol 1982;118(4):253–4.
26. Vircburger MI, Prelevic GM, Brkic S, Andrejevic MM, Peric LA. Transitory alopecia and hypergonadotrophic hypogonadism during cimetidine treatment. Lancet 1981;1(8230):1160–1.
27. Labeeuw M, Cabanne JF, Dubot P. Recurrent myalgias associated with cimetidine. Int J Clin Pharmacol Ther Toxicol 1986;24(7):349–50.
28. UK Committee on Safety of Medicines. Cimetidine and arthropathy. Curr Probl, 1981:7.
29. Spence RW, Celestin LR. Gynaecomastia associated with cimetidine. Gut 1979;20(2):154–7.
30. Potter HP Jr, Byrne EB, Lebovitz S. Fever after cimetidine and ranitidine. J Clin Gastroenterol 1986;8(3 Pt 1):275–6.
31. Rampello L, Nicoletti G. Sindrome da sospension della terapia con H2-antagonisti ipossibile ruolo della iperprolattinemia. [The H2-antagonist therapy withdrawal syndrome: the possible role of hyperprolactinemia.] Medicina (Firenze) 1990;10(3):294–6.
32. Dawson GW, Vestal RE. Cimetidine inhibits the in vitro N-demethylation of methadone. Res Commun Chem Pathol Pharmacol 1984;46(2):301–4.
33. Serlin MJ, Sibeon RG, Mossman S, Breckenridge AM, Williams JR, Atwood JL, Willoughby JM. Cimetidine: interaction with oral anticoagulants in man. Lancet 1979;2(8138):317–19.
34. Cappelli J, Lenaerts A, Lamy V, Ramdani B, Moisse R. Hématome intramural du grèle associé aux anticoagulants, potentialisés par interaction avec la cimétidine. Med Chir Dig 1999;28:71–2.
35. Choonara IA, Cholerton S, Haynes BP, Breckenridge AM, Park BK. Stereoselective interaction between the R enantiomer of warfarin and cimetidine. Br J Clin Pharmacol 1986;21(3):271–7.
36. Niopas I, Toon S, Rowland M. Further insight into the stereoselective interaction between warfarin and cimetidine in man. Br J Clin Pharmacol 1991;32(4):508–11.
37. Macphee GJ, Thompson GG, Scobie G, Agnew E, Park BK, Murray T, McColl KE, Brodie MJ. Effects of cimetidine on carbamazepine auto- and hetero-induction in man. Br J Clin Pharmacol 1984;18(3):411–19.
38. Dalton MJ, Powell JR, Messenheimer JA Jr, Clark J. Cimetidine and carbamazepine: a complex drug interaction. Epilepsia 1986;27(5):553–8.
39. Neuvonen PJ, Tokola RA, Kaste M. Cimetidine-phenytoin interaction: effect on serum phenytoin concentration and antipyrine test. Eur J Clin Pharmacol 1981; 21(3):215–20.
40. Webster LK, Mihaly GW, Jones DB, Smallwood RA, Phillips JA, Vajda FJ. Effect of cimetidine and ranitidine on carbamazepine and sodium valproate pharmacokinetics. Eur J Clin Pharmacol 1984;27(3):341–3.
41. Curry SH, DeVane CL, Wolfe MM. Cimetidine interaction with amitriptyline. Eur J Clin Pharmacol 1985; 29(4):429–33.
42. Steiner E, Spina E. Differences in the inhibitory effect of cimetidine on desipramine metabolism between rapid and slow debrisoquin hydroxylators. Clin Pharmacol Ther 1987;42(3):278–82.
43. Sutherland DL, Remillard AJ, Haight KR, Brown MA, Old L. The influence of cimetidine versus ranitidine on doxepin pharmacokinetics. Eur J Clin Pharmacol 1987;32(2):159–64.
44. Wells BG, Pieper JA, Self TH, Stewart CF, Waldon SL, Bobo L, Warner C. The effect of ranitidine and cimetidine on imipramine disposition. Eur J Clin Pharmacol 1986;31(3):285–90.
45. Henauer SA, Hollister LE. Cimetidine interaction with imipramine and nortriptyline. Clin Pharmacol Ther 1984;35(2):183–7.
46. Leo RJ, Lichter DG, Hershey LA. Parkinsonism associated with fluoxetine and cimetidine: a case report. J Geriatr Psychiatry Neurol 1995;8(4):231–3.
47. Greb WH, Buscher G, Dierdorf HD, Koster FE, Wolf D, Mellows G. The effect of liver enzyme inhibition by cimetidine and enzyme induction by phenobarbitone on the pharmacokinetics of paroxetine. Acta Psychiatr Scand Suppl 1989;350:95–8.
48. Massarella JW, Defeo TM, Liguori J, Passe S, Aogaichi K. The effects of cimetidine and ranitidine on the pharmacokinetics of cifenline. Br J Clin Pharmacol 1991;31(4):481–3.

49. Quart BD, Gallo DG, Sami MH, Wood AJ. Drug interaction studies and encainide use in renal and hepatic impairment. Am J Cardiol 1986;58(5):C104–13.
50. Tjandra-Maga TB, van Hecken A, van Melle P, Verbesselt R, de Schepper PJ. Altered pharmacokinetics of oral flecainide by cimetidine. Br J Clin Pharmacol 1986;22(1):108–10.
51. Berk SI, Gal P, Bauman JL, Douglas JB, McCue JD, Powell JR. The effect of oral cimetidine on total and unbound serum lidocaine concentrations in patients with suspected myocardial infarction. Int J Cardiol 1987;14 (1):91–4.
52. Biollaz J, Shaheen O, Wood AJ. Cimetidine inhibition of ethmozine metabolism. Clin Pharmacol Ther 1985;37 (6):665–8.
53. Bauer LA, Black D, Gensler A. Procainamide–cimetidine drug interaction in elderly male patients. J Am Geriatr Soc 1990;38(4):467–9.
54. Kolb KW, Garnett WR, Small RE, Vetrovec GW, Kline BJ, Fox T. Effect of cimetidine on quinidine clearance. Ther Drug Monit 1984;6(3):306–12.
55. MacKichan JJ, Boudoulas H, Schaal SF. Effect of cimetidine on quinidine bioavailability. Biopharm Drug Dispos 1989;10(1):121–5.
56. North DS, Mattern AL, Kapil RP, Lalonde RL. The effect of histamine-2 receptor antagonists on tocainide pharmacokinetics. J Clin Pharmacol 1988;28(7):640–3.
57. Howes CA, Pullar T, Sourindhrin I, Mistra PC, Capel H, Lawson DH, Tilstone WJ. Reduced steady-state plasma concentrations of chlorpromazine and indomethacin in patients receiving cimetidine. Eur J Clin Pharmacol 1983;24(1):99–102.
58. Hulhoven R, Desager JP, Cox S, Harvengt C. Influence of repeated administration of cimetidine on the pharmacokinetics and pharmacodynamics of adinazolam in healthy subjects. Eur J Clin Pharmacol 1988;35(1):59–64.
59. Pourbaix S, Desager JP, Hulhoven R, Smith RB, Harvengt C. Pharmacokinetic consequences of long term coadministration of cimetidine and triazolobenzodiazepines, alprazolam and triazolam, in healthy subjects. Int J Clin Pharmacol Ther Toxicol 1985; 23(8):447–51.
60. Abernethy DR, Greenblatt DJ, Divoll M, Moschitto LJ, Harmatz JS, Shader RI. Interaction of cimetidine with the triazolobenzodiazepines alprazolam and triazolam. Psychopharmacology (Berl) 1983;80(3):275–8.
61. Desmond PV, Patwardhan RV, Schenker S, Speeg KV Jr. Cimetidine impairs elimination of chlordiazepoxide (Librium) in man. Ann Intern Med 1980;93(2):266–8.
62. Pullar T, Edwards D, Haigh JR, Peaker S, Feely MP. The effect of cimetidine on the single dose pharmacokinetics of oral clobazam and N-desmethylclobazam. Br J Clin Pharmacol 1987;23(3):317–21.
63. Divoll M, Greenblatt DJ, Abernethy DR, Shader RI. Cimetidine impairs clearance of antipyrine and desmethyldiazepam in the elderly J Am Geriatr Soc 1982;30(11): 684–9.
64. Greenblatt DJ, Abernethy DR, Morse DS, Harmatz JS, Shader RI. Clinical importance of the interaction of diazepam and cimetidine. N Engl J Med 1984; 310(25):1639–43.
65. Klotz U, Reimann I. Delayed clearance of diazepam due to cimetidine. N Engl J Med 1980;302(18):1012–14.
66. Greenblatt DJ, Abernethy DR, Koepke HH, Shader RI. Interaction of cimetidine with oxazepam, lorazepam, and flurazepam. J Clin Pharmacol 1984;24(4):187–93.
67. Ochs HR, Greenblatt DJ, Gugler R, Muntefering G, Locniskar A, Abernethy DR. Cimetidine impairs nitrazepam clearance. Clin Pharmacol Ther 1983;34(2):227–30.
68. Houtzagers JJ, Streurman O, Regardh CG. The effect of pretreatment with cimetidine on the bioavailability and disposition of atenolol and metoprolol. Br J Clin Pharmacol 1982;14(1):67–72.
69. Daneshmend TK, Roberts CJ. Cimetidine and bioavailability of labetalol. Lancet 1981;1(8219):565.
70. Durant PA, Joucken K. Bronchospasm and hypotension during cardiopulmonary bypass after preoperative cimetidine and labetalol therapy. Br J Anaesth 1984; 56(8):917–20.
71. Chellingsworth MC, Laugher S, Akhlaghi S, Jack DB, Kendall MJ. The effects of ranitidine and cimetidine on the pharmacokinetics and pharmacodynamics of metoprolol. Aliment Pharmacol Ther 1988;2(6):521–7.
72. Tateishi T, Ohashi K, Fujimura A, Ebihara A. The influence of diltiazem versus cimetidine on propranolol metabolism. J Clin Pharmacol 1992;32(12):1099–104.
73. Boehning W. Effect of cimetidine and ranitidine on plasma theophylline in patients with chronic obstructive airways disease treated with theophylline and corticosteroids. Eur J Clin Pharmacol 1990;38(1):43–5.
74. Fraser IM, Buttoo KM, Walker SE, Stewart JH, Babul N. Effects of cimetidine and ranitidine on the pharmacokinetics of a chronotherapeutically formulated once-daily theophylline preparation (Uniphyl). Clin Ther 1993;15(2): 383–93.
75. Winship LC, McKenney JM, Wright JT Jr, Wood JH, Goodman RP. The effect of ranitidine and cimetidine on single-dose diltiazem pharmacokinetics. Pharmacotherapy 1985;5(1):16–19.
76. Edgar B, Lundborg P, Regardh CG. Clinical pharmacokinetics of felodipine. A summary. Drugs 1987;34(Suppl 3): 16–27.
77. Smith SR, Kendall MJ, Lobo J, Beerahee A, Jack DB, Wilkins MR. Ranitidine and cimetidine; drug interactions with single dose and steady-state nifedipine administration. Br J Clin Pharmacol 1987;23(3):311–15.
78. Muck W, Wingender W, Seiberling M, Woelke E, Ramsch KD, Kuhlmann J. Influence of the H2-receptor antagonists cimetidine and ranitidine on the pharmacokinetics of nimodipine in healthy volunteers. Eur J Clin Pharmacol 1992;42(3):325–8.
79. van Harten J, van Brummelen P, Lodewijks MT, Danhof M, Breimer DD. Pharmacokinetics and hemodynamic effects of nisoldipine and its interaction with cimetidine. Clin Pharmacol Ther 1988;43(3):332–41.
80. Soons PA, Vogels BA, Roosemalen MC, Schoemaker HC, Uchida E, Edgar B, Lundahl J, Cohen AF, Breimer DD. Grapefruit juice and cimetidine inhibit stereoselective metabolism of nitrendipine in humans. Clin Pharmacol Ther 1991;50(4):394–403.
81. Smith MS, Benyunes MC, Bjornsson TD, Shand DG, Pritchett EL. Influence of cimetidine on verapamil kinetics and dynamics. Clin Pharmacol Ther 1984;36(4):551–4.
82. Loi CM, Rollins DE, Dukes GE, Peat MA. Effect of cimetidine on verapamil disposition. Clin Pharmacol Ther 1985;37(6):654–7.
83. Harvey VJ, Slevin ML, Dilloway MR, Clark PI, Johnston A, Lant AF. The influence of cimetidine on the pharmacokinetics of 5-fluorouracil. Br J Clin Pharmacol 1984;18(3):421–30.
84. Komatsubara M, Nagata T, Miyauchi S, Kamo N. Cimetidine enhances the antiproliferative effect of 5-fluorouracil on colon carcinoma SW620. Anticancer Res 1999;19(2A):1153–7.
85. Rogers HJ, Morrison P, House FR, Bradbrook ID. Effect of cimetidine on the absorption and efficacy of orally administered furosemide. Int J Clin Pharmacol Ther Toxicol 1982;20(1):8–11.

86. Archambeaud-Mouveroux F, Nouaille Y, Nadalon S, Treves R, Merle L. Interaction between gliclazide and cimetidine. Eur J Clin Pharmacol 1987;31(5):631.
87. Lewis SM, McCloskey WW. Potentiation of nephrotoxicity by H2-antagonists in patients receiving cyclosporine. Ann Pharmacother 1997;31(3):363–5.
88. Kambam JR, Dymond R, Krestow M. Effect of cimetidine on duration of action of succinylcholine. Anesth Analg 1987;66(2):191–2.
89. Sato Y, Tsuchida H, Harada Y, Namiki A. [Effect of cimetidine on neuromuscular blockade by succinylcholine and pancuronium.] Masui 1990;39(2):168–73.
90. Ulsamer B. Vecuroniumbromid: Beeinflussung der Pharmakodynamik durch Etomidat, Cimetidin und Ranitidin. [Vecuronium bromide: modification of its pharmacodynamics by etomidate, cimetidine and ranitidine.] Anaesthesist 1988;37(8):504–9.
91. McCarthy G, Mirakhur RK, Elliott P, Wright J. Effect of H2-receptor antagonist pretreatment on vecuronium- and atracurium-induced neuromuscular block. Br J Anaesth 1991;66(6):713–15.
92. Caballeria J, Baraona E, Rodamilans M, Lieber CS. Effects of cimetidine on gastric alcohol dehydrogenase activity and blood ethanol levels.. Gastroenterology 1989;96(2 Pt 1): 388–92.
93. Fraser AG, Prewett EJ, Hudson M, Sawyerr AM, Rosalki SB, Pounder RE. The effect of ranitidine, cimetidine or famotidine on low-dose post-prandial alcohol absorption. Aliment Pharmacol Ther 1991; 5(3):263–72.
94. Seitz HK, Bosche J, Czygan P, Veith S, Simon B, Kommerell B. Increased blood ethanol levels following cimetidine but not ranitidine. Lancet 1983;1(8327):760.

Cimetropium bromide

See also Anticholinergic drugs

General Information

Cimetropium bromide is an anticholinergic drug that belongs to a series of scopolamine quaternary salts with strong antimuscarinic effects (1).

Reference

1. Scarpignato C, Bianchi Porro G. Cimetropium bromide, a new antispasmodic compound: pharmacology and therapeutic perspectives. Int J Clin Pharmacol Res 1985;5(6): 467–77.

Cinchocaine

See also Local anesthetics

General Information

Cinchocaine (dibucaine) is an aminoamide local anesthetic. It is ten times more potent than lidocaine and potentially very toxic. It is available in a number of over-the-counter topical formulations, such as antihemorrhoidal drugs.

Organs and Systems

Nervous system

Low concentrations of cinchocaine (0.003 and 0.03% respectively) caused irreversible neurotoxicity in A_β and C rabbit vagus nerve preparations (1). Cinchocaine had the greatest neurotoxic effect and the lowest safety margin compared with tetracaine and bupivacaine.

Cauda equina syndrome has been reported after a spinal anesthetic using cinchocaine (2).

- A 64-year-old man with a history of borderline diabetes who had undergone two previous operations uneventfully under spinal anesthetic received a spinal anesthetic with hyperbaric 0.24% dibucaine 2.2 ml and then a general anesthetic because of unilateral block. The next day he complained of difficulty in defecation and urination, with abnormal anal sensation. A diagnosis of cauda equina syndrome was made. He made a gradual recovery, but mild hypesthesia remained after 4 months.

A possible cause for this adverse event may have been maldistribution in the intrathecal space of the high concentration of cinchocaine, affecting the cauda equina and resulting in nerve damage; the incomplete block achieved in this case is suggestive of this. Elderly patients undergoing urological surgery often have risk factors for cauda equina syndrome, such as intraoperative lithotomy position, frequent spinal anesthetics, old age, and diabetes mellitus. The authors suggested that cinchocaine should be avoided for spinal anesthesia in these patients, because of its high neurotoxicity compared with other local anesthetics.

Hematologic

Cinchocaine inhibits ADP-mediated platelet aggregation (3); it is not known whether this has any clinical significance.

Skin

Two cases of contact dermatitis have been reported after the use of Proctosedyl and Ruscens Llorens, both of which contain cinchocaine. After patch testing, the first case was found to be allergic in origin and the second was due to photosensitivity. Neither showed cross-sensitivity to other local anesthetics (4).

Two cases of allergic contact dermatitis have been described after the use of cinchocaine formulations.

- A 71-year-old Japanese man, who was using an over-the-counter formulation, Makiron, for minor wounds, developed an itchy rash with seropapules and erosions on his right leg at the site of application (5). Makiron contains 0.1% cinchocaine hydrochloride and chlorphenamine maleate as well as naphazoline hydrochloride and benzethonium chloride. On patch testing, he was positive to both chlorphenamine and cinchocaine.
- A 79-year-old man presented with a 10-day history of weeping dermatitis affecting the perianal skin, buttocks, and proximal thighs (6). He had used Proctosedyl ointment topically for the preceding 3 weeks. Proctosedyl is an over-the-counter topical formulation for use as an antihemorrhoidal agent. It contains cinchocaine 5%, hydrocortisone, and lanolin. Patch testing was strongly positive to cinchocaine.

The authors highlighted the potential limitations of the International Contact Dermatitis Research Group (ICDRG) standard series for topical anesthetics. Benzocaine is the only topical anesthetic in the series and it will not detect contact allergy to amide agents; cross-sensitivity can also exist. They suggested that patch testing should include agents from both groups.

DoloPosterine N is an ointment for topical application in the treatment of hemorrhoids. Its active ingredient is cinchocaine. Although cinchocaine is a known contact sensitizer, as described above, systemic contact dermatitis is rare.

- A 62-year-old woman, who had applied DoloPosterine N ointment topically to the perianal skin and rectal mucosa for several days, developed erythematous vesicular lesions in the perianal area and an erythematous edematous rash of the face, axillae, elbow flexures, and inner thighs (7). This abated on withdrawal of the drug and the administration of oral prednisolone for 10 days. Patch testing was positive with cinchocaine.

Immunologic

An anaphylactic reaction to cinchocaine has been described.

- A 71-year-old man received intrathecal anesthesia using 0.3% cinchocaine 2 ml for a transurethral prostatectomy (8). He had a history of allergic rhinitis, and 2 months before had had an uneventful prostate biopsy and cystoscopy, also under spinal anesthesia with isobaric bupivacaine. Within 45 minutes of the spinal injection he complained of periorbital itching, started to shake, and developed muscle rigidity. He rapidly became unconscious, with a systolic blood pressure of 40 mmHg and widespread erythema. He was treated with hydrocortisone and antihistamines and required an infusion of adrenaline. Intradermal testing after full recovery was positive with cinchocaine.

Death

Three deaths after seizures and cardiac arrest have been reported in toddlers who accidentally ingested small amounts of cinchocaine (SEDA-21, 135).

References

1. Ogawa S, Mikuni E, Nakamura T, Noda K, Ito S. [Neurotoxicity of dibucaine on the isolated rabbit cervical vagus nerve.]Masui 1998;47(4):439–46.
2. Yorozu T, Matsumoto M, Hayashi S, Yamada T, Nakaohji T, Nakatsuka I. [Dibucaine for spinal anesthesia is a probable risk for cauda equina syndrome.]Masui 2002;51(10):1151–4.
3. Peerschke EI. Platelet membrane alterations induced by the local anesthetic dibucaine. Blood 1986;68(2):463–71.
4. Lee AY. Allergic contact dermatitis from dibucaine in Proctosedyl ointment without cross-sensitivity. Contact Dermatitis 1998;39(5):261.
5. Hayashi K, Kawachi S, Saida T. Allergic contact dermatitis due to both chlorpheniramine maleate and dibucaine hydrochloride in an over-the-counter medicament. Contact Dermatitis 2001;44(1):38–9.
6. Kearney CR, Fewings J. Allergic contact dermatitis to cinchocaine. Australas J Dermatol 2001;42(2):118–19.
7. Erdmann SM, Sachs B, Merk HF. Systemic contact dermatitis from cinchocaine. Contact Dermatitis 2001;44(4): 260–1.
8. Mizuno Y, Esaki Y, Kato H. [Anaphylactoid reaction to dibucaine during spinal anesthesia.] Masui 2002;51(11): 1254–6.

Cinchophen

General Information

Cinchophen is a uricosuric drug that was formerly used in the treatment of gout (1). In 1991 the Spanish authorities withdrew cinchophen. It had been known for some time that it can cause severe hepatitis (SEDA-17, 114).

Reference

1. Cutrin Prieto C, Nieto Pol E, Batalla Eiras A, Casal Iglesias L, Perez Becerra E, Lorenzo Zuniga V. Hepatitis toxica por cincofeno: descripcion de tres enfermos. [Toxic hepatitis from cinchophen: report of 3 cases.] Med-Clin-(Barc). 1991;97(3):104–6.

Cinmetacin

See also Non-steroidal anti-inflammatory drugs

General Information

Cinmetacin is an NSAID related to indometacin. There has been little experience with its use. In one study, gastrointestinal adverse effects developed in 13 of 30 patients (1).

Reference

1. Lucietti MV, Banchieri G. Studio clinico sulla efficacia e tollerabilita di un nuovo antiflogistico non-steroideo, la cinmetacina. [Clinical study of the efficacy of and tolerance for a new nonsteroidal anti-inflammatory agent, cinmetacin.] G Clin Med 1980;61(7):545–52.

Cinnarizine and flunarizine

See also Antihistamines

General Information

Cinnarizine and flunarizine are piperazine derivatives with antihistaminic properties and calcium channel blocking activity (SEDA-13, 131) (SEDA-14, 136) (SEDA-22, 178). Flunarizine is the difluoro derivative of cinnarizine. Cinnarizine is used to treat motion sickness.

A few controlled clinical trials of flunarizine in patients with intermittent claudication have suggested significant improvements in subjective signs and some objective measurements. Its effectiveness in patients with cerebrovascular insufficiency has not been clearly shown, but its use in the prevention of migraine and other forms of common headache has been studied extensively. Several double-blind controlled studies have suggested that flunarizine in a dosage not over 10 mg/day reduces the frequency of headaches (SEDA-11, 179). Clinical studies of the antiepileptic efficacy of flunarizine have been equivocal (SEDA-20, 191).

With a maintenance dosage of 10 mg/day, the main adverse effects of flunarizine are somnolence, sedation, fatigue, and drowsiness during the first few days in up to 10% of patients. During prolonged treatment some patients note difficulty in sleeping, lethargy, and reduced motivation. A dosage of 20 mg/day or more can cause drowsiness, increased sweating, peripheral edema, and fatigue (SEDA-7, 229).

Organs and Systems

Nervous system

A study in young volunteers has established the effects of cinnarizine 15–45 mg on daytime sleepiness and performance (1). Doses of 30 mg or more caused impaired performance and increased sleepiness. The authors therefore advised that cinnarizine should not be used in aircrew involved in tasks that demand attention.

Insomnia has been described with cinnarizine (SEDA-22, 178).

Blepharospasm has been attributed to flunarizine in an elderly woman (SEDA-22, 178).

Extrapyramidal adverse effects

Several reports have described extrapyramidal reactions and depression associated with the use of cinnarizine and flunarizine (SEDA-14, 136) and worsening of motility in parkinsonian patients (SEDA-13, 391).

In a Spanish study there were 70 reports of tremor and parkinsonism in patients taking cinnarizine and 11 reports of tremor and parkinsonism in patients taking flunarizine (2).

In a Brazilian study carried out to establish whether there are geographic differences in the cause of parkinsonism, the diagnosis of drug-induced parkinsonism was made in 45 of 338 patients (3). Cinnarizine and flunarizine were two of the three most commonly prescribed drugs.

In a retrospective study in 74 patients with cinnarizine-induced parkinsonism over 15 years, cinnarizine-induced parkinsonism was more frequent in women; most of the patients (66/74) recovered completely within 16 months after withdrawal (4). This suggests that cinnarizine-induced parkinsonism is reversible in most cases, but there is still a question of whether cinnarizine predisposes to permanent Parkinson's disease in a few patients. Cinnarizine-induced parkinsonism is a warning against prolonged use of an apparently harmless drug, especially in elderly people.

Parkinsonism, tardive dyskinesia, and depression have been described in some mostly elderly patients taking flunarizine (SEDA-12, 170) (SEDA-13, 169) (SEDA-14, 167) (SEDA-15, 198). These symptoms are resistant to anticholinergic drugs, levodopa, and bromocriptine, but regress within a few weeks to months after withdrawal of flunarizine; however, mild rigidity and bradykinesia persist in some patients. The recommended dosage of 10 mg/day should never be exceeded, and in elderly patients dosages higher than 5 mg/day can lead to an increased risk of extrapyramidal symptoms. Patients who take flunarizine to prevent migraine are usually some 25–30 years younger than those with cerebrovascular and peripheral vascular disease and appear to be at less risk of developing extrapyramidal symptoms with flunarizine (5).

Liver

Drug-induced cholestasis has rarely been reported in patients taking cinnarizine.

- An 87-year-old man took cinnarizine 75 mg/day for tinnitus and developed jaundice 7 weeks later, with dark urine and pale stools (6). He had taken no other drugs. Bile duct obstruction was ruled out and serological tests for viral hepatitis were negative. A liver biopsy 6 weeks later showed distinct centrilobular cholestasis and a slight lymphocytic infiltrate. He recovered completely and the liver tests were normal after another 3 months without cinnarizine. Rechallenge was not performed.

Skin

Various skin lesions have been attributed to cinnarizine and flunarizine.

- A 32-year-old woman developed subacute cutaneous lupus erythematosus after exposure to the sun while taking cinnarizine and thiethylperazine for vertigo (7). A similar eruption had occurred 10 years before, after exposure to the sun, while she was taking cinnarizine only. The problem did not occur when she was not taking the drug.
- A 78-year-old woman developed generalized lichen pemphigoides while taking cinnarizine (225 mg/day) and recovered after withdrawal of the drug and anti-inflammatory drug treatment (8).
- A lichen planus pemphigoides-like eruption following the use of cinnarizine has been reported in a Japanese woman (SEDA-11, 146).

Immunologic

Subacute cutaneous lupus erythematosus has been attributed to cinnarizine.

- A 32-year-old woman developed an erythematous, papulosquamous, annular, polycyclic skin eruption on her neck, trunk, and lateral parts of the limbs after sunbathing while taking cinnarizine and thiethylperazine (a phenothiazine) for vertigo. She had positive antinuclear antibodies (nucleolar pattern, anti-Ro/SSA). The lesions cleared without residual scars within a few weeks after stopping both drugs and starting steroids and chloroquine.

Phenothiazines can induce photosensitivity, but cinnarizine does not. The authors' arguments that cinnarizine was to blame in this case were its structural resemblance to piperazine and a similar episode of skin eruption in the same patient after sunbathing many years before while she was taking cinnarizine only but for which she did not seek medical advice (7).

References

1. Nicholson AN, Stone BM, Turner C, Mills SL. Central effects of cinnarizine: restricted use in aircrew. Aviat Space Environ Med 2002;73(6):570–4.
2. Luria SM, Kinney JA, McKay CL, Paulson HM, Ryan AP. Effects of aspirin and dimenhydrinate (Dramamine) on visual processes. Br J Clin Pharmacol 1979;7(6):585–93.
3. Cardoso F, Camargos ST, Silva Junior GA. Etiology of parkinsonism in a Brazilian movement disorders clinic. Arq Neuropsiquiatr 1998;56(2):171–5.
4. Marti-Masso JF, Poza JJ. Cinnarizine-induced parkinsonism: ten years later. Mov Disord 1998;13(3):453–6.
5. Bono G, Martucci N, Merlo P, et al. Safety profile of flunarizine. A retrospective study in migraine and cerebrovascular disorders. Ann NY Acad Sci 1988;522:712.
6. Colle I, Reynaert H, Naegels S, Hoorens A, Urbain D. Cinnarizine-induced cholestasis. J Hepatol 1999;30(3):553.
7. Toll A, Campo-Pisa P, Gonzalez-Castro J, Campo-Voegeli A, Azon A, Iranzo P, Lecha M, Herrero C. Subacute cutaneous lupus erythematosus associated with cinnarizine and thiethylperazine therapy. Lupus 1998;7(5):364–6.
8. Vlasin Z, Rulcova J, Hlubinka M. Lichenoid eruption resembling lichen pemphigoides after cinnarizine. Cesko-Slov Dermatol 1998;73:11–14.

Ciprofloxacin

See also Fluoroquinolones

General Information

Ciprofloxacin is a fluoroquinolone antibacterial drug with a wider spectrum of activity than nalidixic acid.

Observational studies

Antimicrobial prophylaxis to prevent inhalational anthrax has been recommended for people potentially exposed to *Bacillus anthracis* as a result of recent bioterrorist attacks. Of 3428 people taking ciprofloxacin, 666 (19%) reported severe nausea, vomiting, diarrhea, or abdominal pain; 484 (14%) reported fainting, lightheadedness, or dizziness; 250 (7%) reported heartburn or acid reflux; and 216 (6%) reported rashes, hives, or an itchy skin. Of those taking ciprofloxacin, 287 (8%) stopped taking it, 116 (3%) because of adverse events, 27 (1%) because of fear of possible adverse events, and 28 (1%) because they "did not think it was needed" (1–4).

The imaging of inflammation/infection with ^{99m}Tm-labeled ciprofloxacin in 96 patients had a sensitivity of 81% and specificity of 87%. The positive and negative predictive values were 90 and 75% respectively. No adverse effects were reported (5).

Comparative studies

In a multicenter, double-blind study of 234 patients with acute bacterial exacerbations of chronic bronchitis, ciprofloxacin (500 mg bd) was associated with a trend toward a longer infection-free interval and a significantly higher bacteriological eradication rate compared with clarithromycin (500 mg bd) after 14 days (6).

In a double-blind study, ciprofloxacin (500 mg bd) was associated with an infection-free interval and clinical response that were similar to those achieved with cefuroxime axetil (500 mg bd), but the bacteriological eradication rate associated with ciprofloxacin was significantly higher (7).

Organs and Systems

Cardiovascular

Ciprofloxacin causes prolongation of the QT interval (8,9).

Nervous system

Headache was recorded in 8% of patients taking ciprofloxacin (10)

Ciprofloxacin can cause confusion and general seizures (11,12).

Ciprofloxacin can cause facial dyskinesia (13,14).

Two cases of generalized painful dysesthesia associated with ciprofloxacin have been reported (15).

Sensory systems

Eyes

Bilateral acute visual loss, possibly due to toxic optic neuropathy, was observed after 4 weeks of treatment with ciprofloxacin 1.5 g/day and improved after withdrawal (16).

Ciprofloxacin 0.3% ophthalmic drops can cause microprecipitates of pure ciprofloxacin in the corneal epithelium (17). In four corneal transplantation patients treated preoperatively with ciprofloxacin 0.3% ophthalmic drops, there were microprecipitates associated with damaged corneal epithelium in two patients; another developed a macroprecipitate in a corneal ulcer (18). The crystalline precipitates were pure ciprofloxacin.

Ears

Topical 0.2% ciprofloxacin (0.2 ml od for 7 days) did not significantly affect the auditory brainstem response thresholds of guinea pigs, whereas 4% gentamicin (0.2 ml od for 7 days) resulted in total hearing loss (19).

Topical 0.2% ciprofloxacin solution was effective and well tolerated in 232 patients with chronic suppurative otitis media; the most frequently reported adverse events were pruritus, stinging, and earache. Audiometric tests did not show changes attributable to ciprofloxacin (20).

In children with tympanic membrane perforation, topical ciprofloxacin caused no signs of local intolerance or ototoxicity and did not result in significant serum concentrations (21).

Psychological, psychiatric

The administration of ciprofloxacin has been associated with psychosis (22,23) and hypoactive delirium (24,25).

- A 27-year-old woman developed an acute psychotic reaction following the use of ciprofloxacin eye-drops (1 drop hourly to each eye) (26).

Hematologic

Ciprofloxacin has been associated with hemolysis in combination with a severe skin reaction in a young adult (27).

Fatal ciprofloxacin-associated thrombotic thrombocytopenic purpura (28) and thrombocytopenia (29) have been reported.

Gastrointestinal

In a randomized, double-blind comparison of prulifloxacin 600 mg/day and ciprofloxacin 500 mg bd in 235 patients with acute exacerbations of chronic bronchitis, the most common treatment-related adverse event was gastric pain of mild or moderate intensity, reported in 8.5% of the patients taking prulifloxacin and 6.8% of those taking ciprofloxacin (30).

Ciprofloxacin has been associated with diarrhea due to *Clostridium difficile* (31–33). In 27 patients the only significant risk factor for nosocomial *C. difficile*-associated diarrhea was the use of ciprofloxacin (34).

Liver

Ciprofloxacin causes a mild reversible rise in liver enzymes in 2–3% of patients. Acute hepatitis is rare, but has been reported in a 32-year-old man (35).

Pancreas

A report has suggested that ciprofloxacin can cause pancreatitis (36).

Urinary tract

Two cases of acute renal insufficiency due to necrotizing vasculitis associated with ciprofloxacin were reported in elderly patients (37). In two patients who underwent high-dose chemotherapy with autologous stem cell rescue, acute renal insufficiency developed while they were taking prophylactic ciprofloxacin; withdrawal resulted in prompt reversal of renal insufficiency (38). Ciprofloxacin-induced acute renal insufficiency has been reported in cancer patients undergoing high-dose chemotherapy and autologous stem cell rescue (38). A case report has suggested that ciprofloxacin overdose can lead to acute renal insufficiency characterized by acute tubular necrosis with distal nephron apoptosis (39).

- An 18-year-old woman with cystic fibrosis had pronounced impairment of renal function after taking oral ciprofloxacin 750 mg tds (30 mg/kg/day) for 3 weeks; withdrawal led to normalization of renal function within 10 days (40).

Hemolytic-uremic syndrome has been attributed to ciprofloxacin (41).

- A 53-year-old white man was given chemotherapy for acute lymphoblastic leukemia and after 4 weeks recovered his blood cell count but developed a fever and was given oral ciprofloxacin 500 mg bd. After four doses he developed the typical features of hemolytic–uremic syndrome with microangiopathic hemolytic anemia. The ciprofloxacin was withdrawn, and he received five sessions of plasma exchange. He recovered completely.

Bilateral hydronephrosis and acute renal insufficiency due to urinary tract stones predominantly composed of ciprofloxacin has been reported (42).

Skin

Ciprofloxacin can cause a fixed drug eruption (43,44), purpuric skin lesions (44,45), bullous pemphigoid (46), cutaneous vasculitis (45–47), and ultraviolet recall-like phenomenon (48).

Musculoskeletal

Tendinopathy

Ciprofloxacin can be associated with partial or complete tendinitis. Of 72 lung transplant recipients who received ciprofloxacin, 20 had Achilles tendon involvement (tendinitis 15, rupture 5) (49). Tendon rupture occurred at a lower dosage of ciprofloxacin than tendinitis and the mean recovery duration was significantly longer.

- Achilles tendon rupture without any sudden pain occurred in a 45-year-old female runner who developed bilateral tendinopathy of the Achilles tendon after repeated treatment with ciprofloxacin; histological analysis showed cystic changes with focal necrosis (50).

Arthropathy

The available data suggest that the incidence of arthrotoxicity in children taking ciprofloxacin is the same as in adults; the use of other fluoroquinolones is too rare to obtain clear information about the risks in children (51). In 12 children with sickle cell disease treated successfully for acute osteomyelitis with oral ciprofloxacin, transient bilateral Achilles tendon tendinitis occurred in one 5-year old (52). Another case was reported in a hemodialysis patient with a ciprofloxacin-associated Achilles tendon rupture (53).

In 75 children with typhoid fever, aged under 6 years (mean age 32 months), ciprofloxacin had no adverse effects on growth or joints (54). In another study only 2 of 219 children treated with ciprofloxacin developed arthropathy, in one case transiently (55). In a necropsy study on children treated with ciprofloxacin 20–40 mg/kg/day for an average of 148 days, there were no chondrotoxic effects; however, synovial membranes showed signs of subacute synovitis, which had not been noted in life (56).

Data on more than 1500 children treated with ciprofloxacin suggest that the safety profile of ciprofloxacin in children and adolescents is similar to the profile in adults (57). Adverse events, mostly involving the gastrointestinal tract, were noted in 5–15% of patients. Reversible arthralgia occurred in 36 of 1113 patients, but there was no radiographic evidence of cartilage damage.

An acute reversible arthropathy has been described in a child with cancer treated with a short course of ciprofloxacin for febrile neutropenia (58).

Immunologic

Anaphylactoid reactions occurred in 3 of about 3200 students who took ciprofloxacin 500 mg for chemoprophylaxis of meningococcal meningitis; two had no history of atopic illness (59). Additional adverse reactions were mild skin rashes in three students and nausea and vomiting in two.

Angioimmunoblastic lymphadenopathy is a rare disorder characterized by generalized lymphadenopathy, fever, hepatosplenomegaly, immune hemolytic anemia, and polyclonal hypergammaglobulinemia. Biopsy-proven angioimmunoblastic lymphadenopathy has been reported in a 79-year-old man who had received ciprofloxacin (60).

A Jarisch–Herxheimer reaction to ciprofloxacin has been reported (61).

- A 14-year-old girl developed tachycardia, hypotension, and disseminated intravascular coagulation after her first dose of oral ciprofloxacin 500 mg for presumed pyelonephritis. A peripheral blood smear showed spirochetes consistent with *Borrelia* species.

Susceptibility Factors

Age

Children

In 36 premature infants, delivered at 25–35 weeks and with birth weights of 750–2050 g, ciprofloxacin (13.8 mg/kg/day in two or three divided doses for 3–20 days) had good efficacy in 66% of cases (62). Thrombocytopenia (five cases), raised transaminases (three cases), hyperbilirubinemia (three cases), and raised creatinine concentration (two patients) were reported as adverse events; one child developed femoral osteitis.

In a Russian study of children with cystic fibrosis, the adverse effects of ciprofloxacin were chiefly gastrointestinal (nausea, stomach pain, diarrhea) and increased transaminase activity (63). One episode of arthrotoxicity was transient. There were no negative effects on growth and no chondrotoxicity.

Oral ciprofloxacin (10 mg/kg bd) was as safe and effective as intramuscular ceftriaxone (50 mg/kg/day) in the treatment of acute invasive diarrhea in 201 children (aged 6 months to 10 years) (64). Possible drug-related adverse events occurred in 8% and were mild and transient. Joints were normal during and after the completion of therapy in all patients.

Elderly people

In a retrospective analysis there were no clinically important differences in the safety profile of ciprofloxacin in patients aged under or over 65 years (65). The incidence of drug-related adverse events was higher in those under 65 years (25%) than in those aged 65 years or more (17%); the most common adverse events affected the gastrointestinal and central nervous systems.

Other features of the patient

Ten patients with peripheral arterial occlusive disease were scheduled to undergo elective percutaneous transluminal angioplasty after a single dose of ciprofloxacin 400 mg (66). Antibiotic concentrations were significantly reduced in ischemic lesions compared with healthy adipose tissue. However, improvement of arterial blood flow in the affected limb was associated with increased cure rates of soft tissue infections.

The pharmacokinetics of intravenous ciprofloxacin have been studied in intensive care unit patients during continuous venovenous hemofiltration ($n = 5$) or hemodiafiltration ($n = 5$) (67). Ciprofloxacin clearance was not altered. A dosage of 400 mg/day was sufficient to maintain effective drug plasma concentrations in patients undergoing continuous renal replacement therapy.

Drug Administration

Drug administration route

In a comparison of intravenous and oral ciprofloxacin in children, treatment associated adverse events were reported in 11% of children taking oral ciprofloxacin, compared with 19% of the children who were treated intravenously (68). In 31 children (1.5%) arthralgia occurred, but it was generally mild to moderate and resolved spontaneously.

Drug overdose

A patient developed acute renal insufficiency after ciprofloxacin overdose. This was mediated by tubulointerstitial nephritis with distal nephron apoptosis, as evidenced by renal biopsy (39).

Drug–Drug Interactions

Ciclosporin

In 42 patients who had received a kidney transplant, cases were treated with ciprofloxacin in the first 1–6 months after transplantation, and matched controls (two per case) were not. The proportion of cases with at least one episode of biopsy-proven rejection 1–3 months after transplantation (45%) was significantly higher than in the controls (19%). The authors speculated that ciprofloxacin increases rejection rates in renal transplant recipients by antagonizing ciclosporin-dependent inhibition of interleukin-2 production (69).

Clozapine

Ciprofloxacin can alter plasma clozapine concentrations, perhaps by inhibition of cytochrome P450 enzymes (70).

Didanosine

Didanosine one enteric-coated capsule/day (400 mg/day) did not affect the absorption of ciprofloxacin in 16 patients (71).

Glibenclamide

Hypoglycemia and raised serum concentrations of glibenclamide, which is metabolized by CYP2C9, occurred after treatment with ciprofloxacin for 1 week in a patient taking long-term glibenclamide (72).

Insulin

Hypoglycemia occurred in a patient treated with insulin and ciprofloxacin 500 mg bd (29).

Methadone

Ciprofloxacin, given to a patient who had been successfully treated with methadone for more than 6 years, caused profound sedation, confusion, and respiratory depression (73). This may have been due to inhibition of CYP1A2 and CYP3A4, two of the isozymes involved in the metabolism of methadone.

Methotrexate

Methotrexate elimination can be delayed by ciprofloxacin. Two adolescents with malignant diseases had reduced elimination of methotrexate (12 g/m^2 4-hourly) when they took ciprofloxacin 500 mg bd (74).

Oral contraceptives

Some antibiotics can reduce the efficacy of oral contraceptives. However, there is pharmacokinetic evidence that plasma concentrations of oral contraceptive steroids are unchanged by co-administration of ciprofloxacin (75). Furthermore, ciprofloxacin (500 mg bd) did not interfere with the ovarian suppression produced by the oral contraceptive Marvelon (30 micrograms of ethinylestradiol plus 150 micrograms of desogestrel) in 24 healthy women in a randomized, double-blind, placebo-controlled, crossover trial (76).

Phenytoin

Ciprofloxacin may interact with phenytoin reducing phenytoin concentrations (77).

- A lower than expected phenytoin serum concentration has been measured in a 78-year-old white woman with a grade III astrocytoma of the right parieto-occipital region treated with ciprofloxacin (500 mg bd) (78).

Increased renal excretion has been suggested to be at least partly responsible for the increased clearance.

Besides this kinetic interaction, the possible epileptogenic potential of ciprofloxacin itself may contribute to the development of seizure activity.

Probenecid

The renal excretion of ciprofloxacin was reduced and plasma concentrations increased by probenecid (79).

Quinidine

Serum quinidine concentrations rose during concomitant administration of ciprofloxacin (80). The authors speculated that the mechanism was inhibition of cytochrome P450 by ciprofloxacin.

Rifamycins

Rifampicin-induced lupus-like syndrome is associated with combination therapy with ciprofloxacin, since rifampicin is metabolized by (among others) CYP3A4, which is inhibited by ciprofloxacin, and combined usage may lead to higher rifampicin blood concentrations (81).

Ropinirole

During co-administration of ciprofloxacin with ropinirole in 12 patients there was an increase in the plasma ropinirole concentration, which is metabolized by CYP1A2 (82).

Warfarin

Ciprofloxacin can occasionally cause an exaggerated hypoprothombinemic response and bleeding in patients taking warfarin. In 66 patients (median age 72 years, range 36–94), the mean time to detection of the coagulopathy after ciprofloxacin challenge was 5.5 days (83). Hospitalization was reported in 15 cases, bleeding in 25, and death in one. The median INR was 10.0. Patients in their seventh decade and those requiring polypharmacy were most at risk.

Food–Drug Interactions

The systemic availability of ciprofloxacin is reduced by 30–36% when it is taken with dairy products (84).

References

1. Centers for Disease Control and Prevention (CDC). Update: adverse events associated with anthrax prophylaxis among postal employees—New Jersey, New York City, and the District of Columbia metropolitan area, 2001. MMWR Morb Mortal Wkly Rep 2001;50(47):1051–4.
2. Centers for Disease Control and Prevention (CDC). Update: Investigation of bioterrorism-related anthrax and adverse events from antimicrobial prophylaxis. MMWR Morb Mortal Wkly Rep 2001;50(44):973–6.
3. The Centers for Disease Control and Prevention. Investigation of bioterrorism-related anthrax and adverse events from antimicrobial prophylaxis. JAMA 2001;286(20):2536–7.
4. The Centers for Disease Control and Prevention. Update: investigation of bioterrorism-related anthrax and interim guidelines for exposure management and antimicrobial therapy, October 2001. JAMA 2001;286(18):2226–32.
5. Sundram FX, Wong WY, Ang ES, Goh AS, Ng DC, Yu S. Evaluation of technetium-99m ciprofloxacin (Infecton) in the imaging of infection. Ann Acad Med Singapore 2000;29(6):699–703.
6. Chodosh S, Schreurs A, Siami G, Barkman HW Jr, Anzueto A, Shan M, Moesker H, Stack T, Kowalsky S. Efficacy of oral ciprofloxacin vs. clarithromycin for treatment of acute bacterial exacerbations of chronic bronchitis. The Bronchitis Study Group. Clin Infect Dis 1998;27(4):730–8.
7. Chodosh S, McCarty J, Farkas S, Drehobl M, Tosiello R, Shan M, Aneiro L, Kowalsky S. Randomized, double-blind study of ciprofloxacin and cefuroxime axetil for treatment

of acute bacterial exacerbations of chronic bronchitis. The Bronchitis Study Group. Clin Infect Dis 1998;27(4):722–9.

8. Owens RC Jr, Ambrose PG. Torsades de pointes associated with fluoroquinolones. Pharmacotherapy 2002;22(5):663–8; discussion 668–72.
9. Singh H, Kishore K, Gupta MS, Khetarpal S, Jain S, Mangla M. Ciprofloxacin-induced QTc prolongation. J Assoc Physicians India 2002;50:430–1.
10. McCarty JM, Richard G, Huck W, Tucker RM, Tosiello RL, Shan M, Heyd A, Echols RM. A randomized trial of short-course ciprofloxacin, ofloxacin, or trimethoprim/sulfamethoxazole for the treatment of acute urinary tract infection in women. Ciprofloxacin Urinary Tract Infection Group. Am J Med 1999;106(3):292–9.
11. Tattevin P, Messiaen T, Pras V, Ronco P, Biour M. Confusion and general seizures following ciprofloxacin administration. Nephrol Dial Transplant 1998;13(10):2712–13.
12. Kushner JM, Peckman HJ, Snyder CR. Seizures associated with fluoroquinolones. Ann Pharmacother 2001; 35(10):1194–8.
13. Lee CH, Cheung RT, Chan TM. Ciprofloxacin-induced oral facial dyskinesia in a patient with normal liver and renal function. Hosp Med 2000;61(2):142–3.
14. MacLeod W. Case report: severe neurologic reaction to ciprofloxacin. Can Fam Physician 2001;47:553–5.
15. Zehnder D, Hoigne R, Neftel KA, Sieber R. Painful dysaesthesia with ciprofloxacin. BMJ 1995;311(7014):1204.
16. Vrabec TR, Sergott RC, Jaeger EA, Savino PJ, Bosley TM. Reversible visual loss in a patient receiving high-dose ciprofloxacin hydrochloride (Cipro). Ophthalmology 1990; 97(6):707–10.
17. Madhavan HN, Rao SK. Ciprofloxacin precipitates in the corneal epithelium. J Cataract Refract Surg 2002; 28(6):909.
18. Eiferman RA, Snyder JP, Nordquist RE. Ciprofloxacin microprecipitates and macroprecipitates in the human corneal epithelium. J Cataract Refract Surg 2001; 27(10):1701–2.
19. Ikiz AO, Serbetcioglu B, Guneri EA, Sutay S, Ceryan K. Investigation of topical ciprofloxacin ototoxicity in guinea pigs. Acta Otolaryngol 1998;118(6):808–12.
20. Miro N. Controlled multicenter study on chronic suppurative otitis media treated with topical applications of ciprofloxacin 0.2% solution in single-dose containers or combination of polymyxin B, neomycin, and hydrocortisone suspension. Otolaryngol Head Neck Surg 2000; 123(5):617–23.
21. Claros P, Sabater F, Claros A Jr, Claros A. Determinacion de niveles plasmaticos de ciprofloxacino en niños tratados con ciprofloxacino topico al 0.2% en presencia de perforacion timpanica. [Determination of plasma ciprofloxacin levels in children treated with 0.2% topical ciprofloxacin for tympanic perforation.] Acta Otorrinolaringol Esp 2000;51(2):97–9.
22. Zabala S, Gascon A, Bartolome C, Castiella J, Juyol M. Ciprofloxacino y psicosis aguda. [Ciprofloxacin and acute psychosis.] Enferm Infecc Microbiol Clin 1998;16(1):42.
23. James EA, Demian AZ. Acute psychosis in a trauma patient due to ciprofloxacin. Postgrad Med J 1998; 74(869):189–90.
24. Grassi L, Biancosino B, Pavanati M, Agostini M, Manfredini R. Depression or hypoactive delirium? A report of ciprofloxacin-induced mental disorder in a patient with chronic obstructive pulmonary disease. Psychother Psychosom 2001;70(1):58–9.
25. Imani K, Druart F, Glibert A, Morin T. Troubles neuropsychiatriques induits par la ciprofloxacine. [Neuropsychiatric disorders induced by ciprofloxacin.] Presse Méd 2001;30(27):1356.
26. Tripathi A, Chen SI, O'Sullivan S. Acute psychosis following the use of topical ciprofloxacin. Arch Ophthalmol 2002;120(5):665–6.
27. Kundu AK. Ciprofloxacin-induced severe cutaneous reaction and haemolysis in a young adult. J Assoc Physicians India 2000;48(6):649–50.
28. Mouraux A, Gille M, Pieret F, Declercq I. Purpura thrombotique thrombocytopenique fulminant au decour d'un traitement pas ciprofloxacine. [Fulminant thrombotic thrombocytopenic purpura in the course of ciprofloxacin therapy.] Rev Neurol (Paris) 2002;158(11):1115–17.
29. Kljucar S, Rost KL, Landen H. Ciprofloxacin in der Therapie des nosobomialen pneumonie: Eine Anwendungs beobachtung bei 676 patienten. [Ciprofloxacin in the treatment of hospital-acquired pneumonia: a surveillance study in 676 patients.] Pneumologie 2002;56(10):599–604.
30. Grassi C, Salvatori E, Rosignoli MT, Dionisio P; Prulifloxacin Study Group. Randomized, double-blind study of prulifloxacin versus ciprofloxacin in patients with acute exacerbations of chronic bronchitis. Respiration 2002;69(3):217–22.
31. Fernandez de la Puebla Gimenez RA, Lechuga Varona MT, Garcia Sanchez E. Colitis seudomembranosa por ciprofloxacino. [Pseudomembranous colitis due to ciprofloxacin.] Med Clin (Barc) 1998;111(7):278–9.
32. Zabala Lopez S, Iglesias Quiros E, Gonzalez Heras S, Martinez Navarro C, Gambaro Royo B. Diarrea asociada a *Clostridium difficile* secundaria al uso de ciprofloxacino, complicando un primer brote de enfermedad inflamatoria intestinal. [Diarrhea associated with *Clostridium difficile* secondary to the use of ciprofloxacin, complicating a first occurrence of intestinal inflammatory disease.] Rev Esp Enferm Dig 2000;92(8):539–40.
33. Thomas C, Golledge CL, Riley TV. Ciprofloxacin and *Clostridium difficile*—associated diarrhea. Infect Control Hosp Epidemiol 2002;23(11):637–8.
34. Yip C, Loeb M, Salama S, Moss L, Olde J. Quinolone use as a risk factor for nosocomial *Clostridium difficile*-associated diarrhea. Infect Control Hosp Epidemiol 2001;22(9):572–5.
35. Contreras MA, Luna R, Mulero J, Andreu JL. Severe ciprofloxacin-induced acute hepatitis. Eur J Clin Microbiol Infect Dis 2001;20(6):434–5.
36. Mann S, Thillainayagam A. Is ciprofloxacin a new cause of acute pancreatitis? J Clin Gastroenterol 2000;31(4):336.
37. Shih DJ, Korbet SM, Rydel JJ, Schwartz MM. Renal vasculitis associated with ciprofloxacin. Am J Kidney Dis 1995;26(3):516–19.
38. Raja N, Miller WE, McMillan R, Mason JR. Ciprofloxacin-associated acute renal failure in patients undergoing high-dose chemotherapy and autologous stem cell rescue. Bone Marrow Transplant 1998;21(12):1283–4.
39. Dharnidharka VR, Nadeau K, Cannon CL, Harris HW, Rosen S. Ciprofloxacin overdose: acute renal failure with prominent apoptotic changes. Am J Kidney Dis 1998; 31(4):710–12.
40. Bald M, Ratjen F, Nikolaizik W, Wingen AM. Ciprofloxacin-induced acute renal failure in a patient with cystic fibrosis. Pediatr Infect Dis J 2001;20(3):320–1.
41. Allan DS, Thompson CM, Barr RM, Clark WF, Chin-Yee IH. Ciprofloxacin-associated hemolytic–uremic syndrome. Ann Pharmacother 2002;36(6):1000–2.
42. Chopra N, Fine PL, Price B, Atlas I. Bilateral hydronephrosis from ciprofloxacin induced crystalluria and stone formation. J Urol 2000;164(2):438.
43. Maquirriain Gorriz MT, Merino Munoz F, Tres Belzunegui JC, Sangros Gonzalez FJ. Erupcion fija por farmacos inducida por ciprofloxacino. [Fixed drug eruption induced by ciprofloxacin.] Aten Primaria 1998;21(8):585–6.

44. Rodriguez-Morales A, Llamazares AA, Benito RP, Cocera CM. Fixed drug eruption from quinolones with a positive lesional patch test to ciprofloxacin. Contact Dermatitis 2001;44(4):255.
45. Pons R, Escutia B. Vasculitis por ciprofloxacino con afectacion cutanea y renal. [Ciprofloxacin-induced vasculitis with cutaneous and renal involvement.] Nefrologia 2001;21(2):209–12.
46. Kimyai-Asadi A, Usman A, Nousari HC. Ciprofloxacin-induced bullous pemphigoid. J Am Acad Dermatol 2000;42(5 Pt 1):847.
47. Perez Vazquez A, Gutierrez Perez B, Carreter de Granda E, Zuniga Perez-Lemaur M, Conde Yague R. Vasculitis cutanea por ciprofloxacino. [Cutaneous vasculitis caused by ciprofloxacin.] An Med Interna 2000;17(4):225.
48. Terzano C, Taurino AE, Peona V. Nebulized tobramycin in patients with chronic respiratory infections during clinical evolution of Wegener's granulomatosis. Eur Rev Med Pharmacol Sci 2001;5(4):131–8.
49. Chhajed PN, Plit ML, Hopkins PM, Malouf MA, Glanville AR. Achilles tendon disease in lung transplant recipients: association with ciprofloxacin. Eur Respir J 2002;19(3):469–71.
50. Petersen W, Laprell H. Die "schleichende" Ruptur der Achillessehne nach Ciprofloxacin induzierter Tendopathie. Ein Fallbericht. [Insidious rupture of the Achilles tendon after ciprofloxacin-induced tendopathy. A case report.] Unfallchirurg 1998;101(9):731–4.
51. Gendrel D, Moulin F. Fluoroquinolones in paediatrics. Paediatr Drugs 2001;3(5):365–77.
52. Gbadoe AD, Dogba A, Dagnra AY, Atakouma Y, Tekou H, Assimadi JK. Osteomyelites aïgues de l'enfant drepanocytaire en zone tropicale: interêt de l'utilisation des fluoroquinolones par voie orale. [Acute osteomyelitis in the child with sickle cell disease in a tropical zone: value of oral fluoroquinolones.] Arch Pediatr 2001; 8(12):1305–10.
53. Malaguti M, Triolo L, Biagini M. Ciprofloxacin-associated Achilles tendon rupture in a hemodialysis patient. J Nephrol 2001;14(5):431–2.
54. Doherty CP, Saha SK, Cutting WA. Typhoid fever, ciprofloxacin and growth in young children. Ann Trop Paediatr 2000;20(4):297–303.
55. Singh UK, Sinha RK, Prasad B, Chakrabarti B, Sharma SK. Ciprofloxacin in children: is arthropathy a limitation? Indian J Pediatr 2000;67(5):386–7.
56. Postnikov SS, Nazhimov VP, Semykin SIu, Kapranov NI. [Comparative morphological analysis of the articular cartilage, epiphyseal plate, spongy bone, and synovial membrane of the knee joint in children treated and not treated with ciprofloxacin.]Antibiot Khimioter 2000; 45(11):9–13.
57. Kubin R. Safety and efficacy of ciprofloxacin in paediatric patients—review. Infection 1993;21(6):413–21.
58. Mullen CA, Petropoulos D, Rytting M, Jeha S, Zipf T, Roberts WM, Rolston KV. Acute reversible arthropathy in a pediatric patient with cancer treated with a short course of ciprofloxacin for febrile neutropenia. J Pediatr Hematol Oncol 1998;20(5):516–17.
59. Burke P, Burne SR. Allergy associated with ciprofloxacin. BMJ 2000;320(7236):679.
60. Knoops L, van den Neste E, Hamels J, Theate I, Mineur P. Angioimmunoblastic lymphadenopathy following ciprofloxacin administration. Acta Clin Belg 2002;57(2):71–3.
61. Webster G, Schiffman JD, Dosanjh AS, Amieva MR, Gans HA, Sectish TC. Jarisch–Herxheimer reaction associated with ciprofloxacin administration for tick-borne relapsing fever. Pediatr Infect Dis J 2002;21(6):571–3.
62. Wlazlowski J, Krzyzanska-Oberbek A, Sikora JP, Chlebna-Sokol D. Use of the quinolones in treatment of severe bacterial infections in premature infants. Acta Pol Pharm 2000;57(Suppl):28–31.
63. Postnikov SS, Semykin SIu, Kapranov NI, Perederko LV, Polikarpova SV. [The efficacy and safety of ciprofloxacin in treating children with mucoviscidosis.] Antibiot Khimioter 2000;45(4):14–17.
64. Leibovitz E, Janco J, Piglansky L, Press J, Yagupsky P, Reinhart H, Yaniv I, Dagan R. Oral ciprofloxacin vs. intramuscular ceftriaxone as empiric treatment of acute invasive diarrhea in children. Pediatr Infect Dis J 2000;19(11):1060–7.
65. Heyd A, Haverstock D. Retrospective analysis of the safety profile of oral and intravenous ciprofloxacin in a geriatric population. Clin Ther 2000;22(10):1239–50.
66. Joukhadar C, Klein N, Frossard M, Minar E, Stass H, Lackner E, Herrmann M, Riedmuller E, Muller M. Angioplasty increases target site concentrations of ciprofloxacin in patients with peripheral arterial occlusive disease. Clin Pharmacol Ther 2001;70(6):532–9.
67. Malone RS, Fish DN, Abraham E, Teitelbaum I. Pharmacokinetics of levofloxacin and ciprofloxacin during continuous renal replacement therapy in critically ill patients. Antimicrob Agents Chemother 2001;45(10):2949–54.
68. Hampel B, Hullmann R, Schmidt H. Ciprofloxacin in pediatrics: worldwide clinical experience based on compassionate use—safety report. Pediatr Infect Dis J 1997;16(1):127–9.
69. Wrishko RE, Levine M, Primmett DR, Kim S, Partovi N, Lewis S, Landsberg D, Keown PA. Investigation of a possible interaction between ciprofloxacin and cyclosporine in renal transplant patients. Transplantation 1997;64(7):996–9.
70. Joos AA. Pharmakologische Interaktionen von Antibiotika und Psychopharmaka. [Pharmacologic interactions of antibiotics and psychotropic drugs.] Psychiatr Prax 1998;25(2):57–60.
71. Jablonowski H. Didanosin als Kapsel. Bewahrtes Medikament in neuer Form. [Didanosine as a capsule. A reliable drug in a new dosage form.] MMW Fortschr Med 2001;143(Suppl 1):92–5.
72. Roberge RJ, Kaplan R, Frank R, Fore C. Glyburide–ciprofloxacin interaction with resistant hypoglycemia. Ann Emerg Med 2000;36(2):160–3.
73. Herrlin K, Segerdahl M, Gustafsson LL, Kalso E. Methadone, ciprofloxacin, and adverse drug reactions. Lancet 2000;356(9247):2069–70.
74. Dalle JH, Auvrignon A, Vassal G, Leverger G, Kalifa C. Interaction methotrexate–ciprofloxacine: à propos de deux cas d'intoxication sevère. [Methotrexate–ciprofloxacin interaction: report of two cases of severe intoxication..] Arch Pediatr 2001;8(10):1078–81.
75. Archer JS, Archer DF. Oral contraceptive efficacy and antibiotic interaction: a myth debunked. J Am Acad Dermatol 2002;46(6):917–23.
76. Scholten PC, Droppert RM, Zwinkels MG, Moesker HL, Nauta JJ, Hoepelman IM. No interaction between ciprofloxacin and an oral contraceptive. Antimicrob Agents Chemother 1998;42(12):3266–8.
77. Otero MJ, Moran D, Valverde MP. Interaction between phenytoin and ciprofloxacin. Ann Pharmacother 1999;33(2):251–2.
78. McLeod R, Trinkle R. Comment: unexpectedly low phenytoin concentration in a patient receiving ciprofloxacin. Ann Pharmacother 1998;32(10):1110–11.
79. Jaehde U, Sorgel F, Reiter A, Sigl G, Naber KG, Schunack W. Effect of probenecid on the distribution and elimination of ciprofloxacin in humans. Clin Pharmacol Ther 1995;58(5):532–41.
80. Teppo AM, Haltia K, Wager O. Immunoelectrophoretic "tailing" of albumin line due to albumin-IgG antibody

complexes: a side effect of nitrofurantoin treatment? Scand J Immunol 1976;5(3):249–61.
81. Patel GK, Anstey AV. Rifampicin-induced lupus erythematosus. Clin Exp Dermatol 2001;26(3):260–2.
82. Kaye CM, Nicholls B. Clinical pharmacokinetics of ropinirole. Clin Pharmacokinet 2000;39(4):243–54.
83. Ellis RJ, Mayo MS, Bodensteiner DM. Ciprofloxacin–warfarin coagulopathy: a case series. Am J Hematol 2000;63(1):28–31.
84. Schmidt LE, Dalhoff K. Food–drug interactions. Drugs 2002;62(10):1481–502.

Ciramadol

General Information

Data on the incidence of adverse effects after usual doses of oral ciramadol are conflicting. In one study there was a low incidence of mild adverse effects (1), but in another, in which ciramadol 60 mg was more effective than codeine 60 mg or placebo, there was a high incidence of opioid adverse effects (2); some other workers have had the same experience.

References

1. Graf DF, Pandit SK, Kothary SP, Freeland GR. A double-blind comparison of orally administered ciramadol and codeine for relief of postoperative pain. J Clin Pharmacol 1985;25(8):590–5.
2. van Steenberghe D, Verbist D, Quirynen M, Thevissen E. Double-blind comparison of the analgesic potency of ciramadol, codeine and placebo against postsurgical pain in ambulant patients. Eur J Clin Pharmacol 1986;31(3):355–8.

Cisapride

General Information

Cisapride is structurally similar to metoclopramide, but has no dopamine receptor antagonist activity and hence no central antiemetic effect. However, because it stimulates the release of acetylcholine in the gastrointestinal tract it is effective in conditions such as reflux esophagitis and gastroparesis. During clinical trials, the most frequent unwanted effects were diarrhea (5–11%) and abdominal pain (16% with 20 mg bd).

Observational studies

The effect of cisapride 20 mg bd for 7 days in preventing symptoms of gastro-esophageal reflux disease induced by a provocative meal has been assessed in 122 patients who had had symptoms suggestive of gastro-esophageal reflux for at least 3 months (1). Cisapride prevented or reduced the symptoms of heartburn and related symptoms, such as belching and regurgitation. Mild to moderate diarrhea was the main adverse effect.

Comparative studies

In a randomized, double-blind study in 106 patients with non-ulcer dyspepsia, cinitapride 1 mg tds was as effective as cisapride 5 mg tds in relieving symptoms (2). Adverse events, mainly gastrointestinal, were transient and did not require drug withdrawal. In another randomized study in 28 children (aged 5–17 years) with diabetic gastroparesis, domperidone 0.9 mg/kg/day for 8 weeks was superior to cisapride 0.8 mg/kg/day in reversing gastric emptying delay and gastric electrical abnormalities, as well as in improving dyspeptic symptoms and diabetic control (3). No potentially drug-related adverse effects were reported.

Placebo-controlled studies

The effect of cisapride 10 mg qds for 5 days on the frequency of nocturnal transient lower esophageal sphincter relaxation and esophageal acid exposure has been studied in a double-blind, placebo-controlled, crossover study in 10 patients with gastro-esophageal reflux disease (4). Cisapride significantly reduced the frequency of transient lower esophageal sphincter relaxation during sleep and increased lower esophageal sphincter pressure without changing gastric emptying. However, in a larger double-blind, placebo-controlled, crossover study in 30 patients with gastro-esophageal reflux disease, cisapride 20 mg bd for 4 weeks (despite adequate plasma concentrations) had no significant effects on swallow-induced esophageal peristaltic activity, the basal tone of the lower esophageal sphincter, or the number of transient lower esophageal sphincter relaxations induced by gas distension of the stomach (5). Adverse effects were similar in the two treatment sequences, although there were a few more episodes of abdominal cramps, nausea, and headache with cisapride.

General adverse effects

A comparison of data from prescription event monitoring in over 13 000 recipients of cisapride and from a further 9726 recipients involved in a controlled study showed that diarrhea, in about 2–4% of patients, was the commonest adverse effect reported. Other relatively common adverse effects are headache, abdominal pain, nausea and vomiting, and constipation, all in about 1–1.5% of patients.

A thorough review of the effects of cisapride in patients in intensive care suggested that adverse reactions are not likely to be severe or problematical (6). However, cisapride has been withdrawn because of the risk of prolongation of the QT interval and consequent ventricular dysrhythmias.

Organs and Systems

Cardiovascular

The FDA reported that between September 1993 and April 1996 it received reports of prolonged QT intervals in 23 patients and torsade de pointes or ventricular fibrillation in 34. Some proved fatal (SEDA-21, 361).

Several later studies confirmed the finding of QT interval prolongation during cisapride therapy in children (7).

The effects of cisapride on the QT_c interval, heart rate, and cardiac rhythm were reported in a controlled study of 83 infants aged 2–54 months who received cisapride for a minimum of 4 days for gastro-esophageal reflux and 77 controls, using continuous bipolar limb lead electrocardiography for 8 hours (8). The QT_c interval was significantly prolonged by cisapride in infants under 3 months old. There was no significant difference in heart rates and there were no dysrhythmias. None of the infants was receiving drugs that inhibit the hepatic metabolism of cisapride via CYP3A4.

The effect of cisapride 0.8 mg/kg/day for 14 days on the QT_c interval has been studied prospectively in 50 infants with feeding intolerance, apnea, and bradycardia episodes secondary to gastro-esophageal reflux and gastrointestinal dysmotility (9). In 15 infants there was prolongation of the QT_c interval at some time during the 14 days. Infants with a QT_c interval on day 3 at least two standard deviations above the mean baseline QT_c interval were more likely to develop a prolonged QT_c interval.

Over 30 drugs (for example clarithromycin, erythromycin, and troleandomycin; nefazodone; fluconazole, itraconazole, and ketoconazole; indinavir and ritonavir) and other substances (for example grapefruit juice) can interact with cisapride and enhance its dysrhythmogenic effect. Despite regulatory action, including strengthened warnings in the product information, reports of dysrhythmias have repeatedly appeared. For example, in the UK the Medicines Control Agency received 60 reports of serious cardiac adverse events between 1988 and 2000; five were fatal (10). The corresponding worldwide figures were 386 serious ventricular dysrhythmias with 125 deaths and 50 unexplained deaths.

- An 81-year-old woman, who had a permanent pacemaker for complete heart block with symptomatic bradycardia-dependent torsade de pointes, had breakthrough torsade de pointes during therapy with cisapride 10 mg tds for 22 days and paroxetine for 9 days (11). She made a good recovery on withdrawal of the drugs.

In some countries therefore the product licence was suspended (10) and cisapride was subsequently withdrawn from the market by Janssen Cilag in 2003 (12).

Before its withdrawal in the UK cisapride was specifically contraindicated in premature babies for up to 3 months after birth, because of the risk of QT interval prolongation (10). Between 1988 and 2000 the Medicines Control Agency received 64 reports of suspected adverse effects of cisapride in children under 13 years, of which two were cases of QT prolongation and two were sudden unexplained deaths. Another 106 cardiovascular events were reported from other countries, including 30 cases of QT prolongation, six cases of ventricular fibrillation or tachycardia, and four sudden unexplained deaths.

Electrocardiographic changes and predisposition to cardiac dysrhythmias were investigated in 63 children (mean age 29 months) with gastro-esophageal reflux who had taken cisapride 0.2 mg/kg tds for at least 15 days and 57 control children (mean age 27 months) who were hospitalized for other reasons and were not given cisapride or other oral treatment (13). All the children had an electrocardiogram performed at inclusion, and 24-hour Holter recording was performed in all children with prolonged QT intervals. When a prolonged QT interval was detected cisapride was withdrawn and a new electrocardiogram was recorded. Five children in the treatment group and six controls had prolonged QT intervals, which normalized in three of the five children after cisapride was withdrawn. Holter recording was normal in all children.

The effect of cisapride 0.2 mg/kg tds for 8 weeks on cardiac rhythm was studied in a placebo-controlled, double-blind trial in 49 children aged 0.5–4 years with gastro-esophageal reflux resistant to other medical therapy (14). None had underlying cardiac disease or electrolyte imbalance. Cisapride had no effect on cardiac electrical function. However, in a prospective study cisapride 2 mg/kg qds given for 72 hours to 10 premature infants caused a significant increase in the QT_c interval compared with pretreatment values (15).

The relation between cisapride plasma concentrations, QT_c interval, and cardiac rhythm was evaluated in a controlled study in 211 infants undergoing routine 8-hour polysomnography (16). Cisapride was given for at least 4 days. At comparable doses of cisapride and comparable plasma concentrations, the QT_c was significantly higher in infants below 3 months of age.

In a postmarketing study of the safety of cisapride during 1993–9, 341 patients had cardiac effects, of whom 80 (23%) died, the deaths being directly or indirectly associated with a dysrhythmic event (17). The cardiac effects included QT interval prolongation, torsade de pointes, polymorphous ventricular tachycardia, ventricular fibrillation, ventricular tachycardia, cardiac arrest, unspecified "serious" dysrhythmias, and sudden death. In most instances the dysrhythmia occurred in the presence of risk factors such as other drugs or medical conditions.

Nervous system

Despite the fact that cisapride is not a dopamine receptor antagonist, tardive dyskinesia has been reported.

- Tardive dyskinesia with involuntary movement of muscles of mastication and the tongue has been reported in a 76-year-old man who took cisapride 10 mg tds, with complete resolution on withdrawal (18).

Psychological, psychiatric

In 16% of children given cisapride for intestinal pseudo-obstruction, treatment was followed by mild irritability and hyperactivity (SEDA-18, 370). In one adult, aggressive behavior seemed to be a direct complication of treatment (19).

Gastrointestinal

The effect of cisapride 10 mg bd on gastroduodenal reflux and gall bladder motility has been assessed in 77 patients with gallstones in a double-blind, placebo-controlled study (20). Cisapride increased gallbladder motility but did not have any effect on gastroduodenal reflux. Diarrhea, abdominal cramps, and increased bladder frequency were common adverse effects.

A multicenter trial in 353 patients assessed the efficacy and tolerance of sodium alginate (four 10 ml sachets a day) compared with cisapride (5 mg qds) in the symptomatic treatment of uncomplicated gastro-esophageal reflux without severe esophagitis (21). Sodium alginate, which costs less than cisapride, was more effective in relieving symptoms. Adverse effects were rare and not serious. Constipation was the most common adverse effect of alginate while diarrhea was the commonest adverse effect of cisapride.

Liver

In one elderly man receiving cisapride, hepatitis occurred and resolved rapidly on drug withdrawal; there was no detectable cause other than the use of cisapride (22).

Urinary tract

Cisapride can cause functional changes in the urinary tract because of increased pressure in the bladder, which may be a problem in individuals with hyperactive bladders. In individuals who had complete traumatic spinal cord injury, the increase in reflex bladder contractions was sufficient to reduce compliance markedly (23).

Six cases of pollakiuria have been published (24), reversible when treatment was withdrawn (SEDA-19, 325).

Susceptibility Factors

Age

Children

The use of cisapride and its benefit to harm balance in children has been reviewed (25). Overall it is well tolerated. The most common adverse effects are diarrhea, abdominal cramps, borborygmi, and colic. Serious adverse events are rare and include isolated cases of extrapyramidal reactions, seizures in epileptic patients, cholestasis, QT interval prolongation and ventricular dysrhythmias, anorexia, and enuresis. Interactions of cisapride with other drugs are similar to those reported in adults. Co-administration of drugs that inhibit CYP3A4, such as imidazoles, macrolide antibiotics, the antidepressant nefazodone, and protease inhibitors such as ritonavir, are contraindicated. Furthermore, co-administration of anticholinergic drugs can compromise the beneficial effects of cisapride.

A systematic review of randomized, controlled trials of cisapride for gastro-esophageal reflux in children has been reported (26). Seven comparisons of cisapride with placebo (286 children in all) were included. The reflux index was significantly reduced by cisapride. However, there was no clear evidence that cisapride reduced symptoms of gastro-esophageal reflux. Adverse events (mainly diarrhea) were not significantly more common with cisapride.

The effects of cisapride 0.2 mg/kg tds on acid gastro-esophageal reflux in 32 formerly preterm infants receiving respiratory stimulation with caffeine have been studied using 24-hour esophageal pH monitoring (27). Cisapride significantly reduced the reflux index and the frequency of reflux without impairing the systemic availability or therapeutic effects of caffeine.

The effects of cisapride 0.2–0.3 mg/kg tds on chronic constipation were studied in a double-blind, placebo-controlled trial in 36 children (28). Cisapride was effective in the treatment of chronic constipation without major adverse effects.

The effects of low-dose cisapride (0.1 mg/kg tds) on gastric emptying and the QT interval were studied in a double-blind, placebo-controlled, crossover trial in 20 infants of low birth weights (29). Low-dose cisapride significantly improved gastric emptying without prolonging the QT interval.

Elderly patients

The pharmacokinetics of cisapride have been studied in eight elderly patients (mean age 85 years) (27). There were no adverse effects, apart from a slight increase in stool frequency. There were no changes in the corrected QT interval. However, plasma cisapride concentrations were higher than expected. Thus, in extremely elderly patients cisapride should be given once or twice a day rather than three times.

Other features of the patient

Cisapride should not be prescribed for patients with a history of disturbances of cardiac rhythm or who are at risk of developing frank dysrhythmias, especially individuals with hypokalemia or hypomagnesemia (SEDA-22, 389).

Cisapride should not be used in cases of intestinal obstruction, perforation, or hemorrhage (SEDA-22, 389).

Drug–Drug Interactions

Cimetidine

In eight healthy volunteers oral cimetidine 400 mg tds increased the steady-state C_{max} and AUC of oral cisapride 10 mg tds. Cisapride shortened the t_{max} and reduced the AUC of cimetidine (30). The authors concluded that cimetidine inhibits the metabolism of cisapride, and cisapride enhances the gastrointestinal absorption of cimetidine.

Digoxin

A possible interaction between cisapride and digoxin has been reported (31).

- A 90-year-old woman took cisapride, first in a dose of 5 mg bd and then 5 mg tds. She had been taking digoxin for a long time, but the serum digoxin concentration began to fall gradually after cisapride was given, from 1.1 nmol/l in January to 0.7 nmol/l in March and 0.5 nmol/l in August. The digoxin tablets were of reportedly high dissolution rate, with an onset of action at 30–60 minutes and a peak effect at 4–6 hours after a single dose. The onset of action of cisapride is 30–60 minutes, but the duration of its promotility effect during multiple dose therapy is not clear. The drugs were then separated by 4 hours, with the aim of reducing the promotility effect of cisapride on digoxin absorption, and there was an improvement in both clinical response and digoxin concentration.

The authors speculated that cisapride reduced digoxin absorption by accelerating bowel transit time.

Diltiazem

A possible interaction of cisapride 20 mg/day with diltiazem has been reported in a 45-year-old woman who developed near syncope and had QT interval prolongation (32). The QT interval returned to normal after withdrawal of cisapride. Rechallenge was not attempted. Diltiazem inhibits CYP3A4, and should therefore probably be avoided in combination with cisapride.

Oral anticoagulants

The absorption of the anticoagulants warfarin and phenprocoumon is unaffected by cisapride (SEDA-21, 361).

Propranolol

The absorption of propranolol is unaffected by cisapride (SEDA-21, 361).

References

1. Castell D, Silvers D, Littlejohn T, Orr W, Napolitano J, Oleka N, Jokubaitis L. Cisapride 20 mg b.d. for preventing symptoms of GERD induced by a provocative meal. The CIS-USA-89 Study Group. Aliment Pharmacol Ther 1999;13(6):787–94.
2. Caro L, Curi LA, Giglio NR, Mezzotero O. Cinitapride versus cisapride in the treatment of non-ulcer dyspepsia. Prensa Med Argent 2002;89:95–101.
3. Franzese A, Borrelli O, Corrado G, Rea P, Di Nardo G, Grandinetti AL, Dito L, Cucchiara S. Domperidone is more effective than cisapride in children with diabetic gastroparesis. Aliment Pharmacol Ther 2002;16(5):951–7.
4. Pehlivanov N, Sarosiek I, Whitman R, Olyaee M, McCallum R. Effect of cisapride on nocturnal transient lower oesophageal sphincter relaxations and nocturnal gastro-oesophageal reflux in patients with oesophagitis: a double-blind, placebo-controlled study. Aliment Pharmacol Ther 2002;16(4):743–7.
5. Finizia C, Lundell L, Cange L, Ruth M. The effect of cisapride on oesophageal motility and lower sphincter function in patients with gastro-oesophageal reflux disease. Eur J Gastroenterol Hepatol 2002;14(1):9–14.
6. Goldhill DR. Cisapride and the ICU patient. Care Crit Ill 1997;13:61–4.
7. Vandenplas Y, Benatar A, Cools F, Arana A, Hegar B, Hauser B. Efficacy and tolerability of cisapride in children. Paediatr Drugs 2001;3(8):559–73.
8. Benatar A, Feenstra A, Decraene T, Vandenplas Y. Cisapride and proarrhythmia in childhood. Pediatrics 1999;103(4 Pt 1):856–7.
9. Chhina S, Peverini RL, Deming DD, Hopper AO, Hashmi A, Vyhmeister NR. QTc interval in infants receiving cisapride. J Perinatol 2002;22(2):144–8.
10. Committee on Safety of Medicines Medicines Contol Agency. Cisapride (Prepulsid) withdrawn. Curr Probl Pharmacovig 2000;26:9–10.
11. Ng KS, Tham LS, Tan HH, Chia BL. Cisapride and torsades de pointes in a pacemaker patient. Pacing Clin Electrophysiol 2000;23(1):130–2.
12. Committee on Safety of Medicines. Cisparide: licences withdrawn. Curr Probl Pharmacvig 2004;30:3.
13. Ramirez-Mayans J, Garrido-Garcia LM, Huerta-Tecanhuey A, Gutierrez-Castrellon P, Cervantes-Bustamante R, Mata-Rivera N, Zarate-Mondragon F. Cisapride and QTc interval in children. Pediatrics 2000;106(5):1028–30.
14. Levy J, Hayes C, Kern J, Harris J, Flores A, Hyams J, Murray R, Tolia V. Does cisapride influence cardiac rhythm? Results of a United States multicenter, double-blind, placebo-controlled pediatric study. J Pediatr Gastroenterol Nutr 2001;32(4):458–63.
15. Cools F, Benatar A, Bougatef A, Vandenplas Y. The effect of cisapride on the corrected QT interval and QT dispersion in premature infants. J Pediatr Gastroenterol Nutr 2001;33(2):178–81.
16. Benatar A, Feenstra A, Decraene T, Vandenplas Y. Cisapride plasma levels and corrected QT interval in infants undergoing routine polysomnography. J Pediatr Gastroenterol Nutr 2001;33(1):41–6.
17. Wysowski DK, Corken A, Gallo-Torres H, Talarico L, Rodriguez EM. Postmarketing reports of QT prolongation and ventricular arrhythmia in association with cisapride and Food and Drug Administration regulatory actions. Am J Gastroenterol 2001;96(6):1698–703.
18. Gomez Rodriguez MT, Mugarza Hernandez MD, Marin Perez O. Cisapride and tardive dyskinesia. Revision of one case. Medifam Rev Med Fam Comunitaria 2000;10:119–22.
19. Anonymous. Cisapride-aggressive behaviour. Bull Swed Adverse Drug React Advisory Comm 1991;57:1.
20. Baxter PS, Maddern GJ. Effect of cisapride on gastroduodenal reflux and gall bladder motility in patients with gallstones. Dig Surg 1998;15(1):35–41.
21. Poynard T, Vernisse B, Agostini H. Randomized, multicentre comparison of sodium alginate and cisapride in the symptomatic treatment of uncomplicated gastro-oesophageal reflux. Aliment Pharmacol Ther 1998; 12(2):159–65.
22. Denie C, Gohy P. Hépatite cytolytique attributable au cisapride. [Cytolytic hepatitis induced by cisapride.] Gastroenterol Clin Biol 1992;16(4):368–9.
23. Carone R, Vercelli D, Bertapelle P. Effects of cisapride on anorectal and vesicourethral function in spinal cord injured patients. Paraplegia 1993;31(2):125–7.
24. Wager E, Tooley PJ, Pearce GL, Wilton LV, Mann RD. A comparison of two cohort studies evaluating the safety of cisapride: Prescription-Event Monitoring and a large phase IV study. Eur J Clin Pharmacol 1997; 52(2):87–94.
25. Aronin SI, Peduzzi P, Quagliarello VJ. Community-acquired bacterial meningitis: risk stratification for adverse clinical outcome and effect of antibiotic timing. Ann Intern Med 1998;129(11):862–9.
26. Gilbert RE, Augood C, MacLennan S, Logan S. Cisapride treatment for gastro-oesophageal reflux in children: a systematic review of randomized controlled trials. J Paediatr Child Health 2000;36(6):524–9.
27. Kentrup H, Baisch HJ, Kusenbach G, Heimann G, Skopnik H. Effect of cisapride on acid gastro-oesophageal reflux during treatment with caffeine. Biol Neonate 2000;77(2):92–5.
28. Nurko S, Garcia-Aranda JA, Worona LB, Zlochisty O. Cisapride for the treatment of constipation in children: A double-blind study. J Pediatr 2000;136(1):35–40.
29. Costalos C, Gounaris A, Varhalama E, Kokori F, Alexiou N, Katsarakis I. Effect of low-dose cisapride on gastric emptying and QTc interval in preterm infants. Acta Paediatr 2000;89(12):1446–8.
30. Kirch W, Janisch HD, Ohnhaus EE, van Peer A. Cisapride-cimetidine interaction: enhanced cisapride bioavailability and accelerated cimetidine absorption. Ther Drug Monit 1989;11(4):411–14.

31. Kubler PA, Pillans PI, McKay JR. Possible interaction between cisapride and digoxin. Ann Pharmacother 2001;35(1):127–8.
32. Thomas AR, Chan LN, Bauman JL, Olopade CO. Prolongation of the QT interval related to cisapride-diltiazem interaction. Pharmacotherapy 1998;18(2):381–5.

Cisatracurium besilate

See also Neuromuscular blocking drugs

General Information

Cisatracurium is one of the ten isomers of atracurium. With an ED_{95} of 0.05 mg/kg it is about three times more potent than atracurium (1–3). The duration of action of cisatracurium tends to be slightly longer than that of atracurium. Less cisatracurium is required to achieve a given degree of neuromuscular blockade and so less laudanosine is produced.

Cisatracurium and atracurium share the same metabolic pathways, but Hofmann elimination may have a greater role in the elimination of cisatracurium than in atracurium (2,4–7). Spontaneous in vivo degradation accounts for 77% of total body clearance of cisatracurium (6). Organ clearance is 23% of total body clearance. Major metabolites of cisatracurium are laudanosine and a monoquaternary acrylate.

Clinical problems due to histamine release after bolus administration of cisatracurium have not been observed, even with very large doses up to 0.4 mg/kg (3,8), but in some patients there were considerable increases in plasma histamine concentrations (8–10).

Organs and Systems

Cardiovascular

With doses up to eight times the ED_{95} no cardiovascular adverse effects were observed (8) and in other studies cisatracurium had only minor cardiovascular adverse effects (9,11,12). Patients with coronary artery disease undergoing myocardial revascularization tolerated cisatracurium doses up to several fold the ED_{95} well; hemodynamic changes from pre- to postinjection were minimal (13,14).

Immunologic

Anaphylactic reactions have been reported (15–17).

Susceptibility Factors

Age

In line with its non-organ-dependent elimination pathways, neither the plasma clearance nor the duration of action of cisatracurium differed between young and elderly patients (18).

Renal disease

In patients with or without renal failure, there was no difference in the duration of action of cisatracurium (19).

Hepatic disease

In patients with hepatic failure neither the half-life nor the duration of action of cisatracurium was prolonged when compared with controls (20). In another study, however, the volume of distribution was increased and the plasma clearance reduced in patients with end-stage liver disease (21). Recovery times were not statistically different but the variability was greater in patients with liver disease (21).

Drug–Drug Interactions

General anesthetics

The action of cisatracurium is potentiated by isoflurane, sevoflurane, and enflurane (22).

References

1. Belmont MR, Lien CA, Quessy S, Abou-Donia MM, Abalos A, Eppich L, Savarese JJ. The clinical neuromuscular pharmacology of 51W89 in patients receiving nitrous oxide/opioid/barbiturate anesthesia. Anesthesiology 1995;82(5):1139–45.
2. Lien CA, Schmith VD, Belmont MR, Abalos A, Kisor DF, Savarese JJ. Pharmacokinetics of cisatracurium in patients receiving nitrous oxide/opioid/barbiturate anesthesia. Anesthesiology 1996;84(2):300–8.
3. Lepage JY, Malinovsky JM, Malinge M, Lechevalier T, Dupuch C, Cozian A, Pinaud M, Souron R. Pharmacodynamic dose-response and safety study of cisatracurium (51W89) in adult surgical patients during N_2O-O_2-opioid anesthesia. Anesth Analg 1996;83(4):823–9.
4. Welch RM, Brown A, Ravitch J, Dahl R. The in vitro degradation of cisatracurium, the R, cis-R′-isomer of atracurium, in human and rat plasma. Clin Pharmacol Ther 1995;58(2):132–42.
5. Fisher DM, Canfell PC, Fahey MR, Rosen JI, Rupp SM, Sheiner LB, Miller RD. Elimination of atracurium in humans: contribution of Hofmann elimination and ester hydrolysis versus organ-based elimination. Anesthesiology 1986;65(1):6–12.
6. Kisor DF, Schmith VD, Wargin WA, Lien CA, Ornstein E, Cook DR. Importance of the organ-independent elimination of cisatracurium. Anesth Analg 1996; 83(5):1065–71.
7. Tsui D, Graham GG, Torda TA. The pharmacokinetics of atracurium isomers in vitro and in humans. Anesthesiology 1987;67(5):722–8.
8. Lien CA, Belmont MR, Abalos A, Eppich L, Quessy S, Abou-Donia MM, Savarese JJ. The cardiovascular effects and histamine-releasing properties of 51W89 in patients receiving nitrous oxide/opioid/barbiturate anesthesia. Anesthesiology 1995;82(5):1131–8.
9. Doenicke A, Soukup J, Hoernecke R, Moss J. The lack of histamine release with cisatracurium: a double-blind comparison with vecuronium. Anesth Analg 1997; 84(3):623–8.
10. Doenicke AW, Czeslick E, Moss J, Hoernecke R. Onset time, endotracheal intubating conditions, and plasma

histamine after cisatracurium and vecuronium administration. Anesth Analg 1998;87(2):434–8.
11. Schramm WM, Jesenko R, Bartunek A, Gilly H. Effects of cisatracurium on cerebral and cardiovascular hemodynamics in patients with severe brain injury. Acta Anaesthesiol Scand 1997;41(10):1319–23.
12. Schramm WM, Papousek A, Michalek-Sauberer A, Czech T, Illievich U. The cerebral and cardiovascular effects of cisatracurium and atracurium in neurosurgical patients. Anesth Analg 1998;86(1):123–7.
13. Reich DL, Mulier J, Viby-Mogensen J, Konstadt SN, van Aken HK, Jensen FS, DePerio M, Buckley SG. Comparison of the cardiovascular effects of cisatracurium and vecuronium in patients with coronary artery disease. Can J Anaesth 1998;45(8):794–7.
14. Searle NR, Thomson I, Dupont C, Cannon JE, Roy M, Rosenbloom M, Gagnon L, Carrier M. A two-center study evaluating the hemodynamic and pharmacodynamic effects of cisatracurium and vecuronium in patients undergoing coronary artery bypass surgery. J Cardiothorac Vasc Anesth 1999;13(1):20–5.
15. Clendenen SR, Harper JV, Wharen RE Jr, Guarderas JC. Anaphylactic reaction after cisatracurium. Anesthesiology 1997;87(3):690–2.
16. Toh KW, Deacock SJ, Fawcett WJ. Severe anaphylactic reaction to cisatracurium. Anesth Analg 1999;88(2):462–4.
17. Iannuzzi E, Iannuzzi M, Pedicini MS, Cirillo V, Chiefari M, Sacerdoti G. Anaphylactic reaction after cisatracurium administration. Eur J Anaesthesiol 2002;19(9):691–3.
18. Sorooshian SS, Stafford MA, Eastwood NB, Boyd AH, Hull CJ, Wright PM. Pharmacokinetics and pharmacodynamics of cisatracurium in young and elderly adult patients. Anesthesiology 1996;84(5):1083–91.
19. Boyd AH, Eastwood NB, Parker CJ, Hunter JM. Pharmacodynamics of the 1R cis-1′R cis isomer of atracurium (51W89) in health and chronic renal failure. Br J Anaesth 1995;74(4):400–4.
20. Tullock W, Scott V, Smith DA, Phillips L, Cook DR. Kinetics/dynamics of 51W89 in liver transplant patients and in healthy patients. Anesthesiology 1994;81:A1076.
21. De Wolf AM, Freeman JA, Scott VL, Tullock W, Smith DA, Kisor DF, Kerls S, Cook DR. Pharmacokinetics and pharmacodynamics of cisatracurium in patients with end-stage liver disease undergoing liver transplantation. Br J Anaesth 1996;76(5):624–8.
22. Wulf H, Kahl M, Ledowski T. Augmentation of the neuromuscular blocking effects of cisatracurium during desflurane, sevoflurane, isoflurane or total i.v. anaesthesia. Br J Anaesth 1998;80(3):308–12.

Citalopram and escitalopram

See also Selective serotonin re-uptake inhibitors (SSRIs)

General Information

Citalopram is a racemic bicyclic phthalane derivative and is a highly selective serotonin re-uptake inhibitor with minimal effects on noradrenaline and dopamine neuronal reuptake. Inhibition of 5-HT re-uptake by citalopram is primarily due to the *S*-enantiomer (escitalopram). Its most frequent adverse events (nausea, somnolence, dry mouth, increased sweating) are mainly transient and mostly mild to moderate (1).

The single and multiple-dose pharmacokinetics of citalopram are linear and dose-proportional in the range 10–60 mg/day. Citalopram is metabolized to demethylcitalopram, didemethylcitalopram, citalopram-N-oxide, and a deaminated propionic acid derivative. Citalopram has a mean half-life of about 35 hours (2). Racemic citalopram is several times more potent than its metabolites in inhibiting serotonin reuptake (3).

In a systematic review of clinical trials the therapeutic efficacy of citalopram was significantly greater than that of placebo and comparable with that of other antidepressants (4).

Escitalopram oxalate is the *S*-enantiomer of citalopram (5). The therapeutic activity of citalopram resides in the *S*-isomer and escitalopram binds with high affinity to the human serotonin transporter; *R*-citalopram is about 30-fold less potent. The half-life of escitalopram is 27–32 hours. Citalopram and escitalopram have negligible effects on CYP isozymes.

Escitalopram was efficacious in patients with major depressive disorder in short-term, placebo-controlled trials, three of which included citalopram as an active control, and in a 36-week study in the prevention of relapse in depression (5). It has also been used to treat generalized anxiety disorder, panic disorder, and social anxiety disorder. Results also suggest that, at comparable doses, escitalopram demonstrates clinically relevant and statistically significant superiority to placebo treatment earlier than citalopram. The most common adverse events associated with escitalopram include nausea, insomnia, disorders of ejaculation, diarrhea, dry mouth, and somnolence. Only nausea occurred in more than 10% of patients taking escitalopram.

A meta-analysis of 20 short-term studies of five SSRIs (citalopram, fluoxetine, fluvoxamine, paroxetine, and sertraline) has been published (6). There were no overall differences in efficacy, but fluoxetine had a slower onset of action. Citalopram and sertraline were least likely to cause drug interactions, but citalopram was implicated more often in fatal overdoses.

Organs and Systems

Cardiovascular

There has been some concern about the cardiovascular safety of citalopram, mainly because of animal studies showing effects on cardiac conduction. These most commonly occur in large overdoses, in which a variety of cardiac abnormalities, including QT_c prolongation, have been noted. However, this can occur with therapeutic doses too.

- Bradycardia (34/minute) with a prolonged QT_c interval of 463 ms occurred in a patient taking citalopram 40 mg/day (7). The bradycardia resolved when citalopram was withdrawn. The patient also had alcohol dependence and evidence of cardiomyopathy; presumably this may have potentiated the effect of citalopram on cardiac conduction.
- A 21-year-old woman developed QT_c prolongation (457 ms) after taking a fairly modest overdose (400 mg) of citalopram (usual daily dose 20–60 mg) (8). The QT_c prolongation resolved uneventfully over the next 30 hours.

This suggests that even modest overdoses of citalopram can cause QT_c prolongation and that cardiac monitoring should be considered. Based on the pharmacokinetic profile of citalopram and the temporal pattern of QT_c change, the authors suggested that the effect of citalopram on the QT_c interval was mediated by one of its metabolites, dimethylcitalopram.

Prolongation of the QT_c interval has been reported in five patients who made non-fatal suicide attempts by taking large amounts of citalopram. Their electrocardiograms showed other conduction disorders, including sinus tachycardia and inferolateral repolarization disturbances (SEDA-21, 12).

Nervous system

SSRIs can infrequently cause extrapyramidal movement disorders and can also worsen established Parkinson's disease (SEDA-22, 23) and another case has been reported (9).

- A 68-year-old woman developed major depression. A neurological assessment excluded neurological diseases, including Parkinson's disease. After treatment with citalopram, 20 mg/day for 7 days, she developed severe parkinsonism, with rigidity, tremor, and bradykinesia, and became unable to walk. The citalopram was withdrawn after a further week and nortriptyline was substituted; however, 10 days later parkinsonism was still present. Her symptoms eventually responded to cobeneldopa.

The authors concluded that the citalopram had probably precipitated latent Parkinson's disease. Citalopram is the most highly selective SSRI and, in anecdotal accounts, has been implicated somewhat less often than other SSRIs in extrapyramidal movement disorders. However, this case, together with another report of citalopram-induced worsening of pre-existing Parkinson's disease (10), suggests that it should be used with caution in patients with this disorder.

Psychological, psychiatric

Mania has been reported in six patients, five of whom were taking citalopram and one paroxetine (SEDA-22, 12).

Electrolyte balance

Hyponatremia can sometimes cause severe disturbances of consciousness.

- A 47-year-old woman with multiple sclerosis took citalopram 20 mg/day for 4 weeks and was found unconscious in her apartment (11). The main finding was a low plasma sodium (108 mmol/l). As a result of prolonged coma, she had rhabdomyolysis and required intubation for 3 days as well as sodium replacement therapy. She eventually made a full recovery.

It is possible in this case that the underlying demyelinating disease may have made the patient more susceptible to the sodium-lowering effects of the SSRI.

- A 45-year-old woman developed hyponatremia complicated by rhabdomyolysis while taking citalopram and the antipsychotic drug chlorprothixene for depressive psychosis (12). The hyponatremia became apparent 2 weeks after the dose of citalopram was increased to 40 mg/day, when she complained of weakness and lethargy.

SSRI-induced hyponatremia is unusual in non-geriatric populations, but the chlorprothixene may have played a role in this case.

Gastrointestinal

Gastrointestinal adverse effects are one of the major disadvantages of SSRIs. The most common is nausea, and the incidence is said to be 20% or more for citalopram (13,14).

Sexual function

Citalopram has a relatively modest effect in delaying ejaculation (15).

Sexual disinhibition has been reported in five patients, four of whom were taking citalopram; they had an unusual increase in sexual interest, with preoccupation with sexual thoughts, promiscuity, and excessive interest in pornography (16). In some of the cases symptoms such as diminished need for sleep suggested the possibility of a manic syndrome.

Long-Term Effects

Drug withdrawal

Reports of withdrawal symptoms after citalopram withdrawal are rare, but it is uncertain whether this reflects a truly lower propensity to cause withdrawal symptoms.

- A 30-year-old man with a history of major depression and panic disorder had been in remission for a year with citalopram 20 mg/day, valproate 600 mg/day, and alprazolam 3 mg/day (17). The citalopram was tapered over 3 weeks to 5 mg/day and then withdrawn. The day after the last dose he experienced anxiety and irritability together with frequent short-lasting bursts of dizziness, not having had the latter previously panic and depression did not recur and after a week the symptoms resolved spontaneously.
- A 45-year-old woman achieved remission from an episode of major depression within 2 weeks of taking citalopram (40 mg/day). After about 3 months of treatment she missed her daily dose of citalopram, and 3 hours later had a sudden episode of dizziness while driving. A similar episode occurred 2 weeks later again after a missed dose of citalopram. The dizziness remitted about 1 hour after the citalopram was taken.

These symptoms, particularly dizziness, are characteristic of SSRI withdrawal, and suggest that citalopram, like other SSRIs, can cause a withdrawal syndrome in some patients, despite slow tapering of the dose.

Withdrawal symptoms in the 2 weeks after sudden discontinuation of citalopram have been examined in a double-blind, placebo-controlled study (18). Withdrawal symptoms were overall mild, but neurological and psychiatric disturbances were 2–3 times as common in patients randomized to placebo than in those randomized to continue with citalopram. The authors pointed out that withdrawal symptoms were particularly common in patients who were randomized to placebo who also had depressive relapses. This shows the difficulty of disentangling the effects of depressive relapse from those of pure treatment withdrawal. However, it is also possible that acute withdrawal of medication induces an abnormal neurobiological state, in which both depression and abstinence symptoms are more likely to occur. It would be wise to warn patients about the possible effects of missing doses of the shorter-acting SSRIs.

Second-Generation Effects

Lactation

Citalopram has been reported to cause sleep disturbance in a breast-fed infant (19).

- A 29-year-old woman took citalopram (40 mg/day) while breast feeding her 5-week-old daughter. The maternal citalopram concentrations were 99 ng/ml in the serum and 205 ng/ml in the breast milk. The serum concentration in the infant was 13 ng/ml, and the child's sleep was fitful and disturbed. The dosage of citalopram was reduced to 20 mg/day and the two feeds after each daily dose were replaced by artificial nutrition. One week later the infant was sleeping normally, and the serum citalopram concentrations in mother and infant had fallen to 35 ng/ml and 2 ng/ml, respectively.

These data suggest that although breast feeding during citalopram treatment is possible, careful dosing and close observation of mother and infant are necessary.

Drug Administration

Drug overdose

Six deaths have been reported after overdosage of citalopram. Although five of the six had also taken other substances, these were not thought to have contributed significantly (SEDA-20, 8). Of five patients who made non-fatal suicide attempts by taking large amounts of citalopram (up to 5200 mg), four developed generalized seizures and all had prolonged QT_c intervals. Other conduction disorders included sinus tachycardia and inferolateral repolarization disturbances. Two patients developed rhabdomyolysis and one hypokalemia. These data suggest that citalopram overdose can cause seizures and disturbances of cardiac conduction that might predispose to fatal dysrhythmias (SEDA-21, 12) (20,21).

In another case prolonged sinus bradycardia occurred (22).

- A 32-year-old woman took 800 mg of citalopram, 20 times her usual daily dose, in a suicide attempt. On admission to hospital she had a sinus bradycardia (41/minute) but the electrocardiogram was otherwise normal, with a QT interval of 430 ms. Treatment with atropine failed to increase her heart rate and she had hypotension and syncope. A temporary pacemaker was inserted and was required for the next 6 days before it could be safely removed.

There are concerns that citalopram may be less safe in acute overdose than other SSRIs (SEDA-21, 12). Among all fatal poisonings in one forensic district of Sweden, citalopram was the fourth most commonly used drug (22 of 358 cases) (23). However, when correction was made for prescription rate, citalopram was less toxic than amitriptyline, dextropropoxyphene, or nitrazepam. This study has confirmed that citalopram is less toxic than tricyclic antidepressants such as amitriptyline. However, whether it is more toxic than other SSRIs is still uncertain.

Drug–Drug Interactions

General

Of all the SSRIs citalopram has the least inhibitory effect on cytochrome P450 enzymes and has not been associated with clinically significant interactions with other CNS drugs.

It has been used successfully in combination with the tricyclic antidepressant desipramine in a 45-year-old woman who had previously suffered tricyclic toxicity when desipramine had been combined with paroxetine (24).

Acenocoumarol

When a drug has a relatively narrow therapeutic index, such as acenocoumarol, pharmacokinetic interactions can have serious clinical consequences.

- A 63-year-old woman taking acenocoumarol 18 mg/week (INR 1.8) started to take citalopram 20 mg/day and 10 days later noted spontaneous bleeding from her gums; the INR had risen to more than 15 (25). She was treated with two units of whole blood and the citalopram was withdrawn. Five days later the INR had returned to the target range.

Citalopram is said to be less likely than other SSRIs to cause drug interactions, because it is a relatively weak inhibitor of CYP isozymes. However, even slight inhibition may have produced serious consequences in this case.

Clozapine

The effect of citalopram on plasma concentrations of clozapine have been prospectively studied in 15 patients with schizophrenia taking clozapine 200–400 mg/day (26). The addition of citalopram 40 mg/day did not alter plasma clozapine concentrations.

However, in a 39-year-old man with a schizoaffective disorder, citalopram 40 mg/day appeared to increase plasma clozapine concentrations and increased adverse effects (27). The adverse effects settled within 2 weeks of a reduction in citalopram dosage to 20 mg/day, with a corresponding 25% fall in clozapine concentrations. It is possible that at higher doses, citalopram can increase clozapine concentrations, perhaps through inhibition of CYP1A2 or CYP3A4.

Digoxin

Citalopram 40 mg/day for 4 weeks did not alter the pharmacokinetics of digoxin 1 mg orally (28). Digoxin is not a CYP substrate, so an interaction with SSRIs is unlikely, but the authors cited a report that fluoxetine increased plasma digoxin concentrations (29).

Risperidone

The effect of citalopram on plasma concentrations of risperidone has been prospectively studied in 15 patients with schizophrenia (26). The addition of citalopram did not alter plasma risperidone concentrations.

References

1. Nemeroff CB. Overview of the safety of citalopram. Psychopharmacol Bull 2003;37(1):96–121.
2. Kragh-Sorensen P, Overo KF, Petersen OL, Jensen K, Parnas W. The kinetics of citalopram: single and multiple dose studies in man. Acta Pharmacol Toxicol (Copenh) 1981;48(1):53–60.
3. Sanchez C, Hyttel J. Comparison of the effects of antidepressants and their metabolites on reuptake of biogenic amines and on receptor binding. Cell Mol Neurobiol 1999;19(4):467–89.
4. Parker NG, Brown CS. Citalopram in the treatment of depression. Ann Pharmacother 2000;34(6):761–71.
5. Burke WJ. Escitalopram. Expert Opin Invest Drugs 2002;11(10):1477–86.
6. Edwards JG, Anderson I. Systematic review and guide to selection of selective serotonin reuptake inhibitors. Drugs 1999;57(4):507–33.
7. Favre MP, Sztajzel J, Bertschy G. Bradycardia during citalopram treatment: a case report. Pharmacol Res 1999;39(2):149–50.
8. Catalano G, Catalano MC, Epstein MA, Tsambiras PE. QTc interval prolongation associated with citalopram overdose: a case report literature review. Clin Neuropharmacol 2001;24(3):158–62.
9. Stadtland C, Erfurth A, Arolt V. De novo onset of Parkinson's disease after antidepressant treatment with citalopram. Pharmacopsychiatry 2000;33(5):194–5.
10. Linazasoro G. Worsening of Parkinson's disease by citalopram. Parkinsonism Relat Disord 2000;6(2):111–13.
11. Hull M, Kottlors M, Braune S. Prolonged coma caused by low sodium and hypo-osmolarity during treatment with citalopram. J Clin Psychopharmacol 2002; 22(3):337–8.
12. Zullino D, Brauchli S, Horvath A, Baumann P. Inappropriate antidiuretic hormone secretion and rhabdomyolysis associated with citalopram. Thérapie 2000;55(5):651–2.
13. Dencker SJ, Hopfner Petersen HE. Side effect profile of citalopram and reference antidepressants in depression. In: Montgomery SA, editor. Citalopram: The New Antidepressant from Lundbeck Research. Amsterdam: Excerpta Medica, 1989:31.
14. Shaw DM, Crimmins R. A multicenter trial of citalopram and amitriptyline in major depressive illness. In: Montgomery SA, editor. Citalopram: The New Antidepressant from Lundbeck research. Amsterdam: Excerpta Medica, 1989:43–9.
15. Waldinger MD, Olivier B, Nafziger AN, Bertino JS Jr. Goss-Bley AI, Kashuba ADM. Sexual dysfunction and fluvoxamine therapy. J Clin Psychiatry 2001;62(2):126–7.
16. Greil W, Horvath A, Sassim N, Erazo N, Grohmann R. Disinhibition of libido: an adverse effect of SSRI? J Affect Disord 2001;62(3):225–8.
17. Benazzi F. Citalopram withdrawal symptoms. Eur Psychiatry 1998;13:219.
18. Markowitz JS, DeVane CL, Liston HL, Montgomery SA. An assessment of selective serotonin reuptake inhibitor discontinuation symptoms with citalopram. Int Clin Psychopharmacol 2000;15(6):329–33.
19. Schmidt K, Olesen OV, Jensen PN. Citalopram and breast-feeding: serum concentration and side effects in the infant. Biol Psychiatry 2000;47(2):164–5.
20. Personne M, Persson H, Sjoberg E. Citalopram toxicity. Lancet 1997;350(9076):518–19.
21. Power A. Drug treatment of depression. Citalopram in overdose may result in serious morbidity and death. BMJ 1998;316(7127):307–8.
22. Rothenhausler HB, Hoberl C, Ehrentrout S, Kapfhammer HP, Weber MM. Suicide attempt by pure citalopram overdose causing long-lasting severe sinus bradycardia, hypotension and syncopes: successful therapy with a temporary pacemaker. Pharmacopsychiatry 2000;33(4):150–2.
23. Jonasson B, Saldeen T. Citalopram in fatal poisoning cases. Forensic Sci Int 2002;126(1):1–6.
24. Ashton AK. Lack of desipramine toxicity with citalopram. J Clin Psychiatry 2000;61(2):144.
25. Borras-Blasco J, Marco-Garbayo JL, Bosca-Sanleon B, Navarro-Ruiz A. Probable interaction between citalopram and acenocoumarol. Ann Pharmacother 2002;36(2):345.
26. Avenoso A, Facciola G, Scordo MG, Gitto C, Ferrante GD. No effect of citalopram on plasma levels of clozapine, risperidone and their active metabolites in patients with chronic schizophrenia. Clin Drug Invest 1998;16:393–8.
27. Borba CP, Henderson DC. Citalopram and clozapine: potential drug interaction. J Clin Psychiatry 2000;61(4):301–2.
28. Larsen F, Priskorn M, Overo KF. Lack of citalopram effect on oral digoxin pharmacokinetics. J Clin Pharmacol 2001;41(3):340–6.
29. Leibovitz A, Bilchinsky T, Gil I, Habot B. Elevated serum digoxin level associated with coadministered fluoxetine. Arch Intern Med 1998;158(10):1152–3.

Citric acid and citrates

General Information

Citric acid is used in effervescing mixtures and granules. Formulations that contain citric acid are used in the management of dry mouth and to dissolve renal calculi, alkalinize the urine, and prevent encrustation of urinary catheters. Citric acid is also an ingredient of citrated anticoagulant solutions.

Uses

Urinary calculi

Treatment of complex and large urinary calculi secondary to infection can be difficult, and complete removal of the stone may not always be possible. Residual stone fragment rates are 37% (range 10–57%) after percutaneous nephrolithotomy and 20% after anatrophic nephrolithotomy (1). Technical advances in the management of urinary calculi have resulted in improved stone clearance rates in these cases. Owing to a combination of factors, such as large stone mass, associated infection, abnormal renal anatomy, and poor general health of the patient, infection stones can still pose a difficult treatment problem. This has resulted in the use of alternative (and minimally invasive) treatment options. Dissolution treatment, either alone or as adjuvant therapy, has been used. Citric acid, in various concentrations, has been used in dissolution treatment (2). Citric acid, being a urinary acidifier, inhibits the formation of precipitates of calcium phosphate, calcium carbonate, and magnesium ammonium phosphate, and allows dissolution of stones. It may also help to reduce the size of calculi, allowing spontaneous elimination.

Citric acid has been used to treat 22 patients (10 men and 12 women, mean age 45, range 15–60 years; 23 affected kidneys) with kidney stones (14 staghorn calculi, four partial staghorn calculi, and five large-burden calculi) (3). They underwent irrigation with solution R (citric acid monohydrate 6 g, magnesium carbonate 2.8 g, glucolactone 0.6 g, and water 100 ml) following debulking of the stone with percutaneous nephrolithotomy ($n = 20$), ureteroscopy, and shock wave lithotripsy ($n = 2$) combined with open procedures ($n = 4$). Irrigation was performed through a nephrostomy tube ($n = 20$) or in a retrograde fashion ($n = 3$) using a closed infusion pump system (40 ml/hour). The response to treatment was checked using a nephrostogram and/or plain X-ray. In six kidneys irrigation had to be abandoned because of loin pain, leak, or sepsis after an average duration of 2 (1–5) days. The average duration of irrigation was 6 (1–20) days. At the end of irrigation, four kidneys had complete radiographic clearance, and the stone was reduced to calyceal dust in three. There was a partial response in 11 and no response in five. Following alternative interventions in six cases (four with a partial response and two with no response), further clearance was achieved in three and calyceal dust in three. The response was better if the stone was reduced to less than 10 mm before irrigation. At the mean follow-up of 2.4 (1–4) years, of 13 kidneys with stone clearance or calyceal dust, nine suffered recurrence or re-growth, five of which required further interventions. Only four of the 23 kidneys remained stone-free.

In patients with complex stone disease, adjuvant solution R irrigation can reduce the stone burden, although the overall success rate is limited. However, there is a considerable potential for adverse effects, necessitating close monitoring for sepsis and electrolyte abnormalities.

Anticoagulation

In 2000 the FDA issued an urgent warning to all hospital pharmacies and hemodialysis units that triCitrasol, an unapproved formulation of sodium citrate that has been used as an anticoagulant to keep intravascular lines open, can cause death after intravenous infusion. triCitrasol is marketed in individual sterile 30 ml glass vials, distributed both individually and in hemodialysis kits (4). A patient died of cardiac arrest shortly after the injection of triCitrasol 46.7% into a permanent hemodialysis blood access catheter that had just been implanted. Rapid or excessive infusion of citrate solutions can cause fatal cardiac dysrhythmias, seizures, or bleeding due to sequestration of blood calcium.

triCitrasol is manufactured by Cytosol Laboratories, and is distributed by Medcomp (previously by Citra Anticoagulants, Inc). Both Cytosol Labs and Medcomp have voluntarily recalled triCitrasol for use with blood access catheters. On 9 April 2000, Medcomp announced in a letter to its customers that it was recalling its kits (or trays) containing triCitrasol and the Medcomp Ash Split Catheter II for hemodialysis or apheresis, a blood separation and re-transfusion process. About 3000 Medcomp catheter kits with triCitrasol were distributed nationwide. They were also distributed in Puerto Rico and Canada.

The FDA urged hospital pharmacies and hemodialysis units across the USA to stop using the product. Alternative 4% solutions of citrate are available for use in these and most other medical settings.

Organs and Systems

Cardiovascular

Citric acid toxicity has been reported previously, but only after intravenous administration. It was originally seen with massive transfusion of blood products with citrate as the anticoagulant. Two case reports have described accidental intravenous administration of citrate or citric acid; at a maximum serum concentration of citrate (4.1 mmol/l) there were profound alterations in blood pressure and QT interval; these were reversed by calcium infusion (5).

Metabolism

Although there is a long list of causes of metabolic acidosis with an increased anion gap (6,7), clinical clues can help diagnosis. A case report has illustrated the acute metabolic and hemodynamic effects of ingestion of a massive load of oral citric acid. The principal findings included a metabolic acidosis accompanied by an increase in the plasma anion gap, not due to lactic acidosis, hyperkalemia, and the abrupt onset of hypotension (8).

- A 42-year-old previously healthy male prisoner drank a large volume of a commercial solution of unknown composition. His medical history was non-contributory, except for severe epigastric pain. Within an hour, his condition deteriorated; he was ashen, his blood pressure was 80/40 mmHg, and his pulse rate was 102/minute. His neck vessels were flat and his breath sounds were equal bilaterally, with occasional expiratory wheezes at both bases. There were no cardiac murmurs. The abdomen was soft and the bowel sounds were active. His extremities were warm with no cyanosis or edema. There were no neurological abnormalities. Fortuitously, because of therapy to avoid cardiac complications of hyperkalemia, he was given 1 g of calcium chloride, 50 mmol of sodium bicarbonate, 25 g of glucose, and 10 units of regular insulin intravenously. His blood pressure immediately increased to 116/76 mmHg and his pulse rate fell to 90/minute. By the next morning his plasma acid–base balance was normal, as was his ionized calcium concentration (1.1 mmol/l).

Because of the short duration and severity of the metabolic acidosis, together with a near-normal lactate concentration, acid ingestion was the most likely cause for his acid–base disorder. This diagnosis was confirmed once the composition of the ingested fluid was known.

References

1. Segura JW, Preminger GM, Assimos DG. Nephrolithiasis Clinical Guidelines Panel. Report on the Management of Staghorn Calculi. Baltimore: American Urological Association, 1994.

2. Wang LP, Wong HY, Griffith DP. Treatment options in struvite stones. Urol Clin North Am 1997;24(1):149–62.
3. Joshi HB, Kumar PV, Timoney AG. Citric acid (solution R) irrigation in the treatment of refractory infection (struvite) stone disease: is it useful? Eur Urol 2001;39(5):586–90.
4. Anonymous. Sodium citrate (triCitrasol). Warning: cardiac arrest. WHO Newslett 2000;2:6.
5. Bunker JP, Bendixen HH, Murphy AJ. Hemodynamic effects of intravenously administered sodium citrate. Nord Hyg Tidskr 1962;266:372–7.
6. Emmett M, Narins RG. Clinical use of the anion gap. Medicine (Baltimore) 1977;56(1):38–54.
7. Oh MS, Carroll HJ. The anion gap. N Engl J Med 1977;297(15):814–17.
8. DeMars CS, Hollister K, Tomassoni A, Himmelfarb J, Halperin ML. Citric acid ingestion: a life-threatening cause of metabolic acidosis. Ann Emerg Med 2001;38(5):588–91.

Clarithromycin

See also Macrolide antibiotics

General Information

Clarithromycin is a commonly used macrolide antibiotic and is a regular part of regimens for the eradication of *Helicobacter pylori*, often in combination with a nitroimidazole antibiotic as well, in addition to a proton pump inhibitor. Variable rates of adverse events (4–30%) have been reported with clarithromycin.

Comparative studies

In a double-blind, multicenter trial in 328 patients with *H. pylori* infection and non-ulcer dyspepsia, omeprazole 20 mg bd, amoxicillin 1 g bd, and clarithromycin 500 mg bd were compared with omeprazole alone. The rate of success and quality of life were similar in both groups. There were no serious adverse events. However, there were 12 withdrawals in the group given omeprazole and antibiotics and two in the group given omeprazole alone. Diarrhea occurred in 63 patients in those given omeprazole and antibiotics and in ten patients given omeprazole alone (1). In another double-blind, placebo-controlled trial eradication of *H. pylori* (omeprazole 20 mg, amoxicillin 1 g, and clarithromycin 500 mg bd) in long-term users of NSAIDs with past or current peptic ulcer or troublesome dyspepsia led to impaired healing of gastric ulcers and did not affect the rate of peptic ulcers or dyspepsia over 6 months (2).

Beta-lactam antibiotics

In a multicenter, double-blind, randomized comparison of cefprozil, 500 mg bd for 5 days and clarithromycin 500 mg bd for 10 days in 295 subjects with an acute exacerbation of chronic bronchitis, the most common adverse effects of clarithromycin were nausea (8%), diarrhea (12%), taste disturbance (8%), and dry mouth (5%) (3).

Clarithromycin (250 mg bd for 10 days) was as effective as cefuroxime axetil (250 mg bd for 10 days) in the treatment of acute maxillary sinusitis in a randomized, double-blind, multicenter study in 370 patients; 10% of patients in each group had adverse events (4).

Other macrolides

The incidence of disseminated *Mycobacterium avium* complex (MAC) infection has increased dramatically with the AIDS epidemic. Treatment regimens for patients with a positive culture for MAC from a sterile site should include two or more drugs, including clarithromycin. Prophylaxis against disseminated MAC should be considered for patients with a CD4 cell count of less than 50 x 10^6/l (5). In a randomized, open trial in 37 patients with HIV-associated disseminated MAC infection, treatment with clarithromycin + ethambutol produced more rapid resolution of bacteremia, and was more effective at sterilization of blood cultures after 16 weeks than azithromycin + ethambutol (6).

In a direct comparison of clarithromycin with erythromycin stearate, the rate of adverse events was 19% in 96 patients taking clarithromycin and 35% in 112 patients taking erythromycin (7). Most of the adverse events associated with clarithromycin affect the gastrointestinal tract (7%).

In a prospective, single-blind, randomized study of a 7-day course of clarithromycin (7.5 mg/kg bd) and a 14-day course of erythromycin (13.3 mg/kg tds) in 153 children with pertussis, the incidence of treatment-emergent drug-related adverse events was significantly higher with erythromycin than with clarithromycin (62 versus 45%) (8). Three subjects given erythromycin withdrew prematurely because of adverse events: one because of a rash; one with vomiting and diarrhea; and one with vomiting, abdominal pain, and rash.

Quinolones

In a multicenter, double-blind, randomized comparison of trovafloxacin 200 mg and clarithromycin 500 mg bd in 176 subjects with acute exacerbations of chronic bronchitis, the most common adverse effects of clarithromycin were nausea (3%), diarrhea (4%), and taste disturbances (4%) (9).

Tetracyclines

Clarithromycin (0.75–2 g/day), minocycline (200 mg/day), and clofazimine (100 mg/day) for 15 months were investigated as treatment of MAC lung disease in 30 HIV-negative patients. Eight patients did not complete the study owing to deviations from protocol or adverse effects. Persistently negative cultures were found in 14 of the other patients. There were three cases of hepatic disturbances and three of ototoxicity, which required a reduction in clarithromycin dosage after a short interruption of treatment (10).

Organs and Systems

Cardiovascular

- QT interval prolongation and a ventricular dysrhythmia occurred in an HIV-positive 30-year-old man at the start of intravenous clarithromycin therapy 500 mg 12-hourly (11).

Intravenous clarithromycin caused thrombophlebitis in four patients when it was given inappropriately as a rapid bolus injection instead of a short infusion; the manufacturers have received other reports of similar reactions, even with infusions, but the incidence seems to be considerably lower than with erythromycin (12). In a prospective, non-randomized study, phlebitis occurred in 15 of 19 patients treated with intravenous erythromycin (incidence rate of 0.40 episodes/patient-day) and in 19 of 25 patients treated with intravenous clarithromycin (0.35 episodes/patient-day) (13).

Respiratory

Bronchospasm with clarithromycin occurred in a 44-year-old woman who had no history of respiratory allergies but had had adverse drug reactions to general and regional anesthetics and to ceftriaxone (14). After the administration of a quarter of the therapeutic dose the patient had dyspnea, cough, and bronchospasm throughout the lung.

Nervous system

Adverse events on the nervous system due to clarithromycin have been observed in 3% of patients.

- Progressive loss of strength and difficulty in swallowing and eye opening after the first dose of clarithromycin (2 g/day) occurred in a patient with cerebral toxoplasmosis and AIDS (15). This myasthenic syndrome resolved within 6 hours of withdrawal of clarithromycin and administration of pyridostigmine.

The authors postulated that this adverse effect may have been the consequence of neuromuscular blockade, through inhibition of the presynaptic release of acetylcholine.

Sensory systems

Eyes

Topical clarithromycin can cause self-resolving corneal deposits (16).

Ears

- Ototoxicity was attributed to clarithromycin in a 76-year-old man 4 days after he started to take clarithromycin for atypical pulmonary tuberculosis (17). When the clarithromycin was withdrawn his hearing improved subjectively, but it worsened again on re-exposure.

Taste

Abnormal taste developed in 17 of 175 patients treated with clarithromycin 250 mg bd for 10 days for community-acquired pneumonia, compared with 3 of 167 patients treated with sparfloxacin (18). Mild to moderate gastrointestinal disturbances were the most common adverse events and were reported in 13 and 11% respectively.

Psychological, psychiatric

Two patients, a man aged 74 and a woman aged 56 years, developed delirium after taking clarithromycin (19).

Two patients (aged 21 and 33 years) with late-stage AIDS had acute psychoses shortly after taking clarithromycin (2 g/day) for MAC bacteremia (20). In both cases the psychosis resolved on withdrawal but recurred on rechallenge. In one case treatment with azithromycin was well tolerated.

Of cases of mania attributed to antibiotics and reported to the WHO, 28% were due to clarithromycin (21).

- A 77-year-old man who was HIV-negative developed mania after 6 days treatment with clarithromycin 1 g/day for a soft tissue infection; his mental state resolved on withdrawal (22).
- A 53-year-old Canadian lawyer taking long-term fluoxetine and nitrazepam developed a frank psychosis 1–3 days after starting to take clarithromycin 500 mg/day for a chest infection (23). His symptoms resolved on withdrawal of all three drugs, and did not recur with erythromycin or when fluoxetine and nitrazepam were restarted in the absence of antibiotics.

The symptoms may have been due to a direct effect of clarithromycin or else inhibition of hepatic cytochrome P450 metabolism, leading to fluoxetine toxicity.

Clarithromycin occasionally causes hallucinations.

- Visual hallucinations with marked anxiety and nervousness occurred after the second dose of oral clarithromycin 500 mg in a 32-year-old woman (24). Clarithromycin was withdrawn and the symptoms disappeared a few hours later.
- Visual hallucinations developed in a 56-year-old man with chronic renal insufficiency and underlying aluminium intoxication maintained on peritoneal dialysis 24 hours after he started to take clarithromycin 500 mg bd for a chest infection, and resolved completely 3 days after withdrawal (25).

Hematologic

- Thrombotic thrombocytopenic purpura was reported in a 42-year-old man with no past medical history after he had just completed a 30-day course of clarithromycin 250 mg bd (26).

Gastrointestinal

Erythromycin acts as a motilin receptor agonist (27–29). This mechanism may be at least partly responsible for the gastrointestinal adverse effects of macrolides. Clarithromycin may act on gastrointestinal motility in a similar way. In dogs, clarithromycin caused contractions and discomfort, as did erythromycin (30). In healthy volunteers, oral clarithromycin 250 mg bd caused a statistically significant increase in the number of postprandial antral contractions and antral motility (31). A single oral dose of clarithromycin 3000 mg resulted in severe abdominal pain within 1 hour of administration in two patients (32).

Based on observations made in dogs and rabbits, clarithromycin is significantly less potent than azithromycin and erythromycin as an agonist for stimulation of smooth muscle contraction (33). Therefore, a lower rate of gastrointestinal adverse events would be expected with clarithromycin.

Pseudomembranous colitis is relatively rarely seen with macrolides, but has been reported with clarithromycin (SED-12, 597) (34,35).

Liver

Abnormal liver function tests and hepatomegaly have been described with clarithromycin; in 4291 patients, the frequency of increased alanine transaminase activity was 5% (36). Clarithromycin was also associated with cholestatic hepatitis (30). To date, at least nine cases of hepatotoxicity have been described in HIV-negative patients taking clarithromycin 1–2 g/day for chronic lung disease due to *M. avium* or *Mycobacterium abscessus* (37). The pattern of liver enzyme abnormality was primarily cholestatic, and the patients were typically elderly (all but one aged over 60 years), or of low weight. Only three patients were symptomatic, and the liver function abnormalities resolved on withdrawal. Subsequent rechallenge was successful in four patients, unsuccessful in one, and not performed in four. There was some dispute as to whether toxicity was dose-related or not, but it is wise to recommend that elderly patients should receive an initial daily dose of 1 g in this disease setting.

Although cholestatic hepatitis has been typically described in association with erythromycin, newer macrolides are not totally free of this risk. A gradual increase in bilirubin and transaminases has been reported during treatment of a *Mycobacterium chelonae* infection with clarithromycin. These alterations were quickly reversible after withdrawal, but re-appeared on re-exposure to clarithromycin 1 g (38).

- Fatal drug-induced cholestasis associated with clarithromycin 500 mg bd for 3 days has been reported in a 59-year-old woman with diabetes mellitus and chronic renal insufficiency (39).
- Idiosyncratic drug-induced fatal fulminant hepatic failure has been reported in a 40-year-old woman with end-stage renal insufficiency taking clarithromycin 500 mg bd (40).

Skin

Clarithromycin has been associated with fixed drug eruptions and hypersensitivity reactions (41,42). In one case a clarithromycin-induced fixed drug eruption was reproduced by oral provocation, whereas patch tests on both unaffected and residual pigmented skin were negative (43).

- A 31-year-old woman developed Stevens–Johnson syndrome after she had taken oral erythromycin 333 mg tds for otitis media (44). After two doses she developed oral ulcers, tongue swelling, and a generalized erythematous rash. The diagnosis was confirmed histologically. She recovered slowly after withdrawal of erythromycin.
- Roxithromycin-induced generalized urticaria and tachycardia with a positive prick test and a cross-reaction to erythromycin and clarithromycin has been reported in a 31-year-old woman (45).

Clarithromycin can cause phototoxicity (46).

Drug–Drug Interactions

Antifungal imidazoles

In three patients with pulmonary MAC and aspergillosis infections, itraconazole was suggested to increase the plasma concentration of clarithromycin as well as the clarithromycin:14-hydroxyclarithromycin ratio (47). This effect may have been due to inhibition of CYP3A4 by itraconazole.

Antihistamines

Toxic effects of terfenadine and astemizole have been reported in patients taking concomitant macrolides, especially clarithromycin (48–51), typically resulting in prolongation of the QT interval and cardiac dysrhythmias (torsade de pointes) (52).

Cisapride

Cisapride can prolong the QT interval, with a risk of ventricular dysrhythmias (53,54). Clarithromycin increases serum concentrations of cisapride (55). This potentially dangerous interaction can result in QT interval prolongation and dysrhythmias such as torsade de pointes.

- Torsade de pointes occurred in a 77-year-old woman taking cisapride and clarithromycin (56).

Warnings have been issued by the manufacturers to avoid concomitant administration.

Colchicine

- Fatal colchicine intoxication occurred in a 67-year-old man who had taken clarithromycin 500 mg bd for 4 days (57).

Clarithromycin may have inhibited colchicine metabolism and caused a rise in colchicine concentration.

Digoxin

Clarithromycin has been reported to cause digoxin toxicity (58). Two different mechanisms are involved, inhibition of the renal excretion of digoxin and alteration of intestinal flora, which reduces the presystemic hydrolysis of digoxin.

- A 70-year-old woman taking digoxin for atrial fibrillation developed nausea, vomiting, and dizziness 2 days after starting to take clarithromycin (59). Her serum digoxin concentration was 3.9 ng/ml (target range 0.5–2.0).

Disulfiram

Fatal toxic epidermal necrolysis and fulminant hepatitis occurred shortly after the start of treatment with clarithromycin in a 47-year-old man who was taking disulfiram (60).

- A 47-year-old man with a history of chronic alcoholism took disulfiram 250 mg/day for 1 month. He then took clarithromycin 500 mg bd and paracetamol 500 mg tds and 1 week later noticed non-pruritic cutaneous maculopapular lesions on his legs, extending to the rest of his body, excluding the palms and soles. Previous drug therapy was withdrawn. A skin biopsy showed toxic epidermal necrolysis. During the next several days the skin lesions worsened. Cutaneous blisters became evident, initially covering less than 10% of the body surface, but then extending all over the body. The serum bilirubin concentration was 359 μmol/l (direct bilirubin 213 μmol/l), the partial thromboplastin time longer than 200 seconds, and the prothrombin time 26 seconds. He developed septic shock and, despite supportive measures, died.

Ergot alkaloids

In patients with ergotamine toxicity, vasoconstriction can lead to frank ischemia. Clarithromycin interferes with ergotamine metabolism.

- A 41-year-old woman developed worsening lower leg pain, pallor, and a sensation of coolness aggravated by exertion; there was severe vasospasm in the legs (61). She had taken a caffeine + ergotamine formulation for migraine for many years and had recently been given clarithromycin 500 mg bd for flu-like symptoms.

HIV nucleoside reverse transcriptase inhibitors

Clarithromycin reduced the peak concentration and AUC of zidovudine at steady state by about 12% (32), possibly as a result of reduced zidovudine absorption (62). However, if the two drugs were taken at least 2 hours apart, the pharmacokinetics of zidovudine were unaffected.

In 12 HIV-positive patients there was no statistically significant difference in concentrations of didanosine when clarithromycin was added (63).

Midazolam

In an open, randomized, crossover, pharmacokinetic and pharmacodynamic study in 12 healthy volunteers who took clarithromycin 250 mg bd for 5 days, azithromycin 500 mg/day for 3 days, or no pretreatment, followed by a single dose of midazolam (15 mg), clarithromycin increased the AUC of midazolam by over 3.5 times and the mean duration of sleep from 135 to 281 minutes (64). In contrast, there was no change with azithromycin, suggesting that it is much safer for co-administration with midazolam.

Omeprazole

In 21 healthy volunteers, clarithromycin (400 mg bd) for 3 days before omeprazole (20 mg/day) significantly inhibited the metabolism of omeprazole (65).

Pimozide

Clarithromycin inhibits the metabolism of pimozide, pimozide plasma concentrations increase, and there is an increased risk of cardiotoxicity through prolongation of the QT interval and fatal ventricular dysrhythmias (66).

Rifamycins

Clarithromycin is one of the core drugs for MAC infections in both HIV-infected and non-infected patients. For this indication, doses of up to 2000 mg/day are used, typically in combination with other drugs.

The interaction of clarithromycin with the rifamycins is complex. Clarithromycin inhibits CYP3A4, while both rifampicin and rifabutin induce P450 cytochromes, including CYP3A4, resulting in enhanced metabolism of drugs. The changes in serum concentrations of clarithromycin and its metabolite in the presence of the enzyme inducers rifampicin and rifabutin suggest that metabolism of clarithromycin by CYP3A4 is increased (67).

After the addition of rifampicin, peak serum concentrations of clarithromycin fell markedly, from a mean of 5.8–2.5 μg/ml (67). At the same time the ratio of the serum concentrations of clarithromycin and its 14-OH metabolite was reversed from 3.3:1 to 1:2.7. There were similar, although less marked, changes after the addition of rifabutin 600 mg/day to a regimen that included clarithromycin 1000 mg/day.

Whether these changes in serum clarithromycin concentrations are relevant to its antimicrobial activity is unknown, since prediction of clinical efficacy based on serum concentrations of clarithromycin is probably not justified, given that the macrolides accumulate to a large degree in tissues and macrophages.

In patients with MAC infections taking rifabutin or rifampicin the addition of clarithromycin resulted in rifamycin-related adverse events in 77% of patients (68). These included uveitis (69–72), especially at rifabutin doses of 600 mg/day or more, neutropenia, nausea, vomiting, diarrhea, and abnormal liver enzyme activities. In addition, diffuse polyarthralgia (19%) was observed. Since inhibition of cytochrome P450 by clarithromycin can interfere with rifabutin metabolism, as illustrated by a report of a significant increase in the AUC of rifabutin during treatment with clarithromycin (68), the authors recommended using rifabutin in a dosage of 300 mg/day in regimens that include a macrolide.

The effects of fluconazole and clarithromycin on the pharmacokinetics of rifabutin and 25-*O*-desacetylrifabutin have been studied in ten HIV-infected patients who were given rifabutin 300 mg qds in addition to fluconazole 200 mg qds and clarithromycin 500 mg qds (73). There was a 76% increase in the plasma AUC of rifabutin when either fluconazole or clarithromycin was given alone and a 152% increase when both drugs were given together. The authors concluded that patients should be monitored for adverse effects of rifabutin when it is co-administered with fluconazole or clarithromycin.

Sulfonylureas

- Severe hypoglycemia occurred in two elderly men with type 2 diabetes mellitus and mild to moderate impaired renal function, who took clarithromycin 1000 mg/day for respiratory infections, in addition to a sulfonylurea (glibenclamide 5 mg/day in one case and glipizide 15 mg/day in the other) (74). Both developed severe hypoglycemia within 48 hours of starting clarithromycin.

Tacrolimus

Clarithromycin can increase the steady-state concentrations of drugs that depend primarily on CYP3A metabolism.

- Steady-state tacrolimus concentrations rose in a 32-year-old African-American man who took clarithromycin 500 mg bd for 4 days (75).
- In two women aged 37 and 69, acute and reversible tacrolimus nephrotoxicity developed after the addition of clarithromycin for an upper respiratory tract infection (76).

Theophylline and other xanthines

Inhibition of cytochrome P450 activity by clarithromycin affects the metabolism of theophylline. However, the results of several studies of the effect of clarithromycin on theophylline concentrations are conflicting. While the total body clearance of theophylline fell (77) and plasma theophylline concentrations increased by 18% (78), mean theophylline concentrations remained within the target range (78). Based on these data it is wise to monitor serum theophylline concentrations in patients taking high dosages of theophylline or in patients with theophylline concentrations in the upper target range who start to take clarithromycin (36).

Warfarin

Increases in International Normalized Ratio (INR) have been detected in patients who have previously been stabilized on warfarin when they were simultaneously given clarithromycin. In one case this caused a suprachoroidal hemorrhage (79).

References

1. Blum AL, Talley NJ, O'Morain C, van Zanten SV, Labenz J, Stolte M, Louw JA, Stubberod A, Theodors A, Sundin M, Bolling-Sternevald E, Junghard O. Lack of effect of treating *Helicobacter pylori* infection in patients with nonulcer dyspepsia. Omeprazole plus Clarithromycin and Amoxicillin Effect One Year after Treatment (OCAY) Study Group. N Engl J Med 1998;339(26):1875–81.
2. Hawkey CJ, Tulassay Z, Szczepanski L, van Rensburg CJ, Filipowicz-Sosnowska A, Lanas A, Wason CM, Peacock RA, Gillon KR. Randomised controlled trial of *Helicobacter pylori* eradication in patients on non-steroidal anti-inflammatory drugs: HELP NSAIDs study. Helicobacter Eradication for Lesion Prevention. Lancet 1998;352(9133):1016–21.
3. McCarty JM, Pierce PF. Five days of cefprozil versus 10 days of clarithromycin in the treatment of an acute exacerbation of chronic bronchitis. Ann Allergy Asthma Immunol 2001;87(4):327–34.
4. Stefansson P, Jacovides A, Jablonicky P, Sedani S, Staley H. Cefuroxime axetil versus clarithromycin in the treatment of acute maxillary sinusitis. Rhinology 1998;36(4):173–8.
5. Faris MA, Raasch RH, Hopfer RL, Butts JD. Treatment and prophylaxis of disseminated *Mycobacterium avium* complex in HIV-infected individuals. Ann Pharmacother 1998; 32(5):564–73.
6. Ward TT, Rimland D, Kauffman C, Huycke M, Evans TG, Heifets L. Randomized, open-label trial of azithromycin plus ethambutol vs. clarithromycin plus ethambutol as therapy for *Mycobacterium avium* complex bacteremia in patients with human immunodeficiency virus infection. Veterans Affairs HIV Research Consortium. Clin Infect Dis 1998;27(5):1278–85.
7. Anderson G, Esmonde TS, Coles S, Macklin J, Carnegie C. A comparative safety and efficacy study of clarithromycin and erythromycin stearate in community-acquired pneumonia. J Antimicrob Chemother 1991; 27(Suppl A):117–24.
8. Lebel MH, Mehra S. Efficacy and safety of clarithromycin versus erythromycin for the treatment of pertussis: a prospective, randomized, single blind trial. Pediatr Infect Dis J 2001;20(12):1149–54.
9. Sokol WN Jr, Sullivan JG, Acampora MD, Busman TA, Notario GF. A prospective, double-blind, multicenter study comparing clarithromycin extended-release with trovafloxacin in patients with community-acquired pneumonia. Clin Ther 2002;24(4):605–15.
10. Roussel G, Igual J. Clarithromycin with minocycline and clofazimine for *Mycobacterium avium intracellulare* complex lung disease in patients without the acquired immune deficiency syndrome. GETIM. Groupe d'Etude et de Traitement des Infections a Mycobacteries. Int J Tuberc Lung Dis 1998;2(6):462–70.
11. Vallejo Camazon N, Rodriguez Pardo D, Sanchez Hidalgo A, Tornos Mas MP, Ribera E, Soler Soler J. Taquicardia Ventricular y QT largo asociades a la administracion de claritromycina en un patiente afectado de infeccion por el VIH. [Ventricular tachycardia and long QT associated with clarithromycin administration in a patient with HIV infection.] Rev Esp Cardiol 2002; 55(8):878–81.
12. Cousins D, Upton D. Beware bolus clarithromycin. Pharm Pract 1996;4:443–5.
13. de Dios Garcia-Diaz J, Santolaya Perrin R, Paz Martinez Ortega M, Moreno-Vazquez M. Flebitis relacionada con la administracion intravenosa de antibioticos macrolidos. Estudio comparativo de eritromicina y claritromicina. [Phlebitis due to intravenous administration of macrolide antibiotics. A comparative study of erythromycin versus clarithromycin.] Med Clin (Barc) 2001; 116(4):133–5.
14. Gangemi S, Ricciardi L, Fedele R, Isola S, Purello-D'Ambrosio F. Immediate reaction to clarithromycin. Allergol Immunopathol (Madr) 2001;29(1):31–2.
15. Pijpers E, van Rijswijk RE, Takx-Kohlen B, Schrey G. A clarithromycin-induced myasthenic syndrome. Clin Infect Dis 1996;22(1):175–6.
16. Tyagi AK, Kayarkar VV, McDonnell PJ. An unreported side effect of topical clarithromycin when used successfully to treat *Mycobacterium avium-intracellulare* keratitis. Cornea 1999;18(5):606–7.
17. Kolkman W, Groeneveld JH, Baur HJ, Verschuur HP. Door claritromycine geinduceerde ototoxiciteite. [Ototoxicity induced by clarithromycin.] Ned Tijdschr Geneeskd 2002;146(37):1743–5.
18. Ramirez J, Unowsky J, Talbot GH, Zhang H, Townsend L. Sparfloxacin versus clarithromycin in the treatment of community-acquired pneumonia. Clin Ther 1999;21(1):103–17.
19. Pijlman AH, Kuck EM, van Puijenbroek EP, Hoekstra JB. Acuut delies, waarschijulijk uitgelokt door claritromycine. [Acute delirium, probably precipitated by clarithromycin.] Ned Tijdschr Geneeskd 2001; 145(5):225–8.
20. Nightingale SD, Koster FT, Mertz GJ, Loss SD. Clarithromycin-induced mania in two patients with AIDS. Clin Infect Dis 1995;20(6):1563–4.
21. Abouesh A, Stone C, Hobbs WR. Antimicrobial-induced mania (antibiomania): a review of spontaneous reports. J Clin Psychopharmacol 2002;22(1):71–81.
22. Cone LA, Sneider RA, Nazemi R, Dietrich EJ. Mania due to clarithromycin therapy in a patient who was not infected with human immunodeficiency virus. Clin Infect Dis 1996;22(3):595–6.
23. Pollak PT, Sketris IS, MacKenzie SL, Hewlett TJ. Delirium probably induced by clarithromycin in a patient receiving fluoxetine. Ann Pharmacother 1995;29(5):486–8.
24. Jimenez-Pulido SB, Navarro-Ruiz A, Sendra P, Martinez-Ramirez M, Garcia-Motos C, Montesinos-Ros A. Hallucinations with therapeutic doses of clarithromycin. Int J Clin Pharmacol Ther 2002;40(1):20–2.
25. Steinman MA, Steinman TI. Clarithromycin-associated visual hallucinations in a patient with chronic renal failure

on continuous ambulatory peritoneal dialysis. Am J Kidney Dis 1996;27(1):143–6.
26. Alexopoulou A, Dourakis SP, Kaloterakis A. Thrombotic thrombocytopenic purpura in a patient treated with clarithromycin. Eur J Haematol 2002;69(3):191–2.
27. Lin HC, Sanders SL, Gu YG, Doty JE. Erythromycin accelerates solid emptying at the expense of gastric sieving. Dig Dis Sci 1994;39(1):124–8.
28. Hasler WL, Heldsinger A, Chung OY. Erythromycin contracts rabbit colon myocytes via occupation of motilin receptors. Am J Physiol 1992;262(1 Pt 1):G50–5.
29. Kaufman HS, Ahrendt SA, Pitt HA, Lillemoe KD. The effect of erythromycin on motility of the duodenum, sphincter of Oddi, and gallbladder in the prairie dog. Surgery 1993;114(3):543–8.
30. Nakayoshi T, Izumi M, Tatsuta K. Effects of macrolide antibiotics on gastrointestinal motility in fasting and digestive states. Drugs Exp Clin Res 1992;18(4):103–9.
31. Sifrim D, Janssens J, Vantrappen G. Comparison of the effects of midecamycin acetate and clarithromycin on gastrointestinal motility in man. Drugs Exp Clin Res 1992;18(8):337–42.
32. Polis M, Haneiwich S, Kovacs J, et al. Dose escalation study to determine the safety, maximally tolerated dose and pharmacokinetics of clarithromycin with zidovudine in HIV-infected patients. In: Interscience Conference on Antimicrobial Agents and Chemotherapy American Society for Microbiology, 1991.
33. Nellans H, Petersen A. Stimulation of gastrointestinal motility: clarithromycin significantly less potent than azithromycin. In: Seventh International Congress of Chemotherapy, Berlin, 1991.
34. Teare JP, Booth JC, Brown JL, Martin J, Thomas HC. Pseudomembranous colitis following clarithromycin therapy. Eur J Gastroenterol Hepatol 1995;7(3):275–7.
35. Gantz NM, Zawacki JK, Dickerson WJ, Bartlett JG. Pseudomembranous colitis associated with erythromycin. Ann Intern Med 1979;91(6):866–7.
36. Peters DH, Clissold SP. Clarithromycin. A review of its antimicrobial activity, pharmacokinetic properties and therapeutic potential. Drugs 1992;44(1):117–64.
37. Brown BA, Wallace RJ Jr, Griffith DE, Girard W. Clarithromycin-induced hepatotoxicity. Clin Infect Dis 1995;20(4):1073–4.
38. Yew WW, Chau CH, Lee J, Leung CW. Cholestatic hepatitis in a patient who received clarithromycin therapy for a *Mycobacterium chelonae* lung infection. Clin Infect Dis 1994;18(6):1025–6.
39. Fox JC, Szyjkowski RS, Sanderson SO, Levine RA. Progressive cholestatic liver disease associated with clarithromycin treatment. J Clin Pharmacol 2002; 42(6):676–80.
40. Christopher K, Hyatt PA, Horkan C, Yodice PC. Clarithromycin use preceding fulminant hepatic failure. Am J Gastroenterol 2002;97(2):489–90.
41. Rosina P, Chieregato C, Schena D. Fixed drug eruption from clarithromycin. Contact Dermatitis 1998;38(2):105.
42. Igea JM, Lazaro M. Hypersensitivity reaction to clarithromycin. Allergy 1998;53(1):107–9.
43. Hamamoto Y, Ohmura A, Kinoshita E, Muto M. Fixed drug eruption due to clarithromycin. Clin Exp Dermatol 2001;26(1):48–9.
44. Sullivan S, Harger B, Cleary JD. Stevens–Johnson syndrome secondary to erythromycin. Ann Pharmacother 1999;33(12):1369.
45. Kruppa A, Scharffetter-Kochanek K, Krieg T, Hunzelmann N. Immediate reaction to roxithromycin and prick test cross-sensitization to erythromycin and clarithromycin. Dermatology 1998;196(3):335–6.
46. Parkash P, Gupta SK, Kumar S. Phototoxic reaction due to clarithromycin. J Assoc Physicians India 2002;50:1192–3.
47. Auclair B, Berning SE, Huitt GA, Peloquin CA. Potential interaction between itraconazole and clarithromycin. Pharmacotherapy 1999;19(12):1439–44.
48. Tran HT. Torsades de pointes induced by nonantiarrhythmic drugs. Conn Med 1994;58(5):291–5.
49. Zechnich AD, Hedges JR, Eiselt-Proteau D, Haxby D. Possible interactions with terfenadine or astemizole. West J Med 1994;160(4):321–5.
50. Jurima-Romet M, Crawford K, Cyr T, Inaba T. Terfenadine metabolism in human liver. In vitro inhibition by macrolide antibiotics and azole antifungals. Drug Metab Dispos 1994;22(6):849–57.
51. Honig P, Wortham D, Zamani K, Cantilena L. Comparison of the effect of the macrolide antibiotics erythromycin, clarithromycin and azithromycin on terfenadine steady-state pharmacokinetics and electrocardiographic parameters. Drug Invest 1994;7:148.
52. Botstein P. Is QT interval prolongation harmful? A regulatory perspective. Am J Cardiol 1993;72(6):B50–2.
53. Evans ME, Feola DJ, Rapp RP. Polymyxin B sulfate and colistin: old antibiotics for emerging multiresistant Gram-negative bacteria. Ann Pharmacother 1999; 33(9):960–7.
54. Tonini M, De Ponti F, Di Nucci A, Crema F. Review article: cardiac adverse effects of gastrointestinal prokinetics. Aliment Pharmacol Ther 1999;13(12):1585–91.
55. Wysowski DK, Bacsanyi J. Cisapride and fatal arrhythmia. N Engl J Med 1996;335(4):290–1.
56. Piquette RK. Torsade de pointes induced by cisapride/clarithromycin interaction. Ann Pharmacother 1999;33(1):22–6.
57. Dandekar SS, Laidlaw DA. Suprachoroidal haemorrhage after addition of clarithromycin to warfarin. J R Soc Med 2001;94(11):583–4.
58. Ford A, Smith LC, Baltch AL, Smith RP. Clarithromycin-induced digoxin toxicity in a patient with AIDS. Clin Infect Dis 1995;21(4):1051–2.
59. Dogukan A, Oymak FS, Taskapan H, Guven M, Tokgoz B, Utas C. Acute fatal colchicine intoxication in a patient on continuous ambulatory peritoneal dialysis (CAPD). Possible role of clarithromycin administration. Clin Nephrol 2001;55(2):181–2.
60. Masia M, Gutierrez F, Jimeno A, Navarro A, Borras J, Matarredona J, Martin-Hidalgo A. Fulminant hepatitis and fatal toxic epidermal necrolysis (Lyell disease) coincident with clarithromycin administration in an alcoholic patient receiving disulfiram therapy. Arch Intern Med 2002;162(4):474–6.
61. Xu H, Rashkow A. Clarithromycin-induced digoxin toxicity: a case report and a review of the literature. Conn Med 2001;65(9):527–9.
62. Amsden GW. Macrolides versus azalides: a drug interaction update. Ann Pharmacother 1995;29(9):906–17.
63. Gillum JG, Bruzzese VL, Israel DS, Kaplowitz LG, Polk RE. Effect of clarithromycin on the pharmacokinetics of 2′,3′-dideoxyinosine in patients who are seropositive for human immunodeficiency virus. Clin Infect Dis 1996;22(4):716–18.
64. Yeates RA, Laufen H, Zimmermann T. Interaction between midazolam and clarithromycin: comparison with azithromycin. Int J Clin Pharmacol Ther 1996;34(9):400–5.
65. Furuta T, Ohashi K, Kobayashi K, Iida I, Yoshida H, Shirai N, Takashima M, Kosuge K, Hanai H, Chiba K, Ishizaki T, Kaneko E. Effects of clarithromycin on the metabolism of omeprazole in relation to CYP2C19 genotype status in humans. Clin Pharmacol Ther 1999;66(3):265–74.
66. Desta Z, Kerbusch T, Flockhart DA. Effect of clarithromycin on the pharmacokinetics and pharmacodynamics of pimozide in healthy poor and extensive metabolizers of cytochrome P450 2D6 (CYP2D6). Clin Pharmacol Ther 1999;65(1):10–20.

67. Wallace RJ Jr, Brown BA, Griffith DE, Girard W, Tanaka K. Reduced serum levels of clarithromycin in patients treated with multidrug regimens including rifampin or rifabutin for *Mycobacterium avium–M. intracellulare* infection. J Infect Dis 1995;171(3):747–50.
68. Griffith DE, Brown BA, Girard WM, Wallace RJ Jr. Adverse events associated with high-dose rifabutin in macrolide-containing regimens for the treatment of Mycobacterium avium complex lung disease. Clin Infect Dis 1995;21(3):594–8.
69. Fuller JD, Stanfield LE, Craven DE. Rifabutin prophylaxis and uveitis. N Engl J Med 1994;330(18):1315–16.
70. Shafran SD, Deschenes J, Miller M, Phillips P, Toma E. Uveitis and pseudojaundice during a regimen of clarithromycin, rifabutin, and ethambutol. MAC Study Group of the Canadian HIV Trials Network. N Engl J Med 1994;330(6):438–9.
71. Frank MO, Graham MB, Wispelway B. Rifabutin and uveitis. N Engl J Med 1994;330(12):868.
72. Havlir D, Torriani F, Dube M. Uveitis associated with rifabutin prophylaxis. Ann Intern Med 1994;121(7): 510–12.
73. Jordan MK, Polis MA, Kelly G, Narang PK, Masur H, Piscitelli SC. Effects of fluconazole and clarithromycin on rifabutin and 25-O-desacetylrifabutin pharmacokinetics. Antimicrob Agents Chemother 2000;44(8):2170–2.
74. Bussing R, Gende A. Severe hypoglycemia from clarithromycin–sulfonylurea drug interaction. Diabetes Care 2002;25(9):1659–61.
75. Ibrahim RB, Abella EM, Chandrasekar PH. Tacrolimus-clarithromycin interaction in a patient receiving bone marrow transplantation. Ann Pharmacother 2002; 36(12):1971–2.
76. Gomez G, Alvarez ML, Errasti P, Lavilla FJ, Garcia N, Ballester B, Garcia I, Purroy A. Acute tacrolimus nephrotoxicity in renal transplant patients treated with clarithromycin. Transplant Proc 1999;31(6):2250–1.
77. Niki Y, Nakajima M, Tsukiyama K, et al. Effect of TE-031(A-56268), a new oral macrolide antibiotic on serum theophylline concentration. Chemotherapy 1988;36:515.
78. Ruf F, Chu S, Sonders R, Sennello L. Effect of multiple doses of clarithromycin on the pharmacokinetics of theophylline. In: International Conference on Antimicrobial Agents and Chemotherapy. Atlanta, Georgia, USA: American Society for Microbiology, 1990.
79. Ausband SC, Goodman PE. An unusual case of clarithromycin associated ergotism. J Emerg Med 2001;21(4): 411–13.

Clebopride

General Information

Like alizapride, clebopride is a prokinetic dopamine receptor antagonist that has extrapyramidal effects. These effects were initially overlooked, but a warning was eventually issued in 1988 (1). The problem has continued to be reported, the incidence at effective doses probably being as high as 25%.

In a 1991 report on a crossover trial, a third of the participants had to withdraw because of adverse effects, among which drowsiness, dizziness, tremors, and anxiety were prominent (2).

Organs and Systems

Nervous system

Clebopride can cause extrapyramidal syndromes (3,4). They range from transient dyskinesia to persistent parkinsonism, tardive dyskinesia (5,6), and tardive dystonia (7).

Extrapyramidal symptoms associated with clebopride have been reported in two 17-year-old patients within 10–16 hours of taking clebopride 0.5 mg tds (3).

In one case respiratory dyskinesia, which can easily be mistaken for psychogenic hyperventilation, was described (SEDA-17, 414).

Progressive supranuclear palsy has also been described (8).

References

1. Anonymous. Clebopride: warning on extrapyramidal symptoms. WHO Drug Inf 1988;2(2):69.
2. Durand JM, Quiles N, Kaplanski G, Soubeyrand J. Thrombosis and recombinant interferon-alpha. Am J Med 1993;95(1):115–16.
3. Serrano Serrano ME, Alvarez Frejo M, Tabernero Garcia J, Martin Martin S. Sindrome extrapyramidal por cleboprida. [An extrapyramidal syndrome due to clebopride.] Aten Primaria 1999;23(1):50–1.
4. Cuena Boy R, Macia Martinez MA. Toxicidad extrapiramidal a metoclopramida y a cleboprida: estudio de las notificaciones voluntarias de reacciones adversas al Sistema Espanol de Farmacovigilancia. [Extrapyramidal toxicity caused by metoclopramide and clebopride: study of voluntary notifications of adverse effects to the Spanish Drug Surveillance System.] Aten Primaria 1998; 21(5):289–95.
5. Sempere AP, Duarte J, Palomares JM, Coria F, Claveria LE. Parkinsonism and tardive dyskinesia after chronic use of clebopride. Mov Disord 1994;9(1):114–15.
6. Jimenez-Jimenez FJ, Cabrera-Valdivia F, Ayuso-Peralta L, Tejeiro J, Vaquero A, Garcia-Albea E. Persistent parkinsonism and tardive dyskinesia induced by clebopride. Mov Disord 1993;8(2):246–7.
7. Sempere AP, Mola S, Flores J. Distonia tardia tras la administracion de clebopride. [Tardive dystonia following the administration of clebopride.] Rev Neurol 1997;25 (148):2060.
8. Campdelacreu J, Kumru H, Tolosa E, Valls-Sole J, Benabarre A. Progressive supranuclear palsy syndrome induced by clebopride. Mov Disord 2004;19(4):482–4.

Clemastine

See also Antihistamines

General Information

Clemastine (SEDA-7, 172) (SEDA-21, 173) belongs to the benzhydryl ether group and was developed in the hope of lessening sedative effects. There was no significant difference compared with other first-generation antihistamines.

Organs and Systems

Nervous system

Clemastine caused sedation in 9–50% of patients (1).

Reference

1. Kriz RJ. Patient evaluation of clemastine fumarate and comparison with other antihistamines. Wis Med J 1981;80(12):31–3.

Clenbuterol

See also Beta$_2$-adrenoceptor agonists

General Information

Clenbuterol may cause somewhat more adverse effects than some other beta$_2$-adrenoceptor agonists and its long half-life could perhaps explain this.

Organs and Systems

Cardiovascular

Induction of physiological cardiac hypertrophy has important implications in various clinical settings, particularly in training of the left ventricle in operations for certain types of congenital heart disease. Positive effects of beta$_2$-adrenoceptor overexpression on cardiac function have been shown in experiments in mice (1).

The hypothesis that clenbuterol improves right ventricular systolic function in large mammalian species when given at the time of induction of pressure-overload cardiac hypertrophy has been tested in 15 open-chest operated sheep before and after 6 weeks of pulmonary artery banding (2). The animals were randomly assigned to either saline solution or clenbuterol. There was a highly significant improvement in the slope of the end-systolic pressure–volume loops in the clenbuterol-treated animals, without detrimental hemodynamic effects. No predictions can be made as to the lasting effects of clenbuterol's ability to augment systolic function in a chronically pressure-overloaded, thin-walled ventricle beyond 6 weeks, or the potential for tachyphylaxis.

Nervous system

Dyskinetic movements have been reported in one elderly patient taking clenbuterol (SEDA-17, 164).

Drug Administration

Drug overdose

The effects of overdose with clenbuterol have been described (3).

- A 28-year-old woman developed a sustained sinus tachycardia (140/minute), hypokalemia (2.4 mmol/l), hypophosphatemia (0.29 mmol/l), and hypomagnesemia (0.76 mmol/l) after accidentally ingesting a reportedly small quantity of clenbuterol. She was treated with metoprolol and potassium. Her serum clenbuterol concentration was 2.93 ng/ml 3 hours after ingestion, well above the maximal peak serum concentration of 0.087 ng/ml 2.4 hours after administration of a therapeutic dose of 20 μg of clenbuterol (4).

References

1. Hoffman RJ, Hoffman RS, Freyberg CL, Poppenga RH, Nelson LS. Clenbuterol ingestion causing prolonged tachycardia, hypokalemia, and hypophosphatemia with confirmation by quantitative levels. J Toxicol Clin Toxicol 2001;39(4):339–44.
2. Baselt RC. Clenbuterol. In: Disposition of Toxic Drugs and Chemicals in Man. 5th ed. Foster City, CA: Chemical Toxicology Institute, 2000:189–90.
3. Malolepszy J, Boszormenyi Nagy G, Selroos O, Larsso P, Brander R. Safety of formoterol Turbuhaler at cumulative dose of 90 microg in patients with acute bronchial obstruction. Eur Respir J 2001;18(6):928–34.
4. Nelson HS, Bensch G, Pleskow WW, DiSantostefano R, DeGraw S, Reasner DS, Rollins TE, Rubin PD. Improved bronchodilation with levalbuterol compared with racemic albuterol in patients with asthma. J Allergy Clin Immunol 1998;102(6 Pt 1):943–52.

Clidinium bromide

See also Anticholinergic drugs

General Information

The anticholinergic drug clidinium is best known as a component of Librax (chlordiazepoxide 5 mg plus clidinium bromide 2.5 mg); the dose used is sufficient to produce typical anticholinergic adverse effects. Since here it is combined with a benzodiazepine, it is most unwise to allow patients taking Librax to drive motor vehicles or to ingest alcohol.

Clobazam

See also Benzodiazepines

General Information

Clobazam, a 1,5-benzodiazepine, differs in its chemical structure from most other benzodiazepines. It has been claimed to have less sedative effects for its effective anticonvulsant and anti-anxiety effects (SED-12, 98). Whether because of tolerance or not, clobazam tends to be less sedative than clonazepam. Both the therapeutic and adverse effects of clobazam have been related to its major metabolite *N*-desmethylclobazam, the formation of which depends on CYP2C19 activity. Mutant alleles that confer high CYP2C19 activity, and are therefore associated with high concentrations of the metabolite, are particularly common (30–40%) in Asian populations (1).

Comparative studies

In a randomized double-blind comparison of clobazam, carbamazepine, and phenytoin monotherapy in children with epilepsy, there were no differences in tests of intelligence, memory, attention, psychomotor speed, and impulsivity between clobazam and the other drugs after 6 and 12 months of therapy, suggesting that the adverse effects of clobazam on cognition and behavior may be less common than generally thought (2). However, the authors did not discuss a trend for some scores, particularly items in the Wechsler Intelligence Scale for Children–Revised, to improve significantly only in children taking non-benzodiazepine anticonvulsants. Moreover, many children withdrew from the study before completion of the follow-up, resulting in potential bias.

In a prospective multicenter double-blind comparison of clobazam with phenytoin or carbamazepine monotherapy in children with partial or generalized tonic-clonic seizures, the retention rate after one year did not differ, but exit due to inefficacy tended to be more common with clobazam (19 versus 11% for the other drugs combined), while exit due to adverse effects tended to be more common with carbamazepine or phenytoin (15 versus 4% for clobazam) (3). Although all treatments were claimed to have similar efficacy, detailed descriptions of the changes in seizure frequency and the proportion of patients who gradually achieved seizure control in each treatment group were not given. Behavioral and mood problems tended to be more common with clobazam than with the other drugs (38/119 versus 29/116). Drooling was more common with clobazam (7/119 versus 2/116), whereas rash or vomiting were more common with the other treatments (9/116 versus 4/119 and 10/116 versus 4/119 respectively). Tolerance was reported in 7.5% of patients taking clobazam, in 4.2% of those taking carbamazepine, and in 6.7% of those taking phenytoin; however, the definition of tolerance (no seizures for 3–6 months, followed by seizures sufficiently numerous to require a switch to another drug) was questionable, and no information was given about patients with seizure relapses who required an increase in dosage. Although these results suggest that clobazam is a valuable alternative to phenytoin and carbamazepine in childhood epilepsy, more precise characterization of responses would have been desirable.

Organs and Systems

Respiratory

Patients receiving intravenous benzodiazepines must be monitored for respiratory depression, and may need artificial ventilation during intensive treatment.

Nervous system

Clobazam is better tolerated than other benzodiazepines used in epilepsy (4). Its most common adverse effects are mild and transient drowsiness, dizziness, or fatigue; rather less common are muscle weakness, restlessness, aggressiveness, weight increase, ataxia, mood disorders, psychotic and behavioral disturbances, vertigo, hypotonia, hypersalivation, and edema (SED-13, 152). There may be a loss of therapeutic response over time.

Akathisia has been rarely seen with benzodiazepines (SED-13, 152).

Psychological, psychiatric

Of 63 children with refractory epilepsy given add-on clobazam (mean dosage 0.8 mg/kg/day) and followed for 15–64 months, 15 (24%) had to discontinue treatment owing to adverse effects, which included severe aggressive outbursts, hyperactivity, insomnia, and depression with suicidal ideation (5). Likewise, there were behavioral or mood problems in 38 of 119 children taking clobazam monotherapy over one year of follow-up, while drooling was reported in seven children (3). In another study, 7 of 63 children treated with clobazam developed aggressive agitation, self-injurious behavior, insomnia, and incessant motor activity. All the affected children were relatively young (mean age 6 years) and mentally disabled (6).

In controlled trials with clonazepam, adverse events were recorded in 60–90% of cases, and led to withdrawal rates as high as 36% (7). The most common effects were drowsiness, ataxia, and behavioral and personality changes. Other problems were hypersalivation, tolerance, and sometimes a paradoxical increase in seizure frequency.

Skin

Toxic epidermal necrolysis has been associated with clobazam (SEDA-21, 48). Bullae with sweat gland necrosis rarely complicate coma, but have recently been reported in association with clobazam, used as adjunctive therapy for resistant epilepsy in a 4-year-old girl (8).

Long-Term Effects

Drug tolerance

Clobazam has similar effects on anxiety to other benzodiazepines, but may be better tolerated (SEDA-20, 31). Used as an anticonvulsant, clobazam is generally well tolerated in epileptic patients, many showing little evidence of tolerance (4). On the other hand, children with epilepsy appear unusually prone to adverse behavioral reactions when taking clobazam (SEDA-19, 34).

Drug withdrawal

Withdrawal effects can be troublesome. Of 13 patients taken off clonazepam 0.01–0.5 mg/day because of adverse effects, 8 had withdrawal seizures and 5 had other withdrawal symptoms (SEDA-19, 63). Choreoathetosis was described in one patient completing withdrawal of clonazepam (SED-13, 152).

Epileptic-negative myoclonus status (almost continuous lapses in muscle tone associated with epileptiform discharges and interfering with postural control and motor coordination) rarely occur after rapid withdrawal of clobazam or valproate (9).

Drug–Drug Interactions

Antiepileptic drugs

Several metabolic interactions between clobazam and other antiepileptic drugs have been reported, in particular phenytoin intoxication after the addition of clobazam (SED-12, 98).

Carbamazepine

Negative myoclonus and more typical signs of carbamazepine intoxication (fatigue, ataxia, clumsiness) occurred in a 66-year-old man after he took add-on clobazam (10 mg/day) for 4 weeks (10). Plasma concentrations of carbamazepine (58 μmol/l) and carbamazepine-10,11-epoxide (19 μmol/l) were higher than before clobazam therapy, and his symptoms resolved quickly when carbamazepine dosage was reduced and clobazam was withdrawn. The interaction was confirmed on rechallenge.

This interaction does not occur in most patients.

Stiripentol

After the addition of stiripentol (50 mg/kg) in 20 children treated with clobazam, mean serum clobazam concentrations increased about twofold and norclobazam concentrations increased about threefold; a mean 25% reduction in clobazam dose was required because of adverse effects (11). Serum concentrations of concomitantly administered valproic acid rose by about 20%. These findings are in agreement with evidence that stiripentol is a potent metabolic inhibitor.

References

1. Kosaki K, Tamura K, Sato R, Samejima H, Tanigawara Y, Takahashi T. A major influence of CYP2C19 genotype on the steady-state concentration of N-desmethylclobazam. Brain Dev 2004;26(8):530–4.
2. Bawden HN, Camfield CS, Camfield PR, Cunningham C, Darwish H, Dooley JM, Gordon K, Ronen G, Stewart J, van Mastrigt R. The cognitive and behavioural effects of clobazam and standard monotherapy are comparable. Canadian Study Group for Childhood Epilepsy. Epilepsy Res 1999;33(2–3):133–43.
3. Canadian Study Group for Childhood Epilepsy. Clobazam has equivalent efficacy to carbamazepine and phenytoin as monotherapy for childhood epilepsy. Epilepsia 1998;39(9):952–9.
4. Remy C. Clobazam in the treatment of epilepsy: a review of the literature. Epilepsia 1994;35(Suppl 5):S88–91.
5. Sheth RD, Ronen GM, Goulden KJ, Penney S, Bodensteiner JB. Clobazam for intractable pediatric epilepsy. J Child Neurol 1995;10(3):205–8.
6. Sheth RD, Goulden KJ, Ronen GM. Aggression in children treated with clobazam for epilepsy. Clin Neuropharmacol 1994;17(4):332–7.
7. Sato S. Clonazepam. In: Levy R, Mattson R, Meldrum B, Penry J, Dreifuss F, editors. Antiepileptic Drugs. 3rd ed. New York: Raven Press, 1989:65.
8. Setterfield JF, Robinson R, MacDonald D, Calonje E. Coma-induced bullae and sweat gland necrosis following clobazam. Clin Exp Dermatol 2000;25(3):215–18.
9. Gambardella A, Aguglia U, Oliveri RL, Russo C, Zappia M, Quattrone A. Negative myoclonic status due to antiepileptic drug tapering: report of three cases. Epilepsia 1997;38(7):819–23.
10. Genton P, Nguyen VH, Mesdjian E. Carbamazepine intoxication with negative myoclonus after the addition of clobazam. Epilepsia 1998;39(10):1115–18.
11. Rey E, Tran A, D'Athis P, Chiron C, Dulac O, Vincent J, Pons G. Stiripentol potentiates clobazam in childhood epilepsy: a pharmacological study. Epilepsia 1999;40(Suppl 7): 112–13.

Clobuzarit

See also Non-steroidal anti-inflammatory drugs

General Information

Clobuzarit, a methylpropionic acid derivative, thought to have a penicillamine-like effect, was withdrawn from the market in the 1980s because of several reports of Stevens–Johnson syndrome (1).

Reference

1. Bird HA. Rheumatology and the pharmaceutical industry. J Rheumatol 1983;10(4):663–4.

Clofazimine

See also Antituberculosis drugs

General Information

Clofazimine is weakly bactericidal against *Mycobacterium leprae*. It is active in chronic skin ulcers (Buruli ulcer) and partly against *Mycobacterium avium* intracellulare. The usual adult dosage is 50–100 mg/day. At higher doses, its anti-inflammatory effect seems to prevent the development of acute reactions, such as erythema nodosum leprosum.

Clofazimine is a strongly lipophilic dye and accumulates in tissues, especially fat, bile, macrophages, the reticuloendothelial system, and skin. This is the basis of adverse reactions, including skin discoloration (1). Lymphedema (2), diminished sweating, and reduced tearing have been observed (3).

Observational studies

In 84 patients with leprosy who took clofazimine, the most common adverse effect was a dark red skin pigmentation of varying intensity, which appeared within 10 weeks of the start of therapy (4). The intensity of the colour was proportional to the density of the infiltration. There was ichthyosis in 56 patients. Adverse effects such as anorexia, diarrhea, lymph gland enlargement, liver enlargement, corneal drying, and loss of weight were self-correcting, but nine patients had severe gastrointestinal effects (severe abdominal pain, vomiting, and diarrhea).

Organs and Systems

Respiratory

Clofazimine crystals were observed in macrophages in the respiratory alveoli of a patient with AIDS; this is considered harmless (5).

Nervous system

Intraneural deposition of a ceroid-like pigment has been seen after treatment of lepromatous leprosy with clofazimine (6). This pigment does not affect the healing process. Treatment can be continued, provided that the dose is not too high.

Sensory systems

In 76 patients taking multidrug therapy, including clofazimine, for at least 6 months, 46% had conjunctival deposition, 53% had deposition in the cornea, and crystals were found in the tears of 32% (7). Conjunctival pigmentation has been reported, as well as reversible linear brownish corneal streaks. Two cases of macular pigmentation have also been described (SEDA-5, 294).

Gastrointestinal

Nausea, vomiting, diarrhea, abdominal pain, and anorexia have been reported with clofazimine (8).

Clofazimine can accumulate and precipitate in tissues, such as the wall of the small bowel, after prolonged administration. Enteropathy can develop if crystals are stored in the lamina propria of the jejunal mucosa and the mesenteric lymph nodes. These effects depend on the dosage and duration of therapy. When this complication is suspected jejunal biopsy is indicated. At laparotomy, all organs can have an orange–yellow color (SEDA-9, 272) (1,9). On drug withdrawal, the enteropathy progressively improves. Recognized for the first time in 1967, only 14 cases of this complication have so far appeared in the English-language literature (10). Acute or chronic abdominal pain was the main symptom. In most patients, the diagnosis was made after exploratory laparotomy. Barium meal follow-through or CT scanning of the abdomen showed mucosal thickening in the small intestine. Mesenteric lymph node enlargement was present in the index case. Characteristic eosinophilic clofazimine crystals were demonstrated in the histiocytes of all patients except three. The authors proposed the term "clofazimine-induced crystal-storage histiocytosis" to emphasize causes other than B cell neoplasms for crystal-storage histiocytosis. Awareness of this complication of clofazimine can avoid unnecessary surgical exploration.

Liver

Clofazimine can inhibit the liver damage that is associated with lepromatous leprosy and the leprosy reaction; it has only minimal or no deleterious effects on liver function (11).

Skin

Pigmentation and purple skin discoloration are the most frequent adverse effects of clofazimine. It is therefore unacceptable to most light-skinned patients (12).

Ichthyosis is very frequent at dosages of clofazimine over 100 mg/day (SEDA-8, 290).

Nails

Nail changes, such as brown discoloration of the nail plate and onycholysis, have been described in patients taking high doses (300 mg/day) of clofazimine (13). Clofazimine crystals were demonstrated in the nails and nail beds.

References

1. Merrett MN, King RW, Farrell KE, Zeimer H, Guli E. Orange/black discolouration of the bowel (at laparotomy) due to clofazimine. Aust NZ J Surg 1990;60(8):638–9.
2. Oommen T. Clofazimine-induced lymphoedema. Lepr Rev 1990;61(3):289.
3. Braude AL, Davis Ch E, Fierer J. Infectious Diseases and Medical Microbiology. 2nd ed. Philadelphia: WB Saunders, 1966:1171.
4. Ramu G, Iyer GG. Side effects of clofazimine therapy. Lepr India 1976;48(Suppl 4):722–31.
5. Sandler ED, Ng VL, Hadley WK. Clofazimine crystals in alveolar macrophages from a patient with the acquired immunodeficiency syndrome. Arch Pathol Lab Med 1992;116(5):541–3.
6. McDougall AC, Jones RL. Intra-neural ceroid-like pigment following the treatment of lepromatous leprosy with clofazimine (B663; Lamprene). J Neurol Neurosurg Psychiatry 1981;44(2):116–20.
7. Kaur I, Ram J, Kumar B, Kaur S, Sharma VK. Effect of clofazimine on eye in multibacillary leprosy. Indian J Lepr 1990;62(1):87–90.
8. Lal S, Garg BR, Hameedulla A. Gastro-intestinal side effects of clofazimine. Lepr India 1981;53(2):285–8.
9. Jost JL, Venencie PY, Cortez A, Orieux G, Debbasch L, Chomette G, Puissant A, Vayre P. Entéropathie à la clofazimine. [Enteropathy caused by clofazimine.] J Chir (Paris) 1986;123(1):7–9.
10. Sukpanichnant S, Hargrove NS, Kachintorn U, Manatsathit S, Chanchairujira T, Siritanaratkul N, Akaraviputh T, Thakerngpol K. Clofazimine-induced crystal-storing histiocytosis producing chronic abdominal pain in a leprosy patient. Am J Surg Pathol 2000;24(1):129–35.
11. Bulakh PM, Kowale CN, Ranade SM, Burte NP, Chandorkar AG. The effect of clofazimine on liver function tests in lepra reaction (ENL). Lepr India 1983;55(4):714–18.
12. Burte NP, Chandorkar AG, Muley MP, Balsara JJ, Bulakh PM. Clofazimine in lepra (ENL) reaction, one year clinical trial. Lepr India 1983;55(2):265–77.
13. Dixit VB, Chaudhary SD, Jain VK. Clofazimine induced nail changes. Indian J Lepr 1989;61(4):476–8.

Clofedanol

General Information

Clofedanol is a centrally acting cough suppressant with mild local anesthetic properties. In an open study 30 patients were treated with clofedanol for 14 days. Two were withdrawn from the study because of tiredness and vomiting. These adverse effects disappeared immediately after treatment was withdrawn (1).

Reference

1. Cosmi F, Mollaioli M, Aimi M, et al. Attivatá antitussigena del clofedanolo. Eur Rev Med Pharmacol Sci 1983;5:239–42.

Cloforex

See also Anorectic drugs

General Information

Cloforex is similar in structure to chlorphentermine. It produces adverse effects similar to those of other appetite suppressants. Outstanding among them are sleeplessness or tiredness, headache, diarrhea, increased sweating, and dryness of the mouth; there may also be tolerance to its effects (1).

Reference

1. Bjurulf P, Carlstrom S, Rorsman G. Oberex, a new appetite-reducing agent. Acta Med Scand 1967;182(3):273–80.

Clometacin

See also Non-steroidal anti-inflammatory drugs

General Information

The NSAID clometacin is an indometacin derivative.

Because of the risk of long-term or repeated use of clometacin, the French authorities restricted its use to prescriptions for no more than 8 days. It seems wise to recommend that it be no longer used.

Organs and Systems

Hematologic

Thrombocytopenia has been attributed to clometacin (SEDA-6, 94).

Liver

The hepatotoxic potential of clometacin was first reported in France in 1978. Since then many cases of hepatotoxic effects have been described (SEDA-7, 109). In two retrospective studies the clinical, biochemical, immunological, and histopathological features were outlined in detail (1,2). The patients had jaundice and/or hepatomegaly (90%), weakness (60%), fever (30%), and abdominal pain (20%), with or without diarrhea, nausea, and vomiting, usually presenting after long-term use or shortly after a rechallenge. The biochemical disorders were hepatocellular hepatitis and cholestatic hepatitis. High titers of antitissue antibodies and hypergammaglobulinemia were also present in most patients. Histological findings were characteristic of acute hepatitis or chronic active hepatitis. There was a high prevalence of HLA-antigen B8. These immunological features suggest an autoimmune pathogenesis.

Urinary tract

A retrospective analysis of acute renal insufficiency related to NSAID therapy in France showed that clometacin was most frequently implicated. Cases of functional renal insufficiency and interstitial nephritis with nephrotic syndrome were reported (SEDA-12, 84).

Skin

Skin eruptions, generalized pruritus, and weight loss have been reported (1).

References

1. Pariente EA, Hamoud A, Goldfain D, Latrive JP, Gislon J, Cassan P, Morin T, Staub JL, Ramain JP, Bertrand JL. Hepatites a la clometacine (Duperan). Etude retrospective de 30 cas. Un modèle d'hépatité autoimmune médicamenteuse? [Hepatitis caused by clometacin (Duperan). Retrospective study of 30 cases. A model of autoimmune drug-induced hepatitis?] Gastroenterol Clin Biol 1989;13(10):769–74.
2. Islam S, Mekhloufi F, Paul JM, Islam M, Johanet C, Legendre C, Degott C, Abuaf N, Homberg JC. Characteristics of clometacin-induced hepatitis with special reference to the presence of anti-actin cable antibodies. Autoimmunity 1989;2(3):213–21.

Clomethiazole

General Information

Clomethiazole is a sedative-hypnotic that has been used extensively in the treatment of alcohol withdrawal, as well as for inducing sedation and sleep in the elderly. In addition to GABA enhancement, which it shares with the benzodiazepines, clomethiazole also enhances the activity of another inhibitory amino acid, glycine. Whether this property is clinically important is uncertain. As well as the expected effects of sedation and memory impairment, it produces nasal irritation, especially in younger patients, in whom it has a shorter half-life. Its use in alcohol withdrawal is becoming less common, possibly owing to the demonstrated safety and efficacy of longer-acting benzodiazepines, such as chlordiazepoxide, and alternatives such as carbamazepine.

Hypotension, phlebitis, and respiratory depression can occur after intravenous use. While effects in the elderly may be increased, the incidence of adverse effects is similar to that seen in younger subjects (1).

Clomethiazole, like the benzodiazepines, has an additive effect with other CNS depressants, and can cause profound bradycardia when combined with beta-adrenoceptor antagonists.

Organs and Systems

Nervous system

In a double-blind, double-dummy, placebo-controlled comparison of clomethiazole and gammahydroxybutyrate in ameliorating the symptoms of alcohol withdrawal, alcohol-dependent patients were randomized to receive either clomethiazole 1000 mg or gammahydroxybutyrate 50 mg/kg (2). There was no difference between the three treatments in ratings of alcohol withdrawal symptoms or requests for additional medication. After tapering the active medication, there was no increase in withdrawal symptoms, suggesting that physical tolerance did not develop to either clomethiazole or gammahydroxybutyrate during the 5-day treatment period. The most frequently reported adverse effect of gammahydroxybutyrate was transient vertigo, particularly after the evening double dose.

The effect of clomethiazole on cerebral outcome in patients undergoing coronary artery bypass surgery has been investigated in 245 patients, who were randomized double-blind to placebo or clomethiazole (1800 mg over 45 minutes followed by 800 mg/hour until the end of surgery) (3). A battery of eight neuropsychological tests was administered preoperatively and repeated 4–7 weeks after surgery. There were no differences between the clomethiazole and placebo groups in postoperative neuropsychological tests scores. Thus, clomethiazole did not improve or worsen cerebral outcome after coronary artery bypass surgery.

The efficacy and safety of clomethiazole (75 mg/kg by intravenous infusion over 24 hours), as a neuroprotective drug, were studied in a double-blind, placebo-controlled trial (CLASS, the Clomethiazole Acute Stroke Study) in 1360 patients with acute hemispheric stroke (4). Clomethiazole was generally well tolerated and safe. Sedation was the most common adverse event, leading to treatment withdrawal in 16% of patients compared with 4.2% of placebo-treated patients.

In a small subset of CLASS (95 patients) mortality at 90 days was 19% in the clomethiazole group and 23% in the placebo group (5). Sedation was the most common adverse event (clomethiazole 53%, placebo 17%), followed by rhinitis and coughing. The incidence and pattern of serious adverse events was similar between the groups.

A report has illustrated the dangers of driving a motor vehicle whilst taking clomethiazole (6).

- A 53-year-old male car driver was followed by the police for about 2 km, while he drove in an unsafe manner, until the car crashed into the owner's garage. Analysis of his blood showed a clomethiazole concentration of 3.3 μg/ml. Neither alcohol nor any other drug could be detected. One day later he committed suicide by swallowing at least 60 capsules of clomethiazole.

Liver

Reversible cholestatic jaundice has been attributed to clomethiazole (SEDA-21, 39).

Long-Term Effects

Drug abuse

As with other GABA enhancers, clomethiazole is highly abusable in susceptible individuals and should not be used for outpatient detoxification (7).

Drug dependence

Clomethiazole maintains its efficacy with apparently less dependence than temazepam during prolonged use (7).

Drug–Drug Interactions

Alteplase

The safety of the thrombolytic drug alteplase (tPA) plus clomethiazole in patients with acute ischemic stroke has been assessed in a randomized, double-blind study (8). All received alteplase 0.9 mg/kg, beginning within 3 hours of stroke onset, and then either intravenous clomethiazole 68 mg/kg ($n = 97$) over 24 hours, or placebo ($n = 93$) beginning within 12 hours of stroke onset. During follow-up for 90 days the number of serious adverse event reports was 47 in the clomethiazole group and 48 in the placebo group. There were 15 deaths in those given clomethiazole and nine in those given placebo, but this was not significantly different. Sedation was also greater with clomethiazole (42%) than with placebo (13%).

Cimetidine

Cimetidine can reduce clomethiazole clearance by 60–70% (9).

References

1. Fagan D, Lamont M, Jostell KG, Tiplady B, Scott DB. A study of the psychometric effects of chlormethiazole in healthy young and elderly subjects. Age Ageing 1990;19(6):395–402.
2. Nimmerrichter AA, Walter H, Gutierrez-Lobos KE, Lesch OM. Double-blind controlled trial of gamma-hydroxybutyrate and clomethiazole in the treatment of alcohol withdrawal. Alcohol Alcohol 2002;37(1):67–73.
3. Kong RS, Butterworth J, Aveling W, Stump DA, Harrison MJ, Hammon J, Stygall J, Rorie KD, Newman SP. Clinical trial of the neuroprotectant clomethiazole in coronary artery bypass graft surgery: a randomized controlled trial. Anesthesiology 2002;97(3):585–91.
4. Wahlgren NG, Ranasinha KW, Rosolacci T, Franke CL, van Erven PM, Ashwood T, Claesson L. Clomethiazole acute stroke study (CLASS): results of a randomized, controlled trial of clomethiazole versus placebo in 1360 acute stroke patients. Stroke 1999;30(1):21–8.
5. Wahlgren NG, Diez-Tejedor E, Teitelbaum J, Arboix A, Leys D, Ashwood T. Grossman E. Results in 95 hemorrhagic stroke patients included in CLASS, a controlled trial of clomethiazole versus placebo in acute stroke patients. Stroke 2000;31(1):82–5.
6. Logemann E. Risks for driving under the influence of clomethiazole. Probl Forens Sci 2000;XLIII:144–7.
7. Bayer AJ, Bayer EM, Pathy MS, Stoker MJ. A double-blind controlled study of chlormethiazole and triazolam as

hypnotics in the elderly. Acta Psychiatr Scand 1986;329(Suppl):104–11.
8. Lyden P, Jacoby M, Schim J, Albers G, Mazzeo P, Ashwood T, Nordlund A, Odergren T. The Clomethiazole Acute Stroke Study in Tissue-type Plasminogen Activator-treated Stroke (CLASS-T): final results. Neurology 2001;57(7):1199–205.
9. Shaw G, Bury RW, Mashford ML, Breen KJ, Desmond PV. Cimetidine impairs the elimination of chlormethiazole. Eur J Clin Pharmacol 1981;21(1):83–5.

Clomiphene

General Information

Clomiphene is a very weak non-steroidal estrogen; it blocks the feedback effect of endogenous estrogens on the pituitary, promoting the further secretion of gonadotropins. The primary use of clomiphene in women is in the induction of ovulation. In men, it has been used to treat infertility in view of its ability to increase endogenous production of testosterone (1).

General adverse effects

In one large study, some adverse reactions in treated women were due to its ovulatory effects and others were direct reactions to the substance itself (2). The most common problem was ovarian enlargement (14%), followed by hot flushes (11%), abdominal and pelvic discomfort (7.0%), and nausea and vomiting (2.1%). Incidental symptoms were breast discomfort, vaginal changes, psychological symptoms, headache, heavier menses, and increased urinary frequency. Sporadic case-reports on clomiphene in the literature relate to fetal ovarian dysplasia or maternal psychosis (SEDA-7, 391), either of which may have been coincidental. However, it must be borne in mind that the substance is related structurally to triparanol, an obsolete drug that produced a series of disastrous adverse effects some 40 years ago.

In another study, the adverse effects of the antiestrogenic effects of clomiphene citrate were hot flushes (10%), mood swings, depression, headaches (1%), pelvic pain (5.5%), nausea (2%), breast tenderness (2–5%), dryness and loss of hair (0.3%), visual symptoms, halos and streaks around lights (particularly at night), blurring, and scotoma (1.5%) (3).

Organs and Systems

Nervous system

In a multicenter WHO study, two men withdrew because of visual disturbances, dizziness, and headaches (4).

Reproductive system

In some men taking clomiphene in the hope of improving subfertility, a non-bacterial pyospermia developed and could well have had an adverse effect on the outcome; it appeared more commonly in clomiphene users than controls (5).

Long-Term Effects

Tumorigenicity

Mammary cancer in the mother has been suspected as a risk of clomiphene, but specific investigations into the matter have not supported this suspicion (SED-12, 1034) (6).

A case of testicular seminoma in a man receiving both clomiphene and mesterolone for 15 months for oligospermia has been described (7), but it is unlikely that the drug was responsible.

Malignant melanoma

Concern that the drug treatment of female infertility might predispose the user to malignant melanoma was first engendered by a US study published in 1995 (8). Among women who had used clomiphene citrate for infertility, the incidence of melanoma was higher (RR = 1.8; 95% CI = 0.8, 3.5) than among American women in general. However, in a case-cohort study of nearly 4000 infertile women there was a similar increase in the incidence of melanoma among those who had been treated with human chorionic gonadotropin compared with the rest; there was no association with the use of clomiphene.

Quite apart from the inherent discrepancy in these findings, several pieces of evidence have confused the debate. In the first place, the cohort of melanoma cases was small—barely a handful. In the second place, some earlier papers had suggested that infertility in women might of itself have an association with melanoma. The same impression came from various studies, in which the incidences of cancers in infertile women were examined (9–11). If that were true, it could affect the initial findings in either direction: a high spontaneous incidence might mask a real drug effect, or it might provide a predisposition to melanoma, which the drugs might then more readily trigger.

In the meantime, data from Australia have shown no greater incidence of melanoma among women who had used fertility drugs and undergone in vitro fertilization than in the country's general female population (12). Since then there has been one more significant paper, again from Australia, using data from a specialized fertility clinic in Queensland, relating to all women who attended the center over a decade (13). Whenever possible, the women were traced and their subsequent history noted. Originally intended as a retrospective case-cohort study using a subcohort, the approach had to be amended because no cases of melanoma were found in the subcohort. The work therefore proceeded as a matched case-control study; all the data were taken and set against publicly available figures on melanoma in Queensland. After some necessary exclusions, 3186 women were included; care was taken to minimize recall bias. Fourteen women developed melanoma after fertility treatment, eight cases being invasive. The expected incidence in the general population would have been 15.8

cases in the same period. The incidence actually observed was therefore only 0.89 of that anticipated (95% CI = 0.54, 1.48). The numbers of women who had used clomiphene or human menopausal gonadotropin were too small to make more differentiated calculations, but the incidence of melanoma seemed to correspond to that in the general population.

On current evidence there seems no reason to discourage fertility-promoting drug treatments because of any risk of melanoma; they may even reduce it to some extent. However, this does not alter the fact that the data are deficient in various ways. Quite apart from the small numbers of melanoma cases that have been recorded, all the work to date has been performed in relatively sunny parts of the world; it is not known what would happen in other climates. Within countries there are sharp differences in melanoma figures; in the USA, where about 32 000 new cases of skin melanoma were projected for 1994 (14), the highest melanoma rates occur among light-skinned populations in areas of intense sunlight, for example Arizona; the same applies to Queensland, Australia. In the USA as a whole there is a melanoma incidence among whites of 12.4 per 100 000 (15), while mortality rates vary inversely with latitude (16). Furthermore, in whites, there has been a recent increase in the incidence of melanoma, during the precise period that this type of treatment has become popular, but probably for entirely different reasons, which may be associated with lifestyles and holiday habits; the reported incidence in whites rose by no less than 102% from 1973 to 1991 (16). Finally, as the Australian authors themselves stressed, the fact that the Queensland clinic was a private institution specializing in IVF/GIFT therapy means that women with endocrine-associated or ovulation-associated infertility may not have been referred to it so readily.

All this makes it very difficult to find a baseline incidence for melanoma with which cases treated for infertility can be compared. It is to be hoped that data of this type will continue to arrive from other centers, so that a definitive judgement will become possible.

Second-Generation Effects

Teratogenicity

Suspicions that clomiphene might adversely affect a fetus that has developed as a result of successful ovulation induction are difficult to confirm or allay, since the condition for which clomiphene is being used, that is subfertility, might itself be associated with a risk of malformation. The fear originally arose after 18 cases of trisomy had been reported in the USA; later data on a large series of clomiphene-induced pregnancies (17) indicated that if there was indeed such risk it must be very small; a study of 200 instances of Down's syndrome showed that none of them had been exposed to the drug (SEDA-6, 357). Another report concerned a case of congenital retinopathy (SEDA-7, 391).

Cornel and colleagues concluded in 1989 that there was a relative risk of at least two of an association between disturbed fertility and neural tube defects (18), but others found no evidence for an association between maternal clomiphene use and such defects. The authors of a pooled analysis of all published work concluded that any increase in neural tube defects is likely to be less than two-fold and that there may in fact be no increase at all (1).

One unusual possibility is a change in the sex ratio; in one study the ratio of boys to girls among infants conceived after induction of ovulation with clomiphene was 0.85, significantly different from the normal human sex ratio at birth, which is about 1.06 (19).

An unusual condition that has been tentatively ascribed to clomiphene is persistence of the hyperplastic primary vitreous, that is fetal ophthalmic tissue that normally resolves before birth. If more than a trace of the material persists, ocular complications, including cataract and retinal detachment, can result. In a case reported from Canada, there had been an estimated 3 weeks of exposure to high doses of clomiphene (100 mg/day) after gestation, and the child's vision was severely impaired (20). This is probably not a mere chance association, since several cases of visual defects of various types after exposure to clomiphene have been described before, and in some animal studies the drug does adversely affect ocular development.

References

1. Greenland S, Ackerman DL. Clomiphene citrate and neural tube defects: a pooled analysis of controlled epidemiologic studies and recommendations for future studies. Fertil Steril 1995;64(5):936–41.
2. Kistner RW. The use of clomiphene citrate in the treatment of anovulation. Semin Drug Treat 1973;3(2):159–76.
3. Vollenhoven BJ, Healy DL. Short- and long-term effects of ovulation induction. Endocrinol Metab Clin North Am 1998;27(4):903–14.
4. World Health Organization. A double-blind trial of clomiphene citrate for the treatment of idiopathic male infertility. Int J Androl 1992;15(4):299–307.
5. Matthews GJ, Goldstein M, Henry JM, Schlegel PN. Nonbacterial pyospermia: a consequence of clomiphene citrate therapy. Int J Fertil Menopausal Stud 1995;40(4):187–91.
6. Kimbel HK. Inquiry of the 'Arzneimittelkommission der Deutschen Arzteschaft'. Personal communication, 1978.
7. Neoptolemos JP, Locke TJ, Fossard DP. Testicular tumour associated with hormonal treatment for oligospermia. Lancet 1981;2(8249):754.
8. Rossing MA, Daling JR, Weiss NS, Moore DE, Self SG. Risk of cutaneous melanoma in a cohort of infertile women. Melanoma Res 1995;5(2):123–7.
9. Ron E, Lunenfeld B, Menczer J, Blumstein T, Katz L, Oelsner G, Serr D. Cancer incidence in a cohort of infertile women. Am J Epidemiol 1987;125(5):780–90.
10. Brinton LA, Melton LJ 3rd, Malkasian GD Jr, Bond A, Hoover R. Cancer risk after evaluation for infertility. Am J Epidemiol 1989;129(4):712–22.
11. Modan B, Ron E, Lerner-Geva L, Blumstein T, Menczer J, Rabinovici J, Oelsner G, Freedman L, Mashiach S, Lunenfeld B. Cancer incidence in a cohort of infertile women. Am J Epidemiol 1998;147(11):1038–42.
12. Venn A, Watson L, Lumley J, Giles G, King C, Healy D. Breast and ovarian cancer incidence after infertility and in vitro fertilisation. Lancet 1995;346(8981):995–1000.
13. Young P, Purdie D, Jackman L, Molloy D, Green A. A study of infertility treatment and melanoma. Melanoma Res 2001;11(5):535–41.

14. Boring CC, Squires TS, Tong T, Montgomery S. Cancer statistics, 1994. CA Cancer J Clin 1994;44(1):7–26.
15. Rees LAG, Eisner MP, Kosary CL, Hankey BF, Miller BA, Clegg L, Edwards BK, editors. SEER Cancer Statistics Review, 1973–1999. Bethesda MD: National Cancer Institute, 2002. http./seer.cancer.gov/csr/1973–1999/.
16. Glass AG, Hoover RN. The emerging epidemic of melanoma and squamous cell skin cancer. JAMA 1989;262(15):2097–100.
17. Gysler M, March CM, Mishell DR Jr, Bailey EJ. A decade's experience with an individualized clomiphene treatment regimen including its effect on the postcoital test. Fertil Steril 1982;37(2):161–7.
18. Cornel MC, ten Kate LP, Dukes MN, de Jong-v D Berg LT, Meyboom RH, Garbis H, Peters PW. Ovulation induction and neural tube defects. Lancet 1989;1(8651):1386.
19. James WH. The sex ratio of infants born after hormonal induction of ovulation. Br J Obstet Gynaecol 1985; 92(3):299–301.
20. Bishai R, Arbour L, Lyons C, Koren G. Intrauterine exposure to clomiphene and neonatal persistent hyperplastic primary vitreous. Teratology 1999;60(3):143–5.

Clomipramine

See also Tricyclic antidepressants

General Information

Clomipramine is the imipramine analogue of chlorpromazine. However, while the difference between chlorpromazine and promazine is large, adding a chloride atom to imipramine hardly affects its actions. Most trials have failed to show any superiority of the chlorinated compound over imipramine. The adverse effects profile is similar (1), but drowsiness, confusion, and "feeling awful" are commonly reported (2).

In a controlled comparison between clomipramine and amitriptyline, the former caused adverse effects more often, especially drowsiness (3). Overdose toxicity is the same as with other tricyclic antidepressants (4); fatal interactions with monoamine oxidase (MAO) inhibitors have been reported (SEDA-18, 16) (5). Altogether, toxic effects are not substantially different.

Besides depression, clomipramine is also widely used in the treatment of phobic and obsessive-compulsive disorders (6–8) and in panic disorders (9).

Organs and Systems

Cardiovascular

Venous thrombosis is a recognized complication of tricyclic antidepressants. Thrombosis of the cerebral veins occurred in a 61-year-old woman after intravenous clomipramine, and the authors suggested that the risk may be greater when the intravenous route is used (10).

Intravenous administration invariably produced electrocardiographic changes, sometimes slow to reverse, in elderly patients (11).

At therapeutic doses, tricyclic antidepressants can cause postural hypotension, but they are regarded as being safe in patients who require general anesthesia. However, hypotension during surgery has been associated with clomipramine (12).

- A 57-year-old man due to undergo mitral valve surgery took clomipramine (150 mg at night) up to the night before surgery. His blood pressure before induction with thiopental (250 mg) and fentanyl (250 μg) was 105/65 mmHg, with a heart rate of 70 beats/minute. Anesthesia was maintained with isofluorothane, and 45 minutes after induction, his systolic blood pressure fell to 90 mmHg. Ephedrine (30 mg total), phenylephrine (500 μg total), or dopamine (10 μg/kg/minute) did not increase the blood pressure. After sternotomy, his systolic blood pressure fell to 55 mmHg and his pulse rate to 60 beats/minute, and he had third-degree atrioventricular block. Further ephedrine, phenylephrine, and adrenaline were without effect. During cardiopulmonary bypass, a noradrenaline infusion was started (0.2 μg/kg/minute) and isofluorothane was withdrawn. After he had been weaned from bypass the noradrenaline infusion was continued at a dose of 0.2–0.8 μg/kg/minute, sufficient to maintain the systolic blood pressure at 90–100 mmHg. After the operation, clomipramine was withheld and the noradrenaline infusion tapered off, and 3 days later the hypotension had resolved.

The hypotension in this case was severe and refractory to noradrenergic stimulation, perhaps because of the $alpha_1$-adrenoceptor antagonist properties of clomipramine. The fall in systolic blood pressure was accompanied by a paradoxical fall in heart rate, perhaps because the anticholinergic effect of clomipramine removed the effect of vagal tone on the resting heart rate. It seems likely that the hypotensive effect of clomipramine was potentiated by general anesthesia; however, such a reaction is rare and the underlying cardiac problem may have contributed to this severe adverse reaction. This case reinforces current advice that tricyclic antidepressants are best avoided in patients with significant cardiac disease.

Nervous system

Use of the intravenous route is fraught with danger and without any demonstrable advantages.

- A 31-year-old woman who received clomipramine intravenously 300 mg/day developed seizures and cardiac arrest on the 15th day; she was successfully resuscitated (13).

Seizures occurred in four of 50 patients receiving intravenous treatment. Those vulnerable to this complication were not identified in advance by prescreening electroencephalography (14).

Endocrine

Clomipramine has also aroused interest because of an action on prolactin release, which occurs with major tranquillizers but not with other tricyclic antidepressants (15). This action of clomipramine is related to its chemical structure and reflects a greater effect on dopamine metabolism and serotonin uptake compared with other antidepressants.

Sexual function

Delayed or complete abolition of ejaculation is attributed to strong 5-HT re-uptake blockade but perhaps with additional alpha-adrenoceptor-blocking activity (16). Impotence may be due to a ganglionic blocking action.

Four patients taking up to 100 mg/day developed uncontrollable yawning, in three cases (two men and one woman) associated with sexual arousal, in two instances with spontaneous orgasm (17). In all four patients the symptoms disappeared after withdrawal.

References

1. Collins GH. The use of parenteral and oral chlorimipramine (Anafranil) in the treatment of depressive states. Br J Psychiatry 1973;122(567):189–90.
2. Capstick N. Psychiatric side-effects of clomipramine (Anafranil). J Int Med Res 1973;1:444.
3. Rickels K, Weise CC, Csanalosi I, Chung HR, Feldman HS, Rosenfeld H, Whalen EM. Clomipramine and amitriptyline in depressed outpatients. A controlled study. Psychopharmacologia 1974;34(4):361–76.
4. Haqqani MT, Gutteridge DR. Two cases of clomipramine hydrochloride (Anafranil) poisoning. Forensic Sci 1974; 3(1):83–7.
5. Beaumont G. Drug interactions with clomipramine (Anafranil). J Int Med Res 1973;1:480.
6. Yaryura-Tobias JA, Neziroglu F, Bergman L. Chlorimipramine for obsessive-compulsive neurosis: an organic approach. Curr Ther Res 1976;20:541.
7. Silva FR, Wijewickrama HS. Clomipramine in phobic and obsessional states: preliminary report. NZ Med J 1976; 84(567):4–6.
8. Kelly MW, Myers CW. Clomipramine: a tricyclic antidepressant effective in obsessive compulsive disorder. DICP 1990;24(7–8):739–44.
9. Modigh K, Westberg P, Eriksson E. Superiority of clomipramine over imipramine in the treatment of panic disorder: a placebo-controlled trial. J Clin Psychopharmacol 1992; 12(4):251–61.
10. Eikmeier G, Kuhlmann R, Gastpar M. Thrombosis of cerebral veins following intravenous application of clomipramine. J Neurol Neurosurg Psychiatry 1988;51(11):1461.
11. Symes MH. Cardiovascular effects of clomipramine (Anafranil). J Int Med Res 1973;1:460.
12. Malan TP Jr., Nolan PE, Lichtenthal PR, Polson JS, Tebich SL, Bose RK, Copeland JG 3rd. Severe, refractory hypotension during anesthesia in a patient on chronic clomipramine therapy. Anesthesiology 2001;95(1):264–6.
13. Singh G. Cardiac arrest with clomipramine. BMJ 1972; 3(828):698.
14. Dickson J. Neurological and EEG effects of clomipramine (Anafranil). J Int Med Res 1973;1:449.
15. Jones RB, Luscombe DK, Groom GV. Plasma prolactin concentrations in normal subjects and depressive patients following oral clomipramine. Postgrad Med J 1977; 53(Suppl. 4):166–71.
16. Beaumont G. Sexual side-effects of clomipramine (Anafranil). J Int Med Res 1973;1:469.
17. McLean JD, Forsythe RG, Kapkin IA. Unusual side effects of clomipramine associated with yawning. Can J Psychiatry 1983;28(7):569–70.

Clonazepam

See also Benzodiazepines

General Information

Clonazepam is a benzodiazepine that is used predominantly in epilepsy, panic disorder, and mania, and also appears to be effective in relieving antipsychotic drug-induced akathisia (1). The use of clonazepam in psychiatric disorders is complicated by significant drowsiness in a majority of patients, and additional behavioral problems in children (SEDA-19, 34).

Although they are commonly used in the adjunctive management of chronic pain, benzodiazepines are generally not analgesic per se. One exception may be the stabbing/lancinating neuropathic pain that often responds to anticonvulsants, including clonazepam. Nevertheless, the use of benzodiazepines in pain syndromes is generally contraindicated, and clonazepam, although often effective, should be used with caution (SEDA-17, 42). This is because of the availability of other agents with comparable or superior efficacy and the significant incidence of adverse effects of clonazepam, including depression, self-poisoning, cognitive impairment, and dependence (2), as well as the potential for diversion.

Organs and Systems

Nervous system

In controlled trials with clonazepam, adverse events were recorded in 60–90% of cases and led to withdrawal rates as high as 36% (3). The most common effects were drowsiness, ataxia, and behavioral and personality changes. Other problems were hypersalivation, tolerance, and sometimes a paradoxical increase in seizure frequency.

Psychological, psychiatric

The addition of clonazepam to clomipramine has been reported to have caused acute mania (4).

- A 48-year-old Japanese man with a history of bipolar affective disorder became depressed again. He was already taking lithium carbonate 800 mg/day and carbamazepine 800 mg/day. Clomipramine was added, and the dose was increased to 225 mg/day over 2 months and then maintained for 2 months. Because clomipramine had little effect, clonazepam 3 mg/day was added. On the first day after he took clonazepam, symptoms of hyperthymia, haughtiness, talkativeness, and flight of ideas suddenly appeared once more. Drug-induced delirium was excluded, because orientation was not disrupted and the symptoms did not fluctuate over time. Clomipramine and clonazepam were withdrawn. Because the symptoms were similar to the previous manic episode, the same prescription was reinstated, with the addition of sodium valproate 800 mg/day. After 3 months, he was discharged in remission and had no recurrence. He had not taken other benzodiazepines throughout the treatment.

This report suggests that clonazepam induced a switch to mania, possibly in combination with an effect of clomipramine.

Mouth and teeth

A sensation of a burning mouth has been attributed to clonazepam (5).

- A 52-year-old white woman developed a burning mouth. She had previously taken alprazolam for anxiety, but this was changed to clonazepam because of increased anxiety and panic. Clonazepam relieved her symptoms, but after 4 weeks of therapy she continued to have a constant, mild, oral burning sensation. Examination of the mouth was normal and laboratory tests were unremarkable. The dose of clonazepam was reduced and her symptoms abated but remained intolerable. Clonazepam was withdrawn and her symptoms completely resolved. Since no other medications relieved her anxiety and panic she took clonazepam again, but again developed an intolerable burning mouth. Clonazepam was again withdrawn and her symptoms resolved.

Long-Term Effects

Drug withdrawal

Withdrawal effects can be troublesome. Of 13 patients taken off clonazepam at a rate of 0.016–0.5 mg/day because of adverse effects, 8 had withdrawal seizures and five had other withdrawal symptoms (SEDA-19, 63). Choreoathetosis was described in one patient completing withdrawal of clonazepam (SED-13, 152).

- A 43-year-old man underwent an incomplete transcranial removal of a pituitary growth-hormone-secreting macroadenoma (6). His daily insulin dose was reduced from more than 300–104 U/day and he was given hydrocortisone and levothyroxine replacement therapy, together with lanreotide injections. A month after discharge, he was given high-dose clonazepam. Three months later, the clonazepam was withdrawn abruptly and he developed hypoglycemic coma.

The author concluded that interruption of benzodiazepine treatment had caused reduced growth hormone secretion and insulin requirements.

Drug–Drug Interactions

Carbamazepine

The mutual interaction of clonazepam and carbamazepine has been investigated in 183 children and adults with epilepsy during routine clinical care (7). Carbamazepine increased the clearance of clonazepam by 22% and clonazepam reduced the clearance of carbamazepine by 21%.

The effects of concomitant carbamazepine, phenytoin, sodium valproate, and zonisamide on the steady-state serum concentrations of clonazepam have been investigated in 51 epileptic in-patients under 20 years of age (8). Serum concentrations of clonazepam correlated positively with the dose of clonazepam and negatively with the doses of carbamazepine and valproic acid, but not with phenytoin or zonisamide. These results confirm that as the oral doses of carbamazepine and sodium valproate increase, the serum concentration of clonazepam falls, but there is no interaction with either phenytoin or zonisamide. In the case of carbamazepine the mechanism of action is thought to be enzyme induction, increasing the metabolism of clonazepam. It is not known what the mechanism is with sodium valproate. In patients with epilepsy, the co-administration of either sodium valproate or carbamazepine will reduce the serum concentration of clonazepam and increase the risk of a seizure. When clonazepam is used in the treatment of epilepsy, sodium valproate and carbamazepine should be avoided; phenytoin and zonisamide would be safer alternatives.

Phenelzine

A flushing reaction has been associated with an interaction of phenelzine with clonazepam (SEDA-17, 17).

Sertraline

In a randomized, double-blind, placebo-controlled, crossover study in 13 subjects, sertraline did not affect the pharmacokinetics or pharmacodynamics of clonazepam (9).

Valproate

The effects of concomitant carbamazepine, phenytoin, sodium valproate, and zonisamide on the steady-state serum concentrations of clonazepam have been investigated in 51 epileptic in-patients under 20 years of age (8). Serum concentrations of clonazepam correlated positively with the dose of clonazepam and negatively with the doses of carbamazepine and valproic acid, but not with phenytoin or zonisamide. These results confirm that as the oral doses of carbamazepine and sodium valproate increase, the serum concentration of clonazepam falls, but there is no interaction with either phenytoin or zonisamide. In the case of carbamazepine the mechanism of action is thought to be enzyme induction, increasing the metabolism of clonazepam. It is not known what the mechanism is with sodium valproate. In patients with epilepsy, the co-administration of either sodium valproate or carbamazepine will reduce the serum concentration of clonazepam and increase the risk of a seizure. When clonazepam is used in the treatment of epilepsy, sodium valproate and carbamazepine should be avoided; phenytoin and zonisamide would be safer alternatives.

References

1. Lima AR, Weiser KV, Bacaltchuk J, Barnes TR. Anticholinergics for neuroleptic-induced acute akathisia. Cochrane Database Syst Rev 2004;(1):CD003727.
2. Reddy S, Patt RB. The benzodiazepines as adjuvant analgesics. J Pain Symptom Manage 1994;9(8):510–14.

3. Sato S. Clonazepam. In: Levy R, Mattson R, Meldrum B, Penry J, Dreifuss F, editors. Antiepileptic Drugs. 3rd ed. New York: Raven Press, 1989:765.
4. Ikeda M, Fujikawa T, Yanai I, Horiguchi J, Yamawaki S. Clonazepam-induced maniacal reaction in a patient with bipolar disorder. Int Clin Psychopharmacol 1998;13(4):189–90.
5. Culhane NS, Hodle AD. Burning mouth syndrome after taking clonazepam. Ann Pharmacother 2001;35(7–8):874–6.
6. Shuster J. Benzodiazepines and glucose control; mycophenolate mofetil-induced dyshidrotic eczema; concomitant use of bupropion and amantadine causes neurotoxicity; intra-articular steroids and acute adrenal crisis. Hosp Pharm 2000;35:489–91.
7. Yukawa E, Nonaka T, Yukawa M, Ohdo S, Higuchi S, Kuroda T, Goto Y. Pharmacoepidemiologic investigation of a clonazepam–carbamazepine interaction by mixed effect modeling using routine clinical pharmacokinetic data in Japanese patients. J Clin Psychopharmacol 2001;21(6):588–93.
8. Ikawa K, Eshima N, Morikawa N, Kawashima H, Izumi T, Takeyama M. Influence of concomitant anticonvulsants on serum concentrations of clonazepam in epileptic subjects: an age- and dose-effect linear regression model analysis. Pharm Pharmacol Commun 1999;5:307–10.
9. Bonate PL, Kroboth PD, Smith RB, Suarez E, Oo C. Clonazepam and sertraline: absence of drug interaction in a multiple-dose study. J Clin Psychopharmacol 2000; 20(1):19–27.

Clonidine and apraclonidine

General Information

The presynaptic alpha-adrenoceptor agonists, particularly methyldopa and clonidine, are agonists at presynaptic alpha$_2$-adrenoceptors. Guanabenz, guanfacine, and tiamenidine appear to be qualitatively similar to clonidine; clear evidence of quantitative differences remains to be confirmed.

The mechanism of action of these drugs depends on reducing sympathetic nervous outflow from the nervous system by interference with regulatory neurotransmitter systems in the brainstem. Because none of the drugs was selective or specific for circulatory control systems, the hypotensive effects were invariably accompanied by other nervous system effects. However, the identification of imidazoline receptors has suggested that it may be possible to develop drugs, such as moxonidine and relminidine, with greater selectivity for circulatory control mechanisms and a reduced likelihood of unwanted nervous system depressant effects (1).

Clonidine has been used to treat hypertension and migraine. It ameliorates the opioid withdrawal syndrome by reducing central noradrenergic activity. Its role in the treatment of psychiatric disorders has been the subject of an extensive review, but without new information on its safety (2). Clonidine is also used epidurally, in combination with opioids, neostigmine, and anesthetic and analgesic agents, to produce segmental analgesia, particularly for postoperative relief of pain after obstetrical and surgical procedures.

The use of clonidine in children has been comprehensively reviewed (3,4).

Apraclonidine (*para*-aminoclonidine) is a relatively non-specific alpha$_1$- and alpha$_2$-adrenoceptor agonist, which is less likely to cross the blood–brain barrier than clonidine. Apraclonidine suppresses aqueous humor flow by 39–44% and lowers intraocular pressure by 20–23% (5).

Organs and Systems

Cardiovascular

Clonidine causes sinus bradycardia and atrioventricular block, as illustrated by two cases, one a 10-year-old boy (6) and the other a 71-year-old woman (7), who developed Wenckebach's phenomenon. Clonidine was also studied in seven patients subjected to electrophysiological studies after 5 weeks of therapy (8). It slowed the sinus rate and increased the atrial pacing rate, producing Wenckebach's phenomenon, indicating depressed function of the sinus and AV nodes.

In three patients with chronic schizophrenia and primary polydipsia given clonidine in doses of up to 800 micrograms/day for 2–5 months, blood pressure and pulse fell significantly in a dose-dependent manner, but fluid intake, as assessed by measurements of weight and 24-hour urine volume, was not affected (9). Hypotension and bradycardia limited the extent to which the dose of clonidine could be increased. The lack of effect of clonidine on polydipsia in this small sample and the inconsistent results of two other recent studies have provided little overall support for using clonidine to treat primary polydipsia associated with schizophrenia.

Clonidine-induced hypertension has been reported in a patient with autonomic dysfunction (10).

- A 39-year-old quadriplegic man with poorly controlled pain had many features consistent with autonomic dysfunction (for example a C4 spinal lesion, orthostatic hypotension, hypertension). He routinely used transdermal clonidine and transdermal glyceryl trinitrate as needed for control of acute hypertensive episodes. The clonidine was discontinued, after which his blood pressure fell (maximum systolic and diastolic pressures by about 50 and 25 mmHg respectively).

Because clonidine relies on central alpha$_2$-adrenoceptor agonist activity for its hypotensive effects, it can cause hypertension in patients with autonomic dysfunction. It should therefore be used with great caution when autonomic dysfunction is suspected.

The effect of intrathecal clonidine has been evaluated in a prospective randomized study in 45 children aged 6–15 years, who were randomized to receive either 0.5% hyperbaric bupivacaine or 0.5% hyperbaric bupivacaine plus clonidine 2 micrograms/kg (11). Clonidine was associated with non-significant prolongation of motor block, from an average of 150–190 minutes. Postoperative analgesia was significantly longer with clonidine (490 versus 200 minutes). Clonidine was associated with higher incidences of hypotension (54 versus 36%) and bradycardia (30 versus 0%).

Respiratory

The effects of clonidine and other alpha$_2$-adrenoceptor agonists on respiratory function in asthmatics have been reviewed (12). Inhaled alpha$_2$-adrenoceptor agonists reduce the bronchial response to allergens, and if ingested they can aggravate the bronchial response to histamine.

Nervous system

Treatment with centrally acting agents is characterized by a relatively high incidence (up to 60% in some studies) of nervous system depressant effects (dizziness, drowsiness, tiredness, dry mouth, headache, depression), particularly during the initial period of treatment or after dosage increments. Sedation, lethargy, and tiredness are common with clonidine, particularly at the start of treatment (13).

In a placebo-controlled study of a single oral dose of clonidine 0.25–3 mg in 18 healthy men aged 18–21 years, clonidine caused more sleepiness than placebo; it significantly reduced stage 1 and rapid-eye-movement (REM) sleep and increased stage 2 sleep (14).

Clonidine 300 micrograms was given orally to 30 patients 60 minutes before intrathecal anesthesia with lidocaine 40 mg or 80 mg, and 60 other patients received either plain lidocaine 100 mg or lidocaine 40 mg or 80 mg with clonidine 100 micrograms intrathecally (15). Clonidine, both intrathecally and orally, prolonged the duration of spinal block and allowed a reduction in the dose of lidocaine needed for a given duration of block, but prolongation of motor block, exceeding the duration of sensory block, was a drawback with both routes and doses of clonidine. The smallest hemodynamic changes were seen with lidocaine 40 mg + clonidine 100 micrograms intrathecally, which provided adequate anesthesia for operations lasting up to 140 minutes. All doses of clonidine caused sedation.

Endocrine

Clonidine stimulates the release of growth hormone and has been used as a provocation test of growth hormone reserve (16).

Clonidine reduces plasma renin activity and urinary aldosterone and catecholamine concentrations (17).

Mouth

Dry mouth is common with clonidine, and investigation of the mechanism has come from an experimental study in which the direct effect of clonidine on salivary amylase excretion from rat parotid dispersed cells was measured in vitro (18). Clonidine stimulated calcium influx into the cells and inhibited postsynaptic alpha$_1$-adrenoceptor responses.

Gastrointestinal

Constipation is frequent with clonidine, and one case of pseudo-obstruction of the bowel has been reported (19).

Urinary tract

Epidural clonidine is less likely to produce urinary retention than epidural opioids (20,21).

Skin

Rashes occur in about 4% of patients taking clonidine (22).

Transdermal clonidine formulated in adhesive skin patches has been used for long-term treatment with once-weekly application. When transdermal clonidine is used to lower blood pressure systemic adverse effects seem to be fewer than with oral clonidine (23). However, localized skin reactions are common, and the incidence increases with the dose and duration of use. Common signs include erythema, scaling, vesiculation, excoriation, and induration. Allergic contact dermatitis is less frequent but still common. Hyperpigmentation and depigmentation also occur. Pretreatment with 0.5% hydrocortisone is associated with less skin irritation and higher blood concentrations.

Immunologic

During long-term treatment of glaucoma with apraclonidine allergic reactions can occur. In a retrospective analysis of 64 patients who used apraclonidine 1% for more than 2 weeks, 31 (48%) developed an allergic reaction that led to withdrawal of treatment, with a mean latency of 4.7 months (24). Those who had allergic reactions tended to be older and female.

- A 46-year-old woman, who took clonidine 25 mg bd for menopausal flushing, developed depigmentation and swelling of her forearms (25). A skin biopsy showed a pattern consistent with immune complex disease, with IgG, IgM, Clq, C2c, and C4 complement between muscle fibers and at the dermo-epidermal junctions. All of these abnormalities disappeared after withdrawal.

Long-Term Effects

Drug tolerance

During long-term treatment of glaucoma, apraclonidine 0.5% is effective in reducing intraocular pressure, both in the short term and for up to 24 months. However, efficacy is lost in some patients. Of 174 patients followed for up to 24 months apraclonidine was ineffective in 38 patients (21%), at some point during the study (26).

Drug withdrawal

A withdrawal syndrome with marked rebound hypertension (attributed to increased sympathetic nervous activity as a result of drug-modified receptor responses) is an occasional but well-recognized complication of the abrupt withdrawal of alpha$_2$-adrenoceptor agonists, particularly with clonidine. In its most florid form, the clonidine withdrawal syndrome is characterized by a pronounced increase in blood pressure, tachycardia, tremulousness, and sweating (27). There is an associated marked increase in catecholamine output and the features are reminiscent of pheochromocytoma or accelerated hypertension. Milder cases can pass unnoticed, unless the patient is being carefully monitored. The syndrome begins within 48 hours of withdrawal, and although the exact incidence is unknown it is more likely if the patient has been taking a high dosage. There has even been a case report of rebound hypertension in association with transdermal clonidine (28). Treatment is by combined alpha- and beta-blockade, and it is important to avoid monotherapy with a beta-blocker, since this may exacerbate the syndrome by promoting unopposed alpha-adrenergic effects.

There have been two case reports of other serious complications arising from the acute withdrawal of clonidine. Neuropsychiatric disturbance with self-injury occurred in a child (29) and myocardial infarction developed in a patient with no history of ischemic heart disease (30).

Drug Administration

Drug formulations

Transdermal clonidine (clonidine TTS) has been used with some success for the treatment of mild hypertension. Systemic adverse effects are similar to those seen after oral administration, but are less frequent and milder. They include dry mouth, drowsiness, headache, sexual disturbance, cold extremities, obstipation, and fatigue (31–33). These adverse effects rarely necessitate withdrawal of clonidine TTS.

A high percentage of patients who take clonidine (up to 38%) (34) develop contact allergic reactions, usually due to the active ingredient, at the patch application site (35). This has been reported with a frequency of 15% in 357 African–American hypertensive patients. It can lead to drug discontinuation in 4.2% of patients.

Recurrent maculopapular rash due to both topical and systemic administration of clonidine has been reported (36).

- A 47-year-old woman was given transdermal, oral, and intravenous clonidine at different times, separated by several months. The patches were withdrawn after 2 months because of pruritic erythematous vesiculation at the site of application. Oral clonidine (0.3 mg/day) had to be withdrawn when a generalized maculopapular rash appeared on the third day, and was promptly exacerbated by each dose. Intravenous clonidine 0.150 mg was followed within 30 minutes by a severe, generalized, maculopapular reaction requiring systemic steroids and antihistamines.

The authors interpreted these reactions as being allergic. A patch test was very positive to the commercial formulation. Clonidine is a weak sensitizer, but occlusion and prolonged skin contact during transdermal application can cause delayed hypersensitivity.

Drug administration route

The most common ocular adverse effects of topical apraclonidine are conjunctival hyperemia, itching, foreign body sensation, and lacrimation. The most frequent systemic adverse effects are dry mouth and unusual taste perception (37–39). With *para*-aminoclonidine, headaches, attributable to ocular vasoconstriction, as well as anxiety, vomiting, dry mouth, tremor, and pallor, have been reported (40).

Drug overdose

The effects of exposure to clonidine hydrochloride in children, as reported to US poison centers from 1993 to 1999, have been retrospectively reviewed (41). There were 10 060 reported exposures, of which 57% were in children under 6 years, 34% in children aged 6–12 years, and 9% in adolescents aged 13–18 years. In 1999 there were 2.5 times as many exposures as in 1993. Clonidine was the child's medication in 10% of those under 6 years, 35% of those aged 6–12 years, and 26% of the adolescents. Unintentional overdose was most common in those under 6 years, while therapeutic errors and suicide attempts predominated in those aged 6–12-years and the adolescents. In 6042 symptomatic children (60%), the most common symptoms were lethargy (80%), bradycardia (17%), hypotension (15%), and respiratory depression (5%). Most of the exposures resulted in no effect (40%) or minor effects (39%). There were moderate effects in 1907 children (19%), major effects in 230 (2%), and one death in a 23-month-old child.

- A hypertensive crisis and myocardial infarction occurred in a 62-year-old woman after a combined injection of hydromorphone 48 mg and clonidine 12 mg subcutaneously in an attempt to refill an implanted epidural infusion pump (42). She was immediately treated with naloxone, but she subsequently had accelerated hypertension, a brief tonic-clonic seizure, and an anteroseptal myocardial infarction. Cardiac catheterization showed no coronary narrowing or blockage, but an anterior infarct was confirmed.

It is believed that the reaction was secondary to the vasoconstricting effects of high-dose clonidine through stimulation of peripheral alpha-adrenoceptors.

Drug–Drug Interactions

Mianserin

Mianserin has alpha-adrenoceptor activity and so might interact with clonidine (43). In healthy volunteers, pretreatment with mianserin 60 mg/day for 3 days did not modify the hypotensive effects of a single 300 mg dose of clonidine. In 11 patients with essential hypertension, the addition of mianserin 60 mg/day (in divided doses) for 2 weeks did not reduce the hypotensive effect of clonidine. The results of this study appear to have justified the authors' conclusion that adding mianserin to treatment with clonidine will not result in loss of blood pressure control.

Mirtazapine

Hypertension has been reported with mirtazapine plus clonidine (44).

- A 20-year-old man had had Goodpasture's syndrome for 2.5 years, end-stage renal disease on chronic hemodialysis for 15 months, and hypertension controlled with metoprolol, losartan, and clonidine. He developed dyspnea and hypertension (blood pressure 178/115 mmHg) 2 weeks after his psychiatrist first gave him mirtazapine 15 mg at bedtime to treat depression. His blood pressure did not fall significantly, despite the addition of losartan and minoxidil and the use of intravenous glyceryl trinitrate and labetalol. Only after emergency dialysis and intravenous nitroprusside did his blood pressure fall to 150–180/80–100 mmHg. When mirtazapine was withdrawn, his blood pressure was controlled with minoxidil 5 mg, clonidine 0.1 mg, and metoprolol 10 mg, all bd.

The authors recognized that mirtazapine alone could have caused the hypertensive event. In postmarketing surveillance of mirtazapine, hypertension occurred in at least 1% of patients. However, it is likely that the patient lost antihypertensive control because mirtazapine antagonized the antihypertensive effect of clonidine. Mirtazapine, a tetracyclic antidepressant, stimulates the noradrenergic system through antagonism at central $alpha_2$ inhibitory receptors, which is precisely opposite to the effect of clonidine.

Neostigmine

Clonidine increases the analgesic effect of intrathecal neostigmine without enhancing its adverse effects (45).

References

1. Webster J, Koch HF. Aspects of tolerability of centrally acting antihypertensive drugs. J Cardiovasc Pharmacol 1996;27(Suppl 3):S49–54.
2. Ahmed I, Takeshita J. Clonidine: a critical review of its role in the treatment of psychiatric disorders. Drug Ther 1996;6:53–70.
3. Dollery CT. Advantages and disadvantages of alpha-adrenoceptor agonists for systemic hypertension. Am J Cardiol 1988;61(7):D1–5.
4. Nishina K, Mikawa K, Shiga M, Obara H. Clonidine in paediatric anaesthesia. Paediatr Anaesth 1999;9(3):187–202.
5. Schadlu R, Maus TL, Nau CB, Brubaker RF. Comparison of the efficacy of apraclonidine and brimonidine as aqueous suppressants in humans. Arch Ophthalmol 1998;116(11):1441–4.
6. Dawson PM, Vander Zanden JA, Werkman SL, Washington RL, Tyma TA. Cardiac dysrhythmia with the use of clonidine in explosive disorder. DICP 1989;23(6):465–6.
7. Marini M, Cavani E, Abbatangelo R, Mascelloni R. Periodismo di Luciani Wenckeback e clonidina. Presentazione di un caso. [Luciani-Wenckeback period and clonidine. Presentation of a case.] Clin Ter 1988;126(4):273–6.
8. Roden DM, Nadeau JH, Primm RK. Electrophysiologic and hemodynamic effects of chronic oral therapy with the alpha-agonists clonidine and tiamenidine in hypertensive volunteers. Clin Pharmacol Ther 1988; 43(6):648–54.
9. Delva NJ, Chang A, Hawken ER, Lawson JS, Owen JA. Effects of clonidine in schizophrenic patients with primary polydipsia: three single case studies. Prog Neuropsychopharmacol Biol Psychiatry 2002;26(2):387–92.
10. Backo AL, Clause SL, Triller DM, Gibbs KA. Clonidine-induced hypertension in a patient with a spinal lesion. Ann Pharmacother 2002;36(9):1396–8.
11. Kaabachi O, Ben Rajeb A, Mebazaa M, Safi H, Jelel C, Ben Ghachem M, Ben Ammar M. La rachianesthésie chez l'enfant: étude comparative de la bupivacaïne hyperbare avec et sans clonidine. [Spinal anesthesia in children: comparative study of hyperbaric bupivacaine with or without clonidine.] Ann Fr Anesth Reanim 2002;21(8):617–21.
12. Rosen B, Ovsyshcher IA, Zimlichman R. Complete atrioventricular block induced by methyldopa. Pacing Clin Electrophysiol 1988;11(11 Pt 1):1555–8.
13. Schmitt H, Schwartz J, Blanchot P, Fritel D, Froment A, Traeger J. Expérience française de la clonidine. Nouv Presse Méd 1972;1:877.
14. Carskadon MA, Cavallo A, Rosekind MR. Sleepiness and nap sleep following a morning dose of clonidine. Sleep 1989;(4):338–44.
15. Dobrydnjov I, Samarutel J. Enhancement of intrathecal lidocaine by addition of local and systemic clonidine. Acta Anaesthesiol Scand 1999;43(5):556–62.
16. Morris AH, Harrington MH, Churchill DL, Olshan JS. Growth hormone stimulation testing with oral clonidine: 90 minutes is the preferred duration for the assessment of growth hormone reserve. J Pediatr Endocrinol Metab 2001;14(9):1657–60.
17. Houston MC. Clonidine hydrochloride. South Med J 1982;75(6):713–19.
18. Yamada K, Tanaka K, Aoki M, Banno A, Nakagawa S, Yamaguchi M, Togari A, Matsumoto S. Effect of clonidine on amylase secretion from rat parotid gland. Asia Pacific J Pharmacol 1996;11:19–24.
19. Kellaway GS. Adverse drug reactions during treatment of hypertension. Drugs 1976;11(Suppl 1):91–9.
20. Gentili M, Bonnet F. Spinal clonidine produces less urinary retention than spinal morphine. Br J Anaesth 1996;76(6):872–3.
21. Batra YK, Gill PK, Vaidyanathan S, Aggarwal A. Effect of epidural buprenorphine and clonidine on vesical functions in women. Int J Clin Pharmacol Ther 1996;34(7): 309–11.
22. Onesti G, Bock KD, Heimsoth V, Kim KE, Merguet P. Clonidine: a new antihypertensive agent. Am J Cardiol 1971;28(1):74–83.
23. Prisant LM. Transdermal clonidine skin reactions. J Clin Hypertens (Greenwich) 2002;4(2):136–8.
24. Butler P, Mannschreck M, Lin S, Hwang I, Alvarado J. Clinical experience with the long-term use of 1% apraclonidine. Incidence of allergic reactions. Arch Ophthalmol 1995;113(3):293–6.
25. Petersen HH, Hansen M, Albrectsen JM. Clonidine-induced immune complex disease. Acta Dermatol Venereol 1989;69(6):519–20.
26. Gross RL, Pinyero A, Orengo-Nania S. Clinical experience with apraclonidine 0.5%. J Glaucoma 1997;6(5):298–302.
27. Hansson L, Hunyor SN, Julius S, Hoobler SW. Blood pressure crisis following withdrawal of clonidine (Catapres, Catapresan), with special reference to arterial and urinary catecholamine levels, and suggestions for acute management. Am Heart J 1973;85(5):605–10.
28. Schmidt GR, Schuna AA. Rebound hypertension after discontinuation of transdermal clonidine. Clin Pharm 1988;7(10):772–4.
29. Dillon JE. Self-injurious behavior associated with clonidine withdrawal in a child with Tourette's disorder. J Child Neurol 1990;5(4):308–10.
30. Berge KH, Lanier WL. Myocardial infarction accompanying acute clonidine withdrawal in a patient without a history of ischemic coronary artery disease. Anesth Analg 1991;72(2):259–61.
31. Weber MA, Drayer JI, Brewer DD, Lipson JL. Transdermal continuous antihypertensive therapy. Lancet 1984;1(8367):9–11.
32. Groth H, Vetter H, Knusel J, Boerlin HJ, Walger P, Baumgart P, Wehling M, Siegenthaler W, Vetter W. Clonidin-TTS bei essentieller Hypertonie: Wirkung und Vertr äglichkeit. [Clonidine transdermal therapeutic system in essential hypertension: effect and tolerance.] Schweiz Med Wochenschr 1983;113(49):1841–5.
33. Olivari MT, Cohn JN. Cutaneous administration of nitroglycerin: a review. Pharmacotherapy 1983;3(3):149–57.

34. Carmichael AJ. Skin sensitivity and transdermal drug delivery. A review of the problem. Drug Saf 1994;10(2):151–9.
35. Dias VC, Tendler B, Oparil S, Reilly PA, Snarr P, White WB. Clinical experience with transdermal clonidine in African–American and Hispanic–American patients with hypertension: evaluation from a 12-week prospective, open-label clinical trial in community-based clinics. Am J Ther 1999;6(1):19–24.
36. Crivellaro MA, Bonadonna P, Dama A, Senna G, Passalacqua G. Skin reactions to clonidine: not just a local problem. Case report. Allergol Immunopathol (Madr) 1999;27(6):318–19.
37. Araujo SV, Bond JB, Wilson RP, Moster MR, Schmidt CM Jr, Spaeth GL. Long term effect of apraclonidine. Br J Ophthalmol 1995;79(12):1098–101.
38. Robin AL, Ritch R, Shin D, Smythe B, Mundorf T, Lehmann RP. Topical apraclonidine hydrochloride in eyes with poorly controlled glaucoma. The Apraclonidine Maximum Tolerated Medical Therapy Study Group. Trans Am Ophthalmol Soc 1995;93:421–41.
39. Robin AL, Ritch R, Shin DH, Smythe B, Mundorf T, Lehmann RP. Short-term efficacy of apraclonidine hydrochloride added to maximum-tolerated medical therapy for glaucoma. Apraclonidine Maximum-Tolerated Medical Therapy Study Group. Am J Ophthalmol 1995; 120(4):423–32.
40. Abrams DA, Robin AL, Pollack IP, deFaller JM, DeSantis L. The safety and efficacy of topical 1% ALO 2145 (p-aminoclonidine hydrochloride) in normal volunteers. Arch Ophthalmol 1987;105(9):1205–7.
41. Klein-Schwartz W. Trends and toxic effects from pediatric clonidine exposures. Arch Pediatr Adolesc Med 2002; 156(4):392–6.
42. Frye CB, Vance MA. Hypertensive crisis and myocardial infarction following massive clonidine overdose. Ann Pharmacother 2000;34(5):611–5.
43. Elliott HL, Whiting B, Reid JL. Assessment of the interaction between mianserin and centrally-acting antihypertensive drugs. Br J Clin Pharmacol 1983;15(Suppl 2):S323–8.
44. Abo-Zena RA, Bobek MB, Dweik RA. Hypertensive urgency induced by an interaction of mirtazapine and clonidine. Pharmacotherapy 2000;20(4):476–8.
45. Hood DD, Mallak KA, Eisenach JC, Tong C. Interaction between intrathecal neostigmine and epidural clonidine in human volunteers. Anesthesiology 1996; 85(2):315–25.

Clopidogrel

General Information

Clopidogrel is a thienopyridine compound, structurally related to ticlopidine, which inhibits ADP-induced platelet aggregation (1). Its efficacy in stroke, myocardial infarction, and other vascular causes of death has been demonstrated in the CAPRIE Study (2), a large trial in which 9599 patients were treated with clopidogrel. The most frequent adverse effects were gastrointestinal symptoms, although they were not significantly more frequent than with aspirin. Bleeding disorders were as common with clopidogrel as with aspirin (9.3% with each). More patients withdrew from treatment because of rashes from clopidogrel (0.9%) than from aspirin (0.4%). Neutropenia and thrombocytopenia occurred very rarely and with similar rates in the two groups.

The adverse effects of clopidogrel have been reviewed (3).

Organs and Systems

Hematologic

During active surveillance by medical directors of blood banks, hematologists, and the manufacturers of clopidogrel, 11 patients were identified in whom thrombotic thrombocytopenic purpura developed during or soon after treatment with clopidogrel (4). Of these 11 patients, 10 had taken clopidogrel for 14 days or less before the onset. From this study it is not possible to calculate the frequency of thrombotic thrombocytopenic purpura, since the size of the population from which the 11 cases were drawn is unknown.

- Fatal aplastic anemia has been reported in two patients taking clopidogrel (5,6). Aplastic anemia was diagnosed 5 months after starting clopidogrel in the first patient and after 3 months in the second. Both died from infection (sepsis and pneumonia). Except for allopurinol in the first case, these patients did not take any medications associated with aplastic anemia.

Major bleeding is uncommon with clopidogrel. In a randomized, double-blind, placebo-controlled, 18-month study of the effects of aspirin 75 mg/day in 7599 high-risk patients with recent ischemic stroke or transient ischemic attacks and at least one additional vascular risk factor who were already taking clopidogrel 75 mg/day, life-threatening bleeding was more common in the group who took aspirin and clopidogrel compared with clopidogrel alone: 96 (2.6%) versus 49 (1.3%); absolute risk increase 1.3% (95% CI 0.6, 1.9) (7). Episodes of major bleeding were also more common in those taking aspirin plus clopidogrel, but there was no difference in mortality.

Acquired autoimmune hemophilia has been attributed to clopidogrel (8).

Skin

Clopidogrel can cause pruritus and urticaria (9).

Immunologic

A severe allergic reaction has been associated with clopidogrel (10).

- A 57-year-old man took clopidogrel after a myocardial infarction and after 5 days developed a fever, rash, pruritus, and abdominal pain. Three days later he developed shock. He had thrombocytopenia, lymphopenia, aseptic leukocyturia, and raised serum activities of transaminases, amylase, and gamma-glutamyl transpeptidase. Blood cultures were negative. Clopidogrel was withdrawn and within 1 week he had completely recovered and all blood tests had returned to normal. One month later, he took clopidogrel again; 4 hours later the same symptoms reappeared, with aseptic leukocyturia and raised transaminases and gamma-glutamyl transpeptidase. Drug allergy was suspected and clopidogrel was withdrawn. All the symptoms disappeared within a few days and did not recur during the following year.

It is highly probable that this reaction was provoked by clopidogrel because of the positive rechallenge and because the patient did not take any other drug.

References

1. Coukell AJ, Markham A. Clopidogrel. Drugs 1997;54(5):745–50.
2. CAPRIE Steering Committee. A randomised, blinded, trial of clopidogrel versus aspirin in patients at risk of ischaemic events (CAPRIE). Lancet 1996;348(9038):1329–39.
3. Sharis PJ, Cannon CP, Loscalzo J. The antiplatelet effects of ticlopidine and clopidogrel. Ann Intern Med 1998;129(5):394–405.
4. Bennett CL, Connors JM, Carwile JM, Moake JL, Bell WR, Tarantolo SR, McCarthy LJ, Sarode R, Hatfield AJ, Feldman MD, Davidson CJ, Tsai HM. Thrombotic thrombocytopenic purpura associated with clopidogrel. N Engl J Med 2000;342(24):1773–7.
5. Trivier JM, Caron J, Mahieu M, Cambier N, Rose C. Fatal aplastic anaemia associated with clopidogrel. Lancet 2001;357(9254):446.
6. Meyer B, Staudinger T, Lechner K. Clopidogrel and aplastic anaemia. Lancet 2001;357(9266):1446–7.
7. Diener HC, Bogousslavsky J, Brass LM, Cimminiello C, Csiba L, Kaste M, Leys D, Matias-Guiu J, Rupprecht HJ; MATCH investigators. Aspirin and clopidogrel compared with clopidogrel alone after recent ischaemic stroke or transient ischaemic attack in high-risk patients (MATCH): randomised, double-blind, placebo-controlled trial. Lancet 2004;364(9431):331–7.
8. Haj M, Dasani H, Kundu S, Mohite U, Collins PW. Acquired haemophilia A may be associated with clopidogrel. BMJ 2004;329(7461):323.
9. Khambekar SK, Kovac J, Gershlick AH. Clopidogrel induced urticarial rash in a patient with left main stem percutaneous coronary intervention: management issues. Heart 2004;90(3):e14.
10. Sarrot-Reynauld F, Bouillet L, Bourrain JL. Severe hypersensitivity associated with clopidogrel. Ann Intern Med 2001;135(4):305–6.

Clortermine hydrochloride

See also Anorectic drugs

General Information

Clortermine, an alpha-dimethylphenethylamine chlorine derivative, suppresses food-reinforced behavior without concomitant stimulation or depression of the central nervous system. Headache was the main characteristic complaint in 49 obese people taking clortermine 50 mg/day; in four subjects it was severe enough to stop treatment. In all cases, the complaints were drug-related and not placebo-related (SED-9, 17) (1).

Reference

1. Mizrahi A. Drug profile: Voranil (clortermine). J Int Med Res 1974;2:317.

Clotiapine

See also Neuroleptic drugs

General Information

Clotiapine is a dibenzothiazepine neuroleptic drug.

Organs and Systems

Pancreas

Pancreatitis has been attributed to clotiapine (1).

- A 49-year-old woman started to take clotiapine 200 mg/day for a severe psychotic episode. On the second day, she complained of abdominal pain and nausea, followed by vomiting. Increased activities of serum amylase (1490 U/ml), serum lipase (3855 U/ml), and urinary amylase (3417 U/ml) suggested pancreatitis. There was no evidence of gallstones or tumor. She was given perphenazine instead, and her amylase and lipase activities fell to normal. Six months later, when she had a psychotic relapse, she was again treated with clotiapine and 2 days later had a rapid rise in amylase activity (887 U/ml). When switched to perphenazine, she had new peaks in amylase and lipase. A year later, her amylase and lipase were normal and her psychiatric disorder was stabilized with pimozide.

Reference

1. Francobandiera G, Rondalli G, Telattin P. Acute pancreatitis associated with clothiapine use. Hum Psychopharmacol Clin Exp 1999;14:211–12.

Cloximate

General Information

Cloximate is approved in only a few countries, so experience with its use is limited. The usual adverse effects of NSAIDs (headache, insomnia, drowsiness, anorexia, gastrointestinal symptoms, a transient increase in blood urea, leukopenia, thrombocytopenia, and rashes) have been reported (1).

Reference

1. Kolarz G, Lieni KS, Richel H, Scherak O. Doppelblindstudie zwischen Indometacin und Cloximat, einem neuen nichtsteroidalen Anti-rheumatikum. Therapiewoche 1979; 29:5898.

Clozapine

See also Neuroleptic drugs

General Information

Clozapine is a dibenzodiazepine, an atypical neuroleptic drug with a high affinity for dopamine D_4 receptors and a low affinity for other subtypes (1). It is also an antagonist at alpha-adrenoceptors, 5-HT_{2A} receptors, muscarinic receptors, and histamine H_1 receptors.

Observational studies

Rates of hospitalization with clozapine have been analysed by Novartis, the manufacturers, based on two retrospective studies of hospitalization among patients with treatment-resistant schizophrenia (2). All the patients who began clozapine treatment in Texas State psychiatric facilities during the early 1990s ($n = 299$) were compared with controls who received traditional neuroleptic drugs ($n = 223$), matched for severity, age, and sex. More patients in the latter group required continuous hospitalization: at 4 years, four times as many patients taking a traditional medication had a 6-month period of continuous hospitalization.

In a study in Ohio, patients with chronic borderline personality disorder who were in hospital for an average of 110 days/year were given clozapine (mean daily dosage at time of discharge 334 mg; range 175–550 mg) (3). None stopped taking clozapine and few adverse effects were reported. Among the seven patients who were taking clozapine when they were discharged, hospitalization fell to a mean of 6.3 days per patient per year. There was no control group in this study.

- Of 10 adolescent inpatients (aged 12–17 years) with severe acute manic or mixed episodes, who did not improve after treatment with conventional drugs and who were given clozapine (mean dose 143 mg/day), all responded positively after 15–28 days and adverse effects (increased appetite, sedation, enuresis, sialorrhea) were frequent but not severe enough to require reduced dosages (4). Mean weight gain after 6 months was 7 kg (11%), and neither reduced white cell counts nor epileptic seizures were reported during follow-up for 12–24 months.

In a case series in which clozapine was used as add-on medication, two patients with bipolar disorder and one with schizoaffective disorder had marked reductions in affective symptoms after clozapine had been added to pretreatment with a mood stabilizer; transient and moderate weight gain and fatigue were the only adverse effects (5).

In a retrospective open study of 46 patients taking clozapine for 4 years, clozapine had to be discontinued in 10 patients (21%) and serious adverse effects were rare; no patient had agranulocytosis (6). The most troublesome adverse effects were drooling, sedation, and weight gain, and three patients had seizures.

Experiences in uncontrolled open studies in Chinese patients have been summarized (7). The most common adverse effect of clozapine was hypersalivation, followed by sedation. Mandatory blood monitoring is considered an obstacle in persuading some patients to undergo a trial of clozapine, mainly for cultural reasons, summed up by the Chinese proverb that "a hundred grains of rice make a drop of blood."

Clozapine has been used in some special groups of patients, including patients with severe borderline personality disorder (8), patients with aggressive schizophrenia (9), and mentally retarded adults (10).

Of 12 in-patients with borderline personality disorder treated with clozapine for 16 weeks, 10 developed sedation, which disappeared during the first month of treatment; 9 had hypersialorrhea, and 6 had falls in white blood cell counts, which never reached unsafe values.

Patients with aggressive schizophrenia ($n = 29$) improved when treated with clozapine; one was withdrawn after the development of leukopenia. In 10 mentally retarded patients taking clozapine for 15 days to 46 months improvement was observed. Half of the patients developed sedation and hypersalivation, and one discontinued the drug after 2 weeks because of neutropenia. The putative neurotoxicity of clozapine in moderately to profoundly retarded patients (that is, those with an accentuation of cognitive deficits due to the drug's anticholinergic and sedating properties) was not observed. Fifty special hospitalized patients with schizophrenia associated with serious violence were treated with clozapine (mean dose at 2 years 465 mg) (11). The most frequent adverse effects were hypersalivation ($n = 14$), sedation ($n = 10$), and weight gain ($n = 6$); two patients had tonic-clonic seizures, two others developed mild neutropenia, and in one case treatment was stopped owing to agranulocytosis.

In a retrospective review, 33 mentally retarded patients were evaluated; adverse effects were mild and transient, constipation being the most common ($n = 10$) (12). There were no significant cardiovascular adverse effects and no seizures; no patient discontinued treatment because of agranulocytosis. Small sample sizes, short durations of treatment, and lack of controls in these studies preclude definite conclusions.

A 37-item survey covering a variety of somatopsychic domains has been administered to 130 patients with schizophrenia taking a stable clozapine regimen (mean dose 464 mg/day; mean duration 34 months) (13). Most of them reported an improvement in their level of satisfaction, quality of life, compliance with treatment, thinking, mood, and alertness. Most reported worse nocturnal salivation (88%); weight gain (35%) came second; fewer patients reported a worsening of various gastrointestinal and urinary symptoms.

Clinical predictors of response have been examined in 37 partially treatment-refractory outpatients who had been assigned to clozapine in a double-blind, haloperidol-controlled, long-term (29-week) study (14). Clozapine responders were rated as less severely ill, had fewer negative symptoms, and had fewer extrapyramidal adverse effects at baseline compared with non-responders.

Combination therapy

Of 656 Danish patients who were taking clozapine, 35% were taking concomitant neuroleptic drugs, 28% benzodiazepines, 19% anticholinergic drugs, 11% antidepressants, 8% antiepileptic drugs, and 2% lithium (15). The rationale for supplementing clozapine treatment in refractory schizophrenia in this way has been thoroughly reviewed following a bibliographic search covering 1978–1998 (16). In all, 70 articles were retrieved but only a few were controlled studies, most being case reports/series. Among the many possible drug combinations, the evidence suggests that clozapine plus sulpiride is the most efficacious combination. The combined use of benzodiazepines and clozapine can cause cardiorespiratory collapse; valproate can cause hepatic dysfunction and more so with clozapine; lithium can cause neurotoxicity and seizures and more so with clozapine; and at least some serotonin reuptake inhibitors (SSRIs) appear to raise plasma clozapine concentrations to above the usual target range.

Organs and Systems

Cardiovascular

Clozapine has been associated with cardiomyopathy (SED-14, 142) (SEDA-21, 52) (17), changes in blood pressure (SEDA-21, 52) (SEDA-21, 52) (SEDA-22, 57) (18,19), electrocardiographic changes (SEDA-22, 57) (20–22), and venous thromboembolism (SEDA-20, 47).

Hypertension

Several cases of hypertension have been associated with clozapine (SEDA-22, 57), and alpha$_2$-adrenoceptor blockade has been proposed as a possible mechanism (18). Four patients developed pseudopheochromocytoma syndrome associated with clozapine (23); all had hypertension, profuse sweating, and obesity. The authors suggested that clozapine could increase plasma noradrenaline concentrations by inhibiting presynaptic reuptake mediated by alpha$_2$-adrenoceptors.

Hypotension

Hypotension is the most commonly observed cardiovascular adverse effect of neuroleptic drugs, particularly after administration of those that are also potent alpha-adrenoceptor antagonists, such as chlorpromazine, thioridazine, and clozapine (24). A central mechanism involving the vasomotor regulatory center may also contribute to the lowering of blood pressure.

- A 51-year-old man taking maintenance clozapine developed profound hypotension after cardiopulmonary bypass (19).

Cardiac dysrhythmias

A substantial portion of patients taking clozapine develop electrocardiographic abnormalities; the prevalence was originally estimated at 10% (SEDA-20, 47) (SEDA-22, 57). However, although the prevalence may be higher, most of the effects are benign and do not need treatment. In 61 patients with schizophrenia taking clozapine, in whom a retrospective chart review was conducted to identify electrocardiographic abnormalities, the prevalence of electrocardiographic abnormalities in those who used neuroleptic drugs other than clozapine was 14% (6/44), while in the neuroleptic drug-free patients it was 12% (2/17); when treatment was switched to clozapine, the prevalence of electrocardiographic abnormalities rose to 31% (19/61) (25).

The correlation between plasma clozapine concentration and heart rate variability has been studied in 40 patients with schizophrenia treated with clozapine 50–600 mg/day (21). The patients had reduced heart rate variability parameters, which correlated negatively with plasma clozapine concentration.

Clozapine can cause prolongation of the QT interval (26).

- In a 30-year-old man taking clozapine there were minor electrocardiographic abnormalities, including a prolonged QT interval. A power spectrum analysis of heart rate variability showed marked abnormalities in autonomic nervous system activity. When olanzapine was substituted, power spectrum analysis studies showed that his heart rate had improved significantly and that his cardiovascular parameters had returned to normal. Serial electrocardiograms showed minimal prolongation of the QT interval.

Tachycardia is the most common cardiovascular adverse effect of clozapine, and atrial fibrillation has also been reported (SEDA-22, 57) (20).

The reports of sudden death associated with clozapine and the possibility that it may have direct prodysrhythmic properties have been reviewed (27).

A patient developed ventricular fibrillation and atrial fibrillation after taking clozapine for 2 weeks (22).

- A 44-year-old man with no significant cardiac history was given clozapine and 12 days later had bibasal crackles in the chest and ST segment elevation in leads V2 and V3 of the electrocardiogram. He then developed ventricular tachycardia and needed resuscitation. He also developed atrial fibrillation for 24 hours, which subsequently resolved.

Cardiomyopathy

Cardiomyopathy has been associated with neuroleptic drugs, including clozapine (28–30), and partial data initially suggested an incidence of 1 in 500 in the first month.

A thorough study of the risk of myocarditis or cardiomyopathy in Australia detected 23 cases (mean age 36 years; 20 men) out of 8000 patients treated with clozapine from January 1993 to March 1999 (absolute risk 0.29%; relative risk about 1000–2000) (17). All the accumulated data on previous reports of sudden death, myocarditis, or cardiac disease noted in connection with clozapine treatment were requested from the Adverse Drug Reactions

Advisory Committee (ADRAC); there were 15 cases of myocarditis (five fatal) and 8 of cardiomyopathy (one fatal) associated with clozapine. All cases of myocarditis occurred within 3 weeks of starting clozapine. Cardiomyopathy was diagnosed up to 36 months after clozapine had been started. There were no confounding factors to account for cardiac illness. Necropsy results showed mainly eosinophilic infiltrates with myocytolysis, consistent with an acute drug reaction.

The manufacturers analysed 125 reports of myocarditis with clozapine and found 35 cases with fatal outcomes (31). A total of 53% occurred in the first month of therapy, and a small number (4.8%) occurred more than 2 years after the start of treatment. In this series, 70% of the patients were men.

Taking into account the results from an epidemiological study of deaths in users and former users of clozapine (32), the cardiovascular mortality risk related to clozapine may be outweighed by the overall lower mortality risk associated with its beneficial effects, since the death rate was lower among current users (322 per 100 000 person years) than among past users (696 per 100 000 person years). The reduction in death rate during current use was largely accounted for by a reduction in the suicide rate compared with past use (RR = 0.25; CI = 0.10, 0.30).

Since cardiomyopathy is potentially fatal, some precautions must be taken. If patients taking clozapine present with flu-like symptoms, fever, myalgia, dizziness or faintness, chest pain, dyspnea, tachycardia or palpitation, and other signs or symptoms of heart failure, consideration should always be given to a diagnosis of myocarditis. Suspicion should be heightened if the symptoms develop during the first 6–8 weeks of therapy. It should be noted, however, that flu-like symptoms can also occur during the titration period, supposedly as a result of alpha-adrenoceptor antagonism by clozapine. Patients in whom myocarditis is suspected should be referred immediately to a cardiac unit for evaluation.

Clozapine rechallenge after myocarditis has been described (33).

- A 23-year-old man with no history of cardiac disease was given clozapine 12.5 mg/day, increasing to 200 mg/day over 3 weeks; 5 weeks later he complained of shortness of breath and non-specific aches and pains in his legs and body. There was marked ST-segment depression and T wave inversion in the lateral and inferior leads of the electrocardiogram. There was no eosinophilia, and creatine kinase activity was not raised. An echocardiogram showed a hyperdynamic heart and left ventricular size was at the upper limit of normal. The heart valves were normal. Clozapine was withdrawn, but his mental state and quality of life deteriorated, and 2 years later clozapine was restarted because other drugs had not produced improvement. The dose of clozapine was built up to 225 mg at night and he remained well and free from cardiac adverse effects.

In this case a consultant cardiologist diagnosed myocarditis secondary to clozapine, as no other confounding co-morbidity was identified. However, the negative rechallenge suggests either that the clozapine was not responsible or that there was tolerance to the effect.

Pericarditis

Serositis (pericarditis and pericardial effusion, with or without pleural effusion) has been reported in patients taking clozapine (34–36).

- A 43-year-old man developed a pericardial effusion after taking clozapine for 7 years. The condition resolved when the drug was withdrawn.
- A 16-year-old girl developed pericarditis associated with clozapine. There were electrocardiographic changes and serial rises in serum troponin I, a highly sensitive and specific marker of myocardial injury.

The latter is said to be the first reported case of pericarditis due to clozapine demonstrating rises in troponin I, which resolved despite continuation of therapy. The authors suggested that troponin I is the preferred marker for monitoring the cardiac adverse effects of clozapine.

Venous thromboembolism

Typical neuroleptic drugs have been associated with an increased risk of venous thromboembolism (37). Data from the Swedish Reactions Advisory Committee suggested that clozapine is also associated with venous thromboembolic complications (38). Between 1 April 1989 and 1 March 2000, 12 cases of venous thromboembolism were collected; in 5 the outcome was fatal. Symptoms occurred in the first 3 months of treatment in eight patients; the mean clozapine dose was 277 mg/day (75–500). Although during the study total neuroleptic drug sales, excluding clozapine, accounted for 96% of all neuroleptic drug sales, only three cases of thromboembolism associated with those neuroleptic drugs were reported. The reported risk of thromboembolism associated with clozapine is estimated to be 1 per 2000–6000 treated patients, the true risk being higher owing to under-reporting. These conclusions were consistent with those from an observational study (32).

Between February 1990, when clozapine was first marketed in the USA, and December 1999 the FDA received 99 reports of venous thromboembolism (83 mentioned pulmonary embolism with or without deep vein thrombosis and 16 mentioned deep vein thrombosis alone) (39). In 63 cases death had resulted from pulmonary embolism; 32 were confirmed by necropsy. Of 36 non-fatal cases, only 7 had been documented objectively by such diagnostic techniques as perfusion-ventilation lung scanning and venography. Thus, in 39 of the 99 reports there was objective evidence of pulmonary embolism or deep vein thrombosis. The median age of the 39 individuals was 38 (range 17–70) years and 20 were women. The median daily dose was 400 (range 125–900) mg. The median duration of clozapine exposure before diagnosis was 3 months (range 2 days to 6 years). Information on risk factors for pulmonary embolism and deep vein thrombosis varied; however, 18 of the 39 patients were obese. The frequency of fatal pulmonary embolism in this study is consistent with that described in the labelling for clozapine in the USA.

As of 31 December 1993, there were 18 cases of fatal pulmonary embolism in association with clozapine therapy in users aged 10–54 years. Based on the extent of use recorded in the Clozapine National Registry, the mortality rate associated with pulmonary embolism was 1 death per 3450 person years of use. This rate was about 28 times higher than that in the general population of a similar age and sex (95% CI = 17, 42). Whether pulmonary embolism can be attributed to clozapine or some characteristic(s) of its users is not clear (40).

Fatal pulmonary embolism occurred in a 29-year-old man who was not obese, did not smoke, and had not had recent surgery, after he had taken clozapine 300 mg/day for 6 weeks (41).

Nervous system

Clozapine has been used to treat benign essential tremor refractory to the usual drugs (propranolol, primidone, alprazolam, phenobarbital, and botulinum toxin) in a randomized, double-blind, crossover study in 15 patients with essential tremor (42). Responders with more than 50% improvement after a single dose of clozapine 12.5 mg, compared with placebo, subsequently received 39–50 mg unblinded for a mean of 16 months. Tremor was effectively reduced by a single dose of clozapine in 13 of 15 patients; sedation was the only adverse effect reported.

Sleep

In a study of the effects of clozapine on the electroencephalogram, 13% of patients developed spikes with no relation to dose or serum concentration of clozapine; 53% developed electroencephalographic slowing. Compared with plasma concentrations below 300 ng/ml, a clozapine serum concentration of 350–450 ng/ml led to more frequent and more severe electroencephalographic slowing (43). There were considerable differences in the electroencephalographic patterns between classical neuroleptic drugs and clozapine (44). Clozapine-treated patients showed significantly more stage 2 sleep, more stable non-REM sleep (stages 2, 3, and 4), and less stage 1 than patients treated with haloperidol or flupentixol. In a longitudinal study, clozapine significantly improved sleep continuity and significantly increased REM density, but did not affect the amount of REM sleep (45).

Seizures

Clozapine has a proconvulsant effect. Factors that increase the likelihood of seizures include high doses of clozapine, rapid dose titration, the concurrent use of other epileptogenic agents (such as antidepressants, neuroleptic drugs, and mood stabilizers) and a previous history of neurological abnormalities (46).

The prevalence of seizures with clozapine is higher than average (about 5%) and is dose-dependent (SED-14, 142) (47,48).

- A tonic-clonic seizure occurred in a 30-year-old man 4 weeks after he started to take clozapine 400 mg/day (49). This was followed by a large increase in liver enzymes, which had been normal the week before.

Seizure characteristics and electroencephalographic abnormalities in 12 patients taking clozapine have been identified; there was a surprisingly high incidence of focal epileptiform abnormalities (50). Seizures associated with clozapine are dose-dependent (SEDA-21, 53) (SEDA-22, 57). However, there have been reports of seizure activity in patients taking therapeutic or subtherapeutic doses of clozapine (47,48). Seizures have occasionally been reported in patients taking low doses.

- A 28-year-old woman, with no history of prior seizures and not taking concomitant medication, had seizures while taking clozapine 200 mg/day (48).
- A 75-year-old patient developed seizures while taking clozapine 12.5 mg/day.

However, in the second case the seizure was unlikely to have been due to clozapine, given the very low dose and non-recurrence with rechallenge at higher dosages (51).

Despite the risk of seizures in patients without pre-existing epilepsy, six patients with epilepsy and severe psychosis taking clozapine had no increases in seizure frequency, and three had a substantial reduction (52).

Several anticonvulsants have been shown to be helpful in the prevention and treatment of clozapine-induced seizures.

- A 15-year-old boy with refractory schizophrenia had seizures with clozapine; he was given gabapentin, and several years later was free of seizures (53).

The addition of lamotrigine to clozapine therapy has been associated with rapid improvement of psychiatric symptoms (54); this has been observed in three cases of poor response or resistance to clozapine monotherapy.

Stuttering has been associated with clozapine (SEDA-22, 58). The pathogenesis of developmental stuttering, as well as acquired or neurogenic stuttering, is unclear. However, since clozapine-induced stuttering can precede a seizure (SEDA-25, 64) it may be related to an effect on the brain rather than to a dystonic syndrome, as previously suggested.

- A 28-year-old man taking clozapine 300 mg/day developed severe stuttering and subsequently had a generalized tonic-clonic seizure while taking 425 mg/day (55). There were electroencephalographic abnormalities, especially left-sided slowing.
- A 49-year-old woman had prominent stuttering before a generalized epileptic seizure and recovered after antiepileptic treatment (56).

Extrapyramidal effects

Clozapine has a more favorable extrapyramidal effects profile than other neuroleptic drugs (57) and little or no parkinsonian effect (58).

Akathisia

The low prevalence of akathisia in patients taking clozapine has led to the proposal that clozapine should be used to treat patients with neuroleptic drug-induced chronic akathisia (59,60).

Parkinsonism

The efficacy and safety of treatment with clozapine in patients with Parkinson's disease have been discussed (SEDA-22, 57), and a multicenter retrospective review of the effects of clozapine in 172 patients with Parkinson's disease has been published (61). The mean duration of clozapine treatment was 17 (range 1–76) months. Low-dose clozapine improved the symptoms of psychosis, anxiety, depression, hypersexuality, sleep disturbances, and akathisia. Of the 40 patients, 24% withdrew as a result of adverse events, mostly sedation ($n = 19$). Sedation was reported in 46%, sialorrhea in 11%, and postural hypotension in 9.9%. Neutropenia was detected in four patients (2.3%).

Six patients who met the criteria for a diagnosis of HIV-associated psychosis, and who had previously developed moderate parkinsonism as a result of typical neuroleptic drugs, were treated with clozapine (62). Parkinsonism improved by an average of 77%, but one patient did not complete the trial because of a progressive fall in leukocyte count.

Clozapine has been used to treat psychosis related to Parkinson's disease (SEDA-22, 57) (61). In a randomized, double-blind, placebo-controlled trial of low doses of clozapine (6.25–50 mg/day) in 60 patients (mean age 72 years) with idiopathic Parkinson's disease and drug-induced psychosis, the patients in the clozapine group had significantly more improvement after 14 months than those in the placebo group in all measures used to determine the severity of psychosis (63). Clozapine improved tremor and had no deleterious effect on the severity of parkinsonism, but in one patient it was withdrawn because of leukopenia.

In a randomized, double-blind, placebo-controlled, 4-week trial in 60 patients with similar drug-induced psychosis in Parkinson's disease, assigned to clozapine ($n = 32$) or placebo ($n = 28$), the initial clozapine dose of 6.25 mg/day was titrated over at least 10 days to a maximum of 50 mg/day and was rapidly effective (64). Somnolence and worsening of parkinsonism were significantly more frequent in the clozapine group, seven of whom reported worsening of Parkinson's disease, usually mild or transient, which was confirmed by aggravation of the Schwab and England score by 10–20% in three patients; however, no-one withdrew for this reason.

Tardive dyskinesia

It is said that clozapine causes less tardive dyskinesia than haloperidol and even that it can improve pre-existing tardive dyskinesia (65–69).

Patients with schizophrenia with ($n = 15$) and without ($n = 11$) tardive dyskinesia differed markedly in their dopaminergic response to haloperidol, assessed by means of plasma homovanillic acid variations, which increased, whereas this difference was not observed after clozapine (70).

Nevertheless, 46 patients taking clozapine had higher tardive dyskinesia scores compared with 127 taking typical neuroleptic drugs (71). In a multiple regression analysis, there was a significant relation between the total score on the Abnormal Involuntary Movement Scale (AIMS) as a dependent variable and current neuroleptic drug dose, duration of treatment, age, sex, diagnosis, current antiparkinsonian therapy, and illness duration. There was no beneficial effect of clozapine on the prevalence of tardive dyskinesia, and the authors' conclusion was that certain patients develop tardive dyskinesia despite long-term intensive clozapine treatment; however, since most clozapine users were past users of typical neuroleptic drugs, this conclusion must be regarded with caution.

- A 45-year-old woman developed tardive dyskinesia while taking clozapine (72). She had never had any of the symptoms before she started to take 223 mg/day and first experienced involuntary tongue movements and akathisia 5 months after the start of treatment.
- Tardive dyskinesia has been attributed to clozapine in a 44-year-old man, who had discontinued haloperidol 24 days before the event (73).

Tardive dystonia

It is generally considered that clozapine has little or no potential to cause tardive dystonia; it has even been speculated that it may be an effective therapy for this adverse effect (SEDA-21, 53). The efficacy of clozapine in severe dystonia was therefore assessed in an open trial in five patients (74). All had significant improvement; nevertheless, all had adverse effects, such as sedation and orthostatic hypotension: in one case persistent symptomatic orthostatic hypotension and tachycardia limited treatment.

However, there was no evidence of a beneficial effect of clozapine in primary dystonia, the most common form of dystonia and a difficult disorder to treat, until the report of a 56-year-old woman with severe and persistent primary cranial dystonia (Meige's syndrome), who responded to clozapine (50–100 mg) (75).

Tardive dystonia, probably associated with clozapine, has been described (76).

- A 37-year-old man, who had taken numerous neuroleptic drugs from 1975 to 1990, was switched to clozapine because of breakthrough psychosis. Clozapine was effective and was his only neuroleptic drug treatment from that time. In 1996, when his clozapine dosage was 825 mg/day, he had left torticollis of 60–70°, mild left laterocollis, and superimposed spasmodic head movements jerking his head to the left. He had difficulty rotating his head to the right past the midline.

Tardive tremor

Tardive tremor is a hyperkinetic movement disorder associated with chronic neuroleptic drug treatment. It was first described in 1991 as a symmetrical tremor, of low frequency, present at rest and during voluntary movements but most prominent during maintenance of posture, and often accompanied by tardive dyskinesia. Tetrabenazine is the current treatment. Sequential responsiveness to both tetrabenazine and clozapine has been reported (77).

- A 55-year-old man with a 15-year history of schizophrenia treated with various neuroleptic drugs developed a tremor and was given tetrabenazine 75 mg/day, with complete regression of the tremor. Three months later he developed depression, a known adverse effect of tetrabenazine, which was discontinued, with subsequent partial improvement of his depressive symptoms but reappearance of the tardive tremor. Clozapine 25 mg/day was started and increased to 75 mg/day; his tardive tremor again disappeared.

Neuroleptic malignant syndrome

Neuroleptic malignant syndrome has been associated with clozapine (SEDA-22, 58) (78), although some doubts were expressed about the features of earlier cases. In the light of two cases, a 35-year-old man and a 62-year-old woman, the literature was comprehensively reviewed and the characteristics of neuroleptic malignant syndrome due to clozapine and typical neuroleptic drugs were compared (79). Causation with clozapine was deemed highly probable in 14 cases, of medium probability in 5 cases, and of low probability in 8 cases. The most commonly reported clinical features were tachycardia, changes in mental status, and sweating. Fever, rigidity, and raised creatine kinase activity were less prominent than in the neuroleptic malignant syndrome associated with typical neuroleptic drugs. This suggests that the presentation of clozapine-induced neuroleptic malignant syndrome may be different from that of typical neuroleptic drugs. Two other cases have also illustrated that possibility (80,81).

Neuroleptic malignant syndrome and subsequent acute interstitial nephritis has been reported in a 44-year-old woman (82). This patient met the main criteria for neuroleptic malignant syndrome, although she did not develop rigidity or a rise in creatine kinase activity. On the other hand, abnormal creatine kinase activity and signs of myotoxicity were respectively found in 14% and 2.1% of patients who took clozapine for an average of 18 months ($n = 94$) (83).

Delirium

Toxic delirium caused by neuroleptic drugs with potent anticholinergic properties has been widely reported (SED-11, 107), and has been reported with low-dose clozapine (84).

Psychological, psychiatric

Suicide, suicidality, and suicidal ideation are very serious problems in patients with schizophrenia. Based on general observations that 1–2% of patients with schizophrenia complete suicide within 1 year after initial attempts, the authors of a retrospective study of 295 neuroleptic drug-resistant patients with schizophrenia who had taken clozapine monotherapy for at least 6 months would have expected as many as 10 or 11 successful suicides or suicide attempts, but none was observed (85).

Obsessive-compulsive symptoms during clozapine therapy have been suggested to be more common than first reported (SEDA-21, 54). In a retrospective cohort study, new or worse obsessiveness has been analysed in 121 consecutive young patients with recent-onset schizophrenia or other psychotic disorders taking clozapine and other neuroleptic drugs (86). More clozapine-treated subjects (21%) had new or worse obsessiveness than subjects treated with other neuroleptic drugs (1.3%). However, there was no information on comparability of the groups.

Panic disorder has been attributed to clozapine (87).

- A 34-year-old woman taking clozapine 400 mg/day for psychiatric symptoms had recurrent attacks of sudden chest pressure, dizziness, fear of dying, and intense anxiety; reducing the dose of clozapine to 250 mg/day led to modest improvement. Olanzapine 10 mg/day was then substituted, without recurrence, and her panic symptoms progressively improved.

Metabolism

Diabetes mellitus

Several cases of de novo diabetes mellitus or exacerbation of existing diabetes in patients taking neuroleptic drugs have been reported, including patients taking clozapine (88–91). There was no significant relation to weight gain.

- A 49-year-old man taking olanzapine developed diabetes mellitus and recovered after withdrawal (92).
- Diabetic ketoacidosis occurred in a 31-year-old man who had taken clozapine 200 mg/day for 3 months for refractory schizophrenia (93). Clozapine was withdrawn and he remained metabolically stable. Two months later, clozapine was restarted, and only 72 hours after drug re-exposure he had increased fasting glycemia and insulinemia, suggesting insulin resistance as the underlying mechanism. Apart from slight obesity, he had no predisposing factors.

Hyperglycemia occurs at 2 weeks to 3 months after the start of clozapine treatment and occurs without predisposing factors. Clozapine-induced hyperglycemia can be serious, leading to coma, but it is reversible if clozapine is withdrawn. In some cases, continuation of clozapine is possible by controlling blood glucose concentrations with hypoglycemic drugs. This approach can be useful in refractory schizophrenia responsive to clozapine. All patients should be advised to report altered consciousness, polyuria, or increased thirst.

Glucose metabolism has been studied in 17 patients taking clozapine (94). Six had impaired glucose tolerance and eight had a glycemic peak delay.

Diabetes was also more common in 63 patients taking clozapine than in 67 receiving typical depot neuroleptic drugs (95). The percentages of type 2 diabetes mellitus were 12% and 6% respectively. Nevertheless, the mechanism is not known. In six patients with schizophrenia, clozapine increased mean concentrations of blood glucose, insulin, and C peptide (96). The authors concluded that the glucose intolerance was due to increased insulin resistance.

However, opposite data have been found in a case-control study in 7227 patients with new diabetes and 6780 controls, all with psychiatric disorders (97). Clozapine was not significantly associated with diabetes (adjusted OR = 0.98; 95% CI = 0.74, 1.31) and there was no suggestion of relations between larger dosages or longer durations of clozapine use and an increased risk of diabetes. Among individual non-clozapine neuroleptic drugs, there were significantly increased risks for two phenothiazines: chlorpromazine (OR = 1.31; 95% CI = 1.09, 1.56) and perphenazine (OR = 1.34; 95% CI = 1.11, 1.62). The authors suggested that, in contrast to earlier reports, these results provided some reassurance that clozapine does not increase the risk of diabetes. However, cases of diabetes were identified by the new use of antidiabetic drugs, and it is therefore possible that clozapine was associated with less pronounced glucose intolerance that did not require drug therapy.

Weight gain

Weight gain is often associated with clozapine (SEDA-21, 54). In 42 patients who took clozapine for at least 1 year, men and women gained both weight and body mass, which is more directly related to cardiovascular morbidity (98). Over 10 weeks, leptin concentrations, which correlate with body mass index, increased significantly from baseline in 12 patients taking clozapine (99).

The association between clozapine-related weight gain and increased mean arterial blood pressure has been examined in 61 patients who were randomly assigned to either clozapine or haloperidol in a 10-week parallel-group, double-blind study, and in 55 patients who chose to continue to take clozapine in a subsequent 1-year open study (100). Clozapine was associated with significant weight gain in both the double-blind trial (mean 4.2 kg) and the open trial (mean 5.8 kg). There was no significant correlation between change in weight and change in mean arterial blood pressure.

There were no significant associations between cycle length and weight change during clozapine treatment in 13 premenopausal women with psychoses (101).

Sleep apnea associated with clozapine-induced obesity has been reported (102).

- A 45-year-old woman with schizophrenia who took clozapine 300 mg/day for 16 months gained 18 kg and had hypertriglyceridemia and glucose intolerance. She had daytime sedation, difficulty in sleeping at night, loud snoring, and periods of apnea during sleep.

Nasal continuous positive airway pressure produced improvement.

Phenylpropanolamine 75 mg/day did not promote weight loss in a randomized, placebo-controlled study in 16 patients with schizophrenia who had gained at least 10% of their body weight while taking clozapine (103).

- A 29-year-old man taking clozapine 800 mg/day gained 46 kg in weight after 25 months, and had myoclonic jerks in the hands, arms, and shoulders on both sides (104). He was treated with topiramate (which causes weight loss). The myoclonic jerks disappeared completely. He lost 21 kg over 5 months, with no significant change in eating habits or food consumption, and felt more energetic, more active, and more motivated to exercise.

Hematologic

Neutropenia and agranulocytosis

DoTS classification (BMJ 2003; 327:1222–1225)
Dose-relation: hypersusceptibility effect
Time-course: intermediate or delayed
Susceptibility factors: genetic; age

Incidence

Clozapine-induced agranulocytosis was originally determined to be 0.21% in a selected Finnish population (SED-9, 83) (105), and the drug was withdrawn, only to be cautiously reintroduced in some countries a decade later, with hematological monitoring. With mandatory hematological monitoring by the Clozaril Patient Management System in the USA, the cumulative incidence of agranulocytosis was 0.8% at 1 year and 0.9% at 1.5 years of treatment; the risk was not related to dosage (SEDA-18, 54) (106). In France, the incidences of agranulocytosis and neutropenia in clozapine-treated patients from December 1991 were 0.46 and 2.1% respectively (107). Some of the available postmarketing data on clozapine-induced agranulocytosis are presented in Table 1 (108).

Mechanism

The underlying mechanisms of agranulocytosis are unknown, but hemopoietic cytokines, such as granulocyte colony-stimulating factor (G-CSF), are likely to be involved (109).

- In a 26-year-old woman who developed granulocytopenia twice, first when taking clozapine and again when taking olanzapine, G-CSF concentrations, but not those of other cytokines, closely paralleled the granulocyte count.
- In a 73-year-old patient who developed granulocytopenia while taking clozapine, G-CSF and leukocyte

Table 1 Reported incidences of clozapine-induced agranulocytosis

Country	Period	Number of patients	Incidence (mortality) (%)	Reference
Finland	1975	2260	0.70 (0.35)	(SED-9, 83) (105)
USA	1990–1991	11382	0.80 (0.02)	(SEDA-18, 54)
France	1992	2834	0.46 (ND)	(SEDA-21, 54)
USA	1990–1994	99502	0.38 (0.01)	(SEDA-22, 59)
UK and Ireland	1990–1994	6316	0.80 (0.03)	(SEDA-22, 59)
New Zealand	1988–1995	963	1.15 (0.00)	(SEDA-22, 59)
Australia	1993–1996	4061	0.90 (0.00)	(99)
Spain	1993–1999	6354	0.16 (0.02)	Agencia Española del Medicamento (personal communication)
Total		133402	0.44 (0.018)	

counts were reliable indicators of the evolution of the condition, showing an abortive form of toxic bone-marrow damage with subsequent recovery (110).

Immune-mediated mechanisms of clozapine-induced agranulocytosis have been reviewed in the context of agranulocytosis in a 46-year-old woman (111). Immune and toxic mechanisms have also been explored in patients taking clozapine, three who developed agranulocytosis, seven who developed neutropenia, and five who were asymptomatic. There was no evidence of antineutrophil antibodies in the blood of patients shortly after an episode of clozapine-induced agranulocytosis, and an antibody mechanism seems unlikely, in view of the delay in onset of clozapine-induced agranulocytosis on re-exposure to the drug (112).

Susceptibility factors

Some of the genetic aspects of clozapine-induced agranulocytosis have been evaluated (113). Polymorphisms of specific clozapine metabolizing enzyme systems were determined in 31 patients with agranulocytosis and in 77 without. Genotyping of a recently discovered G-463 A polymorphism of the myeloperoxidase gene and CYP2D6 showed no evidence of an association.

Because of the unusually high incidence of agranulocytosis in Finnish and Jewish patients (SEDA-20, 49), an ethnic susceptibility factor for agranulocytosis has been suggested. Human leukocyte antigen (HLA) B38 phenotype was found in 83% of patients who developed agranulocytosis and in 20% of clozapine-treated patients who did not develop agranulocytosis (114). Gene products contained in the haplotype may be involved. In an open study in 31 German patients with clozapine-induced agranulocytosis and 77 controls with schizophrenia, agranulocytosis was significantly associated with HLA-Cw*7, DQB*0502, DRB1*0101, and DRB3*020 (115). No other antigens were associated with agranulocytosis, but age was another major susceptibility factor. In another study in two groups of Finnish patients (19 "clozapine responders" and 26 patients with a history of non-fatal clozapine-induced granulocytopenia or agranulocytosis), the frequency of the HLA-A1 allele in the latter was low (12%), whereas HLA-A1 was associated with a good therapeutic response at an allele frequency of 58% (the frequency of HLA-A1 being 20% in the Finnish population) (116).

Concordant clozapine-induced agranulocytosis in monozygotic twins also suggested a genetic susceptibility; in both twins there was a low leukocyte count after 9 weeks of treatment (117). Serological typing of the HLA system showed identical patterns in the twins: HLA-A: 28, 26; HLA-B: 49, 63; DR: 2 (versus 16), 12, 52; DQ: 1. The authors pointed out that these data suggest that genetic factors may participate not only in the time of onset of schizophrenia, but also in the emergence and timing of agranulocytosis in response to clozapine.

Clinical features

Careful attention should be paid to possible early warnings of agranulocytosis, such as fever, sore throat, and lymphadenopathy.

Circadian variation in white cell count, with a dip in the morning, has been misdiagnosed as clozapine-induced neutropenia (118).

- A 31-year-old man with resistant schizophrenia took clozapine 500 mg/day. Although this was effective, the granulocyte count fell to 1.2×10^9/l (total count not given) and clozapine was withdrawn. During the subsequent year, several neuroleptic drugs were used, with unsatisfactory results. Careful monitoring showed a pronounced diurnal variation in both total white cell count (2.9–4.2×10^9/l in the morning and 3.6–7.1×10^9/l in the afternoon) and granulocytes (0.8–1.4×10^9/l in the morning and 2.9–5.5×10^9/l in the afternoon).

Thus, an apparently low white cell count may simply reflect the nadir of the diurnal variation and may not indicate a need to withdraw clozapine.

In over 11 000 patients the risk of agranulocytosis was higher in the first 3 months of treatment and is greater among women and elderly patients (119).

Agranulocytosis after very long-term clozapine therapy has been reported (120).

- A 41-year-old man suddenly developed agranulocytosis after taking clozapine nearly continuously for 89 months. During this time, his white blood cell and granulocyte counts remained stable. The white blood cell and granulocyte counts returned to baseline shortly after withdrawal of clozapine and administration of sargramostim.

Rechallenge

Cases of negative or positive rechallenge in patients with agranulocytosis have been reported (SEDA-20, 54) (SEDA-22, 59).

- A 58-year-old man developed agranulocytosis during a second trial of clozapine, despite a successful previous trial (121).
- A 17-year-old boy with severe clozapine-induced neutropenia had a negative rechallenge; because he had had an unsatisfactory response to traditional neuroleptic drugs, clozapine was continued despite a fall in white blood cell count, since concomitant treatment with granulocyte colony-stimulating factor was followed by rapid normalization of the white blood cell count (122).
- A 29-year-old woman developed agranulocytosis after taking clozapine 300 mg/day for 5 years; 4 months after withdrawal, the clozapine was reintroduced (500 mg/day), and after 8 months the leukocyte count was still within the reference range (123).

Monitoring therapy

Over 10 000 patients have been treated with clozapine in Australia since its introduction in 1993, and the Clozaril monitoring system has ensured that since that time there have been no deaths from agranulocytosis in patients taking clozapine (124).

An increase in white blood cell count of at least 15% above previous counts is a sensitive, although not specific, predictor for the development of agranulocytosis within 75 days (119). Clozapine dosage and baseline white cell count do not appear to predict agranulocytosis.

Monitoring G-CSF concentrations, if available, may be useful in following patients in whom clozapine-induced marrow damage is suspected.

An example of a false sense of security gained by relying on monitoring monthly blood counts in patients taking clozapine has been published (125).

- A 61-year-old man who had taken clozapine for 3 years had normal blood counts. However, one day, his hemoglobin was 8.5 g/dl, having previously been 13 g/dl, following a steady asymptomatic fall over 6 months that had been documented but had gone unnoticed. He subsequently underwent investigation and treatment for anemia.

However, it is not clear in this case that clozapine was responsible for the anemia.

Treatment

Withdrawal of clozapine can lead to resolution of agranulocytosis, but not always. Granulocytopenia, presumably induced by clozapine, persisted in a 53-year-old woman after she switched from clozapine to quetiapine (126).

Treatment with granulocyte colony-stimulating factor and granulocyte macrophage colony stimulating factors was helpful in a case of sepsis and neutropenia induced by clozapine (127) and in a case of agranulocytosis in a 45-year-old man (128).

Lithium can be used in combination with clozapine, and in these patients the possibility of inducing leukocytosis and increasing the total leukocyte count and the granulocyte count has been considered (SEDA-20, 50). Lithium has even been used to prevent clozapine-induced neutropenia (SEDA-22, 59). It has also been used in a patient with clozapine-induced neutropenia and in another with complete agranulocytosis: in both cases lithium increased the neutrophil count to within the reference range within 6 days (129). In the patient who had neutropenia, clozapine was restarted in the presence of lithium and the neutrophil count did not fall thereafter. Five other patients who took combined clozapine and lithium had a significant improvement with this combination and there were no cases of agranulocytosis, neuroleptic malignant syndrome, or other adverse effects (130).

Eosinophilia

Clozapine-induced eosinophilia and subsequent neutropenia has been reported (131). As the patient had a high IgE concentration, an allergic cause was proposed. In a previous study in 70 patients there was no predictive value of eosinophilia for clozapine-induced neutropenia (132). Eosinophilia associated with clozapine treatment has been reported in 13% of treated patients in a study in Australia (28).

Platelet count

Thrombocytosis and thrombocytopenia have both been reported.

- Thrombocytosis (774×10^9/l) occurred in a middle-aged man taking clozapine (133).
- A 43-year-old man developed thrombocytopenia (platelet count 60×10^9/l), which persisted for 40 months after clozapine treatment (134). There was increased in vitro platelet serotonin release in the presence of clozapine (135).

In the second case, the authors suggested an immune mechanism and pointed out that the manufacturers recommend withdrawing clozapine when the platelet count falls below 100×10^9/l.

Mouth and teeth

Hypersalivation is a common adverse effect of clozapine (136), which has been estimated to occur in 10–23% of patients (SEDA-20, 49). Salivary gland swelling has been reported in patients treated with clozapine (SEDA-20, 49) (137).

There is evidence implicating alpha-adrenoceptors in hypersalivation caused by clozapine, and it has been hypothesized that a biallelic polymorphism in the promoter region of the alpha$_2$-adrenoceptor gene confers susceptibility to schizophrenia, which is associated with a clozapine-induced favorable therapeutic response and/or clozapine-induced hypersalivation (138). However, the results in 97 patients showed that the alpha$_2$-adrenoceptor gene polymorphism did not play a major role in susceptibility to hypersalivation or the therapeutic response of patients with schizophrenia.

A comprehensive review has been published on the evidence of the benefit of using antimuscarinic agents, adrenoceptor antagonists, and adrenoceptor agonists in treating clozapine-induced hypersalivation (139). There is a lack of good-quality controlled trials, most papers having reported series of uncontrolled cases dependent on subjective measures of improvement reported by patients; however, the authors suggested that the most effective treatment may be a combination of terazosin and benzhexol (140). Ten patients with sialorrhea associated with clozapine, who did not respond to anticholinergic or adrenergic drugs, received intranasal ipratropium bromide; at 6 months, six patients maintained improvement (141).

Gastrointestinal

Reflux esophagitis has been reported in patients taking clozapine (142). It has been speculated that reduced esophageal motility was the mechanism (143).

Constipation is an adverse effect that has often been associated with clozapine; it can be serious and even fatal (SEDA-22, 60).

- A 49-year-old man taking clozapine developed a perforated colon and peritonitis (144). He survived, albeit with a markedly reduced quality of life.

The authors suggested that diet modification and regular exercise should be encouraged in patients taking clozapine, in order to prevent constipation.

- A 43-year-old man took clozapine 750 mg/day for 6 years and developed vomiting and epigastric pain (145). He had ulcerative esophagitis, and a CT scan was reportedly normal "apart from constipation." He was given omeprazole 20 mg/day and twice-daily psyllium. Six months later he developed abdominal pain with feculent vomiting. Emergency laparotomy revealed large-bowel obstruction secondary to severe fecal impaction. He died 3 weeks later with septic shock and progressive multisystem organ failure.

Liver

Transient asymptomatic liver enzyme rises are common with clozapine (146).

Hepatitis associated with clozapine has been reported (SEDA-20, 49) (SEDA-22, 59).

- A 49-year-old woman (147) took clozapine 300 mg/day and developed lethargy, anorexia, fever, eosinophilia, leukocytosis, and abnormal liver function tests. The serum clozapine concentration was 8595 nmol/l. Clozapine was withdrawn and after 8 days her condition stabilized and low-dose clozapine treatment was successfully restarted with serum monitoring.

Obstructive jaundice has been described (148).

- A 48-year-old man with schizophrenia started taking clozapine 12.5 mg/day, increasing over the next 18 days to 150 mg/day. By that time he was icteric, with mild distress and fever and raised bilirubin 149 μmol/l (reference range 5–26), direct bilirubin 92 μmol/l, gamma-glutamyl transpeptidase 446 IU/l (<65), alanine transaminase 100 IU/l (<40), and aspartate transaminase 56 IU/l (<40). Hepatitis serology showed positive hepatitis B surface antibodies, and HBs antigen was negative, as were hepatitis A, hepatitis C, Epstein-Barr virus, and cytomegalovirus. He also had hyperglycemia, pleural effusion, eosinophilia, hematuria, and proteinuria, which also resolved on clozapine withdrawal.

A case of fatal liver failure has been reported (149).

Pancreas

Occasional cases of pancreatitis have been related to clozapine therapy (SEDA-17, 63).

- A 73-year-old woman with a 4-year history of Parkinson's disease developed hallucinations and delusions that were interpreted as secondary effects of levodopa (150). She was given clozapine 25 mg/day and continued to take levodopa. Four days later she complained of abdominal pain. She had raised activities of serum amylase 806 IU/l (reference range <220 IU/l), lipase 2598 IU/l (<190 IU/l), and creatine kinase 464 IU/l (<190 IU/l), and normal concentrations of total and direct bilirubin. Other causes of pancreatitis were ruled out.

Two other cases have been reported in patients with no prior history of alcohol abuse or gallstones (151,152). The authors recommended monitoring serum amylase activity during slow increases in the dosage of clozapine if there is leukocytosis or eosinophilia, which may be associated with asymptomatic pancreatitis.

Urinary tract

Enuresis has been rarely associated with clozapine (0.23% of patients) (SEDA-19, 54) (153), and has been successfully treated with benzatropine in patients taking a variety of psychotropic medications (154).

In a retrospective study, 27 of 61 Chinese patients who took clozapine for more than 3 months developed urinary incontinence, persistent in 15 cases (155). The reaction could not be related to age, sex, clozapine dosage, duration of clozapine use, duration of hospitalization, duration of illness, age at onset of schizophrenia, or concurrent treatment with other psychiatric drugs.

Polymorphisms of the alpha 1a adrenoceptor gene were found to play no major role in the pathogenesis of schizophrenia or in clozapine-induced urinary incontinence (156).

Acute interstitial nephritis has been attributed to clozapine (157).

- A 38-year-old woman developed anorexia, lethargy, and vomiting, and noticed a profound reduction in urine output about 11 days after starting clozapine (125 mg bd). Severe renal insufficiency was confirmed (blood urea 33 mmol/l and creatinine 1200 μmol/l). There was no history of pre-existing renal or other systemic disease.

Musculoskeletal

Clozapine-induced myokymia (weakness and reduced muscle tone, with undulating movements of the muscle and skin, accompanied by involuntary repetitive firing of grouped motor unit action potentials) has been reported (158).

- A 33-year-old woman developed muscle twitching and spasms of the legs and back after having taken clozapine for 3 years (158). Neurological examination showed myokymia in both thighs, calves, and the lower lip. The myokymia disappeared 1 week after withdrawal of clozapine.

In an open study in 41 patients, strength control was evaluated before the start of clozapine therapy and again at the end of the titration period (on average 9 weeks later). The results suggested that the strength deficit was primarily due to clozapine and that there were two distinct effects: an initial transient stage characterized by "drowsiness" and a subsequent stage with dose-dependent myoclonic features (159).

- Rhabdomyolysis occurred in two men, aged 21 and 42 years, taking clozapine (160,161). The first had no risk factors, but calcium-dependent potassium efflux, normally responsible for membrane hyperpolarization and muscle refractoriness, was severely impaired in his erythrocytes. The second had marked hyponatremia, due to psychogenic polydipsia, and developed a marked rise in creatine kinase activity (62 730 U/l) after correction of hyponatremia with hyperosmolar fluids.

Sexual function

The frequency and course of sexual disturbances associated with clozapine have been studied in a prospective open study in 75 men and 25 women, mean age 29 years, and compared with the effects of haloperidol in 41 men and 12 women, mean age 26 years (162). There were no statistically significant differences between the patients taking haloperidol and those taking clozapine. During 1–6 weeks of treatment with clozapine, the most frequent sexual disturbances among women were diminished sexual desire (28%) and amenorrhea (12%), while among men they were diminished sexual desire (57%), erectile dysfunction (24%), orgasmic dysfunction (23%), ejaculatory dysfunction (21%), and increased sexual desire (15%). The mean daily doses were haloperidol 16 mg and clozapine 261 mg.

Retrograde ejaculation has been associated with clozapine (163).

Immunologic

Allergic reactions associated with clozapine are uncommon; however, a case of rash (SEDA-21, 55) and a case of pleural effusion (SEDA-22, 60) have previously been reported. Both rash and pleural effusion have been reported in a 37-year-old woman about 1 week after starting clozapine (164).

Body temperature

Clozapine often causes a benign transient increase in body temperature early in treatment (165).

Long-Term Effects

Drug withdrawal

Rebound psychosis or delirium or both have been reported after withdrawal of clozapine (166–171). Clozapine withdrawal has also been associated with nausea, vomiting, diarrhea, headache, restlessness, agitation, and sweating (172,173), which occur as the result of cholinergic rebound and which may respond to anticholinergic drugs (174), and with dystonias and dyskinesias. Delirium and the return of dyskinetic movements can occur within days after clozapine withdrawal.

Four patients had severe dystonias and dyskinesias on abrupt withdrawal of clozapine (175), and another two had obsessive-compulsive symptoms during withdrawal; resumption of clozapine led to the complete disappearance of the obsessive-compulsive symptoms (176).

Second-Generation Effects

Pregnancy

Clozapine caused no serious complications or developmental abnormalities during pregnancy in two cases (177).

Susceptibility Factors

Age

Data from an open study ($n = 329$) have suggested that patients aged 55–64 years may have a better response to clozapine than those aged 65 and older, but there were no significant differences between the two age groups in the number of patients remaining on clozapine therapy and the number in whom therapy was discontinued ($n = 134$) (178). The mean duration of clozapine therapy was 278 days. The most common adverse effects that required withdrawal were sedation ($n = 12$), hematological adverse effects ($n = 7$), and cardiovascular adverse effects ($n = 6$).

In over 11 000 patients the risk of agranulocytosis was greater among elderly patients (119).

Sex

In over 11 000 patients the risk of agranulocytosis was greater among women (119).

Other features of the patient

Patients with Lewy body dementia may be more intolerant of neuroleptic drugs, including atypical drugs, than other patients with neurodegenerative dementia. However, because hallucinations are common in this form of dementia, it is likely that people with Lewy body dementia will be exposed to neuroleptic drugs. Two patients with Lewy body dementia taking clozapine developed confusion and behavioral symptoms (179).

Drug Administration

Drug formulations

Since clozapine is expensive, it is interesting that generic clozapine (given as 25 and 100 mg tablets) behaves like Clozaril, the branded formulation; bioequivalence has been observed in 30 patients with schizophrenia (180).

Drug dosage regimens

Since up to 17% of patients must discontinue clozapine because of adverse effects, strategies for minimizing and managing the adverse effects of clozapine have been reviewed (181,182). Treatment should begin with a low dosage, 12.5–25 mg/day.

The optimal plasma concentration of clozapine is 200–350 ng/ml, which usually corresponds to a daily dose of 200–400 mg (183,184). A nomogram to predict clozapine steady-state plasma concentrations has been generated using data from 71 patients (185). Clozapine steady-state plasma concentrations and demographic variables were obtained. The model explained 47% of the variance in clozapine concentrations. Two equations were obtained to predict steady-state plasma concentrations, one for men and one for women:

$$\text{clozapine (ng/ml)} = 0.464D + 111S + 145 \text{ (men)}$$
$$\text{clozapine (ng/ml)} = 1.590D + 111S - 149 \text{ (women)}$$

where D = dosage (mg/day), S = 1 for smokers, and S = 0 for non-smokers.

A further model for optimizing individual dosage regimens using Bayesian methods has been proposed (186).

Drug overdose

Fatal overdoses have been reported with clozapine (187).

Seven patients who took large doses of clozapine (mean 3 g, range 0.4–16 g) have been reported (188). All made a full recovery and toxicokinetic modelling suggested that norclozapine was formed by a saturable process but that clozapine kinetics were linear over the estimated doses.

- Clozapine overdose (2.5 g) in a 67-year-old woman resulted in seizures, loss of consciousness, metabolic acidosis, prolonged sedation, and aspiration pneumonia (189). By 9 days after intoxication she had recovered completely.
- A 40-year-old man who took 3–4 g of clozapine became unconscious, with constricted pupils, sinus tachycardia, and twitching; peak clozapine and norclozapine concentrations were 3.5 mg/l and 0.7 mg/l respectively, with secondary peaks at about 36 hours (190). Recovery was uneventful, and he was well 2 days after admission.
- A 41-year-old woman took 12.5 g of clozapine (125 tablets of 100 mg each) in a suicide attempt (191). She developed agitation, hallucinations, diminished distrust, and lethargy; she was given physostigmine 2 mg and recovered completely within 1 week.

Drug–Drug Interactions

Benzodiazepines

Caution has been recommended when starting clozapine in patients taking benzodiazepines (SEDA-19, 55). Three cases of delirium associated with clozapine and benzodiazepines (192) have been reported. There have been several reports of synergistic reactions, resulting in increased sedation and ataxia, when lorazepam was begun in patients already taking clozapine (193).

Hypotension, collapse, and respiratory arrest occurred when low doses (12.5–25 mg) of clozapine were added to a pre-existing diazepam regimen in several patients (SEDA-22, 41).

- A 50-year-old man developed syncope and electrocardiographic changes (sinus bradycardia with deep inverted anteroseptal T waves and minor ST changes in other leads) with the concurrent administration of clozapine (after the dosage was increased to 300 mg/day) and diazepam (30 mg/day) (194).

Caffeine

Caffeine has been associated with changes in the metabolism of clozapine (SEDA-20, 50) (SEDA-22, 61). Seven schizophrenic patients taking clozapine monotherapy participated in a study of the effects of caffeine withdrawal from the diet (195). After a caffeine-free diet for 5 days, clozapine plasma concentrations fell by 50%. The authors suggested that schizophrenic patients treated with clozapine should have their caffeine intake medically supervised, and that monitoring of concentrations of clozapine and its metabolite may be warranted.

Ciprofloxacin

A possible pharmacokinetic interaction between ciprofloxacin, which inhibits CYP1A2, and clozapine, with moderately increased serum concentrations of clozapine, has been reported (196).

Cisplatin

There is a potentially dangerous interaction with cancer treatment in patients with schizophrenia taking clozapine, because of the unpredictable risk of myelotoxicity. However, a 37-year-old patient taking clozapine for schizophrenia was given full-dose cisplatin and concomitant radiotherapy for an undifferentiated nasopharyngeal carcinoma, without significant neutropenia (197).

Cocaine

An interaction between clozapine and cocaine, causing near syncope, has been reported (198).

Erythromycin

Increased clozapine serum concentrations have been reported with erythromycin (199,200) and can cause adverse effects (SEDA-21, 55). However, in 12 healthy men who took a single dose of clozapine 12.5 mg alone or in combination with a daily dose of erythromycin 1.5 g, the metabolism of clozapine was not altered (201). This confirms that CYP3A4 is a relatively minor pathway for clozapine metabolism, in contrast to CYP1A2.

In a case of neutropenia the authors suggested that an interaction of clozapine with erythromycin had been the precipitating factor (202).

Interferon alfa

Agranulocytosis was observed after patients taking clozapine were given interferon alfa (SEDA-22, 404) (203). In one case, agranulocytosis occurred after 7 weeks of combined therapy in a 29-year-old patient who had been taking clozapine for more than 5 years without developing hematological abnormalities (203). Even so, it was not clear in these cases whether the agranulocytosis was due to the combination of clozapine with interferon-alfa or the clozapine alone.

Lithium

Seizures and other neurological effects have been described in a few cases when lithium was added to clozapine (204), but in other instances the combination was beneficial in overcoming treatment resistance or attenuating clozapine-induced leukopenia.

Modafinil

Clozapine toxicity occurred in a 42-year-old man after he was given modafinil 300 mg/day, a central stimulant, to combat sedation associated with clozapine (450 mg/day) (205). He complained of dizziness, had an unsteady gait, and fell twice. His serum clozapine concentration was 1400 ng/ml, which suggested a metabolic interaction between clozapine and modafinil. The authors suspected that inhibition of CYP2C19 by modafinil had reduced clozapine clearance.

Perphenazine

Perphenazine doubled clozapine concentrations in a 46-year-old male smoker, with paradoxical myoclonus, hypersalivation, and worsening of psychosis (206). The mechanism of this effect is not known; perphenazine is a substrate for CYP2D6, but that is not important in the metabolism of clozapine.

Phenobarbital

Phenobarbital can stimulate the metabolism of clozapine, probably by inducing its N-oxidation and demethylation. Seven patients taking clozapine in combination with phenobarbital had significantly lower plasma clozapine concentrations than 15 controls taking clozapine only (207).

Risperidone

Clozapine plasma concentrations increase when risperidone is introduced. The effects of risperidone 3.25 mg/day on cytochrome P450 isozymes have therefore been assessed in eight patients by determination of the metabolism of caffeine (for CYP1A2), dextromethorphan (for CYP2D6), and mephenytoin (for CYP2C19) (220). The results suggested that risperidone is a weak in vivo inhibitor of CYP2D6, CYP2C19, and CYP1A2. The authors concluded that inhibition by risperidone of those isozymes is an unlikely mechanism to explain increased clozapine concentrations.

SSRIs

Some SSRIs increase clozapine plasma concentrations (SEDA-20, 50) (SEDA-21, 55) (SEDA-22, 62) by inhibiting its metabolism.

Citalopram

Citalopram had no effect on plasma concentrations of clozapine ($n = 8$), risperidone ($n = 7$), or their active metabolites over 8 weeks (208). However, a possible interaction of clozapine with citalopram has been reported, with increased serum clozapine concentrations, perhaps dose-related (209).

Fluoxetine

In 10 patients stabilized on clozapine (200–450 mg/day) who took fluoxetine (20 mg/day) for 8 weeks, mean plasma concentrations of clozapine, norclozapine, and clozapine N-oxide increased significantly by 58%, 36%, and 38% respectively (210).

In two cases ingestion of clozapine and fluoxetine had a fatal outcome (211). The blood fluoxetine concentration was 0.7 μg/ml, which would be considered a high therapeutic concentration (usual target range 0.03–0.5 μg/ml). The blood clozapine concentration was 4900 ng/ml, which is within the lethal concentration range (1600–7100 ng/ml).

Dual effects were observed in a 44-year-old schizophrenic patient taking clozapine with both fluoxetine and sertraline for mood stabilization (212). Clinical and motor status improved with both fluoxetine and sertraline; cognitive function improved with clozapine and fluoxetine, but was not sustained with sertraline.

Fluvoxamine

Fluvoxamine increases clozapine plasma concentrations (210,213). In 16 patients taking clozapine monotherapy, fluvoxamine 50 mg was added in the hope of ameliorating the negative symptoms of schizophrenia (214). At steady state the serum concentrations of clozapine and its metabolites increased up to five-fold (average two- to three-fold). However, adverse effects were almost unchanged in frequency and severity, in spite of the pharmacokinetic interaction.

In another study there were similar increases in plasma clozapine concentrations and adverse reactions in 18 patients taking fluvoxamine 50 mg (week 5, mean dose 97 mg) (215).

In nine men who were given a single dose of clozapine 50 mg on two separate occasions with a 2-week interval, fluvoxamine increased clozapine plasma concentrations, and the total mean clozapine AUC was increased by a factor of 2.6; all the patients were sedated during combined therapy (216).

Combined therapy with clozapine and fluvoxamine ($n = 11$) and clozapine monotherapy ($n = 12$) have been monitored before and during the first 6 weeks of medication (217). The co-administration of fluvoxamine attenuated and delayed the clozapine-induced increase in plasma concentrations of tumor necrosis factor-alpha, enhanced and accelerated the clozapine-induced increase in leptin plasma concentrations without a significant effect on clozapine-induced weight gain, and reduced granulocyte counts.

In two studies of short duration (18 patients each) there were benefits of using low doses of clozapine plus fluvoxamine, and the authors suggested taking advantage of this interaction (218). Patients taking fluvoxamine required relatively low doses of clozapine and had clinically significant reductions in the symptoms of their illness while avoiding the sedative adverse effects associated with the usual doses of clozapine.

Paroxetine

The effect of paroxetine on steady-state plasma concentrations of clozapine and its metabolites has been studied in 17 patients taking clozapine (200–400 mg/day), nine of whom took additional paroxetine (20–40 mg/day) (219). Paroxetine, a potent inhibitor of CYP2D6, inhibited the metabolism of clozapine, possibly by affecting a pathway other than N-desmethylation and N-oxidation. After 3 weeks of paroxetine, mean plasma concentrations of clozapine and norclozapine increased significantly by 31% and 20% respectively, while concentrations of clozapine N-oxide were unchanged.

Sertraline

Dual effects were observed in a 44-year-old schizophrenic patient taking clozapine with both fluoxetine and sertraline for mood stabilization (212). Clinical and motor status improved with both fluoxetine and sertraline; cognitive function improved with clozapine and fluoxetine, but was not sustained with sertraline. However, sertraline did not affect steady-state plasma concentrations of clozapine and its metabolites in 17 patients taking clozapine (200–400 mg/day), 8 of whom took additional sertraline (50–100 mg/day) (219).

Tricyclic antidepressants

Nefazodone had minimal effects on clozapine metabolism when co-administered in six patients: mean clozapine concentrations rose by 4% and norclozapine concentrations by 16% (221).

Valproate

Clozapine inhibits the metabolism of valproate (222). Valproic acid has been reported to increase the sedative effects of clozapine (SEDA-20, 50) and alter serum concentrations of clozapine.

- In a 33-year-old woman taking clozapine and valproic acid, the serum concentrations of clozapine fell significantly (223).

The authors suggested that valproic acid had induced the metabolism of clozapine.

However, one study showed only small effects on plasma clozapine concentrations, which were thought to be unlikely to be clinically significant (224).

Smoking

Smoking is highly prevalent among patients with schizophrenia, of whom 70–80% smoke tobacco. In a before-and-after study, 55 smokers smoked less when treatment was switched to clozapine than when they were taking typical neuroleptic drugs (225). Nevertheless, it is probable that heavy smoking can induce CYP1A2, the main enzyme involved in the metabolism of clozapine, and plasma concentrations of clozapine are lower in smokers than in non-smokers. Conversely, sudden cessation of smoking can cause a rise in plasma clozapine concentrations. In one case, seizures have been reported as a result (226).

- A 35-year-old schizophrenic man successfully treated with clozapine 700–725 mg/day for more than 7 consecutive years abruptly stopped chronic heavy cigarette smoking and 2 weeks later suddenly developed tonic-clonic seizures followed by stupor and coma. After recovery, he successfully reduced the daily dose by about 40% before he stopped smoking.

Diagnosis of Adverse Drug Reactions

In an open study in 37 patients (27 men and 10 women; mean age 35 years) with treatment-resistant schizophrenia treated with clozapine for 18 weeks, there was no correlation between plasma clozapine concentrations and percentage improvement on the Positive and Negative Syndrome Scale (227). Plasma clozapine concentrations were not significantly different between those who responded to clozapine ($n = 19$) and those who did not ($n = 18$), nor between patients who smoked ($n = 28$) and those who did not ($n = 9$). Dosages were adjusted according to clinical response, and plasma concentrations of clozapine and its metabolites were measured weekly. The mean endpoint clozapine dosage was 487 mg/day and there was a significant correlation between the daily dosage of clozapine and the plasma concentrations of clozapine and its metabolites. Three patients dropped out of the study owing to adverse effects (two because of significant sedation and one because of hypersalivation); there were no cases of agranulocytosis.

References

1. Kulkarni SK, Ninan I. Dopamine D4 receptors and development of newer antipsychotic drugs. Fundam Clin Pharmacol 2000;14(6):529–39.
2. Reid WH. New vs. old antipsychotics: the Texas experience. J Clin Psychiatry 1999;60(Suppl 1):23–5.
3. Parker GF. Clozapine and borderline personality disorder. Psychiatr Serv 2002;53(3):348–9.
4. Masi G, Mucci M, Millepiedi S. Clozapine in adolescent inpatients with acute mania. J Child Adolesc Psychopharmacol 2002;12(2):93–9.
5. Hummel B, Dittmann S, Forsthoff A, Matzner N, Amann B, Grunze H. Clozapine as add-on medication in the maintenance treatment of bipolar and schizoaffective disorders. A case series. Neuropsychobiology 2002;45(Suppl 1):37–42.
6. Connelly JC, Fullick J. Experience with clozapine in a community mental health care setting. South Med J 1998;91(9):838–41.
7. Chong SA, Mahendran R, Wong KE. Use of atypical neuroleptics in a state mental institute. Ann Acad Med Singapore 1998;27(4):547–51.
8. Benedetti F, Sforzini L, Colombo C, Maffei C, Smeraldi E. Low-dose clozapine in acute and continuation treatment of severe borderline personality disorder. J Clin Psychiatry 1998;59(3):103–7.
9. Hector RI. The use of clozapine in the treatment of aggressive schizophrenia. Can J Psychiatry 1998;43(5):466–72.
10. Buzan RD, Dubovsky SL, Firestone D, Dal Pozzo E. Use of clozapine in 10 mentally retarded adults. J Neuropsychiatry Clin Neurosci 1998;10(1):93–5.
11. Dalal B, Larkin E, Leese M, Taylor PJ. Clozapine treatment of long-standing schizophrenia and serious violence: a two-year follow-up study of the first 50 patients treated with clozapine in Rampton high security hospital. Crim Behav Ment Health 1999;9:168–78.
12. Antonacci DJ, de Groot CM. Clozapine treatment in a population of adults with mental retardation. J Clin Psychiatry 2000;61(1):22–5.
13. Waserman J, Criollo M. Subjective experiences of clozapine treatment by patients with chronic schizophrenia. Psychiatr Serv 2000;51(5):666–8.
14. Umbricht DS, Wirshing WC, Wirshing DA, McMeniman M, Schooler NR, Marder SR, Kane JM. Clinical predictors of response to clozapine treatment in ambulatory patients with schizophrenia. J Clin Psychiatry 2002;63(5):420–4.
15. Peacock L, Gerlach J. Clozapine treatment in Denmark: concomitant psychotropic medication and hematologic monitoring in a system with liberal usage practices. J Clin Psychiatry 1994;55(2):44–9.
16. Chong SA, Remington G. Clozapine augmentation: safety and efficacy. Schizophr Bull 2000;26(2):421–40.
17. Killian JG, Kerr K, Lawrence C, Celermajer DS. Myocarditis and cardiomyopathy associated with clozapine. Lancet 1999;354(9193):1841–5.
18. Shiwach RS. Treatment of clozapine induced hypertension and possible mechanisms. Clin Neuropharmacol 1998;21(2):139–40.
19. Donnelly JG, MacLeod AD. Hypotension associated with clozapine after cardiopulmonary bypass. J Cardiothorac Vasc Anesth 1999;13(5):597–9.

20. Low RA Jr., Fuller MA, Popli A. Clozapine induced atrial fibrillation. J Clin Psychopharmacol 1998;18(2):170.
21. Rechlin T, Beck G, Weis M, Kaschka WP. Correlation between plasma clozapine concentration and heart rate variability in schizophrenic patients. Psychopharmacology (Berl) 1998;135(4):338–41.
22. Varma S, Achan K. Dysrhythmia associated with clozapine. Aust NZ J Psychiatry 1999;33(1):118–19.
23. Krentz AJ, Mikhail S, Cantrell P, Hill GM. Pseudophaeochromocytoma syndrome associated with clozapine. BMJ 2001;322(7296):1213.
24. Bredbacka PE, Paukkala E, Kinnunen E, Koponen H. Can severe cardiorespiratory dysregulation induced by clozapine monotherapy be predicted? Int Clin Psychopharmacol 1993;8(3):205–6.
25. Kang UG, Kwon JS, Ahn YM, Chung SJ, Ha JH, Koo YJ, Kim YS. Electrocardiographic abnormalities in patients treated with clozapine. J Clin Psychiatry 2000;61(6):441–6.
26. Cohen H, Loewenthal U, Matar MA, Kotler M. Reversal of pathologic cardiac parameters after transition from clozapine to olanzapine treatment: a case report. Clin Neuropharmacol 2001;24(2):106–8.
27. Tie H, Walker BD, Singleton CB, Bursill JA, Wyse KR, Campbell TJ, Valenzuela SM, Breit SN. Clozapine and sudden death. J Clin Psychopharmacol 2001;21(6):630–2.
28. Chatterton R. Eosinophilia after commencement of clozapine treatment. Aust NZ J Psychiatry 1997;31(6):874–6.
29. Leo RJ, Kreeger JL, Kim KY. Cardiomyopathy associated with clozapine. Ann Pharmacother 1996;30(6):603–5.
30. Juul Povlsen U, Noring U, Fog R, Gerlach J. Tolerability and therapeutic effect of clozapine. A retrospective investigation of 216 patients treated with clozapine for up to 12 years. Acta Psychiatr Scand 1985;71(2):176–85.
31. Warner B, Schadelin J. Clinical safety and epidemiology. Leponex/Clozaril and myocarditis. Basel, Switzerland: Novartis Pharm AG, 1999.
32. Walker AM, Lanza LL, Arellano F, Rothman KJ. Mortality in current and former users of clozapine. Epidemiology 1997;8(6):671–7.
33. Reid P, McArthur M, Pridmore S. Clozapine rechallenge after myocarditis. Aust NZ J Psychiatry 2001;35(2):249.
34. Catalano G, Catalano MC, Frankel Wetter RL. Clozapine induced polyserositis. Clin Neuropharmacol 1997; 20(4):352–6.
35. Murko A, Clarke S, Black DW. Clozapine and pericarditis with pericardial effusion. Am J Psychiatry 2002;159(3):494.
36. Kay SE, Doery J, Sholl D. Clozapine associated pericarditis and elevated troponin I. Aust NZ J Psychiatry 2002;36(1):143–4.
37. Zornberg GL, Jick H. Antipsychotic drug use and risk of first-time idiopathic venous thromboembolism: a case-control study. Lancet 2000;356(9237):1219–23.
38. Hagg S, Spigset O, Soderstrom TG. Association of venous thromboembolism and clozapine. Lancet 2000;355(9210): 1155–6.
39. Knudson JF, Kortepeter C, Dubitsky GM, Ahmad SR, Chen M. Antipsychotic drugs and venous thromboembolism. Lancet 2000;356(9225):252–3.
40. Kortepeter C, Chen M, Knudsen JF, Dubitsky GM, Ahmad SR, Beitz J. Clozapine and venous thromboembolism. Am J Psychiatry 2002;159(5):876–7.
41. Ihde-Scholl T, Rolli ML, Jefferson JW. Clozapine and pulmonary embolus. Am J Psychiatry 2001;158(3):499–500.
42. Ceravolo R, Salvetti S, Piccini P, Lucetti C, Gambaccini G, Bonuccelli U. Acute and chronic effects of clozapine in essential tremor. Mov Disord 1999;14(3):468–72.
43. Freudenreich O, Weiner RD, McEvoy JP. Clozapine-induced electroencephalogram changes as a function of clozapine serum levels. Biol Psychiatry 1997;42(2):132–7.
44. Wetter TC, Lauer CJ, Gillich G, Pollmacher T. The electroencephalographic sleep pattern in schizophrenic patients treated with clozapine or classical antipsychotic drugs. J Psychiatr Res 1996;30(6):411–19.
45. Hinze-Selch D, Mullington J, Orth A, Lauer CJ, Pollmacher T. Effects of clozapine on sleep: a longitudinal study. Biol Psychiatry 1997;42(4):260–6.
46. Toth P, Frankenburg FR. Clozapine and seizures: a review. Can J Psychiatry 1994;39(4):236–8.
47. Haller E, Binder RL. Clozapine and seizures. Am J Psychiatry 1990;147(8):1069–71.
48. Ravasia S, Dickson RA. Seizure on low-dose clozapine. Can J Psychiatry 1998;43(4):420.
49. Panagiotis B. Grand mal seizures with liver toxicity in a case of clozapine treatment. J Neuropsychiatry Clin Neurosci 1999;11(1):117–8.
50. Silvestri RC, Bromfield EB, Khoshbin S. Clozapine-induced seizures and EEG abnormalities in ambulatory psychiatric patients. Ann Pharmacother 1998;32(11):1147–51.
51. Solomons K, Berman KG, Gibson BA. All that seizes is not clozapine. Can J Psychiatry 1998;43(3):306–7.
52. Langosch JM, Trimble MR. Epilepsy, psychosis and clozapine. Hum Psychopharmacol 2002;17(2):115–19.
53. Usiskin SI, Nicolson R, Lenane M, Rapoport JL. Gabapentin prophylaxis of clozapine-induced seizures. Am J Psychiatry 2000;157(3):482–3.
54. Saba G, Dumortier G, Kalalou K, Benadhira R, Degrassat K, Glikman J, Januel D. Lamotrigine–clozapine combination in refractory schizophrenia: three cases J Neuropsychiatry Clin Neurosci 2002;14(1):86.
55. Duggal HS, Jagadheesan K, Nizamie SH. Clozapine-induced stuttering and seizures. Am J Psychiatry 2002; 159(2):315.
56. Supprian T, Retz W, Deckert J. Clozapine-induced stuttering: epileptic brain activity? Am J Psychiatry 1999; 156(10):1663–4.
57. Miller CH, Mohr F, Umbricht D, Woerner M, Fleischhacker WW, Lieberman JA. The prevalence of acute extrapyramidal signs and symptoms in patients treated with clozapine, risperidone, and conventional antipsychotics. J Clin Psychiatry 1998;59(2):69–75.
58. Pi EH, Simpson GM. Medication-induced movement disorder. In: Sadock BJ, Sadock VA, editors. Comprehensive Textbook of Psychiatry, 7th ed. Philadelphia, Lippincott Williams and Wilkins, 2000:2265–71.
59. Spivak B, Mester R, Abesgaus J, Wittenberg N, Adlersberg S, Gonen N, Weizman A. Clozapine treatment for neuroleptic-induced tardive dyskinesia, parkinsonism, chronic akathisia in schizophrenic patients. J Clin Psychiatry 1997;58(7):318–22.
60. Levine J, Chengappa KN. Second thoughts about clozapine as a treatment for neuroleptic-induced akathisia. J Clin Psychiatry 1998;59(4):195.
61. Trosch RM, Friedman JH, Lannon MC, Pahwa R, Smith D, Seeberger LC, O'Brien CF, LeWitt PA, Koller WC. Clozapine use in Parkinson's disease: a retrospective analysis of a large multicentered clinical experience. Mov Disord 1998;13(3):377–82.
62. Lera G, Zirulnik J. Pilot study with clozapine in patients with HIV-associated psychosis and drug-induced parkinsonism. Mov Disord 1999;14(1):128–31.
63. Friedman J, Lannon M, Cornelia C, Factor S, Kurlan R, Richard I. Low-dose clozapine for the treatment of drug-induced psychosis in Parkinson's disease. New Engl J Med 1999;340:757–63.
64. Pollak P, Destee A, Tison F, Pere JJ, Bordiex I, Agid Y. Clozapine in drug-induced psychosis in Parkinson's disease. The French Clozapine Parkinson Study Group. Lancet 1999;353(9169):2041–2.

65. Littrell KH, Johnson CG, Littrell S, Peabody CD. Marked reduction of tardive dyskinesia with olanzapine. Arch Gen Psychiatry 1998;55(3):279–80.
66. O'Brien J, Barber R. Marked improvement in tardive dyskinesia following treatment with olanzapine in an elderly subject. Br J Psychiatry 1998;172:186.
67. Lykouras L, Malliori M, Christodoulou GN. Improvement of tardive dyskinesia following treatment with olanzapine. Eur Neuropsychopharmacol 1999;9(4):367–8.
68. Casey DE. Effects of clozapine therapy in schizophrenic individuals at risk for tardive dyskinesia. J Clin Psychiatry 1998;59(Suppl 3):31–7.
69. Dalack GW, Becks L, Meador-Woodruff JH. Tardive dyskinesia, clozapine, and treatment response. Prog Neuropsychopharmacol Biol Psychiatry 1998;22(4):567–73.
70. Andia I, Zumarraga M, Zabalo MJ, Bulbena A, Davila R. Differential effect of haloperidol and clozapine on plasma homovanillic acid in elderly schizophrenic patients with or without tardive dyskinesia. Biol Psychiatry 1998;43(1):20–3.
71. Modestin J, Stephan PL, Erni T, Umari T. Prevalence of extrapyramidal syndromes in psychiatric inpatients and the relationship of clozapine treatment to tardive dyskinesia. Schizophr Res 2000;42(3):223–30.
72. Kumet R, Freeman MP. Clozapine and tardive dyskinesia. J Clin Psychiatry 2002;63(2):167–8.
73. Elliott ES, Marken PA, Ruehter VL. Clozapine-associated extrapyramidal reaction. Ann Pharmacother 2000;34(5):615–18.
74. Karp BI, Goldstein SR, Chen R, Samii A, Bara-Jimenez W, Hallett M. An open trial of clozapine for dystonia. Mov Disord 1999;14(4):652–7.
75. Sieche A, Giedke H. Treatment of primary cranial dystonia (Meige's syndrome) with clozapine. J Clin Psychiatry 2000;61(12):949.
76. Molho ES, Factor SA. Worsening of motor features of parkinsonism with olanzapine. Mov Disord 1999;14(6):1014–16.
77. Delecluse F, Elosegi JA, Gerard JM. A case of tardive tremor successfully treated with clozapine. Mov Disord 1998;13(5):846–7.
78. Trayer JS, Fidler DC. Neuroleptic malignant syndrome related to use of clozapine. J Am Osteopath Assoc 1998;98(3):168–9.
79. Karagianis JL, Phillips LC, Hogan KP, LeDrew KK. Clozapine-associated neuroleptic malignant syndrome: two new cases and a review of the literature. Ann Pharmacother 1999;33(5):623–30.
80. Lara DR, Wolf AL, Lobato MI, Baroni G, Kapczinski F. Clozapine-induced neuroleptic malignant syndrome: an interaction between dopaminergic and purinergic systems? J Psychopharmacol 1999;13(3):318–19.
81. Benazzi F. Clozapine-induced neuroleptic malignant syndrome not recurring with olanzapine, a structurally and pharmacologically similar antipsychotic. Hum Psychopharmacol Clin Exp 1999;14:511–12.
82. Doan RJ, Callaghan WD. Clozapine treatment and neuroleptic malignant syndrome. Can J Psychiatry 2000;45(4):394–5.
83. Reznik I, Volchek L, Mester R, Kotler M, Sarova-Pinhas I, Spivak B, Weizman A. Myotoxicity and neurotoxicity during clozapine treatment. Clin Neuropharmacol 2000;23(5):276–80.
84. Wilkins-Ho M, Hollander Y. Toxic delirium with low-dose clozapine. Can J Psychiatry 1997;42(4):429–30.
85. Reinstein MJ, Chasonov MA, Colombo KD, Jones LE, Sonnenberg JG. Reduction of suicidality in patients with schizophrenia receiving clozapine. Clin Drug Invest 2002;22:341–6.
86. de Haan L, Linszen DH, Gorsira R. Clozapine and obsessions in patients with recent-onset schizophrenia and other psychotic disorders. J Clin Psychiatry 1999; 60(6):364–5.
87. Bressan RA, Monteiro VB, Dias CC. Panic disorder associated with clozapine. Am J Psychiatry 2000;157(12):2056.
88. Popli AP, Konicki PE, Jurjus GJ, Fuller MA, Jaskiw GE. Clozapine and associated diabetes mellitus. J Clin Psychiatry 1997;58(3):108–11.
89. Wirshing DA, Spellberg BJ, Erhart SM, Marder SR, Wirshing WC. Novel antipsychotics and new onset diabetes. Biol Psychiatry 1998;44(8):778–83.
90. Rigalleau V, Gatta B, Bonnaud S, Masson M, Bourgeois ML, Vergnot V, Gin H. Diabetes as a result of atypical anti-psychotic drugs—a report of three cases. Diabet Med 2000;17(6):484–6.
91. Wehring H, Alexander B, Perry PJ. Diabetes mellitus associated with clozapine therapy. Pharmacotherapy 2000;20(7):844–7.
92. Melkersson K, Hulting AL. Recovery from new-onset diabetes in a schizophrenic man after withdrawal of olanzapine. Psychosomatics 2002;43(1):67–70.
93. Colli A, Cocciolo M, Francobandiera F, Rogantin F, Cattalini N. Diabetic ketoacidosis associated with clozapine treatment. Diabetes Care 1999;22(1):176–7.
94. Chae BJ, Kang BJ. The effect of clozapine on blood glucose metabolism. Hum Psychopharmacol 2001;16(3):265–71.
95. Hagg S, Joelsson L, Mjorndal T, Spigset O, Oja G, Dahlqvist R. Prevalence of diabetes and impaired glucose tolerance in patients treated with clozapine compared with patients treated with conventional depot neuroleptic medications. J Clin Psychiatry 1998; 59(6):294–9.
96. Yazici KM, Erbas T, Yazici AH. The effect of clozapine on glucose metabolism. Exp Clin Endocrinol Diabetes 1998;106(6):475–7.
97. Wang PS, Glynn RJ, Ganz DA, Schneeweiss S, Levin R, Avorn J. Clozapine use and risk of diabetes mellitus. J Clin Psychopharmacol 2002;22(3):236–43.
98. Frankenburg FR, Zanarini MC, Kando J, Centorrino F. Clozapine and body mass change. Biol Psychiatry 1998;43(7):520–4.
99. Bromel T, Blum WF, Ziegler A, Schulz E, Bender M, Fleischhaker C, Remschmidt H, Krieg JC, Hebebrand J. Serum leptin levels increase rapidly after initiation of clozapine therapy. Mol Psychiatry 1998;3(1):76–80.
100. Baymiller SP, Ball P, McMahon RP, Buchanan RW. Weight and blood pressure change during clozapine treatment. Clin Neuropharmacol 2002;25(4):202–6.
101. Feldman D, Goldberg JF. A preliminary study of the relationship between clozapine-induced weight gain and menstrual irregularities in schizophrenic, schizoaffective, and bipolar women. Ann Clin Psychiatry 2002; 14(1):17–21.
102. Wirshing DA, Pierre JM, Wirshing WC. Sleep apnea associated with antipsychotic-induced obesity. J Clin Psychiatry 2002;63(4):369–70.
103. Borovicka MC, Fuller MA, Konicki PE, White JC, Steele VM, Jaskiw GE. Phenylpropanolamine appears not to promote weight loss in patients with schizophrenia who have gained weight during clozapine treatment. J Clin Psychiatry 2002;63(4):345–8.
104. Dursun SM, Devarajan S. Clozapine weight gain, plus topiramate weight loss. Can J Psychiatry 2000;45(2):198.
105. de la Chapelle A, Kari C, Nurminen M, Hernberg S. Clozapine-induced agranulocytosis. A genetic and epidemiologic study. Hum Genet 1977;37(2):183–94.
106. Alvir JM, Lieberman JA, Safferman AZ, Schwimmer JL, Schaaf JA. Clozapine-induced agranulocytosis. Incidence

and risk factors in the United States. N Engl J Med 1993;329(3):162–7.
107. Lamarque V. Effets hématologiques de la clozapine: bilan de l'experience internationale. [Hematologic effects of clozapine: a review of the international experience.] Encephale 1996;22(Spec No 6):35–6.
108. Copolov DL, Bell WR, Benson WJ, Keks NA, Strazzeri DC, Johnson GF. Clozapine treatment in Australia: a review of haematological monitoring. Med J Aust 1998;168(10):495–7.
109. Schuld A, Kraus T, Hinze-Selch D, Haack M, Pollmacher T. Granulocyte colony-stimulating factor plasma levels during clozapine- and olanzapine-induced granulocytopenia. Acta Psychiatr Scand 2000;102(2):153–5.
110. Jauss M, Pantel J, Werle E, Schroder J. G-CSF plasma levels in clozapine-induced neutropenia. Biol Psychiatry 2000;48(11):1113–15.
111. van de Loosdrecht AA, Faber HJ, Hordijk P, Uges DR, Smit A. Clozapine-induced agranulocytosis: a case report. Immunopathophysiological considerations. Neth J Med 1998;52(1):26–9.
112. Guest I, Sokoluk B, MacCrimmon J, Uetrecht J. Examination of possible toxic and immune mechanisms of clozapine-induced agranulocytosis. Toxicology 1998;131(1):53–65.
113. Dettling M, Sachse C, Muller-Oerlinghausen B, Roots I, Brockmoller J, Rolfs A, Cascorbi I. Clozapine-induced agranulocytosis and hereditary polymorphisms of clozapine metabolizing enzymes: no association with myeloperoxidase and cytochrome P4502D6. Pharmacopsychiatry 2000;33(6):218–20.
114. Lieberman JA, Yunis J, Egea E, Canoso RT, Kane JM, Yunis EJ. HLA-B38, DR4, DQw3 and clozapine-induced agranulocytosis in Jewish patients with schizophrenia. Arch Gen Psychiatry 1990;47(10):945–8.
115. Dettling M, Schaub RT, Mueller-Oerlinghausen B, Roots I, Cascorbi I. Further evidence of human leukocyte antigen-encoded susceptibility to clozapine-induced agranulocytosis independent of ancestry. Pharmacogenetics 2001;11(2):135–41.
116. Lahdelma L, Ahokas A, Andersson LC, Suvisaari J, Hovatta I, Huttunen MO, Koskimies S. Mitchell B. Balter Award. Human leukocyte antigen-A1 predicts a good therapeutic response to clozapine with a low risk of agranulocytosis in patients with schizophrenia. J Clin Psychopharmacol 2001;21(1):4–7.
117. Horacek J, Libiger J, Hoschl C, Borzova K, Hendrychova I. Clozapine-induced concordant agranulocytosis in monozygotic twins. Int J Psychiatry Clin Pract 2001;5:71–3.
118. Ahokas A, Elonen E. Circadian rhythm of white blood cells during clozapine treatment. Psychopharmacology (Berl) 1999;144(3):301–2.
119. Hu RJ, Malhotra AK, Pickar D. Predicting response to clozapine: status of current research. CNS Drugs 1999;11:317–26.
120. Patel NC, Dorson PG, Bettinger TL. Sudden late onset of clozapine-induced agranulocytosis. Ann Pharmacother 2002;36(6):1012–15.
121. Gupta S, Noor-Khan N, Frank B. Agranulocytosis in a second clozapine trial. Psychiatr Serv 1998;49(8):1094.
122. Sperner-Unterweger B, Czeipek I, Gaggl S, Geissler D, Spiel G, Fleischhacker WW. Treatment of severe clozapine-induced neutropenia with granulocyte colony-stimulating factor (G-CSF). Remission despite continuous treatment with clozapine. Br J Psychiatry 1998;172:82–4.
123. Silvestrini C, Arcangeli T, Biondi M, Pancheri P. A second trial of clozapine in a case of granulocytopenia. Hum Psychopharmacol 2000;15(4):275–9.
124. Stewart P, Ezzy J. CPMSPlus, an innovative, web-based patient monitoring system for Clozaril centres. Aust J Hosp Pharm 2001;31:56.
125. Davies RH. Late awareness of anaemia in a patient receiving clozapine. Psychiatr Bull 2001;25:194–5.
126. Diaz P, Hogan TP. Granulocytopenia with clozapine and quetiapine. Am J Psychiatry 2001;158(4):651.
127. Melzer M, Hassanyeh FK, Snow MH, Ong EL. Sepsis and neutropenia induced by clozapine. Clin Microbiol Infect 1998;4(10):604–5.
128. Marcos F, Solano F, Arbol F, Caballero L, Maldonado G, Lopez P, Duran A. Clozapine-induced agranulocytosis. SN 2000;5:27–9.
129. Blier P, Slater S, Measham T, Koch M, Wiviott G. Lithium and clozapine-induced neutropenia/agranulocytosis. Int Clin Psychopharmacol 1998;13(3):137–40.
130. Moldavsky M, Stein D, Benatov R, Sirota P, Elizur A, Matzner Y, Weizman A. Combined clozapine–lithium treatment for schizophrenia and schizoaffective disorder. Eur Psychiatry 1998;13:104–6.
131. Lucht MJ, Rietschel M. Clozapine-induced eosinophilia: subsequent neutropenia and corresponding allergic mechanisms. J Clin Psychiatry 1998;59(4):195–7.
132. Ames D, Wirshing WC, Baker RW, Umbricht DS, Sun AB, Carter J, Schooler NR, Kane JM, Marder SR. Predictive value of eosinophilia for neutropenia during clozapine treatment. J Clin Psychiatry 1996;57(12):579–81.
133. Hampson ME. Clozapine-induced thrombocytosis. Br J Psychiatry 2000;176:400.
134. Gonzales MF, Elmore J, Luebbert C. Evidence for immune etiology in clozapine-induced thrombocytopenia of 40 months' duration: a case report. CNS Spectr 2000;5:17–18.
135. Dunayevich E, McElroy SL. Atypical antipsychotics in the treatment of bipolar disorder: pharmacological and clinical effects. CNS Drugs 2000;13:433–41.
136. Szabadi E. Clozapine-induced hypersalivation. Br J Psychiatry 1997;171:89.
137. Patkar AA, Alexander RC. Parotid gland swelling with clozapine. J Clin Psychiatry 1996;57(10):488.
138. Tsai SJ, Wang YC, Yu, Younger WY, Lin CH, Yang KH, Hong CJ. Association analysis of polymorphism in the promoter region of the alpha$_{2a}$-adrenoceptor gene with schizophrenia and clozapine response. Schizophr Res 2001;49(1–2):53–8.
139. Cree A, Mir S, Fahy T. A review of the treatment options for clozapine-induced hypersalivation. Psychiatr Bull 2001;25:114–16.
140. Reinstein MJ, Sirotovskaya LA, Chasanov MA, Jones LE, Mohan S. Comparative efficacy and tolerability of benzatropine and terazosin in the treatment of hypersalivation secondary to clozapine. Clin Drug Invest 1999;17:97–102.
141. Calderon J, Rubin E, Sobota WL. Potential use of ipratropium bromide for the treatment of clozapine-induced hypersalivation: a preliminary report. Int Clin Psychopharmacol 2000;15(1):49–52.
142. Laker MK, Cookson JC. Reflux oesophagitis and clozapine. Int Clin Psychopharmacol 1997;12(1):37–9.
143. Baker RW, Chengappa KN. Gastroesophageal reflux as a possible result of clozapine treatment. J Clin Psychiatry 1998;59(5):257.
144. Freudenreich O, Goff DC. Colon perforation and peritonitis associated with clozapine. J Clin Psychiatry 2000;61(12):950–1.
145. Levin TT, Barrett J, Mendelowitz A. Death from clozapine-induced constipation: case report and literature review. Psychosomatics 2002;43(1):71–3.
146. Hummer M, Kurz M, Kurzthaler I, Oberbauer H, Miller C, Fleischhacker WW. Hepatotoxicity of clozapine. J Clin Psychopharmacol 1997;17(4):314–17.

147. Larsen JT, Clemensen SV, Klitgaard NA, Nielsen B, Brosen K. Clozapin-udlost toksisk hepatitis. [Clozapine-induced toxic hepatitis.] Ugeskr Laeger 2001; 163(14):2013–4.
148. Thompson J, Chengappa KN, Good CB, Baker RW, Kiewe RP, Bezner J, Schooler NR. Hepatitis, hyperglycemia, pleural effusion, eosinophilia, hematuria and proteinuria occurring early in clozapine treatment. Int Clin Psychopharmacol 1998;13(2):95–8.
149. Macfarlane B, Davies S, Mannan K, Sarsam R, Pariente D, Dooley J. Fatal acute fulminant liver failure due to clozapine: a case report and review of clozapine-induced hepatotoxicity. Gastroenterology 1997;112(5):1707–9.
150. Gatto EM, Castronuovo AP, Uribe Roca MC. Clozapine and pancreatitis. Clin Neuropharmacol 1998;21(3):203.
151. Cerulli TR. Clozapine-associated pancreatitis. Harv Rev Psychiatry 1999;7(1):61–3.
152. Bergemann N, Ehrig C, Diebold K, Mundt C, von Einsiedel R. Asymptomatic pancreatitis associated with clozapine. Pharmacopsychiatry 1999;32(2):78–80.
153. Poyurovsky M, Modai I, Weizman A. Trihexyphenidyl as a possible therapeutic option in clozapine-induced nocturnal enuresis. Int Clin Psychopharmacol 1996;11(1):61–3.
154. Costa JF, Sramek J, Bera RB, Brenneman M, Cristobal M. Control of bed-wetting with benztropine. Am J Psychiatry 1990;147(5):674.
155. Lin CC, Bai YM, Chen JY, Lin CY, Lan TH. A retrospective study of clozapine and urinary incontinence in Chinese in-patients. Acta Psychiatr Scand 1999;100(2):158–61.
156. Hsu JW, Wang YC, Lin CC, Bai YM, Chen JY, Chiu HJ, Tsai SJ, Hong CJ. No evidence for association of alpha 1a adrenoceptor gene polymorphism and clozapine-induced urinary incontinence. Neuropsychobiology 2000;42(2):62–5.
157. Elias TJ, Bannister KM, Clarkson AR, Faull D, Faull RJ. Clozapine-induced acute interstitial nephritis. Lancet 1999;354(9185):1180–1.
158. David WS, Sharif AA. Clozapine-induced myokymia. Muscle Nerve 1998;21(6):827–8.
159. Vrtunski PB, Konicki PE, Jaskiw GE, Brescan DW, Kwon KY, Jurjus G. Clozapine effects on force control in schizophrenic patients. Schizophr Res 1998;34(1–2):39–48.
160. Koren W, Koren E, Nacasch N, Ehrenfeld M, Gur H. Rhabdomyolysis associated with clozapine treatment in a patient with decreased calcium-dependent potassium permeability of cell membranes. Clin Neuropharmacol 1998;21(4):262–4.
161. Wicki J, Rutschmann OT, Burri H, Vecchietti G, Desmeules J. Rhabdomyolysis after correction of hyponatremia due to psychogenic polydipsia possibly complicated by clozapine. Ann Pharmacother 1998;32(9):892–5.
162. Hummer M, Kemmler G, Kurz M, Kurzthaler I, Oberbauer H, Fleischhacker WW. Sexual disturbances during clozapine and haloperidol treatment for schizophrenia. Am J Psychiatry 1999;156(4):631–3.
163. Jeffries JJ, Vanderhaeghe L, Remington GJ, Al-Jeshi A. Clozapine-associated retrograde ejaculation. Can J Psychiatry 1996;41(1):62–3.
164. Stanislav SW, Gonzalez-Blanco M. Papular rash and bilateral pleural effusion associated with clozapine. Ann Pharmacother 1999;33(9):1008–9.
165. Tremeau F, Clark SC, Printz D, Kegeles LS, Malaspina D. Spiking fevers with clozapine treatment. Clin Neuropharmacol 1997;20(2):168–70.
166. Shiovitz TM, Welke TL, Tigel PD, Anand R, Hartman RD, Sramek JJ, Kurtz NM, Cutler NR. Cholinergic rebound and rapid onset psychosis following abrupt clozapine withdrawal. Schizophr Bull 1996; 22(4):591–5.
167. Verghese C, DeLeon J, Nair C, Simpson GM. Clozapine withdrawal effects and receptor profiles of typical and atypical neuroleptics. Biol Psychiatry 1996;39(2):135–8.
168. Ekblom B, Eriksson K, Lindstrom LH. Supersensitivity psychosis in schizophrenic patients after sudden clozapine withdrawal. Psychopharmacology (Berl) 1984;83(3):293–4.
169. Perenyi A, Kuncz E, Bagdy G. Early relapse after sudden withdrawal or dose reduction of clozapine. Psychopharmacology (Berl) 1985;86(1–2):244.
170. Eklund K. Supersensitivity and clozapine withdrawal. Psychopharmacology (Berl) 1987;91(1):135.
171. Goudie AJ. What is the clinical significance of the discontinuation syndrome seen with clozapine? J Psychopharmacol 2000;14(2):188–92.
172. Simpson GM, Varga E. Clozapine—a new antipsychotic agent. Curr Ther Res Clin Exp 1974;16(7):679–86.
173. Lieberman JA, Kane JM, Johns CA. Clozapine: guidelines for clinical management. J Clin Psychiatry 1989;50(9):329–38.
174. de Leon J, Stanilla JK, White AO, Simpson GM. Anticholinergics to treat clozapine withdrawal. J Clin Psychiatry 1994;55(3):119–20.
175. Ahmed S, Chengappa KN, Naidu VR, Baker RW, Parepally H, Schooler NR. Clozapine withdrawal-emergent dystonias and dyskinesias: a case series. J Clin Psychiatry 1998;59(9):472–7.
176. Poyurovsky M, Bergman Y, Shoshani D, Schneidman M, Weizman A. Emergence of obsessive–compulsive symptoms and tics during clozapine withdrawal. Clin Neuropharmacol 1998;21(2):97–100.
177. Stoner SC, Sommi RW Jr, Marken PA, Anya I, Vaughn J. Clozapine use in two full-term pregnancies. J Clin Psychiatry 1997;58(8):364–5.
178. Sajatovic M, Ramirez LF, Garver D, Thompson P, Ripper G, Lehmann LS. Clozapine therapy for older veterans. Psychiatr Serv 1998;49(3):340–4.
179. Burke WJ, Pfeiffer RF, McComb RD. Neuroleptic sensitivity to clozapine in dementia with Lewy bodies. J Neuropsychiatry Clin Neurosci 1998;10(2):227–9.
180. Sramek JJ, Anand R, Hartman RD, Schran HF, Hourani J, Barto S, Wardle TS, Shiovitz TM, Cutler NR. A bioequivalence study of brand and generic clozapine in patients with schizophrenia. Clin Drug Invest 1999;17:51–8.
181. Young CR, Bowers MB Jr, Mazure CM. Management of the adverse effects of clozapine. Schizophr Bull 1998; 24(3):381–90.
182. Lieberman JA. Maximizing clozapine therapy: managing side effects. J Clin Psychiatry 1998;59(Suppl 3):38–43.
183. Conley RR. Optimizing treatment with clozapine. J Clin Psychiatry 1998;59(Suppl 3):44–8.
184. Olesen OV. Therapeutic drug monitoring of clozapine treatment. Therapeutic threshold value for serum clozapine concentrations. Clin Pharmacokinet 1998; 34(6):497–502.
185. Perry PJ, Bever KA, Arndt S, Combs MD. Relationship between patient variables and plasma clozapine concentrations: a dosing nomogram. Biol Psychiatry 1998; 44(8):733–8.
186. Guitton C, Kinowski JM, Gomeni R, Bressolle F. A kinetic model for simultaneous fit of clozapine and norclozapine concentrations in chronic schizophrenic patients during long-term treatment. Clin Drug Invest 1998;16:35–43.
187. Keller T, Miki A, Binda S, Dirnhofer R. Fatal overdose of clozapine. Forensic Sci Int 1997;86(1–2):119–25.
188. Reith D, Monteleone JP, Whyte IM, Ebelling W, Holford NH, Carter GL. Features and toxicokinetics of clozapine in overdose. Ther Drug Monit 1998;20(1):92–7.
189. Hagg S, Spigset O, Edwardsson H, Bjork H. Prolonged sedation and slowly decreasing clozapine serum

concentrations after an overdose. J Clin Psychopharmacol 1999;19(3):282–4.
190. Renwick AC, Renwick AG, Flanagan RJ, Ferner RE. Monitoring of clozapine and norclozapine plasma concentration-time curves in acute overdose. J Toxicol Clin Toxicol 2000;38(3):325–8.
191. Sartorius A, Hewer W, Zink M, Henn FA. High-dose clozapine intoxication. J Clin Psychopharmacol 2002; 22(1):91–2.
192. Jackson CW, Markowitz JS, Brewerton TD. Delirium associated with clozapine and benzodiazepine combinations. Ann Clin Psychiatry 1995;7(3):139–41.
193. Cobb CD, Anderson CB, Seidel DR. Possible interaction between clozapine and lorazepam. Am J Psychiatry 1991;148(11):1606–7.
194. Tupala E, Niskanen L, Tiihonen J. Transient syncope and ECG changes associated with the concurrent administration of clozapine and diazepam. J Clin Psychiatry 1999;60(9):619–20.
195. Carrillo JA, Herraiz AG, Ramos SI, Benitez J. Effects of caffeine withdrawal from the diet on the metabolism of clozapine in schizophrenic patients. J Clin Psychopharmacol 1998;18(4):311–16.
196. Raaska K, Neuvonen PJ. Ciprofloxacin increases serum clozapine and N-desmethylclozapine: a study in patients with schizophrenia. Eur J Clin Pharmacol 2000;56(8):585–9.
197. Bareggi C, Palazzi M, Locati LD, Cerrotta A, Licitral L. Clozapine and full-dose concomitant chemoradiation therapy in a schizophrenic patient with nasopharyngeal cancer. Tumori 2002;88(1):59–60.
198. Hameedi FA, Sernyak MJ, Navui SA, Kosten TR. Near syncope associated with concomitant clozapine and cocaine use. J Clin Psychiatry 1996;57(8):371–2.
199. Taylor D. Pharmacokinetic interactions involving clozapine. Br J Psychiatry 1997;171:109–12.
200. Cohen LG, Chesley S, Eugenio L, Flood JG, Fisch J, Goff DC. Erythromycin-induced clozapine toxic reaction. Arch Intern Med 1996;156(6):675–7.
201. Hagg S, Spigset O, Mjorndal T, Granberg K, Persbo-Lundqvist G, Dahlqvist R. Absence of interaction between erythromycin and a single dose of clozapine. Eur J Clin Pharmacol 1999;55(3):221–6.
202. Usiskin SI, Nicolson R, Lenane M, Rapoport JL. Retreatment with clozapine after erythromycin-induced neutropenia. Am J Psychiatry 2000;157(6):1021.
203. Hoffmann RM, Ott S, Parhofer KG, Bartl R, Pape GR. Interferon-alpha-induced agranulocytosis in a patient on long-term clozapine therapy. J Hepatol 1998;29(1):170.
204. Edge SC, Markowitz JS, DeVane CL. Clozapine drug–drug interactions: a review of the literature. Hum Psychopharmacol 1997;12:5–20.
205. Dequardo JR. Modafinil-associated clozapine toxicity. Am J Psychiatry 2002;159(7):1243–4.
206. Cooke C, de Leon J. Adding other antipsychotics to clozapine. J Clin Psychiatry 1999;60(10):710.
207. Facciola G, Avenoso A, Spina E, Perucca E. Inducing effect of phenobarbital on clozapine metabolism in patients with chronic schizophrenia. Ther Drug Monit 1998;20(6):628–30.
208. Avenoso A, Facciolà G, Scordo MG, Gitto C, Ferrante GD, Madia AG, Spina E. No effect of citalopram on plasma levels of clozapine, risperidone and their active metabolites in patients with chronic schizophrenia. Clin Drug Invest 1998;16:393–8.
209. Borba CP, Henderson DC. Citalopram and clozapine: potential drug interaction. J Clin Psychiatry 2000;61(4):301–2.
210. Spina E, Avenoso A, Facciola G, Fabrazzo M, Monteleone P, Maj M, Perucca E, Caputi AP. Effect of fluoxetine on the plasma concentrations of clozapine and its major metabolites in patients with schizophrenia. Int Clin Psychopharmacol 1998;13(3):141–5.
211. Ferslew KE, Hagardorn AN, Harlan GC, McCormick WF. A fatal drug interaction between clozapine and fluoxetine. J Forensic Sci 1998;43(5):1082–5.
212. Purdon SE, Snaterse M. Selective serotonin reuptake inhibitor modulation of clozapine effects on cognition in schizophrenia. Can J Psychiatry 1998;43(1):84–5.
213. Markowitz JS, Gill HS, Lavia M, Brewerton TD, DeVane CL. Fluvoxamine–clozapine dose-dependent interaction. Can J Psychiatry 1996;41(10):670–1.
214. Szegedi A, Anghelescu I, Wiesner J, Schlegel S, Weigmann H, Hartter S, Hiemke C, Wetzel H. Addition of low-dose fluvoxamine to low-dose clozapine monotherapy in schizophrenia: drug monitoring and tolerability data from a prospective clinical trial. Pharmacopsychiatry 1999;32(4):148–53.
215. Lammers CH, Deuschle M, Weigmann H, Hartter S, Hiemke C, Heese C, Heuser I. Coadministration of clozapine and fluvoxamine in psychotic patients—clinical experience. Pharmacopsychiatry 1999;32(2):76–7.
216. Chang WH, Augustin B, Lane HY, ZumBrunnen T, Liu HC, Kazmi Y, Jann MW. In-vitro and in-vivo evaluation of the drug–drug interaction between fluvoxamine and clozapine. Psychopharmacology (Berl) 1999;145(1):91–8.
217. Hinze-Selch D, Deuschle M, Weber B, Heuser I, Pollmacher T. Effect of coadministration of clozapine and fluvoxamine versus clozapine monotherapy on blood cell counts, plasma levels of cytokines and body weight. Psychopharmacology (Berl) 2000;149(2):163–9.
218. Prior TI. Is there a way to overcome over-sedation in a patient being treated with clozapine? J Psychiatry Neurosci 2002;27:224.
219. Spina E, Avenoso A, Salemi M, Facciola G, Scordo MG, Ancione M, Madia A. Plasma concentrations of clozapine and its major metabolites during combined treatment with paroxetine or sertraline. Pharmacopsychiatry 2000; 33(6):213–17.
220. Eap CB, Bondolfi G, Zullino D, Bryois C, Fuciec M, Savary L, Jonzier-Perey M, Baumann P. Pharmacokinetic drug interaction potential of risperidone with cytochrome p450 isozymes as assessed by the dextromethorphan, the caffeine, and the mephenytoin test. Ther Drug Monit 2001;23(3):228–31.
221. Taylor D, Bodani M, Hubbeling A, Murray R. The effect of nefazodone on clozapine plasma concentrations. Int Clin Psychopharmacol 1999;14(3):185–7.
222. Costello LE, Suppes T. A clinically significant interaction between clozapine and valproate. J Clin Psychopharmacol 1995;15(2):139–41.
223. Conca A, Beraus W, Konig P, Waschgler R. A case of pharmacokinetic interference in comedication of clozapine and valproic acid. Pharmacopsychiatry 2000; 33(6):234–5.
224. Facciola G, Avenoso A, Scordo MG, Madia AG, Ventimiglia A, Perucca E, Spina E. Small effects of valproic acid on the plasma concentrations of clozapine and its major metabolites in patients with schizophrenic or affective disorders. Ther Drug Monit 1999;21(3):341–5.
225. McEvoy JP, Freudenreich O, Wilson WH. Smoking and therapeutic response to clozapine in patients with schizophrenia. Biol Psychiatry 1999;46(1):125–9.
226. Skogh E, Bengtsson F, Nordin C. Could discontinuing smoking be hazardous for patients administered clozapine medication? A case report. Ther Drug Monit 1999; 21(5):580–2.
227. Llorca PM, Lancon C, Disdier B, Farisse J, Sapin C, Auquier P. Effectiveness of clozapine in neuroleptic-resistant schizophrenia: clinical response and plasma concentrations. J Psychiatry Neurosci 2002;27(1):30–7.

Clusiaceae

See also Herbal medicines

General Information

The genera in the family of Clusiaceae (Table 1) include St. John's wort.

Hypericum perforatum

Hypericum perforatum (devil's scourge, goat weed, rosin rose, St. John's wort, Tipton weed, witch's herb) contains the naphthodianthrones hypericin and pseudo-hypericin, flavonoids, such as hyperoside, isoquercitin, and rutin, and phloroglucinols, such as adhyperforin and hyperforin. It is effective in mild to moderate depression (1).

Adverse effects

A meta-analysis of 23 randomized, controlled trials of St. John's wort showed that the herbal extract is more effective than placebo for mild to moderate depression, but that current evidence was inadequate to establish whether St. John's wort is as effective as standard antidepressants (2). In clinical trials, St. John's wort appeared to have fewer short-term adverse effects than some conventional antidepressants, but information on long-term adverse effects is lacking.

Two reviews have systematically addressed the safety of St. John's wort. One showed that the most common adverse events were gastrointestinal symptoms, dizziness, confusion, tiredness, sedation, and dry mouth (3). A second review compared the adverse effect profile of St. John's wort with those of conventional antidepressants (4). The adverse effects of St. John's wort were fewer and less serious than those associated with conventional antidepressant drugs.

A review of all reported adverse effects associated with St. John's wort has shown that it has an encouraging safety profile (3). Adverse effects reported in clinical trials were invariably mild and transient: gastrointestinal symptoms (8.5%), dizziness/confusion (4.5%), tiredness/sedation (4.5%), and dry mouth (4.0%). Synthetic drugs used in comparative trials were burdened with significantly higher rates of adverse effects. Data obtained from the WHO Collaborating Center for International Drug Monitoring are summarized in Table 2.

Cardiovascular

A 41-year-old man who had taken St. John's wort had a hypertensive crisis after taking cheese with red wine (5).

Table 1 The genera of Clusiaceae

Calophyllum (calophyllum)
Clusia (attorney)
Garcinia (sap tree)
Hypericum (St. John's wort)
Mammea (mammea)
Pentadesma (pentadesma)
Platonia (platonia)
Triadenum (marsh St. John's wort)

Table 2 Reports of adverse effects of formulations of St. John's wort (up to May 1998)

System	Number of cases
Cardiovascular (edema)	2
Cardiovascular (bradycardia)	1
Respiratory	4
Nervous system	5
Nervous system (stroke)	1
Psychiatric	15
Hematological (coagulation)	4
Gastrointestinal	2
Liver	4
Urinary tract (interstitial nephritis)	1
Skin (allergic reactions)	16
Skin (conjunctivitis)	1
Reduced therapeutic response	1

St. John's wort is a monoamine oxidase inhibitor, and the authors believed that this explained how the concomitant use of a tyramine-rich food with St. John's wort had caused this problem.

Nervous system

The mechanism of action of St. John's wort in depression is not understood, but serotonin re-uptake inhibition is one possibility, for which evidence is increasing. In one case this may have led to the serotonin syndrome in a 33-year-old woman who developed extreme acute anxiety after taking only three doses of extracts of St. John's wort and recovered after withdrawal (6).

- A 40-year-old man with a history of anxiety disorder and depression presented with flushing, sweating, agitation, weakness of the legs, dry mouth, tightness in the chest, and inability to focus (7). He was taking clonazepam (0.5 mg bd) and had started to take St. John's wort 10 days before. He had previously had two similar episodes after having taken sertraline.

The authors concluded that self-medication with St. John's wort, which has SSRI activity, had caused the serotonin syndrome.

Psychiatric

Delirium has been attributed to St. John's wort.

- A 76-year-old woman began taking an extract of St. John's wort (75 mg/day) and developed delirium and psychosis 3 weeks later (8). She had no relevant medical history and did not take any other medications. She was given risperidone and donepezil hydrochloride, and her paranoid delusions and visual hallucinations improved.

The final diagnosis was acute psychotic delirium associated with St. John's wort in a woman with underlying Alzheimer's dementia.

Hypomania has been reported with St. John's wort (9).

- A 47-year-old woman with an 8-year history of nocturnal panic attacks and a recent history of major depression had a poor response to SSRIs and instead took a 0.1% tincture of St. John's wort. After 10 days she noted racing and distorted thoughts, increased irritability, hostility, aggressive behavior, and a reduced need for sleep. After discontinuing the herbal treatment, her symptoms resolved within 2 days.

The author suggested that St. John's wort had caused this episode of hypomania.

Two cases of mania have been associated with the use of St. John's wort (10). The authors pointed out that St. John's wort, like all antidepressants, can precipitate hypomania, mania, or increased cycling of mood states, particularly in patients with occult bipolar disorder. Alternatively, the mania experienced by these patients could simply be the expression of the natural cause of their psychiatric illness.

Endocrine

In a retrospective case-control study, 37 patients with raised TSH concentrations were compared with 37 individuals with normal TSH concentrations (11). Exposure to St. John's wort during the previous 3–6 months increased the odds of a raised TSH concentration by a factor of 2.12 (95% CI = 0.36, 12). The authors concluded that an association between St. John's wort and raised TSH concentrations is probable.

Skin

Photosensitivity has been attributed to St. John's wort (12).

- A 35-year-old woman took ground whole St. John's wort (500 mg/day) for mild depression. After 4 weeks she developed stinging pain on her face and the backs of both hands, which worsened with sun exposure. She was seen after the area of pain had spread following exposure to the sun. After withdrawal of St. John's wort, the symptoms gradually disappeared during the next 2 months.

The authors thought that photoactive hypericins had caused demyelination of cutaneous nerve axons. If they are correct, then this would be the first human case of photosensitivity after St. John's wort, a condition previously only reported in animals.

Of 43 users of St. John's wort surveyed by telephone, 47% reported adverse effects that they related to the remedy (13). The only potentially serious complaint was photosensitivity, which was noted by four individuals.

An Australian dermatologist has reported three cases of phototoxic reactions to St. John's wort (14). The patients were fair-skinned and had had significant exposure to ultraviolet light. In two cases St. John's wort was applied topically. In all cases complete recovery occurred after withdrawal of St. John's wort and cessation of exposure to ultraviolet light.

Hair

Alopecia has been attributed to St. John's wort.

- A 24-year-old woman with schizophrenia who self-medicated with St. John's wort while also taking olanzapine (5–10 mg/day) developed hair loss on her scalp and eyebrows 5 months later; it persisted for 12 months (7). Her medical history was otherwise unremarkable.

The authors speculated that, like SSRIs, St. John's wort can cause hair loss.

Pregnancy

Like all herbal remedies, there is insufficient evidence that it is safe to take St. John's wort during pregnancy. Two women who took St. John's wort during pregnancy in order to avoid potential harmful effects of synthetic antidepressants to the fetus also discontinued their prescribed medications and did not discuss their decisions with their doctor (15). Although the effects of St. John's wort on the fetus are not known, the authors cautioned against using it under these circumstances and argued that tricyclic antidepressants or fluoxetine would be safer.

Drug interactions

Interactions of St. John's wort with prescribed drugs are due to its ability to induce the activity of both CYP3A4 and the P glycoprotein transporter system (16). Prescribed drugs that interact with St. John's wort include ciclosporin, digoxin, HIV protease inhibitors, oral contraceptives, serotonin re-uptake inhibitors, theophylline, and warfarin (17).

The mechanism of hepatic enzyme induction by St. John's wort has been intensively researched (18,19). Treatment of human hepatocytes with extracts of St. John's wort or with hyperforin (one of its active constituents) resulted in induction of CYP3A4 expression (20).

Following reports about the potential for herb–drug interactions, many national regulatory agencies issued warnings about the use of St. John's wort and its safety was reviewed (21,22).

Ciclosporin

St. John's wort is a hepatic enzyme inducer (23) and can lower the plasma concentrations of various prescribed drugs, including oral anticoagulants and ciclosporin.

In 30 patients a fall in ciclosporin concentrations by 33–62% after self-medication with St. John's wort necessitated a gradual increase in the dose of ciclosporin of 187% (range 84–292%) (24). No patient suffered any permanent consequences as a result.

There have also been anecdotal reports of interactions of ciclosporin with St. John's wort.

- A 29-year-old woman, who had received a cadaveric kidney and pancreas transplant, had stable organ function with ciclosporin when she decided to take St. John's wort (25). Subsequently her ciclosporin concentrations became subtherapeutic and she developed signs of organ rejection. St. John's wort was withdrawn and her ciclosporin concentrations returned to the target range. However, she developed chronic kidney rejection and had to return to dialysis.
- A 63-year-old patient with a liver allograft developed severe acute rejection 14 months after transplantation (26). Two weeks before he had taken St. John's wort, which significantly reduced his ciclosporin concentration. The dose of ciclosporin was doubled, at the expense of adverse effects. He recovered fully after St. John's wort was withdrawn.
- A 55-year-old woman, who had received a kidney transplant and had stable organ function with ciclosporin, took St. John's wort and 4 weeks later her ciclosporin concentration fell sharply (27). The concentration rose again on withdrawal of St. John's wort and fell on

rechallenge. As the problem was identified early enough, the patient incurred no serious consequences.

- Two patients who took ciclosporin after kidney transplantation self-medicated with St. John's wort, and their ciclosporin concentrations became subtherapeutic (28). One subsequently had an acute transplant rejection. Withdrawal of St. John's wort resulted in normalization of ciclosporin concentrations.
- After a kidney transplant for end-stage renal insufficiency a 58-year-old man was given ciclosporin, azathioprine, and prednisolone (29). Four years later he started to take St. John's wort (300 mg bd) for depression, and 2 weeks later his previously stable ciclosporin concentrations had halved. Withdrawal of the St. John's wort resulted in normalization of his ciclosporin concentrations.

In a systematic review of all reports of interactions of St. John's wort with ciclosporin, 11 case reports and two case series were found (30). In most cases there was little doubt about causality.

Digoxin

In a randomized, placebo-controlled, double-blind study volunteers with steady-state digoxin concentrations took either placebo, a standardized extract of St. John's wort, encapsulated St. John's wort powder, St. John's wort tea, or an encapsulated fatty oil formulation of St. John's wort (31). The extract and the powder caused marked reductions in digoxin concentrations but the tea and the fatty oil formulation did not. The mechanism was not discussed, and it is not clear why the different formulations had different effects.

Irinotecan

In a randomized, crossover study five patients with cancer taking irinotecan were given St. John's wort (32). The plasma concentrations of irinotecan significantly fell in the presence of the herbal remedy. The authors pointed out that this is likely to reduce the effectiveness of the anticancer drug.

Oral contraceptives

- A 36-year-old woman became pregnant whilst taking an oral contraceptive, ethinylestradiol/dienogest (doses not stated) (33). She had also taken St. John's wort extract.

As no other cause for contraceptive failure could be identified, the authors concluded that the St. John's wort had been responsible.

Selective serotonin re-uptake inhibitors

Inhibition of serotonin re-uptake by St. John's wort can lead to interactions with SSRIs (34).

- A 28-year-old man without a previous psychiatric history was given sertraline 50 mg/day for depression after bilateral orchidectomy. Against medical advice, he also took St. John's wort and subsequently became manic.

The authors suggested that inhibition of serotonin re-uptake by sertraline had been potentiated by the use of St. John's wort.

Warfarin

In an open, crossover, randomized study in 12 healthy men St. John's wort significantly induced the apparent clearance of both *S*-warfarin and *R*-warfarin (by 29 and 23% respectively), which in turn resulted in a significant reduction in the pharmacological effect of racemic warfarin (35).

References

1. Stevinson C, Ernst E. Hypericum for depression. An update of the clinical evidence. Eur Neuropsychopharmacol 1999; 9(6):501–5.
2. Linde K, Ramirez G, Mulrow CD, Pauls A, Weidenhammer W, Melchart D. St. John's wort for depression—an overview and meta-analysis of randomised clinical trials. BMJ 1996;313(7052):253–8.
3. Ernst E, Rand JI, Barnes J, Stevinson C. Adverse effects profile of the herbal antidepressant St. John's wort (*Hypericum perforatum* L.). Eur J Clin Pharmacol 1998;54(8):589–94.
4. Stevinson C, Ernst E. Safety of *Hypericum* in patients with depression. A comparison with conventional antidepressants CNS Drugs 1999;11(2):125–32.
5. Patel S, Robinson R, Burk M. Hypertensive crisis associated with St. John's wort. Am J Med 2002;112(6):507–8.
6. Brown TM. Acute St. John's wort toxicity. Am J Emerg Med 2000;18(2):231–2.
7. Parker V, Wong AH, Boon HS, Seeman MV. Adverse reactions to St. John's wort. Can J Psychiatry 2001;46(1):77–9.
8. Laird RD, Webb M. Psychotic episode during use of St. John's wort J Herbal Pharmacother 2001;1:81–7.
9. Schneck C. St. John's wort and hypomania. J Clin Psychiatry 1998;59(12):689.
10. Nierenberg AA, Burt T, Matthews J, Weiss AP. Mania associated with St. John's wort. Biol Psychiatry 1999;46(12):1707–8.
11. Ferko N, Levine MA. Evaluation of the association between St. John's wort and elevated thyroid-stimulating hormone. Pharmacotherapy 2001;21(12):1574–8.
12. Bove GM. Acute neuropathy after exposure to sun in a patient treated with St. John's Wort. Lancet 1998;352(9134):1121–2.
13. Beckman SE, Sommi RW, Switzer J. Consumer use of St. John's wort: a survey on effectiveness, safety, and tolerability Pharmacotherapy 2000;20(5):568–74.
14. Lane-Brown MM. Photosensitivity associated with herbal preparations of St. John's wort (*Hypericum perforatum*). Med J Aust 2000;172(6):302.
15. Grush LR, Nierenberg A, Keefe B, Cohen LS. St. John's wort during pregnancy. JAMA 1998;280(18):1566.
16. Karyekar CS, Eddington ND, Dowling TC. Effect of St. John's wort extract on intestinal expression of cytochrome P4501A2: studies in LS180 cells. J Postgrad Med 2002;48(2):97–100.
17. Henderson L, Yue QY, Bergquist C, Gerden B, Arlett P. St. John's wort (*Hypericum perforatum*): drug interactions and clinical outcomes Br J Clin Pharmacol 2002; 54(4):349–56.
18. Budzinski JW, Foster BC, Vandenhoek S, Arnason JT. An in vitro evaluation of human cytochrome P450 3A4 inhibition by selected commercial herbal extracts and tinctures. Phytomedicine 2000;7(4):273–82.
19. Obach RS. Inhibition of human cytochrome P450 enzymes by constituents of St. John's wort, an herbal preparation used in the treatment of depression. J Pharmacol Exp Ther 2000;294(1):88–95.
20. Moore LB, Goodwin B, Jones SA, Wisely GB, Serabjit-Singh CJ, Willson TM, Collins JL, Kliewer SA. St. John's wort induces hepatic drug metabolism through activation of the pregnane X receptor. Proc Natl Acad Sci USA 2000;97(13):7500–2.

21. Biffignandi PM, Bilia AR. The growing knowledge of St. John's wort (*Hypericum perforatum* L.) drug interactions and their clinical significance. Curr Ther Res Clin Exp 2000;61:389–94.
22. Schulz V. Häufigkeit und klinische Relevanz der Interaktionen und Nebenwirkungen von *Hypericum-Präparaten.* Perfusion 2000;13:486.
23. Ernst E. Second thoughts about safety of St. John's wort. Lancet 1999;354(9195):2014–16.
24. Breidenbach T, Kliem V, Burg M, Radermacher J, Hoffmann MW, Klempnauer J. Profound drop of cyclosporin A whole blood trough levels caused by St. John's wort (*Hypericum perforatum*). Transplantation 2000;69(10): 2229–30.
25. Barone GW, Gurley BJ, Ketel BL, Lightfoot ML, Abul-Ezz SR. Drug interaction between St. John's wort and cyclosporine. Ann Pharmacother 2000;34(9):1013–16.
26. Karliova M, Treichel U, Malago M, Frilling A, Gerken G, Broelsch CE. Interaction of *Hypericum perforatum* (St. John's wort) with cyclosporin A metabolism in a patient after liver transplantation. J Hepatol 2000;33(5):853–5.
27. Mai I, Kruger H, Budde K, Johne A, Brockmoller J, Neumayer HH, Roots I. Hazardous pharmacokinetic interaction of Saint John's wort (*Hypericum perforatum*) with the immunosuppressant cyclosporin. Int J Clin Pharmacol Ther 2000;38(10):500–2.
28. Turton-Weeks SM, Barone GW, Gurley BJ, Ketel BL, Lightfoot ML, Abul-Ezz SR. St. John's wort: a hidden risk for transplant patients. Prog Transplant 2001; 11(2):116–20.
29. Moschella C, Jaber BL. Interaction between cyclosporine and *Hypericum perforatum* (St. John's wort) after organ transplantation. Am J Kidney Dis 2001;38(5):1105–7.
30. Ernst E. St. John's wort supplements endanger the success of organ transplantation. Arch Surg 2002;137(3):316–19.
31. Uehleke B, Mueller SC, Woehling H, Petzsch M, Riethling AK, Drewelow B. Interaction of St. John's wort with digoxin in relation to dosage and formulation. Phytomedicine 2000;SII:20.
32. Mathijssen RH, Verweij J, de Bruijn P, Loos WJ, Sparreboom A. Effects of St. John's wort on irinotecan metabolism. J Natl Cancer Inst 2002;94(16):1247–9.
33. Schwarz UI, Buschel B, Kirch W. Failure of oral contraceptive because of St. John's wort. Eur J Clin Pharmacol 2001;57:A25.
34. Barbenel DM, Yusufi B, O'Shea D, Bench CJ. Mania in a patient receiving testosterone replacement postorchidectomy taking St. John's wort and sertraline. J Psychopharmacol 2000;14(1):84–6.
35. Jiang X, Williams KM, Liauw WS, Ammit AJ, Roufogalis BD, Duke CC, Day RO, McLachlan AJ. Effect of St. John's wort and ginseng on the pharmacokinetics and pharmacodynamics of warfarin in healthy subjects. Br J Clin Pharmacol 2004;57(5):592–9.

Coagulation proteins

See also Individual agents

General Information

The major coagulation and fibrinolytic proteins are listed in Table 1.

Coagulation protein concentrates became available in the 1970s, a significant step in the prevention and management of bleeding. The factors that are currently available are factor VII, factor VIIa, factor VIII, factor IX, factor XI, and factor XIII. There is also a factor VIII inhibitor bypassing factor, activated prothrombin

Table 1 Proteins involved in coagulation and fibrinolysis

Protein (synonym)	Function
Coagulation proteins	
Factor I (fibrinogen)	Activated to fibrin
Factor II* (prothrombin)	Activated to thrombin
Factor III (tissue thromboplastin)	Extrinsic pathway
Factor IV (calcium)	Co-factor
Factor V (Ac-globulin; proaccelerin)	Converts prothrombin to thrombin
Factor VI (unassigned)	
Factor VII* (proconvertin)	Extrinsic pathway
Factor VIII (antihemophilic factor)	Intrinsic pathway
Factor IX* (Christmas factor)	Intrinsic pathway
Factor X* (Stuart–Prower factor)	Extrinsic pathway
Factor XI (plasma thromboplastin antecedent)	Intrinsic pathway
Factor XII (Hageman factor)	Intrinsic pathway
Factor XIII (fibrin stabilizing factor)	Stabilizes fibrin
Von Willebrand factor (factor VIII-related antigen; vWF)	
High molecular weight kininogen (Fitzgerald factor)	Intrinsic pathway
Prekallikrein (Fletcher factor)	Intrinsic pathway
Fibrinolytic proteins	
Plasminogen	Converted to fibrinolysin
Prourokinase	Precursor of urokinase
Tissue plasminogen activator	Activates plasminogen
Antithrombin III	Inhibits thrombin, IXa, Xa, XIa, XIIa
Protein C*	Inhibits factors Va, VIIIa
Protein S*	Co-factor for protein C
α_2-Antiplasmin	Inhibits binding of fibrinolysin

*Vitamin K-dependent factor; the intrinstic and extrinsic pathways converge with the activation of factor X to Xa by factor VIII and IX.

complex concentrate. Fresh frozen plasma and prothrombin complex concentrate, which contain mixtures of coagulation proteins, are also available.

Two major classes of complications in the use of these proteins have emerged (1). First, transfusion-related infections with various blood-borne viruses, such as hepatitis B and C and human immunodeficiency virus (HIV). Secondly, alloimmune antibodies (inhibitors) against the deficient coagulation factors.

Organs and Systems

Cardiovascular

Two factor XI products, both containing antithrombin III and heparin, have been associated with evidence of coagulation activation and thrombotic events in patients with pre-existing vascular disease (2). It has been recommended that doses of more than 30 U/kg and factor XI peak concentrations in severely deficient patients of more than 500–700 U/l should be avoided. In addition, the concurrent use of tranexamic acid or other antifibrinolytic drugs should be avoided.

Immunologic

Patients with bleeding disorders are at risk of developing antibodies against the protein that is absent, present in reduced amounts, or present in an inactive form in their blood. Such coagulation inhibitors make treatment very difficult. Inhibitors of factor VIII are the most common and develop in 5–20% of patients with hemophilia A. Inhibitors of factor IX develop in 1–4% of patients with hemophilia B (3,4). Patients with factor VIII inhibitors present clinically either as "high responders" who show a strong anamnestic response and a sharp rise in inhibitor concentrations after exposure to factor VIII, or "low responders," who show little or no anamnestic response (5).

Because of the difference in prevalence of inhibitors in hemophilia B and hemophilia A, it has been postulated that there is a correlation between mutation type and inhibitor risk (6). Of the patients with gross deletion, nonsense, or frameshift mutations, 11% developed inhibitors compared with 0% and 0.36% of patients with hemophilia B with mis-sense or other mutations.

Recombinant and high-purity coagulation factor products appear to have a greater tendency to induce inhibitors than human-derived concentrates of intermediate or low purity (7). These intermediate-purity or low-purity human-derived concentrates are probably more suitable for inducing immune tolerance in patients with hemophilia with inhibitors. It has been suggested that for immune tolerance a high content of Von Willebrand factor in factor VIII concentrates is required, although direct comparisons of different products have not been made (8).

Risk factors for developing an inhibitor are the severity of the hemophilia, age (under 30 years), genetic predisposition, antigenicity of factor replacement therapy, and race (increased prevalence among black people) (9). In addition, it has been suggested that changing from one product to another can also stimulate the development of inhibitors (10).

Inhibitor formation has been observed in only a few patients with factor XI deficiency. Like patients with hemophilia A and B, these patients may be treated with prothrombin complex concentrates or recombinant factor VIIa (2).

Drug Administration

Drug contamination

In the past, plasma factor VIII products have exposed patients with hemophilia to foreign proteins as well as blood-borne viruses, including hepatitis B, hepatitis C, human parvovirus B19, and human immunodeficiency virus (11,12). Before the introduction of heat-treated concentrates in 1985, about 20% of patients with hemophilia in the UK became infected with HIV (13) and virtually all patients with hemophilia who were exposed to large-pool coagulation factor concentrates before the introduction of viral inactivation procedures developed hepatitis C (14). Studies using a second-generation enzyme-linked immunosorbent assay showed 89% anti-HCV positivity in a heterogeneous group of patients in the USA and in 98% of Dutch patients with hemophilia who had been exposed to large-pool, non-virally inactivated coagulation factor concentrates (14). In the UK and the Netherlands increased mortality due to liver disease in patients with hemophilia has been reported (14). In patients co-infected with HIV, liver disease was more severe, probably because of higher amounts of hepatitis C viral RNA (13). In addition, patients infected with hepatitis C virus genotype 1 had a more rapid course of disease due to HIV (14).

Since viral inactivation methods, such as solvent detergent and heat pasteurization, were implemented in the production process, the risks of HIV and hepatitis have virtually been eliminated. Dry heating at 60°C is insufficient to eliminate all hepatitis C virus, which requires dry heating at 80°C, pasteurization, or treatment with mixtures of solvents and detergents (14). Nevertheless, many viral inactivation methods currently used do not completely eliminate certain (non-enveloped) viruses, for example parvovirus and hepatitis A (11,15); removal of the small, non-lipid-enveloped parvovirus B19 requires 15 nm nanofiltration. HIV appears to progress more rapidly in patients co-infected with hepatitis B and cytomegalovirus (11). In addition, hepatitis C replicated more rapidly in patients infected with HIV (11).

In a mortality study amongst patients with hemophilia in the UK in 1977–91, AIDS was far the commonest cause of death, and liver disease ranked as the third commonest cause of death (15).

It has been postulated that transfusion-transmitted virus (TT virus) can be transmitted through heat-treated blood products (16). Transfusion-transmitted virus is a common DNA virus in healthy Japanese, and it lacks a lipid envelope, similar to parvovirus B19 (16,17). Transmission of transfusion-transmitted virus often occurs with blood transfusion and it can cause post-transfusion hepatitis with high postoperative peak alanine transaminase activity (17). No patients with hepatitis due to transfusion-transmitted virus have clinically apparent hepatitis (17). The incidence of transfusion-transmitted virus viremia in patients with hemophilia was 43% of those who received only virus-inactivated concentrates and 78% in those who received non-inactivated products before 1984 (16).

Bacterial growth in infusion bags has not been detected, and complications such as infections during the postoperative period have not been observed (18).

Although transmission of classic Creutzfeldt–Jakob disease has never been observed, manufacturers have withdrawn plasma-derived products prepared from plasma obtained from donors who were subsequently found to have classic Creutzfeldt–Jakob disease (19). Although leukocytes are believed to play a key role in the pathogenesis of variant CJD, there may also be a theoretical risk of transmission by plasma products. However, various steps used in the manufacture of plasma-derived factors also contribute to reduced infectivity by bovine spongiform encephalopathy (20). The risk of transmission of nvCJD by recombinant products is unknown, as the cell cultures used for manufacturing them sometimes contain bovine proteins (21).

References

1. Ingerslev J. Efficacy and safety of recombinant factor VIIa in the prophylaxis of bleeding in various surgical procedures in hemophilic patients with factor VIII and factor IX inhibitors. Semin Thromb Hemost 2000;26(4):425–32.
2. Bolton-Maggs PH. The management of factor XI deficiency. Haemophilia 1998;4(4):683–8.
3. Hasegawa DK, Edson JR. Detection of factor VIII and IX inhibitors after first exposure to heat-treated concentrates. Lancet 1987;1(8530):449.
4. Pasi KJ, Hamon MD, Perry DJ, Hill FG. Factor VIII and IX inhibitors after exposure to heat-treated concentrates. Lancet 1987;1(8534):689.
5. Van Leeuwen EF, Mauser-Bunschoten EP, Van Dijken PJ, Kok AJ, Sjamsoedin-Visser EJ, Sixma JJ. Disappearance of factor VIII:C antibodies in patients with haemophilia A upon frequent administration of factor VIII in intermediate or low dose. Br J Haematol 1986;64(2):291–7.
6. Parquet A, Laurian Y, Rothschild C, Navarro R, Guerois C, Gay V, Durin A, Peynet J, Sultan Y. Incidence of factor IX inhibitor development in severe haemophilia B patients treated with only one brand of high purity plasma derived factor IX concentrate. Thromb Haemost 1999;82(4):1247–9.
7. Penner JA. Haemophilic patients with inhibitors to factor VIII or IX: variables affecting treatment response. Haemophilia 2001;7(1):103–8.
8. Berntorp E. Immune tolerance induction: recombinant vs. human-derived product. Haemophilia 2001;7(1):109–13.
9. Penner JA. Management of haemophilia in patients with high-titre inhibitors: focus on the evolution of activated prothrombin complex concentrate AUTOPLEX T. Haemophilia 1999;5(Suppl 3):1–9.
10. Zanon E, Zerbinati P, Girolami B, Bertomoro A, Girolami A. Frequent but low titre factor VIII inhibitors in haemophilia A patients treated with high purity concentrates. Blood Coagul Fibrinolysis 1999;10(3):117–20.
11. Hoots K, Canty D. Clotting factor concentrates and immune function in haemophilic patients. Haemophilia 1998;4(5):704–13.
12. Seremetis S, Lusher JM, Abildgaard CF, Kasper CK, Allred R, Hurst D. Human recombinant DNA-derived antihaemophilic factor (factor VIII) in the treatment of haemophilia A: conclusions of a 5-year study of home therapy. The KOGENATE Study Group. Haemophilia 1999;5(1):9–16.
13. Sabin CA, Yee TT, Devereux H, Griffioen A, Loveday C, Phillips AN, Lee CA. Two decades of HIV infection in a cohort of haemophilic individuals: clinical outcomes and response to highly active antiretroviral therapy. AIDS 2000;14(8):1001–7.
14. Meijer K, Smid WM, van der Meer J. Treatment of chronic hepatitis C in haemophilia patients. Haemophilia 2000;6(6):605–13.
15. Giangrande PL. Hepatitis in haemophilia. Br J Haematol 1998;103(1):1–9.
16. Sumazaki R, Yamada-Osaki M, Kajiwara Y, Shirahata A, Matsui A. Transfusion transmitted virus. Lancet 1998;352(9136):1308–9.
17. Fujiwara T, Iwata A, Iizuka H, Tanaka T, Okamoto H. Transfusion transmitted virus. Lancet 1998;352(9136): 1310–1.
18. Tagariello G, Davoli PG, Gajo GB, De Biasi E, Risato R, Baggio R, Traldi A. Safety and efficacy of high-purity concentrates in haemophiliac patients undergoing surgery by continuous infusion. Haemophilia 1999; 5(6):426–30.
19. White GC 2nd. Seventeen years' experience with Autoplex/Autoplex T: evaluation of inpatients with severe haemophilia A and factor VIII inhibitors at a major haemophilia centre. Haemophilia 2000;6(5):508–12.
20. Cervenakova L, Brown P, Hammond DJ, Lee CA, Saenko EL. Factor VIII and transmissible spongiform encephalopathy: the case for safety. Haemophilia 2002; 8(2):63–75.
21. Mauser-Bunschoten EP, Roosendaal G, van den Berg HM. Product choice and haemophilia treatment in the Netherlands. Haemophilia 2001;7(1):96–8.

Cobalt

General Information

Cobalt is a metallic element (symbol Co; atomic no. 27). It is an important constituent of the cobalamins (vitamin B_{12}) and is found as arsenates and arsenides in naturally occurring minerals such as erythrite, skutterudite, and smaltite.

Cobalt has been used in the treatment of anemia, because of its erythropoietic action. However, it is toxic to many organs, and its medicinal benefits have repeatedly been questioned. In most countries the use of cobalt in anemia has been abandoned, although it is possible that in very rare cases there may be a need for it. If it is still to be used at all, the administration of cobalt ought to be entrusted to an experienced clinical hematologist.

Occupational exposure is mainly due to cobalt powders. Its main other uses are in metal alloys and medical devices (for example aneurysm clips) (1).

The toxicity of cobalt has been reviewed (SEDA-1, 185) (SED-9, 370) (2).

One tragic case in 1989 concerned a 13-month-old baby treated with a commercial iron–cobalt formulation that was still on sale, resulting in hypothyroidism, cardiomyopathy, polycythemia, and hypertrichosis (SEDA-16, 231).

Cobalt in metal implants and prostheses

Complications from the use of metal implants and prostheses can arise because of biochemical and histological reactions to some of the materials used (SEDA-22, 250). These include titanium, stainless steel (10–14% nickel, 17–20% chromium), and cobalt chrome alloys (27–30% chromium, 57–68% cobalt, and up to 2.5% nickel). All of these metals can produce sensitization or elicit toxic reactions when they are solubilized and come into contact with tissues; it can be difficult or even impossible to differentiate between hypersensitivity and toxic reactions.

Nickel plays a major role in sensitization of patients. Even the small amount present in cobalt chrome alloys often suffices to elicit allergic reactions. Reactions to cobalt are more generally toxic in nature (3). An increased rate of allergy to cobalt and nickel has been found in those patients bearing metallic implants who have developed bone infection in the surroundings of osteosynthesis material.

Metals from prostheses can continue to be released into the system for many years. The development of hypersensitivity takes time, and allergic reactions are usual delayed for weeks, months, or 1–2 years. The symptoms can assume a variety of forms. Local reactions can cause loosening of the device or local pain. Dermatological reactions include eczema, bullous pemphigoid, urticaria, and "muscle tumors."

Attempts continue to predict metal sensitivity in the individual patient so that the choice of material can be made accordingly. In vitro tests for metal allergies have been developed on the basis of lymphokine (MIF) release from sensitized T lymphocytes exposed to metal–protein complexes (4). About 6% of patients without a previous metal implant had positive reactions to nickel, chromium, or cobalt. However, it is still not clear whether such a positive reaction is a reliable predictor of clinical problems. In practice few patients have either local or systemic reactions; when symptoms occur and other causes are ruled out, the implant should be removed. Some workers recommend removal of an implant whenever there is both a positive MIF test and a positive skin test, even in the current absence of a serious reaction. Allergic dermatitis will clear up as soon as the metal has begun to be cleared from the tissue. The type of metal and the amount released into the tissue will affect the time taken for the disappearance of toxic dermatological phenomena.

Catastrophic failure of two cemented cobalt-containing femoral stems that had been used in conjunction with the impacting bone-grafting technique has been reported in two cases (5).

- A-59-year-old woman with degenerative arthritis of the hip was managed with bipolar arthroplasty and later with total hip replacement. A long-stem component, manufactured from forged cobalt-chromium, was later used for revision. She developed acute pain in the thigh and buttock, with tenderness and swelling in the thigh and hip and pain on movement. Hip X-rays showed catastrophic failure of the femoral component of the prosthesis, and at operation the prosthesis and the femur were fractured at the same level.
- A 51-year old woman sustained a fracture of the left femoral neck, later treated by total hip arthroplasty, which was revised several times with the impaction bone grafting technique and insertion of a prosthesis with cement. She developed a persistent weakness of the hip in flexion and abduction. Later the left hip buckled and she fell while walking. X-rays showed a periprosthetic fracture with bending of the femoral component.

It was thought that the mechanism of failure had been cantilever bending secondary to good distal fixation in the presence of poor proximal bone support resulting from poor proximal incorporation of the impacted allograft. In essence, a fatigue fracture had occurred in a forged cobalt–chromium stem that did not have an obvious manufacturing defect at the site of failure. Both failures were apparently related to implant design and operative technique rather than to defects introduced during the manufacturing process.

References

1. Steiger HJ, van Loon JJ. Virtues and drawbacks of titanium alloy aneurysm clips. Acta Neurochir Suppl 1999;72:81–8.
2. Barceloux DG. Cobalt. J Toxicol Clin Toxicol 1999;37(2):201–6.
3. Waterman AH, Schrik JJ. Allergy in hip arthroplasty. Contact Dermatitis 1985;13(5):294–301.
4. Hierholzer S, Hierholzer G. Untersuchungen zur Metalallergie nach Osteosynthesen. [Allergy to metal following osteosynthesis.] Unfallchirurgie 1982;8(6):347–52.
5. Jazrawi LM, Della Valle CJ, Kummer FJ, Adler EM, Di Cesare PE. Catastrophic failure of a cemented, collarless, polished, tapered cobalt-chromium femoral stem used with impaction bone-grafting. A report of two cases. J Bone Joint Surg Am 1999;81(6):844–7.

Cocaine

General Information

Cocaine is an alkaloid derived from the plant *Erythroxylon coca* and other *Erythroxylon* species in South America. The leaves contain cocaine as the principal alkaloid, plus a variety of minor alkaloids. Only decocainized coca products are legal in the USA, but some commercially available tea products have been found in the past to contain cocaine in a concentration normally found in coca leaves (about 5 mg of cocaine per 1 g tea-bag). This results in only mild symptoms when package directions to drink a few cups per day are followed, but massive overdosing can result in severe agitation, tachycardia, sweating, and raised blood pressure.

Cocaine, as the leaf or as an extracted substance in different forms, has been used for different purposes. Andean Indians have long chewed leaves of the coca plant to reduce hunger and increase stamina. Pure cocaine was first extracted from coca in the 19th century; it was used to treat exhaustion, depression, and morphine addiction and was available in many patent medicines, tonics, and soft drinks. In the USA, after the Harrison Narcotic Act of 1914 and the Narcotic Drugs Import and Export Act of 1922, the use of cocaine fell, and the National Commission on Marihuana and Drug Abuse in 1973 reported that cocaine was little used. Since then, however, use has grown and there is now an epidemic in many countries. There may be about 5 million regular cocaine users in the USA, and users who have significant difficulties, including serious as well as fatal medical complications, continue to be reported frequently (1,2). Deaths occur not only from overdosage but also from drug-induced mental states, which can lead to serious injuries (3).

Cocaine was also the first aminoester local anesthetic, and its adverse effects differ from those of other local anesthetics. Owing to its rapid absorption by mucous membranes, cocaine applied topically can cause systemic toxic effects. There is a wide variation in the rate and amount of cocaine that is systemically absorbed. This variability can be affected by the type and concentration of vasoconstrictor used with cocaine and also accounts for the differences in cocaine pharmacokinetics in cocaine abusers (SEDA-20, 128).

As a recreational drug cocaine can be snorted (sniffed), swallowed, injected, or smoked. The street drug comes in the form of a white powder, cocaine hydrochloride. The hydrochloride salt and the cutting agents are removed to create the free base, which is smoked. The inexpensive widely available crack formulation is prepared by alkalinizing cocaine hydrochloride and precipitating the resultant alkaloidal free-base cocaine, which, unlike the hydrochloride, is not destroyed by heat when smoked. Smoking crack provides a rapid effect, comparable to that of intravenous injection. Intense euphoria, followed within minutes by dysphoria, leads to frequent dosing and a greater potential for rapid addiction (4). As with amphetamines, the euphoric effect can enhance craving, and repeated reinforcement can lead to conditioned drug responses, which facilitate dependence. Facilitated conditioned effects with cocaine may be due to its rapid elimination and the development of acute tolerance. Frequent repeated dosing becomes necessary to sustain euphoria, thereby promoting a tight temporal juxtaposition of euphoria with recent drug-taking (5).

Rapid intravenous or inhalational administration of cocaine can cause very high concentrations in areas of high vascular perfusion, for example the heart and brain, before eventual distribution to other tissues. Under these conditions there is a catecholaminergic storm in the heart and a local anesthetic effect, with prolongation of conduction. Once beyond the immediate period of vulnerability, accumulation (for example through frequent overdosing or accidents from body packing of condom-filled stimulants to avoid detection) leads to a different cascade of events over a period of hours, leading to death. This cascade includes a catecholaminergic hypermetabolic state, with hyperpyrexia and acidosis, anorexia, and repeated seizures, usually ending in cardiac collapse (1,6). On the other hand, chronic dosing can cause catecholaminergic cardiomyopathy, for example contraction bands, cardiomegaly (7,8), and repeated vasospastic insults to cerebral and coronary arteries (9). Whether these chronic effects predispose to increased sensitivity to acute toxicity has not been systematically explored, but autopsy studies suggest that they do.

In addition to other chronic changes in abusers, personality deterioration carries a significant association with high-risk behaviors, which are a source of physical and psychiatric morbidity and mortality. These include suicide, violent trauma and aggressive behavior, high-risk methods of drug use (for example needle sharing), and high-risk sexual behavior, with increased risks of HIV, hepatitis B, and other infections.

The stimulant properties of cocaine are similar to those of amphetamines, although the differences are notable, in part because of the very short half-life of cocaine. However, cocaine has the same problem of abuse potential as other stimulants, and at high doses causes stimulant psychosis (10). In addition, even when it is used as a local nasopharyngeal anesthetic, it has toxic, even fatal, effects in high doses.

Death from cocaine often occurs within 2–3 minutes, suggesting direct cardiac toxicity, fatal dysrhythmias, and depression of medullary respiratory centers as common causes of death (11,12). Thus, cocaine's local anesthetic properties can contribute additional hazards when high doses are used, reminiscent of deaths reported in the era when it was used as a mucous membrane paste for nasopharyngeal surgery (13).

Periods of increased cocaine use, especially intravenous administration, inhalation of the free base, and high-dose use, are associated with cocaine-related deaths. For example, according to the Drug Abuse Warning Network, there was a three-fold increase in such deaths from 195 to 580 per year in the USA between 1981 and 1985. Despite the importance of these mortality data, relatively little is known of the types of pathophysiological sequences involved in the cascade of events leading to death. More important, there is a paucity of guidelines to appropriate diagnostic and treatment strategies for the various prefatal conditions.

General adverse effects

Cocaine has a spectrum of pharmacological effects. It initially causes excitement and euphoria; later, with higher doses, lower centers become involved, producing reduced coordination, tremors, hyper-reflexia, increased respiratory rate, and at times nausea, vomiting, and convulsions. These symptoms are eventually followed by CNS depression.

Cardiovascular effects include tachycardia, hypertension, and increased cardiac irritability; large intravenous doses can cause cardiac failure. Cardiac dysrhythmias have been ascribed to a direct toxic effect of cocaine and a secondary sensitization of ventricular tissue to catecholamines (14), along with slowed cardiac conduction secondary to local anesthetic effects. Myocardial infarction has increased as a complication of cocaine abuse (7,8). Dilated cardiomyopathies, with subsequent recurrent myocardial infarction, have been associated with long-term use of cocaine, raising the possibility of chronic effects on the heart (15). Many victims have evidence of pre-existing fixed coronary artery disease precipitated by cocaine (SEDA-9, 35) (16–18). However, myocardial infarction has been noted even in young intranasal users with no evidence of coronary disease (19), defined by autopsy or angiography (20,21). If applied to mucous membranes, cocaine causes local vasoconstriction, and, with chronic use, necrosis.

As a general rule, mortality is higher when cocaine is used intravenously or as smoked free base than if taken nasally or orally (22). The symptoms of acute cocaine poisoning include agitation, sweating, tachycardia, tonic-clonic seizures, severe respiratory and metabolic acidosis, apnea, and ventricular dysrhythmias. Seizures occur at high doses, and may be a major determinant of fatal outcomes; their control with sedatives is important to reduce lethality (23). Associated hyperthermia can contribute as a primary cause in cases of fatal hyperpyrexia, and can potentiate the hypoxic cardiovascular events in cardiac deaths in those who survive the initial acute dose (24,25). A study of a very large number of cocaine deaths showed that the morbidity rate increased by four times on days on which the ambient temperature rose above 31.1°C (26). The final agonal events in cocaine deaths involve the combination of sympathomimetic myocardial responses and/or cardiac conduction slowing, secondary to cocaine's local anesthetic effect, leading to dysrhythmias (27). In reported fatal overdoses, convulsions and death have usually occurred within minutes. Most patients who have survived for the first 3 hours after an initial acute overdose have been likely to recover. Treatment includes respiratory and cardiovascular resuscitative measures. Short-acting barbiturates, benzodiazepines, beta-blockers, and phentolamine have all been used with some success (20,28). Because of a possible risk of coronary vasodilatation with the use of propranolol to manage dysrhythmias in cocaine overdose, the use of labetalol for this indication is recommended, if a beta-blocker is required (29,30). In one study of 60 cocaine-related deaths, autopsy findings were non-specific but typical of those found in respiratory depression of central origin (31).

Organs and Systems

Cardiovascular

Cocaine abuse is a risk factor for myocardial ischemia, infarction, and dysrhythmias, as well as pulmonary edema, ruptured aortic aneurysm, infectious endocarditis, vascular thrombosis, myocarditis, and dilated cardiomyopathy (32). Acutely, cocaine suppresses myocardial contractility, reduces coronary caliber and coronary blood flow, induces electrical abnormalities in the heart, and increases heart rate and blood pressure. These effects can lead to myocardial ischemia (33,34). However, intranasal cocaine in doses used medicinally or recreationally does not have a deleterious effect on intracardiac pressures or left ventricular performance (35).

Tachycardia and vasoconstriction from cocaine can exacerbate coronary insufficiency, complicated by dysrhythmias and hypertensive and vascular hemorrhage (1). Sudden deaths have been reported in patients with angina (36). Chronic dosing includes cardiomyopathy and cardiomegaly; other chronic conditions include endocarditis and thrombophlebitis. Crack smoking has led to pneumopericardium (37).

The cardiac effects of intracoronary infusion of cocaine have been studied in dogs and humans (38). The procedure can be performed safely and does not alter coronary arterial blood flow. The effects of direct intracoronary infusion of cocaine on left ventricle systolic and diastolic performance have been studied in 20 patients referred for cardiac catheterization for evaluation of chest pain. They were given saline or cocaine hydrochloride (1 mg/minute) in 15-minute intracoronary infusions, and cardiac measurements were made during the final 2–3 minutes of each infusion. The blood cocaine concentration obtained from the coronary sinus was 3.0 μg/ml, which is similar in magnitude to the blood–cocaine concentration reported in abusers who die of cocaine intoxication. Minimal systemic effects were produced. The overall results were that cocaine caused measurable deterioration of left ventricular systolic and diastolic performance.

Possible predictors of cardiovascular responses to smoked cocaine have been studied in 62 crack cocaine users (24 women and 38 men, aged 20–45 years) who used a single dose of smoked cocaine 0.4 mg/kg (39). Physiological responses to smoked cocaine, such as changes in heart rate and blood pressure, were monitored. The findings suggested that higher baseline blood pressure and heart rate, a greater amount and frequency of current cocaine use, and current cocaine snorting predicted a reduced cardiovascular response to cocaine. By contrast, factors such as male sex, African-American race, higher body weight, and current marijuana use were associated with a greater cardiovascular response.

Fatal pulmonary edema developed in a 36-year-old man shortly after injecting free-base cocaine intravenously (40).

Symptoms of cardiac ischemia

Cocaine users often present with complaints suggestive of acute cardiac ischemia (chest pain, dyspnea, syncope, dizziness, and palpitation). Two studies have shown that the risk of actual acute cardiac ischemia among cocaine users with such symptoms was low. The first study reviewed the clinical database from the Acute Cardiac Ischemia–Time Insensitive Predictive Instrument Clinical Trial, a multicenter prospective clinical trial conducted in the USA in 1993 (41). Among 10 689 enrolled patients, 293 (2.7%) had cocaine-associated complaints. This rate varied from 0.3% to 8.4% in the 10 participating hospitals. Only six of these patients had a diagnosis of acute cardiac ischemia (2.0%), four with unstable angina and two with acute myocardial infarction. The cocaine users were admitted to the coronary care unit as often as other study participants (14 versus 18%), but were much less likely to have confirmed unstable angina (1.4 versus 9.3%). A second study also suggested that cocaine users who present with chest pain have a very low risk of adverse cardiac events (42). Emergency departments have instituted centers for the evaluation and treatment of patients with chest pain who are at low to moderate risk of acute coronary syndromes. In this particular study, patients with a history of coronary artery disease or presentations that included hemodynamic instability, electrocardiographic changes consistent with ischemia, or clinically unstable angina were directly admitted to hospital. In a retrospective study of 179 patients with reliable 30-day follow-up in chest pain centers, there was one cardiac complication due to cocaine use.

Coronary artery disease

By one estimate, since the first report in 1982, over 250 cases of myocardial infarction due to cocaine have been reported, mostly in the USA. The first report from the UK was published in 1999 (43).

In a review of 114 cases, coronary anatomy, defined either by angiography or autopsy, was normal in 38% of chronic cocaine users who had had a myocardial infarction (20). The authors of another review concluded that "the vast majority of patients dying with cocaine toxicity, either have no pathological changes in the heart, or only minimal changes" (21). There can be a delay between the use of cocaine and the development of chest pain (44). The results of a study of 101 consecutive patients admitted with acute chest pain related to cocaine suggested that it commonly causes chest pain that may not be secondary to myocardial ischemia (45). The use of intranasal cocaine for therapeutic purposes (to treat epistaxis) was associated with myocardial infarction in a 57-year-old man with hypertension and stable angina (46).

In a review of the literature, 91 patients with cocaine-induced myocardial infarction were identified (47). Myocardial infarction occurred in 44 patients after intranasal use, in 27 after smoking, and in 19 after intravenous use. Almost half had a prior episode of chest pain. Two-thirds had their myocardial infarction within 3 hours of use. There were acute complications related to the myocardial infarction in 18 patients. Of 24 patients followed up, 58% had subsequent cardiac complications. Two-phase myocardial imaging with ^{99m}Tc-sestamibi can be helpful in the definitive diagnosis of cocaine-induced myocardial infarction in patients with a history of cocaine use, chest pain, and a non-diagnostic electrocardiogram (48). Damage to the myocardium associated with cocaine can be unrecognized by the abuser (49). Major electrocardiographic findings (including myocardial infarction, myocardial ischemia, and bundle branch block) were recorded during a review of 99 electrocardiograms of known cocaine abusers. None of the 11 patients with major electrocardiographic changes had a past history of cardiac disease or had complained of chest pain. The mechanism by which cocaine causes acute myocardial damage is unclear. Of 20 healthy cocaine abusers given intravenous cocaine, in doses commonly self-administered, or placebo, none developed myocardial ischemia or ventricular dysfunction on two-dimensional echocardiography during the test (50).

Myocardial infarction has been documented in 6% of patients who present to emergency departments with cocaine-associated chest pain (51,52). Treatment of cocaine-associated myocardial infarction has previously generally been conservative, using benzodiazepines, aspirin, glyceryl trinitrate, calcium channel blockers, and thrombolytic drugs. In the context of 10 patients with cocaine-associated myocardial infarction, who were treated with percutaneous interventions, including angioplasty, stenting, and AngioJet mechanical extraction of thrombus, the authors suggested that percutaneous intervention can be performed in such patients safely and with a high degree of procedural success (53). Patients with cocaine-associated chest pain and electrocardiographic ST-segment elevation should first undergo coronary angiography, if available, followed by percutaneous intervention. Alternatively, thrombolytic drugs can be used. However, the relative safety and efficacy of thrombolytic drugs compared with percutaneous intervention is undefined in patients with cocaine-associated myocardial infarction.

Other vascular disease

Dissection of the aorta has been reported during cocaine use (54,55). The authors of these two reports noted that all six cases of this rare complication reported in the past 5 years were in men with pre-existing essential hypertension. In a review of emergency visits to a hospital during a 20-year period, 14 of 38 cases of acute aortic dissection involved cocaine use; 6 were of type A and 8 of type B (56). Crack cocaine had been smoked in 13 cases and powder cocaine had been snorted in one case. The mean time of onset of chest pain was 12 hours after cocaine use. The chronicity of cocaine use was not known in most of the cases. The cocaine users were typically younger than the non-cocaine users. Chronic untreated hypertension and cigarette smoking were often present.

- A 43-year-old man with untreated hypertension developed transient mild chest pressure followed by shortness of breath for 4 hours (57). He had long used tobacco, alcohol, and cocaine and admitted to having used cocaine within the last 12 hours. He had a tachycardia with a pansystolic murmur suggesting mitral regurgitation. Urine drug screen was positive for cocaine metabolites. A chest X-ray showed mild cardiomegaly and prominent upper lobe vasculature. An electrocardiogram showed atrial flutter at a rate of 130/minute and non-specific T wave changes. The diagnoses were myocardial infarction due to cocaine, with mild congestive heart failure, mitral regurgitation and atrial flutter. However, transesophageal echocardiography showed severe aortic insufficiency and a dissection flap in the ascending aorta. He underwent emergency repair of the aortic root and resuspension of the aortic valve.

Intramural hematoma of the ascending aorta has been reported in a cocaine user (58).

- A healthy 39-year-old man developed retrosternal chest pain radiating to the back with nausea and sweating. About 10–15 minutes before, he had inhaled cocaine for 2 hours and then smoked crack cocaine. He had an aortic dissection, which was repaired surgically.

The authors identified hypertension secondary to the use of cocaine as the risk factor for this complication.

Coronary artery dissection associated with cocaine is rare. The first case was reported in 1994 (59) and two other cases have been reported (60,61).

- A healthy 33-year-old man with prior cocaine use had a small myocardial infarction and, 36 hours later, having inhaled cocaine, developed a dissection of the left main coronary artery, extending distally to the left anterior descending and circumflex arteries. There was marked anterolateral and apical hypokinesis.
- A 23-year-old man with a history of intravenous drug abuse and hepatitis C was found unconscious, hypoxic, and hypotensive. A urine drug screen was positive for cocaine metabolites, benzodiazepines, and opiates. An electrocardiogram suggested a myocardial infarction, verified by raised troponin I and the MB fraction of creatine kinase. He had severe hypokinesia with a left ventricular ejection fraction of 10%, falling to less than 5%. He became septic, developed multiorgan system failure, and died. The postmortem findings included dissection of the left anterior descending artery with complete occlusion of the true lumen and thrombosis of the false lumen. The left ventricle showed extensive transmural myocardial necrosis with adjacent contraction band necrosis. He also had deep vein thromboses in veins in the neck and abdomen and multiple pulmonary infarctions.

Peripheral vascular disease in the fingers has been attributed to cocaine.

- A 48-year-old man who smoked cigarettes and used cocaine developed ischemia of the right index finger due to occlusion of the distal ulnar artery (62). He had a history of recurrent deep vein thrombosis. A venous bypass graft was performed. Two years later he had non-healing gangrene of the left index finger. His blood pressure was normal in both arms. Urine toxicology was positive for cocaine. Angiography of the left arm showed small-vessel vasculitis.
- A healthy 36-year-old man, who had used intranasal crack cocaine daily in increasing doses for 2 weeks, developed pain, numbness, swelling, and cyanosis of the fingers and toes aggravated by cold and an ulcer on one finger (63). Ultrasound Doppler of the hand confirmed ischemic finger necrosis. He was treated unsuccessfully with aspirin, diltiazem, and heparin, but responded to intravenous infusions of iloprost for 5 days.

Another less common complication of cocaine use is cerebral vasculitis (64), and benign cocaine-induced cerebral angiopathy has been reported (65). (Stroke is discussed under the section Nervous system in this monograph).

Cardiac dysrhythmias

Dysrhythmias seem to be the most likely cause of sudden death from cocaine, but cardiac conduction disorders are more common in patients with acute cocaine toxicity. Severe cocaine toxicity also causes acidemia and cardiac dysfunction (66). Four patients developed seizures, psychomotor agitation, and cardiopulmonary arrest; two of these are briefly summarized here.

- A 43-year-old man injected a large dose of cocaine in a suicide attempt and had a seizure and cardiopulmonary arrest, from which he was resuscitated. His arterial blood pH was 6.72 and his electrocardiogram showed a wide complex tachycardia. An infusion of sodium bicarbonate maintained the blood pH at 7.50 and the electrocardiogram became normal. The bicarbonate infusion was discontinued after 12 hours.
- A 25-year-old man had a cardiac arrest after taking one "knot" or sealed bag of crack cocaine (2.5 g) and was resuscitated. His arterial blood pH was 6.92 and an electrocardiogram showed sinus rhythm, QRS axis 300°, and terminal 40 msec of the QRS axis 285°. After an infusion of sodium bicarbonate, his blood pH was 7.30, his QRS axis 15°, and the terminal 40 msec QRS axis 30°. He passed the bag of cocaine rectally within 12 hours of admission.

These patients' initial laboratory values showed acidosis, prolongation of the QRS complex and QT_c interval, and right axis deviation. Appropriate treatment included hyperventilation, sedation, active cooling, and sodium bicarbonate, which led to correction of the blood pH and of the cardiac conduction disorders. The authors suggested that when intracellular pH is lowered, myocardial contractility is depressed as a result of reduced calcium availability. During acidosis, there are abnormalities of repolarization and depolarization, which potentiate dysrhythmias.

The electrocardiographic PR interval increased with increasing abstinence from crack cocaine in a study of 441 chronic cocaine users who had smoked at least 10 g of cocaine in the 3 months before enrollment (67). The authors suggested that this may have reflected the normalization of a depolarization defect. Chronic cocaine users have shortened PR intervals, indicative of rapid cardiac depolarization.

Cardiovascular effects of cocaine as a local anesthetic

Cardiovascular effects due to enhanced sympathetic activity include tachycardia, increased cardiac output, vasoconstriction, and increased arterial pressure. Myocardial infarction is the most common adverse cardiac effect (39), and there is an increased risk of myocardial depression when amide-type local anesthetics, such as bupivacaine, levobupivacaine, lidocaine, or ropivacaine are administered with antidysrhythmic drugs.

- A woman who inappropriately used cocaine on the nasal mucosa to treat epistaxis had a myocardial infarction (49).
- A patient who was treated with intranasal cocaine and phenylephrine during a general anesthetic had a myocardial infarction and a cardiac arrest due to ventricular fibrillation (SEDA-20, 128).
- Myocardial ischemia was reported in a fit 29-year-old patient after the nasal application of cocaine for surgery. No relief was gained from vasodilators or intracoronary verapamil, and there were no other signs of cocaine toxicity. Although coronary vasoconstriction and platelet activation are systemic effects of cocaine, pre-existing thrombus may also have played a part (SEDA-22, 142).

Previous cocaine abuse has also been implicated in increasing the risk of myocardial ischemia when other local anesthetics are used.

Cardiac dysrhythmias have also been described in patients after the use of topical cocaine for nasal surgery (SEDA-20, 128).

- A patient who was treated with intranasal cocaine and submucosal lidocaine during general anesthesia developed ventricular fibrillation (SEDA-17, 142).

These events do not appear to have been related to the concomitant use of a vasoconstrictor, but more to excessive doses of cocaine.

Substantial systemic absorption of cocaine can cause severe cardiovascular complications (68).

- An 18-year-old man had both nasal cavities prepared with a pack soaked in 3–5 ml of Brompton solution (3% cocaine, about 3 mg/kg, plus adrenaline 1:4000) 2 hours preoperatively. In the anesthetic room he was anxious and withdrawn, with a mild tachycardia. Ten minutes later the nasal pack was removed and polypectomy was begun, with immediate sinus tachycardia and marked ST depression on lead II of the electrocardiogram. Increasing the depth of anesthesia and giving fentanyl had little effect, and the procedure was terminated. After extubation a further electrocardiogram showed T wave flattening in leads II, III, aVF, and aVL. Further cardiac investigations ruled out a myocardial infarction, an anatomical defect, or other pathological or metabolic processes. On day 4 a stress electrocardiogram showed no ischemic changes.

Absorption of cocaine from the nasal mucosa in eight patients using cotton pledglets soaked in 4 ml of 4% cocaine and applied for 10 or 20 minutes resulted in an absorption rate four times higher than expected, but was not associated with any cardiovascular disturbance; however, one of four patients who received 4 ml of 10% cocaine for 20 minutes developed intraoperative hypertension and another transient ventricular tachycardia (69). The authors advised against topical use of 10% cocaine.

Respiratory

The respiratory effects of cocaine are well known (70). In healthy crack cocaine users, there is evidence of cocaine-related injury to the pulmonary microcirculation, from fiberoptic bronchoscopy and examination of the bronchoalveolar fluid in 10 cocaine-only smokers, six cocaine-plus-tobacco smokers, 10 tobacco smokers, and 10 non-smokers, all with normal respiratory function (71). The percentages of hemosiderin-positive alveolar macrophages (a marker of recent alveolar hemorrhage) were markedly increased in the cocaine smokers compared with the others. Furthermore, the concentrations of endothelin (ET-1), an indicator of cell damage, were significantly raised in the cocaine smokers and to a lesser extent in the cocaine-and-tobacco smokers. These findings suggest that many asymptomatic healthy crack users have chronic alveolar hemorrhage that is not clinically evident.

In 177 heavy cocaine users (compared with 75 non-cocaine users), some of whom were also tobacco or marijuana users, cocaine use was associated with a higher prevalence of acute respiratory symptoms, including black sputum and chest pain. However, chronic respiratory symptoms occurred at similar frequencies in both groups. In cocaine-only smokers, mild impairment in carbon monoxide diffusing capacity suggested pulmonary capillary membrane damage, and abnormal airway conductance suggested injury to the upper airway or the large intrathoracic bronchi. Reported pulmonary complications of crack cocaine range from acute symptoms (coughing, chest pain, and palpitation) to acute syndromes (end-stage lung disease, eosinophilic infiltrates of the lung, and pulmonary infarction). The single-breath carbon monoxide diffusing capacity after the use of crack cocaine was reduced in three of six reports (70). If confirmed, a reduced carbon monoxide diffusing capacity after crack may signify damage to the alveolar capillary membrane or the pulmonary vasculature. It has been suggested that a well-designed controlled study to investigate the true impact of crack on the lung is necessary, since several confounding factors may account for the discrepancy in results (72).

Reports of acute pulmonary syndromes after the inhalation of cocaine have long been familiar.

- A 32-year-old woman rapidly developed progressive deterioration of respiratory function leading to end-stage lung disease (73). An open lung biopsy showed an inflammatory process with extensive accumulation of free silica.

The authors cautioned that some cocaine may contain silica, which could lead to severe pulmonary complications after smoking.

- A 27-year-old man twice developed inflammatory lung disease (with a predominance of eosinophils) after inhaling crack cocaine (74). Glucocorticoid treatment led to prompt resolution on both occasions.
- A 23-year-old woman developed pulmonary infarction associated with the use of crack (75).

Passive inhalation of free-base cocaine in small children can lead to serious consequences.

- A previously healthy 3-week-old boy developed pulmonary edema and autonomic manifestations of cocaine exposure from passive use (76). The urinary drug screen was positive for benzoylecgonine, a cocaine metabolite.
- Fatal pulmonary edema developed in a 36-year-old man shortly after he injected free-base cocaine intravenously (43).

A case of severe bullous emphysema in a cocaine smoker has been described (77).

- A 40-year-old man with cough, shortness of breath, and fever progressed to respiratory failure. He had smoked cocaine for the previous 17 years. His tobacco history was not known. His medical history included recurrent respiratory tract infections. A chest X-ray and CT scan showed findings consistent with bilateral bullous emphysema with a right lung abscess. He was ventilated and given antibiotics but died from respiratory failure secondary to pneumonia. Sputum cultures were positive for *Enterobacter cloacae* and *Streptococcus* species. Alpha-1 antitrypsin deficiency was ruled out.

Spontaneous pneumomediastinum has been reported (78).

- A 20-year-old obese Hispanic man awoke with severe, continuous retrosternal chest pain radiating to the neck and back (79). The pain was aggravated by deep breathing and local chest pressure. He denied substance abuse and gave a history of a flu-like illness 2 months before. His respiratory rate was 19/minute. He had a two-component pericardial rub. Laboratory blood testing ruled out myocardial infarction. His arterial blood gases and pH, electrocardiogram, chest X-ray, and echocardiogram were unremarkable. A later chest X-ray showed air in the mediastinum and chest CT confirmed the diagnosis of pneumomediastinum. Urine toxicology was positive for cocaine and cannabinoids. On further questioning, he admitted to substance use and performing a Valsalva maneuver during inhalation.

Handling cocaine pipes can cause thermal injury to the fingertips. The presence of bilateral thumb burns raised suspicion of crack lung in a young woman with suspected community-acquired pneumonia (80). When confronted with urine toxicology positive for cocaine, she admitted to having smoked large quantities of free-base cocaine only a few hours before the onset of symptoms.

Pneumothorax and pneumomediastinum

Two cases of spontaneous pneumothorax in intranasal cocaine users have been reported from Italy (81).

- A 30-year-old man, a cocaine sniffer, who had used cocaine more than five times a month for 4 years, complained of shortness of breath and acute chest pain. He had episodic cough and bloody sputum. A chest X-ray showed an 80% pneumothorax on the left side. On thoracoscopy the entire lung visceral pleura seemed to be covered by fibrinous exudate. After yttrium aluminium garnet (YAG) laser pleurodesis surgery, which abrades the pleura, he made a full recovery within 4 days.
- A 24-year-old man who had been inhaling cocaine nasally 4–5 times a month for a year developed respiratory distress and chest pain 2 days after the last use, because of a right-sided pneumothorax. He underwent video-assisted thoracoscopic surgery with laser pleurodesis and responded rapidly.

In both cases, pneumothorax occurred with a delay after cocaine inhalation. The authors suggested that it was therefore unlikely that these cases of pneumothorax were due to direct traumatic effects of the drug powder inhaled, to barotrauma due to exaggerated inspiration, or to a Valsalva maneuver. Histological examination in both cases showed small foreign body granulomas with polarized material in the subpleural parenchyma. The authors proposed that the pleural damage could have been directly caused by a filler substance known as mannite (a fine white powder comprised of insoluble cellulose fibers).

Spontaneous pneumomediastinum has been reported with the inhalation of free-base cocaine (78).

Asthma

Cocaine can cause exacerbation of asthma. All adult visits to an urban emergency room for an asthma attack during a 7-month period were reviewed (82). Of 163 patients (aged 18–55 years), 116 agreed to participate in a facilitated questionnaire and 103 provided urine samples for drug screening. African-Americans made up 89% of the group and 35% were cigarette smokers. Urine toxicology was positive for cocaine in 13% and for opiates in 5.8%. The severity of the exacerbation of asthma was greatest in the cocaine-positive group, 38% of whom were admitted to hospital (compared with 20% of the non-cocaine users). The length of stay was significantly longer in the cocaine-positive patients. Most of the patients did not use inhaled corticosteroids according to the treatment guidelines.

Ear, nose, throat

Intranasal use, a common method of cocaine abuse, can damage the sinonasal tract, causing acute and chronic inflammation, necrosis, and osteocartilaginous erosion (SEDA-17, 36). These conditions occur secondary to the combined effects of direct trauma from instrumentation, vasoconstriction of small blood vessels with resultant ischemic necrosis, and chemical irritation from adulterants. Intranasal cocaine users can develop septal perforation, saddle-nose deformities, and sinonasal structural damage.

- A 43-year-old woman with a past history of chronic heavy cocaine use and osteomyelitis of the hard palate and nasal cavity 10 years before had required continuous follow-up for recurrent ethmoid and sphenoid sinusitis (83). Endoscopy showed an absent nasal septum, middle turbinates, anterior two-thirds of the inferior turbinates, and lateral nasal wall.
- Pott's puffy tumor, a subperiosteal infection of the frontal bone, has been described in a 34-year-old man with a history of chronic intranasal cocaine use (84).

This rare complication of frontal sinusitis appeared to develop secondary to the insertion of foreign bodies into the nose to facilitate inhalation of cocaine. Local trauma plus cocaine-induced vasoconstriction may have led to the complication.

Midline nasal and hard palate destruction have been reported in two chronic users of intranasal cocaine (85). The pathophysiology of these lesions is multifactorial, including ischemia secondary to vasoconstriction, chemical irritation from adulterants, impaired mucociliary transport, reduced immunity, and infection secondary to trauma.

In another case there was progression of septal perforation to secondary bone infection in a chronic cocaine user (86).

- A 56-year-old chronic intranasal cocaine abuser with a visible nasal defect presented with a hole in the roof of his mouth. He had been reportedly drug free for 2 weeks. He had an oronasal fistula with adjacent black necrotic areas and erosive destruction of the nasal septum, turbinates, and antrum, with mucoperiosteal thickening of the sphenoid and maxillary sinuses. Treatment included antibiotics and a prosthesis plate construction to cover the defect. Two years later, having continued to inhale cocaine, he had progressive destruction of his sinonasal tract, a fistula between his oral and nasal cavity, a saddle-nose deformity with total cartilage loss, and a complete palatal defect. Biopsy of the nasal septum showed acute osteomyelitis and extensive bacterial overgrowth (including anerobic *Actinomyces*-like organisms). He was given intravenous antibiotics for 6 weeks followed by long-term oral antibiotics.

Cocaine-related erosion of the external nasal structures has been described (87).

- A 43-year-old woman with a T12 paraplegia due to a car accident 24 years earlier and a sublabial abscess 2 years before developed progressive erosion of both the internal and external portions of her nose over 6 months, with nasal crusting and nose bleeds. Several antibiotics were unhelpful. There was partial destruction of the external nasal structure and two oronasal fistulae in the upper gingival sulcus. Intranasal biopsy showed acute and chronic inflammation. On two occasions urine drug screening was positive for cocaine, although she denied using cocaine.

Nervous system

Research in 21 cocaine users and 13 non-drug-using, age-matched controls has suggested that chronic cocaine use may be associated with specific neurochemical changes in the brains of habitual users (88). All the subjects underwent a spectral brain scan in a proton MRS scanner. The significant finding was that the concentration of *N*-acetylaspartate in the left thalamus (but not in the basal ganglia) was significantly lower (17%) in the chronic cocaine users than in the controls. *N*-acetylaspartate is found in adult neurons and not in glia; it is often used as a marker of neuronal viability; a reduction suggests neuronal damage and/or loss.

Assessment of smooth pursuit eye movements has been used in the study of neurophysiological effects of a variety of clinical and subclinical disorders. In 126 patients who met DSM-IIIR criteria for dependence on alcohol, cocaine, or heroin, or dual alcohol and cocaine abuse, there was a significant reduction in tracking accuracy in the heroin-dependent and the dually-dependent subjects relative to controls (89). However, eye movement dysfunction in the drug-dependent groups was not detectable when the effects of antisocial personality disorder were statistically removed. The magnitude of the dysfunction correlated significantly with several antisocial personality-related features, including an increased number of criminal charges, months of incarceration, increased problems associated with drug abuse, and lower intellectual functioning. The findings suggested that there may be an association between premorbid personality traits and eye movement impairment.

Cocaine use has been associated with a reduced inhibitory response of the P50 auditory evoked response, attributed to increased catecholaminergic and reduced cholinergic neurotransmission secondary to cocaine (90). In a double-blind, placebo-controlled study, 11 cocaine users in the first and third weeks of detoxification had electrophysiological testing 10 minutes before and 30 minutes after taking nicotine gum 6 mg. Nicotine briefly reversed the inhibitory deficit.

Chronic substance use has been associated with long-lasting changes in brain function (91). Five brain regions that may be affected (the orbitofrontal gyrus, rectal gyrus, anterior cingulate gyrus, basal ganglia, and thalamus) were selected for analyses of cerebral glucose metabolism by positron emission scanning in controls, cocaine users, and alcoholics (17 in each group), who performed the Stroop test, which assesses cognitive interference and response inhibition. In controls, higher brain glucose metabolism in the orbitofrontal gyrus correlated with poorer performance. In contrast, in substance users, higher brain glucose metabolism was associated with better performance. Chronic abuse appears to be associated with altered function of the orbitofrontal gyrus.

Cerebellar dysfunction

Cocaine has been associated with movement disorders, such as acute dystonias, choreoathetosis, and akathisia. Chronic pancerebellar dysfunction occurred in a cocaine user with schizophrenia treated with risperidone (92).

- A 38-year-old man was found comatose in a crack house. The ambient temperature was 13°C. He had earlier abused cocaine. His temperature was 43°C, heart rate 115, blood pressure 144/89 mmHg, and oxygen saturation 97% on air. His general muscle tone was flaccid. He had a mild leukocytosis and hypophosphatemia. Urine toxicology was positive for benzoylecgonine, a cocaine metabolite. He was mechanically ventilated, cooled, and given intravenous fluids. His temperature fell to 38°C, but he later developed acute disseminated intravascular coagulation and rhabdomyolysis. After 5 days he developed nystagmus, intention tremor, truncal ataxia, dysarthria, ocular dysmetria, and dysmetria of the arms and legs. There were no sensory or motor deficits. Finger-to-nose and heel-to-knee tests were slowed and uncoordinated. He could not stand. Brain imaging studies (CT and MRI scans) were unremarkable. He was given thiamine, propranolol, clonazepam, primidone, and baclofen every 8 hours without improvement. After 1 year he still had nystagmus, intention tremor, ataxic gait, and dysmetria. He could walk short distances slowly.

Cocaine and neuroleptic drugs can both cause hyperthermia and the authors proposed that the combination of cocaine and risperidone may have caused this problem.

Migraine

About 60–75% of chronic cocaine abusers report severe headaches (93), which can resemble migraine; migraine-like symptoms can include auras, visual field changes, and paraphasia (94). About 60–75% of chronic cocaine abusers report severe headaches (93,94). Of 21 patients who were admitted to hospital from January 1985 to December 1988 for acute headache associated with cocaine intoxication 15 had headaches with migrainous features in the absence of neurological or systemic complications (93). None had a history of cocaine-unrelated headaches or a family history of migraine, and all had a favourable outcome. The authors discussed three possible mechanisms of cocaine-related vascular headaches, depending on the interval between cocaine ingestion and development of the headache. They postulated that acute headaches after cocaine use may relate to the sympathomimetic or vasoconstrictive effects of cocaine, while headaches after cocaine withdrawal or exacerbated during a cocaine binge may relate to cocaine-induced effects on the serotoninergic system.

Movement disorders

The effects of cocaine or its withdrawal on neurotransmitter activity have been evaluated in several studies. Although changes in dopaminergic activity appear to be associated with early cocaine abstinence, extrapyramidal symptoms (due to alterations in dopamine functioning) have only infrequently been reported in cocaine users. However, in a recent report, extrapyramidal symptoms of classic muscle stiffness and cogwheel rigidity at the elbow occurred during the "crash" phase of a 40-year-old man's cocaine withdrawal (95).

Cocaine can cause other movement disorders (96). Motor and vocal tics, pre-existing tremors, and generalized dystonia were induced or exacerbated by drug use, and continued even after cocaine use ended. Lastly, dopamine dysregulation (that is reduced dopamine receptor availability in association with reduced frontal metabolism) was demonstrated by positive emission tomography in 20 chronic cocaine abusers (97). The findings were prominent in the orbitofrontal, cingulate, and prefrontal cortex 3–4 months after detoxification. The author hypothesized that dysregulation of these brain areas may result in compulsive drug-taking behavior.

Dystonia has been described shortly after the use of cocaine (SEDA-16, 24). In a retrospective study of 116 patients taking neuroleptic drugs, 42% of cocaine users versus 14% of non-users developed dystonia (98). This suggests that the use of cocaine may be a major risk factor for acute dystonic reactions secondary to the use of neuroleptic drugs.

Cocaine-induced chronic tics have been reported (99), and cocaine has reportedly exacerbated Gilles de la Tourette syndrome (100).

Myasthenia gravis

A 24-year-old woman developed myasthenia gravis during cocaine use (101). The authors speculated that while cocaine did not cause impairment of motor axons for neuromuscular transmission, a reduction in the number of acetylcholine receptors per neuromuscular junction (as occurs in myasthenia gravis) could have increased the susceptibility to an effect of cocaine.

A rare case of polysubstance abuse, which unmasked myasthenia and caused complete external ophthalmoplegia, has been reported (102).

- A 29-year-old woman, who used cocaine 2 g/day, heroin 1 g/day, and methadone 40 mg/day, developed abscesses caused by drug injection. She had had generalized weakness, difficulty in swallowing, and lagging eyelids for 1 week. There was bilateral ptosis, and a diagnosis of myasthenia was made. Edrophonium 10 mg relieved the ptosis and improved ocular movements.

Seizures

Cocaine lowers the seizure threshold and may therefore be dangerous to patients already at risk of seizures (40). Exacerbation of generalized tonic-clonic seizures (which occurred initially during the use of crack but later continued independently of the drug) has been described, with progressive electroencephalographic abnormalities (103). In this case, the development of the seizures suggested that cocaine can stimulate kindling, with progressive intensification of after-discharges and the eventual emergence of seizure activity.

Cerebrovascular vasoconstriction and a sudden increase in blood pressure probably underlie the many reports of cocaine-induced strokes, CNS hemorrhage, and migraine (SEDA-17, 1).

Three cases of generalized seizures occurring shortly after the intravenous use of cocaine (104).

Sleep disturbance

The disruption of normal sleeping patterns during cocaine withdrawal may be related to effects on the cholinergic system. In a study of nine patients undergoing cocaine withdrawal, rapid eye movement (REM) latency was markedly shortened, REM sleep percentage was increased, REM density was very high, and the total sleep period was long during the first week (105). Changes in REM sleep are thought to be related to changes in cholinergic activity. At week 3, characteristic chronic insomnia was observed.

Stroke

Cocaine has been associated with cerebrovascular events, such as transient ischemic attacks (SEDA-24, 24), cerebral hemorrhage (106,107), and cerebral infarction (SEDA-22, 23) (SEDA-20, 26) (SEDA-20, 21).

Regional cerebral blood flow was assessed using single photon emission computed tomography (SPECT) and tracer HMPAO in 10 cocaine abusers within 72 hours of last cocaine use and then after 21 days of abstinence (108). Compared with controls, recent cocaine abusers had significantly reduced cerebral blood flow in 11 of 14 brain regions, with the largest reductions in the frontal cortex and parietal cortex and greater cerebral blood flow in the brain stem. These perfusion defects appeared to be primarily due to combined abuse of alcohol and cocaine. Frontal but not parietal defects appeared to resolve partially during 21 days of abstinence.

In a review of ischemic stroke in young American adults (aged 15–44 years) admitted to 46 regional hospitals between 1988 and 1991, illicit drug use was noted in 12% and was the probable cause of stroke in 4.7% (109). Multidrug use was common among users: 73% used cocaine, 29% used heroin, and 14% used phencyclidine. Drug-associated stroke in these young adults appeared to be related to vascular mechanisms (such as large and small vessel occlusive disease) rather than to hypertension or to diabetes. Cerebral infarction is significantly more common among users of cocaine alkaloid (crack) than cocaine hydrochloride (110).

Ischemic stroke has been attributed to combined use of cocaine and amphetamine (111).

- A previously healthy 16-year-old man developed an unsteady gait and double vision. His symptoms began 5 minutes after intranasal "amfetamine" (actually amfetamine cut with cocaine). He had a left-sided internuclear ophthalmoplegia, an incomplete fascicular paresis of the left oculomotor nerve, and saccadic vertical smooth pursuit. Cranial MRI showed a left-sided hyperintense lesion near the midline of the mesencephalon. A repeat MRI scan 9 days later showed that the lesion was much smaller. He made a full recovery within 3 weeks.

The cause of cocaine-related stroke and transient ischemic attacks has been studied by transcranial Doppler sonography, a continuous measure of cerebral blood flow velocity, to monitor the course of cerebral hemodynamic changes during acute intravenous injection of placebo, and of cocaine 10, 25, and 50 mg in seven cocaine abusers (112). There was a significant increase in mean and systolic velocity (lasting about 2 minutes) with all doses of cocaine but not with placebo. Cocaine produced an immediate brief period of vasoconstriction (as demonstrated by an increase in systolic velocity) in the large arteries of the brain.

"Spontaneous" acute subdural hematoma related to cocaine abuse has been described (113).

- A 38-year-old man with a 10-year history of cocaine use became comatose. He had had an acute severe headache and progressive deterioration after abusing cocaine. His Glasgow Coma Scale was 3 and his pupils were dilated but reactive to light. He had hypertension and bradycardia. Routine toxicology was positive for cocaine. Blood tests, including coagulation profile, were normal. A CT scan of the brain showed a left acute subdural hematoma with midline shift and obliteration of the basal cisterns. During emergency craniotomy the source of the bleed was identified as a pinhole rupture of a parietal cortical artery. The patient had no history of head injury and there were no intraoperative findings of head injury. He died 24 hours later without evidence of clot reaccumulation. An autopsy was not performed.

Hypertensive encephalopathy can follow the use of cocaine (114).

Brown–Séquard syndrome after esophageal sclerotherapy and recent crack cocaine abuse has been reported (115).

- A 44-year-old man with hepatitis C and cirrhosis, esophageal varices, and poorly controlled hypertension, who was also a chronic alcoholic and crack cocaine abuser, had his varices injected at endoscopy and developed right-sided weakness and numbness up to T4. There was flaccid right leg weakness, right T4-6 hypalgesia, left leg hypalgesia up to L1, and reduced sweating on the left up to T4-6. An MRI scan of the thoracic spine showed a lesion at T4-6 involving the anterior and central portions of the spinal cord. A urine screen was positive for cocaine. He recovered spontaneously 2 weeks later.

Cocaine-induced ischemia was the most likely cause of this adverse outcome.

Subarachnoid hemorrhage

There is an association between cocaine use and aneurysmal subarachnoid hemorrhage (SEDA-18, 36) (SEDA-21, 26) (116). Subarachnoid hemorrhage was temporally related to cocaine abuse in 12 young adult abusers who had underlying cerebral aneurysms; hypertension was a probable contributing factor (117) and cocaine is a risk factor for cerebral vasospasm after aneurysmal subarachnoid hemorrhage (118). In a retrospective analysis of the medical records of 440 patients who presented to a neurosurgery unit between 1992 and 1999 with aneurysmal subarachnoid hemorrhage, 27 patients (6.1%) had either a positive urine screen for cocaine metabolites ($n = 20$) or a history of cocaine use within 72 hours of subarachnoid hemorrhage ($n = 7$). Cocaine users were more likely to have cerebral vasospasm from 3 to 16 days after subarachnoid hemorrhage than non-exposed patients (63 versus 30%). They were also more likely to be younger and to have aneurysms of the anterior circulation than the control group (97 versus 84%).

Sensory systems

Ophthalmic effects associated with cocaine can occur during both active drug use and early abstinence. Cocaine abuse has been associated with ophthalmic complications, including ulceration of the cornea, vasoconstrictor effects on the retinal vasculature, irregularities in oculomotor performance, and secondary optic neuropathy.

Corneal ulceration secondary to smoking crack cocaine has been reported in a 27-year-old woman (119).

Cases of the "crack eye syndrome" continue to be reported. Of 14 crack cocaine users with corneal problems, 10 had corneal ulcers infected with both bacterial and fungal organisms; 4 had corneal epithelial defects (120). All were actively smoking crack daily. The authors suggested that crack smoking predisposes users, through an unknown mechanism, to corneal epithelial changes, infection, and perforation. Typical presentations include loss of vision with or without pain.

- A 29-year-old woman with a painful corneal ulcer related to cocaine abuse was found to be putting cocaine powder directly into the affected eye to reduce the pain (121). Her history included prior corneal perforations.

Such topical use of cocaine may aggravate the condition.

Acute iritis has been reported after intranasal use (122).

There has been a report of retinal changes in 60 users of crack (123). Microtalc retinopathy and retinal nerve fiber layer "rake" or "slit" defects were detected by threshold visual field testing and fundus photography.

Orbital infarction has been described after cocaine use (124).

- A 36-year-old woman drank alcohol and snorted cocaine and heroin at a party. She lost consciousness, with her head positioned down with her left face pressed against a desk. She awoke 3 hours later with severe left orbital pain. Her right eye was normal but there was complete visual loss in the left eye and a nearly complete left ptosis. The left pupil did not react to light but reacted consensually. Movements in the right eye were full, but movements in the left eye were severely limited in all directions. In the left fundus there was retinal edema and retinal pigment epithelium disruption. An orbital MRI scan showed diffuse swelling of all the extraocular muscles in the left orbit. A week later the pain had abated and there was mild improvement in the eye movements and ptosis, but no change in vision. She was instructed to wear protective polycarbonate lenses at all times.

Central retinal artery occlusion has previously been reported in cases of intravenous and intranasal cocaine abuse and has also been reported in a man who smoked crack cocaine (125).

- A 42-year-old man smoked crack and developed sudden painless loss of vision in his right eye for 9 hours. He had smoked cigarettes for 20 years and crack cocaine twice a week for the previous 4 years. Visual acuity in the right eye was counting fingers at one meter, and in the left eye 6/4. There was a right relative afferent papillary defect. In the right fundus there was evidence of central retinal artery occlusion and the left fundus was unremarkable. Treatment included intravenous acetazolamide, intermittent ocular massage, and rebreathing into a paper bag. He was found to have sickle cell trait, a risk factor for central retinal artery occlusion.

Psychological, psychiatric

Single photon emission computerized tomography (SPECT) has suggested that some psychiatric symptoms in cocaine users are associated with changes in blood flow (126). Multiple scalloped areas of reduced cerebral blood flow (especially periventricular regions and deep portions of the brain) have been seen. Hypoperfusion has also been noted in the frontal lobes of cocaine users with mania.

Cognitive function

The effects of cocaine on cognitive functions have been measured in controlled studies. The preliminary results of a study of 20 heavy cocaine abusers and a group of matched controls showed impaired function on neuropsychological tests in 50% of the abusers compared with 15% of the controls (127). There were problems with concentration, memory, problem-solving, and abstract thinking in the cocaine users. The heavy users had the greatest loss of memory. Recent cocaine use was associated with poorer oral fluency and arithmetic scores.

The effect of cocaine on cognitive functioning has been studied in 20 crack users, 37 crack and alcohol users, and 29 controls at 6 weeks and 6 months of abstinence (128). The two substance-dependent groups had significant cognitive impairment in a range of neuropsychological tests compared with the controls at both times. Drug dose was strongly associated with the extent of impairment. Abstinent substance users were more depressed than controls during the test period, but depression had only a slight effect on neuropsychological performance.

Neuropsychological performance was examined in 355 incarcerated adult male felons, who were classified by DSM-IV criteria into four subgroups: alcohol dependence or abuse ($n = 101$), cocaine dependence or abuse ($n = 60$), multisubstance dependence or abuse ($n = 56$), and no history of drug abuse ($n = 138$) (129). The cocaine and control groups had similar neuropsychological test scores. However, both the multisubstance and alcohol groups performed significantly worse on nearly all measures. The multisubstance group had worse short-term memory, long-term memory, and visuomotor ability. Correlations between neuropsychological performance and length of abstinence from drug use showed that after abstinence the alcohol group had the greatest improvement on tests. Although the cocaine group had the least amount of improvement with abstinence, their overall performance was not significantly different from controls.

Even after 4 weeks of abstinence, chronic heavy cocaine users have poor cognitive functioning compared with non-drug-using controls (130). A battery of neuropsychological tests was administered to 30 abstinent chronic cocaine abusers and 21 non-drug-using matched controls. Decrements in areas such as executive functioning, visuoperception, psychomotor speed, and manual dexterity were associated with heavier use of cocaine. Neither frequency nor duration of cocaine use was a strong predictor of performance.

Neurolinguistic functioning has been assessed in six African-American male cocaine abusers undergoing drug rehabilitation (131). A test battery to assess language, cognition, and memory skills was administered at 1 week and 1 month of cocaine abstinence. Participants' performances were compared with the normative data for each test. There was reduced ability for general language knowledge, memory, and verbal learning ability during the period of early abstinence. However, the sample size was small and the duration of study short.

Mood disorders

The rate of co-morbidity has been studied in 208 female African-American crack cocaine users; 148 were in treatment, 54 were active crack users, and 61% reported a history of sexual abuse (132). Many had co-morbid depression (48%) and eating disorders (11%).

Delirium

Cocaine-induced delirium with severe acidosis has been reported (133).

- A 25-year-old man with agitation and paranoia who had consumed a lot of alcohol with cocaine the night before had a clonic seizure lasting 1 minute. In the emergency room, he responded to pain and made incomprehensible sounds. His pulse rate was 116/minute, blood pressure 100/40 mmHg, respiratory rate 28/minute, and temperature 38.3°C. He was acidotic (pH 6.53), with a $PaCO_2$ of 13.1 kPa, a base deficit of 36 mmol/l, a serum potassium concentration of 7 mmol/l, and sodium 153 mmol/l. He was hyperventilated and given sodium bicarbonate, dantrolene, and passive cooling. His acidosis quickly corrected and his temperature fell to 37.6°C within 1 hour.

Obsessive-compulsive disorder

Suspected risk factors for obsessive-compulsive disorder were investigated in a prospective epidemiological study, using data from the Epidemiologic Catchment Area surveys (1980–1984) (134). Users of both cocaine and marijuana were at increased risk of obsessive-compulsive disorder compared with non-users of illicit drugs, but cocaine use alone was not associated with an increased risk, within the limited sample size.

Panic disorder

As with several other drugs, for example marijuana, PCP, and LSD, cocaine can precipitate panic disorder, which continues long after drug withdrawal (135). Among 280 patients in a methadone maintenance clinic, the prevalence of panic disorder increased from 1% to 6% over a decade (136). A marked rise in the frequency of cocaine abuse coincided with this outbreak. The authors suggested that episodes of panic occurring in cocaine users can result in hospitalization for either psychiatric or medical illnesses.

Paranoid psychoses

Of 55 individuals with cocaine dependence, 53% reported transient cocaine-induced psychotic symptoms (137). Paranoid delusions (related to drug use) and auditory hallucinations were often reported. In addition, almost one-third (all of whom also described psychotic symptoms) reported transient behavioral stereotypes.

Paranoid psychosis has also been described in a 64-year-old man who had first begun to use crack cocaine 6 months before. The paranoid symptoms continued for 3 weeks after he stopped using crack.

The author suggested that the man's age may have made him particularly sensitive to the psychiatric effects of cocaine (138).

The possible genetic basis of cocaine-induced paranoia has been studied in 45 European Americans with cocaine dependency (139). Low activity of the enzyme dopamine β-hydroxylase (the enzyme that catalyses the conversion of dopamine to noradrenaline) in the serum or cerebrospinal fluid was positively associated with the occurrence of positive psychotic symptoms in several psychiatric disorders. The activity of dopamine β-hydroxylase is a stable, genetically determined trait that is regulated by genes located at the DBH locus. The haplotype associated with low dopamine β-hydroxylase activity, Del-a, occurred more often in 29 subjects with cocaine-induced paranoia than in 16 without. These findings may have implications for the pharmacological treatment of cocaine dependence.

Endocrine

Blood sugar concentrations can become labile in people with diabetes mellitus who use cocaine, not only because their diet changes, but also because adrenaline concentrations affect the mobilization of glucose (36).

In a prospective study, endocrine responses to hyperthermic stress were assessed in 10 male cocaine users after 4 weeks of abstinence and again after 1 year of abstinence (140). They sat in a sauna for 30 minutes at a temperature of 90°F and a relative humidity of 10%. At the end of the sauna, they rested for another 30 minutes at room temperature. Sublingual temperature, pulse rate, and blood pressure were recorded just before and immediately after the sauna and 30 minutes after the period at room temperature. Venous β-erythropoietin, ACTH, metenkephalin, prolactin, and cortisol were also measured. There were no significant differences between the two groups in heart rate and blood pressure. At baseline and after 1 year of abstinence, plasma prolactin concentrations were higher in the cocaine users than in the controls. Moreover, the hormonal responses in the cocaine users were different from those in controls. Concentrations of all the hormones, except for metenkephalin, were significantly lower in the cocaine users than in the controls at the end of the sauna; the cocaine users did not have significant hormonal changes to hyperthermia after either 4 weeks or 1 year of abstinence. The authors concluded that cocaine abuse produces alterations in the hypothalamic-pituitary axis, which persist during abstinence.

Electrolyte balance

Cocaine-induced periodic paralysis with hypokalemia has been reported (141).

- A healthy 33-year-old man suddenly developed generalized weakness and became unable to walk or lift his limbs; he also had mild chest pain. He had had similar episodes 10 days and 5 years before, with spontaneous resolution. He had no spontaneous motor activity and his strength was 2/5 in all major muscle groups with a very mild left upper limb predominance. Cardiac enzymes and neuroimaging of the brain and spinal cord were normal. Creatinine kinase was raised (395 IU/l). Acetylcholine receptor antibodies were in the reference range. His serum potassium concentration was 1.9 mmol/l. Urine toxicology screen showed cocaine, cannabinoids, and benzodiazepines and he admitted to cocaine binge use the previous night and also before the previous two episodes. With potassium supplements his strength gradually improved.

Such severe generalized weakness and hypokalemia may be due to intracellular shift of potassium due to adrenergic stimulation by cocaine or a direct effect on potassium channels.

Hematologic

In an attempt to replicate the conclusions of an earlier study, there was no association between cocaine use during pregnancy and acute thrombocytopenia in 326 patients (142). There were similar prevalences of thrombocytopenia in cocaine-using women (13/160) and non-using women (11/160) during pregnancy. Thrombocytopenia occurred more often in the third trimester in both groups.

Gastrointestinal

Gastrointestinal symptoms, especially diarrhea, occur after cocaine use. Cases of more severe abdominal distress have required surgical intervention and have been due to bowel infarction (1,143) or pneumoperitoneum (144).

Esophageal damage

The esophagus can undergo thermal injury, in which the inner esophageal wall has a "candy-cane" appearance (alternating pink and white linear bands), when boiling-hot liquids are consumed. This reversible condition is associated with chest pain, difficulty in swallowing, odynophagia, and abdominal pain. Candy-cane esophagus secondary to smoking crack cocaine has been reported (145).

- A 55-year-old man accidentally sucked into his mouth and swallowed a portion of boiling water during his last smoke of free base cocaine and 2 days later developed sudden constant pain in the left shoulder and arm accompanied by sweating. He had melena, a hematocrit of 30%, a blood urea nitrogen of 35 mmol/l, and a serum creatinine of 1.1 mmol/l. The initial electrocardiogram showed sinus rhythm, left atrial enlargement, and borderline left ventricular hypertrophy. However, 2 hours later he started to sweat and became hypotensive (blood pressure 85/50 mmHg). An electrocardiogram showed new biphasic T waves and T wave inversion. Urgent cardiac catheterization showed patent coronary arteries. Esophagogastroduodenoscopy within the hour showed a candy-cane appearance in the distal esophagus, patchy erythema and erosions in the gastric antrum, and an ulcer in the base of the duodenal bulb. Biopsies of the esophagus tissue showed parakeratosis, squamous hyperplasia with regeneration, and minimal inflammation. Biopsies of the stomach showed chronic gastritis and bacteria consistent with *Helicobacter pylori*. Later that day, the electrocardiogram normalized.

The most likely cause of the chest pain was microvascular spasm of the epicardial coronary arteries, due to either thermal injury to the esophagus or a direct effect of cocaine.

Peptic ulceration

There is a higher incidence of gastric ulcers in cocaine users, both perforated ulcers and giant gastroduodenal ulcers, thought to be due to localized ischemia secondary to vasoconstriction (146,147). Two reports have afforded data on gastrointestinal ulcers and cocaine. In one study the authors observed that since the advent of crack cocaine they had seen more than 70 cases of crack-related perforated ulcers (146). They suggested that an ischemic process rather than an acid-producing mechanism was to blame. They described three patients, all of whom had laparoscopic omental patches for ulcers, with good results. In a longitudinal assessment of patients with endoscopically diagnosed gastric ulcers ($n = 98$) or duodenal ulcers ($n = 116$) users of cocaine or metamfetamine were nearly 10 times more likely to have giant gastric or duodenal ulcers (over 2.5 cm) compared with non-users (147). The authors speculated that cocaine and amfetamine-induced catecholamine stimulation of α-adrenoceptors may cause intense vasoconstriction and thus a reduced blood supply to an ulcer, resulting in a giant ulcer.

Five cases of gastric perforation (rather than the more common duodenal perforation) have been reported in young male smokers of crack, all of whom had only brief histories of prodromal symptoms and none of whom had long-standing peptic ulcer disease (148).

Intestinal ischemia

Two women developed chronic mesenteric ischemia, successfully managed by revascularization (149). The authors concluded that in both cases chronic mesenteric ischemia had been caused by intravenous cocaine abuse.

Ischemia of the small bowel and colon after the use of cocaine has been reported (SEDA-22, 33).

- A 38-year-old man presented with a 2-day history of severe abdominal pain and bloody stools after smoking cocaine 48 hours earlier (150). He had abdominal pain, guarding, rebound tenderness, and high-pitched, hypoactive bowel sounds. His white blood cell count was 31×10^9/l. Radiography showed thumb-printing in the transverse colon. Endoscopy showed friable edematous mucosa with submucosal hemorrhage and patches of yellowish fibrinous material. He recovered fully with intravenous nutrition and supportive measures after 30 days.
- A 36-year-old man who had injected cocaine the day before admission and who occasionally sniffed, smoked, or injected cocaine, presented with a 3-day history of severe abdominal pain and bloody diarrhea (151). His mid-abdomen was very tender, with rebound tenderness and guarding; bowel sounds were absent. Radiography showed a dilated transverse colon and dilated small bowel loops. He underwent emergency surgery and an edematous dilated transverse colon was removed. The pathology was consistent with ischemic colitis. The blood vessels were dilated but showed no structural abnormalities or thrombosis.

Liver

Cocaine has been associated with liver toxicity (SEDA-14, 32) (SEDA-13, 27).

- A 23-year-old man became unresponsive and had a seizure after taking cocaine and alcohol (152). Severe liver necrosis developed and hepatocellular damage was documented with ^{99m}Tc-PYP imaging.

Acute hepatitis induced by intranasal cocaine, with transient increases in liver enzymes, has been reported in three HIV-positive patients (153). All had non-active chronic viral hepatitis with normal immunological status; one was seropositive for hepatitis B virus and two were positive for hepatitis C virus. A few days after intranasal cocaine use, serum transaminases rose to high values, and two of the patients had fever, stiffness, sweats, and hepatomegaly. Alcohol and hepatotoxic agents were ruled out. Within a few days, the clinical and laboratory signs of hepatitis improved in all three cases.

Urinary tract

Cocaine can cause acute renal insufficiency (SEDA-21,19) (SEDA-24, 38). Acute renal insufficiency, with malignant hypertension, apparently precipitated by cocaine-induced vasoconstriction, has been described in a 33-year-old woman who had pre-existing scleroderma and normal renal function (154). She was successfully treated with hemodialysis.

Cocaine can also cause chronic renal insufficiency (155). Of hemodialysis patients from an urban center in California, 55 who reported a history of significant cocaine use were compared with 138 non-users. A diagnosis of hypertension-related end-stage renal disease was reported in 49 of the 55 cocaine users (89%) and 64 of the 138 non-users (46%). Of 113 patients with end-stage renal disease, 49 had a history of cocaine use. The patients who had used cocaine had hypertension for a shorter duration (5.3 versus 12.7 years). They were also younger (41 versus 54 years). The authors proposed that this outcome had been caused by several mechanisms: renal vasoconstriction or stenosis, resulting in ischemic nephropathy and secondary hypertension, direct renal damage with progressive renal insufficiency, and recurrent episodes of accelerated hypertension, vasculitis, acute tubular necrosis, and rhabdomyolysis.

Chronic cocaine use can exacerbate pre-existing hypertension, when renal blood vessels narrow secondary to cocaine-induced intimal fibrosis. Acute renal insufficiency with concomitant rhabdomyolysis after cocaine use has been reported (156,157), but it can also occur, albeit rarely, in the absence of rhabdomyolysis (158).

- A healthy 31-year-old man developed acute renal insufficiency 18 hours after inhaling cocaine 5 g. His blood pressure was 150/100 mmHg, his serum creatinine 177 μmol/l, creatine phosphokinase activity 107 U/l, and serum potassium concentration 3.8 mmol/l. The urinary sodium concentration was 30 mmol/l and there was a trace of protein and 1–2 red blood cells per high-power field. Immunological studies were unremarkable. Ultrasound showed kidneys of normal size with hyperechogenity of the right kidney. Over the next 10 days he recovered spontaneously.

The authors suggested that intense cocaine-induced renal vasoconstriction had been the likely underlying mechanism.

Renal infarction is an uncommon adverse effect of cocaine (159).

- After using intranasal cocaine, a 25-year-old African man developed fever and progressive right flank pain over 4 days. He had a temperature of 38.3°C, a blood pressure of 106/54 mmHg, and severe tenderness in the right flank and right lower quadrant of the abdomen. His urine contained cocaine. A CT scan showed reduced uptake in the lower pole of the kidney, confirming renal infarction. Other causes were ruled out.

Sexual function

The practice of trading sex for drugs in places where there is a high prevalence of cocaine abuse has been noted in both metropolitan areas and smaller communities along major interstate highways. In Baltimore, there was a 97% increase in the number of primary and secondary cases of syphilis from 1993 to 1995 (160).

Priapism has been reported in men who have used cocaine by inhalation or applied it topically to the glans penis or intraurethrally (SEDA-19, 26).

- Three men developed priapism and delayed seeking treatment (161). Cocaine use within the previous 24 hours was the singular contributing factor in all three cases. Two of the men had had previous episodes of priapism, which had resolved spontaneously. Initial duplex ultrasonography confirmed low penile blood flow. Manual aspiration and irrigation failed in all three cases. Surgical shunting failed in the first two cases. One man required partial penile amputation for infected, gangrenous, distal penile tissue; one responded to angiographic embolization; and one had only a partial response to angiographic embolization, but then refused further intervention; his erection resolved during the next 24 hours.

The authors suggested that acute sexual excitement during cocaine intoxication can cause penile erection, with impaired detumescence. Cocaine can inhibit the reuptake of noradrenaline (by blocking transport in presynaptic sympathetic neurons), thus preventing sinusoidal contraction and the efflux of penile blood.

- A 44-year-old black man developed priapism 2 hours after having overdosed on 30–40 trazodone tablets 50 mg and 10 Tylenol No. 3 (paracetamol plus codeine) tablets (162). Toxicology analysis was positive for cocaine and opiates. The priapism required detumescence twice, on initial presentation and then 6 hours later, and 8 hours after presentation he again developed painless priapism, which resolved spontaneously after 1.5 hours.

Trazodone-induced priapism may be mediated by alpha-adrenoceptor antagonism. While the mechanism for cocaine-induced priapism is unclear, it may result from vasospasm, venous pooling, and sludging of blood in the penis. The authors proposed that the two drugs may act in an additive or synergistic manner, posing a greater hazard than either alone.

Priapism associated with intracavernosal injection of cocaine has also been reported.

- A 43-year-old man developed persistent painful erection after intracavernosal injection of cocaine (163). He had previously administered cocaine in this way to prolong erections. Cavernosal aspiration resulted in partial detumescence, but the condition recurred. Urine screen was positive for cocaine. Aspiration and irrigation fully alleviated the condition.

During penile erection, nitric oxide is released from the endothelium of the cavernous spaces and from nerve endings (non-adrenergic and non-cholinergic). Nitric oxide stimulates guanylate cyclase, which is involved in the conversion of guanosine triphosphate to cyclic guanosine monophosphate (cGMP); the latter relaxes the smooth muscle in the corpora cavernosa, allowing influx of blood for erection. The authors suggested that cocaine directly applied to the cavernosal endothelium can cause nitric oxide production.

Immunologic

The prevalence of infection with the human immunodeficiency virus (HIV) among drug abusers, including cocaine users, is increasing (164). Two separate reports have suggested that cocaine may compromise immunological function. In one study, human mononuclear cells were stimulated in vitro with mitogens in the presence and absence of cocaine; cocaine inhibited the proliferation of the mononuclear cells (165). In a second study, cocaine amplified HIV-1 replication in co-cultures containing cytomegalovirus-activated peripheral blood mononuclear cells (166).

Two cases of connective tissue disease have been reported (167).

A case of urticarial vasculitis, a type III hypersensitivity reaction, has been reported after cocaine use (168).

- A 24-year-old man with acute malaise and fever had a pruritic rash with multiple erythematous circumscribed weals on the trunk, arms, legs, neck, and scalp. He admitted to using intranasal cocaine 6 months, 4 days, and 1 day before the onset of the symptoms. His temperature was 39°C. His erythrocyte sedimentation rate was 80 mm in the first hour, C-reactive protein was 283 mg/l (reference range below 10), and the white blood cell count was 12.4×10^9/l with 89% neutrophils. A biopsy of an urticarial lesion showed a perivascular inflammatory infiltrate in the upper and middle dermis. Bed rest, oral prednisone, oral hydroxyzine, and topical polidocanol led to improvement within 24 hours.

Two cases of cocaine-induced type I hypersensitivity reactions, have been reported (169).

- A 23-year-old woman developed tongue swelling and difficulty in breathing immediately after having sniffed cocaine. The anterior half of her tongue was edematous with bleeding lesions caused by her fingernails. There were cocaine metabolites in the urine. The diagnosis was angioedema of the tongue induced by cocaine or its contaminants, and it resolved with subcutaneous adrenaline, H_1 receptor antihistamines, and intravenous glucocorticoids.
- A 19-year-old man developed generalized urticaria, intense pruritus, and mild bronchospasm 30 minutes after injecting cocaine for the third time. He had weals on the face, neck, arms, and chest, and scattered wheezing in the lungs. Urine toxicology screen was positive for cocaine metabolites. His symptoms resolved several hours after the administration of H_1 receptor antihistamines and intravenous glucocorticoids.

Body temperature

Cocaine can cause hyperthermia, primarily in hot weather, perhaps through a hypermetabolic state; impaired heat dissipation may be another contributing factor. Seven healthy, cocaine-naïve subjects participated in tests of progressive passive heat stress, during which each received intranasal cocaine or lidocaine as placebo (170). Esophageal temperature, skin blood flow, sweat rate, and perceived thermal sensation were measured. Cocaine augmented the temperature increase during heat stress and also increased the temperature threshold for the onset of both cutaneous vasodilatation and sweating. It also impaired the perception of heat. This study elicited commentary, in which it was pointed out that measured effects of small doses of cocaine may not be reflective of true cocaine poisoning (171). Also, the subjects in the study did not have psychomotor agitation, which is often prominent in cocaine toxicity and which improves with sedatives.

Death

Poisoning can occur with doses of cocaine as low as 20 mg (10 drops of cocaine 4%). Victims generally collapse and die after associated cardiovascular abnormalities, dysrhythmias, and respiratory failure. Signs and symptoms of intoxication include excitement, restlessness, headache, nausea, vomiting, abdominal pain, convulsions, and delirium.

In a retrospective study of 48 men who suffered cocaine-related deaths and a control group of 51 male cocaine users who died of trauma, the blood cocaine concentrations measured in the two groups were similar (172). However, concentrations of the cocaine metabolite benzoylecgonine were higher in those with cocaine-related deaths. This group also had a significantly lower body mass index, with larger hearts and heavier lungs, livers, and spleens than the control subjects. Reduced body weight, an adverse effect of long-term cocaine use, is probably related to its effects on the serotonergic system and therefore appetite. Cardiomegaly is thought to result from chronic cocaine-induced excessive catecholamine stimulation, with circulatory overload, and increased organ weight is a result of passive visceral congestion in cocaine-induced heart failure. Cardiac alterations may explain why similar blood cocaine concentrations can be lethal in some cases but benign in others. This study shows that isolated measurements of postmortem cocaine and benzoylecgonine blood concentrations cannot be used to assess or predict cocaine toxicity.

The increasing prevalence of multisubstance abuse can influence morbidity and mortality (173).

- An 18-year-old man experienced sudden and severe chest pain while drinking alcohol. He vomited, collapsed, and died. On postmortem examination, thrombosis of the left coronary artery, dilated cardiomyopathy with congestive heart failure, and pulmonary embolism were noted. Blood analysis showed raised cocaine and marijuana concentrations and a trace of alcohol.

The author's opinion was that although multidrug use had played a part, the high blood concentration of cocaine had been the main cause of death. He also noted that marijuana can interact with cocaine to produce pronounced sympathomimetic effects.

The smuggling of illicit drugs by the technique called "body packing" carries medical risks. Drug packages can rupture and digestive secretions can seep into packets and allow drug absorption. Consequently, drug intoxication, intestinal obstruction, peritonitis, and death can occur. A man carrying 99 cocaine powder packages weighing 10 g died as a result (174), and the death of a drug dealer has been reported (175).

- A 17-year-old man swallowed a small plastic bag of cocaine in order to avoid arrest. After 1 hour he complained of a headache and 30 minutes later developed palpitation and agitation and collapsed. Histological examination of his heart showed myocardial necrosis. The blood concentration of cocaine was high at 98 μg/ml. The tissue concentrations of cocaine and its metabolites in various organs and fluids were recorded; the highest concentrations of cocaine and metabolites were detected in the liver, lungs, brain, and blood (in descending order).

The cause of sudden death in this case was probably a cardiac dysrhythmia.

Long-Term Effects

Drug tolerance

Chronic cocaine exposure and long-term adaptation at the molecular level have been investigated; changes in transcription factor gene expression may be involved (176). NURR1 is a key factor that regulates transcription of the gene that encodes the cocaine-sensitive dopamine transporter and functions in the development of dopamine neurons. In a recent study, postmortem human midbrain specimens from cocaine users and controls underwent various analyses. Human NURR1 gene expression was markedly reduced in dopamine neurons in the cocaine users and normal in the controls. NURR1-deficient cocaine abusers also had dopamine neurons with markedly reduced dopamine transporter gene expression. NURR1 appears to have a critical role in the brain's adaptation to repeated cocaine exposure and in maintenance of dopamine neurons.

Drug dependence

There has been considerable interest in evaluating drugs such as amfepramone (diethylpropion) for attenuating the negative emotional state induced by craving for cocaine, in the hope of finding a drug for long-term treatment of cocaine dependence. However, in 50 cocaine-dependent patients amfepramone was ineffective and caused significant adverse effects (177). Of the patients who took amfepramone 25–75 mg/day, 12% were withdrawn from the study: one developed coronary vasospasm and another atrial fibrillation. These poor results are comparable to those of earlier studies with methylphenidate in cocaine addicts (178,179).

Drug withdrawal

There have been reports of the effects of cocaine withdrawal on cognition. There was impairment of memory, visuospatial abilities, and concentration in 16 cocaine abusers during the first 2 weeks of abstinence (55). Measured deficits were independent of withdrawal-related depression.

Tumorigenicity

Chronic cocaine use, which is associated with immunosuppression, may be carcinogenic. The possible association between chronic cocaine exposure and pancreatic adenocarcinoma has been investigated (180,181). A study of hospital records in Brazil for the years 1986–1998 showed that of 198 patients with pancreatic adenocarcinoma, 13 (6.5%) were younger than 40 years; of these, five had a history of chronic cocaine inhalation and one had abused marijuana.

Second-Generation Effects

Pregnancy

Some of the risks run by the pregnant cocaine-using mother and her child (such as preterm labor and premature delivery) have been reported (182). However, the literature on maternal cocaine use and its possible outcomes is problematic, because many studies have been methodologically flawed (183).

A retrospective study of data from a large perinatal registry showed that there was an increased risk of placenta previa among women who used cocaine, compared with those who did not use drugs or alcohol (184).

Another apparent obstetric risk of cocaine use is rupture of a uterine scar (from a previous cesarean section).

- There was extensive laceration of the maternal urinary bladder after a vaginal birth in a 34-year-old woman whose urine tested positive for cocaine (185).

The authors postulated that the injury may have resulted from a cocaine-augmented contractile response of the pregnant uterus.

A "pre-eclampsia–like" syndrome has been described, characterized by acute hypertension and a low platelet count, in a 33-year-old cocaine user; her 20-week-old fetus died (186).

One of the serious medical conditions linked with cocaine use during pregnancy is premature delivery, with an incidence in cocaine users of 17–27%. The mechanism of the effect of cocaine on both spontaneous and agonist-induced contractility of pregnant human myometrium has been evaluated (187). Myometrium samples from 42 women who were undergoing cesarean section at term were examined after exposure to various pharmacological probes in combination with cocaine. The results suggested that cocaine augments the contractility of uterine tissue by both adrenergic and non-adrenergic mechanisms. Cocaine increased spontaneous myometrial contractility over three-fold. Prazosin, an alpha-adrenoceptor antagonist, blocked this effect, but only for the first 35 minutes. Cocaine increased both the sensitivity and maximal tissue response to the alpha-adrenoceptor agonist methoxamine. The maximal response to oxytocin, but not sensitivity, was increased by cocaine; prazosin did not inhibit this effect.

Cocaine has been associated with both preterm delivery and premature rupture of the membranes (188). Among 85 of 604 expectant mothers with premature rupture of the membranes with documented cocaine exposure compared with women with no drug exposure for six conditions of major neonatal morbidity, cocaine users were older and of higher parity. The non-cocaine users had more morbidity, in particular neonatal infection and sepsis. The authors proposed that the mechanism of premature rupture of the membranes in the presence of cocaine may not be related to infection. Instead, cocaine may have a direct effect on the myometrium, stimulating uterine contractility.

The Maternal Lifestyle Study has reported that the prevalence of adverse perinatal complications associated with the use of cocaine or opiates during pregnancy was lower than has been previously reported (189). In 11 811 mother–infant pairs followed prospectively, 11% of the exposed and non-exposed groups were hospitalized at least once. However, violence was a factor (20%) in admissions among the cocaine-exposed women.

Teratogenicity

The data suggest that cocaine-exposed infants may be at increased risk of congenital malformations (190). However, it is unclear by what mechanism cocaine affects the fetus. Interruption of the intrauterine blood supply, with subsequent destruction of fetal structures, may account for some of its effects (191).

There are frequent reports of intrauterine growth retardation, neurobehavioral abnormalities, cerebral injury, and cardiac anomalies in "coke babies" (SEDA-14, 15) (SEDA-21, 4) (SEDA-21, 129) (192,193). Brain hemorrhages (194) and asymmetrical growth retardation (195) associated with maternal cocaine abuse have been discussed.

In 500 neonates ankyloglossia, a defect in the attachment of the tongue within the mouth, was 3.5 times more common in cocaine-exposed neonates than in others (196). Other facial, vertebral, and cardiovascular defects have been described (SEDA-17, 4) (19).

Two other clinical syndromes involving anomalies of multiple organ systems in fetuses of cocaine-abusing women have been described.

- An infant with Pena–Shokeir phenotype (including facial, musculoskeletal, pulmonary, and cardiac malformations accompanied by extensive brain damage) was born to a cocaine-abusing mother (197). The infant died shortly after birth.
- An infant exposed to cocaine in utero had a combination of facial, ear, eye, and vertebral anomalies, accompanied by cardiac, central nervous system, and other malformations (198).

In contrast, in 34 light-to-moderate cocaine users compared with 600 non-users attending a public prenatal care clinic, pronounced untoward effects on the fetus were reportedly less common than in other studies (199). In all cases the cocaine had been taken intranasally, and the majority of users reduced their intake during pregnancy; none had been referred for drug abuse counseling and none was taking drug treatment. There was no significant difference in obstetric complications among these mild cocaine users compared with non-users, and no significant differences in infant growth, morphology, or behavior. However, the cocaine users had histories of more fetal losses and during pregnancy they suffered more infectious diseases, such as hepatitis, *Herpes simplex*, and gonorrhea.

Fetal growth

Among the adverse outcomes of prenatal cocaine exposure, low birth weight and reduced length and head circumference have been reported. In a prospective study in New York City, 386 pairs of cocaine- and crack-using mothers and their infants and 130 matched control pairs were followed during the course of pregnancy and delivery (200). The neonates were assessed by physical and neurological examination, the Brazelton Neonatal Behavioral Assessment Scale (BNBAS), and the Neonatal Stress Scale during the first 48 hours of life. The results corroborated earlier findings of reduced fetal growth in cocaine-exposed infants. Significantly more (17%) of the babies of cocaine users had a head circumference less than the tenth percentile compared with the controls (3%). They performed less well on the BNBA Scale and had higher measures on the Neonatal Stress Scale. They had clinically significant neurological impairment, with jitteriness, increased tone, and an exaggerated Moro reflex. However, some of these findings may have reflected a direct neurotoxic effect of cocaine, since testing was done during the first 48 hours of life. The authors observed that crack had a more adverse outcome than cocaine. They concluded that the most important predictor of neonatal outcome may be the frequency, quantity, and type of cocaine used.

The effect of maternal cocaine use on infant outcome has been prospectively assessed in 224 women, of whom 105 were cocaine users and 119 were controls (201). The infants were of gestational age 34 weeks or more and were not asphyxiated. The infants exposed to cocaine were more likely to be admitted to the newborn intensive care unit, to be treated for congenital syphilis or presumed sepsis, to have a greater length of stay, to have lower birth weight and head circumference, and to be discharged to the care of someone other than the mother. However, the two groups were similar in the incidence of abnormal cranial and renal ultrasonography and abnormal pneumocardiography. Moreover, when controlled for cigarette use and other confounders, there were no significant differences in the groups on growth retardation factors.

Cardiovascular

Intrauterine cocaine exposure is associated with neonatal cardiovascular dysfunction and malformations. The long-term effects of cocaine on the neonate's cardiovascular system and development are unknown. The effect of cocaine on the infant's autonomic function and subsequent development has been reported (202). Heart rate variability, a non-invasive test of autonomic function, was evaluated in 77 prenatally cocaine-exposed infants, 77 healthy controls, and 89 infants who had been exposed prenatally to drugs other than cocaine (alcohol, marijuana, and/or nicotine). Within the first 72 hours of life, the cocaine-exposed infants were asymptomatic but had lower heart rate variability and lower vagal tone than the two comparison groups. At follow-up, the cocaine-exposed infants had recovered at 2–6 months of age and now had higher heart rate variability and vagal tone than the two non-exposed groups. Most of the increase in heart rate variability and vagal tone was seen in the infants who had had light cocaine exposure and was not apparent in those who had had heavy exposure.

The same researchers have published two reports on the cardiovascular effects of intrauterine cocaine. In the first study, 82 healthy neonates with intrauterine cocaine exposure, 108 exposed to drugs other than cocaine, and 87 healthy controls were evaluated for global and segmental systolic and diastolic cardiac function (203). During the first 48 hours of life, the neonates with intrauterine cocaine exposure had significant left ventricular diastolic segmental abnormalities. They had a higher index of asynchrony and global and segmental fractional area changes in contrast to the other two groups. The degree of abnormality in the index of asynchrony was greater in the neonates with heavier cocaine exposure. In a second study at 2–6 months of age, 56 cocaine-exposed infants were compared with 72 who had been exposed to drugs other than cocaine and 60 healthy controls (204). The cocaine-exposed infants had recovered left ventricular diastolic function. Only in infants with heavy cocaine exposure was there an alteration in septal wall diastolic filling.

- A 6-month-old fetus who had been exposed to cocaine had a single-ventricle heart; the authors suggested that coronary spasm, resulting in infarction, may have destroyed the right ventricle (205).

Nervous system

In two reports it was suggested that brain hemorrhage (194) and asymmetrical growth retardation (195,206) can occur.

Cognitive effects

The influence of exposure to cocaine in utero on the developing human nervous system is not yet clearly understood (SEDA-22, 21). Prenatal cocaine exposure has been associated with neurobehavioral effects in infancy, ranging from no effect to effects on arousal and state regulation, as well as on neurophysiological and neurological functions. A prospective controlled study in 154 cocaine-using pregnant mothers and suitable matched controls from a rural community produced neurobehavioral effects that supported those from previous controlled studies (207). The mothers underwent drug testing and medical examination during each trimester. Their infants were assessed as near to 40 weeks after conception as possible, using the BNBA Scale. When controlled for the effects of marijuana, alcohol, and tobacco use, the use of cocaine in the third trimester was negatively related to state regulation, attention, and responsiveness among the exposed infants. Twice as many cocaine-exposed infants as controls failed to come to and maintain the quiet alert state required for orientation testing.

It is unclear whether abnormalities in early infancy are associated with neurodevelopmental impairment at a later age. Several studies have suggested that the findings are limited to early childhood. The possible effects of prenatal cocaine exposure on later cognitive functioning and difficulties have been reported in three studies. In the first, 236 infants at 8 and 18 months of age were evaluated; 37 had heavy exposure to cocaine in utero, 30 had light exposure, and 169 had no exposure (208). Cognitive functioning was assessed with the Bayley Scales of Infant Development. Information processing was tested with an infant-controlled habituation procedure. At 8 months, cocaine-exposed infants and controls had no differences in cognitive functioning. Their abilities to process information indexed by habituation and response to novelty were comparable. However, at 18 months the infants with high cocaine exposure performed poorly on the Mental Development Index (MDI). The 18-month index covers a wider range of cognitive tasks requiring integrated learning, responsiveness to environmental cues, and memory than the 8-month index. These results suggest that the effects of cocaine are more likely to show up when more challenging measures are used. Infants raised in high-risk environments, with stressors and low support, scored lower at both 8 and 18 months.

In a second study, intellectual functioning at 6–9 years was measured in 88 cocaine-exposed children and 96 unexposed children in New York City (209). The participants were interviewed and underwent medical and neurological examination and psychological assessment. Child intelligence was measured with the Wechsler Intelligence Scale for Children-III (WISC-III). Intelligence quotient scores did not differ between the two groups of children, even when adjustments for co-variables were made.

In a third study the Robert Wood Johnson database of published literature on prenatal cocaine exposure and child outcome was examined (210). Only 8 of 101 studies focused on school-age children. Intelligence quotient (IQ), receptive language, and expressive language were measured. This meta-analysis showed an average difference of 3.12 IQ points between cocaine-exposed and control groups. When the IQ distribution is shifted downwards by this amount, there is a 1.6-fold increase in the number of children with IQs under 70. The authors noted that the calculated decrement in IQ in exposed children is subtle and does not include the possible effect of the drug on domains of function such as language abilities.

Research on the relation between prenatal cocaine exposure and childhood behavior also continues. In a pilot study, 27 children exposed to cocaine in utero and 75 control children were assessed (211). The children had a mean age of 80 months and most were first-grade students. The child's first-grade teacher (blinded to exposure status and study design) rated the children's behavior with the Conners' Teacher Rating Scale (CTRS) and the Problem Behavior Scale (PROBS 14), an investigator-developed scale that measures behaviors associated with cocaine exposure. The drug-exposed children had higher CTRS scores (that is more problematic behavior), but the difference was not significant. On subscales of the PROBS 14, the drug-exposed group had significantly more problematic behavior. These results appear to substantiate teachers' reports of problematic behavior in children with prenatal cocaine exposure.

The effects of prenatal cocaine exposure on information processing and developmental assessment have been studied in 108 infants aged 3 months, 61 of whom had been exposed to cocaine, and 47 controls using an infant-control habituation and novelty responsiveness procedure in a developmental assessment using the Bayley Scales of Infant Development (212). Infants exposed to cocaine prenatally were significantly more likely than controls to fail to start the habituation procedure, and those who did were significantly more likely than controls to react with irritability early in the procedure. Cocaine-exposed infants had a comparatively depressed performance on the motor but not the mental Bayley scales. This information was obtained by raters blind to the history and was controlled for both perinatal and sociodemographic factors. Most of the infants in both groups reached the habituation criteria, and among those who did there were no significant differences between cocaine-exposed and non-exposed infants in habituation or in recovery to a novel stimulus. Thus, differences in reactivity to novelty, but not information processing, between cocaine-exposed and non-cocaine-exposed infants suggested that the effects of prenatal cocaine exposure may be on arousal and attention regulation, rather than on early cognitive processes.

Developmental correlates have been assessed in three groups of children aged 4–6 years (213). In 18 children there had been prenatal exposure to cocaine and the mothers had continued to use crack. Another 28 children had had no prenatal exposure but their mothers had used crack after the children were born. The control group were 28 children whose mothers had never used cocaine. Prenatally exposed children performed significantly worse than the others in tests of receptive language and visual motor drawing. Prenatal crack exposure was associated with poor visual motor performance, even after controlling for intrauterine alcohol and marijuana exposure, age, birth weight, and duration of maternal crack use.

There have been two studies of the neurodevelopmental effects of cocaine during the first 48 hours of life. In the first, 23 cocaine-exposed and 29 non-exposed infants were prospectively assessed within the first 48 hours of life; infant meconium was used to detect cocaine and the BNBA Scale was used for clinical assessment (214). One-third of the cocaine-exposed neonates were born to women who denied cocaine use. In six of the seven clusters assessed, cocaine-exposed infants fared badly compared with control infants. The cocaine-exposed infants had poor autonomic stability and there was a dose–response relation between meconium cocaine concentration and poor performance in relation to orientation and so-called "regulation of state," which refers to how the infant responds when aroused. The authors concluded that cocaine exposure is independently related to poor behavioral performance in areas that are central to optimal infant development. They emphasized the value of the identification and quantification of cocaine in infants.

In another blinded study, neurodevelopmental and neurobehavioral performance were prospectively assessed in 131 neonates (mean age 43 hours) exposed in utero to cocaine, with or without other drugs (215). Cocaine-exposed neonates were developmentally at risk in the tests compared with infants exposed to other drugs alone or in combination. As in the previous study, larger amounts of cocaine were associated with higher neurobehavioral risk scores.

In a study of immediate and late dose–response effects of cocaine exposure in utero on neurobehavioral performance, 251 full-term urban neonates were examined by blinded raters at 2 and 17 days (216). The babies were classified as having been heavily exposed, lightly exposed, or not exposed to cocaine. After controlling for covariates, in contrast to the studies mentioned above (211,215), there were no neurobehavioral effects of exposure at 2 days of age. However, at 17 days there was a significant dose-related effect: heavily exposed infants had poorer state regulation and greater excitability, implying impairment of their ability to modulate arousal. The authors postulated that these late effects might be expected if cocaine exposure in utero is associated with evolving neuroanatomical damage or disruption of the monoaminergic neurotransmitter systems. These effects did not appear to be related to intrauterine growth retardation, as has been suggested by others.

Arousal and attention have been investigated in 180 healthy nursery infants before hospital discharge and at 1 month of age (217). Cocaine-exposed infants showed a lack of arousal-modulated attention and preferred faster frequencies of stimulation, regardless of arousal condition compared with non-exposed infants. There were similar differences 1 month after birth, showing that these effects persisted beyond the period of presence of cocaine or its metabolites at birth. These effects were independent of absence of prenatal care, alcohol use, minority status, or sex, suggesting a direct and even chronic effect of intrauterine cocaine exposure on arousal-modulated attention and presumably on the developing nervous system of the infants.

The behavioral and hormonal responses in 30 preterm cocaine-exposed infants were compared with the responses in 30 non-cocaine-exposed infants of similar gestational age (218). The mothers of cocaine-exposed infants were more often single, had higher parity and more obstetric complications, and were less likely to visit, touch, hold, and feed their infants than the other mothers. Cocaine-exposed infants had smaller head circumferences at birth, spent more time in the neonatal intensive care unit, and had a greater incidence of periventricular or intraventricular hemorrhages. They also had poorer state regulation and difficulty in maintaining alert states and in regulating their own behavior. They spent more time in indeterminate sleep (suggesting nervous system immaturity), with reduced periods of quiet sleep and increased amounts of agitation, tremulousness, mouthing, multiple limb movements, and clenched fists. There were higher urinary noradrenaline, dopamine, and cortisol concentrations and lower plasma insulin concentrations in the cocaine-exposed infants, suggesting that they may have experienced a high degree of stress in the perinatal period.

In a study of 464 inner-city black infants, whose mothers were recruited prenatally based on alcohol and cocaine use during pregnancy, gestational age of less than 38 weeks was significantly correlated with cocaine use in the mothers (219). The infants were tested at 6.5, 12, and 13 months of age; the cocaine-exposed infants were more excitable, preferred faster frequencies of stimulation, had more difficulty habituating, were more reactive, and showed a greater startle response to noise. Moreover, these effects of cocaine on cognitive function were documented beyond the neonatal period, thus eliminating effects from acute cocaine exposure or withdrawal. The authors suggested that two separate mechanisms may underlie the effects of cocaine on gestational age and cognition. The nervous system deficits, poorer cognitive performance, and faster reactivity are probably mediated by a direct action of cocaine (requiring heavy exposure) on neurotransmitters, whereas shortened gestation may be mediated by vasoconstriction, which occurs at lower exposure. Timing of exposure during pregnancy may also play a critical role in determining the type of deficits.

The effects of prenatal maternal cocaine use on neurobehavior have been reported in 2-week old infants (220). The BNBA Scale was administered to the infants of mothers who had a reported high frequency of cocaine use during pregnancy: ($n = 23$, >75th percentile reported days of use) or a low frequency ($n = 32$, <75th percentile).

Infants with high intrauterine exposure had higher scores on the BNBAS excitability cluster than infants with low exposure. Infants with a high BNBAS excitability score had poorer tone and motor movement, were more irritable and hard to console, and had difficulties in self-quieting.

In a meta-analysis of 18 published reports (1985–1988, 13 of which failed to meet the inclusion criteria and were excluded) on the effect of in utero exposure to cocaine on infant neurobehavioral outcome, cocaine-exposed infants were compared to non-exposed infants on BNBAS cluster scales at birth and at 3–4 weeks of age (221). Although the sample size was large enough to detect statistical significance in most of the tests of difference between the two groups, the magnitude of all the effects was small. This was true for differences in the motor performance and abnormal reflex clusters in the infant groups (with a slight trend toward increasing standard differences over time) and in the orientation and autonomic regular clusters (with a trend toward a reduced effect size over time). However, the main finding of the study was the small magnitude of the neurobehavior dysfunction at both times. The authors cautioned that these data may not be generalizable, since polydrug exposure, the amount of cocaine exposure, and other variables could have confounded the data.

In 158 cocaine-exposed (82 heavily and 76 lightly exposed) and 161 non-cocaine exposed infants, neurobehavioral function was assessed at 43 weeks after conception (222). Mediating factors (the timing and amount of drug exposure) and maternal psychological distress as a confounding factor were considered in the design and statistical analysis. The infants with heavy cocaine exposure had significantly more jitteriness and attentional difficulties. They were also more likely to be identified with an abnormality and less likely to cooperate with testing procedures than infants in the other groups. Higher concentrations of cocaine metabolites, cocaethylene and benzoylecgonine, were associated with a higher incidence of movement and tone abnormalities, jitteriness, and the presence of any abnormality. Higher cocaethylene concentrations were associated with attentional abnormalities; higher concentrations of metahydroxybenzoylecgonine were associated with jitteriness.

Cognitive, motor, and behavior development, as measured by the Mullen Scales of Early Learning and the Bayley Scales of Infant Development-II, were compared in 56 prenatally cocaine-exposed infants and toddlers (aged 1–3 years) and 56 non-exposed matched controls (223). There were developmental problems in expressive and receptive language areas in those who had been exposed prenatally.

The effect of intrauterine cocaine exposure on visual attention, cognition, and behavior has been investigated in 14 cocaine-exposed children and 20 controls aged 14–60 months (224). The cocaine-exposed children were slower in tests of disengagement and sustained attention. They also had greater difficulties in behavioral regulation.

Research on the effects of prenatal cocaine exposure on development in the first 2 years of life has been reported in 203 full-term infants (225). The infants, who were defined as having had no cocaine exposure, light exposure, or heavy exposure, were tested with the Bayley Scales of Infant Development at 6, 12, and 24 months. Assays of neonatal meconium for cocaine metabolites along with mothers' self-reports were used to evaluate the dose–response relation. There were no significant adverse effects due to cocaine exposure on scores in the major tests up to 24 months of age. Cocaine-exposed infants with the lowest 10th percentile birth weight and those placed with kinship caregivers had less optimal development. Cocaine-exposed infants who participated in child-focused early intervention programs scored higher than the others.

The behavioral effects of prenatal cocaine exposure at age 5 years have been studied in 140 children exposed to cocaine, 61 exposed to alcohol, tobacco, and/or marijuana, and 120 not exposed to any drugs (226). They were evaluated with the Achenbach Child Behavior Checklist. There was no association between behavior and intrauterine cocaine exposure. However, the current behavioral health of the mother, including recent drug use and psychological functioning, did affect the child's internalizing and externalizing behavior.

Gastrointestinal

Cocaine exposure in utero can affect various fetal organs. Gastrointestinal disorders, including ten cases of necrotizing enterocolitis (227), one of intestinal atresia, and one of spontaneous colonic perforation, have been reported (228).

Reproductive system

An increased incidence of genital malformations has often been noted (229).

Fetotoxicity

The prevalence rate of cocaine use during pregnancy is 10–45% in some centers in North America. As cocaine use is increasing and widespread, information on the possible adverse effects secondary to fetal cocaine exposure continues to amass in case reports and studies.

However, in a prospective, large-scale, longitudinal study there was no association between prenatal cocaine exposure and congenital anomalies in 272 offspring of 154 cocaine-using mothers and 154 non-using matched controls (230). The cocaine-exposed group had significantly more premature infants, who were significantly smaller in birth weight, length, and head circumference than the control infants. However, there were no differences in the type or number of abnormalities.

The impact of prenatal exposure to cocaine on fetal growth and fetal head circumference has been studied in 476 African-American neonates, including 253 full-term infants prenatally exposed to cocaine (with or without alcohol, tobacco, or marijuana) and 223 non-cocaine exposed infants (147 drug-free, 76 exposed to alcohol, tobacco, or marijuana) (231). The cocaine-associated deficit in fetal growth was 0.63 standard deviations and for gestational age 0.33 standard deviations. There were also cocaine-associated deficits in birth weight and length, but no evidence of a disproportionate effect on head circumference.

The relation between prenatal cocaine exposure and early childhood outcome has been reviewed (232). Prospective longitudinal studies of perinatal cocaine exposure and associated outcomes were studied in a survey of 36 of 74 reports, published from 1984 to October 2000, in which the examiners were blinded to cocaine exposure. Prenatal cocaine exposure did not alter physical growth, developmental test scores, or receptive and expressive language among children aged 6 years or less. The authors concluded that there is no convincing evidence that prenatal cocaine exposure is associated with effects on a child's physical or behavioral development, and that many findings once thought to be specific effects of in utero cocaine exposure instead correlated with factors such as the quality of the child's environment and prenatal exposure to tobacco, marijuana, or alcohol.

This review generated responses from other authorities in the field. Some commented that the conclusions may be premature, given the age of the subjects, and drew attention to several studies that have shown subtle but consistent deficits in cognitive and attentional processes in 6- and 7-year-old children (233). These effects may become more prominent as development continues and may persist into adulthood. Others criticized the attempt to isolate cocaine exposure from all other associated risk factors; from a public health perspective, prenatal cocaine exposure clusters with other risk factors, such as poor caregiving, child maltreatment, domestic violence, and prenatal exposure to other substances (234). Furthermore, the selection criteria narrowed the total articles reviewed to under half of the 74 articles found. Others suggested that the study had been misinterpreted (235).

The effects of prenatal cocaine exposure have been assessed prospectively in 217 infants, 95 (44%) of whom had benzoylecgonine, a cocaine metabolite, in their meconium (214). Among these infants, benzoylecgonine concentration was inversely related to fetal growth (birth weight, length, and head circumference), whereas maternal self-report of days of cocaine use did not correlate with either fetal growth or meconium benzoylecgonine concentration. The report suggested a dose–response relation between the magnitude of prenatal cocaine exposure and impaired fetal growth.

In 39 cocaine-exposed infants and 39 control infants aged 35 weeks or older, head size was smaller and birth weight tended to be lower in the cocaine-exposed infants (236). Moreover, the head circumference of the cocaine-exposed infants was significantly smaller at any given birth weight than in the control infants. The behavioral scores were significantly higher (on days 1 and 2) in the cocaine-exposed infants; the higher scores were most frequently attributed to increased jitteriness, a hyperactive Moro response, and excessive sucking. Lastly, cocaine-exposed infants had an increase in flow velocity in the anterior cerebral arteries between days 1 and 2; however, there was no increased propensity to ischemic and/or hemorrhagic cerebral injury in the infants exposed to cocaine. The blood flow changes on the second day may have reflected falling infant cocaine concentrations after birth.

In a longitudinal evaluation of 28 infants exposed to cocaine in utero and 22 unexposed controls for 15 months, the cocaine-exposed infants weighed significantly less at birth than the control infants, but not subsequently (237). Compared with controls, motor development was compromised in the cocaine-exposed infants at 4 and 7 months, but not at 1 and 15 months, suggesting that compromised motor performance in the exposed group normalized for later milestones, probably through a self-righting process. A disturbing aspect of this study was the extremely poor performance in all-motor assessments at every age by every infant (including the controls). The investigators postulated that in an inner-city population (such as that studied here), once an infant accumulates three or more risk points (as most infants in the study did), additional risk factors (including exposure to cocaine) have little further negative impact on their development.

The complex interplay between the relative effects of prenatal cocaine exposure and the perinatal and environmental factors on development has been evaluated, using a structural model to describe the direct and indirect effects of prenatal drug exposure on developmental outcome from birth to age 6 months (238). Key variables included prenatal drug exposure, perinatal medical characteristics, maternal/caregiver/family characteristics, the home environment, and neurobehavioral outcomes. The study was based on 154 predominantly crack-using women and 154 control subjects matched for pregnancy risk, parity, race, and socioeconomic status. Prior exclusion criteria included age under 18 years, a major illness diagnosed before pregnancy, chronic use of legal drugs, and any use of illicit drugs other than cocaine and marijuana. Urine specimens were collected at two unanticipated times and positive serum samples were confirmed by gas chromatography/mass spectroscopy. Measures analysed by blinded evaluators included medical assessment at birth and developmental assessments at birth, 1 month, and 6 months, as well as caregiver characteristics and environmental factors at birth and 1 month.

Exposure to cocaine affected development at birth. Increasing exposure was significantly related to poor developmental outcomes, as measured by the Brazelton qualifier scores. Although no direct effects of cocaine were found at either 1 month or 6 months analysed separately, time-dependent analysis showed an effect on development at 6 months. The indirect effects of cocaine exposure were mediated through maternal psychosocial well-being at delivery and birth head circumference. In addition, indirect effects of prenatal cocaine exposure were also related to concomitant alcohol and tobacco use and the birth head circumference. Neither maternal nor caregiver factors at 1 month was directly related to developmental outcome at any time. These findings support previous findings (239–241) that suggest that cocaine is a mild teratogen with regard to neurodevelopmental outcome.

The presence of cocaine during the prenatal period disrupts the development of neural systems involved in mediating visual attention. Of 14 cocaine-exposed children and 20 control children aged 14–60 months, whose visual attention, cognition, and behavior were assessed, the cocaine-exposed children had slower reaction times, supporting the hypothesis that impairment in disengagement and sustained attention are associated with prenatal cocaine exposure (242). There was a trend to slower reaction times to targets presented in the right visual field, but not the left visual field. Cocaine-exposed children also had greater difficulties in behavioral regulation, especially related to an ability to cope with heightened levels of positive and negative emotions (243).

An association between prenatal cocaine exposure and deficits in total language functioning was found in 236 cocaine-exposed and 207 non-cocaine exposed full-term children (244). The link between prenatal cocaine exposure and language deficits during early childhood was not related to cocaine-associated deficits in birth weight, length, or head circumference. Three different but potentially interacting mechanisms whereby maternal cocaine use might affect early language development have been proposed (245):

- subtle dysregulation of attentional systems, with potential for disrupting an infant's ability to extract and process available linguistic information;
- disruptions in parent–child linguistic interactions due to cocaine and other drug use;
- impoverished, unstable, and endangering social and care-giving environments.

Early detection of language deficits allowed ameliorative intervention aimed at improving academic performance and social adaptation in preschool and school-aged children.

Cardiovascular

In a retrospective review of all dysrhythmias in children with prenatal cocaine exposure, 18 cases were detected in 554 infants who had positive urine screens for cocaine (246). In 13 neonates the dysrhythmia occurred beyond the period of direct cocaine exposure and six of the children had dysrhythmias after the neonatal period. Most of the dysrhythmias were supraventricular extra beats. Overall, the rate of consultations for dysrhythmias was higher among cocaine-exposed neonates than expected. Some cocaine-exposed children had symptomatic dysrhythmias that were persistent or recurrent and required treatment to maintain cardiac output and restore normal cardiac rhythm. Children who were exposed prenatally to cocaine appeared to be at increased risk of abnormal responses to stress, manifested by symptomatic dysrhythmias beyond the period of cocaine exposure.

- A child presented at 12 months of age with status epilepticus, sustained ventricular tachycardia, and a positive urine screen for cocaine. At 22 months he returned with a cardiac arrest, a history of a fall, a head injury, and a positive test for cocaine in the urine. He died soon after.

There has been a recent report of a myocardial infarct in a full-term infant born to a 28-year-old woman who had used cocaine 2–3 times per week and methadone 40 mg/day (247).

Respiratory

Respiratory rates in the 3-week-old babies of mothers who had used cocaine during pregnancy were higher than expected; in addition newborn babies who had been exposed prenatally to both cocaine and narcotic analgesics had abnormal control of breathing (following hypercapnia challenge) during the first few months of life (248). The preliminary results of another study are also of some interest; this prospective study of maternal drug abuse showed a reduced incidence of respiratory distress syndrome among premature infants prenatally exposed to cocaine (249). The authors noted that while this finding needs to be confirmed, it may suggest that fetal lung maturation can be accelerated by exposure to cocaine.

Prenatal cocaine exposure appears to have short-term effects on respiratory function in very low birth weight infants. In a retrospective study of 149 such infants, 48 cocaine-exposed and 101 non-exposed, the cocaine-exposed infants had transiently improved respiratory status at time of delivery; they needed surfactant treatment in lower doses and at a lower frequency and intubation less often (250). At 24 and 48 hours there was no significant difference between the treatment requirements in the two groups. The development of bronchopulmonary dysplasia was also similar. The authors suggested that prenatal cocaine exposure affects the fetus by two mechanisms: indirectly through reduced uterine blood flow with placental insufficiency and directly through an adrenergic effect on the fetus. The fetus may experience cocaine as a stressor that leads to accelerated fetal lung maturity.

Nervous system

Fetal microcephaly has been attributed to cocaine abuse during pregnancy (251). Urine toxicology confirmed the presence of morphine, benzoylecgonine, barbiturates, paracetamol, and propoxyphene. Analyses of amniotic fluid, placenta, and fetal serum and urine were also positive for these substances. The authors suggested that vascular disruption was the likely major mechanism of anomalies, both behavioral and malformative, due to prolonged exposure to cocaine in utero.

- An infant born at 37 weeks gestation to a mother who had engaged in discontinuous cocaine abuse during the first and second trimesters of pregnancy had microcrania (below the 10th percentile), a closed anterior fontanelle, and overlapping of all sutures (252). The infant was of low birth weight (2290 g; 25th percentile). There were deep scalp rugae, a prominent occipital bone, and normal hair pattern. An MRI scan of the brain showed enlargement of the lateral ventricles and pericerebral spaces, with severe reduction of the cerebral and cerebellar parenchyma and white matter abnormalities.

These findings are part of the recognizable pattern of defects in the rare condition termed fetal brain disruption sequence. The presence of a normal hair pattern suggests normal brain development during the first 18 weeks of gestation. At a later stage partial destruction of the brain results in reduced intracranial pressure and subsequent collapse of the fetal skull.

Prenatal cocaine exposure has been associated with subependymal hemorrhage and subependymal cyst formation in term neonates and more recently in preterm neonates (<36 weeks of gestation) (253). Medical records and cranial sonograms obtained during 1 year on 122 premature infants showed an increased incidence of subependymal cysts in preterm cocaine-exposed infants (8 of 18) compared with non-exposed infants (8 of 99). There was no increase in the incidence of major structural abnormalities. All subependymal cysts resolved by 4 months of age. The authors noted that the neurodevelopmental implications of such cyst formation are unknown.

An unusual congenital malformation, the cloverleaf skull, has been associated with cocaine exposure in utero (254). In this condition, the cranium is trilobed, with severe brain deformity and hydrocephalus, because of premature fusion of the coronal and lambdoid sutures.

- A girl born by cesarean section at 38 weeks gestation weighed 3515 g and measured 54 cm in length and needed cardiopulmonary resuscitation. She had feeding and respiratory problems. Cranial sonography on day 11 showed a trilobed cranial mass with ventricular enlargement. She was discharged on day 35. The mother, a 24-year-old cocaine user, had engaged in active drug use for the 2 years before and during the first 2 months of pregnancy; she had also used alcohol (three units per day) and smoked marijuana (1–2 joints per day) during the first 5 months, and she had smoked 10 joints per day throughout the entire pregnancy. The father was also a marijuana smoker. The infant failed to thrive (body weight at 6 months 3120 g, height 57 cm), developed sepsis, and died. Autopsy showed adrenal infarction secondary to systemic infection.

Psychological

A study in 105 African-American infants suggested that infants exposed prenatally to cocaine are at a high risk of significant problems in arousal and attention (255). The 8-week-old infants had their heart rates recorded when presented with a series of stimuli. The order of the stimuli was as follows: auditory (rattle), visual (red ring), and social (examiner's face and voice). There were four groups of infants: preterm drug-exposed ($n = 25$), full-term drug-exposed ($n = 32$), preterm non-exposed ($n = 22$), and full-term non-exposed ($n = 26$). Preterm infants' ages were corrected to match those of the full-term infants. There were significant differences in the responses to social stimuli. Drug-exposed infants had an accelerated heart rate (indicating distress or arousal), whereas non-drug exposed infants had a slowed response (indicating focused attention). However, there were no heart rate differences among the groups in the auditory or visual conditions.

There have been two studies of the adverse effect of prenatal cocaine on behavior of the offspring. In the first, 31 cocaine-exposed, very low birth weight infants and matched very low birth weight controls followed longitudinally were assessed at 3 years (256). The cocaine-exposed children had delayed cognitive, motor, and language development compared with the controls. Of the exposed children 45% scored in the range of mental retardation compared with 16% of the controls. Infants in the exposed group during the neonatal period were less responsive in their interactions and their mothers were less nurturing and less emotionally available.

In contrast, in a second study there were few differences in interactive behaviors between prenatally cocaine-exposed and non-exposed 12-month-old infants and their mothers (257). Videotapes recorded African-American infants and their mothers engaged in interactions (49 cocaine-exposed, 63 non-exposed). Children who were prenatally exposed to cocaine ignored their mother's departure during separation significantly more often than controls. Mothers who abused cocaine used more verbal behavior with their children than non-abusers.

The effects of prenatal cocaine exposure on later learning abilities, including language, have been further investigated in 265 infants aged 1 year (134 cocaine-exposed and 131 matched non-exposed), who were tested using the Preschool Language Scale-3 (PLS-3) by blinded examiners (258). The infants were assigned to three cocaine exposure groups (as defined by maternal self-report and infant meconium assay): non-exposure ($n = 131$), heavier exposure ($n = 66$), and lighter exposure ($n = 68$). Fetal cocaine exposure was associated with deficits in developmental precursors of speech/language skills. At 1 year of age, more heavily exposed infants had poorer auditory comprehension than the non-exposed infants and worse total language performance than lighter and non-exposed infants. The more heavily exposed infants were also more likely to be classified as mildly delayed than non-exposed infants. Moreover, the degree of cocaine exposure had an inverse relation to auditory comprehension.

Drug Administration

Drug administration route

With the use of cocaine eye-drops, poisoning can occur with doses as small as 20 mg (10 drops of cocaine 4%). Victims generally collapse and die after associated cardiovascular abnormalities, dysrhythmias, and respiratory failure. Signs and symptoms of intoxication include excitement, restlessness, headache, nausea, vomiting, abdominal pain, convulsions, and delirium.

Drug overdose

Body packing, the act of swallowing packets holding illegal drugs in order to hide the evidence from legal authorities, can cause symptoms of drug intoxication or overdose (SEDA-22, 44) (259). In an analysis of all cases of cocaine body packers reported to a metropolitan poisons control center from January 1993 to May 1994, 34 of 46 individuals were symptom-free. Eight had mild symptoms (hypertension and tachycardia) that resolved with decontamination (activated charcoal or whole body irrigation) or tranquilizers (one received benzodiazepines). Two had severe symptoms, including seizures and cardiac dysrhythmias, and both died.

An increase in the number of deaths of all body packers in New York has been associated with an increase in deaths among opiate body packers: of 50 deaths among body packers from 1990 to 2001, 42 were due to opiates (260). Four were related to cocaine and four to both opiates and cocaine. In 37 cases open or leaking drug packets in the gastrointestinal tract resulted in acute intoxication and death. Five cases involved intestinal obstruction or perforation, one a gunshot wound, one an intracerebral hemorrhage due to hypertensive disease, and one was undetermined. The number of packets recovered was 1–111 (average 46).

- A 49-year-old man became ill during a plane flight (261). He admitted to having swallowed 102 latex packages of cocaine 5 g each and 20 tablets of activated charcoal 125 mg. After stabilization in an emergency room, he suffered a seizure. After restabilization he had not defecated and was given a laxative of a mineral oil liquid paraffin. During the next 24 hours his condition worsened. His serum cocaine concentration increased from 1.95 to 2.2 μg/ml. During preparation for surgery he developed an untreatable dysrhythmia and died. Autopsy showed cocaine packages in the gut, 71 ruptured and 95 intact.

The reported lethal oral dose of cocaine is 1–3 g. In this case, paraffin may have contributed to rupture of the packages by dissolving the latex.

In another cocaine body packer, non-surgical management was followed by the development of a giant gastric ulcer (262).

- A 35-year-old man presented to the emergency room 5 days after swallowing 35 latex-wrapped packages of cocaine. He was asymptomatic but concerned that only 10 of the 35 packets had passed in his stools. He was treated with laxatives and passed only 8 packages during the next 8 days. Radiography showed that 10–15 foreign bodies remained clustered in the stomach 14 days after ingestion. Several fragments of latex wrapping were found in his stools. On exploratory laparotomy, 15 latex packages were found impacted in the antrum just proximal to the pylorus. Beneath the packages there was a giant gastric ulcer, 2.5 cm in diameter. He had an uneventful postoperative course.

Fatal crack cocaine ingestion has been reported in an infant (263).

- A 10-month-old girl developed apnea, ventricular fibrillation, and a metabolic acidosis, and died shortly afterwards. Her 2-year-old brother had fed her crack cocaine. At autopsy the brain had a thinned corpus callosum, ranging in thickness from 0.2 to 0.5 cm. There were two pieces of crack cocaine in the duodenum and high concentrations of cocaine in the blood and other tissues.

The authors noted that the thinned corpus callosum suggested that the infant had been exposed to cocaine in utero or during the early postnatal period.

Drug–Drug Interactions

Alcohol

Cocaine abusers have reported that alcohol prolongs the euphoriant properties of cocaine, while ameliorating the acutely unpleasant physical and psychological sequelae, primarily paranoia and agitation. It may also lessen the dysphoria associated with acute cocaine abstinence. It has also been proposed that concurrent alcohol abuse may be an integral part of cocaine abuse. The combination of cocaine with alcohol can cause enhanced hepatotoxicity and enhanced cardiotoxicity (264). Trauma in patients who use cocaine plus alcohol has been reported (265). Those who use cocaine plus alcohol are 3–5 times more likely to have homicidal ideation and plans; this is particularly prominent in patients with antisocial personality disorder (266). A large high school survey by the Centers for Disease Control and Prevention showed that illicit substance abuse, prevalence of weapon carrying, and physical fighting were higher among the adolescents who reported recent use of cocaine, marijuana, alcohol, and corticosteroids. Among 215 female homicide offenders, 70% had been regular drug users at some time before imprisonment. Alcohol, crack, and powdered cocaine were the drugs most likely to be related to these homicides (267).

In a double-blind study, subjects meeting DSM-IV criteria for cocaine dependence and alcohol abuse participated in three drug administration sessions, involving intranasal cocaine with oral alcohol, cocaine with oral placebo alcohol, and cocaine placebo with oral alcohol (268). Cocaine plus alcohol produced greater euphoria and increased perception of well-being than cocaine alone. Heart rate was significantly higher with cocaine plus alcohol than with either alone. Cocaine concentrations were higher after cocaine plus alcohol than after cocaine alone. Metabolism of cocaine to cocaethylene was observed only during administration of cocaine plus alcohol. The authors concluded that enhanced psychological effects during abuse of cocaine plus alcohol may encourage the ingestion of larger amounts of these substances, placing users at increased risk of toxicity than with either drug alone.

The adverse effects of the combined use of alcohol and cocaine have been reviewed (269). There is little evidence that this combination acts synergistically or that either drug enhances the negative effects of the other. However, the combination leads to the formation of cocaethylene, which may potentiate cardiotoxic effects and the combination has a greater than additive effect on heart rate. Lastly, cocaine antagonizes the learning and psychomotor performance deficits and driving impairment caused by alcohol.

Reports of liver complications after cocaine use are infrequent. However, fulminant hepatitis with acute renal insufficiency requiring liver transplantation occurred after the use of cocaine and alcohol (270).

- A 33-year-old chronic alcoholic with hepatitis C developed acute liver and renal insufficiency with grade III encephalopathy. Hemodialysis was begun and emergency liver transplantation was performed. The explanted liver showed marked diffuse macrovesicular steatosis with massive coagulative-type necrosis. The postoperative course included a persistently raised gamma-glutamyltransferase, but he recovered fully after 60 days.

Macrovesicular steatosis can be attributed to alcohol or cocaine, but massive liver necrosis is more probably due to cocaine. The mechanisms of cocaine hepatotoxicity, such as increased lipid peroxidation, free radical activity, and impaired calcium sequestration, may be potentiated by alcohol.

Atropine

Anticholinergic poisoning involving adulterated cocaine has been reported (271).

- A 39-year-old man who was a recreational user of alcohol and cocaine presented with agitation, hallucinations, and delirium. He had a dry flushed skin, tachycardia, dilated, minimally reactive pupils, urinary retention, and absent bowel sounds. He was treated with intravenous fluids and a sedative. There were cocaine metabolites in the urine. Reanalysis of a urine sample by thin layer chromatography confirmed the presence of the anticholinergic drug atropine.

Clozapine

An interaction of clozapine with cocaine has been reported (272). Eight male cocaine addicts underwent four oral challenges with increasing doses of clozapine (12.5, 25, and 50 mg) and placebo, followed 2 hours later by cocaine 2 mg/kg intranasally (273). Subjective and physiological responses, and serum cocaine concentrations were measured over 4 hours. Clozapine pretreatment increased cocaine concentrations during the study and significantly increased the peak serum cocaine concentrations dose-dependently. Despite this rise in blood concentrations, clozapine pretreatment significantly reduced subjective responses to cocaine, including "expected high," "high," and "rush" effects, notably at the 50 mg dose. There were also significant effects on "sleepiness," "paranoia" and "nervousness." Clozapine caused a significant near-syncopal episode in one subject, requiring withdrawal. Clozapine had no significant effect on baseline pulse rate or systolic blood pressure, but it attenuated the significant pressor effects of a single dose of intranasal cocaine. These data suggested a possible therapeutic role for clozapine in the treatment of cocaine addiction in humans, but also suggest caution due to the near-syncopal event and the increase in serum cocaine concentrations.

Diamorphine

Rhabdomyolysis and ventricular fibrillation has been attributed to cocaine plus diamorphine (heroin) ingestion (274).

- A 28-year-old man went into cardiorespiratory arrest after using intravenous cocaine and diamorphine. He was intubated and ventilated and given adrenaline, naloxone, and sodium bicarbonate. During a thoracotomy he developed ventricular fibrillation and was electrically converted to sinus rhythm. He had hyperkalemia and myoglobinuria. He developed acute renal insufficiency, disseminated intravascular coagulopathy, and a right leg compartment syndrome. There were cocaine metabolites and opioids in his urine. Hemodialysis and fasciotomy were performed, but he died 2 months later with a complicating bronchopneumonia.

The authors discussed the possibility that naloxone, an effective opioid antidote, may have been harmful in this case.

Ephedrine

Chronic cocaine use sensitizes coronary arterial α-adrenoceptors to agonists (SEDA-22, 154).

Indometacin

Cocaine combined with indometacin in a 23-year-old pregnant woman at 34 weeks gestation may have caused fetal anuria and neonatal gastric hemorrhage (275).

Monoamine oxidase inhibitors

The combination of monoamine oxidase inhibitors with cocaine can cause hyperpyrexia (270).

Neuroleptic drugs

Cocaine-abusing psychiatric patients significantly more often develop neuroleptic drug-induced acute dystonia according to a 2-year study carried out on the island of Curaçao, Antilles, where cocaine and cannabis are often abused (277). The sample consisted of 29 men with neuroleptic drug-induced acute dystonia aged 17–45 years who had received high potency neuroleptic drugs in the month before admission; nine were cocaine users and 20 non-users. Cocaine use was a major risk factor for neuroleptic drug-induced acute dystonia and should be added to the list of well-known risk factors, such as male sex, younger age, neuroleptic drug dosage and potency, and a history of neuroleptic drug-induced acute dystonia. The authors suggested that high-risk cocaine-using psychiatric patients who start to take neuroleptic drugs should be provided with an anticholinergic drug as a prophylactic measure to prevent neuroleptic drug-induced acute dystonia.

Nimodipine

It has been suggested that calcium channel blockers can be used to treat cocaine dependence, and some studies have shown reductions in cocaine-induced subjective and cardiovascular responses with nifedipine and diltiazem. The cardiovascular and subjective responses to cocaine have been evaluated in a double-blind, placebo-controlled, crossover study in five subjects pretreated with two dosage of nimodipine (278). Nimodipine 60 mg attenuated the rise in systolic, but not diastolic, blood pressure after cocaine. In three subjects nimodipine 90 mg produced greater attenuation than 60 mg. The subjective effects of cocaine were not altered by either dose of nimodipine.

Suxamethonium

Procaine and cocaine are esters that are hydrolysed by plasma cholinesterase and may therefore competitively enhance the action of suxamethonium (succinylcholine) (279). Chloroprocaine may have a similar action. Lidocaine also interacts, although the mechanism is not clear unless very high doses are used (280).

References

1. Stein R, Ellinwood EH Jr Medical complication of cocaine abuse. Drug Ther 1990;10:40.
2. Rowbotham MC. Neurologic aspects of cocaine abuse. West J Med 1988;149(4):442–8.

3. Marzuk PM, Tardiff K, Leon AC, Hirsch CS, Stajic M, Portera L, Hartwell N, Iqbal MI. Fatal injuries after cocaine use as a leading cause of death among young adults in New York City. N Engl J Med 1995; 332(26):1753–7.
4. Gawin FH, Ellinwood EH Jr, Cocaine and other stimulants. Actions, Abuse, Treatment. N Engl J Med 1988;318(18):1173–82.
5. Clayton RR. Cocaine use in the United States: in a blizzard or just being snowed? NIDA Res Monogr 1985;61:8–34.
6. Lathers CM, Tyau LS, Spino MM, Agarwal I. Cocaine-induced seizures, arrhythmias and sudden death. J Clin Pharmacol 1988;28(7):584–93.
7. Karch SB, Billingham ME. The pathology and etiology of cocaine-induced heart disease. Arch Pathol Lab Med 1988;112(3):225–30.
8. Jiang JP, Downing SE. Catecholamine cardiomyopathy: review and analysis of pathogenetic mechanisms. Yale J Biol Med 1990;63(6):581–91.
9. Hong R, Matsuyama E, Nur K. Cardiomyopathy associated with the smoking of crystal methamphetamine. JAMA 1991;265(9):1152–4.
10. Ellinwood EH Jr, Petrie WM. Dependence on amphetamine, cocaine, and other stimulants. In: Pradhan SN, editor. Drug Abuse: Clinical and Basic Aspects. New York: CV Mosby, 1977:248.
11. Barinerd H, Krupp M, Chatton J, et al. Current Medical Diagnosis and Treatment. Los Altos CA. Lange. Medical Publishers, 1970.
12. Moe GK, Akildskov JA. Antiarrhythmic drugs. In: Gilman AG, Goodman LS, editors. The Pharmacological Basis of Therapeutics. New York: MacMillan, 1970.
13. Ellinwood EH Jr, Petrie WM. Drug induced psychoses. In: Pickens RW, Heston LL, editors. Psychiatric Factors in Drug Abuse. New York: Grune & Stratton, 1979:301.
14. Nanji AA, Filipenko JD. Asystole and ventricular fibrillation associated with cocaine intoxication. Chest 1984;85(1):132–3.
15. Wiener RS, Lockhart JT, Schwartz RG. Dilated cardiomyopathy and cocaine abuse. Report of two cases. Am J Med 1986;81(4):699–701.
16. Wodarz N, Boning J. "Ecstasy"-induziertes psychotisches Depersonalisationssyndrom. ["Ecstasy"-induced psychotic depersonalization syndrome.] Nervenarzt 1993;64(7):478–80.
17. McCann UD, Ricaurte GA. MDMA ("ecstasy") and panic disorder: induction by a single dose. Biol Psychiatry 1992;32(10):950–3.
18. Williams H, Meagher D, Galligan P. MDMA. ("Ecstasy"); a case of possible drug-induced psychosis. Ir J Med Sci 1993;162(2):43–4.
19. Isner JM, Estes NA3rd 3rd, Thompson PD, Costanzo-Nordin MR, Subramanian R, Miller G, Katsas G, Sweeney K, Sturner WQ. Acute cardiac events temporally related to cocaine abuse. N Engl Med 1986;315(23):1438–43.
20. Minor RL Jr, Scott BD, Brown DD, Winniford MD. Cocaine-induced myocardial infarction in patients with normal coronary arteries. Ann Intern Med 1991; 115(10):797–806.
21. Virmani R. Cocaine-associated cardiovascular disease: clinical and pathological aspects. NIDA Res Monogr 1991;108:220–9.
22. Stark TW, Pruet CW, Stark DU. Cocaine toxicity. Ear Nose Throat J 1983;62(3):155–8.
23. Jonsson S, O'Meara M, Young JB. Acute cocaine poisoning. Importance of treating seizures and acidosis. Am J Med 1983;75(6):1061–4.
24. Catravas JD, Waters IW. Acute cocaine intoxication in the conscious dog: studies on the mechanism of lethality. J Pharmacol Exp Ther 1981;217(2):350–6.
25. Covino BG, Vasalla HG. Local Anesthetics: Mechanism of Action and Clinical Use. New York: Grune and Stratton, 1976:127.
26. Marzuk PM, Tardiff K, Leon AC, Hirsch CS, Portera L, Iqbal MI, Nock MK, Hartwell N. Ambient temperature and mortality from unintentional cocaine overdose. JAMA 1998;279(22):1795–800.
27. Jaffe JH. Drug Addiction and Drug Abuse. In: Gilman AG, Goodman LS, Rall TW, Murad F, editors. The Pharmacological Basis of Therapeutics. 7th edn. New York: McMillan, 1985:54.
28. Hollander JE, Carter WA, Hoffman RS. Use of phentolamine for cocaine-induced myocardial ischemia. N Engl J Med 1992;327(5):361.
29. Lange RA, Cigarroa RG, Flores ED, McBride W, Kim AS, Wells PJ, Bedotto JB, Danziger RS, Hillis LD. Potentiation of cocaine-induced coronary vasoconstriction by beta-adrenergic blockade. Ann Intern Med 1990;112(12):897–903.
30. Boehrer JD, Moliterno DJ, Willard JE, Hillis LD, Lange RA. Influence of labetalol on cocaine-induced coronary vasoconstriction in humans. Am J Med 1993; 94(6):608–10.
31. Mittleman RE, Wetli CV. Death caused by recreational cocaine use. An update. JAMA 1984; 252(14):1889–93.
32. Cregler LL. Cocaine: the newest risk factor for cardiovascular disease. Clin Cardiol 1991;14(6):449–56.
33. Kloner RA, Hale S, Alker K, Rezkalla S. The effects of acute and chronic cocaine use on the heart. Circulation 1992;85(2):407–19.
34. Thadani P. Cardiovascular toxicity of cocaine: underlying mechanisms. NIDA Res Monogr 1991;108:1–238.
35. Boehrer JD, Moliterno DJ, Willard JE, Snyder RW2nd 2nd, Horton RP, Glamann DB, Lange RA, Hillis LD. Hemodynamic effects of intranasal cocaine in humans. Am Coll Cadiol 1992;20(1):90–3
36. Cohen S. Reinforcement and rapid delivery systems: understanding adverse consequences of cocaine. NIDA Res Monogr 1985;61:151–7.
37. Cregler LL, Mark H. Medical complications of cocaine abuse. N Engl J Med 1986;315(23):1495–500.
38. Pitts WR, Vongpatanasin W, Cigarroa JE, Hillis LD, Lange RA. Effects of the intracoronary infusion of cocaine on left ventricular systolic and diastolic function in humans. Circulation 1998;97(13):1270–3.
39. Sofuoglu M, Nelson D, Dudish-Poulsen S, Lexau B, Pentel PR, Hatsukami DK. Predictors of cardiovascular response to smoked cocaine in humans. Drug Alcohol Depend 2000;57(3):239–45.
40. Allred RJ, Ewer S. Fatal pulmonary edema following intravenous "freebase" cocaine use. Ann Emerg Med 1981;10(8):441–2.
41. Feldman JA, Fish SS, Beshansky JR, Griffith JL, Woolard RH, Selker HP. Acute cardiac ischemia in patients with cocaine-associated complaints: results of a multicenter trial. Ann Emerg Med 2000;36(5):469–76.
42. Kushman SO, Storrow AB, Liu T, Gibler WB. Cocaine-associated chest pain in a chest pain center. Am J Cardiol 2000;85(3):394–6.
43. Inyang VA, Cooper AJ, Hodgkinson DW. Cocaine induced myocardial infarction. J Accid Emerg Med 1999;16(5):374–5.
44. Amin M, Gabelman G, Karpel J, Buttrick P. Acute myocardial infarction and chest pain syndromes after cocaine use. Am J Cardiol 1990;66(20):1434–7.

45. Sharkey SW, Glitter MJ, Goldsmith SR. How serious is cocaine-associated acute chest pain syndromes after cocaine use. Cardiol Board Rev 1992;9:58–66.
46. Ross GS, Bell J. Myocardial infarction associated with inappropriate use of topical cocaine as treatment for epistaxis. Am J Emerg Med 1992;10(3):219–22.
47. Hollander JE, Hoffman RS. Cocaine-induced myocardial infarction: an analysis and review of the literature. J Emerg Med 1992;10(2):169–77.
48. Yuen-Green MS, Yen CK, Lim AD, Lull RJ. Tc-99m sestamibi myocardial imaging at rest for evaluation of cocaine-induced myocardial ischemia and infarction. Clin Nucl Med 1992;17(12):923–5.
49. Tanenbaum JH, Miller F. Electrocardiographic evidence of myocardial injury in psychiatrically hospitalized cocaine abusers. Gen Hosp Psychiatry 1992;14(3):201–3.
50. Eisenberg MJ, Mendelson J, Evans GT Jr, Jue J, Jones RT, Schiller NB. Left ventricular function immediately after intravenous cocaine: a quantitative two-dimensional echocardiographic study. J Am Coll Cardiol 1993;22(6):1581–6.
51. Rejali D, Glen P, Odom N. Pneumomediastinum following Ecstasy (methylenedioxymetamphetamine, MDMA) ingestion in two people at the same "rave". J Laryngol Otol 2002;116(1):75–6.
52. Morgan MJ, McFie L, Fleetwood H, Robinson JA. Ecstasy (MDMA): are the psychological problems associated with its use reversed by prolonged abstinence? Psychopharmacology (Berl) 2002;159(3):294–303.
53. Fox HC, McLean A, Turner JJ, Parrott AC, Rogers R, Sahakian BJ. Neuropsychological evidence of a relatively selective profile of temporal dysfunction in drug-free MDMA ("ecstasy") polydrug users. Psychopharmacology (Berl) 2002;162(2):203–14.
54. Cohle SD, Lie JT. Dissection of the aorta and coronary arteries associated with acute cocaine intoxication. Arch Pathol Lab Med 1992;116(11):1239–41.
55. Berry J, van Gorp WG, Herzberg DS, Hinkin C, Boone K, Steinman L, Wilkins JN. Neuropsychological deficits in abstinent cocaine abusers: preliminary findings after two weeks of abstinence. Drug Alcohol Depend 1993; 32(3):231–7.
56. Hsue PY, Salinas CL, Bolger AF, Benowitz NL, Waters DD. Acute aortic dissection related to crack cocaine. Circulation 2002;105(13):1592–5.
57. Riaz K, Forker AD, Garg M, McCullough PA. Atypical presentation of cocaine-induced type A aortic dissection: a diagnosis made by transesophageal echocardiography. J Investig Med 2002;50(2):140–2.
58. Neri E, Toscano T, Massetti M, Capannini G, Frati G, Sassi C. Cocaine-induced intramural hematoma of the ascending aorta. Tex Heart Inst J 2001;28(3):218–19.
59. Jaffe BD, Broderick TM, Leier CV. Cocaine-induced coronary-artery dissection. N Engl J Med 1994; 330(7):510–11.
60. Eskander KE, Brass NS, Gelfand ET. Cocaine abuse and coronary artery dissection. Ann Thorac Surg 2001;71(1):340–1.
61. Steinhauer JR, Caulfield JB. Spontaneous coronary artery dissection associated with cocaine use: a case report and brief review. Cardiovasc Pathol 2001;10(3):141–5.
62. Kumar PD, Smith HR. Cocaine-related vasculitis causing upper-limb peripheral vascular disease. Ann Intern Med 2000;133(11):923–4.
63. Balbir-Gurman A, Braun-Moscovici Y, Nahir AM. Cocaine-induced Raynaud's phenomenon and ischaemic finger necrosis. Clin Rheumatol 2001;20(5):376–8.
64. Morrow PL, McQuillen JB. Cerebral vasculitis associated with cocaine abuse. J Forensic Sci 1993;38(3):732–8.
65. Martin K, Rogers T, Kavanaugh A. Central nervous system angiopathy associated with cocaine abuse. J Rheumatol 1995;22(4):780–2.
66. Wang RY. pH-dependent cocaine-induced cardiotoxicity. Am J Emerg Med 1999;17(4):364–9.
67. Kajdasz DK, Moore JW, Donepudi H, Cochrane CE, Malcolm RJ. Cardiac and mood-related changes during short-term abstinence from crack cocaine: the identification of possible withdrawal phenomena. Am J Drug Alcohol Abuse 1999;25(4):629–37.
68. Laffey JG, Neligan P, Ormonde G. Prolonged perioperative myocardial ischemia in a young male: due to topical intranasal cocaine? J Clin Anesth 1999;11(5):419–24.
69. Liao BS, Hilsinger RL Jr, Rasgon BM, Matsuoka K, Adour KK. A preliminary study of cocaine absorption from the nasal mucosa. Laryngoscope 1999;109(1):98–102.
70. Tashkin DP, Gorelick D, Khalsa ME, Simmons M, Chang P. Respiratory effects of cocaine freebasing among habitual cocaine users. J Addict Dis 1992;11(4):59–70.
71. Baldwin GC, Choi R, Roth MD, Shay AH, Kleerup EC, Simmons MS, Tashkin DP. Evidence of chronic damage to the pulmonary microcirculation in habitual users of alkaloidal ("crack") cocaine. Chest 2002;121(4):1231–8.
72. Ettinger NA, Albin RJ. A review of the respiratory effects of smoking cocaine. Am J Med 1989;87(6):664–8.
73. O'Donnell AE, Mappin FG, Sebo TJ, Tazelaar H. Interstitial pneumonitis associated with "crack" cocaine abuse. Chest 1991;100(4):1155–7.
74. Oh PI, Balter MS. Cocaine induced eosinophilic lung disease. Thorax 1992;47(6):478–9.
75. Delaney K, Hoffman RS. Pulmonary infarction associated with crack cocaine use in a previously healthy 23-year-old woman. Am J Med 1991;91(1):92–4.
76. Batlle MA, Wilcox WD. Pulmonary edema in an infant following passive inhalation of free-base ("crack") cocaine. Clin Pediatr (Phila) 1993;32(2):105–6.
77. van der Klooster JM, Grootendorst AF. Severe bullous emphysema associated with cocaine smoking. Thorax 2001;56(12):982–3.
78. Hunter JG, Loy HC, Markovitz L, Kim US. Spontaneous pneumomediastinum following inhalation of alkaloidal cocaine and emesis: case report and review. Mt Sinai J Med 1986;53(6):491–3.
79. Goel P, Flaker GC. Cardiovascular complications of cocaine use. N Engl J Med 2001;345(21):1575–6.
80. Gatof D, Albert RK. Bilateral thumb burns leading to the diagnosis of crack lung. Chest 2002;121(1):289–91.
81. Torre M, Barberis M. Spontaneous pneumothorax in cocaine sniffers. Am J Emerg Med 1998;16(5):546–9.
82. Rome LA, Lippmann ML, Dalsey WC, Taggart P, Pomerantz S. Prevalence of cocaine use and its impact on asthma exacerbation in an urban population. Chest 2000;117(5):1324–9.
83. Gupta A, Hawrych A, Wilson WR. Cocaine-induced sinonasal destruction. Otolaryngol Head Neck Surg 2001;124(4):480.
84. Noskin GA, Kalish SB. Pott's puffy tumor: a complication of intranasal cocaine abuse. Rev Infect Dis 1991;13(4):606–8.
85. Smith JC, Kacker A, Anand VK. Midline nasal and hard palate destruction in cocaine abusers and cocaine's role in rhinologic practice. Ear Nose Throat J 2002; 81(3):172–7.
86. Talbott JF, Gorti GK, Koch RJ. Midfacial osteomyelitis in a chronic cocaine abuser: a case report. Ear Nose Throat J 2001;80(10):738–43.
87. Vilela RJ, Langford C, McCullagh L, Kass ES. Cocaine-induced oronasal fistulas with external nasal erosion but without palate involvement. Ear Nose Throat J 2002;81(8):562–3.

88. Li SJ, Wang Y, Pankiewicz J, Stein EA. Neurochemical adaptation to cocaine abuse: reduction of N-acetyl aspartate in thalamus of human cocaine abusers. Biol Psychiatry 1999;45(11):1481–7.
89. Costa L, Bauer LO. Smooth pursuit eye movement dysfunction in substance-dependent patients: mediating effects of antisocial personality disorder. Neuropsychobiology 1998;37(3):117–23.
90. Adler LE, Olincy A, Cawthra E, Hoffer M, Nagamoto HT, Amass L, Freedman R. Reversal of diminished inhibitory sensory gating in cocaine addicts by a nicotinic cholinergic mechanism. Neuropsychopharmacology 2001;24(6):671–9.
91. Goldstein RZ, Volkow ND, Wang GJ, Fowler JS, Rajaram S. Addiction changes orbitofrontal gyrus function: involvement in response inhibition. Neuroreport 2001;12(11):2595–9.
92. Tanvetyanon T, Dissin J, Selcer UM. Hyperthermia and chronic pancerebellar syndrome after cocaine abuse. Arch Intern Med 2001;161(4):608–10.
93. Dhuna A, Pascual-Leone A, Belgrade M. Cocaine-related vascular headaches. J Neurol Neurosurg Psychiatry 1991;54(9):803–6.
94. Mossman SS, Goadsby PJ. Cocaine abuse simulating the aura of migraine. J Neurol Neurosurg Psychiatry 1992;55(7):628.
95. Satel SL, Swann AC. Extrapyramidal symptoms and cocaine abuse. Am J Psychiatry 1993;150(2):347.
96. Cardoso FE, Jankovic J. Cocaine-related movement disorders. Mov Disord 1993;8(2):175–8.
97. Volkow ND, Fowler JS, Wang GJ, Hitzemann R, Logan J, Schlyer DJ, Dewey SL, Wolf AP. Decreased dopamine D_2 receptor availability is associated with reduced frontal metabolism in cocaine abusers. Synapse 1993;14(2):169–77.
98. Hegarty AM, Lipton RB, Merriam AE, Freeman K. Cocaine as a risk factor for acute dystonic reactions. Neurology 1991;41(10):1670–2.
99. Attig E, Amyot R, Botez T. Cocaine induced chronic tics. J Neurol Neurosurg Psychiatry 1994;57(9):1143–4.
100. Mesulam MM. Cocaine and Tourette's syndrome. N Engl J Med 1986;315(6):398.
101. Berciano J, Oterino A, Rebollo M, Pascual J. Myasthenia gravis unmasked by cocaine abuse. N Engl J Med 1991;325(12):892.
102. Valmaggia C, Gottlob IM. Cocaine abuse, generalized myasthenia, complete external ophthalmoplegia, and pseudotonic pupil. Strabismus 2001;9(1):9–12.
103. Dhuna A, Pascual-Leone A, Langendorf F. Chronic, habitual cocaine abuse and kindling-induced epilepsy: a case report. Epilepsia 1991;32(6):890–4.
104. Myers JA, Earnest MP. Generalized seizures and cocaine abuse. Neurology 1984;34(5):675–6.
105. Kowatch RA, Schnoll SS, Knisely JS, Green D, Elswick RK. Electroencephalographic sleep and mood during cocaine withdrawal. J Addict Dis 1992;11(4):21–45.
106. Yapor WY, Gutierrez FA. Cocaine-induced intratumoral hemorrhage: case report and review of the literature. Neurosurgery 1992;30(2):288–91.
107. Ramadan NM, Levine SR, Welch KM. Pontine hemorrhage following "crack" cocaine use. Neurology 1991;41(6):946–7.
108. Kosten TR, Cheeves C, Palumbo J, Seibyl JP, Price LH, Woods SW. Regional cerebral blood flow during acute and chronic abstinence from combined cocaine–alcohol abuse. Drug Alcohol Depend 1998;50(3):187–95.
109. Sloan MA, Kittner SJ, Feeser BR, Gardner J, Epstein A, Wozniak MA, Wityk RJ, Stern BJ, Price TR, Macko RF, Johnson CJ, Earley CJ, Buchholz D. Illicit drug-associated ischemic stroke in the Baltimore-Washington Young Stroke Study. Neurology 1998;50(6):1688–93.
110. Levine SR, Brust JC, Futrell N, Brass LM, Blake D, Fayad P, Schultz LR, Millikan CH, Ho KL, Welch KM. A comparative study of the cerebrovascular complications of cocaine: alkaloidal versus hydrochloride—a review. Neurology 1991;41(8):1173–7.
111. Strupp M, Hamann GF, Brandt T. Combined amphetamine and cocaine abuse caused mesencephalic ischemia in a 16-year-old boy—due to vasospasm? Eur Neurol 2000;43(3):181–2.
112. Herning RI, Better W, Nelson R, Gorelick D, Cadet JL. The regulation of cerebral blood flow during intravenous cocaine administration in cocaine abusers. Ann NY Acad Sci 1999;890:489–94.
113. Alves OL, Gomes O. Cocaine-related acute subdural hematoma: an emergent cause of cerebrovascular accident. Acta Neurochir (Wien) 2000;142(7):819–21.
114. Grewal RP, Miller BL. Cocaine induced hypertensive encephalopathy. Acta Neurol (Napoli) 1991;13(3):279–81.
115. Mueller D, Gilden DH. Brown–Sequard syndrome after esophageal sclerotherapy and crack cocaine abuse. Neurology 2002;58(7):1129–30.
116. Chadan N, Thierry A, Sautreaux JL, Gras P, Martin D, Giroud M. Rupture anéurysmale et toxicomanie à la cocaïne. [Aneurysm rupture and cocaine addiction.] Neurochirurgie 1991;37(6):403–5.
117. Oyesiku NM, Colohan AR, Barrow DL, Reisner A. Cocaine-induced aneurysmal rupture: an emergent negative factor in the natural history of intracranial aneurysms? Neurosurgery 1993;32(4):518–26.
118. Conway JE, Tamargo RJ. Cocaine use is an independent risk factor for cerebral vasospasm after aneurysmal subarachnoid hemorrhage. Stroke 2001;32(10):2338–43.
119. Zagelbaum BM, Tannenbaum MH, Hersh PS. *Candida albicans* corneal ulcer associated with crack cocaine. Am J Ophthalmol 1991;111(2):248–9.
120. Sachs R, Zagelbaum BM, Hersh PS. Corneal complications associated with the use of crack cocaine. Ophthalmology 1993;100(2):187–91.
121. Zagelbaum BM, Donnenfeld ED, Perry HD, Buxton J, Buxton D, Hersh PS. Corneal ulcer caused by combined intravenous and anesthetic abuse of cocaine. Am J Ophthalmol 1993;116(2):241–2.
122. Wang ES. Cocaine-induced iritis. Ann Emerg Med 1991;20(2):192–3.
123. Rofsky JE, Townsend JC, Ilsen PF, Bright DC. Retinal nerve fiber layer defects and microtalc retinopathy secondary to free-basing "crack" cocaine. J Am Optom Assoc 1995;66(11):712–20.
124. Van Stavern GP, Gorman M. Orbital infarction after cocaine use. Neurology 2002;59(4):642–3.
125. Michaelides M, Larkin G. Cocaine-associated central retinal artery occlusion in a young man. Eye 2002; 16(6):790–2.
126. Miller BL, Mena I, Giombetti R, Villanueva-Meyer J, Djenderedjian AH. Neuropsychiatric effects of cocaine: SPECT measurements. J Addict Dis 1992;11(4):47–58.
127. O'Malley S, Adamse M, Heaton RK, Gawin FH. Neuropsychological impairment in chronic cocaine abusers. Am J Drug Alcohol Abuse 1992;18(2):131–44.
128. Di Sclafani V, Tolou-Shams M, Price LJ, Fein G. Neuropsychological performance of individuals dependent on crack-cocaine, or crack-cocaine and alcohol, at 6 weeks and 6 months of abstinence. Drug Alcohol Depend 2002;66(2):161–71.
129. Selby MJ, Azrin RL. Neuropsychological functioning in drug abusers. Drug Alcohol Depend 1998;50(1):39–45.

130. Bolla KI, Rothman R, Cadet JL. Dose-related neurobehavioral effects of chronic cocaine use. J Neuropsychiatry Clin Neurosci 1999;11(3):361–9.
131. Butler LF, Frank EM. Neurolinguistic function and cocaine abuse. J Med Speech-Lang Path 2000;8:199–212.
132. Ross-Durow PL, Boyd CJ. Sexual abuse, depression, and eating disorders in African American women who smoke cocaine. J Subst Abuse Treat 2000;18(1):79–81.
133. Allam S, Noble JS. Cocaine-excited delirium and severe acidosis. Anaesthesia 2001;56(4):385–6.
134. Crum RM, Anthony JC. Cocaine use and other suspected risk factors for obsessive-compulsive disorder: a prospective study with data from the Epidemiologic Catchment Area surveys. Drug Alcohol Depend 1993; 31(3):281–95.
135. Aronson TA, Craig TJ. Cocaine precipitation of panic disorder. Am J Psychiatry 1986;143(5):643–5.
136. Rosen MI, Kosten T. Cocaine-associated panic attacks in methadone-maintained patients. Am J Drug Alcohol Abuse 1992;18(1):57–62.
137. Brady KT, Lydiard RB, Malcolm R, Ballenger JC. Cocaine-induced psychosis. J Clin Psychiatry 1991;52(12):509–12.
138. Nambudiri DE, Young RC. A case of late-onset crack dependence and subsequent psychosis in the elderly. J Subst Abuse Treat 1991;8(4):253–5.
139. Cubells JF, Kranzler HR, McCance-Katz E, Anderson GM, Malison RT, Price LH, Gelernter J. A haplotype at the DBH locus, associated with low plasma dopamine beta-hydroxylase activity, also associates with cocaine-induced paranoia. Mol Psychiatry 2000; 5(1):56–63.
140. Vescovi PP. Cardiovascular and hormonal responses to hyperthermic stress in cocaine addicts after a long period of abstinence. Addict Biol 2000;5:91–5.
141. Lajara-Nanson WA. Cocaine induced hypokalaemic periodic paralysis. J Neurol Neurosurg Psychiatry 2002;73(1):92.
142. Miller JM Jr, Nolan TE. Case-control study of antenatal cocaine use and platelet levels. Am J Obstet Gynecol 2001;184(3):434–7.
143. Nalbandian H, Sheth N, Dietrich R, Georgiou J. Intestinal ischemia caused by cocaine ingestion: report of two cases. Surgery 1985;97(3):374–6.
144. Chan YC, Camprodon RA, Kane PA, Scott-Coombes DM. Abdominal complications from crack cocaine. Ann R Coll Surg Engl 2005;87(1):72–3.
145. Cohen ME, Kegel JG. Candy cocaine esophagus. Chest 2002;121(5):1701–3.
146. Arrillaga A, Sosa JL, Najjar R. Laparoscopic patching of crack cocaine-induced perforated ulcers. Am Surg 1996;62(12):1007–9.
147. Pecha RE, Prindiville T, Pecha BS, Camp R, Carroll M, Trudeau W. Association of cocaine and methamphetamine use with giant gastroduodenal ulcers. Am J Gastroenterol 1996;91(12):2523–7.
148. Abramson DL, Gertler JP, Lewis T, Kral JG. Crack-related perforated gastropyloric ulcer. J Clin Gastroenterol 1991;13(1):17–19.
149. Myers SI, Clagett GP, Valentine RJ, Hansen ME, Anand A, Chervu A. Chronic intestinal ischemia caused by intravenous cocaine use: report of two cases and review of the literature. J Vasc Surg 1996;23(4):724–9.
150. Simmers TA, Vidakovic-Vukic M, Van Meyel JJ. Cocaine-induced ischemic colitis. Endoscopy 1998;30(1):S8–9.
151. Papi C, Candia S, Masci P, Ciaco A, Montanti S, Capurso L. Acute ischaemic colitis following intravenous cocaine use. Ital J Gastroenterol Hepatol 1999;31(4):305–7.
152. Whitten CG, Luke BA. Liver uptake of Tc-99m PYP. Clin Nucl Med 1991;16(7):492–4.
153. Peyriere H, Mauboussin JM. Cocaine-induced acute cytologic hepatitis in HIV-infected patients with nonactive viral hepatitis. Ann Intern Med 2000;132(12):1010–11.
154. Lam M, Ballou SP. Reversible scleroderma renal crisis after cocaine use. N Engl J Med 1992;326(21):1435.
155. Norris KC, Thornhill-Joynes M, Robinson C, Strickland T, Alperson BL, Witana SC, Ward HJ. Cocaine use, hypertension, and end-stage renal disease. Am J Kidney Dis 2001;38(3):523–8.
156. Singhal P, Horowitz B, Quinones MC, Sommer M, Faulkner M, Grosser M. Acute renal failure following cocaine abuse. Nephron 1989;52(1):76–8.
157. Roth D, Alarcon FJ, Fernandez JA, Preston RA, Bourgoignie JJ. Acute rhabdomyolysis associated with cocaine intoxication. N Engl J Med 1988;319(11):673–7.
158. Amoedo ML, Craver L, Marco MP, Fernandez E. Cocaine-induced acute renal failure without rhabdomyolysis. Nephrol Dial Transplant 1999;14(12):2970–1.
159. Saleem TM, Singh M, Murtaza M, Singh A, Kasubhai M, Gnanasekaran I. Renal infarction: a rare complication of cocaine abuse. Am J Emerg Med 2001;19(6):528–9.
160. Anonymous. Outbreak of primary and secondary syphilis—Baltimore City, Maryland, 1995. MMWR Morb Mortal Wkly Rep 1996;45(8):166–9.
161. Altman AL, Seftel AD, Brown SL, Hampel N. Cocaine associated priapism. J Urol 1999;161(6):1817–18.
162. Myrick H, Markowitz JS, Henderson S. Priapism following trazodone overdose with cocaine use. Ann Clin Psychiatry 1998;10(2):81–3.
163. Mireku-Boateng AO, Tasie B. Priapism associated with intracavernosal injection of cocaine. Urol Int 2001;67(1):109–10.
164. Robinson AJ, Gazzard BG. Rising rates of HIV infection. BMJ 2005;330(7487):320–1.
165. Delafuente JC, DeVane CL. Immunologic effects of cocaine and related alkaloids. Immunopharmacol Immunotoxicol 1991;13(1–2):11–23.
166. Peterson PK, Gekker G, Chao CC, Schut R, Verhoef J, Edelman CK, Erice A, Balfour HH Jr. Cocaine amplifies HIV-1 replication in cytomegalovirus-stimulated peripheral blood mononuclear cell cocultures. J Immunol 1992;149(2):676–80.
167. Trozak DJ, Gould WM. Cocaine abuse and connective tissue disease. J Am Acad Dermatol 1984;10(3):525.
168. Hofbauer GF, Hafner J, Trueb RM. Urticarial vasculitis following cocaine use. Br J Dermatol 1999;141(3):600–1.
169. Castro-Villamor MA, de las Heras P, Armentia A, Duenas-Laita A. Cocaine-induced severe angioedema and urticaria. Ann Emerg Med 1999;34(2):296–7.
170. Crandall CG, Vongpatanasin W, Victor RG. Mechanism of cocaine-induced hyperthermia in humans. Ann Intern Med 2002;136(11):785–91.
171. Schier JG, Hoffman RS, Nelson LS. Cocaine and body temperature regulation. Ann Intern Med 2002;137(10):855–6.
172. Karch SB, Stephens B, Ho CH. Relating cocaine blood concentrations to toxicity—an autopsy study of 99 cases. J Forensic Sci 1998;43(1):41–5.
173. Daisley H, Jones-Le Cointe A, Hutchinson G, Simmons V. Fatal cardiac toxicity temporally related to poly-drug abuse. Vet Hum Toxicol 1998;40(1):21–2.
174. Furnari C, Ottaviano V, Sacchetti G, Mancini M. A fatal case of cocaine poisoning in a body packer. J Forensic Sci 2002;47(1):208–10.
175. Fineschi V, Centini F, Monciotti F, Turillazzi E. The cocaine "body stuffer" syndrome: a fatal case. Forensic Sci Int 2002;126(1):7–10.
176. Bannon MJ, Pruetz B, Manning-Bog AB, Whitty CJ, Michelhaugh SK, Sacchetti P, Granneman JG, Mash DC,

Schmidt CJ. Decreased expression of the transcription factor NURR1 in dopamine neurons of cocaine abusers. Proc Natl Acad Sci USA 2002;99(9):6382–5.
177. Alim TN, Rosse RB, Vocci FJ Jr, Lindquist T, Deutsch SI. Diethylpropion pharmacotherapeutic adjuvant therapy for inpatient treatment of cocaine dependence: a test of the cocaine-agonist hypothesis. Clin Neuropharmacol 1995;18(2):183–95.
178. Grabowski J, Roache JD, Schmitz JM, Rhoades H, Creson D, Korszun A. Replacement medication for cocaine dependence: methylphenidate. J Clin Psychopharmacol 1997;17(6):485–8.
179. Gawin F, Riordan C, Kleber H. Methylphenidate treatment of cocaine abusers without attention deficit disorder: a negative report. Am J Drug Alcohol Abuse 1985;11(3–4):193–7.
180. Duarte JG, do Nascimento AF, Pantoja JG, Chaves CP. Chronic inhaled cocaine abuse may predispose to the development of pancreatic adenocarcinoma. Am J Surg 1999;178(5):426–7.
181. Nahrwold DL. Editorial comment. Am J Surg 1999;178:427.
182. Spence MR, Williams R, DiGregorio GJ, Kirby-McDonnell A, Polansky M. The relationship between recent cocaine use and pregnancy outcome. Obstet Gynecol 1991;78(3 Pt 1):326–9.
183. Chasnoff IJ. Methodological issues in studying cocaine use in pregnancy: a problem of definitions. NIDA Res Monogr 1991;114:55–65.
184. Handler A, Kistin N, Davis F, Ferre C. Cocaine use during pregnancy: perinatal outcomes. Am J Epidemiol 1991;133(8):818–25.
185. Hsu CD, Chen S, Feng TI, Johnson TR. Rupture of uterine scar with extensive maternal bladder laceration after cocaine abuse. Am J Obstet Gynecol 1992; 167(1):129–30.
186. Abramowicz JS, Sherer DM, Woods JR Jr, Acute transient thrombocytopenia associated with cocaine abuse in pregnancy. Obstet Gynecol 1991;78(3 Pt 2):499–501.
187. Hurd WW, Betz AL, Dombrowski MP, Fomin VP. Cocaine augments contractility of the pregnant human uterus by both adrenergic and nonadrenergic mechanisms. Am J Obstet Gynecol 1998;178(5):1077–81.
188. Refuerzo JS, Sokol RJ, Blackwell SC, Berry SM, Janisse JJ, Sorokin Y. Cocaine use and preterm premature rupture of membranes: improvement in neonatal outcome. Am J Obstet Gynecol 2002;186(6):1150–4.
189. Bauer CR, Shankaran S, Bada HS, Lester B, Wright LL, Krause-Steinrauf H, Smeriglio VL, Finnegan LP, Maza PL, Verter J. The Maternal Lifestyle Study: drug exposure during pregnancy and short-term maternal outcomes. Am J Obstet Gynecol 2002;186(3):487–95.
190. Chasnoff IJ, Burns WJ, Schnoll SH, Burns KA. Cocaine use in pregnancy. N Engl J Med 1985;313(11):666–9.
191. Jones KL. Developmental pathogenesis of defects associated with prenatal cocaine exposure: fetal vascular disruption. Clin Perinatol 1991;18(1):139–46.
192. Napiorkowski B, Lester BM, Freier MC, Brunner S, Dietz L, Nadra A, Oh W. Effects of in utero substance exposure on infant neurobehavior. Pediatrics 1996; 98(1):71–5.
193. Tsay CH, Partridge JC, Villarreal SF, Good WV, Ferriero DM. Neurologic and ophthalmologic findings in children exposed to cocaine in utero. J Child Neurol 1996;11(1):25–30.
194. Kapur RP, Shaw CM, Shepard TH. Brain hemorrhages in cocaine-exposed human fetuses. Teratology 1991; 44(1):11–18.
195. Little BB, Snell LM. Brain growth among fetuses exposed to cocaine in utero: asymmetrical growth retardation. Obstet Gynecol 1991;77(3):361–4.
196. Harris EF, Friend GW, Tolley EA. Enhanced prevalence of ankyloglossia with maternal cocaine use. Cleft Palate Craniofac J 1992;29(1):72–6.
197. Lavi E, Montone KT, Rorke LB, Kliman HJ. Fetal akinesia deformation sequence (Pena–Shokeir phenotype) associated with acquired intrauterine brain damage. Neurology 1991;41(9):1467–8.
198. Lessick M, Vasa R, Israel J. Severe manifestations of oculoauriculovertebral spectrum in a cocaine exposed infant. J Med Genet 1991;28(11):803–4.
199. Richardson GA, Day NL. Maternal and neonatal effects of moderate cocaine use during pregnancy. Neurotoxicol Teratol 1991;13(4):455–60.
200. Datta-Bhutada S, Johnson HL, Rosen TS. Intrauterine cocaine and crack exposure: neonatal outcome. J Perinatol 1998;18(3):183–8.
201. Hurt H, Brodsky NL, Braitman LE, Giannetta J. Natal status of infants of cocaine users and control subjects: a prospective comparison. J Perinatol 1995;15(4):297–304.
202. Mehta SK, Super DM, Connuck D, Kirchner HL, Salvator A, Singer L, Fradley LG, Kaufman ES. Autonomic alterations in cocaine-exposed infants. Am Heart J 2002;144(6):1109–15.
203. Mehta SK, Super DM, Salvator A, Singer L, Connuck D, Fradley LG, Harcar-Sevcik RA, Thomas JD, Sun JP. Diastolic filling abnormalities by color kinesis in newborns exposed to intrauterine cocaine. J Am Soc Echocardiogr 2002;15(5):447–53.
204. Mehta SK, Super DM, Connuck D, Kirchner HL, Salvator A, Singer L, Fradley LG, Thomas JD, Sun JP. Diastolic alterations in infants exposed to intrauterine cocaine: a follow-up study by color kinesis. J Am Soc Echocardiogr 2002;15(11):1361–6.
205. Shepard TH, Fantel AG, Kapur RP. Fetal coronary thrombosis as a cause of single ventricular heart. Teratology 1991;43(2):113–17.
206. Kosofsky BE. The effect of cocaine on developing human brain. NIDA Res Monogr 1991;114:128–43.
207. Eyler FD, Behnke M, Conlon M, Woods NS, Wobie K. Birth outcome from a prospective, matched study of prenatal crack/cocaine use: II. Interactive and dose effects on neurobehavioral assessment. Pediatrics 1998;101(2):237–41.
208. Alessandri SM, Bendersky M, Lewis M. Cognitive functioning in 8- to 18-month-old drug-exposed infants. Dev Psychol 1998;34(3):565–73.
209. Wasserman GA, Kline JK, Bateman DA, Chiriboga C, Lumey LH, Friedlander H, Melton L, Heagarty MC. Prenatal cocaine exposure and school-age intelligence. Drug Alcohol Depend 1998;50(3):203–10.
210. Lester BM, LaGasse LL, Seifer R. Cocaine exposure and children: the meaning of subtle effects. Science 1998;282(5389):633–4.
211. Delaney-Black V, Covington C, Templin T, Ager J, Martier S, Sokol R. Prenatal cocaine exposure and child behavior. Pediatrics 1998;102(4 Pt 1):945–50.
212. Mayes LC, Bornstein MH, Chawarska K, Granger RH. Information processing and developmental assessments in 3-month-old infants exposed prenatally to cocaine. Pediatrics 1995;95(4):39–45.
213. Bender SL, Word CO, Di Clemente RJ, Crittenden MR, Persaud NA, Ponton LE. The developmental implications of prenatal and/or postnatal crack cocaine exposure in preschool children: a preliminary report. J Dev Behav Pediatr 1995;16(6):418–24.
214. Mirochnick M, Frank DA, Cabral H, Turner A, Zuckerman B. Relation between meconium concentration

of the cocaine metabolite benzoylecgonine and fetal growth. J Pediatr 1995;126(4):636–8.
215. Martin JC, Barr HM, Martin DC, Streissguth AP. Neonatal neurobehavioral outcome following prenatal exposure to cocaine. Neurotoxicol Teratol 1996;18(6):617–25.
216. Tronick EZ, Frank DA, Cabral H, Mirochnick M, Zuckerman B. Late dose-response effects of prenatal cocaine exposure on newborn neurobehavioral performance. Pediatrics 1996;98(1):76–83.
217. Karmel BZ, Gardner JM, Freedland RL. Arousal-modulated attention at four months as a function of intrauterine cocaine exposure and central nervous system injury. J Pediatr Psychol 1996;21(6):821–32.
218. Scafidi FA, Field TM, Wheeden A, Schanberg S, Kuhn C, Symanski R, Zimmerman E, Bandstra ES. Cocaine-exposed preterm neonates show behavioral and hormonal differences. Pediatrics 1996;97(6 Pt 1):851–5.
219. Jacobson SW, Jacobson JL, Sokol RJ, Martier SS, Chiodo LM. New evidence for neurobehavioral effects of in utero cocaine exposure. J Pediatr 1996;129(4):581–90.
220. Schuler ME, Nair P. Brief report: frequency of maternal cocaine use during pregnancy and infant neurobehavioral outcome. J Pediatr Psychol 1999;24(6):511–14.
221. Held JR, Riggs ML, Dorman C. The effect of prenatal cocaine exposure on neurobehavioral outcome: a meta-analysis. Neurotoxicol Teratol 1999;21(6):619–25.
222. Singer LT, Arendt R, Minnes S, Farkas K, Salvator A. Neurobehavioral outcomes of cocaine-exposed infants. Neurotoxicol Teratol 2000;22(5):653–66.
223. Chapman JK. Developmental outcomes in two groups of infants and toddlers: prenatal cocaine exposed and noncocaine exposed part 1. Infant-Toddler Interv 2000; 10:19–36.
224. Heffelfinger AK, Craft S, White DA, Shyken J. Visual attention in preschool children prenatally exposed to cocaine: implications for behavioral regulation. J Int Neuropsychol Soc 2002;8(1):12–21.
225. Frank DA, Jacobs RR, Beeghly M, Augustyn M, Bellinger D, Cabral H, Heeren T. Level of prenatal cocaine exposure and scores on the Bayley Scales of Infant Development: modifying effects of caregiver, early intervention, and birth weight. Pediatrics 2002;110(6):1143–52.
226. Accornero VH, Morrow CE, Bandstra ES, Johnson AL, Anthony JC. Behavioral outcome of preschoolers exposed prenatally to cocaine: role of maternal behavioral health. J Pediatr Psychol 2002;27(3):259–69.
227. Downing GJ, Horner SR, Kilbride HW. Characteristics of perinatal cocaine-exposed infants with necrotizing enterocolitis. Am J Dis Child 1991;145(1):26–7.
228. Spinazzola R, Kenigsberg K, Usmani SS, Harper RG. Neonatal gastrointestinal complications of maternal cocaine abuse. NY State J Med 1992;92(1):22–3.
229. Greenfield SP, Rutigliano E, Steinhardt G, Elder JS. Genitourinary tract malformations and maternal cocaine abuse. Urology 1991;37(5):455–9.
230. Behnke M, Eyler FD, Garvan CW, Wobie K. The search for congenital malformations in newborns with fetal cocaine exposure. Pediatrics 2001;107(5):E74.
231. Bandstra ES, Morrow CE, Anthony JC, Churchill SS, Chitwood DC, Steele BW, Ofir AY, Xue L. Intrauterine growth of full-term infants: impact of prenatal cocaine exposure. Pediatrics 2001;108(6):1309–19.
232. Frank DA, Augustyn M, Knight WG, Pell T, Zuckerman B. Growth, development, and behavior in early childhood following prenatal cocaine exposure: a systematic review. JAMA 2001;285(12):1613–25.
233. Stanwood GD, Levitt P. Prenatal cocaine exposure as a risk factor for later developmental outcomes. JAMA 2001;286(1):45.
234. Singer LT, Arendt RE. Prenatal cocaine exposure as a risk factor for later developmental outcomes. JAMA 2001;286(1):45–6.
235. Delaney-Black V, Covington CY, Nordstrom-Klee B, Sokol RJ. Prenatal cocaine exposure as a risk factor for later developmental outcomes. JAMA 2001; 286(1):46–7.
236. King TA, Perlman JM, Laptook AR, Rollins N, Jackson G, Little B. Neurologic manifestations of in utero cocaine exposure in near-term and term infants. Pediatrics 1995;96(2 Pt 1):259–64.
237. Fetters L, Tronick EZ. Neuromotor development of cocaine-exposed and control infants from birth through 15 months: poor and poorer performance. Pediatrics 1996;98(5):938–43.
238. Behnke M, Eyler FD, Garvan CW, Wobie K, Hou W. Cocaine exposure and developmental outcome from birth to 6 months. Neurotoxicol Teratol 2002;24(3):283–5.
239. Bauer CR. Perinatal effects of prenatal drug exposure. Neonatal aspects. Clin Perinatol 1999;26(1):87–106.
240. Lutiger B, Graham K, Einarson TR, Koren G. Relationship between gestational cocaine use and pregnancy outcome: a meta-analysis. Teratology 1991;44940:405–14.
241. Singer LT, Arendt R, Minnes S, Farkas K, Salvator A. Neurobehavioural outcomes of cocaine-exposed infants. Neurotoxicol Teratol 2000;22(5):653–66.
242. Lidow MS. Prenatal cocaine exposure adversely affects development of the primate cerebral cortex. Synapse 1995;21(4):332–41.
243. Heffelfinger AK, Craft S, White DA, Shyken J. Visual attention in preschool children prenatally exposed to cocaine: implications for behavioural regulation. J Int Neuropsychol Soc 2002;8:12–21.
244. Bandstra ES, Morrow CE, Vogel AL, Fifer RC, Ofir AY, Dausa AT, Xue L, Anthony JC. Longitudinal influence of prenatal cocaine exposure on child language functioning. Neurotoxicol Teratol 2002;24(3):297–308.
245. Malakoff ME, Mayes LC, Schottenfeld R, Howell S. Language production in 24-month-old inner-city children of cocaine- and other drug-using mothers. J Appl Dev Psychol 1999;20:159–80.
246. Frassica JJ, Orav EJ, Walsh EP, Lipshultz SE. Arrhythmias in children prenatally exposed to cocaine. Arch Pediatr Adolesc Med 1994;148(11):1163–9.
247. Bulbul ZR, Rosenthal DN, Kleinman CS. Myocardial infarction in the perinatal period secondary to maternal cocaine abuse. A case report and literature review. Arch Pediatr Adolesc Med 1994;148(10):1092–6.
248. McCann EM, Lewis K. Control of breathing in babies of narcotic- and cocaine-abusing mothers. Early Hum Dev 1991;27(3):175–86.
249. Zuckerman B, Maynard EC, Cabral H. A preliminary report of prenatal cocaine exposure and respiratory distress syndrome in premature infants. Am J Dis Child 1991;145(6):696–8.
250. Hand IL, Noble L, McVeigh TJ, Kim M, Yoon JJ. The effects of intrauterine cocaine exposure on the respiratory status of the very low birth weight infant. J Perinatol 2001;21(6):372–5.
251. Kesrouani A, Fallet C, Vuillard E, Jacqz-Aigrain E, Sibony O, Oury JF, Blot P, Luton D. Pathologic and laboratory correlation in microcephaly associated with prenatal cocaine exposure. Early Hum Dev 2001;63(2):79–81.
252. Bellini C, Massocco D, Serra G. Prenatal cocaine exposure and the expanding spectrum of brain malformations. Arch Intern Med 2000;160(15):2393.
253. Smith LM, Qureshi N, Renslo R, Sinow RM. Prenatal cocaine exposure and cranial sonographic findings in preterm infants. J Clin Ultrasound 2001;29(2):72–7.

254. Esmer MC, Rodriguez-Soto G, Carrasco-Daza D, Iracheta ML, Del Castillo V. Cloverleaf skull and multiple congenital anomalies in a girl exposed to cocaine in utero: case report and review of the literature. Childs Nerv Syst 2000;16(3):176–80.
255. Coles CD, Bard KA, Platzman KA, Lynch ME. Attentional response at eight weeks in prenatally drug-exposed and preterm infants. Neurotoxicol Teratol 1999;21(5):527–37.
256. Singer LT, Hawkins S, Huang J, Davillier M, Baley J. Developmental outcomes and environmental correlates of very low birthweight, cocaine-exposed infants. Early Hum Dev 2001;64(2):91–103.
257. Ukeje I, Bendersky M, Lewis M. Mother–infant interaction at 12 months in prenatally cocaine-exposed children. Am J Drug Alcohol Abuse 2001;27(2):203–24.
258. Singer LT, Arendt R, Minnes S, Salvator A, Siegel AC, Lewis BA. Developing language skills of cocaine-exposed infants. Pediatrics 2001;107(5):1057–64.
259. June R, Aks SE, Keys N, Wahl M. Medical outcome of cocaine bodystuffers. J Emerg Med 2000;18(2):221–4.
260. Gill JR, Graham SM. Ten years of "body packers" in New York City: 50 deaths. J Forensic Sci 2002;47(4):843–6.
261. Visser L, Stricker B, Hoogendoorn M, Vinks A. Do not give paraffin to packers. Lancet 1998;352(9137):1352.
262. Miller JS, Hendren SK, Liscum KR. Giant gastric ulcer in a body packer. J Trauma 1998;45(3):617–19.
263. Havlik DM, Nolte KB. Fatal "crack" cocaine ingestion in an infant. Am J Forensic Med Pathol 2000;21(3):245–8.
264. Sands BF, Ciraulo DA. Cocaine drug-drug interactions. J Clin Psychopharmacol 1992;12(1):49–55.
265. Signs SA, Dickey-White HI, Vanek VW, Perch S, Schechter MD, Kulics AT. The formation of cocaethylene and clinical presentation of ED patients testing positive for the use of cocaine and ethanol. Am J Emerg Med 1996; 14(7):665–70.
266. Salloum IM, Daley DC, Cornelius JR, Kirisci L, Thase ME. Disproportionate lethality in psychiatric patients with concurrent alcohol and cocaine abuse. Am J Psychiatry 1996;153(7):953–5.
267. Spunt B, Brownstein HH, Crimmins SM, Langley S. Drugs and homicide by women. Subst Use Misuse 1996; 31(7):825–45.
268. McCance-Katz EF, Kosten TR, Jatlow P. Concurrent use of cocaine and alcohol is more potent and potentially more toxic than use of either alone—a multiple-dose study. Biol Psychiatry 1998;44(4):250–9.
269. Pennings EJ, Leccese AP, Wolff FA. Effects of concurrent use of alcohol and cocaine. Addiction 2002; 97(7):773–83.
270. Hurtova M, Duclos-Vallee JC, Saliba F, Emile JF, Bemelmans M, Castaing D, Samuel D. Liver transplantation for fulminant hepatic failure due to cocaine intoxication in an alcoholic hepatitis C virus-infected patient. Transplantation 2002;73(1):157–8.
271. Weiner AL, Bayer MJ, McKay CA Jr, DeMeo M, Starr E. Anticholinergic poisoning with adulterated intranasal cocaine. Am J Emerg Med 1998;16(5):517–20.
272. Hameedi FA, Sernyak MJ, Navui SA, Kosten TR. Near syncope associated with concomitant clozapine and cocaine use. J Clin Psychiatry 1996;57(8):371–2.
273. Farren CK, Hameedi FA, Rosen MA, Woods S, Jatlow P, Kosten TR. Significant interaction between clozapine and cocaine in cocaine addicts. Drug Alcohol Depend 2000;59(2):153–63.
274. Cann B, Hunter R, McCann J. Cocaine/heroin induced rhabdomyolysis and ventricular fibrillation. Emerg Med J 2002;19(3):264–5.
275. Carlan SJ, Stromquist C, Angel JL, Harris M, O'Brien WF. Cocaine and indomethacin: fetal anuria, neonatal edema, and gastrointestinal bleeding. Obstet Gynecol 1991;78(3 Pt 2):501–3.
276. Tordoff SG, Stubbing JF, Linter SP. Delayed excitatory reaction following interaction of cocaine and monoamine oxidase inhibitor (phenelzine). Br J Anaesth 1991; 66(4):516–18.
277. van Harten PN, van Trier JC, Horwitz EH, Matroos GE, Hoek HW. Cocaine as a risk factor for neuroleptic-induced acute dystonia. J Clin Psychiatry 1998;59(3):128–30.
278. Kosten TR, Woods SW, Rosen MI, Pearsall HR. Interactions of cocaine with nimodipine: a brief report. Am J Addict 1999;8(1):77–81.
279. Matsuo S, Rao DB, Chaudry I, Foldes FF. Interaction of muscle relaxants and local anesthetics at the neuromuscular junction. Anesth Analg 1978;57(5):580–7.
280. Usubiaga JE, Wikinski JA, Morales RL, Usubiaga LE. Interaction of intravenously administered procaine, lidocaine and succinylcholine in anesthetized subjects. Anesth Analg 1967;46(1):39–45.

Cocamidopropyl betaine

General Information

Cocamidopropyl betaine is the most commonly used amphoteric surfactant in shampoos, bath products, and other cosmetic products. It is popular because of its relatively low irritation potential.

Organs and Systems

Immunologic

Contact allergic reactions are infrequent and have been attributed to sensitizing intermediates rather than cocamidopropyl betaine itself. Of 30 patients who were allergic to cocamidopropyl betaine, all reacted to 3-dimethylaminopropylamine (1). Two studies have shown that cocamidopropylamine is the more relevant impurity (2,3).

References

1. Angelini G, Foti C, Rigano L, Vena GA. 3-Dimethylaminopropylamine: a key substance in contact allergy to cocamidopropylbetaine? Contact Dermatitis 1995;32(2):96–9.
2. Fowler JF, Fowler LM, Hunter JE. Allergy to cocamidopropyl betaine may be due to amidoamine: a patch test and product use test study. Contact Dermatitis 1997; 37(6):276–81.
3. McFadden JP, Ross JS, White IR, Basketter DA. Clinical allergy to cocamidopropyl betaine: reactivity to cocamidopropylamine and lack of reactivity to 3-dimethylaminopropylamine. Contact Dermatitis 2001;45(2):72–4.

Codeine

See also Opioid analgesics

General Information

The pharmacodynamic and adverse effects of codeine are mainly due to *O*-demethylation by CYP2D6 to morphine or a metabolite of morphine (SEDA-21, 86) (SEDA-22, 5). Poor metabolizers may lack the analgesic effect of codeine.

In a retrospective study of patients with chronic rheumatological conditions, 290 of 644 clinic patients had received either codeine or oxycodone analgesia, of whom 137 had been given opioids for a continuous period of over 3 months (1). Adverse effects were described in 38% of both long-term and short-term opioid users, of which the most common were constipation, nausea, and sedation. Headache, dizziness, rash or itching, confusion, insomnia, depression, diarrhea, and myoclonic jerking were also reported. No significant differences in the adverse effects profile were reported between the groups and no subjects discontinued medication because of adverse effects. There were opioid abuse behaviors in 3% of the long-term users, but no association with a history of substance misuse was established.

A prospective double-blind, randomized study in 184 patients with cancers involved three treatment regimens (2): diclofenac alone (50 mg qds), diclofenac plus codeine (40 mg qds), or diclofenac plus imipramine (10–25 mg tds). There was no significant difference between the different treatments in terms of their analgesic effects, as measured on a visual analogue scale after 4 days. However, 10 of 61 subjects taking codeine withdrew because of adverse effects, compared with three taking imipramine group and two taking diclofenac alone. Gastrointestinal disturbances, dry mouth, and central nervous system disturbances were all more frequent in those taking codeine. These results suggest that the addition of a low-potency opioid to diclofenac fails to give enhanced analgesia while the frequency of opioid-related adverse effects increases.

Organs and Systems

Nervous system

Patients with migraine who use daily codeine or other opioids can be more susceptible to chronic daily headaches; this is evident in opiate overuse. In a pilot questionnaire study of 32 patients who used codeine or other opioids for control of their bowel motility after colectomy, chronic daily headaches occurred in those who were misusing opioids, but only if they had pre-existing migraine (3). The study had significant limitations, including the small sample size, diagnosis by means of a mailed questionnaire, a short duration of overuse of opioids, and the fact that it was uncontrolled.

Twelve cases of analgesic-related headache have been reported in children aged 6–16 years, half of whom were taking paracetamol in combination with codeine (4). Headaches occurred on at least 4 days per week and analgesic withdrawal led to symptom resolution in 50% and some improvement in the other cases.

Sensory systems

Reduced pupil size has been related to plasma codeine concentration (5).

Pancreas

Acute pancreatitis has been attributed to codeine (SEDA-21, 86), in one case in a patient taking co-codamol (paracetamol plus codeine) (6).

- A 20-year-old woman, who had previously taken paracetamol without adverse effects, took paracetamol 1 g and codeine 60 mg for a headache. After 3 hours she developed severe upper abdominal pain radiating to the back. The abdominal pain resolved within 24 hours of the administration of phloroglucinol and tiemonium. Her serum amylase activity was raised 3-fold and the serum lipase 15-fold. Other biochemical parameters, abdominal ultrasound, and an MRI scan were normal. Contrast-enhanced computed tomography showed pancreatic edema.

The previous use of paracetamol without adverse reactions supports the theory that the reaction was linked to the addition of codeine.

Four other cases of acute pancreatitis related to codeine have been reported (7).

- A 65-year-old man presented with severe abdominal pain 90 minutes after taking codeine and low-dose paracetamol. Serum amylase and lipase were significantly raised. Liver function tests were moderately abnormal. Abdominal ultrasound and CT scan showed edematous pancreatitis. Endoscopic retrograde cholangiography showed a papilla with a spastic appearance and an abnormal bile duct. He recovered completely, but 3 months later took codeine and paracetamol after a hemorrhoidectomy; abdominal pain recurred 1 hour later and acute pancreatitis was confirmed.
- A 26-year-old woman developed abdominal pain 2 days after taking codeine for a respiratory tract infection. Three hours later she complained of epigastric pain and vomiting. Her serum amylase and lipase were raised. Her symptoms resolved and the diagnosis was mild idiopathic pancreatitis. One week later she took codeine for similar respiratory symptoms. Two hours later she developed similar symptoms and a CT scan showed an enlarged and heterogeneous pancreas, with necrosis of the tail of the pancreas involving the left kidney. She responded to conservative treatment.
- A 53-year-old woman developed severe central abdominal and epigastric pain 90 minutes after taking codeine for migraine. Pancreatic amylase, lipase, and liver function tests were mildly raised. Abdominal ultrasound was consistent with acute pancreatitis.
- A 57-year-old woman developed severe abdominal pain 2 hours after taking codeine. She had had two similar episodes in the past, once with loperamide and once with codeine. An abdominal CT scan showed edematous acute pancreatitis.

In three of these cases unintentional rechallenge with codeine resulted in recurrence of the symptoms, and the diagnosis was confirmed radiologically and biochemically. All the patients had previously had a cholecystectomy, suggesting that this may increase the likelihood of codeine-induced pancreatitis. The authors speculated that codeine could cause a rise in biliary and/or pancreatic sphincter pressure in cholecystectomized patients, either by exacerbating pre-existing disease of the sphincter of Oddi or as a consequence of reduced storage capacity of the biliary tract, initiating acute pancreatitis. They cautioned that codeine-associated acute pancreatitis can be misconstrued—it may seem as if patients are taking codeine for pancreatic pain when in fact the codeine is producing the pain.

Skin

Rashes have been attributed to codeine.

- A 72-year-old man developed a generalized maculopapular rash 12 hours after taking co-codamol (codeine 10 mg plus paracetamol 500 mg) (8). The lesions persisted for 7 days, became scaly, and disappeared. He later reported a similar skin condition after having taken a combination of acetylsalicylic acid, codeine, and caffeine. Patch tests gave a positive result for codeine, suggesting a type IV allergic reaction.
- A 58-year-old man developed a maculopapular rash on the dorsal aspects of the hand and upper body 6 days after taking codeine as an analgesic for hemoptysis secondary to tuberculosis; on withdrawal of codeine, the rash subsided after 48 hours (9).

Two reports have highlighted the importance of using an oral provocation test and not a patch test to determine if codeine is the causative agent in non-urticarial skin lesions (10,11).

- A 58-year-old man developed a pruritic rash on the body and face, with periorbital swelling 3 hours after taking codeine 20 mg, acetylcysteine 600 mg, and acetylsalicylic acid 500 mg. An oral provocation test over 2 hours with codeine phosphate (1 mg, 4 mg, and 8 mg) precipitated a pruritic scarlatiniform rash for 24 hours, with swelling of the arms, starting 7 hours after the 8 mg dose. A rechallenge test confirmed the effect of codeine. Throughout this period, histamine release tests (CAST-ELISA with codeine) were negative.
- A 57-year-old patient presented with generalized malaise, fever, pruritus, and palpebral and labial angioedema 6 hours after taking a tablet containing paracetamol 500 mg, saccharin 10 mg, and codeine phosphate 30 mg. There was complete resolution in 8 hours, after treatment with prednisolone, hydroxyzine, and metamizole. Later a patch test with 1% codeine and an oral provocation test with paracetamol were both negative. Following an oral provocation test with codeine 5 mg, the patient developed similar symptoms.

Immunologic

True allergy to opioids is extremely rare. However, a near anaphylactic reaction in a patient taking codeine has been reported; the management of true codeine allergy was discussed and agents with different structures, such as phenylpiperidines or methadone-like compounds, are recommended (SEDA-17, 80).

Long-Term Effects

Drug abuse

Recreational use and abuse of codeine cough syrup is becoming more frequent. In a literature search of scientific journals and news media, complemented with in-depth interviews of 12 professionals working in the law enforcement or treatment aspects of drug abuse and 25 adults who reported using codeine syrup in the 30 days before their interview, the information provided useful insights into the different types of cough formulations, the reported reasons for their use, and the various types of administration (12). The effects of cough syrup, including their adverse effects, were reported. The most frequently mentioned negative effects included taste disturbance, prolonged sedation beyond the desired effect, loss of co-ordination, lethargy, constipation, and urinary retention. This qualitative study cannot be described as authoritative or representative, because of its limited nature, involving as it did only a small number of individuals living in the Houston area.

Drug dependence

In an exploratory survey among long-term codeine users recruited via newspaper advertisements in Toronto, Canada, more than 300 individuals who used codeine on at least 3 days per week for a minimum of 6 months and were older than 16 years were studied (13). Those who used codeine for pain related to malignancy were excluded. The mean age of the respondents included in the final analysis ($n = 339$) was 44 years and 51% were women. On average, the total number of years of regular codeine use was 12, with a current mean daily dose of 115 mg. About 60% ($n = 213$) had sought help for mental health problems, most commonly for depression (70%), followed by generalized anxiety (55%) and panic attacks (24%). One-third of the subjects ($n = 339$) identified at least one family member as having a mental health problem, with depression as the most frequent. Current antidepressant use was reported by 14% of the whole sample. Men used significantly higher doses of codeine than women; they also used the drug for a longer period and more commonly took it for pleasurable effects and under social pressure. Regular codeine users, in addition to having high rates of drug dependence, had raised scores on general measures of psychological distress and depressive symptoms. From the survey it was not clear to what extent these symptoms preceded codeine use and may have initiated the use and to what extent they were caused by codeine. The authors speculated that many respondents used codeine to modulate mood, particularly dysphoria, in the absence of more appropriate interventions. They suggested that understanding long-term codeine use and its relation to dysphoria may be important in designing both preventive and secondary treatment interventions.

The same investigators further analysed the data according to codeine abuse/dependent and non-dependent status (14). There was codeine abuse/dependence in 41% of the subjects. The most common psychological and physical problems attributed to codeine use in the dependent/abuse group ($n = 124$) were depression (23%), anxiety (22%), gastrointestinal disturbances (15%), constipation (6%), and headache/migraine (5%). The codeine-dependent subjects were younger than those who were not dependent. The mean age of the respondents when they first started using codeine was 26 (range 2–78) years. A total of 563 codeine products had been used on a regular basis; the most common combination involved codeine with paracetamol (70%). Codeine was used for headaches (41%), back pain (22%), and other types of pain (25%). Those in the dependent group were more likely to have used codeine initially for other reasons, for example for pleasure and to relax or reduce stress. Most subjects said that they had obtained their codeine from one physician (66%) or by purchasing it over the counter (54%). Subjects in the dependent group also obtained codeine from friends (32%), from family (11%), "off the street" (19%), and through prescriptions from more than one physician (11%). Overall, more subjects in the dependent group considered themselves to have problems with a larger number of substances (3.3: range 0–15) compared with those in the non-dependent group (1.2: range 0–8). In the dependent group, more subjects said that their physical or mental health problems interfered with normal social activities at least "quite a bit." Significantly more subjects in the dependent group had sought help for a mental health problem, had had an inpatient psychiatric admission, or had sought help for a substance-use disorder, especially alcohol and stimulants. A larger number of subjects in the dependent group identified at least one family member (usually male) with substance-use problems compared with those in the non-dependent group.

This study suggests that codeine dependence may be more common in the general population than has been previously thought. The authors suggested that it is important to identify those with codeine abuse or codeine dependence, since they may be using substantial doses of codeine for apparently little benefit compared to the risks. Furthermore, there are also health risks of associated chronic use of paracetamol and a potential for analgesic rebound headache.

Drug Administration

Drug dosage regimens

In a comparison of the adverse effects of 30, 60, and 90 mg codeine the most frequent adverse effects, headache, drowsiness, nausea, thirst, and a feeling of strangeness, occurred after 60 and 90 mg doses only. Visuomotor co-ordination was altered with 60 and 90 mg and dynamic visual acuity with 90 mg only (15).

Drug–Drug Interactions

Amitriptyline

There were signs of opiate toxicity, reversible with naloxone, in an 80-year-old woman after concomitant treatment with amitriptyline and co-codamol (codeine plus paracetamol) (SEDA-18, 79).

Inhibitors of CYP2D6

Inhibitors of CYP2D6 can reduce or abolish the analgesic effects of codeine (16).

Quinidine

Quinidine inhibits the hepatic metabolism of codeine to morphine. Whether this diminishes or abolishes the analgesic effect of codeine is uncertain (17,18).

References

1. Ytterberg SR, Mahowald ML, Woods SR. Codeine and oxycodone use in patients with chronic rheumatic disease pain. Arthritis Rheum 1998;41(9):1603–12.
2. Minotti V, De Angelis V, Righetti E, Celani MG, Rossetti R, Lupatelli M, Tonato M, Pisati R, Monza G, Fumi G, Del Favero A. Double-blind evaluation of short-term analgesic efficacy of orally administered diclofenac, diclofenac plus codeine, and diclofenac plus imipramine in chronic cancer pain. Pain 1998;74 (2–3):133–7.
3. Wilkinson SM, Becker WJ, Heine JA. Opiate use to control bowel motility may induce chronic daily headache in patients with migraine. Headache 2001; 41(3):303–9.
4. Symon DN. Twelve cases of analgesic headache. Arch Dis Child 1998;78(6):555–6.
5. Peacock JE, Henderson PD, Nimmo WS. Changes in pupil diameter after oral administration of codeine. Br J Anaesth 1988;61(5):598–600.
6. Renkes P, Trechot P. Acetaminophen–codeine combination induced acute pancreatitis. Pancreas 1998; 16(4):556–7.
7. Hastier P, Buckley MJ, Peten EP, Demuth N, Dumas R, Demarquay JF, Caroli-Bosc FX, Delmont JP. A new source of drug-induced acute pancreatitis: codeine. Am J Gastroenterol 2000;95(11):3295–8.
8. Estrada JL, Puebla MJ, de Urbina JJ, Matilla B, Prieto MA, Gozalo F. Generalized eczema due to codeine. Contact Dermatitis 2001;44(3):185.
9. Rodriguez Arroyo LA, Ortiz de Saracho J, Pantoja Zarza L, Gonzalez Valle O. Reacción adversa cutánea tras administración de codeina. [Adverse cutaneous side-effect of codeine administration.] Aten Primaria 2001; 27(6):444–6.
10. Mohrenschlager M, Glockner A, Jessberger B, Worret WI, Ollert M, Rakoski J, Ring J. Codeine caused pruritic scarlatiniform exanthemata: patch test negative but positive to oral provocation test. Br J Dermatol 2000;143(3):663–4.
11. Vidal C, Perez-Leiros P, Bugarin R, Armisen M. Fever and urticaria to codeine. Allergy 2000;55(4):416–17.
12. Elwood WN. Sticky business: patterns of procurement and misuse of prescription cough syrup in Houston. J Psychoactive Drugs 2001;33(2):121–33.

13. Romach MK, Sproule BA, Sellers EM, Somer G, Busto UE. Long-term codeine use is associated with depressive symptoms. J Clin Psychopharmacol 1999; 19(4):373–6.
14. Sproule BA, Busto UE, Somer G, Romach MK, Sellers EM. Characteristics of dependent and nondependent regular users of codeine. J Clin Psychopharmacol 1999; 19(4):367–72.
15. Bradley CM, Nicholson AN. Effects of a mu-opioid receptor agonist (codeine phosphate) on visuo-motor coordination and dynamic visual acuity in man. Br J Clin Pharmacol 1986;22(5):507–12.
16. Sindrup SH, Brosen K, Bjerring P, Arendt-Nielsen L, Larsen U, Angelo HR, Gram LF. Codeine increases pain thresholds to copper vapor laser stimuli in extensive but not poor metabolizers of sparteine. Clin Pharmacol Ther 1990;48(6):686–93.
17. Desmeules J, Gascon MP, Dayer P, Magistris M. Impact of environmental and genetic factors on codeine analgesia. Eur J Clin Pharmacol 1991;41(1):23–6.
18. Sindrup SH, Arendt-Nielsen L, Brosen K, Bjerring P, Angelo HR, Eriksen B, Gram LF. The effect of quinidine on the analgesic effect of codeine. Eur J Clin Pharmacol 1992;42(6):587–91.

Co-dergocrine

General Information

Co-dergocrine is the British Approved Name for a formulation that contains a combination of dihydrogenated ergot alkaloids: dihydroergocornine mesilate, dihydroergocristine mesilate, and (in the ratio 2:1) α- and β-dihydroergocryptine mesilates. It has been used for its supposed therapeutic effects on mood depression, confusion, and lack of self-care in the elderly, and purportedly acts by improving cerebral blood flow. The basis of these indications has been reviewed and has not been fully validated (1)(2)(3).

Surprisingly few adverse effects have been reported. They include sinus bradycardia, nausea, and a single report of vasospastic angiitis (4).

References

1. Hollister LE, Yesavage J. Ergoloid mesylates for senile dementias: unanswered questions. Ann Intern Med 1984;100(6):894–8.
2. Anonymous. Deapril-ST for senile dementia. Med Lett Drugs Ther 1977;19(15):61–2.
3. Olin J, Schneider L, Novit A, Luczak S. Hydergine for dementia. Cochrane Database Syst Rev 2001; (2):CD000359.
4. O'Cayley AC, Macpherson A, Wedgwood J. Sinus bradycardia following treatment with hydergine for cerebrovascular insufficiency. BMJ 1975;4(5993):384–5.

Colchicine

General Information

Colchicine is an antimitotic agent, highly effective in the treatment of gout, but associated with considerable toxicity. Diarrhea is used as a criterion for adequate dosage. Accidental overdosage occurs relatively often and can be dangerous. For these reasons, NSAIDs (except aspirin) are often used in acute gout instead of colchicine.

There is controversy about the long-term toxicity of colchicine. In familial Mediterranean fever, low dosages of colchicine (1–2 mg/day) for 15–18 years have been well tolerated, even by young patients (SEDA-16, 114).

Organs and Systems

Nervous system

Neuropathy, polyneuritis, toxic encephalitis, delirium, and coma have occurred only in severe colchicine intoxication. During prolonged treatment, neuritis, muscular weakness and myopathy occur more commonly than was previously thought in patients with impaired renal function. In some cases the neuromyopathy was part of multiorgan system failure, but in others the syndrome was not accompanied by other features of colchicine toxicity. Patients taking long-term colchicine should take low dosages (probably no more than 0.6 mg/day) and have their serum creatine kinase monitored (SEDA-12, 94).

Metabolism

Transient diabetes and hyperlipidemia have been reported. Metabolic acidosis is probably a consequence of heavy, cholera-like diarrhea. Progressive reduction of libido was attributed to colchicine in patients with familial Mediterranean fever (1).

Electrolyte balance

Water and electrolyte disturbances, including inappropriate antidiuresis, can occur in patients who have taken high doses of colchicine (2,3), including hypernatremia and polyuria (4).

Hematologic

Bone marrow depression is common after colchicine overdose and intoxication and less common in therapeutic doses. Fatal cases of agranulocytosis are more often associated with bone marrow aplasia (SEDA-4, 70) (5). Bone marrow depression usually occurs between the third and sixth days of acute intoxication. Cytoplasmic inclusions in neutrophils and megaloblastic anemia have been described. Administration of therapeutic doses intravenously and orally to two patients with reduced renal function caused profound prolonged neutropenia complicated by septicemia, which ended in death (SEDA-13, 84).

Gastrointestinal

Gastrointestinal symptoms often develop after therapeutic doses and are even used for dose titration. Diarrhea is often followed by nausea, vomiting, and abdominal pain. Long-term therapy can provoke steatorrhea, malabsorption, and defects in intestinal enzyme activity (6).

Urinary tract

Acute renal insufficiency has been associated with colchicine intoxication (7).

Skin

Blood dyscrasias are associated with ecchymosis and purpura. Allergic skin changes are rare. Alopecia is common after acute intoxication and prolonged treatment (SEDA-5, 109). A fixed drug eruption has been reported (SEDA-21, 109).

Musculoskeletal

Acute rhabdomyolysis with fever, muscle cramps, rises in creatine phosphokinase and lactic acid dehydrogenase activity, phlebitis at the injection site, and transitory leukopenia and thrombocytopenia have been reported (8).

Second-Generation Effects

Fertility

Reversible azoospermia (later not confirmed) was observed after long-term treatment with colchicines (9).

Pregnancy

Owing to its antimitotic properties, colchicine should not be given during pregnancy (SED-9, 158) (10).

Susceptibility Factors

Renal disease

The dosage of colchicine should be adjusted according to creatinine clearance during long-term use to avoid the risk of myoneuropathy (SEDA-16, 114). Colchicine should not be used in patients undergoing hemodialysis, since it cannot be removed by either dialysis or exchange transfusion (11).

Drug Administration

Drug administration route

Intravenous administration is potentially much more toxic than oral administration; because of its unfavorable benefit to harm, balance and the availability of less dangerous treatments, colchicine should not be given intravenously (SEDA-5, 109) (SEDA-13, 84) (SEDA-16, 115).

Drug overdose

Acute intoxication with colchicine occurs relatively often, because the therapeutic dose is close to the toxic dose. Gastrointestinal, hematological, and neurological reactions are the most frequent effects (SEDA-7, 118). An accidental overdose of colchicine by nasal insufflation has been reported in a young male drug abuser who had mistaken it for metamfetamine. The effects included gastrointestinal distress, myalgia, thrombocytopenia, hypocalcemia, and hypophosphatemia (12). Electrolyte disturbances can occur (2–4). Deaths have been reported (3).

Drug–Drug Interactions

Ciclosporin

Acute reversible ciclosporin toxicity occurred in a renal transplant patient a few days after colchicine was administered for an acute attack of gout (SEDA-16, 115). Other potential adverse effects of combining colchicine with ciclosporin include diarrhea, increases in serum liver enzymes, bilirubin, and creatinine, and less often severe myalgia (SEDA-19, 101). Acute myopathy, associated with neuropathy in one case, has been observed in two young renal transplant recipients (SEDA-22, 119).

References

1. Peters RS, Lehman TJ, Schwabe AD. Colchicine use for familial Mediterranean fever. Observations associated with long-term treatment. West J Med 1983;138(1):43–6.
2. Gaultier M, Bismuth C, Autret A, Pillon M. Anti-diurèse inappropriée après intoxication aiguë par la colchicine. 2 cas. [Inappropriate antidiuresis after acute colchicine poisoning. 2 cases.] Nouv Presse Méd 1975;4(44):3132–4.
3. Milne ST, Meek PD. Fatal colchicine overdose: report of a case and review of the literature. Am J Emerg Med 1998;16(6):603–8.
4. Usalan C, Altun B, Ulusoy S, Erdem Y, Yasavul U, Turgan C, Caglar S. Hypernatraemia and polyuria due to high-dose colchicine in a suicidal patient. Nephrol Dial Transplant 1999;14(6):1556–7.
5. Liu YK, Hymowitz R, Carroll MG. Marrow aplasia induced by colchicine. A case report. Arthritis Rheum 1978;21(6):731–5.
6. Ben-Chetrit E, Levy M. Colchicine: 1998 update. Semin Arthritis Rheum 1998;28(1):48–59.
7. Rosset L, Descombes E, Fellay G, Regamey C. Toxicité multisystèmique de la colchicine et insuffisance rènale: à propos d'un cas. [Multi-systemic toxicity of colchicine and renal failure: apropos of a case.] Schweiz Med Wochenschr 1998;128(49):1953–7.
8. Letellier P, Langeard M, Agullo M. Rhabdomyolise secondaire à une série d'injections intraveineuses de colchicine. J Med Caen 1979;14:157.
9. Merlin HE. Azoospermia caused by colchicine—a case report. Fertil Steril 1972;23(3):180–1.
10. Wallace SL, Ertel NH. Colchicine: current problems. Bull Rheum Dis 1969;20(4):582–7.
11. Rieger EH, Halasz NA, Wahlstrom HE. Colchicine neuromyopathy after renal transplantation. Transplantation 1990;49(6):1196–8.
12. Baldwin LR, Talbert RL, Samples R. Accidental overdose of insufflated colchicine. Drug Saf 1990;5(4):305–12.

Collagen and gelatin

General Information

Collagen is a natural fibrous protein found in human cartilage, connective tissue, and bone. Glutaraldehyde cross-linked bovine collagen is a sterile, biocompatible, biodegradable, purified bovine dermocollagen cross-linked with glutaraldehyde, mixed in a phosphate-buffered saline solution.

Purified solubilized bovine collagen is used as biomaterial for the treatment of soft tissue defects and has been used for the treatment of stress urinary incontinence since the late 1980s (1). Injected material precipitates at body temperature, forming a matrix allowing fibroblastic infiltration and formation of new tissue. It has been used for cosmetic purposes by injection in the dermis to correct scars and other contour deformities of the skin.

Urethral injection of bovine collagen under local anesthesia is considered safe and effective, with minimal complications (2,3). It has low antigenicity and is associated with a minimal inflammatory response, although foreign body reactions have occasionally been reported (4). However, antibody formation is not impossible (5). Patients with a history of allergic reactions to bovine collagen-derived products should be investigated because of the widespread use of collagen-derived therapeutic devices, the potential for immunological cross-reactivity with dietary collagen (gelatin), and the potential for anaphylaxis.

Gelatin is an important constituent of many drug formulations, including capsules and suppositories. It is also found in some volume replacement solutions (for example Gelofusine). Gelofusine is a colloidal plasma volume expander used in the treatment of hypotension. It is prepared from bovine collagen. Severe anaphylactoid reactions after gelofusine occur with an incidence that has been reported at between 0.066 and 0.345% of cases. They are more common in those with known drug allergy and in men. The mechanism may be triggering of non-immune complement C3 activation by colloid particles in the gelatine formulation or by combination with components in the patient's blood (6).

Organs and Systems

Cardiovascular

Hypotension has been described in a patient who received 500 ml of gelofusine during surgery for an infrarenal abdominal aneurysm (7). Within 5 minutes there was a significant fall in blood pressure, in the absence of surgical bleeding and ischemic changes on the electrocardiogram. There was no change in oxygenation. A further 500 ml of gelofusine was rapidly infused, with an additional fall in blood pressure to 50/30. Subsequently, after recovery, a small test dose (100 ml) of gelofusine reproduced the transient hypotension.

A patient undergoing anesthesia for coronary artery bypass surgery developed a probable anaphylactic reaction to Gelofusine (8). The principal feature of the reaction was cardiovascular depression. An infusion of the angiotensin analogue angiotensinamide was effective in treating the reaction.

Urinary tract

Few complications of urethral injection of collagen have been reported, including urinary tract infection, bleeding, and transient urinary retention. During a prospective, cohort study in 337 women to determine the effectiveness of and adverse effects associated with transurethral collagen injection for treatment of stress urinary incontinence, there were three cases of delayed allergic reactions at the skin test site associated with arthralgia (9). Delayed reactions at the skin test site occurred in three patients (0.9%), and were associated with arthralgias in two. The incidence and systemic nature of this type of reaction led the authors of the study to conclude that glutaraldehyde cross-linked collagen injection is not as innocuous as previously believed, and clinicians were advised to consider double skin testing before treatment. The overall risk of complications in any given individual of this study population was 20% (1), although irritating lower urinary tract symptoms after collagen injection could be related to local inflammatory changes, persistence and eventually worsening of these symptoms should suggest the presence of iatrogenic bladder outlet obstruction (10). Urethral prolapse (11) and unusually long collagen persistence (12) after periurethral collagen injection have also been reported.

Immunologic

Bovine collagen is contraindicated in patients with immunological disorders and reports of delayed allergic reactions underline the need for adequate follow-up when collagen implants are used. Patients should be tested with bovine collagen and reassessed at 4 weeks. About 3% of the patients tested in this way developed hypersensitivity reactions to collagen, whereas 1% of treated patients have symptoms of hypersensitivity at treatment sites (13). In this series, erythema was the sole symptom in 24%, and erythema and induration occurred in an additional 42%. Of the patients with complications, 45% reported an onset of symptoms within 10 days while in 22% the onset was more than 30 days following treatment with collagen. Abscesses as a manifestation of hypersensitivity to bovine collagen occur rarely (four in 10 000 cases), but the possibility of contamination should always be considered. Local tissue necrosis occurs rarely after implantation (nine reported in 10 000 cases) and this is thought to be the result of local vascular interruption rather than a hypersensitivity reaction. The incidence varies widely according to the site of implantation, but more than one-half of the cases involve the glabellar region, probably because of its special vascular distribution (14).

Anaphylactic reactions to collagen have been described (15). Despite pretreatment collagen testing, anaphylactic shock has been reported in one patient, necessitating adrenergic agents and glucocorticoids.

An allergic rash has been described after collagen injection (16).

Delayed hypersensitivity reactions after bovine collagen injection for stress urinary incontinence have been reported.

- A 50-year-old woman had a negative collagen skin test for 4 weeks (9). After an injection of transurethral collagen, she developed a flare-up at the skin test site and subsequently had recurrent flares at 21–26 day intervals for six cycles, which corresponded to her menses and were thought to be hormone-related.
- A 64-year-old woman with recurrent urinary leakage elected to undergo conservative therapy with collagen injection, had no reaction to a collagen skin test, and had an uneventful transurethral injection of collagen 30 days later (17). Her postoperative course was complicated by urethritis, trigonitis, severe urge, bilateral leg arthralgias, leg pain relieved by massage, and leg edema at 6 weeks. She had a total voided volume of 300 ml and a postvoid residual of 180 ml, and was started on intermittent self-catheterization for urinary retention. Induration at the skin injection test site was noticeable 9 weeks after the injection. Her severe urge, leg edema, and pain gradually resolved after 13 months, but her stress incontinence continued without relief.
- A 50-year-old woman with stress urinary incontinence chose a trial of transurethral injection of collagen (18). A skin test showed no evidence of allergy at 1 month and collagen 2.5 ml was injected transurethrally without problems but with little improvement. A second injection of 2.5 ml 5 weeks later was again uneventful, but 2 weeks later she began to have difficulty in emptying her bladder, with a poor stream and a sense of incomplete emptying. At the same time she noticed redness and firmness at the initial skin test site on her arm, which had previously been benign.

Several reports have highlighted the importance of gelatin allergy in young children, with some deaths due to anaphylaxis. Elsewhere, anaphylactoid reactions have been reported to gelatin-containing injectables (SEDA-20, 310).

- A 2-year-old and a 4-year-old boy developed anaphylactic symptoms after being given a chloral hydrate suppository, which contained gelatin, for sedation before electroencephalography (19).

The authors suggested using gelatin-free formulations in children.

References

1. Stothers L, Goldenberg SL, Leone EF. Complications of periurethral collagen injection for stress urinary incontinence. J Urol 1998;159(3):806–7.
2. Winters JC, Appell R. Periurethral injection of collagen in the treatment of intrinsic sphincteric deficiency in the female patient. Urol Clin North Am 1995;22(3):673–8.
3. Appell RA. Collagen injection therapy for urinary incontinence. Urol Clin North Am 1994;21(1):177–82.
4. Moody BR, Sengelmann RD. Self-limited adverse reaction to human-derived collagen injectable product. Dermatol Surg 2000;26(10):936–8.
5. Bonnet C, Charriere G, Vaquier J, Bertin P, Vergne P, Treves R. Bovine collagen induced systemic symptoms: antibody formation against bovine and human collagen. J Rheumatol 1996;23(3):545–7.
6. Laxenaire MC, Charpentier C, Feldman L. Reactions anaphylactoïdes aux substituts colloidaux du plasma: incidence, facteurs de risque, mécanismes. Enquête prospective multicentrique française. Groupe français d'Etude de la Tolerance des Substituts Plasmatiques. [Anaphylactoid reactions to colloid plasma substitutes: incidence, risk factors, mechanisms. A French multicenter prospective study.] Ann Fr Anesth Reanim 1994;13(3):301–10.
7. Walker SR, MacSweeney ST. Plasma expanders used to treat or prevent hypotension can themselves cause hypotension. Postgrad Med J 1998;74(874):492–3.
8. McKinnon RP, Sinclair CJ. Angiotensinamide in the treatment of probable anaphylaxis to succinylated gelatin (Gelofusine). Anaesthesia 1994;49(4):309–11.
9. Stothers L, Goldenberg SL. Delayed hypersensitivity and systemic arthralgia following transurethral collagen injection for stress urinary incontinence. J Urol 1998;159(5):1507–9.
10. Bernier PA, Zimmern PE, Saboorian MH, Chassagne S. Female outlet obstruction after repeated collagen injections. Urology 1997;50(4):618–21.
11. Harris RL, Cundiff GW, Coates KW, Addison WA, Bump RC. Urethral prolapse after collagen injection. Am J Obstet Gynecol 1998;178(3):614–15.
12. Lee SS, Robichaux W, Elsergany RE, Ghoniem GM. Persistence of injectable collagen in human urethra: case report. Urology 1996;47(6):940–1.
13. DeLustro F, Smith ST, Sundsmo J, Salem G, Kincaid S, Ellingsworth L. Reaction to injectable collagen: results in animal models and clinical use. Plast Reconstr Surg 1987;79(4):581–94.
14. Hanke CW, Higley HR, Jolivette DM, Swanson NA, Stegman SJ. Abscess formation and local necrosis after treatment with Zyderm or Zyplast collagen implant. J Am Acad Dermatol 1991;25(2 Pt 1):319–26.
15. Mullins RJ, Richards C, Walker T. Allergic reactions to oral, surgical and topical bovine collagen. Anaphylactic risk for surgeons. Aust NZ J Ophthalmol 1996;24(3):257–60.
16. Lipsky H. Endoscopic treatment of vesicoureteral reflux with collagen. Pediatr Surg Int 1991;6:301–3.
17. Echols KT, Chesson RR, Breaux EF, Shobeiri SA. Persistence of delayed hypersensitivity following transurethral collagen injection for recurrent urinary stress incontinence. Int Urogynecol J Pelvic Floor Dysfunct 2002;13(1):52–4.
18. Ginsberg DA, Boyd SD. Permanent urinary retention after transurethral injection of collagen. J Urol 2002;167(2 Pt 1):648.
19. Yamada A, Ohshima Y, Tsukahara H, Hiraoka M, Kimura I, Kawamitsu T, Kimura K, Mayumi M. Two cases of anaphylactic reaction to gelatin induced by a chloral hydrate suppository. Pediatr Int 2002;44(1):87–9.

Complementary and alternative medicine

General Information

Complementary and alternative medicine (also referred to as "non-orthodox," "unconventional," "holistic," and "integrative" medicine) comprises a heterogeneous array of treatments, from acupuncture to spinal manipulation and from herbal medicine to homeopathy. The techniques covered in this monograph are:

- Acupuncture
- Aromatherapy
- Cell therapy
- Homeopathy
- Hypnosis
- Manipulation
- Massage.

Herbal products and animal products are covered in separate monographs.

Complementary medicine continues to be a growth area (1). A survey conducted in South Australia showed that almost half of the 3004 respondents had used at least one type of complementary remedy in the previous 12 months and that one-fifth had consulted a practitioner of complementary medicine (2). In European countries for which estimates on the annual utilization of complementary medicine are available, estimates range from 20 to 50% of the population (3). In the UK, retail sales of complementary medicines (licensed herbal medicines, homoeopathic remedies, essential oils used in aromatherapy) were estimated to be £72 million in 1996, an increase of 36% in real terms since 1991 (4). This, however, is likely to be a gross underestimate as popular products sold as food supplements, including *Ginkgo biloba* and garlic, were not included. According to a detailed analysis of the herbal medicines market in Germany and France, total sales of herbal products in those countries in 1997 were US$1.8 billion and US$1.1 billion respectively (5). In 1994, annual retail sales of botanical medicines in the US were estimated to be around US$1.6 billion; in 1998, the figure was closer to US$4 billion (6).

Some of the most useful data on trends in complementary medicine use come from two surveys of US adults carried out in 1991 and 1997/8, which involved over 1500 and over 2000 individuals respectively (7,8). The use of at least one form of complementary therapy in the 12 months preceding the survey increased significantly from 34% in 1990 to 42% in 1997 (8) and in November 1998 all 10 journals of the American Medical Association published theme issues on the subject.

The reasons for the popularity of complementary medicine are many and diverse. It appears that complementary medicine is not usually used because of an outright rejection of conventional medicine, but more because users desire to control their own health (9) and because they find complementary medicine to be more congruent with their own values, beliefs, and philosophical orientations toward health and life (10). Also, users may consult different practitioners for different reasons (9). An important reason for the increase in use is that consumers (often motivated by the lay press) consider complementary medicine to be "natural" and assume it is "safe." Of all patients attending an emergency department in the USA 43% had used at least one complementary therapy at some time and 24% were current users (11). All complementary treatments were considered to be safe by 16% of the patients and 33% of all users failed to tell their physicians. Furthermore, 15% of the women and 7% of the men believed that complementary therapies do not interact with other medications. As the popularity of complementary medicine rises, so does the research interest in this subject (12), including research into direct and indirect risks (13–15).

However, this notion is dangerously misleading; adverse effects have been associated with the use of complementary therapies (16). Furthermore, complementary therapies may not only be directly harmful (for example adverse effects of herbal formulations), but like other medical treatments have the potential to be indirectly harmful (for example through being applied incompetently, by delaying appropriate effective treatment, or by causing needless expense) (17).

The efficacy of many complementary therapies is largely unknown, and more definitive evidence is urgently needed (18). Like any other interventions, complementary therapies are associated with adverse effects, and for responsible therapeutic decision-making, the balance of benefits and harms must be considered (19).

Incidence of adverse effects

Most of the data on adverse effects associated with complementary therapies is anecdotal, and assessment and classification of causality is often not possible. Likewise, there have been few attempts to determine systematically the incidence of adverse effects of non-orthodox therapies.

Two prospective interview surveys have generated incidence figures for adverse effects associated with chiropractic treatment. In a Norwegian investigation (20), 102 chiropractors were asked to monitor 1058 new patients. At least one adverse effect was reported by 55% of the patients at some time during the course of a maximum of six treatments. The most common adverse effects were local discomfort (53% of total), headache (12%), tiredness (11%), or radiating discomfort (10%). A Swedish survey used similar methods to monitor 1858 chiropractic consultations and demonstrated an incidence rate for adverse effects of 44% (21). In both studies, all effects noted were mild and transient; no serious effects were recorded.

In a prospective Japanese survey of adverse effects of acupuncture, 55 291 treatments were monitored between 1992 and 1997 (22). There were 64 adverse events in all; none was serious or led to permanent damage.

General adverse effects

Even a perfectly safe remedy (mainstream or unorthodox) can become unsafe when used incompetently. Medical competence can be defined as doing everything in the best interest of the patient according to the best available evidence. There are numerous circumstances, both in orthodox and complementary medicine, when competence is jeopardized:

- missed diagnosis
- misdiagnosis
- disregarding contraindications
- preventing/delaying more effective treatments (for example misinformation about effective therapies, loss of herd immunity through negative attitude towards immunization)

- clinical deterioration not diagnosed
- adverse reaction not diagnosed
- discontinuation of prescribed drugs
- self-medication.

The most obvious danger is that some patients (or their parents) may elect to abandon conventional therapies for serious diseases in favor of alternative approaches. This can have fatal consequences (23). Survey data suggest that a sizeable proportion of complementary practitioners advise their clients to reduce their prescribed medication (24).

Diagnostic techniques can also cause serious risks; an example is the apparent over-use of X-rays by chiropractors (25). Although this practice seems to be in decline, it can put patients at risk through the mutagenic effects of X-rays.

The attitude of consumers towards complementary medicine may also constitute a risk. When 515 users of herbal remedies were interviewed about their behavior vis-a-vis adverse effects of herbal versus synthetic over-the-counter drugs, a clear difference emerged. While 26% would consult their doctor for a serious adverse effect of a synthetic medication, only 0.8% would do the same in relation to an herbal remedy (26). A further risk might lie in the plethora of lay books on complementary medicine now available in every High Street bookstore. A pilot project has attempted to evaluate the value of a random selection of such books and concluded that the lay literature on complementary medicine is far from adequate and has the potential to put the health of the reader at risk (27).

The fear has been expressed that "with the increased interest in alternative medicine, we [shall] see a reversion to irrational approaches to medical practice" (28). The only way to minimize incompetence is proper education and training, combined with responsible regulatory control. While training and control are self-evident features of mainstream medicine they are often not fully incorporated in complementary medicine. Thus the issue of indirect health risk is particularly pertinent to complementary medicine. Whenever complementary practitioners take full responsibility for a patient, this should be matched with full medical competence; if on the other hand, competence is not demonstrably complete, the practitioner in question should not assume full responsibility (29).

Misinformation

More and more patients seek advice on complementary medicine via the Internet. It is therefore important to monitor the validity of such advice. In one survey, most of the 13 most popular websites on complementary medicine for cancer recommended cancer therapies for which there was no evidence of efficacy (30). Three of the sites overtly discouraged cancer patients from using conventional therapies. When the study was repeated, this time focussing on HIV instead of cancer, the results were virtually identical (31). These findings were similar to those of another study of 61 popular websites on herbal medicines for cancer (32). Most of these sites were commercial by nature and claimed cancer cures through herbal medicines, with little regard for current regulations.

Herbalists readily volunteer advice about the administration of herbal medicines during pregnancy, but the nature of their advice is misleading at best and dangerous at worst (33). Others have studied the impact of herbal medicine on the use of conventional treatments (34). Their results showed that 32% of female patients in internal medicine delayed obtaining conventional care while waiting for an herbal medicine to work.

Attitudes to immunization

The indirect risks of complementary medicine are grossly under-researched, and at present we can but guess the size of the problem (35). There are, however, particular aspects on which some data do exist. One is the attitude of practitioners towards immunization. The majority of homeopaths (36–38) and chiropractors (39) are unconvinced of the benefit of immunization. They claim that it causes more illness than it prevents disease and advise, in many instances successfully, their patients against it (40).

When 1593 visitors to a "health fair" were surveyed on their use of complementary medicine, it emerged that elderly users were significantly less likely to use influenza immunization (41). Students of a Canadian chiropractic college were questioned about whether they agreed with immunization in general. The longer they had attended college, the less favorable their attitude toward immunization became (42). An analysis of the contents of 22 leading anti-immunization websites showed that about 70% of these sites claimed that homeopathy represented an alternative to conventional vaccination (43). In a similar study it was found that 39% of the anti-immunization websites claimed that natural lifestyle conveys immunity to infections, thus allegedly rendering immunization unnecessary, and 45% claimed that "alternative health" is superior to immunization (44). In another study homeopaths and chiropractors were specifically asked about their advice regarding MMR immunization; 40% of the homeopaths and 19% of the chiropractors admitted advising mothers against it (45).

This attitude not only exposes individual patients to unjustifiable risks, but also jeopardizes herd immunity, thus representing a threat to public health. A homeopathic remedy might be totally safe, but the homeopath might not be (46).

Acupuncture

On a global basis, acupuncture is one of the most commonly used forms of complementary and alternative medicine. It is used predominantly to alleviate pain, but many other indications have been proposed. Contrary to prevailing public opinion it is not entirely risk free (47). Several review articles have addressed this issue, and it has been pointed out that tissue trauma (for example pneumothorax) and infections (for example hepatitis B) are the most common complications of acupuncture (48). Both are rare and both could be avoidable with adequate training and experience of acupuncturists.

Acupuncture can cause various minor adverse effects (49) and there have been many reports of serious complications (Table 1). The authors of a review of the risks

Table 1 The most common serious complications of acupuncture

Condition	Number of cases in the world literature
Cardiac trauma	<10
Contact dermatitis	<10
Drowsiness	~100
Endocarditis	<10
Erythema	<10
Hepatitis	~130
Perichondritis	~10
Peripheral nerve injury	<10
Pneumothorax	>90
Renal injury	~20
Retained needle	~10
Septicemia	<10
Spinal cord injury	~20
Syncope	~50

associated with acupuncture mentioned pneumothorax (more than 90 cases on record), cardiac tamponade ($n = 6$), injuries of the spinal cord ($n = 10$), and infections ($n = 126$), particularly hepatitis (50).

Some reports of complications after acupuncture are summarized in Table 2.

Acupuncture keeps being associated with serious adverse events (61), and several attempts to define the size of this problem more closely have been published.

In a prospective investigation of the adverse effects of Japanese acupuncture, all adverse effects experienced by patients in an acupuncture clinic seen between November 1992 and October 1997 were recorded (22). There were 64 adverse events. Failure to remove the needles, dizziness, discomfort, and sweating were the most frequent adverse reactions. There were no serious adverse events. These data suggest that superficial needling as used in Japanese acupuncture is relatively safe.

A Japanese survey of 391 patients who received acupuncture in 1441 treatment sessions involving a total of 30 338 needle insertions showed the following systemic adverse effects: tiredness (8.2%), drowsiness (2.8%), aggravation of the presenting condition (2.8%), itching in the punctured region (1.0%), dizziness or vertigo (0.8%), faintness or nausea during treatment (0.8%), headache (0.5%), and chest pain (0.3%) (62). The incidences of local reactions were: minor bleeding after withdrawal of the needle (2.6%), pain on insertion of the needle (0.7%), petechiae or ecchymoses (0.3%), local pain after treatment (0.1%), subcutaneous hematomas (0.1%).

Norwegian researchers sent questionnaires about acupuncture to a random sample of the Norwegian general population (63). Of the 653 respondents, 7% claimed to have had adverse effects. The most common were dizziness, fatigue, and pain from the needles. No serious adverse effects were reported.

In a prospective UK survey of members of the medical and physiotherapy acupuncture organizations in Britain the preliminary data included 25 500 treatments given by 77 acupuncturists (64). There were 29 major events, including four episodes of loss of consciousness and one tonic-clonic seizure. The most common minor events were bleeding or hematoma (3%), aggravation of symptoms (1%), and pain during needling (0.9%).

In a survey of 1100 Australian providers of traditional Chinese medicine the adverse events of acupuncture were also monitored (65). There were 3222 events, including 64 cases of pneumothorax and 80 convulsions. No deaths were recorded.

A systematic review of case reports from the Japanese literature yielded 105 cases of suspected acupuncture adverse effects not previously reported in Western publications (66). These included 21 spinal lesions, 21 cases of pneumothorax, 19 infections, 15 cases of foreign bodies in organs, 10 instances of argyria, 10 neural injuries, and 11 other adverse events, including two cases of cardiac tamponade.

A systematic review of all prospective studies of adverse effects associated with acupuncture included nine primary investigations (67). The most commonly reported adverse events were needle pain (1–45%), tiredness (2–41%), and bleeding (0.03–38%). Pneumothorax was the only serious complication in these studies; it was reported twice in about 250 000 patients.

Table 2 Reports of adverse events associated with acupuncture

Indications	Adverse event	Site of acupuncture	Causality	Reference
Presumably local pain	A closed ankle fracture was converted to an open fracture and open joint by acupuncture	Local	Likely, but insufficient details reported	(51)
Intermittent claudication	Occlusion of the popliteal artery	Local	Likely	(52)
Back pain	Rupture of a pseudoaneurysm	Local	Likely	(53)
Arthritis	Pneumothorax	The neck	Likely	(54)
Shoulder stiffness	High cervical epidural abscess and vertebral osteomyelitis	Posterior nuchal region	Fairly certain	(55)
Not stated	Peritemporomandibular abscess	Local	Fairly certain	(56)
Back pain	Unilateral septic sacroileitis	Local	Likely	(57)
Arthritis	Death due to streptococcal toxic shock-like syndrome	Right shoulder	Probable	(58)
Back pain	Argyria 10 years after acupuncture with a silver needle	Ear	Possible	(59)
Stroke (2 cases)	Angina pectoris during electroacupuncture	Scalp	Possible	(60)

Two prospective UK studies with a total of about 70 000 consultations have confirmed that serious adverse events of acupuncture are true rarities in Britain (68,69). Bleeding and needle pain were the most frequent adverse events, with a prevalence of about 1:1000.

A systematic review of all adverse events associated with acupuncture in the Japanese medical literature located 124 cases (70). These included 25 cases of pneumothorax, 18 cases of spinal cord injury, 11 cases of hepatitis B, and 10 cases of localized argyria.

- An 82-year-old woman was scheduled for gastrectomy with an epidural anesthetic (71). She had previously had many acupuncture treatments with a Japanese technique (okibari), in which small needles are left in situ. Her preoperative chest and abdominal X-rays showed hundreds of needles around the vertebrae. The anesthesiologists feared that an epidural anesthetic might lead to spinal cord injury or pneumothorax, and general anesthesia was chosen instead.

Cardiovascular

Acupuncture has been associated with hemopericardium due to ventricular puncture (72).

- An 83-year-old Austrian woman developed syncope and cardiogenic shock shortly after acupuncture over the sternum. Echocardiography showed cardiac tamponade and pericardiocentesis revealed hemopericardium. At operation a small bleeding perforation of the right ventricle was found and closed. The acupuncture at the point "Ren 17" was above a sternal foramen, which allowed the needle to penetrate the heart.

A case in which acupuncture was apparently responsible for cardiac dysrhythmias has been reported (73).

Respiratory

Pneumothorax has been reported in association with acupuncture (74,75).

- A 28-year-old Chinese woman developed bilateral pneumothoraces after receiving acupuncture in the upper thoracic and paraspinal regions (75). She was treated conservatively and was discharged after 2 days.
- A 30-year-old woman developed bilateral chest pain and dyspnea after paraspinal acupuncture resulted in bilateral pneumothorax; she recovered fully within 2 days (76).

Nervous system

Acupuncture has been associated with subarachnoid hemorrhage due to arterial puncture (77).

- A 44-year-old Chinese man had severe occipital headache, nausea, and vomiting during acupuncture in the posterior neck. A CT scan showed hemorrhage in the third, fourth, and lateral ventricles, and blood was found in the lumbar fluid. The problem was due to puncture of a branch of the vertebral artery at the "feng fu" point, which coincides with the site for performing cisternal puncture. The patient made a spontaneous full recovery within 28 days.

Convulsions, inadvertent anesthesia, loss of co-ordination, and tinnitus have been associated with acupuncture (78).

Endocrine

Galactorrhea has been associated with acupuncture.

- A 41-year-old woman with breast cancer was treated with acupuncture for pain control (79). She had an episode of galactorrhea 6 days after the first treatment and also during the second acupuncture treatment. No reason for this unusual phenomenon other than acupuncture could be found.

The authors pointed out that in Chinese medicine acupuncture at the points used in this patient promotes lactation.

Skin

Acupuncture needles can cause local reactions (80).

- A 55-year-old Japanese woman developed papules at sites where she had had acupuncture 4 years and 3 weeks before. Histological examination showed that the papules were silicone granulomas.

The authors postulated that the papules were reactions to the silicone from the coating of the acupuncture needles.

Skin malignancy (78) and Koebner phenomenon (81) have been associated with acupuncture.

- A 52-year-old man received acupuncture in the backs of both hands for chronic back pain and subsequently developed bilateral swelling of both hands and fingers (82).

No reason for this adverse effect could be found, and the authors considered infection or allergy as the most likely cause, but without finding strong evidence of either.

- A 59-year-old woman presented with a 1-month history of non-pruritic papules on the dorsa of both feet (83). During the previous year she had repeatedly received acupuncture in this area. A biopsy showed mixed lichenoid, spongiotic, and granulomatous dermatitis. Ultrastructural examination showed macrophages containing silicone. At follow-up new lesions on her mid calves were noted, and again she explained she had recently received acupuncture at these sites.

It was discovered that the acupuncturist used silicone-coated needles and silicone deposition was thus caused by acupuncture.

Immunologic

Allergies to the various metals used in acupuncture needles have been described (84).

Infection risk

Acupuncture needles must be handled meticulously to guarantee sterility of the needle on insertion. If such safety rules are not strictly adhered to, there is a high risk of transmitting infectious diseases. In principle one can assume that any blood-borne infection is transmittable through the misuse of acupuncture needles.

Bacterial infections
Osteomyelitis (85), endocarditis (86,87), or generalized *Staphylococcus aureus* infections (88) have been associated with acupuncture.

- A 67-year-old Japanese man was treated with "depot acupuncture," an unusual technique involving the implantation of a sheep gut thread through a spinal anesthesia needle into the abdomen (89). He subsequently developed intractable pain, high fever, and other signs of infection. A CT scan showed a low density mass in the left psoas muscle and the ventral portion of the distal aorta, corresponding to an abscess and a false infected aneurysm. The affected part of the aorta was replaced with a Gore-Tex graft and the patient was treated with antibiotics. He eventually made a full recovery.

In a review of serious complications there were three cases of infection, one of auricular perichondritis that resulted in permanent disfigurement, one of bacterial meningitis with full recovery, and one of pyarthrosis also with full recovery (90).

Microbiologists from Hong Kong have reported four cases of mycobacterial infections within 2 years (91). All the patients had lesions at acupuncture points. Acid-fast bacilli were present in two cases. Gene sequencing identified the strain from two patients as *Mycobacterium chelonae* and from two patients as *Mycobacterium nonchromogenium*.

- A 37-year-old man with diabetes had septicemia and compartment syndrome of the leg after acupuncture in the calf area (92). Decompression fasciotomy was performed and Gram-positive cocci were grown from the wound swab and group A streptococci from blood cultures. He required intensive care, including intravenous antibiotics, and eventually recovered.
- Endophthalmitis occurred in a patient from Singapore (93). Group B streptococci were isolated from the blood. Despite aggressive intravitreal antibiotic therapy the affected eye lost its light perception.
- A 79-year-old woman presented with induration of the right leg three months after receiving acupuncture in this area (94). Radiography showed a focal dystrophic calcification at this point and histological studies showed suppurative granulomatous inflammation with microabscesses and caseous necrosis due to infection with *Mycobacterium chelonae*. She made a full recovery after antibiotic treatment.
- A 42-year-old woman with Marfan's syndrome, who had previously had an aortic root and valve replacement, presented with fever and polyarthralgia 6 days after receiving acupuncture for back pain (95). Examination of the valve showed no abnormalities, but *S. aureus* was grown from blood cultures. Extensive investigations did not identify a cause for the infection. Her condition deteriorated despite antibiotic therapy, and emergency aortic root and valve replacement became necessary. She eventually made a full recovery.

Virus infections
In at least three published case reports, acupuncture was the only plausible explanation for infections with HIV (96,97).

Hepatitis infections may be transmitted in this way (98–100). A retrospective cohort serological study identified five confirmed cases of acute hepatitis B virus infection within 3.5 years related to one London acupuncture clinic (101). The acupuncturist was hepatitis B-positive and the strain of his virus was identical to that from the patient. Nine further patients of his had antibodies to the hepatitis B core antigen but had other risk factors for hepatitis B infection.

After a patient of a London doctor (who practiced an unusual acupuncture technique involving re-injection of native blood) acquired hepatitis B, 352 of his patients treated by this method were investigated; 33 were positive for hepatitis B antigen and 30 showed complete nucleotide identity in the DNA segments derived from the surface and core genes (102). Contaminated saline used in the treatment was identified as the probable vehicle of transmission.

An epidemiological screening program in 2231 subjects in Japan was aimed at defining the risk factors of hepatitis C infection (103). It showed that the relative risk was increased (1.30, CI = 0.65, 2.61) in those participants who had received acupuncture. A newspaper article reported that 21 confirmed cases of hepatitis B were related to a London-based physician who practiced an obscure variation of acupuncture (104).

A nationwide community-based survey in Taiwan has been carried out in seven locations in a total of 11 904 men tested for antibodies against hepatitis C virus. Exposure to acupuncture was a risk factor for hepatitis C positivity (105).

Korean epidemiologists have studied the prevalence of hepatitis C virus infection in a rural population (n = 1033) with a high incidence of liver cancer (106). They noted that the strongest associations in a multivariate analysis were with anti-HCV positivity and the use of acupuncture (OR = 2.2, 95% CI = 1.0, 4.7).

French investigators have evaluated the presence of serum markers of hepatitis A, B, and C viruses in a rural population of 303 volunteers (107). The main risk factors for positivity were past hospitalizations (72%), acupuncture (18%), conjugal unfaithfulness (11%), blood transfusion (9.4%), tattoos (5.8%), homosexuality (1.1%), and intravenous drug addiction (0.73%).

Trauma
If acupuncture, which entails tissue trauma, is performed properly and on the correct acupuncture points, trauma will affect only the skin and the connective tissue below. If, however, acupuncture needles are inserted at the wrong site or penetrate too deeply, other tissues or organs can be affected. Traumatic complications of acupuncture have been reviewed (108). They have been described in relation to the thoracic and abdominal viscera, in the peripheral and central nervous systems, and in blood vessels. Several deaths have been reported from pneumothorax and cardiac tamponade. The anatomical tissues at several acupuncture points are such that needles can injure vulnerable structures. Thus, good knowledge of anatomy is an essential precondition for acupuncturists.

One review identified 32 cases of pneumothorax and two of hemothorax (109). Damage to the middle ear (following auriculoacupuncture), injury to the spinal cord (49), and cardiac tamponade have been other serious traumatic complications (110,111). Needles can also break while in situ, and parts of acupuncture needles have been found in patients' kidneys (112), carpal tunnel (113), cervical spine (114), spinal cord (115), and heart (116). Petechiae and other forms of bleeding have also been reported (109). If a nerve is punctured the patient might experience unnecessary pain and even sustain minor nerve damage, which in extreme cases can be persistent. In another case there was a delayed traumatic effect of an acupuncture needle fragment (117).

- A 43-year-old man developed a false aneurysm of the popliteal artery after a penetrating injury from an acupuncture needle (118). The aneurysm ruptured spontaneously, but the patient was successfully managed by vascular surgery.

A review of serious complications included one case of cardiac tamponade (with full recovery of the patient after surgery), one case of peripheral nerve damage (foot drop with residual weakness after 6 years), and three cases of pneumothorax (all with full recovery) (90).

A further case of pneumothorax has been reported (119).

- A 60-year-old woman was treated by a non-medically qualified acupuncturist for chronic rib pain. About 15 needles were inserted along either side of her back, and one (in the right lower thoracic region) caused immediate discomfort. After removal of the needle she noted pain and breathlessness. A chest X-ray 2 days later confirmed a small right pneumothorax, which resolved spontaneously within one week.

Pregnancy
Abortion and miscarriage (49) have been associated with acupuncture.

Fetotoxicity
Acupuncture in pregnant women might carry a risk for the fetus, since it is postulated that acupuncture can increase oxytocin release in the mother, which might harm the unborn child (120).

Aromatherapy

Aromatherapy is a highly popular form of complementary medicine usually entailing the application of essential plant oils to the skin by gentle massage. It has been shown to have relaxing effects but other claims have not been substantiated by reliable trial evidence (121). Allergic airborne contact dermatitis occurred in a patient who had previously used several essential oils for aromatherapy (122). The toxicity of essential oils has been reviewed (123).

Four cases of allergic contact dermatitis caused by essential oils used in aromatherapy have been described (124). A survey of UK aromatherapists (no details provided) yielded 11 reports of adverse effects (125). Most of these cases seemed to relate to allergic reactions to the essential oils. A therapist also reportedly developed an allergy to ylang-ylang oil used in aromatherapy (126).

Japanese dermatologists have reported an increase in positive patch tests to lavender oil from 1.1% in 1990 to 14% in 1998 (127). The authors argued that this rise coincided with a similar increase in the use of lavender aromatherapy in Japan and that the latter had caused the former.

See also monographs on substances that affect the skin.

Cell therapy

Cell therapy consists of the parenteral or enteral administration of cells or parts of cell obtained from animal organs and/or tissues from cattle, sheep, pigs, or rabbits. Two different types of cell preparations are in use: fresh cells, which are administered in fresh form, and dried cells or so-called sicca cells, which are prepared for later use. The most prevailing risks of cell therapy are local and generalized allergic reactions (fever, nausea, vomiting, urticaria, and anaphylactic shock). Other untoward consequences include fatal and non-fatal encephalomyelitis, polyneuritis, Landry–Guillain–Barré syndrome, fatal serum sickness, perivenous leukoencephalitis, and immune-complex vasculitis.

Homeopathy

Most, although not all, homeopathic remedies are too dilute to cause toxic effects. However, potentially toxic concentrations of arsenic (128) and cadmium (129) in homeopathic remedies have been described. Concern has also been voiced about potentially carcinogenic effects of low potencies of *Aristolochia* (130). Acute pancreatitis has been reported after the administration of a complex homeopathic formulation containing 19 different ingredients (131). Low potencies can also cause allergic reactions (132,133) and cases of severe allergic and anaphylactic reactions have been reported. In cases of concomitant drug treatments, interactions are conceivable, even though there is no published evidence on this matter. Generally speaking, adverse reactions to homeopathic medications are probably rare. However, we cannot at present tell their true incidence, as no definitive study of this has been carried out.

A systematic review of all data on the safety of such medicines has challenged the view that because homeopathic remedies are often highly dilute they are therefore devoid of adverse effects (134). It showed that in placebo-controlled trials the mean incidence of adverse effects of homeopathic remedies was 9.4%, higher than that of placebo (6.1%). All the adverse effects were minor and transient. Anecdotal reports of more serious adverse effects mainly related to aggravation of presenting symptoms, which, from the homeopathic point of view, can be looked on as confirmation that the optimal remedy has been found, and thus interpreted as a positive event. Since the homeopathic principle is that like cures like, exacerbation of symptoms by what can be presumed to be toxic doses of a supposed remedy confirms that the remedy causes the problem and will therefore cure it if given in homeopathic doses.

Harm can also be done when an ineffective homeopathic intervention replaces an effective conventional one (135).

- A 40-year-old woman travelling to a malaria-infested region took her homeopath's advice and was "immunized" with homeopathic remedies (*Ledum palustre* 5CH and *Malaria officinalis* 4CH) instead of taking conventional protection. She contracted malaria and had to be treated for 2 months in intensive care for multiple organ system failure due to *Plasmodium falciparum*.

Seven Israeli children were seriously harmed when their parents used homeopaths and other providers of complementary medicine instead of conventional doctors; four died (136). Similarly, it has been reported that seeing a traditional healer in Kenya increased the risk of dying from an acute pneumonia by 5.3 times (137).

The author of a review of the safety of homeopathic products concluded that they are usually safe, but that continued vigilance is in order, not least because of the currently high popularity of homeopathy (138). In response, it was pointed out that under-reporting is high, that homeopathic products are often mistaken for herbal medicines, and that the main risks of homeopathy relate to the prescriber rather than the medicine (139).

Hypnosis

Hypnosis is not usually seen as a treatment burdened with adverse effects. However, an authoritative review has reminded us that it is by no means completely safe (140). Complications include amnesia, catharsis, paralysis, disorientation, literalness of response, accelerated transference, and memory contamination. A further unwanted effect of hypnosis is an inability to dehypnotize the patient. A review of the literature has shown several such cases and has contributed two new such incidents (141).

Manipulation

Manipulative therapies (chiropractic and osteopathy) are amongst the most prevalent of complementary treatments. Spinal manipulation is carried out by chiropractors, osteopaths, physiotherapists, and other healthcare professionals to treat back and neck pain as well as other (predominantly musculoskeletal) disorders.

A literature review has provided reassurance about the relative safety of spinal manipulation (142). When the serious adverse effects of non-steroidal anti-inflammatory drugs were compared with those of spinal manipulation, both used for neck pain, manipulation emerged as being safer by more than two orders of magnitude. However, these procedures can be associated with serious complications, particularly when they involve the cervical spine (143).

In a survey of UK physiotherapists trained in spinal manipulation, 19% reported having encountered complications of spinal manipulation (144). These related mostly to the upper spine and were mostly not serious. A further survey of 686 general practitioners in the UK disclosed 28 serious adverse effects related to spinal manipulation (145).

An authoritative summary of all cases of complications of spinal manipulation of the cervical spine published since 1925 has appeared (146). There were 177 cases of severe injury. The most common injuries involved arterial dissection or spasm and brain stem lesions. In 32 instances (18%) they were fatal. The author concluded that high velocity thrusts of the cervical spine are not demonstrably associated with more benefit than harm and should therefore be avoided.

In the UK 108 consecutive patients of chiropractors were asked to complete a questionnaire, which 80% of them returned (147). Of the questionnaires 68% were suitable for analysis. Adverse effects at 1 hour after treatment were reported by 28 patients and eight had adverse effects the morning after treatment. The most common adverse effects were extra local pain or radiating pain. No serious adverse effects were reported.

Some chiropractors tend to advise clients against any type of immunization. The basis of this attitude seems to lie in early chiropractic philosophy. Eschewing the germ theory of infectious disease, this philosophy considered any disease to be the result of spinal nerve dysfunction caused by misalignment of vertebrae (148). When 150 US chiropractors were questioned about their attitude towards immunization, only 30% reported recommending childhood immunizations (149).

A systematic review of all prospective studies of the risks associated with spinal manipulation included five primary investigations (150). The most valid studies suggested that about half of all patients who see a chiropractor will have adverse effects, which are usually mild and transient. No reliable data about serious adverse events were uncovered. However, a review of recent case reports has shown that spinal manipulation was associated with several serious adverse effects, including dissection of the vertebral and internal carotid arteries, resulting in strokes and at least one death (151). Other instances relate to epidural hematoma, intracranial aneurysm, cauda equina syndrome, contusion of the spinal cord, myelopathy, radiculopathy, and palsy of the long thoracic nerve.

A report on malpractice suits in the USA has shown that in 1990–96 claims against chiropractors have been constant (between 2.3 and 3.0 claims per 100 policy holders per year) (152). There were about four times more claims against primary care physicians. The percentage of claims paid varied between 46 and 57% for the chiropractors and 29 and 33% for the physicians. The three most frequent reasons for the claims against chiropractors were disc herniation, failure to diagnose, and bone fractures produced through treatment.

The frequency with which chiropractors use radiology of the spine might be a cause for concern. Among Dutch chiropractors 40% have been reported to use X-rays "often or always" (153). In the USA, 96% of chiropractors use X-rays routinely on all new patients, and 80% use them in follow-up (154).

Cardiovascular

The Stroke Council of the American Heart Association registered 359 cases of vascular accidents until 1981 (155). In Switzerland 1255 such incidents were recorded in 1 535 000 manipulations (156). Others estimated the incidence of reported vascular accidents at 1–4 per million treatments (157–159). The mortality/severe long-term impairment rate is 28% (160). The incidence is higher if minor symptoms are included and specifically searched for: out of a total of 75 500 procedures applied, 25 such cases were reported (161). The reported incidence rates are probably a gross under-estimation of the true figures; in a series of 13 cases of clinically and radiologically verified vertebral artery dissection, eight were spontaneous, two occurred after manipulation, and three occurred after minor injury (162).

The mechanisms of vascular complications of cervical manipulations involve vertebral artery dissection, intramural bleeding or pseudo-aneurysm leading to thrombosis or embolism (160) as well as transient cerebral ischemia through mechanical artery compression during cervical rotation (163) and vasospasm (164). The vertebral artery at the C1/C2 segment is most often affected. Combined rotation, extension and traction movements apparently create the highest risk, particularly when executed forcefully (165). The most frequent clinical findings are Wallenberg's syndrome (28%), other brain stem syndromes (49%), cerebellar syndromes (8%), occipital lobe syndromes (5%) and unclassified syndromes (160). They usually occur during or promptly after the intervention, but delays of hours or days have also been observed (159,166,167). Symptoms can start as headache and neck pain, which are frequent reasons for applying manipulative therapies in the first place. In at least one case neck pain was the first sign of dissection, which was treated by manipulation, resulting in a fatal stroke (168).

- Two patients had oculosympathetic palsy after self-treatment with a "shiatsu massager" (169). A thorough diagnostic work-up, including MRI and MRA scans, identified dissection of the carotid artery as the cause of the problem. In the absence of other causes, the authors believed that the self-treatment had caused dissection.
- A 32-year-old woman who had seen a traditional American "bone-setter" for shoulder problems was subjected to a "sudden thrusting of the head upward and to the right" (170). She had neck discomfort immediately afterwards. The pain persisted for 6 days, when she noted vertigo and left-sided ataxia. An MRI scan showed acute infarction in the middle left cerebellar hemisphere and vermis. An MRA scan showed left vertebral artery dissection with a probable embolus.

When all 26 cases of vertebral artery dissection during the period 1989–99 were retrospectively analysed in a tertiary Canadian academic center, possible precipitating factors were identified in 14 patients (171). Chiropractic spinal manipulation and sporting activity were the most common factors (11% and 15% respectively).

Nervous system

Several reports of nervous system adverse effects after spinal manipulation have been published (172–174). They are summarized in Table 3.

Of 13 consultant neurologists in the Republic of Ireland 11 had seen a total of 16 patients with neurological complications after chiropractic spinal manipulation within 5 years; strokes were the most frequently reported problem, and in 13 cases had led to persistent neurological deficits (175).

A survey of 177 members of the American Academy of Neurology aimed to find out how many adverse events related to chiropractice had been noted by these doctors within a 2-year period. Chiropractic interventions were associated with 55 strokes, 16 cases of myelopathy, and 30 cases of radiculopathy (176).

A Ukrainian doctor has reported a series of 49 additional cases with neurological complications after spinal manipulation (177).

Swedish authors have summarized cases reported to three Swedish insurance companies within 2 years (178). They found 21 cases associated with the cervical spine, six associated with the thoracic spine, 13 with the lumbar spine, and 14 with the sacro-iliac joints. Cervical spinal manipulation had caused damage to the vertebral artery with subsequent paralysis in three cases and disk herniation in three cases. Lumbar spinal manipulation had caused disk herniation in six cases, three of whom suffered severe and persistent problems.

German neurologists have reported 10 cases of ischemic stroke due to either vertebral arterial dissection ($n = 8$) or internal carotid artery dissection ($n = 2$) after chiropractic spinal manipulation (179). There were no identifiable predisposing factors. In three cases the dissections were bilateral. The onset of symptoms was immediate ($n = 5$) or delayed by up to 2 days. Neurological deficits developed during up to 3 weeks. In five patients the eventual clinical outcome was good while marked deficits persisted in three patients. One patient continued to suffer from a locked-in syndrome and another was in a persistent vegetative state.

- A 34-year-old woman had pain, dizziness, vomiting, and diplopia immediately after cervical spinal manipulation (180). An MRI scan showed a left cerebellar infarction, and duplex sonography showed dissection of both vertebral arteries leading to 50% occlusion on the right side and total occlusion on the left side.
- A 46-year-old man consulted a traditional Chinese "bone setter" for persistent neck pain (181). The healer had "forcefully rotated his head to one side and then to the other side." The patient immediately developed numbness of the whole body and dyspnea. An MRI

Table 3 Reports of adverse events associated with spinal manipulation

Indication	Adverse event	Site of manipulation	Therapist	Causality	Reference
Back pain	Cauda equina syndrome	Lumbar	Traditional healer	Likely	(172)
Cervical pain	Brown–Séquard syndrome due to contusion of the spinal cord	Cervical	Chiropractor	Fairly certain	(173)
Neck pain	Vertigo, profuse vomiting	Cervical	Chiropractor	Certain	(174)

scan showed incomplete cervical cord injury with mild cervical cord swelling. He was treated with high-dose methylprednisolone and made a good recovery with only minimal persistent deficits.

- A 67-year-old woman had spinal manipulation for neck pain and experienced severe pain (182). She subsequently noted weakness of her left side, which worsened rapidly and also affected bladder function. She had a left-sided ptosis, all sensation was impaired below C6, and she had urinary incontinence. An MRI scan showed an epidural hematoma in the left posterolateral aspect of the spinal cord at C3–C5. Laminectomy was performed and a large epidural hematoma was removed. She subsequently made a full recovery.
- A 34-year-old man with a whiplash injury consulted a chiropractor for his neck pain, and 36 hours after one particularly painful treatment he experienced throbbing, positional headache, dizziness, diplopia, otorrhea, and rhinorrhea (183). After thorough neurological examination the author concluded that the patient had suffered a dural tear due to cervical manipulation.
- A 34-year-old woman had memory loss, ataxia, and poor co-ordination of the right arm associated with right neck pain after consulting a chiropractor (184). An MRI scan confirmed a right cerebellar infarct, most probably caused by upper spinal manipulation. She made a full recovery within 1 month.
- A 41-year-old man with neck pain sought chiropractic care and the evening after felt unable to breathe in the recumbent position (185). Diaphragmatic paralysis was attributed to phrenic nerve injury during cervical manipulation. He remained short of breath and had persistent difficulties breathing in the supine position.

A highly unusual case of thoracic epidural hematoma after spinal manipulation of the lumbar spine has been reported (186).

- A 64-year-old woman experienced acute severe pain and progressive neurological defects for the first time during spinal manipulation. Swift surgical intervention was initiated and a thoracic epidural hematoma was evacuated. This resulted in complete recovery.

A survey of 323 UK neurologists disclosed 35 previously unreported cases of serious neurological complications of spinal manipulation (187). This means that in this particular series, under-reporting of adverse events had been 100%.

Musculoskeletal

Dislocations and fractures of vertebrae have also been reported and are not confined to the upper spine (188,189). Patients with osteoporosis are at high risk; manipulation is therefore contraindicated in these individuals. Nerve lesions range from plexus paralysis and ophthalmoplegia to tetraplegia, disk herniation, and phrenic nerve palsy (188,190). A review of the English language literature included 89 neurological complications after manipulation; the number of unreported cases could be considerably higher.

Massage

There are many different forms of massage therapy, which are not normally associated with serious adverse effects. However, trauma can occur (191).

- A 39-year-old woman with an unremarkable medical history underwent deep body massage, including the abdomen. Within 24 hours she experienced discomfort and nausea and after 72 hours she had a CT scan, which showed a large hematoma in the right hepatic lobe. There was no evidence of a plausible cause for this. In spite of adequate medical treatment, her recovery was slow and she had nausea and low-grade fever for about 6 months.
- An 80-year-old Japanese man with a recent history of cerebral infarction received a shiatsu massage in the neck area to relieve a headache (192). Immediately after he had right visual field impairment. Thorough ophthalmological and neurological show multiple branch occlusions of the central retinal artery and multiple small infarctions in the right frontoparietal lobe. He was given urokinase for 7 days, and made an almost complete recovery.

The authors of the second report concluded that forceful neck massage had caused the problem.

References

1. Ernst E, White A. The BBC survey of complementary medicine use in the UK. Complement Ther Med 2000;8(1):32–6.
2. MacLennan AH, Wilson DH, Taylor AW. Prevalence and cost of alternative medicine in Australia. Lancet 1996;347(9001):569–73.
3. Fisher P, Ward A. Complementary medicine in Europe. BMJ 1994;309(6947):107–11.
4. Anonymous. Complementary Medicines. London: Mintel International Group, 1997:13.
5. Institute of Medical Statistics Self-Medication International. Herbals in Europe. London: IMS Self-Medication International, 1998.
6. Brevoort P. The booming US botanical market. A new overview. Herbalgram 1998;44:33–46.
7. Eisenberg DM, Kessler RC, Foster C, Norlock FE, Calkins DR, Delbanco TL. Unconventional medicine in the United States. Prevalence, costs, and patterns of use. N Engl J Med 1993;328(4):246–52.
8. Eisenberg DM, Davis RB, Ettner SL, Appel S, Wilkey S, Van Rompay M, Kessler RC. Trends in alternative medicine use in the United States, 1990–1997: results of a follow-up national survey. JAMA 1998;280(18):1569–75.
9. Knowledge, attitudes and beliefs of patients of complementary practitioners. In: Vincent C, Furnham A, editors. Complementary Medicine: A Research Perspective. Chicester: Wiley, 1997:97–117.
10. Astin JA. Why patients use alternative medicine: results of a national study. JAMA 1998;279(19):1548–53.
11. Weiss SJ, Takakuwa KM, Ernst AA. Use, understanding, and beliefs about complementary and alternative medicines among emergency department patients. Acad Emerg Med 2001;8(1):41–7.
12. Ernst E, Pittler MH, Stevinson C, White AR, Eisenberg D. The Desktop Guide to Complementary and Alternative Medicine. Edinburgh: Mosby, 2001.

13. Ernst E. Investigating the safety of complementary medicine. In: Lewith G, Jonas W, Walach H, editors. Clinical Research in Complementary Therapies. London: Churchill Livingstone, 2001:171–86.
14. Ernst E. Complementary medicine: its hidden risks. Diabetes Care 2001;24(8):1486–8.
15. Rhodes-Kropf J, Lantz MS; American Association for Geriatric Psychiatry. Alternative medicine. Achieving balance between herbal remedies and medical therapy. Geriatrics 2001;56(8):44–7.
16. Abbot NC, White AR, Ernst E. Complementary medicine. Nature 1996;381(6581):361.
17. De Smet PA. Health risks of herbal remedies. Drug Saf 1995;13(2):81–93.
18. Ernst E. Phytomedicine research. BMJ 1994;308:673–4.
19. Jonas WB, Ernst E. Evaluating the safety of complementary and alternative products and practices. In: Jonas WB, Levin JS, editors. Essentials of Complementary and Alternative Medicine. Philadelphia: Lippincott Williams Wilkins, 1999:89–107.
20. Senstad O, Leboeuf-Yde C, Borchgrevink C. Frequency and characteristics of side effects of spinal manipulative therapy. Spine 1997;22(4):435–41.
21. Leboeuf-Yde C, Hennius B, Rudberg E, Leufvenmark P, Thunman M. Side effects of chiropractic treatment: a prospective study. J Manipulative Physiol Ther 1997;20(8):511–15.
22. Yamashita H, Tsukayama H, Tanno Y, Nishijo K. Adverse events related to acupuncture. JAMA 1998; 280(18):1563–4.
23. Arthur P, Bahl P, Bhan MK, Kirkwood BR, Martines J, Moulton LH, Panny ME, Ram M, Ram M, Underwood B. Randomised trial to assess benefits and safety of vitamin A supplementation linked to immunisation in early infancy. WHO/CHD Immunisation-Linked Vitamin A Supplementation Study Group. Lancet 1998;352(9136):1257–63.
24. Budd GT, Adamson PC, Gupta M, Homayoun P, Sandstrom SK, Murphy RF, McLain D, Tuason L, Peereboom D, Bukowski RM, Ganapathi R. Phase I/II trial of all-trans retinoic acid and tamoxifen in patients with advanced breast cancer. Clin Cancer Res 1998;4(3):635–42.
25. Ernst E. Chiropractors' use of X-rays. Br J Radiol 1998;71(843):249–51.
26. Nicolls MR, Terada LS, Tuder RM, Prindiville SA, Schwarz MI. Diffuse alveolar hemorrhage with underlying pulmonary capillaritis in the retinoic acid syndrome. Am J Respir Crit Care Med 1998;158(4):1302–5.
27. Boros LG, Brandes JL, Lee WN, Cascante M, Puigjaner J, Revesz E, Bray TM, Schirmer WJ, Melvin WS. Thiamine supplementation to cancer patients: a double edged sword. Anticancer Res 1998;18(1B):595–602.
28. Rothman KJ, Moore LL, Singer MR, Nguyen US, Mannino S, Milunsky A. Teratogenicity of high vitamin A intake. N Engl J Med 1995;333(21):1369–73.
29. Ernst E. Competence in complementary medicine. Comp Ther Med 1995;3:6–8.
30. Ernst E, Schmidt K. "Alternative" cancer cures via the Internet? Br J Cancer 2002;87(5):479–80.
31. Schmidt K, Ernst E. "Alternative" therapies for HIV/AIDS: how safe is Internet advice? A pilot study. Int J STD AIDS 2002;13(6):433–5.
32. Bonakdar RA. Herbal cancer cures on the Web: noncompliance with The Dietary Supplement Health and Education Act. Fam Med 2002;34(7):522–7.
33. Ernst E, Schmidt K. Health risks over the Internet: advice offered by "medical herbalists" to a pregnant woman. Wien Med Wochenschr 2002;152(7–8):190–2.
34. Brienza RS, Stein MD, Fagan MJ. Delay in obtaining conventional healthcare by female internal medicine patients who use herbal therapies. J Womens Health Gend Based Med 2002;11(1):79–87.
35. Bostrom H, Rossner S. Quality of alternative medicine—complications and avoidable deaths. Qual Assur Health Care 1990;2(2):111–17.
36. Sulfaro F, Fasher B, Burgess MA. Homoeopathic vaccination. What does it mean? Immunisation Interest Group of the Royal Alexandra Hospital for Children. Med J Aust 1994;161(5):305–7.
37. Rasky E, Freidl W, Haidvogl M, Stronegger WJ. Arbeits- und Lebensweise von homöopathisch tätigen Arztinnen und Arzten in Österreich. Eine deskiptive studie. [Work and life style of homeopathic physicians in Austria. A descriptive study.] Wien Med Wochenschr 1994;144(17):419–24.
38. Ernst E, White AR. Homoeopathy and immunization. Br J Gen Pract 1995;45(400):629–30.
39. Colley F, Haas M. Attitudes on immunization: a survey of American chiropractors. J Manipulative Physiol Ther 1994;17(9):584–90.
40. Simpson N, Lenton S, Randall R. Parental refusal to have children immunised: extent and reasons. BMJ 1995;310(6974):227.
41. Robinson AR, Crane LA, Davidson AJ, Steiner JF. Association between use of complementary/alternative medicine and health-related behaviors among health fair participants. Prev Med 2002;34(1):51–7.
42. Busse JW, Kulkarni AV, Campbell JB, Injeyan HS. Attitudes toward vaccination: a survey of Canadian chiropractic students. CMAJ 2002;166(12):1531–4.
43. Wolfe RM, Sharp LK, Lipsky MS. Content and design attributes of antivaccination web sites. JAMA 2002;287(24):3245–8.
44. Davies P, Chapman S, Leask J. Antivaccination activists on the world wide web. Arch Dis Child 2002;87(1):22–5.
45. Schmidt K, Ernst E. Aspects of MMR. Survey shows that some homoeopaths and chiropractors advise against MMR. BMJ 2002;325(7364):597.
46. Ernst E. The safety of homoeopathy. Br Homoeopathy J 1995;84:193–4.
47. Ernst E. The risks of acupuncture. Int J Risk Safety Med 1995;6:179–86.
48. Jonas WB, Ernst E. Adverse effects of acupuncture. In: Jonas WB, Levin JS, editors. Essentials of Complementary and Alternative Medicine. Philadelphia: Lippincott Williams Wilkins, 1999:172–5.
49. Peacher WG. Adverse reactions, contraindications and complications of acupuncture and moxibustion. Am J Chin Med (Gard City NY) 1975;3(1):35–46.
50. White AR, Ernst E. Risks associated with acupuncture. Perfusion 2002;15:153–8.
51. Kelsey JH. Pneumothorax following acupuncture is a generally recognized complication seen by many emergency physicians. J Emerg Med 1998;16(2):224–5.
52. Bergqvist D, Berggren AL, Bjorck M, Bostrom A, Karacagil S. Akupunktur kan ge kärlskador. [Acupuncture can cause vascular injury.] Lakartidningen 1998;95(3):180–1.
53. Matsuyama H, Nagao K, Yamakawa GI, Akahoshi K, Naito K. Retroperitoneal hematoma due to rupture of a pseudoaneurysm caused by acupuncture therapy. J Urol 1998;159(6):2087–8.
54. Fulde GW. Chest pain and breathlessness after acupuncture—again. Med J Aust 1998;169(1):64.
55. Yazawa S, Ohi T, Sugimoto S, Satoh S, Matsukura S. Cervical spinal epidural abscess following acupuncture: successful treatment with antibiotics. Intern Med 1998; 37(2):161–5.

56. Matsumura Y, Inui M, Tagawa T. Peritemporomandibular abscess as a complication of acupuncture: a case report. J Oral Maxillofac Surg 1998;56(4):495–6.
57. Lau SM, Chou CT, Huang CM. Unilateral sacroiliitis as an unusual complication of acupuncture. Clin Rheumatol 1998;17(4):357–8.
58. Onizuka T, Oishi K, Ikeda T, Watanabe K, Senba M, Suga K, Nagatake T. [A fatal case of streptococcal toxic shock-like syndrome probably caused by acupuncture.] Kansenshogaku Zasshi 1998;72(7):776–80.
59. Legat FJ, Goessler W, Schlagenhaufen C, Soyer HP. Argyria after short-contact acupuncture. Lancet 1998;352(9123):241.
60. Chang-du L, Zhen-ya J. Angina pectoris induced by electric scalp acupuncture: report on two cases. Int J Clin Acupunct 1998;9:53–4.
61. Ernst E, White AR. Acupuncture may be associated with serious adverse events. BMJ 2000;320(7233):513–14.
62. Yamashita H, Tsukayama H, Hori N, Kimura T, Tanno Y. Incidence of adverse reactions associated with acupuncture. J Altern Complement Med 2000;6(4):345–50.
63. Norheim AJ, Fonnebo V. A survey of acupuncture patients: results from a questionnaire among a random sample in the general population in Norway. Complement Ther Med 2000;8(3):187–92.
64. White AR, Ernst E. Survey of adverse events following acupuncture (SAFA). Forsch Komplementarmed 2000;7:29–58.
65. Bensoussan A, Myers SP, Carlton AL. Risks associated with the practice of traditional Chinese medicine: an Australian study. Arch Fam Med 2000;9(10):1071–8.
66. Yamashita H, Tsukayama H, White AR, Ernst E, Tanno Y, Sugishita C. Systematic review of case reports on acupuncture adverse events in the Japanese literature. Forsch Komplementarmed 2000;7:57.
67. Ernst E, White AR. Prospective studies of the safety of acupuncture: a systematic review. Am J Med 2001;110(6):481–5.
68. White A, Hayhoe S, Hart A, Ernst E. Adverse events following acupuncture: prospective survey of 32 000 consultations with doctors and physiotherapists. BMJ 2001;323(7311):485–6.
69. MacPherson H, Thomas K, Walters S, Fitter M. The York acupuncture safety study: prospective survey of 34 000 treatments by traditional acupuncturists. BMJ 2001;323(7311):486–7.
70. Yamashita H, Tsukayama H, White AR, Tanno Y, Sugishita C, Ernst E. Systematic review of adverse events following acupuncture: the Japanese literature. Complement Ther Med 2001;9(2):98–104.
71. Koga K, Shigematsu A, Noguchi T, Shiga Y. Should epidurals be avoided in acupunctured patients? Anaesthesia 2001;56(3):291–2.
72. Kirchgatterer A, Schwarz CD, Holler E, Punzengruber C, Hartl P, Eber B. Cardiac tamponade following acupuncture. Chest 2000;117(5):1510–11.
73. White AR, Abbot NC, Barnes J, Ernst E. Self-reports of adverse effects of acupuncture included cardiac arrhythmia. Acupunc Med 1996;14:121.
74. Shen D, Zhang M. A case of pneumothorax caused by acupuncture. Int J Clin Acupunct 2001;12:79.
75. Kao CL, Chang JP. Bilateral pneumothorax after acupuncture. J Emerg Med 2002;22(1):101–2.
76. Ramnarain D, Braams R. Dubbelzijdige pneumothorax na acupunctuur bij een jonge vrouw. [Bilateral pneumothorax in a young woman after acupuncture.] Ned Tijdschr Geneeskd 2002;146(4):172–5.
77. Choo DC, Yue G. Acute intracranial hemorrhage caused by acupuncture. Headache 2000;40(5):397–8.
78. Tsukerman IM. Redkii sluchai voznikoveniia kartsinom kozhi posle igloterapii (odno nabliudenie). [A rare case of carcinoma of the skin arising after acupuncture (case report).] Vopr Onkol 1970;16(6):88.
79. Jenner C, Filshie J. Galactorrhoea following acupuncture. Acupunct Med 2002;20(2–3):107–8.
80. Yanagihara M, Fujii T, Wakamatu N, Ishizaki H, Takehara T, Nawate K. Silicone granuloma on the entry points of acupuncture, venepuncture and surgical needles. J Cutan Pathol 2000;27(6):301–5.
81. Kirschbaum JO. Koebner phenomenon following acupuncture. Arch Dermatol 1972;106(5):767.
82. McCartney CJ, Herriot R, Chambers WA. Bilateral hand oedema related to acupuncture. Pain 2000;84(2–3):429–30.
83. Alani RM, Busam K. Acupuncture granulomas. J Am Acad Dermatol 2001;45(Suppl 6):S225–6.
84. Tanii T, Kono T, Katoh J, Mizuno N, Fukuda M, Hamada T. A case of prurigo pigmentosa considered to be contact allergy to chromium in an acupuncture needle. Acta Derm Venereol 1991;71(1):66–7.
85. Jones RO, Cross G 3rd. Suspected chronic osteomyelitis secondary to acupuncture treatment: a case report. J Am Podiatry Assoc 1980;70(3):149–51.
86. Scheel O, Sundsfjord A, Lunde P. Bakteriell endokarditt etter behandling hos naturmedisiner. [Bacterial endocarditis after treatment by a natural healer.] Tidsskr Nor Laegeforen 1991;111(22):2741–2.
87. Scheel O, Sundsfjord A, Lunde P, Andersen BM. Endocarditis after acupuncture and injection—treatment by a natural healer. JAMA 1992;267(1):56.
88. Baltimore RS, Moloy PJ. Perichondritis of the ear as a complication of acupuncture. Arch Otolaryngol 1976; 102(9):572–3.
89. Origuchi N, Komiyama T, Ohyama K, Wakabayashi T, Shigematsu H. Infectious aneurysm formation after depot acupuncture. Eur J Vasc Endovasc Surg 2000;20(2):211–13.
90. Ernst E, White AR. Indwelling needles carry greater risks than acupuncture techniques. BMJ 1999;318(7182):536.
91. Woo PC, Leung KW, Wong SS, Chong KT, Cheung EY, Yuen KY. Relatively alcohol-resistant mycobacteria are emerging pathogens in patients receiving acupuncture treatment. J Clin Microbiol 2002;40(4):1219–24.
92. Shah N, Hing C, Tucker K, Crawford R. Infected compartment syndrome after acupuncture. Acupunct Med 2002;20(2–3):105–6.
93. Lee SY, Chee SP. Group B Streptococcus endogenous endophthalmitis : case reports and review of the literature. Ophthalmology 2002;109(10):1879–86.
94. Woo PC, Li JH, Tang W, Yuen K. Acupuncture mycobacteriosis. N Engl J Med 2001;345(11):842–3.
95. Nambiar P, Ratnatunga C. Prosthetic valve endocarditis in a patient with Marfan's syndrome following acupuncture. J Heart Valve Dis 2001;10(5):689–90.
96. Castro KG, Lifson AR, White CR, Bush TJ, Chamberland ME, Lekatsas AM, Jaffe HW. Investigations of AIDS patients with no previously identified risk factors. JAMA 1988;259(9):1338–42.
97. Vittecoq D, Mettetal JF, Rouzioux C, Bach JF, Bouchon JP. Acute HIV infection after acupuncture treatments. N Engl J Med 1989;320(4):250–1.
98. Kent GP, Brondum J, Keenlyside RA, LaFazia LM, Scott HD. A large outbreak of acupuncture-associated hepatitis B. Am J Epidemiol 1988;127(3):591–8.
99. Michitaka K, Horiike N, Ohta Y. [An epidemiological study of hepatitis C virus infection in a local district in Japan.] Rinsho Byori 1991;39(6):586–91.
100. Boxall EH. Acupuncture hepatitis in the West Midlands, 1977. J Med Virol 1978;2(4):377–9.

101. Walsh B, Maguire H, Carrington D. Outbreak of hepatitis B in an acupuncture clinic. Commun Dis Public Health 1999;2(2):137–40.
102. Webster GJ, Hallett R, Whalley SA, Meltzer M, Balogun K, Brown D, Farrington CP, Sharma S, Hamilton G, Farrow SC, Ramsay ME, Teo CG, Dusheiko GM. Molecular epidemiology of a large outbreak of hepatitis B linked to autohaemotherapy. Lancet 2000;356(9227):379–84.
103. Kayaba K, Igarashi M, Okamoto H, Tsuda F. Prevalence of anti-hepatitis C antibodies in a rural community without high mortality from liver disease in Niigata prefecture. J Epidemiol 1998;8(4):250–5.
104. Burrell I. Acupuncture remedy linked to hepatitis outbreak. Independent Newspaper 1998;April 6.
105. Sun CA, Chen HC, Lu CF, You SL, Mau YC, Ho MS, Lin SH, Chen CJ. Transmission of hepatitis C virus in Taiwan: prevalence and risk factors based on a nationwide survey. J Med Virol 1999;59(3):290–6.
106. Shin HR, Kim JY, Ohno T, Cao K, Mizokami M, Risch H, Kim SR. Prevalence and risk factors of hepatitis C virus infection among Koreans in rural area of Korea. Hepatol Res 2000;17(3):185–96.
107. Nalpas B, Zylberberg H, Dubois F, Presles MA, Gillant JC, Lienard M, Delemotte B, Brechot C. Prévalence des infections par les virus hépatotropes en milieu rural. [Prevalence of infection by hepatitis viruses in a rural area. Analysis according to risk factors and alcohol consumption.] Gastroenterol Clin Biol 2000;24(5):536–40.
108. Peuker ET, White A, Ernst E, Pera F, Filler TJ. Traumatic complications of acupuncture. Therapists need to know human anatomy. Arch Fam Med 1999;8(6):553–8.
109. Rampes H, James R. Complications of acupuncture. Acupunct Med 1995;13:26–33.
110. Schiff AF. A fatality due to acupuncture. Med Times 1965;93:630–1.
111. Cheng TO. Pericardial effusion from self-inserted needle in the heart. Eur Heart J 1991;12(8):958.
112. Keller WJ, Parker SG, Garvin JP. Possible renal complications of acupuncture. JAMA 1972;222(12):1559.
113. Southworth SR, Hartwig RH. Foreign body in the median nerve: a complication of acupuncture. J Hand Surg [Br] 1990;15(1):111–12.
114. Murata K, Nishio A, Nishikawa M, Ohinata Y, Sakaguchi M, Nishimura S. Subarachnoid hemorrhage and spinal root injury caused by acupuncture needle—case report. Neurol Med Chir (Tokyo) 1990;30(12):956–9.
115. Shiraishi S, Goto I, Kuroiwa Y, Nishio S, Kinoshita K. Spinal cord injury as a complication of an acupuncture. Neurology 1979;29(8):1188–90.
116. Hasegawa J, Noguchi N, Yamasaki J, Kotake H, Mashiba H, Sasaki S, Mori T. Delayed cardiac tamponade and hemothorax induced by an acupuncture needle. Cardiology 1991;78(1):58–63.
117. Abumi K, Anbo H, Kaneda K. Migration of an acupuncture needle into the medulla oblongata. Eur Spine J 1996;5(2):137–9.
118. Lord RV, Schwartz P. False aneurysm of the popliteal artery complicating acupuncture. Aust NZ J Surg 1996;66(9):645–7.
119. Halvorsen R. Another acupuncture pneumothorax. Acupunct Med 1999;17:71.
120. Chiu DT. The use of acupuncture during pregnancy. Intern J Med 1984;1:19–21.
121. Cooke B, Ernst E. Aromatherapy: a systematic review. Br J Gen Pract 2000;50(455):493–6.
122. Schaller M, Korting HC. Allergic airborne contact dermatitis from essential oils used in aromatherapy. Clin Exp Dermatol 1995;20(2):143–5.
123. Tisserand R, Balacs T. Essential Oil Safety. A Guide For Health Care Professionals. Edinburgh: Churchill Livingstone, 1995.
124. Bleasel N, Tate B, Rademaker M. Allergic contact dermatitis following exposure to essential oils. Australas J Dermatol 2002;43(3):211–13.
125. Smith I. Suspected adverse reaction to essential oils. Aromatherapy World 2000;September:7.
126. Romaguera C, Vilaplana J. Occupational contact dermatitis from ylang-ylang oil. Contact Dermatitis 2000;43(4):251.
127. Sugiura M, Hayakawa R, Kato Y, Sugiura K, Hashimoto R. Results of patch testing with lavender oil in Japan. Contact Dermatitis 2000;43(3):157–60.
128. Kerr HD, Saryan LA. Arsenic content of homeopathic medicines. J Toxicol Clin Toxicol 1986;24(5):451–9.
129. De Smet PAGM. Giftige metalen in homeopathische preparaten Pharm Weekbl 1992;127:125–6
130. Oepen I. Kritische Argumente zur Homöopathie. Dtsch Apoth Ztg 1983;123:1105.
131. Kerr HD, Yarborough GW. Pancreatitis following ingestion of a homeopathic preparation. N Engl J Med 1986;314(25):1642–3.
132. van Ulsen J, Stolz E, van Joost T. Chromate dermatitis from a homeopathic drug. Contact Dermatitis 1988;18(1):56–7.
133. Forsman S. Homeopati kan vara farling vid hudsjukdomar och allergier. [Homeopathy can be dangerous in skin diseases and allergies.] Lakartidningen 1991;88(18):1672.
134. Dantas F, Rampes H. Do homeopathic medicines provoke adverse effects? A systematic review. Br Homeopath J 2000;89(Suppl 1):S35–8.
135. Delaunay P, Cua E, Lucas P, Marty P. Homoeopathy may not be effective in preventing malaria. BMJ 2000;321(7271):1288.
136. Luder AS, Friedman G. The mortality and morbidity of non-medical (alternative) treatment for minors. Int J Adolesc Med Health 2000;12:295–305.
137. Scott JA, Hall AJ, Muyodi C, Lowe B, Ross M, Chohan B, Mandaliya K, Getambu E, Gleeson F, Drobniewski F, Marsh K. Aetiology, outcome, and risk factors for mortality among adults with acute pneumonia in Kenya. Lancet 2000;355(9211):1225–30.
138. Kirby BJ. Safety of homeopathic products. J R Soc Med 2002;95(5):221–2.
139. Fisher P, Dantas F, Rampes H. The safety of homeopathic products. J R Soc Med 2002;95(9):474–5.
140. Barber J. When hypnosis causes trouble. Int J Clin Exp Hypn 1998;46(2):157–70.
141. Gravitz MA. Inability to dehypnotize-implications for management. Hypnosis 1998;25:93–7.
142. Dabbs V, Lauretti WJ. A risk assessment of cervical manipulation vs. NSAIDs for the treatment of neck pain. J Manipulative Physiol Ther 1995;18(8):530–6.
143. Jonas WB, Ernst E. Adverse effects of spinal manipulation. In: Jonas WB, Levin JS, editors. Essentials of Complementary and Alternative Medicine. Philadelphia: Lippincott Williams Wilkins, 1999:176–9.
144. Adams G, Sim J. A survey of UK manual therapists' practice of and attitudes towards manipulation and its complications. Physiother Res Int 1998;3(3):206–27.
145. Abbot NC, Hill M, Barnes J, Hourigan PG, Ernst E. Uncovering suspected adverse effects of complementary and alternative medicine. Int J Risk Saf Med 1998;11:99–106.
146. Di Fabio RP. Manipulation of the cervical spine: risks and benefits. Phys Ther 1999;79(1):50–65.
147. Barrett AJ, Breen AC. Adverse effects of spinal manipulation. J R Soc Med 2000;93(5):258–9.

148. Campbell JB, Busse JW, Injeyan HS. Chiropractors and vaccination: a historical perspective. Pediatrics 2000; 105(4):E43.
149. Lee AC, Li DH, Kemper KJ. Chiropractic care for children. Arch Pediatr Adolesc Med 2000; 154(4):401–7.
150. Ernst E. Prospective investigations into the safety of spinal manipulation. J Pain Symptom Manage 2001; 21(3):238–42.
151. Ernst E. Life-threatening complications of spinal manipulation. Stroke 2001;32(3):809–10.
152. Studdert DM, Eisenberg DM, Miller FH, Curto DA, Kaptchuk TJ, Brennan TA. Medical malpractice implications of alternative medicine. JAMA 1998; 280(18):1610–15.
153. Assendelft WJ, Pfeifle CE, Bouter LM. Chiropractic in The Netherlands: a survey of Dutch chiropractors. J Manipulative Physiol Ther 1995;18(3):129–34.
154. Plamondon RL. Summary of 1994 ACA Annual Statistical Study. J Am Chiropract Assoc 1995;32:57–63.
155. Robertson JT. Neck manipulation as a cause of stroke. Stroke 1981;12(1):1.
156. Dvorakj J. Manuelle Medizin. Stuttgart: Thieme, 1983.
157. Hosek RS, Schram SB, Silverman H, Myers JB, Williams SE. Cervical manipulation. JAMA 1981; 245(9):922.
158. Gutmann G. Injuries to the vertebral artery caused by manual therapy. Mannuelle Ther 1983;21:2–14.
159. Hamann G, Felber S, Haas A, Stristtmatter M, Kujat C, Schimrigk K, Piepgras U. Cervicocephalic artery dissections due to chiropractic manipulations. Lancet 1993; 341(8847):764–5.
160. Frisoni GB, Anzola GP. Vertebrobasilar ischemia after neck motion. Stroke 1991;22(11):1452–60.
161. Michaeli A. Dizziness testing of the cervical spine: can complications of manipulations be prevented? Physiother Theory Pract 1991;7:243–50.
162. Mas JL, Bousser MG, Hasboun D, Laplane D. Extracranial vertebral artery dissections: a review of 13 cases. Stroke 1987;18(6):1037–47.
163. Green D, Joynt RJ. Vascular accidents to the brain stem associated with neck manipulation. JAMA 1959; 170(5):522–4.
164. Smith RA, Estridge MN. Neurologic complications of head and neck manipulations. JAMA 1962;182:528–31.
165. Stevens AJJE. Zur Dopplersonographie der A. vertebralis bei Rotation des Kopfes. In: Gutman G, editor. Arteria Vertebralis Traumatologie und Funktionelle Pathologie. Berlin: Springer, 1985:90.
166. Okawara S, Nibbelink D. Vertebral artery occlusion following hyperextension and rotation of the head. Stroke 1974;5(5):640–2.
167. Frumkin LR, Baloh RW. Wallenberg's syndrome following neck manipulation. Neurology 1990;40(4):611–15.
168. Mas JL, Henin D, Bousser MG, Chain F, Hauw JJ. Dissecting aneurysm of the vertebral artery and cervical manipulation: a case report with autopsy. Neurology 1989;39(4):512–15.
169. Elliott MA, Taylor LP. "Shiatsu sympathectomy": ICA dissection associated with a shiatsu massager. Neurology 2002;58(8):1302–4.
170. Quintana JG, Drew EC, Richtsmeier TE, Davis LE. Vertebral artery dissection and stroke following neck manipulation by Native American healer. Neurology 2002;58(9):1434–5.
171. Saeed AB, Shuaib A, Al-Sulaiti G, Emery D. Vertebral artery dissection: warning symptoms, clinical features and prognosis in 26 patients. Can J Neurol Sci 2000; 27(4):292–6.
172. Balblanc JC, Pretot C, Ziegler F. Vascular complication involving the conus medullaris or cauda equina after vertebral manipulation for an L4-L5 disk herniation. Rev Rhum Engl Ed 1998;65(4):279–82.
173. Lipper MH, Goldstein JH, Do HM. Brown-Séquard syndrome of the cervical spinal cord after chiropractic manipulation. AJNR Am J Neuroradiol 1998; 19(7):1349–52.
174. Hillier CE, Gross ML. Sudden onset vomiting and vertigo following chiropractic neck manipulation. Postgrad Med J 1998;74(875):567–8.
175. Lynch P. Incidence of neurological injury following neck manipulation. Irish Med J 1998;91:130.
176. Lee KP, Carlini WG, McCormick GF, Albers GW. Neurologic complications following chiropractic manipulation: a survey of California neurologists. Neurology 1995;45(6):1213–15.
177. Turyk O. Nevrolohichni uskladnennia, obumovleni manual'noiu terapiieiu, pry osteokhondrozi khrebta. [The neurological complications caused by manual therapy in spinal osteochondrosis.] Lik Sprava 1999;(6):79–82.
178. Rydell N, Raf L. Spinal manipulation-behandling med stor komplikationsrisk. [Spinal manipulation—treatment associated with a high risk of complications.] Lakartidningen 1999;96(34):3536–40.
179. Hufnagel A, Hammers A, Schonle PW, Bohm KD, Leonhardt G. Stroke following chiropractic manipulation of the cervical spine. J Neurol 1999;246(8):683–8.
180. Leweke F, Teschendorf U, Stolz E, Kern A, Hahn M, Dorndorf W. Doppelsietige Dissektionen der Vertebralarterien nach chiropraktischer Behandlung der Halswirbelsäule. Aktuel Neurol 1999;26:35–9.
181. Chung OM. MRI confirmed cervical cord injury caused by spinal manipulation in a Chinese patient. Spinal Cord 2002;40(4):196–9.
182. Tseng SH, Chen Y, Lin SM, Wang CH. Cervical epidural hematoma after spinal manipulation therapy: case report. J Trauma 2002;52(3):585–6.
183. Jeret JS. More complications of spinal manipulation. Stroke 2001;32(8):1936–7.
184. Ng KP, Doube A. Stroke after neck manipulation in the post partum period. NZ Med J 2001;114(1143):498.
185. Schram DJ, Vosik W, Cantral D. Diaphragmatic paralysis following cervical chiropractic manipulation: case report and review. Chest 2001;119(2):638–40.
186. Ruelle A, Datti R, Pisani R. Thoracic epidural hematoma after spinal manipulation therapy. J Spinal Disord 1999;12(6):534–6.
187. Stevinson C, Honan W, Cooke B, Ernst E. Neurological complications of cervical spine manipulation. J R Soc Med 2001;94(3):107–10.
188. Schmitt HP. Risiken und Komplikationen der Manualtherapie der Wirbelsäule aus neurologischer Sicht. [Risks and complications of manual therapy of the spine from the neuropathologic viewpoint.] Nervenarzt 1988; 59(1):32–5.
189. Haldeman S, Rubinstein SM. Compression fractures in patients undergoing spinal manipulative therapy. J Manipulative Physiol Ther 1992;15(7):450–4.
190. Tolge C, Iyer V, McConnell J. Phrenic nerve palsy accompanying chiropractic manipulation of the neck. South Med J 1993;86(6):688–90.
191. Trotter JF. Hepatic hematoma after deep tissue massage. N Engl J Med 1999;341(26):2019–20.
192. Tsuboi K, Tsuboi K. Retinal and cerebral artery embolism after "shiatsu" on the neck. Stroke 2001;32(10):2441.

Conorfone

See also Opioid analgesics

General Information

Conorfone is an opioid analgesic, a codeine derivative, with mixed agonist–antagonist activity (SED-11, 150). It has adverse effects similar to those of codeine, but causes more drowsiness (1).

Reference

1. Dionne RA, Wirdezk PR, Butler DP, Fox PC. Comparison of conorphone, a mixed agonist-antagonist analgesic, to codeine for postoperative dental pain. Anesth Prog 1984;31(2):77–81.

Contact lenses and solutions

General Information

There are two types of contact lenses, soft and hard; most are manufactured from methacrylate polymer (http://www.eyecarecontacts.com/contact_lenses_reports.html).

Soft lenses are made of hydrophilic hydrogel polymers that contain 36–74% water. Other plastics and co-polymers are added to alter the physical characteristics of the lens. The diameter is 10.5–15.5 mm and the thickness at the center 0.03–20 mm. Soft lenses can correct most optical defects, including myopia, hyperopia, and astigmatism. Bifocal lenses are also available. They can be colored with either transparent hues or opaque patterns to change apparent eye color or to mask malformations of the cornea or iris. They are available for daily, weekly, and twice-weekly disposable use, 1–3 months frequent replacement, and annual replacement.

Hard lenses are made from gas-permeable materials that contain silicon and fluorine. They can correct most optical defects and have diameters of 8–10 mm.

Some lenses combine soft and hard materials, including hard lenses with soft surfaces and lenses with a hard center and a soft periphery.

The ocular risks related to the use of contact lenses are due not only to the lenses themselves, but also to the toxic or allergic effects of cleaning solutions (1) and the preservatives that they contain. The latter are also found in various eye-drops. Preservatives have adverse effects on the corneal epithelium and endothelium. Eye-drops that contain preservatives should not be used during surgery or in patients with ocular surface disease, in cases of perforating injury.

Organs and Systems

Sensory systems

Ulcerative keratitis is considered the most serious adverse effect of the use of soft contact lenses.

The risk can be greatly reduced by avoiding overnight wear of the lenses (2,3). In one study extended wear was associated with a 5–6 times higher risk of keratitis than daily wear was (4).

Soft contact lenses, especially extended-wear lenses, carry a significantly higher risk of keratitis than hard lenses do. In a case-control study, the relative risk for overnight wear soft lenses was 21, for daily-wear soft lenses 3.6, and for polymethylmethacrylate hard lenses 1.3, as compared with gas-permeable hard lenses (5).

Microorganisms can infiltrate into soft hydrophilic lenses, causing infection and possibly corneal ulcers. *Acanthamoeba* is the most common cause. In a case-control study there was an increased risk of *Acanthamoeba* infection largely attributable to lack of disinfection or the use of chlorine-based disinfection (the latter having little protective effect against the organism). Around 80% of cases of *Acanthamoeba* keratitis could have been avoided by the use of lens disinfection systems that are effective against this organism (6). *Pseudomonas aeruginosa* adherence to corneal epithelial cells was also enhanced in those who used extended-wear soft contact lenses (7). Because acanthamoebae are more commonly found in stagnant water tanks, contact lens wearers should be advised to use water from downstairs kitchen taps rather than upstairs bathroom taps.

Oxygen deficiency can occur under the lens. The dimension of the lens, duration of wear, and hygiene are determining factors. Tolerance is individual, and less hydrophilic materials produce a higher degree of corneal hypoxia. This is manifested by edema, and sometimes by vascularization and even limbus hyperemia and pannus corneae (8,9). Tear-film disruption can be a contributing factor.

Cases of allergic conjunctivitis and blepharitis have been reported with the preservatives benzalkonium chloride and mercurial salts, although benzalkonium at the commonly used concentration of 0.01% produces no evident damage. These adverse reactions can be prevented by rinsing hard lenses in clean water before insertion in the eye and by boiling soft lenses in normal saline after cleaning.

Chlorhexidine digluconate is a biguanide surfactant with low toxicity, but it is a strong contact sensitizer. Its mucus-binding capacity limits its use: it binds to hydrophilic (soft) contact lenses. Build-up of proteinaceous debris in lenses may greatly increase the binding of chlorhexidine to the lens.

The use of chlorobutanol is limited to pHs below 6. It is subject to thermal degradation and can be adsorbed on to the walls of containers. However, it has no major adverse effects. Chlorobutanol has no effect on wetting of the cornea or contact lenses, as surface-active agents do. When tested with soft lenses, chlorobutanol, concentrated in the lenses, causes mild conjunctivitis.

References

1. Polak BCP, Beekhuis WH. Risk and safety of contact lenses. Int J Risk Safety Med 1990;1:219–23.
2. Schein OD, Glynn RJ, Poggio EC, Seddon JM, Kenyon KR. The relative risk of ulcerative keratitis among users of

daily-wear and extended-wear soft contact lenses. A case-control study. Microbial Keratitis Study Group. N Engl J Med 1989;321(12):773–8.
3. Schein OD, Buehler PO, Stamler JF, Verdier DD, Katz J. The impact of overnight wear on the risk of contact lens-associated ulcerative keratitis. Arch Ophthalmol 1994;112(2):186–90.
4. Nilsson SE, Montan PG. The annualized incidence of contact lens induced keratitis in Sweden and its relation to lens type and wear schedule: results of a 3-month prospective study. CLAO J 1994;20(4):225–30.
5. Dart JK, Stapleton F, Minassian D. Contact lenses and other risk factors in microbial keratitis. Lancet 1991;338 (8768):650–3.
6. Radford CF, Bacon AS, Dart JK, Minassian DC. Risk factors for acanthamoeba keratitis in contact lens users: a case-control study. BMJ 1995;310(6994):1567–70.
7. Fleiszig SM, Efron N, Pier GB. Extended contact lens wear enhances *Pseudomonas aeruginosa* adherence to human corneal epithelium. Invest Ophthalmol Vis Sci 1992;33(10): 2908–16.
8. Marechal-Coutois CH, Delcourt JC. Klinische Resultate einer Untersuchung mit einer 70%ig hydratisierten Linse: die Linse Tp 70 (Yumecon). Contactologie 1981;3D:89.
9. Pickering CAC, Bainbridge B, Birtwistle IH. Occupational asthma due to methylmethacrylate in an orthopedic theater sister. BMJ (Clin Res Ed) 1986;292:1362.

Continuous ambulatory peritoneal dialysis

General Information

One complication of long-term CAPD is peritoneal calcification. The cause is unclear, but it may be associated with multiple bouts of peritonitis combined with hyercalcemia. In one case there was evidence that the effect may be reversible (1).

- A 48-year-old woman undergoing CAPD had several bouts of peritonitis, with four admissions for treatment between 1988 and 1993. In 1993, moderate amounts of calcification surrounding the small bowel were identified by CT scan, and this progressively increased over the following year. CAPD was discontinued and hemodialysis with a low dialysate calcium concentration was used instead. After a further admission 4 months later, parenteral nutrition was begun. Over the following three years, CT scans showed a progressive reduction in the extent of peritoneal calcification surrounding the small bowel.

The authors speculated that hemodialysis and long-term parenteral nutrition may result in reversal of peritoneal calcification caused by CAPD.

Reference

1. Najem ES, Webel M, Ailinani JM. Reversibility of peritoneal calcification in a dialysis patient maintained on hemodialysis and total parenteral nutrition. Am J Roentgenol 1999;172(1):247–8.

Convolvulaceae

See also Herbal medicines

General Information

The genera in the family of Convolvulaceae (Table 1) include bindweed and morning glory.

Table 1 The genera of Convolvulaceae

Aniseia (aniseia)
Argyreia (argyreia)
Bonamia (lady's nightcap)
Calystegia (false bindweed)
Convolvulus (bindweed)
Cressa (alkaliweed)
Dichondra (pony's foot)
Evolvulus (dwarf morning glory)
Ipomoea (morning glory)
Jacquemontia (cluster vine)
Merremia (wood rose)
Operculina (lidpod)
Poranopsis (poranopsis)
Stictocardia (stictocardia)
Stylisma (dawn flower)
Turbina (turbina)
Xenostegia (morning vine)

Convolvulus scammonia

Convolvulus scammonia (Mexican scammony) contains alkaloids that are drastic purgatives with irritant properties. It has now been superseded.

Ipomoea purga

Ipomoea purga (jalap) is a drastic cathartic with irritant action, which has been superseded by less toxic laxatives.

Copper

General Information

Copper is a reddish metallic element (symbol Cu; atomic no. 29). Its symbol derives from the Latin word cuprum, because it was originally discovered in Cyprus. It is widely found as different salts in minerals such as atacamite (chloride); azurite and malachite (carbonates); bornite, chalcocite, chalcopyrite, stannite, tennantite, and tetrahedrite (sulfides); chalcanthite (sulfate); dioptase (silicate); erinite and olivenite (arsenates); tenorite (oxide); torbernite (phosphate); and zorgite (selenide). Copper is an essential constituent of several enzymes. It is carried in the blood by a specific copper-binding protein, ceruloplasmin.

The bulk of publications on copper deal with its metabolism as an essential trace element, its role in Menkes' disease (associated with copper deficiency) and

Wilson's disease (associated with copper excess) (1,2), and its possible role in Alzheimer's disease (3), prion disease (4), and familial amyotrophic lateral sclerosis (5). Copper metabolism and toxicity have been reviewed (6). The potential use of novel chelating agents for copper isotopes with short half-lives in radiopharmacy has been discussed (7).

Copper histidine is increasingly being used in Menkes' disease and allows survival into adolescence (8). The neurological abnormalities respond better than the connective tissue abnormalities.

A boy with Menkes' disease and low plasma concentrations of copper (3.6 μmol/l) and ceruloplasmin (50 mg/l) received copper histidine and died aged 10. Postmortem examination showed significant pathology of the mesenchymal tissues, including skeletal abnormalities, vascular degeneration, and bladder diverticula. The central nervous system, in contrast, showed minimal pathology of copper metabolism compared with classical Menkes' disease.

The differential sensitivity of central nervous system and mesenchymal tissues to copper histidine may be due to heterogeneity in the responses of different copper-dependent enzymes.

There is also contact with copper in daily life. When copper comes into contact with biological materials it becomes corroded, and the compounds that are formed can produce irritation and other reactions.

Some copper compounds have been used therapeutically in the past. Small quantities of copper salts enhance the physiological utilization of iron and are thus often present in hemopoietic formulations. Copper chloride and copper sulfate are used in parenteral nutrition solutions. The artificial radioactive copper isotope ^{64}Cu has been used in mineral metabolic studies. Excess accumulation of copper can occur due to an abnormality of ceruloplasmin and causes Wilson's disease and Menkes' disease, which are both characterized by copper accumulation (SEDA-22, 244) (9).

Copper-containing intrauterine contraceptive devices

Copper-containing intrauterine contraceptive devices (10–12) became popular because local inflammatory reactions in the endometrium are more marked and the contraceptive effect is thus more pronounced (SEDA-21, 234) (13). In addition, copper ions released from intrauterine contraceptive devices reach concentrations in the luminal fluids of the genital tract that are toxic to spermatozoa and embryos. The ability of copper to induce the generation of free radicals and the formation of malonaldehyde may be involved in its contraceptive effect.

There is a positive correlation between high copper loss from an intrauterine contraceptive device and the development of menorrhagia or pathological lesions, such as cervical dysplasia and endometrial cytopathology (14). Evidence of endometrial carcinoma was not found in endometrial aspirates from 189 women who had used Copper-T-200 devices for 1–10 years, but five cases of endometrial hyperplasia (2.67%) were encountered in women in the series, all of whom had worn copper devices for 6 years or more. Inflammatory changes in the endometrial cells were found in 12 cases (6.2%), 11 of 12 having worn the device for over 3 years. It is possible that constant exposure to copper may be responsible for persistence of chronic inflammatory changes in endometrial cells, which could be the precursors of hyperplastic changes. It is not clear whether the dissolved copper is also responsible for the temporarily increased predisposition to bacterial contamination and the somewhat increased risk of pelvic inflammatory disease, seen especially in young nulliparous women using this type of contraceptive method.

Migration of intrauterine contraceptive devices is relatively rare, although they have been found in the omentum, rectosigmoid, peritoneum, bladder, appendix, small bowel, adnexa, and iliac vein. Most authors have recommended removal of copper-containing devices, because of the potential for inflammatory reactions, which can cause bowel obstruction and perforation (15). Two cases of migration of intrauterine contraceptive devices to the bowel have been reported.

- A Copper-T intrauterine contraceptive device migrated to the rectal lumen in a 36-year-old woman with menorrhagia for 3 months and a history of Copper-T insertion 6 years before (16).
- A 28-year-old pregnant woman developed an ileal perforation 4 weeks after the insertion of a Multiload-Cu 375 intrauterine contraceptive device (17).

The second report documents the shortest interval between insertion and proven bowel injury by an intrauterine contraceptive device.

Immunological and hypersensitivity reactions beyond the uterus are uncommon, but they can occur. Rashes, including generalized urticaria and eczematoid eruptions, have occurred as a result of allergy to the copper released from intrauterine contraceptive devices, although they are extremely rare (SEDA-11, 204) (SEDA-12, 186) (SEDA-21, 235). One woman who had worn a copper-containing device for 12 months developed widespread urticaria and angioedema of the eyelids and the labia majora and minora for about 6 months (18). She also had persistent symptoms of premenstrual and postmenstrual spotting and leukorrhea for about 6 months. A patch test was positive with 1% copper sulfate, as was an in vitro lymphocyte stimulating test with copper. An endometrial biopsy showed vulvovaginitis, with hyperplasia of the cervical canal and T cell and eosinophilic granulocyte infiltration. Removal of the device caused complete remission.

Genital tract actinomycosis has come increasingly to the fore (19,20). In one study in Britain, the pelvic smears of nearly one-third of women using plastic devices were positive for *Actinomyces*-like organisms, compared with two of 165 women using copper-loaded IUCDs and none in a series of oral contraceptive users. There was a highly significant correlation between the presence of these organisms on smear and pain and other symptoms of pelvic inflammatory disease.

- A 32-year-old woman, who had had a copper intrauterine contraceptive device for more than 5 years, developed acyclic menstrual bleedings and had a uterine biopsy after removal of the intrauterine device (21). Histology of the abraded tissue showed an actinomycotic endometritis, with brown to black deposits in or around typical *Actinomyces druses*, but there was no carcinoma. Electron microscopy showed copper deposits in the shell and matrix of the druses and inside the bacteria. Electron-dense accumulations showed high signals for copper and sulfur, and to a lesser extent also for phosphorus and oxygen.

Copper accumulation in this case may have been caused by active uptake and concentration by the *Actinomycetes*.

If copper-containing fragments of intrauterine contraceptive devices perforate the uterine wall and enter the peritoneal cavity, acute inflammatory reactions and peritoneal adhesions can occur. Laparoscopic removal is then not only as a rule impossible but may also be dangerous because of the marked peritoneal reaction surrounding the copper part of the device. Laparotomy has therefore been suggested as the primary measure in such cases. Whether copper devices result more commonly in perforation than non-copper devices is not entirely clear, nor is the question answered whether copper increases the risk of extrauterine pregnancies, although older evidence suggested this as a risk (SED-9, 371).

Although copper-containing intrauterine contraceptive devices are very effective, pregnancies do occur and the question of possible second-generation effects has to be considered. In one case the neonate showed significantly increased copper and ceruloplasmin concentrations, whereas maternal concentrations were within the reference range. Whether such exposure to copper can cause harm is not clear; because of the pharmacological effects of copper, it has been suspected of having mutagenic and carcinogenic potential. Until now, there is no clear evidence that harm is actually done. Five published cases scattered throughout the literature in which incomplete closure of the neural tube was found (22) could have been coincidental, bearing in mind the large number of pregnancies in which exposure to copper must occur in this way. In various species of animals which have been studied (rat, rabbit, hamster, sheep) no teratogenicity of intrauterine copper was detected (SED-11, 442).

Organs and Systems

Nervous system

It has been suggested that copper-mediated toxicity in some neurodegenerative diseases (Alzheimer's disease and familial amyotrophic lateral sclerosis) may contribute to neurodegeneration (23). It should be borne in mind that similar but unproven theories have been raised regarding other metals, notably aluminium.

Sensory systems

Penetration of the eye by copper wire has been reported to produce a recurrent chronic uveitis (24).

Ocular chalcosis has been attributed to injury with a copper-containing foreign body (25).

- After having suffered an open-globe injury, presumably due to a small foreign body after a grenade explosion, a 30-year-old man presented 6 years later with ocular chalcosis, including sunflower cataract, a multitude of tiny brownish particles in the anterior vitreous, fibrillar degeneration of the posterior vitreous, and brilliant patches overriding the foveal region. The patches were measured by confocal scanning laser tomography and optical coherence tomography. Besides acquired cyan-dyschromatopsia, psychophysical and electrophysiological tests were unremarkable. Vision was 20/20. The central patches measured 200–700 μm in diameter and 150–200 μm in height above the inner retinal surface. With the exception of a Kayser–Fleischer ring of the cornea the patient presented all the morphological signs of ocular chalcosis. Since signs of inflammation were absent no further therapy was planned.

This man had probably suffered from a penetrating damage of the left eye caused by a copper-containing body, which had eventually dissolved. Although the observed patches on the central retina in ocular chalcosis have previously been described, their nature is not known.

Hematologic

The effects of combined oral contraceptives, depot medroxyprogesterone acetate injections, levonorgestrel subdermal implants (Norplant), copper-containing intrauterine contraceptive devices (IUCDs), and Chinese stainless steel ring IUCDs on hemoglobin and ferritin have been studied in 2507, non-pregnant non-lactating women, aged 18–40 years, in seven countries (Bangladesh, Chile, China, the Dominican Republic, Pakistan, Thailand, and Tunisia) (26). In 1295 current users of the contraceptive methods hemoglobin and ferritin concentrations were higher than in 1212 women who were starting to use contraceptives. The current users of copper IUCDs had higher hemoglobin concentrations (difference in mean concentrations of 0.3 g/dl), but lower ferritin concentrations (difference of 10 g/l) than non-users. Current use of the stainless steel ring had an adverse effect on both hemoglobin and ferritin. In 285 anemic women there were significant mean increases of hemoglobin at 12 months among the users of the hormonal contraceptives, but not among users of copper or stainless steel ring IUCDs. The authors concluded that hemoglobin and ferritin concentrations are affected by contraceptives and that the hormonal contraceptives included in this study have a beneficial effect, while the effects of copper IUCDs should be studied further.

Liver

Copper poisoning can cause hepatic cirrhosis in Wilson's disease (SEDA-21, 234) (27), but no cases appear to be known in which this resulted from medicinal exposure. Apart from Wilson's disease and Menkes' disease, much attention has been given to copper-associated liver disease in infancy and childhood, in which excessive dietary copper overload and a genetic predisposition can lead to high liver copper concentrations and progressive liver disease (28).

Skin

Perimenstrual dermatitis has been attributed to a copper-containing intrauterine contraceptive device (29).

- A 41-year-old woman had a 2-year history of a recurrent, self-healing skin rash associated with abdominal pain. She had had cholinergic urticaria since 1995 and had had a copper-containing intrauterine contraceptive device inserted 12 years before. The eruption followed a cyclical pattern, invariably appearing 3–7 days before the menses and tending to improve spontaneously with the onset of bleeding. This non-itchy rash was associated with abdominal distension and cramps that followed a similar course. She had multiple non-itchy symmetrical erythematous papules on the upper trunk, neck, and arms. Patch-testing was positive for copper sulfate. The intrauterine contraceptive device was removed and the abdominal symptoms subsided at the following cycle. Progressive resolution of the dermatitis was observed. No cutaneous eruption was observed after 8 months and no new lesions developed after a further 5 months.

Hair

A remarkable (although non-medical) case reported in 1996 concerned a man who developed green hair as a result of drinking tap water with a high copper concentration (30). The discoloration disappeared promptly after the use of a shampoo containing penicillamine.

Reproductive system

The fibrinolytic activity of menstrual blood in wearers of Lippes loops exceeds that of patients with menorrhagia, while the values in users of the Cu-T (200) are in the same range as in normally menstruating and untreated women. In users of Lippes loops no fibrin was found in the endometrial stroma. This may explain the increased blood loss associated with the use of the Lippes loop, which can be severe enough to cause anemia (31).

Susceptibility Factors

Hepatic disease

In primary sclerosing cholangitis there is increased hepatic retention of both copper and selenium (32)

Drug Administration

Drug overdose

Overdose of copper sulfate can cause nephrotoxicity.

- A 21-year-old pharmacist developed acute renal insufficiency (33). Three days before he had dissolved a small quantity of copper sulfate in 5 ml of tap water and injected it intravenously in a suicide attempt. The serum copper concentration was 1.950 μg/ml (31 μmol/l). He was dialysed and gradually improved over 6 weeks. His serum copper concentration a month after the incident was 0.5 μg/ml (8 μmol/l). At 8 weeks a renal biopsy showed marked patchy tubular atrophy with interstitial fibrosis and mild focal chronic interstitial inflammation. Some tubules showed regenerating epithelial cells with multilayering and mitosis, with a predominant loss of proximal tubules. The findings were suggestive of chronic tubulointerstitial nephritis.

References

1. Fatemi N, Sarkar B. Molecular mechanism of copper transport in Wilson disease. Environ Health Perspect 2002;110(Suppl 5):695–8.
2. Harada M. Wilson disease. Med Electron Microsc 2002;35(2):61–6.
3. Strausak D, Mercer JF, Dieter HH, Stremmel W, Multhaup G. Copper in disorders with neurological symptoms: Alzheimer's, Menkes, and Wilson diseases. Brain Res Bull 2001;55(2):175–85.
4. Brown DR. Copper and prion disease. Brain Res Bull 2001;55(2):165–73.
5. Llanos RM, Mercer JF. The molecular basis of copper homeostasis copper-related disorders. DNA Cell Biol 2002;21(4):259–70.
6. Barceloux DG. Copper. J Toxicol Clin Toxicol 1999;37(2):217–30.
7. Ma D, Lu F, Overstreet T, Milenic DE, Brechbiel MW. Novel chelating agents for potential clinical applications of copper. Nucl Med Biol 2002;29(1):91–105.
8. George DH, Casey RE. Menkes disease after copper histidine replacement therapy: case report. Pediatr Dev Pathol 2001;4(3):281–8.
9. Loudianos G, Gitlin JD. Wilson's disease. Semin Liver Dis 2000;20(3):353–64.
10. Fortney JA, Feldblum PJ, Raymond EG. Intrauterine devices. The optimal long-term contraceptive method? J Reprod Med 1999;44(3):269–74.
11. Thonneau P, Goulard H, Goyaux N. Risk factors for intrauterine device failure: a review. Contraception 2001;64(1):33–7.
12. Bilian X. Intrauterine devices. Best Pract Res Clin Obstet Gynaecol 2002;16(2):155–68.
13. Ortiz ME, Croxatto HB, Bardin CW. Mechanisms of action of intrauterine devices. Obstet Gynecol Surv 1996;51(Suppl 12):S42–51.
14. Engineer AD, Misra JS, Tandon P. Copper loss & cytopathological changes associated with copper IUD use. Indian J Med Res 1983;78:42–8.
15. Kassab B, Audra P. Le sterilet migrateur. A propos d'un cas et revue de la litterature. [The migrating intrauterine device. Case report and review of the literature.] Contracept Fertil Sex 1999;27(10):696–700.
16. Banerjee N, Kriplani A, Roy KK, Bal S, Takkar D. Retrieval of lost Copper-T from the rectum. Eur J Obstet Gynecol Reprod Biol 1998;79(2):211–12.
17. Chen CP, Hsu TC, Wang W. Ileal penetration by a Multiload-Cu 375 intrauterine contraceptive device. A case report with review of the literature. Contraception 1998;58(5):295–304.
18. Purello D'Ambrosio F, Ricciardi L, Isola S, Gangemi S, Cilia M, Levanti C, Marcazzo A. Systemic contact dermatitis to copper-containing IUD. Allergy 1996; 51(9):658–9.

19. Duguid HL, Parratt D, Traynor R. *Actinomyces*-like organisms in cervical smears from women using intrauterine contraceptive devices. BMJ 1980; 281(6239):534–7.
20. Leeton J. Female genital actinomycosis and the intrauterine device. Med J Aust 1980;1(11):518.
21. Jonas L, Baguhl F, Wilken HP, Haas HJ, Nizze H. Copper accumulation in *Actinomyces druses* during endometritis after long-term use of an intrauterine contraceptive device. Ultrastruct Pathol 2002;26(5):323–9.
22. Graham D, Enkin M, deSa D. Neural tube defects in association with copper intrauterine devices. Int J Gynaecol Obstet 1980;18(6):404–5.
23. Multhaup G. Amyloid precursor protein, copper and Alzheimer's disease. Biomed Pharmacother 1997; 51(3):105–11.
24. Billi B, Lesnoni G, Scassa C, Giuliano MA, Coppe AM, Rossi T. Copper intraocular foreign body: diagnosis and treatment. Eur J Ophthalmol 1995;5(4):235–9.
25. Budde WM, Junemann A. Chalcosis oculi. [Chalcosis oculi.] Klin Monatsbl Augenheilkd 1998;212(3):184–5.
26. Bathija H, Lei ZW, Cheng XQ, Xie L, Wang Y, Rugpao S, Lipisam S, Suwanarach C, Akhter H, Ahmed Y, Islam Z, Sen A, Bahman S, Khan SA, Rabbani A, Khan T, Sued EM, Lumbiganon P, Weerawattrakul Y, Pinitsoontorn P, Bierschwale H, Silva P, Bravo C, Gajardo R, Meta N, Lavin F, Tuane R, Chong E, Hajri S, Siala N, Bessioud M, Boukhris R. Effects of contraceptives on hemoglobin and ferritin. Task Force for Epidemiological Research on Reproductive Health, United Nations Development Programme/United Nations Population Fund/World Health Organization/World Bank Special Programme of Research, Development and Research Training in Human Reproduction, World Health Organization, Geneva, Switzerland. Contraception 1998;58(5):262–73.
27. Price LA, Walker NI, Clague AE, Pullen ID, Smits SJ, Ong TH, Patrick M. Chronic copper toxicosis presenting as liver failure in an Australian child. Pathology 1996;28(4):316–20.
28. Rodeck B, Kardoff R, Melter M. Treatment of copper associated liver disease in childhood. Eur J Med Res 1999;4(6):253–6.
29. Pujol RM, Randazzo L, Miralles J, Alomar A. Perimenstrual dermatitis secondary to a copper-containing intrauterine contraceptive device. Contact Dermatitis 1998;38(5):288.
30. Munkvad S, Weismann K. Kobberinduceret gront haar. Behandling med en penicillaminshampoo. [Copper-induced green hair. Treatment with a penicillamine containing shampoo.] Ugeskr Laeger 1996; 158(26):3791–2.
31. Hefnawi F, Saleh A, Kandil O, El-Sheikha Z, Hassanein M, Askalani H. Fibrinolytic activity of menstrual blood in normal and menorrhagic women and in women wearing the Lippes Loop and the Cu-T (200). Int J Gynaecol Obstet 1979;16(5):400–7.
32. Aaseth J, Thomassen Y, Aadland E, Fausa O, Schrumpf E. Hepatic retention of copper and selenium in primary sclerosing cholangitis. Scand J Gastroenterol 1995;30(12):1200–3.
33. Bhowmik D, Mathur R, Bhargava Y, Dinda AK, Agarwal SK, Tiwari SC, Dash SC. Chronic interstitial nephritis following parenteral copper sulfate poisoning. Ren Fail 2001;23(5):731–5.

Coriariaceae

See also Herbal medicines

General Information

The family of Coriariaceae contains the single genus *Coriaria*.

Coriaria species

Coriaria arborea (tutu) plant is a traditional Maori medicine. It contains various sesquiterpenoids, including a toxin, tutin, that is allied to picrotoxin (1).

Adverse effects

Ingestion of portions or concoctions of *Coriaria* plants can result in tonic-clonic seizures, respiratory arrest, and death.

Three sisters who ate berries of *Coriaria myrtifolia* (redoul) suffered from acute poisoning; the adverse effects affected the gastrointestinal tract (nausea, vomiting, abdominal pain), the nervous system (obnubilation, convulsions, and their complications), and respiratory function (hyperpnea, apnea, short and superficial respiration), together with myositis of the pupils; one died (2).

Of 25 children who ate the fruits of *C. myrtifolia*, 13 had gastrointestinal digestive symptoms and nine had nervous system toxicity, including seizures and coma (3).

References

1. Anonymous. Twenty-fifth Annual Report of the National Toxicoloy Group. Dunedin: New Zealand National Poisons and Hazardous Chemicals Information Centre, 1990:4.
2. Skalli S, David JM, Benkirane R, Zaid A, Soulaymani R. Intoxication aigue par le redoul (*Coriaria myrtifolia* L.). [Acute intoxication by redoul (*Coriaria myrtifolia* L.). Three observations.] Presse Méd 2002;31(33):1554–6.
3. Garcia Martin A, Masvidal Aliberch RM, Bofill Bernaldo AM, Rodriguez Alsina S. Intoxicacion por ingesta de *Coriaria myrtifolia* Estudio de 25 casos. [Poisoning caused by ingestion of *Coriaria myrtifolia*. Study of 25 cases.] An Esp Pediatr 1983;19(5):366–70.

Corticorelin (corticotropin-releasing hormone (CRH))

General Information

For complete functional evaluation of the hypothalamic–hypophyseal–adrenal axis one can use synthetic corticorelin (corticotropin-releasing hormone), which is available in both human (hCRH) and ovine (oCRH) forms (1).

Single bolus injections in standard doses (for example 200 μg of hCRH or oCRH), whether given on a single occasion or at fixed intervals, have a very low rate of complications. At higher doses adverse effects occur in almost 40% of patients (2). At a dose of 1 mg/kg they mainly comprise flushing or a feeling of warmth (30%), a sensation of discomfort (5%), palpitation (3%), and dyspnea (1%). Higher doses (more than 200 mg) can cause hypotension or coronary ischemia. Patients with brain injury are more susceptible to adverse reactions (2). No serious allergic reactions have been reported. Continuous infusions of hCRH or oCRH for several hours have also been well tolerated, but adverse effects occurred with cumulative doses of 200–300 μg/hour.

High doses can provoke marked adverse effects in patients with neurological disorders, coronary heart disease, or disorders of the pituitary–adrenal axis, especially if the blood–brain barrier has been damaged (for example by a head injury or during intracranial surgery). Non-standard doses should only be used in experimental work with well-designed safety precautions.

References

1. Anonymous. Corticorelin: ACTH RF, corticoliberin, corticotrophin-releasing hormone, corticotropin-releasing factor, human corticotropin-releasing hormone, ovine corticotrophin-releasing factor, Xerecept. Drugs R D 2004;5(4):218–19.
2. Nink M, Krause U, Lehnert H, Beyer J. Safety and side effects of human and ovine corticotropin-releasing hormone administration in man. Klin Wochenschr 1991; 69(5):185–95.

Corticosteroids—glucocorticoids

General Information

Nomenclature

The two main classes of adrenal corticosteroids are properly known as glucocorticoids and mineralocorticosteroids. The former are often known by shorter names and are commonly referred to as "glucocorticoids", "corticosteroids", "corticoids", or even simply "steroids"; the latter are often referred to as "mineralocorticoids". Here we shall use the terms "glucocorticoids" and "mineralocorticoids". When referring to both we shall use the term "corticosteroids".

Relative potencies

The main human anti-inflammatory corticosteroid, the glucocorticoid cortisol (hydrocortisone), as secreted by the adrenal gland, has generally been replaced by related glucocorticoids of synthetic origin for therapeutic purposes. These Δ^1-dehydrated glucocorticoids are designed to imitate the physiological hormone. They have marked glucocorticoid potency but only minor effects on sodium retention and potassium excretion; the relative glucocorticoid and mineralocorticoid potencies of the best-known compounds, insofar as these potencies are agreed, are compared in Table 1.

Over many years, a great deal of research has been devoted to producing better glucocorticoids for therapeutic use. Those endeavors have succeeded only in part; from the start the mineralocorticoid effects were sufficiently minor to be nonproblematic; the fact that successive synthetic glucocorticoids had an increasing potency in terms of weight was not of direct therapeutic significance; and the most hoped-for aim, that of dissociating wanted from unwanted glucocorticoid effects has not been achieved (1). Most untoward effects, such as those due to the catabolic and gluconeogenic activities of the glucocorticoid family, probably cannot be dissociated entirely from the anti-inflammatory activity (2) it is possible that myopathy and muscle wasting are actually more common when triamcinolone or dexamethasone are used, but this may merely reflect overdosage of these potent drugs. However, some progress in achieving a dissociation of effects has been made. Beclomethasone does have a relatively greater local than systemic effect. Deflazacort, one of the few new glucocorticoids to have been developed in recent years, originally promised reduced intensity of adverse effects, for example on bone mineral density, but the early promise has not held up (SEDA-18, 389). Cloprednol seems to affect the hypothalamic–pituitary–adrenal axis much less than other glucocorticoids, and to cause less excretion of nitrogen and calcium (3).

Uses

Most patients who are treated therapeutically with glucocorticoids do not have glucocorticoid deficiency. Adverse

Table 1 Relative potencies of glucocorticoids

Compound	Glucocorticoid potency relative to hydrocortisone	Mineralocorticoid potency	Equivalent doses (mg)
Cortisone	0.8	++	25
Hydrocortisone	1.0	++	20
Prednisone	4	+	5
Prednisolone	4	+	5
Methylprednisolone	5	0	4
Triamcinolone	5	0	4
Paramethasone	10	0	2
Fluprednisolone	10	0	1.5
Dexamethasone	30	0	0.75
Betamethasone	30	0	0.6

reactions to glucocorticoids depend very largely on the ways in which, and the purposes for which, they are used. There are four groups of uses.

(1) Substitution therapy is used in cases of primary and secondary adrenocortical insufficiency; the aim is to provide glucocorticoids and mineralocorticoids in physiological amounts, and the better the dosage regimen is adapted to the individual's needs, the less the chance of adverse effects (1).
(2) Anti-inflammatory and immunosuppressive therapy exploits the immunosuppressive, anti-allergic, anti-inflammatory, anti-exudative, and anti-proliferative effects of the glucocorticoids (2). The desired pharmacodynamic effects reflect a general influence of these substances on the mesenchyme, where they suppress reactions that result in the symptoms of inflammation, exudation, and proliferation; the nonspecific effects of glucocorticoids on the mesenchyme are part of their physiological actions, but they can only be obtained to a clinically useful extent by using dosages at which the more specific (and unwanted) physiological effects also occur. High doses sufficient to suppress immune reactions are used in patients who have undergone organ transplantation.
(3) Hormone suppression therapy can be used, for example, to inhibit the adrenogenital syndrome (3). Higher doses are used. The treatment of the adrenogenital syndrome is only partly substitutive and has to be adapted to the individual case, but doses are needed at which various hormonal effects of the glucocorticoids and mineralocorticoids are likely to become troublesome.
(4) Massive doses of glucocorticoids, far exceeding physiological amounts, are given in the immediate management of anaphylaxis, although their beneficial effects are delayed for several hours. This is because, in severely ill patients, early administration of hydrocortisone 100–300 mg as the sodium succinate salt can gradually enhance the actions of adrenaline (4). Glucocorticoids have been used as an adjunct to the use of inotropic and vasopressor drugs for septic shock. Their efficacy, as well as their proposed mechanisms of action, is controversial; inhibition of complement-mediated aggregation and resultant endothelial injury, and inhibition of the release of beta-endorphin are current theories of their mechanism of action. However, controlled studies have not indicated a beneficial effect of high-dose glucocorticoid therapy in treating septic shock (5,6). Hence, there is no established role for glucocorticoids in the treatment of shock, except shock caused by adrenal insufficiency.

Routes of administration

Glucocorticoids can be given by the following routes:

- oral
- rectal
- intravenous
- intramuscular
- inhalation
- nasal
- topical (skin, eyes, ears)
- intradermal
- intra-articular and periarticular
- intraspinal (epidural, intrathecal)
- intracapsular (breast)

All of these routes are covered in this monograph, except the inhalation route, which is the subject of a separate monograph.

Therapeutic studies

Although there have been several trials of early dexamethasone to determine whether it would reduce mortality and chronic lung disease in infants with respiratory distress, the optimal duration and adverse effects of such therapy are unknown. The purpose of one study was: (a) to determine if a 3-day course of early dexamethasone therapy would reduce chronic lung disease and increase survival without chronic lung disease in neonates who received surfactant therapy for respiratory distress syndrome and (b) to determine the associated adverse effects (7). This was a prospective, placebo-controlled, multicenter, randomized study of a 3-day course of early dexamethasone therapy, beginning at 24–48 hours of life in 241 neonates, who weighed 500–1500 g, had received surfactant therapy, and were at significant risk of chronic lung disease or death. Infants randomized to dexamethasone received a 3-day tapering course (total dose 1.35 mg/kg) given in six doses at 12-hour intervals. Chronic lung disease was defined by the need for supplementary oxygen at a gestational age of 36 weeks. Neonates randomized to early dexamethasone were more likely to survive without chronic lung disease (RR = 1.3; CI = 1.0, 1.7) and were less likely to develop chronic lung disease (RR = 0.6; CI = 0.3, 0.98). Mortality rates were not significantly different. Subsequent dexamethasone therapy was less in early dexamethasone-treated neonates (RR = 0.8; CI = 0.70, 0.96). Very early (before 7 days of life) intestinal perforations were more common among dexamethasone-treated neonates (8 versus 1%). The authors concluded that an early 3-day course of dexamethasone increases survival without chronic lung disease, reduces chronic lung disease, and reduces late dexamethasone therapy in high-risk, low birthweight infants who receive surfactant therapy for respiratory distress syndrome. The potential benefits of early dexamethasone therapy in the regimen used in this trial need to be weighed against the risk of early intestinal perforation.

In another randomized trial, the effects and adverse effects of early dexamethasone on the incidence of chronic lung disease have been evaluated in 50 high-risk preterm infants (8). The treated infants received dexamethasone intravenously from the fourth day of life for 7 days (0.5 mg/kg/day for the first 3 days, 0.25 mg/kg/day for the next 3 days, and 0.125 mg/kg/day on the seventh day). The incidence of chronic lung disease at 28 days of life and at 36 weeks of postconceptional age was significantly lower in the infants who were given dexamethasone, who also remained intubated and required oxygen therapy for a shorter period. Hyperglycemia, hypertension, growth failure, and left ventricular hypertrophy were the transient adverse effects associated with early glucocorticoid administration. Early dexamethasone administration may be useful in preventing chronic lung disease, but its use should be restricted to preterm high-risk infants.

A systematic review of randomized controlled trials has been performed to determine whether dexamethasone therapy in the first 15 days of life prevents chronic lung disease in premature infants (9). Studies were identified by a literature search using Medline (1970–97) supplemented by a search of the Cochrane Library (1998, Issue 4). Inclusion criteria were: (a) prospective randomized design with initiation of dexamethasone therapy within the first 15 days of life; (b) report of the outcome of interest; and (c) less than 20% crossover between the treatment and control groups during the study period. The primary outcomes were mortality at hospital discharge and the development of chronic lung disease at 28 days of life and 36 weeks postconceptional age. The secondary outcomes were the presence of a patent ductus arteriosus and treatment adverse effects. Dexamethasone reduced the incidence of chronic lung disease by 26% at 28 days (RR = 0.74; CI = 0.57, 0.96) and 48% at 36 weeks postconceptional age (RR = 0.52; CI = 0.33, 0.81). These reductions were more significant when dexamethasone was started in the first 72 hours of life. The 24% relative risk reduction of deaths was marginally significant (RR = 0.76; CI = 0.56, 1.04). The 27% reduction in patent ductus arteriosus and the 11% increase in infections were not statistically significant, nor were any other changes. The conclusion from this meta-analysis was that systemic dexamethasone given to at-risk infants soon after birth may reduce the incidence of chronic lung disease. There was no evidence of significant short-term adverse effects.

Although dexamethasone is commonly associated with transient adverse effects, several randomized trials have shown that it rapidly reduces oxygen requirements and shortens the duration of ventilation. A randomized study was designed to evaluate the effects of two different dexamethasone courses on growth in preterm infants (10). The first phase included 30 preterm infants at high risk of chronic lung disease, of whom 15 (8 boys) were given dexamethasone for 14 days, from the tenth day of life; they received a total dose of 4.75 mg/kg; 15 babies were assigned to the control group (8 boys). The second phase included 30 preterm infants at high risk of chronic lung disease, of whom 15 babies (7 boys) were treated with dexamethasone for 7 days, from the fourth day of life; they received a total dose of 2.38 mg/kg; 15 babies were assigned to the control group (9 boys). Infants given dexamethasone had significantly less weight gain than controls, but they caught up soon after the end of treatment. At 30 days of life, the gains in weight and length in each group were similar to those in control infants, but those given dexamethasone had significantly less head growth. There were no differences between the groups at discharge. The longer-term impact of postnatal dexamethasone on mortality and morbidity is less clear. Better data, from larger clinical trials with longer follow-up, will determine whether this kind of treatment enhances lives, makes little difference, causes significant harm, or does several of these things (11).

General adverse effects

The incidence and severity of adverse reactions to glucocorticoids depend on the dose and duration of treatment. Even the very high single doses of glucocorticoids, such as methylprednisolone, which are sometimes used, do not cause serious adverse effects, whereas an equivalent dose given over a long period of time can cause many long-term effects.

The two major risks of long-term glucocorticoid therapy are adrenal suppression and Cushingoid changes. During prolonged treatment with anti-inflammatory doses, glucose intolerance, osteoporosis, acne vulgaris, and a greater or lesser degree of mineralocorticoid-induced changes can occur. In children, growth can be retarded, and adults who take high doses can have mental changes. There may be a risk of gastroduodenal ulceration, although this is much less certain than was once thought. Infections and abdominal crises can be masked. Some of these effects reflect the catabolic properties of the glucocorticoids, that is their ability to accelerate tissue breakdown and impair healing. Allergic reactions can occur.

Anyone who prescribes long-term glucocorticoids should have a checklist in mind of the undesired effects that they can exert, both during treatment and on withdrawal, so that any harm that occurs can be promptly detected and countered. The main groups of risks arising from long-term treatment with glucocorticoids are summarized in Table 2.

The adverse reactions that were reported in a study of 213 children are listed in Table 3 (12).

Table 2 Risks of long-term glucocorticoid therapy

1. Exogenous hypercorticalism with Cushing's syndrome
Moon face (facial rounding)
Central obesity
Striae
Hirsutism
Acne vulgaris
Ecchymoses
Hypertension
Osteoporosis
Proximal myopathy
Disorders of sexual function
Diabetes mellitus
Hyperlipidemia
Disorders of mineral and fluid balance (depending on the type of glucocorticoid)
2. Adrenal insufficiency
Insufficient or absent stress reaction
Withdrawal effects
3. Unwanted results accompanying desired effects
Increased risk of infection
Impaired wound healing
Peptic ulceration, bleeding, and perforation
Growth retardation
4. Other adverse effects
Mental disturbances
Encephalopathy
Increased risk of thrombosis
Posterior cataract
Increased intraocular pressure and glaucoma
Aseptic necrosis of bone

Table 3 Adverse reactions in 213 children given intravenous methylprednisolone

Adverse effect	Number
Behavioral changes	21
Abdominal disorders	11
Pruritus	9
Urticaria	5
Hypertension	5
Bone pain	3
Dizziness	3
Fatigue	2
Fractures	2
Hypotension	2
Lethargy	2
Tachycardia	2
Anaphylactoid reaction	1
"Grey appearance"	1

Drug interactions that affect the efficacy of glucocorticoids have been reviewed (13).

Organs and Systems

Cardiovascular

The considerable body of evidence that glucocorticoids can cause increased rates of vascular mortality and the underlying mechanisms (increased blood pressure, impaired glucose tolerance, dyslipidemia, hypercoagulability, and increased fibrinogen production) have been reviewed (14). In view of their adverse cardiovascular effects, the therapeutic options should be carefully considered before long-term glucocorticoids are begun; although they can be life-saving, dosages should be regularly reviewed during long-term therapy, in order to minimize complications.

Hypertension

The secondary mineralocorticoid activity of glucocorticoids can lead to salt and water retention, which can cause hypertension. Although the detailed mechanisms are as yet uncertain, glucocorticoid-induced hypertension often occurs in elderly patients and is more common in patients with total serum calcium concentrations below the reference range and/or in those with a family history of essential hypertension (SEDA-20, 368) (15).

Hemangioma is the most common tumor of infancy, with a natural history of spontaneous involution. Some hemangiomas, however, as a result of their proximity to vital structures, destruction of facial anatomy, or excessive bleeding, can be successfully treated with systemic glucocorticoids between other therapies. The risk of hypertension is poorly documented in this setting. In one prospective study of 37 infants (7 boys, 17 girls; mean age 3.5 months, range 1.5–10) with rapidly growing complicated hemangiomas treated with oral prednisone 1–5 mg/kg/day, blood pressure increased in seven cases (16). Cardiac ultrasound examination in five showed two cases of myocardial hypertrophy, which was unrelated to the hypertension and which regressed after withdrawal of the prednisone.

Myocardial ischemia

Cortisone-induced cardiac lesions are sometimes reported and electrocardiographic changes have been seen in patients taking glucocorticoids (17). Whereas abnormal myocardial hypertrophy in children has perhaps been associated more readily with corticotropin, it has been seen on occasion during treatment with high dosages of glucocorticoids, with normalization after dosage reduction and withdrawal.

Fatal myocardial infarction occurred after intravenous methylprednisolone for an episode of ulcerative colitis (18).

- A day after a dose of intravenous methylprednisolone 60 mg a 79-year-old woman developed acute thoracic pain and collapsed. An electrocardiogram showed signs of a myocardial infarction and her cardiac enzyme activities were raised. She died within several hours. Autopsy showed an anterior transmural myocardial infarction and mild atheromatous lesions in the coronary arteries.

This report highlights the risk of cardiovascular adverse effects with short courses of glucocorticoid therapy in elderly patients with inflammatory bowel disease, even with rather low-dosage regimens. Acute myocardial infarction occurred in an old man with coronary insufficiency and giant cell arteritis after treatment with prednisolone (SEDA-10, 343) but could well have been coincidental.

Myocardial ischemia has been reportedly precipitated by intramuscular administration of betamethasone (SEDA-21, 413) (19). It has been suggested that long-term glucocorticoid therapy accelerates atherosclerosis and the formation of aortic aneurysms, with a high risk of rupture (SEDA-20, 369) (20).

Patients with seropositive rheumatoid arthritis taking long-term systemic glucocorticoids are at risk of accelerated cardiac rupture in the setting of transmural acute myocardial infarction treated with thrombolytic drugs (21).

- Two women and one man, aged 53–74 years, died after they received thrombolytic therapy for acute myocardial infarction. All three had a long history of seropositive rheumatoid arthritis treated with prednisone 5–20 mg/day for many years.

Cardiomyopathy

Postnatal exposure to glucocorticoids has been associated with hypertrophic cardiomyopathy in neonates. Such an effect has not previously been described in infants born to mothers who received antenatal glucocorticoids. Three neonates (gestational ages 36, 29, and 34 weeks), whose mothers had been treated with betamethasone prenatally in doses of 12 mg twice weekly for 16 doses, 8 doses, and 5 doses respectively, developed various degrees of hypertrophic cardiomyopathy diagnosed by echocardiography (22). There was no maternal evidence of diabetes, except for one infant whose mother had a normal fasting and postprandial blood glucose before glucocorticoid therapy, but an abnormal 1-hour postprandial glucose after 8 weeks of betamethasone therapy, with a normal HbA_{1C} concentration. There was no family history of hypertrophic cardiomyopathy, no history of maternal intake of other relevant medications, no hypertension, and none of the infants received glucocorticoids postnatally. Follow-up echocardiography showed complete resolution in all infants. The authors suggested that repeated antenatal maternal glucocorticoids might cause hypertrophic cardiomyopathy in neonates. These changes appear to be dose- and duration-related and are mostly reversible.

Transient hypertrophic cardiomyopathy is a rare sequel of the concurrent administration of glucocorticoid and insulin excess (SEDA-21, 412) (23). The heart is also almost certainly a site for myopathic changes analogous to those that affect other muscles.

Transient hypertrophic cardiomyopathy has been attributed to systemic glucocorticoid administration for a craniofacial hemangioma (24).

- A 69-day-old white child presented with a rapidly growing 2.5 × 1.5 cm hemangioma of the external left nasal side wall. He was normotensive and there was no family history of cardiomyopathy or maternal gestational diabetes. Because of nasal obstruction and possible visual obstruction, he was given prednisolone 3 mg/kg/day. After 10 weeks his weight had fallen from 7.6 to 7.1 kg and 2 weeks later he became tachypneic with a respiratory rate of 40/minutes. A chest X-ray showed cardiomegaly and pulmonary venous congestion. An echocardiogram showed hypertrophic cardiomyopathy. The left ventricular posterior wall thickness was 10 mm (normal under 4 mm), and the peak left ventricular outflow gradient was 64 mmHg. He was given a beta-blocker and a diuretic and the glucocorticoid dose was tapered. The cardiomyopathy eventually resolved.

Dilated cardiomyopathy caused by occult pheochromocytoma has been described infrequently.

- A 34-year-old woman had acute congestive heart failure 12 hours after administration of dexamethasone 16 mg for an atypical migraine (25). The authors postulated that the acute episode had been induced by the dexamethasone, which increased the production of adrenaline, causing $beta_2$-adrenoceptor stimulation, peripheral vasodilatation, and congestive heart failure.

In an addendum the authors reported another similar case.

Cardiac dysrhythmias

Serious cardiac dysrhythmias and sudden death have been reported with pulsed methylprednisolone. Oral methylprednisolone has been implicated in a case of sinus bradycardia (26).

- A 14-year-old boy received an intravenous dose of methylprednisolone 30 mg/kg for progressive glomerulonephritis. After 5 hours, his heart rate had fallen to 50/minute and an electrocardiogram showed sinus bradycardia. His heart rate then fell to 40/minutes and a temporary transvenous pacemaker was inserted and methylprednisolone was withdrawn. His heart rate increased to 80/minutes over 3 days. After a further 3 days, he was treated with oral methylprednisolone 60 mg/m^2/day and his heart rate fell to 40/minutes in 5 days. Oral methylprednisolone was stopped on day 8 of treatment and his heart rate normalized.

Hypokalemia, secondary to mineralocorticoid effects, can cause cardiac dysrhythmias and cardiac arrest.

Recurrent cardiocirculatory arrest has been reported (27).

- A 60-year-old white man was admitted for kidney transplantation. Immediately after reperfusion and intravenous methylprednisolone 500 mg, he developed severe bradycardia with hypotension and then cardiac arrest. After resuscitation, his clinical state improved quickly, but on the morning of the first postoperative day directly after the intravenous administration of methylprednisolone 250 mg, he had another episode of severe bradycardia, hypotension, and successful cardiopulmonary resuscitation. A third episode occurred 24 hours later after intravenous methylprednisolone 100 mg, again followed by rapid recovery after resuscitation. Two weeks later, during a bout of acute rejection, he was given intravenous methylprednisolone 500 mg, after which he collapsed and no heartbeat or breathing was detectable; after cardiopulmonary resuscitation he was transferred to the intensive care unit, where he died a few hours later.

If patients at risk are identified, glucocorticoid bolus therapy should be avoided or, if that is not possible, should only be done under close monitoring.

Pericarditis

- Disseminated *Varicella* and staphylococcal pericarditis developed in a previously healthy girl after a single application of triamcinolone cream 0.1% to relieve pruritus associated with *Varicella* skin lesions (SEDA-22, 443) (28).

Vasculitis

Long-term treatment with glucocorticoids can cause arteritis, but patients with rheumatoid arthritis have a special susceptibility to vascular reactions, and cases of periarteritis nodosa after withdrawal of long-term glucocorticoids have been reported (29).

Respiratory

Local adverse effects are common in patients with asthma who use inhaled glucocorticoids, as suggested by a survey of the prevalence of throat and voice symptoms in patients with asthma using glucocorticoids by metered-dose pressurized aerosol (SEDA-20, 369) (30).

There have been no reports of an increased frequency of lower respiratory tract infections. However, patients with aspiration of gastric material who were treated with glucocorticoids did not have improved survival but had a higher incidence of pneumonia (SED-12, 982).

In cases of pneumothorax with closed thoracotomy tube drainage, chronic glucocorticoid treatment has been reported to delay and impede re-expansion of the lung (SED-8, 820).

Hiccup is a rare complication of glucocorticoid therapy; five cases have been published at various times (31).

- A 59-year-old man had intractable hiccups during treatment with dexamethasone for multiple myeloma (32).
- Persistent hiccupping has been described in a 30-year-old man after the administration of a single

intravenous dose of dexamethasone (16 mg) (33). The symptom was resistant to metoclopramide and resolved spontaneously after 4 days. On rechallenge, the hiccups recurred within 2 hours and disappeared after 36 hours.

Low-dose metoclopramide can be effective and may allow a patient to continue beneficial therapy without the discomfort and exhaustion that can accompany intractable hiccups.

Ear, nose, throat

Atrophic changes and fungal and other infections can alter the nasal mucosa after aerosol treatment (34), and since most systematic published documentation on these intranasal products is limited to 1–2 years of experience (although they have been in use for a far longer period), some reserve is warranted with respect to their long-term safety and the wisdom of continual use.

Nervous system

Cerebral venous thrombosis associated with glucocorticoid treatment has rarely been reported. A relation between glucocorticoids and venous thrombosis has already been suggested but has never been clearly understood. Three young patients, two women (aged 28 and 45) and one man (aged 38 years), developed cerebral venous thrombosis after intravenous high-dose glucocorticoids (35). All presented with probable multiple sclerosis according to clinical, CSF, and MRI criteria. All had a lumbar puncture and were then treated with methylprednisolone 1 g/day for 5 days. All the usual causes of cerebral venous thrombosis were systematically excluded. The authors proposed that glucocorticoids interfere with blood coagulation and suggested that the administration of glucocorticoids after a lumbar puncture carries a particular risk of complications.

Dexamethasone is widely used for the prevention and treatment of chronic lung disease in premature infants, in whom follow-up studies have raised the possibility of an association with alterations in neuromotor function and somatic growth. In 159 survivors (mean age 53 months) of a previous placebo-controlled study, the children who had received dexamethasone had a significantly higher incidence of cerebral palsy (39/80 versus 12/79; OR = 4.62; 95% CI = 2.38, 8.98) (36). The most common form of cerebral palsy was spastic diplegia. Developmental delay was more frequent in the dexamethasone group (44/80 versus 23/79; OR = 2.9; CI = 1.5, 5.4).

Long-term treatment with glucocorticoids can cause cerebral atrophy (37).

Severe organic brain syndrome has been seen in six patients taking long-term glucocorticoids (SEDA-3, 304). The manifestations included confusion, disorientation, apathy, confabulation, irrelevant speech, and slow thinking; the symptoms occurred abruptly.

Latent epilepsy can be made manifest by glucocorticoid treatment. Seizures in patients with lung transplants were related to glucocorticoids, which had been used in high dosages to prevent organ rejection. There was an increased risk of seizures in younger patients (under 25 years) and with intravenous methylprednisolone (SEDA-21, 413) (38).

Long-term glucocorticoid treatment can result in papilledema and increased intracranial pressure (the syndrome of pseudotumor cerebri or so-called "benign intracranial hypertension"), particularly in children.

- Benign intracranial hypertension occurred in a 7-month-old child after withdrawal of topical betamethasone ointment and in a 7-year-old boy treated with a 1% cortisol ointment in large amounts.
- A 6-year-old girl, who had taken prednisone for 2.5 years for nephrotic syndrome with seven relapses in 3 years, developed symptoms of benign intracranial hypertension after oral glucocorticoid dosage reduction over 10 months from 30 mg/day to 2.5 mg/every other day (39). Laboratory studies and head CT scan were normal, but there was bilateral papilledema and the cerebrospinal fluid pressure was increased. She was given prednisone 1 mg/kg/day initially, with acetazolamide, and 25 ml of cerebrospinal fluid was removed. All her symptoms resolved and treatment was gradually withdrawn. She developed no further visual failure.

The symptoms can simulate those of an intracranial tumor. All patients taking large doses of glucocorticoids who complain of headache or blurred vision, particularly after a reduction in dosage, should have an ophthalmoscopic examination to exclude this complication. Paradoxically, cerebral edema occurring during a surgical procedure can be partly prevented by glucocorticoids (40).

An encephalopathy can occur at any age (SEDA-18, 387), not necessarily in association with intracranial hypertension.

There have been repeated reports of epidural lipomatosis, which can lead to spinal cord compression (41,42) or spinal fracture (43); in one instance, the excised lipomata contained brown fat, a phenomenon that may prove to be not unusual in glucocorticoid-induced lipomata (SEDA-16, 451).

- A 40-year-old woman with ulcerative colitis took cortisone 20 mg/day and developed progressive paraplegia (43). There was kyphosis of the thoracic spine from T7 to T9, with pathological fractures. An MRI scan showed massive epidural fat extending from T1 to T9. She recovered 3 months after surgical removal of the epidural fat.
- A 78-year-old man was given methylprednisolone (60 mg/day reducing to 8 mg/day) for temporal arteritis (44). After 4 months, he developed numbness and paresis of the legs and hyperalgesia at dermatomes T3 and T4. After 10 months he had marked disturbance of proprioception combined with spinal ataxia and an increasing loss of motor bladder control. There was an intraspinal epidural lipoma in the dorsal part of the spine from T1-10. The fat was removed surgically and within 4 weeks his gait disturbance and proprioception improved, the sensory deficit abated, and the bladder disorder disappeared completely.
- A 57-year-old man took prednisone 20–30 mg/day for 13 years for rheumatoid arthritis (45). He had been treated unsuccessfully with gold, azathioprine, hydroxychloroquine, and sulfasalazine; tapering his glucocorticoid dosage had been unsuccessful. He developed worsening back pain in his thoracic spine and lateral

leg weakness. He was unable to walk. He was Cushingoid and had marked thoracic kyphosis associated with multiple vertebral body fractures in T5-8. An MRI scan at T5-6 showed displacement and compression of the spinal cord by high-signal epidural fat, which had caused anterior thecal displacement and total effacement of cerebrospinal fluid.

The authors of the last report commented on the high dose of prednisone used.

In the past there was reason to think that glucocorticoids might precipitate multiple sclerosis. However, this has not been confirmed, and there is evidence that a special glucocorticoid regimen can actually be capable of retarding deterioration in multiple sclerosis (SEDA-18, 387).

A Guillain–Barré-like syndrome occurred in a patient receiving high-dose intravenous glucocorticoid therapy (SEDA-16, 449). Although glucocorticoids have been used successfully to treat weakness due to chronic inflammatory demyelinating sensorimotor neuropathy, other types of acquired chronic demyelinating neuropathies can be impaired by these drugs.

- In four patients with a pure motor demyelinating neuropathy treated with oral prednisolone (60 mg/day) motor function rapidly deteriorated within 4 weeks of starting prednisolone (SEDA-19, 375) (46). Intravenous immunoglobulin some months later in two of them produced clear improvement in strength and motor nerve conduction.

Sensory systems

The eye can be involved in generalized adverse reactions to systemically administered glucocorticoids. For example, conjunctivitis can occur as part of an allergic reaction and infections of the eye can be masked as a result of anti-inflammatory and analgesic effects. Ophthalmoplegia can occur as one of the consequences of glucocorticoid myopathy (SEDA-16, 450). Two complications that require special discussion are cataract and glaucoma.

Cataract

Oral glucocorticoid treatment is a risk factor for the development of posterior subcapsular cataract. A review of nine studies including 343 asthmatics treated with oral glucocorticoids showed a prevalence of posterior subcapsular cataracts of 0–54% with a mean value of 9% (47). In a 1993 study in children taking low-dose prednisone there were cataracts in seven of 23 cases (48). Some studies have shown a clear correlation with the duration of treatment and total dosage, others have not (SEDA-17, 449). The use of inhaled glucocorticoids was associated with a dose-dependent increased risk of posterior subcapsular and nuclear cataracts in 3654 patients aged 49–97 years (SEDA-22, 446) (49). Data on glucocorticoid use were available for 3313 of these patients; glucocorticoid use was classified as none in 2784 patients, inhaled only in 241, systemic only in 177, and both inhaled and systemic in 111. Compared with nonuse, current or prior use of inhaled glucocorticoids was associated with a significant increase in the prevalence of nuclear cataracts (adjusted relative prevalence = 1.5; 95% CI = 1.2, 1.9) and posterior subcapsular cataracts (1.9; 1.3, 2.8), but not cortical cataracts. The increased prevalence of posterior subcapsular cataracts was significantly associated with current use of inhaled glucocorticoids (2.6; 1.7, 4.0); there was no association with past use. Current use of inhaled glucocorticoids was also associated with an increased prevalence of cortical cataracts (1.4; 1.1, 1.7). The highest prevalences of posterior subcapsular and grade 4 or 5 nuclear cataracts were found in patients who had taken a cumulative dose of beclomethasone over 2000 mg.

It has been suggested that the risk of cataract is higher in patients with rheumatoid arthritis than in patients with bronchial asthma, and it is also higher in children. The reversibility of the lenticular changes has often been discussed (50,51), but even without glucocorticoid withdrawal regression has been found in children taking long-term treatment (52). Nevertheless, some 7% of the patients who develop cataract caused by glucocorticoid treatment have to be operated on. A change in permeability of the lens capsule, followed by altered electrolyte concentrations in the lens and a change in the mucopolysaccharides in the lens have been advanced as reasons for the development of cataract.

Increased intraocular pressure and glaucoma

Ocular hypertension and open-angle glaucoma are well-known adverse effects of ophthalmic administration of glucocorticoids (SEDA-17, 449).

Frequency

A total of 113 patients with angiographically proven subretinal neovascularization were enrolled into a prospective study of the effects of intravitreal triamcinolone (53). About 30% developed a significant rise in intraocular pressure (at least 5 mmHg) above baseline during the first 3 months.

A large case-control study, in which 9793 elderly patients with ocular hypertension or open-angle glaucoma were compared with 38 325 controls, has shown an increased risk of these complications with oral glucocorticoids (SEDA-22, 446) (54). The risk of ocular hypertension or open-angle glaucoma increased with increasing dose and duration of use of the oral glucocorticoid. There was no significant increase in the risk of ocular hypertension or open-angle glaucoma in patients who had stopped taking oral glucocorticoids 15–45 days before. The authors estimated that the excess risk of ocular hypertension or open-angle glaucoma with current oral glucocorticoid use is 43 additional cases per 10 000 patients per year. However, in patients taking over 80 mg/day of hydrocortisone equivalents, the excess risk is 93 additional cases per 10 000 patients per year. Monitoring of intraocular pressure may be justified in long-term users of oral glucocorticoids, as it is in long-term users of topical glucocorticoids.

Prolonged use of high doses of inhaled glucocorticoids also increases the risk of ocular hypertension and open-angle glaucoma (SEDA-22, 446) (55). In a case-control study of the records of 9793 elderly patients with ocular hypertension or open-angle glaucoma over a 6-year period, there was a significantly increased risk of ocular hypertension and open-angle glaucoma in patients who had taken high doses of inhaled glucocorticoids

(1500–1600 micrograms) for 3 months or longer (OR = 1.44; 95% CI = 1.01, 2.06). Both a high dosage of inhaled glucocorticoid and prolonged continuous duration of therapy had to be present to increase the risk.

Glaucoma and ocular hypertension have been reported after dermal application of glucocorticoids for facial atopic eczema (SEDA-19, 376) (56), and after treatment with beclomethasone by nasal spray and inhalation (SEDA-20, 373) (57).

The effects of topical dexamethasone on intraocular pressure have been compared with those of fluorometholone (SEDA-22, 446) (58). The ocular hypertensive response to topical dexamethasone in children occurs more often, more severely, and more rapidly than that reported in adults. It should be avoided in children if possible and it is desirable to monitor the intraocular pressure when it is being used. Fluorometholone may be more acceptable.

Pathogenesis

The pathogenesis of glucocorticoid-induced glaucoma is still unknown, but there is reduced outflow, and excessive accumulation of mucopolysaccharides may be a major factor. An association with cataract and papilledema has often been observed. The rise in intraocular pressure is variable: in the pediatric study of low dose cited above there was a reversible effect in only two of 23 subjects compared with controls, but in other studies serious increases in pressure have occurred, with a risk of blindness.

There is almost certainly a genetic predisposition to glucocorticoid-induced glaucoma, as there is to glaucoma in general.

Chorioretinopathy

Systemic glucocorticoid treatment can cause severe exacerbation of bullous exudative retinal detachment and lasting visual loss in some patients with idiopathic central serous chorioretinopathy (SEDA-20, 374) (59). The atypical presentation of this condition can include peripheral retinal capillary nonperfusion and retinal neovascularization. The treatment of choice in patients with idiopathic central serous chorioretinopathy is laser photocoagulation.

Keratopathy and keratitis

Band-shaped keratopathy is caused by the deposition of calcium salts in the basement membrane of the corneal epithelium and superficial stroma. It is typically a chronic process that develops over a period of months and years, and is associated with chronic corneal or intraocular inflammation.

- Infectious crystalline keratopathy developed in a 73-year-old woman with noninsulin-dependent diabetes mellitus after the use of topical prednisolone 1% eye-drops, for conjunctival injection over 12 months (SEDA-20, 372) (60).
- Acute-onset calcific band keratopathy has been reported in a woman using topical prednisolone (SEDA-20, 372) (61).

Patients with severe keratoconjunctivitis sicca are at definite risk of this complication, and the addition of phosphate-containing eye-drops tilted the precariously balanced situation toward precipitation of calcium in the cornea and bandage contact lens. Acetate-containing rather than phosphate-containing glucocorticoid eye drops may be a safer alternative in patients with such predisposing factors.

Bacterial keratitis is one of the most frequent ophthalmic infections. In a meta-analysis of publications from 1950 to 2000, the use of a topical glucocorticoid before the diagnosis of bacterial keratitis significantly predisposed to ulcerative keratitis in eyes with pre-existing corneal disease (OR = 2.63; 95% CI = 1.41, 4.91). Previous glucocorticoid use significantly increased the risk of antibiotic failure or other infectious complications (OR = 3.75; 95% CI = 2.52, 5.58). The use of glucocorticoids with an antibiotic for the treatment of bacterial keratitis did not increase the risk of complications, but neither did it improve the outcome of treatment.

Retinal damage

An apparent association between severe retinopathy of prematurity and dexamethasone therapy has been shown in a retrospective study (SEDA-20, 372) (62). Infants treated with dexamethasone required longer periods of mechanical ventilation (44 versus 26 days), had a longer duration of supplemental oxygen (57 versus 29 days), had a higher incidence of patent ductus arteriosus (28/38 versus 18/52), and required surfactant therapy more often for respiratory distress syndrome (17/38 versus 11/52). Prospective, randomized, controlled studies are needed to correct for differences in severity of cardiorespiratory disease. Until such studies are available, careful consideration must be given to indications, dosage, time of initiation, and duration of treatment with dexamethasone in infants of extremely low birthweight.

Retinal hemorrhage occurred in four women after they had received epidural methylprednisolone for chronic back and hip pain (SEDA-20, 373) (63). Retinal and choroidal vascular occlusions are a serious and sometimes lasting complication of periocular and facial injections of glucocorticoids (SEDA-21, 416).

Toxic optic neuropathy

Toxic optic neuropathy can occur and may underlie various reports of sudden blindness in patients taking glucocorticoids. In one case, transient visual loss occurred on several occasions, each time after administration of a glucocorticoid (SEDA-17, 447). In another case, blindness occurred suddenly and paradoxically after glucocorticoid injections into the nasal turbinates (64). Although glucocorticoids are sometimes used successfully to relieve pre-existing optic neuritis, a number of such patients react adversely with increased episodes of visual loss.

Exophthalmos

Exophthalmos has been described incidentally as a complication of long-term glucocorticoid therapy and there has been a series of 21 cases (65).

Psychological, psychiatric

The psychostimulant effects of the glucocorticoids are well known (66), and their dose dependency is recognized (SED-11, 817); they may amount to little more than euphoria or comprise severe mental derangement, for example mania in an adult with no previous psychiatric history (SEDA-17, 446) or catatonic stupor demanding electroconvulsive therapy (67). In their mildest form, and especially in children, the mental changes may be detectable only by specific tests of mental function (68). Mental effects can occur in patients treated with fairly low doses; they can also occur after withdrawal or omission of treatment, apparently because of adrenal suppression (69,70).

- A 32-year-old woman developed irritability, anger, and insomnia after taking oral prednisone (60 mg/day) for a relapse of ileal Crohn's disease (71). The prednisone was withdrawn and replaced by budesonide (9 mg/day), and the psychiatric adverse effects were relieved after 3 days. A good clinical response was maintained, with no relapse after 2 months of budesonide therapy.

Development

Dexamethasone has been used in ventilator-dependent preterm infants to reduce the risk and severity of chronic lung disease. Usually it is given in a tapering course over a long period (42 days). The effects of dexamethasone on developmental outcome at 1 year of age has been evaluated in 118 infants of very low birthweights (47 boys and 71 girls, aged 15–25 days), who were not weaning from assisted ventilation (72). They were randomly assigned double-blind to receive placebo or dexamethasone (initial dose 0.25 mg/kg) tapered over 42 days. A neurological examination, including ultrasonography, was done at 1 year of age. Survival was 88% with dexamethasone and 74% with placebo. Both groups obtained similar scores in mental and psychomotor developmental indexes. More dexamethasone-treated infants had major intracranial abnormalities (21 versus 11%), cerebral palsy (25 versus 7%; OR = 5.3; CI = 1.3, 21), and unspecified neurological abnormalities (45 versus 16%; OR = 3.6; CI = 1.2, 11). Although the authors suggested an adverse effect, they added other possible explanations for these increased risks (improved survival in those with neurological injuries or at increased risk of such injuries).

Behavioral disorders

Children have marked increases in behavioral problems during treatment with high-dose prednisone for relapse of nephrotic syndrome, according to the results of a study conducted in the USA (73). Ten children aged 2.9–15 years (mean 8.2 years) received prednisone 2 mg/kg/day, tapering at the time of remission, which was at week 2 in seven patients. At baseline, eight children had normal behavioral patterns and two had anxious/depressed and aggressive behavior using the Child Behaviour Checklist (CBCL). During high-dose prednisone therapy, five of the eight children with normal baseline scores had CBCL scores for anxiety, depression, and aggressive behavior above the 95th percentile for age. The two children with high baseline CBCL scores had worsening behavioral problems during high-dose prednisone. Behavioral problems occurred almost exclusively in the children who received over 1 mg/kg every 48 hours. Regression analysis showed that prednisone dosage was a strong predictor of increased aggressive behaviour.

Intravenous methylprednisolone was associated with a spectrum of adverse reactions, most frequently behavioral disorders, in 213 children with rheumatic disease, according to the results of a US study (12). However, intravenous methylprednisolone was generally well tolerated. The children received their first dose of intravenous methylprednisolone 30 mg/kg over at least 60 minutes, and if the first dose was well tolerated they were given further infusions at home under the supervision of a nurse. There was at least one adverse reaction in 46 children (22%) of whom 18 had an adverse reaction within the first three doses. The most commonly reported adverse reactions were behavioral disorders (21 children), including mood changes, hyperactivity, hallucinations, disorientation, and sleep disorders. Several children had serious acute reactions, which were readily controlled. Most of them were able to continue methylprednisolone therapy with premedication or were given an alternative glucocorticoid. The researchers emphasized the need to monitor treatment closely and to have appropriate drugs readily available to treat adverse reactions.

Large doses are most likely to cause the more serious behavioral and personality changes, ranging from extreme nervousness, severe insomnia, or mood swings to psychotic episodes, which can include both manic and depressive states, paranoid states, and acute toxic psychoses. A history of emotional disorders does not necessarily preclude glucocorticoid treatment, but existing emotional instability or psychotic tendencies can be aggravated by glucocorticoids. Such patients as these should be carefully and continuously observed for signs of mental changes, including alterations in the sleep pattern. Aggravation of psychiatric symptoms can occur not only during high-dose oral treatment, but also after any increase in dosage during long-term maintenance therapy; it can also occur with inhalation therapy (74). The psychomotor stimulant effect is said to be most pronounced with dexamethasone and to be much less with methylprednisolone, but this concept of a differential psychotropic effect still has to be confirmed.

Memory

The effects of prednisone on memory have been assessed (SEDA-21, 413) (75). Glucocorticoid-treated patients performed worse than controls in tests of explicit memory. Pulsed intravenous methylprednisolone (2.5 g over 5 days, 5 g over 7 days, or 10 g over 5 days) caused impaired memory in patients with relapsing-remitting multiple sclerosis, but this effect is reversible, according to the results of an Italian study (76). Compared with ten control patients, there was marked selective impairment of explicit memory in 14 patients with relapsing-remitting multiple sclerosis treated with pulsed intravenous methylprednisolone. However, this memory impairment completely resolved 60 days after methylprednisolone treatment.

Glucocorticoids can regulate hippocampal metabolism, physiological functions, and memory. Despite evidence of memory loss during glucocorticoid treatment (SEDA-23, 428), and correlations between memory and cortisol concentrations in certain diseases, it is unclear whether exposure to the endogenous glucocorticoid cortisol in amounts seen during physical and psychological stress in humans can inhibit memory performance in otherwise healthy individuals. In an elegant experiment on the effect of cortisol on memory, 51 young healthy volunteers (24 men and 27 women) participated in a double-blind, randomized, crossover, placebo-controlled trial of cortisol 40 mg/day or 160 mg/day for 4 days (77). The lower dose of cortisol was equivalent to the cortisol delivered during a mild stress and the higher dose to major stress. Cognitive performance and plasma cortisol were evaluated before and until 10 days after drug administration. Cortisol produced a dose-related reversible reduction in verbal declarative memory without effects on nonverbal memory, sustained or selective attention, or executive function. Exposure to cortisol at doses and plasma concentrations associated with physical and psychological stress in humans can reversibly reduce some elements of memory performance.

Prednisone, 10 mg/day for 1 year, has been evaluated in 136 patients with probable Alzheimer's disease in a double-blind, randomized, placebo-controlled trial (78). There were no differences in the primary measures of efficacy (cognitive subscale of the Alzheimer Disease Assessment Scale), but those treated with prednisone had significantly greater memory impairment (Clinical Dementia sum of boxes), and agitation and hostility/suspicion (Brief Psychiatric Rating Scale). Other adverse effects in those who took prednisone were reduced bone density and a small rise in intraocular pressure.

In healthy individuals undergoing acute stress, there was specifically impaired retrieval of declarative long-term memory for a word list, suggesting that cortisol-induced impairment of retrieval may add significantly to the memory deficits caused by prolonged treatment (79).

Sleep

The effects of acute systemic dexamethasone administration on sleep structure have been investigated. Dexamethasone caused significant increases in REM latency, the percentage time spent awake, and the percentage time spent in slow-wave sleep. There were also significant reductions in the percentage time spent in REM sleep and the number of REM periods (SEDA-21, 413) (80).

Psychoses

Mania has been attributed to glucocorticoids (81).

- A 46-year-old man, with an 8-year history of cluster headaches and some episodes of endogenous depression, took glucocorticoids 120 mg/day for a week and then a tapering dosage at the start of his latest cluster episode. His headaches stopped but then recurred after 10 days. He was treated prophylactically with verapamil, but a few days later, while the dose of glucocorticoid was being tapered, he developed symptoms of mania. The glucocorticoids were withdrawn, he was given valproic acid, and his mania resolved after 10 days. Verapamil prophylaxis was restarted and he had no more cluster headaches.

The authors commented that the manic symptoms had probably been caused by glucocorticoids or glucocorticoid withdrawal. They concluded that patients with cluster headache and a history of affective disorder should not be treated with glucocorticoids, but with valproate or lithium, which are effective in both conditions. Lamotrigine, an anticonvulsive drug with mood-stabilizing effects, may prevent glucocorticoid-induced mania in patients for whom valproate or lithium are not possible (82).

Glucocorticoids can cause neuropsychiatric adverse effects that dictate a reduction in dose and sometimes withdrawal of treatment. Of 32 patients with asthma (mean age 47 years) who took prednisone in a mean dosage of 42 mg/day for a mean duration of 5 days, those with past or current symptoms of depression had a significant reduction in depressive symptoms during prednisone therapy compared with those without depression (83). After 3–7 days of therapy there was a significant increase in the risk of mania, with return to baseline after withdrawal.

The management of a psychotic reaction in an Addisonian patient taking a glucocorticoid needs special care (SED-8, 820). Psychotic reactions that do not abate promptly when the glucocorticoid dosage is reduced to the lowest effective value (or withdrawn) may need to be treated with neuroleptic drugs; occasionally these fail and antidepressants are needed (SEDA-18, 387). However, in other cases, antidepressants appear to aggravate the symptoms.

- Two patients with prednisolone-induced psychosis improved on giving the drug in three divided daily doses. Recurrence was avoided by switching to enteric-coated tablets.

This suggests that in susceptible patients the margin of safety may be quite narrow (SED-12, 982). It is possible that reduced absorption accounted for the improvement in this case, but attention should perhaps be focused on peak plasma concentrations rather than average steady-state concentrations.

In one case, glucocorticoid-induced catatonic psychosis unexpectedly responded to etomidate (84).

- A 27-year-old woman with myasthenia gravis taking prednisolone 100 mg/day became unresponsive and had respiratory difficulties. She was given etomidate 20 mg intravenously to facilitate endotracheal intubation. One minute later she became alert and oriented, with normal muscle strength, and became very emotional. Eight hours later she again became catatonic and had a similar response to etomidate 10 mg. Glucocorticoid-induced catatonia was diagnosed, her glucocorticoid dosage was reduced, and she left hospital uneventfully 4 days later.

The effect of etomidate on catatonia, similar to that of amobarbital, was thought to be due to enhanced GABA receptor function in patients with an overactive reticular system.

A case report has suggested that risperidone, an atypical neuroleptic drug, can be useful in treating adolescents with glucocorticoid-induced psychosis and may hasten its resolution (85).

- A 14-year-old African-American girl with acute lymphocytic leukemia was treated with dexamethasone

24 mg/day for 25 days. Four days after starting to taper the dose she had a psychotic reaction with visual hallucinations, disorientation, agitation, and attempts to leave the floor. Her mother refused treatment with haloperidol. Steroids were withdrawn and lorazepam was given as needed. Nine days later the symptoms had not improved. She was given risperidone 1 mg/day; within 3 days the psychotic reaction began to improve and by 3 weeks the symptoms had completely resolved.

Obsessive-compulsive disorder

Obsessive-compulsive behavior after oral cortisone has been described (86).

- A 75-year-old white man, without a history of psychiatric disorders, took cortisone 50 mg/day for 6 weeks for pulmonary fibrosis and developed severe obsessive-compulsive behavior without affective or psychotic symptoms. He was given risperidone without any beneficial effect. The dose of cortisone was tapered over 18 days. An MRI scan showed no signs of organic brain disease and an electroencephalogram was normal. His symptoms improved 16 days after withdrawal and resolved completely after 24 days. Risperidone was withdrawn without recurrence.

Endocrine

The endocrine effects of the glucocorticoids variously involve the pituitary–adrenal axis, the ovaries and testes, the parathyroid glands, and the thyroid gland.

Pituitary gland

Empty sella syndrome occurred in a boy who developed hypopituitarism after long-term pulse therapy with prednisone for nephrotic syndrome (87).

- A 16-year-old Japanese boy's growth and development was normal until the age of 2 years. He then developed nephrotic syndrome and was treated with pulsed glucocorticoid therapy nine times over the next 14 years. After the age of 3 years, his rate of growth had fallen. At 16 years, when he was taking prednisone 60 $mg/m^2/day$ he was given prednisone on alternate days and the dose was gradually tapered. The secretion of pituitary hormones, except antidiuretic hormone, was impaired and an MRI scan of his brain showed an empty sella and atrophy of the pituitary gland.

When markedly impaired growth is noted in patients treated with glucocorticoids long-term or in pulses, it is necessary to assess pituitary function and the anatomy of the pituitary gland. Children who receive glucocorticoid pulse therapy may develop an empty sella more frequently than is usually recognized.

Pituitary–adrenal axis

Raised glucocorticoid plasma concentrations usually result, after 2 weeks, in the first signs of iatrogenic Cushing's syndrome. The characteristic symptoms can occur individually or in combination. Whereas in Cushing's disease or corticotropin-induced Cushing's syndrome, the predominant symptoms are in part determined by hyperandrogenicity and tend to comprise hypertension, acne, impaired sight, disorders of sexual function, hirsutism or virilism, striae of the skin, and plethora, Cushing's syndrome due to glucocorticoid therapy is likely to cause benign intracranial hypertension, glaucoma, subcapsular cataract, pancreatitis, aseptic necrosis of the bones, and panniculitis. Obesity, facial rounding, psychiatric symptoms, edema, and delayed wound healing are common to these different forms of Cushing's syndrome.

It has been said that Cushing-like effects are to be expected if the function of the adrenal cortex is suppressed by daily doses of more than 50 mg hydrocortisone or its equivalent. However, pituitary–adrenal suppression has been described at lower dosage equivalents, for example during prolonged intermittent therapy with dexamethasone (88). The secondary adrenal insufficiency caused by therapeutically effective doses can be observed even after giving prednisone 5 mg tds for only 1 week; after withdrawal, adrenal suppression lasts for some days. If one continues this treatment for about 20 weeks, maximal atrophy of the adrenal cortex results, and lasts for some months. This effect begins with inhibition of the hypothalamus, and culminates in true atrophy of the adrenal cortex. It can occur even with glucocorticoids given by inhalation (89). Inhaled fluticasone is associated with at least a twofold greater suppression of adrenal function than inhaled budesonide microgram for microgram, according to the results of a crossover study (SEDA-21, 415) (90). Patients with liver disease may experience adrenal suppression with lower doses of glucocorticoids (91). It is advisable to use alternate-day therapy to avoid suppression of corticotropin secretion in patients who will need long-term therapy; it will produce the same therapeutic effect as daily dosage. It can be helpful to measure the degree of suppression of corticotropin secretion during long-term glucocorticoid treatment of asthmatic children, as a means of optimizing therapy and avoiding excessive dosage (92). The period of time during which the patient should be considered at risk of adrenal insufficiency after withdrawal of oral prednisolone treatment in childhood nephrotic syndrome is still controversial. A study in such patients has suggested that adrenal insufficiency may occur up to 9 months after treatment has ended (SEDA-19, 376) (93).

Many protocols for treating children with early B cell acute lymphoblastic leukemia involve 28 consecutive days of high-dose glucocorticoids during induction. The effect of this therapy on adrenal function has been prospectively evaluated (94) in 10 children by tetracosactide stimulation before the start of dexamethasone therapy and every 4 weeks thereafter until adrenal function returned to normal. All had normal adrenal function before dexamethasone treatment and impaired adrenal responses 24 hours after completing therapy. Each child felt ill for 2–4 weeks after completing therapy. Seven patients recovered normal adrenal function after 4 weeks, but three did not have normal adrenal function until 8 weeks after withdrawal. Thus, high-dose dexamethasone therapy can cause adrenal insufficiency lasting more than 4 weeks after the end of treatment. This problem might be avoided by tapering doses of glucocorticoids and providing supplementary glucocorticoids during periods of increased stress.

Tolerance to glucocorticoids in this, as in some other respects, varies from individual to individual; some patients tolerate 30 mg of prednisone for a long time without developing Cushing's syndrome, while others develop symptoms at 7.5 mg; the doses recommended today to avoid Cushing's syndrome in most patients are usually equivalent to hydrocortisone 20 mg. Cushing's syndrome and other systemic adverse effects can occur not only from oral and injected glucocorticoids, but also from topical and intranasal treatment (95) and intrapulmonary or epidural administration (SEDA-19, 376) (SEDA-20, 370) (96,97).

- Two patients developed hypopituitarism and empty sella syndrome during glucocorticoid pulse therapy for nephrotic syndrome (SEDA-22, 444) (98).

Glucocorticoid-treated patients with inadequate adrenal function who have an intercurrent illness or are due to undergo surgery will have an inadequate reaction to the resulting stress and need to be temporarily protected by additional glucocorticoid (99).

Pseudohyperaldosteronism has been reported even after intranasal application of 9-alpha-fluoroprednisolone (SEDA-11, 340).

Parathyroid function

There is antagonism between the parathyroid hormone and glucocorticoids (100). Latent hyperparathyroidism can be unmasked by glucocorticoids (101).

Thyroid function

Even a single dose of corticotropin briefly inhibits the secretion of thyrotrophic hormone. The uptake of radioactive iodine is also suppressed by corticotropin and by glucocorticoids, but this has no clinical relevance. Pathological changes in thyroid function induced by glucocorticoid treatment are reportedly rare.

Metabolism

Glucose metabolism

All glucocorticoids increase gluconeogenesis. The turnover of glucose is increased, more being metabolized to fat, and blood glucose concentration is increased by 10–20%. Glucose tolerance and sensitivity to insulin are reduced, but provided pancreatic islet function is normal, carbohydrate metabolism will not be noticeably altered. So-called "steroid diabetes," a benign diabetes without a tendency to ketosis, but with a low sensitivity to insulin and a low renal threshold to glucose, only develops in one-fifth of patients treated with high glucocorticoid dosages. Even in patients with diabetes, ketosis is not to be expected, since glucocorticoids have antiketotic activity, presumably through suppression of growth hormone secretion.

Glucocorticoid treatment of known diabetics normally leads to deregulation, but this can be compensated for by adjusting the dose of insulin. The increased gluconeogenesis induced by glucocorticoids mainly takes place in the liver, but glucocorticoid treatment is especially likely to disturb carbohydrate metabolism in liver disease.

When hyperglycemic coma occurs it is almost always of the hyperosmolar nonketotic type. After termination of glucocorticoid treatment, steroid diabetes normally disappears. An apparent exception to these findings is provided by the case of a patient in whom glucocorticoid treatment was followed by severe diabetes with diabetic nephropathy, but this was a seriously ill individual who had already undergone renal transplantation (SEDA-17, 449). Gestational diabetes mellitus was more common in women who had received glucocorticoids with or without beta-adrenoceptor agonists for threatened preterm delivery compared with controls (SEDA-22, 445) (102).

Glucocorticoids probably have more than one effect on carbohydrate metabolism. An increase in fasting glucagon concentration has been observed in volunteers given prednisolone 40 mg/day for 4 days, and this effect may be involved, alongside gluconeogenesis, in glucocorticoid-induced hyperglycemia. Some newer glucocorticoids have been claimed to have smaller effects on blood glucose (as well as less salt and water retention), but further studies are needed to confirm whether this interesting therapeutic approach has been successful (SEDA-13, 353).

Deflazacort, an oxazoline derivative of prednisolone, was introduced as a potential substitute for conventional glucocorticoids in order to ameliorate glucose intolerance. In a randomized study in kidney transplant recipients with pre- or post-transplantation diabetes mellitus, 42 patients who switched from prednisone to deflazacort (in the ratio 5:6 mg) were prospectively compared with 40 patients who continued to take prednisone (SEDA-22, 445) (103). During the mean follow-up period of 13 months, neither graft dysfunction nor acute rejection developed in the conversion group, and there was improvement in blood glucose control. When the conversion group was stratified into those with pre- or post-transplantation diabetes, there were promising effects in the patients with post-transplantation diabetes. More than a 50% dosage reduction of hypoglycemic drugs was possible in 42% of those with post-transplantation diabetes.

The risk of hyperglycemia requiring treatment in patients receiving oral glucocorticoids has been quantified in a case-control study of 11 855 patients, 35 years of age or older, with newly initiated treatment with a hypoglycemic drug (SEDA-19, 375) (104). The risk for initiating hypoglycemic therapy increased with the recent use of a glucocorticoid. The risk grew with increasing average daily glucocorticoid dosage (in mg of hydrocortisone equivalents): 1.77 for 1–39 mg/day, 3.02 for 40–79 mg/day, 5.82 for 80–119 mg/day, and 10.34 for 120 mg/day or more.

Lipid metabolism

High-dose glucocorticoid therapy can cause marked hypertriglyceridemia, with milky plasma (SEDA-15, 421) (SEDA-16, 450). It has been suggested that this is caused by abnormal accumulation of dietary fat, reduced postheparin lipolytic activity, and glucose intolerance (105). An association between glucocorticoid exposure and hypercholesterolemia has been found in several studies (106) and can contribute to an increased risk of atherosclerotic vascular disease.

Most premature neonates need intravenous lipids during the first few weeks of life to acquire adequate energy intake and prevent essential fatty acid deficiency before they can tolerate all nutrition via enteral feeds. Dexamethasone is associated with multiple adverse effects in neonates, including poor weight gain and impairment of glucose and protein metabolism. In ten neonates (four boys, mean age 17.3 days) taking dexamethasone for bronchopulmonary dysplasia, intravenous lipids (3 g/kg/day) caused hypertriglyceridemia in the presence of hyperinsulinemia and increased free fatty acid concentrations (107). Because of concomitant hyperinsulinemia, the authors speculated that dexamethasone reduced fatty acid oxidation, explaining poor weight gain.

Altered fat deposition has been repeatedly reported. Fat can be deposited epidurally and at other sites. Adiposis dolora, which involves the symmetrical appearance of multiple painful fat deposits in the subcutaneous tissues, has on one occasion been attributed to glucocorticoids (SEDA-16, 451).

Tumor lysis syndrome

Acute tumor lysis syndrome is a life-threatening metabolic emergency that results from rapid massive necrosis of tumor cells. There have been repeated reports of an acute tumor lysis syndrome when glucocorticoids are administered in patients with pre-existing lymphoid tumors (108).

- A 60-year-old woman took dexamethasone 4 mg 8-hourly for dyspnea due to a precursor T lymphoblastic lymphoma-leukemia with bilateral pleural effusions and a large mass in the anterior mediastinum (109). She developed acute renal insufficiency and laboratory evidence of the metabolic effects of massive cytolysis. She received vigorous hydration, a diuretic, allopurinol, and hemodialysis. She recovered within 2 weeks and then underwent six courses of CHOP chemotherapy. The mediastinal mass regressed completely. She remained asymptomatic until she developed full-blown acute lymphoblastic leukemia, which was resistant to treatment.

Electrolyte balance

The severity of potassium loss due to glucocorticoids depends partly on the amount of sodium in the diet; the most widely used synthetic glucocorticoids cause less potassium excretion than natural hydrocortisone does. Prednisone and prednisolone have a glucocorticoid activity 4–5 times that of hydrocortisone, but their mineralocorticoid activity is less (see Table 1); even at high dosages they do not cause noteworthy sodium and water retention. Of the major synthetic glucocorticoids, dexamethasone has the strongest anti-inflammatory, hyperglycemic, and corticotropin-inhibitory activity; sodium retention is completely absent; the degree of glucocorticoid-induced metabolic alkalosis may also be less with dexamethasone than with hydrocortisone or methylprednisolone (SEDA-10, 343).

Mineral balance

There can be increases in calcium and phosphorus loss because of effects on both the kidney and the bowel, with increased excretion and reduced resorption (110). Tetany, which has been seen in patients receiving high-dose long-term intravenous glucocorticoids, has been explained as being due to hypocalcemia, and there are also effects on bone. Tetany has also been reported in a patient with latent hyperparathyroidism after the administration of a glucocorticoid (101).

Hypocalcemic encephalopathy occurred in a 35-year-old woman with hypoparathyroidism. It was believed that the administration of methylprednisolone intramuscularly had precipitated severe hypocalcemia, which had led to a metabolic encephalopathy (SEDA-20, 371) (111).

The administration of large doses of glucocorticoids to patients with major burns presenting with low cardiac output has been reported to produce a reversible drop in serum zinc, which might lead to impaired tissue repair (SED-8, 824), but it is not clear whether this has clinical effects.

Metal metabolism

Glucocorticoids increase chromium losses and glucocorticoid-induced diabetes can be reversed by chromium supplementation (112). Doses of hypoglycemic drugs were also reduced by 50% in all patients when they were given supplementary chromium.

Hematologic

Erythrocytes

Polycythemia is a symptom of Cushing's syndrome, and conversely anemia correlates with Addison's disease, but polycythemia is not generally encountered as a consequence of treatment with glucocorticoids, perhaps because there is no increased secretion of androgens; an increase in hemoglobin was nevertheless the most frequent adverse effect observed in a study over 8 years of 77 patients treated for hyperergic-allergic reactions. At the beginning of treatment more than 40% (and during continuous therapy more than 70%) of patients showed this change in erythrocytes (113). There was leukocytosis in more than 60% in the early phases and in more than 40% later (113). Thrombocytosis occurred in 5–10% during continuous treatment. This report agrees fairly well with some older publications, but it has been noted in the past that in the long run very high-dose glucocorticoid treatment can result in suppression of the activity of the bone marrow with fatty infiltration replacing hemopoietic tissue.

Leukocytes

Not all classes of leukocytes are affected by glucocorticoids in the same way. The total leukocyte count is increased, but the number of eosinophilic leukocytes falls, as does the lymphocyte count. The number of monocytes is reduced, as is their capacity to perform phagocytosis.

In children, a leukemoid reaction has been induced by betamethasone treatment (114); this possibility must always be borne in mind, since glucocorticoids can actually be used to treat leukemia or its complications. A case of very high white blood cell count with neutrophilia in a preterm infant whose mother had received two doses of betamethasone prenatally to enhance fetal lung maturation is one of a short list of leukemoid reactions possibly attributable to antenatal glucocorticoid treatment (115).

It is possible that in children with acute lymphoblastic leukemia, glucocorticoid therapy adversely affects the duration of remissions, and it has therefore been suggested that leukemia should be ruled out in children before starting long-term therapy with glucocorticoids (SEDA-11, 340). Depression of the lymphocyte count seems to be a general and direct action of the glucocorticoids (116), but the mechanism is still incompletely understood; certainly, lymphocytolysis seems to be increased by glucocorticoids. Studies of lymphocyte subpopulations show a preferential reduction in T cells, while B cells are constant or slightly reduced. B lymphocyte function (measured as immunoglobulin synthesis) falls, suppressor T lymphocyte activity is suppressed, and helper T lymphocyte function is unaffected by glucocorticoids (SEDA-3, 308) (117).

- Fever and leukopenia with methylprednisolone and prednisolone has been reported in a 29-year-old woman with systemic lupus erythematosus (118).

The authors commented that fever associated with glucocorticoids occurs frequently, whereas leukopenia is rare. Fever and leukopenia are important signs of an exacerbation of systemic lupus erythematosus, and it would be difficult to distinguish between an exacerbation of the disease and an adverse effect of glucocorticoids.

Platelets and coagulation

In heart transplant recipients, intramuscular glucocorticoids can impair fibrinolysis, producing susceptibility to thrombotic disease (SEDA-22, 443) (119). They can also increase the platelet count. In one patient the blue toe syndrome occurred repeatedly when glucocorticoids were used to increase the platelet count (SEDA-16, 451).

Mouth and teeth

Oral candidiasis is seen in some 5–10% of patients who use inhaled glucocorticoids, particularly when oral hygiene is poor, but is rarely symptomatic. The risk can be reduced by the use of a large-volume spacer (120,121).

Hypertrophy of the tongue has been attributed to inhaled beclomethasone and may have been related to edema of the buccal mucosa and tongue from direct contact with the glucocorticoid, infection, glossitis caused by glucocorticoid therapy, a direct effect of glucocorticoids on the tongue muscle, or excess localized deposition of fat, as is seen in patients given systemic glucocorticoids (SEDA-20, 371) (122).

Gastrointestinal

Peptic ulceration

It is no longer seriously believed that glucocorticoid treatment in adults markedly increases the risk of peptic ulceration (123,124). However, the symptoms of an existing peptic ulcer can certainly be masked. There may also be a genuine risk of ulcerative disorders in premature children. The issue has often been complicated by the simultaneous (sometimes unrecorded) use of ulcerogenic non-steroidal anti-inflammatory agents. A meta-analysis of whether glucocorticoid therapy caused peptic ulcer and other putative complications of glucocorticoid therapy was negative: peptic ulcers occurred in nine of 3267 patients in the placebo group (0.03%) and 13 of 3335 patients in the glucocorticoid group (0.04%).

Peptic ulcer should not be considered a contraindication when glucocorticoid therapy is indicated (SEDA-19, 376) (125). However, the risk of a fatal outcome due to ulcer complications was increased about fourfold in a previous case-control study. Gastrointestinal hemorrhage occurred more often in glucocorticoid-treated patients (2.25%) than in controls (1.6%) (126). The frequency of gastrointestinal bleeding in these studies compares well with earlier observations in the Boston Collaborative Surveillance Program's 1978 report, according to which 0.5% of a large series of medical inpatients taking glucocorticoids had gastrointestinal bleeding sufficiently severe to require transfusions and 28% had minor bleeding (SED-12, 986).

- A 47-year-old woman developed a gastrocolic fistula during treatment with aspirin (dosage and duration of therapy not stated) and prednisone for chronic rheumatoid arthritis (127).

The author commented that 50–75% of gastrocolic fistulas are related to benign gastric ulcers secondary to the use of NSAIDs. The use of aspirin plus prednisone, as in this patient, increases the risk of complication of peptic ulcer disease two- to fourfold.

The mechanism of whatever harm glucocorticoids may do to the stomach is not clear; cortisol neither consistently increases acid or pepsinogen secretion, nor reduces the protective production of mucin by the gastric mucosa. Serum gastrin concentrations are raised in Cushing's syndrome and in patients taking prolonged glucocorticoid treatment. On the other hand, the secretion of prostaglandin E_2 in gastric juice in response to pentagastrin was impaired during glucocorticoid therapy in children. Since PGE_2 has a cytoprotective effect on the gastric mucosa, impaired secretion in response to increased acid secretion during glucocorticoid therapy may be related to the development of peptic ulcer (SEDA-19, 376) (128).

Some reports suggest that people with hepatic cirrhosis or nephrotic syndrome are particularly at risk. Whatever the degree of risk, patients taking long-term glucocorticoids should be regularly checked to detect peptic ulcers, which can bleed and even perforate without producing pain. There do not seem to be differences in gastric tolerance between the various synthetic glucocorticoids.

Regional ileitis

While glucocorticoids may have a beneficial effect on regional ileitis, perforation of the ileum, lymphatic dilatation, and microscopic fistulae have been observed after treatment.

Ischemic colitis

Glucocorticoids should be used with caution in progressive systemic sclerosis, and concomitant administration of anticoagulants to prevent ischemic colitis is recommended when administering glucocorticoids in high doses, especially by pulse therapy (SEDA-21, 415) (129).

Ulcerative colitis

A possible risk of glucocorticoid treatment of ulcerative colitis is the development of toxic megacolon or colonic perforation. A change from ulcerative colitis to Crohn's disease may have been induced by prolonged treatment with glucocorticoids (SEDA-19, 376) (130). This case provides further evidence for the view that ulcerative colitis and Crohn's disease may represent a continuous spectrum of inflammatory bowel disease and raises the possibility that reduced polymorphonuclear leukocyte function caused by glucocorticoids may have provoked the development of granulomata.

Diverticular disease

Existing diverticula can perforate during glucocorticoid therapy (SEDA-18, 387). Abdominal tenderness is the most common and often the only early sign of perforated diverticula in patients taking glucocorticoids. However, in some cases, even abdominal tenderness is absent (SEDA-22, 445) (131).

- Perforation of the sigmoid colon occurred in a 61-year-old Caucasian man with colonic diverticular disease and rheumatoid arthritis treated with pulses of methylprednisolone 1 g (132).

The authors suggested that methylprednisolone pulses should be used carefully in patients over 50 years of age and/or people with demonstrated or suspected diverticular disease.

Liver

The process of gluconeogenesis, which is promoted by glucocorticoids, takes place mainly in the liver. The glycolytic enzymes of the liver are also activated by these glucocorticoids. The synthesis of ribonucleic acid and of enzymes involved in protein catabolism is increased, but the process of protein catabolism takes place outside the liver as well, for example in the muscles. There is experimental evidence for glucocorticoid-induced enhancement of hepatic lipid synthesis (SEDA-3, 308), but the main effect of glucocorticoids in this connection is lipid mobilization from adipose tissue. The influence of long-term glucocorticoid treatment on liver function is still unknown. If pathological changes are diagnosed, the possible influence of the disease which is being treated has to be borne in mind.

Liver damage from glucocorticoids is rarely severe, but fatal liver failure has been reported.

- A 71-year-old white woman with a compressive optic neuropathy was given five cycles of intravenous methylprednisolone 1 g/day for 3 days followed by tapering oral cortisone for 10–14 days (133). The intervals between cycles were 14 days to 6 weeks. She was otherwise healthy and had no history of liver disease. Her liver function tests were normal or only slightly raised during the first five cycles. She then developed raised liver enzymes, a prolonged prothrombin time, and fatal liver failure. Postmortem examination showed necrosis of the liver parenchyma. Hepatitis serology (A, B, and C) was negative as was in situ hybridization for immunohistochemical proof of hepatitis Bs and Bc or delta virus antibodies in the liver.
- A 53-year-old woman who took prednisolone 20 mg/day for systemic lupus erythematosus for 38 days developed increased aspartate transaminase and alanine transaminase activities (175 and 144 IU/l respectively on day 38 and 871 and 658 IU/l on day 69) (134). She denied taking hepatotoxic drugs. Serological tests for hepatitis viruses were all negative. Autoantibodies against mitochondria and smooth muscle were not detected. Ultrasound and CT scan were consistent with fatty infiltration. Histology showed macrovesicular fat infiltration, periportal cell infiltration with fibrosis, and a few Mallory bodies. The glucocorticoid was gradually tapered and the transaminases gradually fell.
- A 67-year-old teetotaler was given intravenous prednisolone 25 mg tds for primary dermatomyositis and 8 days later developed painless icteric hepatitis, with daily progressive marked deterioration of liver biochemistry (135). She had not taken any other hepatotoxic drugs, and serological tests for hepatitis and hepatotropic viruses were all negative. Antinuclear, antimitochondrial, and smooth muscle autoantibodies were negative. Ultrasound and CT scan of the upper abdomen showed liver fatty infiltration. Prednisolone was tapered gradually, and she gradually improved. However, on day 26 she developed pneumonia and died 6 days later.

Glucocorticoid treatment in the early phase of acute viral hepatitis carries the risk of transition to chronic active hepatitis (SEDA-3, 308).

Three children developed hepatomegaly and raised liver enzymes after receiving high-dose dexamethasone therapy (0.66–1.09 mg/kg/day) (136).

Pancreas

Pancreatitis and altered pancreatic secretion can occur at any time during long-term glucocorticoid treatment (SED-12, 986) (SEDA-14, 339) (137). Necrosis of the pancreas during glucocorticoid treatment has been described and can be lethal. Impairment of pancreatic function can predispose to glucocorticoid-induced pancreatitis. Two other cases of glucocorticoid-induced pancreatitis have been reported (138).

- A 74-year-old woman with seronegative rheumatoid arthritis was given sulfasalazine followed by methotrexate, both of which were withdrawn because of adverse effects. She also took prednisone 10 mg/day. She developed acute abdominal pain and fever (38.7°C) with no chills. Her serum amylase was 269 IU/l, serum lipase 300 IU/l, and urinary amylase 2895 IU/l. There was no evidence of tumor, hypertriglyceridemia, or lithiasis. In addition to prednisone, she was taking amlodipine, bromazepam, and omeprazole, none of which have been reported to cause pancreatitis. A marked improvement was noted after prednisone withdrawal.
- A 68-year-old woman who had taken prednisone 30 mg/day for polymyalgia rheumatica for 6 months developed sharp stabbing abdominal pain, fever (39°C), and vomiting. Her serum amylase was 310 IU/l, serum lipase 340 IU/l, and urinary amylase 1560 IU/l.

Other causes of pancreatitis were ruled out. She had been taking a thiazide diuretic therapy for the past 10 years. Her symptoms improved noticeably after prednisone withdrawal.

Although the literature suggests a causal relation between glucocorticoid therapy and these various pancreatic complications there is still no certainty; glucocorticoid treatment is, after all, often given simultaneously with other forms of therapy which can cause pancreatitis (SED-11, 82). The strongest evidence that there is a causal relation is provided by a Japanese report on 52 autopsies, which showed marked changes in pancreatic histology in glucocorticoid-treated patients compared with controls (SEDA-17, 449).

Urinary tract

Urinary calculi are more likely during glucocorticoid treatment because of increased excretion of calcium and phosphate (110).

Prednisolone can cause an abrupt rise in proteinuria in patients with nephrotic syndrome. A placebo-controlled study in 26 patients aged 18–68 years with nephrotic syndrome has clarified the mechanisms responsible for this (139). Systemic and renal hemodynamics and urinary protein excretion were measured after prednisolone (125 mg or 150 mg when body weight exceeded 75 kg) and after placebo. Prednisolone increased proteinuria by changing the size-selective barrier of the glomerular capillaries. Neither the renin–angiotensin axis nor prostaglandins were involved in these effects of prednisolone on proteinuria.

Changes resembling diabetic nodular glomerular sclerosis have been seen in glucocorticoid-treated nephrosis.

Treatment with glucocorticoids can result in minor increases in the urinary content of leukocytes and erythrocytes without clear renal injury (140).

The use of high doses of glucocorticoids to counter rejection of renal transplants is still a matter of intensive study; the optimal dose to ensure an effect without undue risk of complications has yet to be agreed on (141).

Vasopressin-resistant polyuria induced by intravenous administration of a therapeutic dose of dexamethasone has been reported (SEDA-20, 370) (142) and nocturia is fairly common during glucocorticoid treatment (143).

The administration of glucocorticoids should be undertaken with caution in progressive systemic sclerosis and the concomitant administration of anticoagulants to prevent scleroderma renal crisis is recommended when administering glucocorticoids in high doses, especially by pulse therapy (SEDA-21, 415) (129).

Skin

Acne is common during treatment, particularly after topical application, and is said to be correlated with the use of compounds that have a particularly strong local effect (144), although this is not proven.

Leukoderma can occur, accompanied by normal melanocyte function but reduced phagocytic activity of the keratinocytes to eliminate the melanosomes (145). Depigmentation can occur at the site of injection of glucocorticoids.

Three cases of severe lipoatrophy, one also with leukoderma, occurring within the same family after intramuscular injection of triamcinolone, suggested genetic susceptibility to this adverse effect (SEDA-3, 303).

Inhibition of the function of the sebaceous glands in the skin is caused by glucocorticoids whilst androgens stimulate their function (146).

A delayed hypersensitivity reaction, characterized by a skin rash, due to dexamethasone has been reported (147). These kinds of reactions to systemic glucocorticoids are rarely reported.

- A 59-year-old woman, who had not used glucocorticoids before, developed an exfoliative rash on her face, upper chest, and skin folds after 3 days treatment with oral dexamethasone (dosage not stated) for an acute episode of encephalomyelitis disseminata. Dexamethasone was immediately withdrawn and her skin lesions resolved over several days. Patch tests were positive to dexamethasone, betamethasone, and clobetasol, but negative to other glucocorticoids, including prednisolone, hydrocortisone butyrate, methylprednisolone, and triamcinolone. Prick tests with all of these glucocorticoids were negative. She tolerated oral methylprednisolone without adverse effects.

Reduced skin thickness and bruising

The glucocorticoids reduce subcutaneous collagen and cause atrophic changes in the skin (148). Subcutaneous atrophy after intramuscular and intra-articular injection has often been reported. Ecchymosis and paper-thin skin folds recall those seen in old people. An increased incidence of subcutaneous ecchymosis in older women has been observed during treatment with triamcinolone acetate (149). Purpura has been observed during glucocorticoid treatment and an increased fragility of the capillaries is thought to occur in about 60% of these patients. There have been reports of cutaneous bruising after the use of high doses of inhaled glucocorticoids (budesonide and beclomethasone), suggesting systemic absorption (SEDA-21, 416) (150).

Prednicarbate is a topical glucocorticoid that seems to have an improved benefit–harm balance, as has been shown in 24 healthy volunteers (7 men, 17 women, aged 25–49 years) in a double-blind, randomized, placebo-controlled study of the effects of prednicarbate, mometasone furoate, and betamethasone 17-valerate on total skin thickness over 6 weeks (151). On day 36, total skin thickness was reduced by a mean of 1% in test fields treated with vehicle; the relative reductions were 13, 17, and 24% for prednicarbate, mometasone furoate, and betamethasone 17-valerate respectively. There were visible signs of atrophy or telangiectasia in two subjects each with betamethasone 17-valerate and mometasone furoate, but not with prednicarbate or its vehicle.

Contact allergy

Topical glucocorticoids are well-known contact sensitizers. Immediate allergic or allergic-like reactions to systemic glucocorticoids also occur, but less often. Two atopic patients developed urticaria, possibly IgE-mediated, from a hydrocortisone injection or infusion (152) and other reactions have been reported.

- A 50-year-old woman developed contact dermatitis on her legs after she applied hydrocortisone aceponate cream (Efficort) to psoriatic lesions on her lower back (153). Similar lesions also occurred on her legs after she used topical betamethasone cream (Diprosone). However, no eczema developed on or around the site of application. Patch tests were negative to a range of glucocorticoids, including Efficort and Diprosone creams. However, a repeated open application test was positive with Efficort cream, hydrocortisone aceponate 0.127% in petroleum, and tixocortol pivalate 1% in petroleum.
- A 42-year-old woman developed a nonpigmented fixed drug eruption after skin testing and an intra-articular injection of triamcinolone acetonide, which has not been previously reported (154).

Contact allergy to glucocorticoids was evaluated in 7238 patients in a multicenter multinational study of five drugs: budesonide, betamethasone-17-valerate, clobetasol-17-propionate, hydrocortisone-17-butyrate, and tixocortol-21-pivalate. There was a positive patch-test reaction to at least one of the glucocorticoids in 189 patients (2.6%). The incidence ranged from 0.4% in Spain to 6.4% in Belgium. Positive reactions were more frequent with budesonide (100 results) and tixocortol (98 reactions) (SEDA-21, 415) (155). Contact allergic reactions to intranasal budesonide and fluticasone propionate have been described. Many of these cases were characterized by perinasal eczema, often with vesicles, and edema as the initial symptoms. Lesions sometimes spread to the upper lip, cheeks, and eyelids. For fluticasone propionate, analysis of data on adverse events from the Spontaneous Reporting System of the US FDA Division of Epidemiology and Surveillance showed that, in the first 5 months after its introduction into the USA in 1995, 46 patients reported 89 adverse events suspected to be caused by fluticasone propionate intranasal spray. Central nervous system symptoms occurred in 46%, cardiac symptoms in 28%, dermatological symptoms in 39%, and epistaxis in 6.5%. These numbers may underestimate the problem, since no cases reported by the drug manufacturer were included. These results suggest that safety issues may differentiate budesonide and fluticasone propionate from other intranasal glucocorticoids, such as beclomethasone dipropionate (SEDA-21, 415) (156).

Budesonide is advocated as a marker molecule for glucocorticoid contact allergy. When patch testing glucocorticoids, one must consider both their sensitizing potential and their anti-inflammatory properties, as well as the possibility of different time courses of such properties. The dose–response relation for budesonide has therefore been investigated with regard to dose, occlusion time, and reading time in 10 patients (ages not stated) who were patch tested with budesonide in ethanol in serial dilutions from 2.0% down to 0.0002%, with occlusion times of 48, 24, and 5 hours (157). Readings were on days 2, 4, and 7. The 48-hour occlusion detected most positive reactors (8/10) at a reading time of 4 days and 0.002% detected most contact allergies. The "edge effect" (reactions with a peripheral ring due to suppression of the allergic reaction under the patch because of the intrinsic anti-inflammatory effect of the glucocorticoid itself) was noted with several concentrations at early readings. That lower concentrations can detect budesonide allergy better at early readings and that patients with an "edge reaction" can have positive reactions to lower concentrations can be explained by individual glucocorticoid reactivity, the dose–response relation, and the time-courses of the elicitation and the anti-inflammatory capacity.

- A 36-year-old man, who had a long history of atopic dermatitis of the neck, chest, and arms, developed allergic contact dermatitis after topical administration of clobetasone ointment 0.05% (Kindavate) and prednisolone ointment 0.3% (Lidomex) (158). Patch tests with both ointments showed a positive reaction only to Kindavate. Further testing with the separate ingredients of Kindavate showed positive reactions to 0.05, 0.01, and 0.005% clobetasone on day 7.
- A 40-year-old woman had a flare-up of her eczema (159). She had had previous negative patch tests 10 years before. She had taken topical glucocorticoids and emollients for a few months, but had not used budesonide. Patch testing with the European standard series showed a positive reaction to budesonide 0.1% at 3 days. All other allergens were negative. The only antecedent exposure was that she had three children with asthma, all of whom regularly used inhaled budesonide and occasionally nebulizers. She had not used the inhaler but had helped her children to manage the devices. A subsequent patch test with powdered budesonide from the inhaler was positive.
- A 14-year-old girl with newly diagnosed systemic lupus erythematosus developed a pruritic bullous eruption while taking prednisone 20 mg/day (160). She was given a single daily dose of intravenous methylprednisolone 60 mg with rapid improvement. In preparation for discharge, the glucocorticoid was changed to oral prednisone 60 mg/day, to which she developed a pruritic bullous eruption consistent with erythema multiforme. She underwent immediate and delayed hypersensitivity tests. Intradermal and patch tests to liquid prednisone were positive. She was given oral methylprednisolone 48 mg/day and has not had recurrence of the skin lesions.
- A 27-year-old woman, a pharmacist, had dermatitis on three separate occasions a few hours after she started to take oral deflazacort 6 mg for vesicular hand eczema (161). On each occasion, her symptoms included a widespread macular rash mainly on the inner aspects of her arms and legs and buttocks. She also had severe scaling, fever, nausea, vomiting, malaise, and hypotension. A skin biopsy was consistent with erythema multiforme, and direct immunofluorescence showed granular deposits at the dermoepidermal junction. Patch tests to the commercial formulation of deflazacort 6 mg (1% aqueous solution) and to pure deflazacort (1% aqueous solution) were positive, but there were no cross-reactions to other glucocorticoids.

The author of the last report commented that the patient probably developed hypersensitivity to deflazacort as a result of occupational exposure.

Other cases of erythema multiforme-like contact dermatitis after topical budesonide have been reported (SEDA-21, 415) (162). In a large case-control study, potential cases of severe forms of erythema multiforme, toxic epidermal necrolysis and Stevens–Johnson syndrome, were collected in four European countries (France, Portugal, Italy, and Germany) (SEDA-20, 371) (163). There was a significant relation with glucocorticoid use in the preceding week (multivariate analysis relative risk = 4.4; 95% CI = 1.9, 10), or when prescribed for long-term therapy (crude relative risk for use less than 2 months = 54; 95% CI = 23, 124). The estimates of excess risks associated with glucocorticoids or sulfonamides (which are well-known to cause these syndromes), expressed as the number of cases attributable to the drug per million users in 1 week, were 1.5 and 4.5 respectively.

Cross-reactivity between glucocorticoids and progestogens has been described (164).

- A 68-year-old woman, with a prolonged history of pityriasis lichenoides chronica treated with topical glucocorticoids, including hydrocortisone, took a formulation containing conjugated estrogens 0.625 mg and hydroxyprogesterone acetate 5 mg (frequency of administration not stated) for late menopausal syndrome. Years later she started to have pruritus, a maculopapular rash, and flu-like symptoms for several days before menstruation. On this occasion, she presented with a severe, pruritic, papulovesicular eruption on her chest, back, abdomen, and legs. The eruption had developed after treatment for 7 days with the estrogen–progestogen formulation; she had developed similar symptoms on several previous occasions after taking the same medication. She was treated with antihistamines and her skin eruption resolved within a few days. Patch tests were positive to 17-OH-progesterone, tixocortol pivalate, and budesonide.

The authors hypothesized that this patient, who had taken topical glucocorticoids for several years, had become sensitive and that the recurrent episodes of autoimmune progestogen dermatitis were related to endogenous progestogen sensitivity following cross-sensitivity to glucocorticoids. This hypothesis was supported by the development of recurrent eczema several times after she took an estrogen–progestogen preparation.

Musculoskeletal

Osteoporosis

The use of glucocorticoids is associated with reduced bone mineral density, bone loss, osteoporosis, and fractures. This has been described during the long-term use of glucocorticoid by any route of administration (SEDA-19, 377) (SEDA-20, 374). The effects of glucocorticoids on bone have been reviewed (SEDA-21, 417) (165). Biochemical markers of bone mineral density are listed in Table 4. In patients with secondary hypoadrenalism, hydrocortisone 30 mg/day for replacement produced a significant fall in osteocalcin, indicating bone loss. Lower doses of hydrocortisone (10 mg and 20 mg) produced similar efficacy in terms of quality of life but smaller effects on osteocalcin concentrations and therefore a reduction in bone loss (166).

The fluorinated glucocorticoids are said to have relatively more catabolic activity than others and might have a greater effect on the skeleton but such impressions may merely reflect the general potency of some newer glucocorticoids and a tendency to use them in inappropriate doses. A relatively new glucocorticoid, deflazacort, has been proposed to have less effect on bone metabolism, but a double-blind study has failed to show an advantage compared with prednisolone (SEDA-21, 417) (167).

Table 4 Biochemical markers of bone mineral density

Bone formation
Blood
Alkaline phosphatase (bone-specific)
Osteocalcin
Procollagen type I carboxy-terminal propeptide (PICP)
Procollagen type I amino-terminal propeptide (PINP)
Procollagen type III amino-terminal propeptide (PIIINP)
Bone resorption
Blood
Acid phosphatase (acid-resistant)
Type I collagen carboxy-terminal telopeptide (ICTP)
Urine
Calcium
Hydroxyproline
Cross-linked peptides (pyridinium and deoxypyridinoline)

Osteoporosis induced by chronic glucocorticoid therapy has been reviewed in patients with obstructive lung diseases (168) and patients with skin diseases (169).

Presentation

Of the effects of glucocorticoids on the skeleton, osteoporosis is the most important clinically; manifestations can include vertebral compression fractures, scoliosis resulting in respiratory embarrassment, and fractures of the long bones. The risk of vertebral fractures is not different in patients taking or not taking glucocorticoids in whom bone mineral density is similar (170).

Glucocorticoids can even cause osteoporosis when they are used for long-term replacement therapy in the Addison's disease, as has been shown by a study of 91 patients who had taken glucocorticoids for a mean of 10.6 years, in whom bone mineral density was reduced by 32% compared with age-matched controls (SEDA-19, 377) (171). However, these results contrasted with the results of a Spanish study in patients with Addison's disease, in which no direct relation was found between replacement therapy and either bone density or biochemical markers of bone turnover of calcium metabolism (alkaline phosphatase, osteocalcin, procollagen I type, parathormone, and 1,25-dihydroxycolecalciferol) (SEDA-19, 377) (172).

Atraumatic posterior pelvic ring fractures that simulate the form of presentation of metastatic diseases can be produced by glucocorticoid administration (SEDA-19, 377) (173).

Accelerated bone loss, with an increased risk of first hip fracture, occurred in elderly women taking oral glucocorticoids (174). At baseline, 122 (1.5%) women were taking inhaled glucocorticoids only (median dose equivalent to inhaled beclomethasone 168 micrograms/day), 228 (2.8%) were taking oral glucocorticoids (median dose equivalent to prednisone 5 mg/day) with or without inhaled glucocorticoids, and 7718 were not taking any glucocorticoids. The women who were taking oral glucocorticoids had lower mean bone mineral density at 3.6 years than nonusers, with an interim fall that was twice as fast. First hip fracture occurred in 4.8% of the women who were taking oral glucocorticoids and in 2.8% of the women who were not (RR = 2.1; CI = 1.0, 4.4). The researchers said that the power of the study was not sufficient to determine the relative risk of hip fracture in women taking inhaled glucocorticoids.

A reduction in bone mineral density has been described in 23 patients (19 men) with chronic fatigue syndrome taking low-dose glucocorticoids in a double-blind, randomized, placebo-controlled study (175). The patients took hydrocortisone 25–35 mg/day or matched placebo for 3 months. Mean bone mineral density in the spine fell by 2% with hydrocortisone and increased by 1% with placebo.

A group of 367 patients with lung disease taking oral glucocorticoids (177 women, mean age 68 years, 190 men, mean age 70 years) and 734 matched controls completed a questionnaire about lifestyle, fractures, and other possible adverse effects of glucocorticoids (176). The cumulative incidence of fractures from the time of diagnosis was 23% in patients taking oral glucocorticoids and 15% in the controls (OR = 1.8; 95% CI = 1.3, 2.6). Fractures of the vertebrae were more likely (OR = 10; 95% CI = 2.9, 35). The adverse effects were dose-related, with a higher risk of all fractures (OR = 2.22; 95% CI = 1.04, 4.8) and vertebral fractures (OR = 9.2; 95% CI = 2.4, 36) in those who took the highest compared with the lowest cumulative doses (61 versus 5 g).

Systemic glucocorticoids are often prescribed for rheumatoid arthritis. Even in low doses they can have clinical benefits and can inhibit joint damage, but they can cause osteoporotic fractures. In a 2-year double-blind, randomized, placebo-controlled trial in 81 patients (29 men, mean age 62 years) with early active rheumatoid arthritis who had not been treated with disease-modifying antirheumatic drugs, 41 were assigned to oral prednisone 10 mg/day and 40 to placebo. NSAIDs were allowed in both groups and after 6 months, sulfasalazine (2 g/day) could be prescribed as rescue medication. Those who took prednisone had more clinical improvement with less use of concomitant drugs. After month 6, radiological scores had progressed significantly less in those who took prednisone. After 24 months, seven patients had new vertebral fractures, five in the prednisone group and two in the placebo group (177).

Mechanisms

Several mechanisms underlie the effect of glucocorticoids on bone, both biochemical and cellular. Effects on calcium are:

(a) increased excretion of calcium into the bowel and inhibition of its absorption;
(b) inhibition of the tubular re-absorption of calcium in the kidney;
(c) increased mobilization of calcium from the skeleton.

When calcium homeostasis cannot be maintained, the resulting hypocalcemia can have serious consequences (SEDA-18, 388) (178,179). This so-called "glucocorticoid hyperparathyroidism" was the explanation traditionally most prominently advanced for glucocorticoid osteoporosis, but it is not the only one and may not be the most central. Other biochemical effects include:

(a) a catabolic effect on protein metabolism, causing a reduction in the bone matrix;
(b) altered vitamin D metabolism, with reduced concentrations of vitamin D metabolites (180);
(c) a dose-dependent reduction of serum osteocalcin, a bone matrix protein that appears to correlate with bone formation.

Measurement of serum osteocalcin is a useful marker for glucocorticoid-induced osteoporosis, and can be used alongside other measures noted below.

Various cellular mechanisms are involved in the production of glucocorticoid-induced osteoporosis (SEDA-20, 375) (181). The major change is a reduction in osteoblast activity that results in a reduced working rate (mean appositional rate), and a reduced active life-span of osteoblasts. The cellular mechanism seems to be related to diminished production of cytokines and other locally acting factors. Increased bone resorption and reduced calcium absorption have also been described. A sophisticated mathematical model has been used to describe changes in calcium kinetics in patients treated with glucocorticoids (SEDA-20, 375) (182). Plasma calcium concentrations were higher than in controls, with a marked reduction in calcium flow into the irreversible stable bone compartment in glucocorticoid-treated patients. The authors concluded that prednisone has direct effects on osteoblast function.

Osteoprotegerin (osteoclastogenesis inhibitory factor, OCIF) has been identified as a novelly secreted cytokine receptor that plays an important role in the negative regulation of osteoclastic bone resorption. There are reports that suggest that glucocorticoids promote osteoclastogenesis by inhibiting osteoprotegerin production in vitro, thereby enhancing bone resorption. However, there are only a few clinical reports in which the regulatory functions of osteoprotegerin have been explored. In order to clarify the potential role of osteoprotegerin in the pathogenesis of glucocorticoid-induced osteoporosis, Japanese investigators have measured serum osteoprotegerin and other markers of bone metabolism before and after glucocorticoid therapy in patients with various renal diseases (183). The findings suggested that short-term administration of glucocorticoids significantly suppresses serum osteoprotegerin and osteocalcin. This might be relevant to the development of glucocorticoid-induced osteoporosis via enhancement of bone resorption and suppression of bone formation. Further long-term studies are needed to elucidate the mechanism of the glucocorticoid-induced reduction in circulating osteoprotegerin and its participation in the pathogenesis of osteoporosis.

Although glucocorticoids can cause changes in trabecular microarchitecture, loss of bone (reduced bone density) seems to be the major determinant of osteoporosis (184).

Although glucocorticoid use seems to be an important factor for low mineral density, sex hormones have also been suggested as an important determinant of bone mineral content. Bone mineral density and sex hormone status have been studied in 99 men with rheumatoid arthritis and 68 age-matched controls (SEDA-20, 375) (185). There were significant reductions in lumbar and femoral density, and salivary testosterone, androstenedione, and dehydroepiandrosterone in the patients. Salivary testosterone correlated with femoral density. By multiple regression analysis, weight, serum testosterone concentrations, and cumulative dose of glucocorticoid were significant predictors of lumbar bone density. Weight, age, androstenedione concentrations, and cumulative dose of glucocorticoids were significant predictors of femoral bone density.

Dose relation

Lumbar spine bone mineral density has been assessed in 76 prepubertal asthmatics (mean age 7.7 years, 26 girls) using glucocorticoids (186). After stratification for dose and route of administration, the children who used over 800 micrograms/day of inhaled glucocorticoids, with or without intermittent oral glucocorticoids, had a significant lower weight-adjusted bone density than children who used 400–800 micrograms/day of inhaled glucocorticoids (mean difference –0.05 g/cm^2; 95% CI = –0.02, –0.09). Bone mass was similar in children who did not use inhaled glucocorticoids and those who used 400–800 micrograms/day.

In kidney transplant recipients, lumbar bone loss was significantly higher in 20 patients who took daily prednisone (5.9%, mean dosage 0.19 mg/kg/day) than in 27 patients who used alternate-day prednisone (1.1%, mean dosage 0.15 mg/kg/day) (187).

Time course

The loss of bone mineral after organ and tissue transplant associated with immunosuppressive therapy follows a delayed time course. The long-term effects of immunosuppressive therapy on bone density have been determined in 25 cardiac transplant patients (SEDA-20, 375) (188). As expected, there was bone loss in the spine during the first year, but this was not maintained during the second and third years after transplantation, despite continuing maintenance immunosuppression with prednisolone. Only four patients, all of whom were hypogonadal, continued to lose bone.

Susceptibility factors

The overall effect of glucocorticoids on bone mineral content differs between patients on comparable treatments, which suggests that some patients are more predisposed than others (SEDA-3, 306), and probably also that the standards of evaluation used in different clinics are not comparable. This variability and the wide range of products and dosage schemes used mean that one does not have a clear impression of what constitutes a safe regimen as far as the skeleton is concerned (SEDA-20, 374), or whether any regimen is safe in this respect. Certainly, in a series of men with rheumatoid arthritis, even a very low dose of glucocorticoids (for example 10 mg or less of prednisolone daily) has proved to have a significant effect on bone mineral density (189); other work has provided similar results (SEDA-20, 374) (190). In another published study, patients who took 1–4 mg/day had the same density as those who were not taking glucocorticoids. Patients who took 5–9 mg/day and those who took more than 10 mg/day had significantly lower bone density (84 and 81% of control values respectively) (SEDA-20, 374) (191).

Glucocorticoid-related complications have been described in 748 adult kidney transplant recipients, followed for at least 1 year. For bone/joint complications, the multivariate analysis showed that the only significant variable was the cumulative duration of glucocorticoid therapy. For avascular necrosis, no variables were significant (SEDA-19, 377) (192).

In a similar study of 65 renal transplant patients treated with immunosuppressive drugs for at least 6 months, multivariate analysis showed that cumulative glucocorticoid dose and female sex were the major predictors of low vertebral bone density (SEDA-19, 377) (193).

In another study, the loss of bone density correlated with the cumulative dose of prednisolone (21 g total dose at 11.4 mg/day) and renal function (SEDA-21, 417) (194).

In a review of renal transplantation during 1974–94, 166 patients were classified into those with osteonecrosis of the femoral head (22 patients) and those without (47 patients) (SEDA-21, 417) (195). The total dose of methylprednisolone was higher in those with osteonecrosis. All five patients who had received intravenous pulse doses over 2000 mg had osteonecrosis.

The risk of vertebral deformity is increased by the combination of an oral glucocorticoid and advanced age, according to the findings in 229 patients (69% women) taking long-term oral glucocorticoids (prednisone equivalents of 5 mg/day or more) and 286 untreated controls (196). The duration of treatment was 0.5–37 (median 4.8) years. More than 60% of the treatment group were aged over 60 years, and most (62%) had been treated for rheumatoid arthritis. Bone mineral density data were analysed in 194 patients. The researchers identified at least one vertebral deformity (defined as a more than 20% reduction in anterior, middle, or posterior vertebral height) in 65 (28%) of the patients in the treatment group, and two or more fractures were identified in 25 (11%). In the treatment group, vertebral deformities were significantly more common in men than in women, and the prevalence of deformities increased with age. Compared with patients aged under 60 years, glucocorticoid-treated patients aged 70–79 years had a five-fold increased risk of vertebral deformity (OR = 5.1; 95% CI = 2.0, 13). The prevalence of vertebral deformities increased significantly with age in the glucocorticoid group. While the mean spine and femoral bone mineral density scores were lower in the glucocorticoid group, logistic regression analysis showed that bone mineral density was only a modest predictor of deformity. Age is an important independent risk factor, with very high prevalence rates in those over 70 years. Increasing duration of glucocorticoid use may increase the risk of fracture.

Comparisons of glucocorticoids

Bone loss induced by glucocorticoids has been assessed in three different populations. A group of 374 subjects (mean age 35 years, 55% women) with mild asthma taking beta-adrenoceptor agonists only, were randomized to inhaled glucocorticoids (budesonide or beclomethasone) or non-glucocorticoid treatment for 2 years (197). Bone mineral density was measured blind after 6, 12, and 24 months. Mean doses of budesonide and beclomethasone were 389 micrograms/day and 499 micrograms/day, respectively. At the end of follow-up, the subjects who had used glucocorticoids had better asthma control. The mean changes in bone density over 2 years in the budesonide, beclomethasone, and control groups were 0.1%, –0.4%, and 0.4% for the lumbar spine and –0.9%, –0.9%, and –0.4% for the neck of the femur. The daily dose of inhaled glucocorticoid was related to the reduction in bone mineral density only at the lumbar spine. Low to moderate doses of inhaled glucocorticoids caused little change in bone mineral density over 2 years and provided better asthma control.

Diagnosis

Several techniques are used to measure bone density. Cortical bone can be assessed in peripheral sites by single-photon absorptiometry and a combination of cortical and trabecular bone in central sites by dual X-ray absorptiometry. Trabecular bone can be assessed by quantitative computer tomography scanning of the lumbar spine. Since single-photon absorptiometry and dual X-ray absorptiometry give a negligible dose of radiation, they are useful for population screening. However, these two techniques are not sensitive enough to show subtle changes in bone density over short periods of time. Quantitative computed tomography gives a significant dose of radiation (of the order of one-tenth of a lateral X-ray of the spine) but can focus on trabecular bone, which has a tenfold greater turnover, compared with cortical bone. Quantitative computed tomography is more sensitive to changing bone density over time.

Other methods, such as the fasting urinary hydroxyproline/creatinine ratio, alkaline phosphatase activity, dual-absorption photometry of the hip, and serum osteocalcin measurements, can also be used, depending on an individual clinic's equipment and experience (SEDA-17, 447).

Management

The prevention and treatment of glucocorticoid bone loss in patients with skin diseases have been reviewed (169). Strategies for the management of this problem have been discussed (SEDA-22, 184) and the clinical implications of trials in the management of glucocorticoid-induced osteoporosis have been reviewed (198). Provided no fractures have occurred, loss of bone mineral density seems to be reversible when treatment is withdrawn (SEDA-18, 389). The management of glucocorticoid-induced osteoporosis has been revised by the UK Consensus Group Meeting on Osteoporosis (SEDA-20, 376) (183) and by the American College of Rheumatology (SEDA-21, 417) (199).

Guidelines for the prevention and treatment of glucocorticoid-induced osteoporosis have been published (200). Although there are several consensus statements and recommendations for prophylactic measures against glucocorticoid-induced osteoporosis in patients with rheumatoid arthritis, prophylaxis is commonly underprescribed. In two recent studies of 191 and 92 patients taking long-term glucocorticoids, relatively few were taking primary prevention, although some were taking vitamin D and calcium tablets. Around 65–68% of all those who qualified for prophylaxis for glucocorticoid-induced osteoporosis did not receive therapy, and only 9% of those in one study and 21% in the other were taking bisphosphonates (201,202).

Low availability compounds

Bone loss in patients taking oral budesonide has been evaluated in a longitudinal study in which bone mineral density was measured annually for 2 years in 138 patients (67 men, mean age 36 years old) with quiescent Crohn's disease (203). They took budesonide (8.5 mg/day; $n = 48$), prednisone (10.5 mg/day, $n = 45$), or non-steroidal drugs ($n = 45$). After 1 year, the bone mineral density in the lumbar spine fell by 2.36% in those who took budesonide, by 0.61% in those who took prednisone, and by 0.09% in those who took non-steroidal drugs. In the second year, the largest fall occurred in those who took budesonide (1.97%), but the differences between the groups were not significant. After 2 years, bone mineral density in the femoral neck fell by 2.94% with budesonide, 0.36% with prednisone, and 1.05% with the non-steroidal drugs. These results suggest that budesonide can cause bone loss, but the non-randomized design of the study limits conclusions about the comparison between budesonide and prednisone.

Pulse administration

The administration of glucocorticoids in sporadic pulses has been shown not to reduce bone density in patients with multiple sclerosis. In a prospective study, 30 patients were given 1000 mg/day of methylprednisolone intravenously for 3 days, followed by oral prednisone in tapering dosage for 2 weeks. Bone density was determined in the lumbar spine and femoral neck before and at 2, 4, and 6 months after therapy. At baseline, the patients had a reduced bone mass compared with controls; this reduction did not correlate with previous exposure to glucocorticoids. Ambulant patients during follow-up after glucocorticoid pulse therapy had an increase in lumbar bone density (+1.7% at 6 months). Average femoral density did not change; however, in patients who required a walking stick or other aid, femoral density fell (–1.6%), while in those with better ambulation it increased (+2.9%). These results suggest that inactivity is the main factor causing bone loss in patients treated with sporadic pulses of glucocorticoids (SEDA-21, 417) (204).

Calcium and vitamin D

Infusion of ionic calcium has sometimes been used to counteract the malabsorption of calcium in patients taking long-term glucocorticoids, particularly in patients who develop secondary hypoparathyroidism (SEDA-3, 306). There is also evidence that in amenorrheic or menopausal women requiring glucocorticoids, the adverse effects on the vertebrae can be countered by hormonal replacement therapy with estrogen and progesterone (205); progestogens similarly seem to have a promising effect in men, and while they cause a fall in serum testosterone they apparently do not undermine the desired effects of glucocorticoids (SEDA-16, 449).

The administration of calcium and vitamin D3 can prevent bone loss induced by glucocorticoids, and trials have confirmed its efficacy when given for 2 years. Patients taking prednisone and placebo lost bone density in the lumbar spine at a rate of 2% per year. Those taking prednisone and calcium plus vitamin D3 gained bone mineral density at a rate of 0.72% per year. Calcium plus vitamin D3 did not improve bone mineral density in patients who were not taking prednisone (SEDA-21, 417) (206).

In a similar randomized double-blind study, the effects of vitamin D (50 000 units/week) and calcium (1000 mg/day) were evaluated in 62 patients with different rheumatic diseases treated with prednisone (10–100 mg/day) (SEDA-21, 418) (207). The primary outcome was bone mineral density in the lumbar spine at 36 months. Patients taking placebo had reductions of 4.1, 3.8, and 1.5% at 12, 24, and 36 months respectively. Patients taking calcium and vitamin D had reductions of 2.6, 3.7, and 2.2% respectively. The results suggested that preventive therapy could be beneficial early in the prevention of glucocorticoid-induced bone loss, but there was no evidence of long-term beneficial effects. In kidney transplant patients, the preventive administration of 25-hydroxycolecalciferol and calcium reduced bone loss in the spine and femoral neck and the number of new vertebral crush fractures (SEDA-21, 418) (208). In children with rheumatic diseases taking glucocorticoids, calcium and vitamin D supplementation improved spinal bone density, although osteocalcin concentrations remained low (SEDA-19, 378) (209).

Calcitonin

Less clear are the results observed after the administration of salmon calcitonin. The usefulness of intranasally administered salmon calcitonin for 2 years has been evaluated in 44 glucocorticoid-dependent asthmatics (SEDA-19, 378) (210). All were taking calcium supplements (1000 mg/day), but one group also took calcitonin (100 IU every other day). Calcitonin increased spinal bone mass during first year of treatment, and maintained bone mass in a steady state during the second year. However, the rate of vertebral fractures was similar in the two groups. The addition of salmon calcitonin did not increase the efficacy of calcium plus vitamin D in the prevention of bone loss in 48 newly diagnosed patients taking glucocorticoids for temporal arteritis and polymyalgia rheumatica in a double-blind, randomized, placebo-controlled trial (SEDA-21, 418) (211). However, salmon calcitonin nasal spray prevented bone loss in the lumbar spine of 31 patients treated with prednisone for polymyalgia rheumatica (SEDA-22, 448) (212). They were randomized to salmon calcitonin nasal spray (200 IU/day) or matched placebo for 1 year. Both groups were treated with calcium supplements if their dietary intake was below 800 mg/day. With calcitonin, the mean bone mineral density in the lumbar spine fell by 1.3% and with placebo by 5% after 1 year. There were no differences in the hip, including the femoral neck and trochanter, or in total body bone density.

Bisphosphonates

There have been several studies of the use of bisphosphonates in preventing glucocorticoid-induced osteoporosis.

Intermittent cyclical etidronate prevented bone loss induced by prednisone in 10 postmenopausal women with temporal arteritis (SEDA-19, 378) (213). Cyclical etidronate (400 mg/day for 2 weeks every 3 months) plus ergocalciferol (0.5 mg/week) was given to 15 postmenopausal women (mean age 63 years) starting glucocorticoid therapy (prednisone 5–20 mg/day). A control group of 11 postmenopausal women (mean age 60 years) with glucocorticoid-induced osteoporosis were treated with calcium supplements only (1 g/day). During the first year, the cyclical regimen significantly increased lumbar and femoral neck bone density compared with placebo (7 and 2.5% for spine and femur respectively). After the second year of cyclical therapy, femoral neck bone density continued to increase while lumbar spine density remained stable (SEDA-20, 376) (214). The effect of intermittent cyclical therapy with etidronate has been investigated in the prevention of bone loss in 117 patients taking high-dose glucocorticoid therapy (a mean daily dose of at least 7.5 mg for 90 days followed by at least 2.5 mg/day for at least 12 months) (215). The patients were randomized to oral etidronate 400 mg/day or placebo for 14 days, followed by 76 days of oral calcium carbonate (500 mg elemental calcium), cycled over 12 months. The mean lumbar spine bone density changed 0.30% and –2.79% in the etidronate and placebo groups respectively. The mean difference between the groups after 1 year (3.0%) was significant. The changes in the femoral neck and greater trochanter were not different between the groups. There was a reduction in pyridinium cross-links, significant from baseline at both 6 and 12 months, in the etidronate group. Osteocalcin increased in the placebo group, and the differences between the groups at 6 and 12 months were –25% and –35% respectively. There was no significant difference between the groups in the number of adverse events, including gastrointestinal disorders. In a placebo-controlled study of the effects of 104 weeks of intermittent cyclical etidronate therapy in 49 patients, the same dose and cycles were used as in the previous study, but calcium (97 mg/day) was given with vitamin D (400 IU) (216). Intermittent cyclical etidronate therapy with vitamin D supplementation significantly increased lumbar spine bone mineral density by 4.5 in patients with osteoporosis resulting from long-term treatment with glucocorticoids.

Contradictory results have been published about the prophylactic use of two other bisphosphonates in patients treated with glucocorticoids. There were no bone losses after therapy, and no differences in bone density or biochemical bone markers between placebo and clodronate (SEDA-22, 447) (217).

Pamidronate disodium has been compared with calcium supplementation in an open trial of primary prevention of glucocorticoid-induced osteoporosis in 27 patients with different rheumatic conditions, randomly assigned to pamidronate (90 mg intravenously every 3 months) plus calcium (800 mg calcium carbonate) or calcium only for 1 year (SEDA-22, 448) (218). The glucocorticoids were given in a starting dosage of 10–80 mg/day. With pamidronate there was a significant increase in bone density (3.6% lumbar, 2.2% femoral neck), but there was a significant reduction with calcium (–5.3% in both spine and femoral neck).

The effects of risedronate on bone density and vertebral fracture have been studied in 518 patients (mean age 59 years, 40% with rheumatoid arthritis, 56% men, 64% of the women postmenopausal) taking moderate to high doses of oral glucocorticoids (equivalent to prednisone 7.5 mg/day or more) (219). The patients were randomized double-blind to placebo, or risedronate 2.5 or 5 mg/day for 1 year. All took elemental calcium 1000 mg/day and vitamin D 400 IU/day. The mean density of the lumbar spine fell by 1% in the placebo group and increased by 1.3% and 1.9% with risedronate 2.5 and 5 mg respectively. There was a significant reduction of 70% in the risk of vertebral fracture with risedronate 5 mg compared with placebo. There were similar incidences of adverse effects in all the groups.

Similar results have been reported in a clinical trial in 290 patients (38% men, 55% of the women postmenopausal) taking high-dose glucocorticoid therapy (prednisone over 7.5 mg/day or equivalent) (220). The subjects were randomized to receive placebo or risedronate 2.5 or 5 mg/day for 1 year. All took elemental calcium 1000 mg/day and vitamin D 400 IU/day. Risedronate 5 mg increased bone mineral density at 1 year by a mean of 2.9% in the lumbar spine, 1.8% in the femoral neck, and 2.4% in the trochanter. The values for placebo were 0.4%, –0.3%, and 1.0% respectively. The results for risedronate 2.5 mg were positive but not significant compared with placebo. The incidence of spinal fractures was reduced by 70% in the combined risedronate treatment groups compared with placebo. Risedronate and placebo caused similar adverse effects.

In a 1-year extension of a previous double-blind, randomized, placebo-controlled study, two doses of alendronate (5 and 10 mg/day) were compared in 66 men and 142 women taking glucocorticoids (at least 7.5 mg/day of prednisone or equivalent) (221). The extension was also double-blind, but those who had taken alendronate 2.5 mg/day in the previous study were given 10 mg/day. All the patients took supplementary calcium and vitamin D. The primary end-point was the mean percentage change in lumbar spine bone mineral density from baseline to 2 years. In those who took alendronate 5, 10, and 2.5/10 mg/day, bone mineral density increased significantly by 2.8, 3.9, and 3.7% respectively, and fell by –0.8% with placebo. There were significantly fewer patients with new vertebral fractures in the alendronate group compared with placebo (0.7 versus 6.8%). Adverse events were similar across the groups.

Fluoride

Fluoride is a potent stimulator of trabecular bone formation. Sodium monofluorophosphate was given to 48 patients with osteoporosis due to glucocorticoids (more than 10 mg of prednisone equivalents/day). Patients were randomly allocated to 1 g of calcium carbonate (control) or 200 mg of sodium monofluorophosphate plus 1 g of calcium carbonate for 18 months. At the end of the study lumbar spine bone density had increased by 7.8% in the fluoride group versus 3.3% in the controls. There were no changes in femoral neck density (SEDA-20, 376) (222).

Growth hormone

Growth hormone is a potent anabolic agent that stimulates protein synthesis, cell growth, and osteoblast activity. Recombinant human growth hormone has been used in patients taking long-term glucocorticoid treatment with suppressed endogenous growth hormone responses to GH-releasing hormone (SEDA-20, 376) (223). A single daily dose of 0.1 IU/kg of human growth hormone was given subcutaneously to nine nonobese patients. There was a significant increase in nitrogen balance, osteocalcin, carboxy-terminal propeptide of type I procollagen, and carboxy-terminal telopeptide of type I collagen. Growth hormone also lowered total high density lipoprotein, and low density lipoprotein cholesterol. These preliminary data suggest that growth hormone could ameliorate some adverse effects induced by long-term glucocorticoids.

Others

Other agents are effective in special populations. Vitamin K prevented bone loss in 20 patients with chronic glomerulonephritis treated with prednisolone (224) and ciclosporin 4.8 mg/kg/day prevented glucocorticoid-induced osteopenia in 52 patients taking prednisone 10 mg/day after kidney transplantation (225).

Avascular necrosis

Avascular aseptic necrosis of bone (SEDA-19, 377) (226,227) is a well-recognized adverse effect related to high-dose glucocorticoid therapy (equivalent to more than 4000 mg of prednisone) for extended periods (3 months or longer) but can occur after short-term glucocorticoid therapy. It occurs in a wide range of patients with many different disorders and is particularly likely to involve the femoral and humeral heads. The first lesions are often localized small osteolytic areas in the subchondral bone, where they can be diagnosed early by X-radiography. Magnetic resonance imaging (MRI) is one of the more sensitive techniques to diagnose avascular necrosis of the femoral head. The development and changes in avascular necrosis of the femoral head had been studied by MRI in patients with systemic lupus erythematosus treated with long-term prednisolone administration (SEDA-19, 377) (SEDA-19, 164). MRI abnormalities could be detected soon after the start of glucocorticoid therapy or were associated with increased dosages for treating exacerbation of the disease. Normal hips are rarely involved in avascular osteonecrosis. However, aseptic osteonecrosis of the femoral head is often seen in young patients; the lunate, capitate, and patella are their locations. Usually only one joint is involved, although lesions can be multiple. Whether intra-articular injections of glucocorticoids can cause necrosis of bone is still uncertain.

Femoral head necrosis in kidney transplant recipients who receive postoperative immunosuppression with prednisone can be prevented, at least to some extent, by minimizing the dosage of prednisone whenever feasible (228). Of 750 patients (445 men and 305 women) who had undergone kidney transplantation in 1968–95, 374 had received an average of 12.5 g of prednisone during the first year after surgery (high-dose prednisone group) and 276 had received an average of 6.5 g during this time (low-dose prednisone group) plus ciclosporin. Femoral head necrosis occurred in 42/374 patients (11%) in the high-dose prednisone group, an average of 26 months after transplantation. In contrast, femoral head necrosis occurred in only 19/376 patients (5.1%) in the low-dose group an average of 21 months after transplantation. The difference between the high- and low-dose groups was highly significant.

The risk of avascular necrosis has been assessed in a nested case-control study using computer records (229). There were 31 cases during 720 000 person-years Avascular necrosis was strongly associated with glucocorticoid exposure (RR = 16). When total prednisone exposure over 35 months was stratified into three levels (under 440 mg, 440–1290 mg, and over 1290 mg), there was no excess risk for cumulative doses of up to 440 mg (RR = 0; 95% CI = 0, 5). The relative risk was increased for doses between 440 and 1290 mg (RR = 6; CI = 1, 43) and indeterminately increased at doses over 1290 mg (CI = 26, infinity).

In 15 men with osteonecrosis of the femoral head after short-term therapy the mean duration of therapy was 21 (range 7–39) days and the mean dose in milligram equivalents of prednisone was 850 (range 290–3300) mg (230). The time from administration of glucocorticoids to hip pain was 17 (range 6–33) months. A new case of bilateral avascular necrosis of the femoral heads after high-dose short-term dexamethasone therapy as an antiemetic in cancer chemotherapy has been reported (231).

Myopathy

The presence of physiological amounts of glucocorticoids is necessary for the normal functioning of muscle. Excessive glucocorticoid concentrations, in contrast, result in protein catabolism and a reduced rate of muscle protein synthesis (232), and hence in muscle atrophy and fibrosis. The molecular and biochemical basis of myopathy has been widely studied, and the mechanism has been attributed to impairment of glycogen synthesis. Muscle glycogen synthase protein content and activity was measured in samples from 14 patients taking glucocorticoids after kidney transplantation and from 20 healthy subjects (SEDA-21, 418) (233). The patients had impaired activation of glycogen synthase and reduced enzyme activity. Muscular weakness can of course also result from glucocorticoid-induced hypokalemia. In spontaneous Cushing's syndrome, there is muscle involvement in some 50% of cases (234).

Among reports of myopathy in patients taking glucocorticoids, involvement of the respiratory muscles is often mentioned (235,236), possibly because this is particularly likely to have clinical consequences. Patients on mechanically assisted ventilation may be particularly at risk of myopathy (SEDA-18, 390). However, any muscle can be affected; one often sees weakness and atrophy of the hip muscles and (in about half the cases) the shoulder muscles and the proximal muscles of the limbs.

The myopathy usually develops gradually, without pain, and symmetrically. However, a single epidural injection of a glucocorticoid for lumbar radicular pain has caused Cushing's syndrome and myopathy (SEDA-20, 370) (97).

There is a suggestion that the incidence of myopathy is greatest during treatment with compounds that are fluorinated at the 9-alpha position, such as triamcinolone, but this may simply reflect its general potency. In children, the risk of effects on muscles is relatively high.

Biopsy is not justified as a routine, but it is useful as a diagnostic tool in distinguishing suspected corticoid myopathy from diseases of the muscles or vascular system with inflammation that may have been the indication for giving glucocorticoids in the first place; electromyographic measurements cannot confirm the diagnosis.

After termination of treatment the myopathy normally improves over a period of several months.

Damage to tendons and fascia

Tendons can be injured by glucocorticoids and can rupture (237). Ten cases of Achilles tendon rupture were seen in a single clinic over a 10-year period (SEDA-17, 448). The risk seems to be greater if local (for example intra-articular) injections are used.

Rupture of the plantar fascia induced by glucocorticoids has usually been reported in athletes. However, a case of spontaneous degenerative rupture has been reported in a 72-year-old man who had received four glucocorticoid injections over 1 year for plantar fasciitis (SEDA-21, 418) (238).

Growth in children

The possibility that inhaled glucocorticoids may impair growth in children is of concern, but difficult to assess, as severe chronic asthma can impair growth. If not adequately controlled, asthma modifies the prepubertal growth spurt, the pubertal growth spurt, and the catch-up phase, which allows the child to attain adult height. There is a wide range of individual responses and some children have adverse effects with relatively small doses of glucocorticoids. It is still not clear whether this is a transient phenomenon, causing a slowing of growth and maturational delay with no adverse effect on adult height, or whether growth can be permanently impaired. Ideally studies should establish the effect of asthma treatments on final adult height (compared with predicted values for sex and parental height). Such studies pose considerable logistic problems. For this reason most studies have measured growth over shorter time spans. Outcome measures have been expressed as the height velocity or growth rate, that is changes in height over a defined time. Alternatively height is measured and compared with that of age- and sex-matched controls. Such relatively short-term studies do not necessarily predict the effects of treatment on eventual adult height.

The growth-inhibiting effects of glucocorticoids in children are related not only to inhibition of growth hormone secretion, but also to the sensitivity of the peripheral tissues to the effects of growth hormone. By means of overnight profile analysis it was shown that glucocorticoid treatment reduces the amplitude but not the number of pulses of the physiological growth hormone secretion (SEDA-14, 335) (239).

Effects on growth occur early in treatment: with sensitive testing methods they can be detected in growing children within a few weeks of starting therapy. The effects can be produced by any route of administration, including even inhalation therapy (at least with dexamethasone) (SEDA-18, 391). Comparisons of attained heights with expected heights in children who have used inhaled or oral glucocorticoids have been summarized in a meta-analysis (SEDA-19, 375) (240). There was a significant but small tendency for glucocorticoid therapy in general to be associated with reduced final height. However, this effect varied according to the route of administration. As expected, there was significant impairment of growth with prednisone and other oral glucocorticoids. On the other hand, inhaled beclomethasone dipropionate was associated with normal stature, even when it was used in higher dosages, for longer durations, or in patients with more severe asthma. In another study in 94 children aged 7–9 years, beclomethasone in a dosage taken by many children with mild asthma (400 micrograms/day) significantly reduced growth (SEDA-20, 369) (241). In children with growth suppression during therapy with inhaled beclomethasone or budesonide (200–400 micrograms/day) there was catch-up growth when they switched to equipotent dosages of inhaled fluticasone (100–200 micrograms/day) (SEDA-21, 414) (242). However, in six children with severe asthma, treatment with inhaled high-dosage fluticasone 1000 micrograms/day was associated with growth retardation and adrenal insufficiency (SEDA-21, 414) (243). In one child, growth rate and adrenal function normalized 9 months after the fluticasone dosage was reduced to 500 micrograms/day.

It is generally agreed that the use of single doses of prednisone on alternate mornings minimizes growth retardation but does not avoid it; in children it has been shown that biochemical markers of growth are lower in patients receiving daily glucocorticoid therapy than in patients treated with an alternate-day regimen or not receiving glucocorticoids (SED-12, 988) (244).

It has long been thought by some physicians that the impairment of growth caused by glucocorticoids can be lessened by switching to corticotropin, but this is uncertain. Compensatory treatment with anabolic hormones is definitely not recommended today, since they do not stimulate growth but actually impede it by promoting closure of the epiphyses. Recombinant growth hormone (rGH) treatment of poorly growing children with glucocorticoid-dependent renal disease has often been observed to improve linear growth. However, the dosage of prednisone has been reported to be a critical factor in determining the efficacy of rGH therapy in glucocorticoid-dependent children (SEDA-19, 375) (245). When the dose of prednisone was greater than 0.35 mg/kg/day, rGH did not increase the linear growth rate. At lower doses, the response was inversely related to the amount of prednisone.

Provided glucocorticoid treatment is terminated before the end of puberty, total growth may catch up with the physiological norm (SEDA-17, 448). Concern has been expressed that fear of growth retardation can result in unjustifiable denial of glucocorticoid therapy. It does, however, seem highly advisable to keep doses as low as possible and to switch to a therapeutic regimen that excludes glucocorticoids as children approach the expected onset of puberty (SEDA-14, 335).

Serum osteocalcin determinations appear to be a helpful marker to evaluate the effects of glucocorticoids on growth in children.

One unanswered question is whether the growth suppression that occurs in children during glucocorticoid treatment persists after treatment is withdrawn and affects final adult height. In an attempt to answer this question, growth 6–7 years after withdrawal of alternate-day prednisone has been evaluated in children (aged 6–14 years) with cystic fibrosis who had participated in a multicenter trial from 1986 to 1991 (246). Of 224 children, 161 had been randomized to prednisone (1 or 2 mg/kg) and 73 to placebo. At the time of the study, 68% were aged 18 years or more. Height fell during prednisone therapy, but catch-up growth began 2 years after withdrawal. However, the heights of the boys treated with prednisone remained significantly lower by 4 cm than those who took placebo. In contrast, in the girls there were no differences in height at 2–3 years after prednisone withdrawal.

Reproductive system

Reduced sperm count and motility and inhibition of the secretory function of the testicles during glucocorticoid treatment have been reported and discussed in relation to the suppression of adrenal androgen production. These reports still await confirmation.

Since amenorrhea is a symptom of Cushing's syndrome, disorders of menstruation are common in fertile women taking higher doses of glucocorticoids (SEDA-3, 305). On the other hand, plasma cortisol concentrations in normally menstruating women have marked circadian variation, the extent of which can reach 200% or more (247), with the peak of the cortisol plasma concentrations at mid-cycle and near its end. Inhibition of ovulation by triamcinolone 25 mg has been reported when the drug is given on day 1 or 2 of the cycle. How glucocorticoids interfere with the hormonal control of the menstrual cycle is still unknown (248).

Women should be warned about the possibility of menstrual disorders after local triamcinolone injections (249). When premenopausal women received their first injection of triamcinolone intra-articularly ($n = 46$), injected into soft tissue ($n = 24$), or epidurally ($n = 7$) they were specifically asked to report flushing or menstrual irregularities during a mean follow-up period of 6 weeks. Of the 77 women in the study, 39 reported menstrual disorders. The onset of menstruation was later than expected in ten women and earlier in 16 women. There was reduced loss of blood and/or a shorter duration of menstruation in four women and increased loss of blood and/or a longer duration of menstruation in 18. Also, 22 women had flushing. Menstrual disorders occurred significantly less often in women who were taking oral contraceptives.

Immunologic

Since the glucocorticoids have immunosuppressive and anti-inflammatory properties, one would not expect allergic reactions to be a problem, except when excipients act as allergens. Nevertheless, allergic reactions to glucocorticoids themselves have been reported (SEDA-21, 419) (250). Urticaria after glucocorticoid treatment has been explained as a reaction of the mesenchyme. Also, an increase in eosinophilic leukocytes (which normally are diminished by glucocorticoids) has been reported as a first reaction to treatment with glucocorticoids.

Class I immune reactions

Anaphylactic shock has been described after intranasal hydrocortisone acetate, intramuscular methylprednisolone (SEDA-21, 419) (251), intravenous methylprednisolone (SEDA-22, 448) (252), intramuscular dexamethasone (SEDA-22, 448) (253), and intra-articular methylprednisolone (SEDA-22, 449) (254). A life-threatening anaphylactic-like reaction to intravenous hydrocortisone has been described in patients with asthma (255). Acute laryngeal obstruction has been described for the first time after the intravenous administration of hydrocortisone (SEDA-22, 449) (256). There is some reason to believe that sodium succinate esters are more likely to cause hypersensitivity reactions (SEDA-17, 449), but unconjugated glucocorticoids can definitely produce allergy in some cases (SEDA-16, 452).

- A 64-year-old woman with a history of bronchial asthma developed increasing shortness of breath after an upper respiratory tract infection (257). Her medication included inhaled salbutamol as necessary, theophylline 300 mg bd, and aspirin 325 mg/day. She was given nebulized salbutamol and ipratropium and hydrocortisone 200 mg intravenously. Within 30 minutes, she developed a generalized rash, fever (38.3°C), and respiratory distress. She was promptly intubated and mechanical ventilation was started. No further doses of glucocorticoid were given. Skin testing with various parenteral formulations of glucocorticoids produced a 5 mm wheal at the site of hydrocortisone and methylprednisolone injections. She was subsequently given a challenge dose of triamcinolone using a metered-dose inhaler with no reaction, and was therefore continued on this medication.
- An anaphylactoid reaction (angioedema, generalized urticaria, worsening bronchospasm, and marked hypotension) occurred in a 35-year-old man with multiple sclerosis who became allergic to methylprednisolone (dose not stated) after starting treatment with interferon beta-1b (258). He had previously been treated with different courses of methylprednisolone. Clinicians should be aware that the complexity of the effects of interferon beta-1b on the immune system can lead to unexpected outcomes. It is uncertain whether the sequence of events here was due to an effect of interferon beta-1b or to coincidence.
- A 17-year-old boy, with an 11-year history of asthma, had anaphylaxis with respiratory distress shortly after he received intravenous methylprednisolone for an exacerbation of asthma while taking a tapering course of oral prednisone 15 mg/day (259). He had been glucocorticoid-dependent for at least 1 year. He reported having received intravenous glucocorticoids previously. He was treated with inhaled salbutamol and then intravenous methylprednisolone 125 mg over 15–30 seconds, and 3–4 minutes later became flushed and dyspneic, and developed diffuse urticarial lesions on his trunk and face and an undetectable blood pressure. He was treated with adrenaline, but required intubation. Sinus bradycardia developed and then asystole. He was successfully resuscitated and a 10–15 seconds period of generalized tonic-clonic activity was treated with diazepam. He remained unresponsive to stimulation for 30 minutes. However, he awoke 1 hour after his respiratory arrest and was extubated and discharged the following day taking a tapering dosage of prednisone.
- An anaphylactoid reaction occurred in a 68-year-old woman after treatment with intravenous methylprednisolone for asthma. She had developed urticaria with methylprednisolone 1 year earlier, but the reaction had been thought to be related to the solvent in the formulation (260).
- Forty minutes after a first dose of prednisone 25 mg, a 17-year-old girl with a history of aspirin intolerance had generalized flushing, hives, hypogastric pain, and abdominal cramps, followed by vomiting and diarrhea (261). She lost consciousness and developed arterial hypotension. She responded to intravenous diphenhydramine and hydrocortisone. Intradermal skin tests were positive for prednisone and negative for methylprednisolone and hydrocortisone. An oral challenge test with prednisone led to flushing, nausea, dizziness, tachycardia, and hypotension and responded to intravenous diphenhydramine and hydrocortisone. Challenge tests with intravenous methylprednisolone and hydrocortisone were negative.
- A 30-year-old man with recurrent atopic eczema of the head and neck, generalized xerosis, keratosis pilaris of the arms, and a history of dyshidrosis was initially treated with prednisolone-21-acetate ointment (262). His skin eruption became worse. He was given oral prednisolone 25 mg, and 5 hours after the first dose developed intense generalized pruritus with erythema and swelling of the face. After 24 hours there was generalized erythema with disseminated partly follicular papules. There was an eosinophilia (1.1×10^9/l). Total IgE was not raised. Patch tests showed delayed reactions to hydrocortisone 1%, prednisolone 1%, prednisolone-21-acetate ointment, and prednisolone 2.5%. Prick and intradermal tests with methylprednisolone succinate, hydrocortisone succinate, betamethasone, and triamcinolone acetonide in concentrations up to 1 : 10 were negative at 15 minutes. However, 4 hours after intradermal testing, generalized pruritus developed and 24 hours later there was a disseminated partly follicular eczematous reaction with involvement of the flexural areas. Biopsy of the eruptions caused by prednisolone and of the positive skin reaction to methylprednisolone succinate showed superficial dermatitis with a perivascular infiltration consisting predominantly of CD4+ cells and some eosinophils. Immunofluorescence showed increased expression of HLA-DR molecules on the CD4+ and CD8+ cells. During the exanthema caused by prednisolone, interleukin-5 (14 pg/ml), interleukin-6 (38 pg/ml), and interleukin-10 (26 pg/ml) were detected in the blood; 2 months after recovery these cytokines were not detectable.

The authors of the last report commented that generalized delayed type hypersensitivity to systemic administration of a glucocorticoid is rare. Despite the potent immunosuppressive effect of glucocorticoids on immunocompetent cells, the clinical features, the skin biopsy specimen, and the positive delayed skin test reactions strongly suggested an immunological mechanism: T cells were clearly involved and the high concentrations of interleukins 5, 6, and 10 were consistent with a T helper type 2 reaction. The raised concentrations of interleukin-5 were probably responsible for the blood and tissue eosinophilia.

Budesonide has been marketed in oral form for intestinal inflammatory disease. An non-IgE-mediated anaphylactic reaction has been associated with oral budesonide (263).

- A 32-year-old woman with Crohn's disease, who had taken prednisone 20 mg/day and azathioprine 150 mg/day, switched to budesonide 9 mg/day because of weight gain, and 5 minutes after the first capsule her tongue and throat swelled, accompanied by wheeziness and diarrhea. She was given clemastine and recovered after 4 ays. Intracutaneous tests with diluted budesonide suggested a non-IgE-mediated reaction. She had a previous history of a similar reaction to mesalazine. One year later her tongue and throat swelled after intravenous dexamethasone.

Urticaria with angioedema has been described in a patient taking deflazacort (264).

- A 64-year-old woman with allergic alveolitis caused by parakeet feathers improved with intravenous methylprednisolone, and was given oral deflazacort 60 mg/day, to be reduced progressively. After 30 days she developed generalized itchy blotches and lip edema. At that time she was mistakenly taking deflazacort in a dose of 120 mg/day. She was given an antihistamine, without any improvement. Deflazacort was then replaced by prednisolone and her symptoms disappeared immediately. Skin tests (a prick test and an epicutaneous test) were positive with deflazacort. Oral provocation with deflazacort 30 mg was positive, with the immediate appearance of the same symptoms as in the initial episode.

Vasculitis

Exacerbation of giant cell arteritis, with clinical signs of an evolving vertebrobasilar stroke, has been attributed to prednisolone (265).

- A 64-year-old man with giant cell arteritis was given prednisolone 60 mg/day. Within 5 days he developed double vision and agitation and became drowsy and confused. A cranial MRI scan showed recent cerebral lesions and a Doppler scan showed high-resistant blood flow in both vertebral arteries. He had an episode of complete loss of vision and was given dexamethasone and intravenous heparin followed by warfarin. He gradually improved over the next few weeks but was left with cognitive and memory deficits.

Immunosuppression

Glucocorticoids inhibit the formation of antibodies. Of 111 consecutive heart transplant recipients taking oral prednisone (mean 13.8 months), 57% developed hypogammaglobulinemia (IgG below 7 g/l) (266). Those with severe hypogammaglobulinemia (IgG below 3.5 g/l) were at increassed risk of opportunistic infections compared with those with IgG concentrations over 3.5 g/l (55 versus 5%, OR = 23). Parenteral glucocorticoid pulse therapy was associated with a significantly increased risk of severe hypogammaglobulinemia (OR = 15).

With long-term treatment, IgG subclass deficiencies can become marked (267). There is suppression of the antigen–antibody reaction, and since this reaction itself normally results in liberation of kinins, the latter is also suppressed. Failure of kinin liberation leads in turn to inhibition of invasion of sensitized leukocytes and reduced production and maturation of phagocytes. Undoubtedly, it is true that using minimal effective doses will avoid the most serious consequences, but the problem cannot be fully circumvented, since the anti-inflammatory effects themselves involve some inhibition of the migration of leukocytes and phagocytosis.

Dexamethasone significantly affected the antibody response of preterm infants with chronic lung disease to immunization against *Haemophilus influenzae* (268). Serum samples were obtained before and after immunization from an unselected cohort of 59 preterm infants (30 boys; gestational age 175–208 days). *Haemophilus influenzae* antibodies were measured using ELISA. IgG antibody concentrations in 16 infants who received no dexamethasone were 0.16 and 4.63 microgram/ml before and after immunization respectively. The corresponding values for those who received dexamethasone were 0.10 and 0.51 microgram/ml.

Infection risk

The consequence of this interference with immune responses can be multiplication of bacteria and an increased risk of bacterial intoxication when infection does occur; hence, the frequency and severity of clinical infections tend to increase during glucocorticoid therapy. Aggravation of existing tuberculosis and reactivation of completely quiescent cases of this infection are classic consequences demanding prophylactic measures; atypical mycobacteria have also caused tissue infections (SEDA-17, 449). Other bacterial infections, some severe and proceeding to sepsis, have followed glucocorticoid treatment. There is little evidence that glucocorticoids, even in high dosages and early in the course of infection, significantly alter the ultimate outcome (269). Use of glucocorticoids in the treatment of septic shock is not recommended in the absence of adrenal suppression.

It has been suggested that there are some differences between drugs. The use of fluticasone nasal spray to control polyp recurrence after functional endoscopic sphenoethmoidectomy should be viewed with caution, as it has been said to be associated with a high incidence of severe postoperative infection compared with beclomethasone (SEDA-21, 375) (270).

Acute generalized exanthematous pustulosis due to a glucocorticoid has been reported (SEDA-21, 416) (271).

Bacterial infections

Infections with *Clostridium difficile*, *Pseudomonas aeruginosa*, and *Listeria monocytogenes* (SEDA-22, 450) (272) have occasionally been precipitated or aggravated by glucocorticoids, as has tuberculous peritonitis (SEDA-20, 377) (273).

The cumulative and mean daily dosages of glucocorticoids in patients with systemic lupus erythematosus, inflammatory myopathy, overlap syndrome, or mixed connective tissue disease were the most important risk factors for the development of tuberculosis, according to a study conducted in Korea (274). Records were analysed from 269 patients who had been hospitalized during a 5-year period. In 21 patients active tuberculosis developed after a mean duration of 27 months from diagnosis of their rheumatic disease, an incidence rate of 20 cases per 1000 patient-years. The mean cumulative and daily dosages of prednisolone during the follow-up period were 31 594 and 25 mg respectively in patients who developed tuberculosis, compared with 17 043 and 18 mg in patients who did not. Glucocorticoid pulse therapy was a risk factor for the development of tuberculosis.

- A 43-year-old woman developed cavitary lung tuberculosis after she received methotrexate and glucocorticoid pulse therapy for rheumatoid arthritis (275).

The authors commented that the onset of the lung infection appeared to be closely related to methotrexate and glucocorticoid pulse therapy, because of the interval between drug administration and the onset of tuberculosis, and the lack of other risk factors for opportunistic infections.

In a retrospective study, the use of glucocorticoids during *Pneumocystis jiroveci* pneumonia (mean total dose methylprednisolone 420 mg, mean treatment duration 12 days) did not increase the risk of development or relapse of tuberculosis or other AIDS-related diseases (SEDA-20, 377) (276). The study included 129 patients (72 who took glucocorticoids and 57 who did not) who were followed up at 6, 12, 18, and 24 months of glucocorticoid therapy. The rates of infections were similar in both groups, and the cumulative rate of tuberculosis at 2 years was 12–13%.

Mycobacterium avium septic arthritis has been reported in two patients with pre-existing rheumatic disease (scleroderma and polymyositis) who were taking prednisolone and azathioprine; the infection was in the left shoulder in one patient and in the knee in the other (277).

The use of glucocorticoids in patients with hematological diseases is a factor that facilitates the occurrence of *Legionella pneumophila* pneumonia, and 10 episodes of this infection were possibly related to glucocorticoids in a series of 67 cases of Legionnaires' disease diagnosed in a single institution during 2.5 years (278).

Viral infections

Infections such as chickenpox can have serious consequences, including death, in patients taking systemic glucocorticoids (SEDA-19, 378) (SEDA-20, 377) (279,280). It has been suggested that *Varicella zoster* immunoglobulin should be given to patients in contact with chickenpox if they have taken glucocorticoids in dosages over 0.5 mg/kg/day during the preceding 3 months, in the context of near-fatal chickenpox in a child receiving prednisolone (SEDA-20, 377) (281). Smallpox vaccination has in the past resulted in vaccinia gangrenosum in patients taking glucocorticoids, and the current type of *Varicella* vaccine is much more likely to produce rashes in children who are already taking glucocorticoids than in controls (SEDA-16, 452).

Herpes simplex virus encephalitis after myxedema coma has been described in an 81-year-old man treated with hydrocortisone (100 mg 8-hourly) and levothyroxine (282). In renal transplantation, two cases of death from *Herpes simplex* as a result of glucocorticoid treatment are on record (SED-8, 827) (SEDA-17, 449).

Fungal and yeast infections

Fungal and yeast infections (including cases of fulminant fungal pericarditis, mucormycosis, *Aspergillus fumigatus* infection, and cutaneous alternariosis) can be precipitated or aggravated by glucocorticoid treatment (SEDA-17, 449) (SEDA-18, 390) (SEDA-20, 377) (SEDA-21, 418) (SEDA-22, 449) (283–286).

Primary esophageal histoplasmosis must be considered in patients who have a history of gastroesophageal reflux disease and are immunosuppressed by long-term glucocorticoids (SEDA-22, 450) (287). Oropharyngeal candidiasis is a well-described adverse effect of inhaled glucocorticoids. However, few cases of esophageal candidiasis have been reported (SEDA-22, 179).

Invasive pulmonary aspergillosis with cerebromeningeal involvement has been described after short-term intravenous administration of methylprednisolone (SEDA-22, 449) (288). Of 473 HIV-infected children, 7 (1.5%) developed invasive aspergillosis during the study period (1987–95) (SEDA-22, 449) (289). Sustained neutropenia or glucocorticoid therapy as predisposing factors for invasive aspergillosis were found in only two patients.

- Fatal pulmonary infection with *Aspergillus fumigatus* and *Nocardia asteroides* has been described in a patient who took prednisone 1 mg/kg/day for 1 month for bronchiolitis obliterans (290).
- Fatal *Aspergillus* myocarditis, probably related to short-term administration of glucocorticoids, has been described in a 58-year-old man, who had an acute exacerbation of his chronic obstructive pulmonary disease and received oxygen, bronchodilators, omeprazole, co-amoxiclav, and intravenous methylprednisolone 40 mg 8-hourly; he died 5 days later and postmortem examination showed a fungal myocarditis (291).
- Fatal aspergillosis with a thyroid gland abscess occurred in a 74-year-old man after treatment with prednisolone for polymyalgia rheumatica (292).

Scedosporium apiospermum infection occurred in the left forearm of an 81-year-old man who was taking chronic oral prednisone (increased to 40 mg/day 1 month before presentation) for lung fibrosis (293).

Cutaneous alternariosis (infection with *Alternaria alternata*) has been described in a 78-year-old farmer with idiopathic pulmonary fibrosis taking oral prednisone 20 mg/day (294).

The effect of dexamethasone has been assessed in a retrospective chart review study in neonates weighing less than 1200 g, both with ($n = 65$) and without ($n = 269$) *Candida* sepsis; dexamethasone therapy and prolonged antibiotic therapy were associated with *Candida* infection (295).

Helminth infections
Strongyloidiasis (SEDA-20, 377) (SEDA-21, 419) (SEDA-22, 449) (296–298) has been precipitated or aggravated by glucocorticoids.

Protozoal infections
Toxoplasmosis has been precipitated by glucocorticoids (299,300).

Pneumocystis jiroveci pneumonia has been precipitated or aggravated by glucocorticoids (SEDA-20, 377) (SEDA-22, 450) (272,301,302). There is some concern about the use of glucocorticoids as adjunctive therapy in patients with AIDS who develop *Pneumocystis jiroveci* pneumonia. The immunosuppressant properties of glucocorticoids have been reported to enhance the risk of tuberculosis and other AIDS-related diseases (for example Kaposi's sarcoma or cytomegalovirus infection).

Amebic dysentery has been precipitated by glucocorticoids (303).

Death

Mortality associated with glucocorticoid has been retrospectively studied in 556 patients with chronic obstructive pulmonary disease admitted to a rehabilitation center (304). Median survival was 38 months and 280 patients died during follow-up. On multivariate analysis, oral glucocorticoid use at a prednisone equivalent of 10 mg/day without inhaled glucocorticoid was associated with an increased risk of death (RR = 2.34; 95% CI = 1.24, 4.44), and 15 mg/day increased the risk further (RR = 4.03; 95% CI = 1.99, 8.15). The risk of death was not increased in those using 5 mg/day or when patients used any oral dose in combination with inhaled glucocorticoids.

Long-Term Effects

Drug withdrawal

Suppression of adrenocortical function is one of the consequences of repeated administration of glucocorticoids; after termination of treatment a withdrawal syndrome can occur. In many cases this is unpleasant rather than acutely dangerous; in such instances the patients may have headache, nausea, dizziness, anorexia, weakness, emotional changes, lethargy, and perhaps fever; in some cases severe mental disorders occur and there are repeated reports of benign intracranial hypertension (305). The glucocorticoid withdrawal syndrome also seems to underlie the "glucocorticoid pseudorheumatism" that can occur when the drugs are withdrawn in rheumatic patients.

Withdrawal symptoms disappear if the glucocorticoid is resumed, but as a rule they will in any case vanish spontaneously within a few days. More serious consequences can ensue, however, in certain types of cases and if adrenal cortical atrophy is severe. In patients treated with corticoids for the nephrotic syndrome and apparently cured, the syndrome is particularly likely to relapse on withdrawal of therapy if the adrenal cortex is atrophic (SEDA-3, 305). In some cases, acute adrenocortical insufficiency after glucocorticoid treatment has actually proved fatal. It is advisable to withdraw long-term glucocorticoid therapy gradually so that the cortex has sufficient opportunity to recover. Table 5 lists methods of withdrawing prednisolone after long-term therapy in different circumstances (306).

Table 5 Suggested methods of withdrawing prednisolone

Circumstances	Change in daily dose
The problem has resolved and treatment has been given for only a few weeks	Reduce by 2.5 mg every 3 or 4 days down to 7.5 mg/day; then reduce more slowly, for example by 2.5 mg every week, fortnight, or month
There is uncertainty about disease resolution and/or therapy has been given for many weeks	Reduce by 2.5 mg every fortnight or month down to 7.5 mg/day then reduce by 1 mg every month
Symptoms of the disease are likely to recur on withdrawal (for example rheumatoid arthritis)	Reduce by 1 mg every month

Anorexia nervosa has been precipitated by withdrawal of oral prednisolone for asthma (SEDA-21, 414) (307).

A case of papilledema as a manifestation of raised intracranial pressure has been reported following withdrawal of topical glucocorticoids (SEDA-3, 305).

Panniculitis, which causes erythematous, firm, warm subcutaneous nodules, can occur within 2 weeks of withdrawal of large doses of glucocorticoids, but case reports confirm that resolution without scarring is the rule and that reintroduction of glucocorticoids is not necessary for improvement (308).

Churg–Strauss syndrome has come into prominence with the introduction of the leukotriene receptor antagonists, because they allow glucocorticoid-dependent asthmatics to discontinue their oral prednisolone. Five patients developed Churg–Strauss syndrome when their oral glucocorticoids were withdrawn (309). The duration of oral glucocorticoid therapy was 3–216 months and the dosage of prednisolone was 2.5–25.5 mg/day. The diagnosis of Churg–Strauss syndrome was made from 6 to 83 months after withdrawal of the oral glucocorticoids. These case reports support the hypothesis that it is the withdrawal of glucocorticoids that unmasks the underlying systemic vasculitis in these patients with asthma, rather than an effect of the new therapeutic agents that permits the reduction (and withdrawal) of prednisolone. Case-control studies are needed to determine the respective roles of the new therapeutic agents, prednisolone withdrawal, or other factors in the emergence of Churg–Strauss syndrome in these asthmatic patients

Tumorigenicity

Direct tumor-inducing effects of the glucocorticoids are not known, but the particular risk that malignancies in patients undergoing immunosuppression with these or other drugs will spread more rapidly is a well-recognized problem.

- Progressive endometrial carcinoma associated with azathioprine and prednisone therapy has been reported (310).

- Rapid progression of Kaposi's sarcoma 10 weeks after combined treatment with glucocorticoids and cyclophosphamide has been described; marked improvement of the skin lesions was noted after discontinuation of prednisone therapy (311).

Patients (mean age 39 years, $n = 1862$) who underwent 1924 renal transplantations from March 1995 to May 1997 were followed for 3–150 months. They received one of the following regimens: prednisolone plus azathioprine (group 1; $n = 100$); prednisolone plus azathioprine plus ciclosporin (group 2; $n = 1464$); and the same therapy as group 2 plus either muromonab-CD3 or antithymocyte globulin as induction or antirejection therapy (group 3; $n = 298$). The mean time to appearance of neoplasia after renal transplantation was 48 months. Malignancies developed earlier in group 3 patients (mean time to appearance 31 months) than in group 2 (39 months) and in group 1 (90 months). Seven of the patients who developed malignancies had also received pulse methylprednisolone for acute rejection. The authors concluded that the treatment of acute rejection with pulsed methylprednisolone and the use of muromonab-CD3 and antithymocyte globulin may lead to an increased incidence of malignancies after renal transplantation. They recommended that strategies be implemented for the early detection of malignancy (312)

In seven patients, accelerated growth of Kaposi's sarcoma lesions during glucocorticoid therapy suggested that glucocorticoids can alter the biological behavior of this malignant disease (313). Hydrocortisone accelerates the growth of cell lines derived from Kaposi's sarcoma cells cultured in vitro and this may partially explain these findings. Reports continue to point to the reversibility of the condition when glucocorticoids are withdrawn (314).

Kaposi's sarcoma has been associated with prednisolone therapy in two elderly women (315).

- An 84-year-old woman with polymyalgia rheumatica and a 79-year-old woman with undifferentiated connective tissue disease and leukocytoclastic vasculitis were given prednisolone 20 mg/day with subsequent dosage reductions. The first patient developed a raised purpuric rash and lymphedema of the left leg within 5 months and the second developed large purple nodules on the soles of her feet and the backs of her hands accompanied by periorbital and peripheral edema. Skin biopsies showed Kaposi's sarcoma, and both patients had raised IgG antibody titers to human herpesvirus-8.

Prior infection with herpesvirus-8 is a requisite for the development of Kaposi's sarcoma. The question arises as to how glucocorticoid treatment alone can lead to the emergence of this malignancy. In vitro evidence supports the hypothesis that glucocorticoids have a direct role in stimulating tumor development and the activation of herpesvirus-8.

A possible relation between systemic glucocorticoid use and a risk of esophageal cancer has been described in a population-based study in Denmark, in which the prescriptions database and the Danish cancer registry were linked (316). There was an increase in the number of cases observed ($n = 36$) compared with the number expected ($n = 19$), with a standardized incidence ratio of 1.92 (95% CI = 1.34, 2.65).

Second-Generation Effects

Pregnancy

In a statement, the American Academy of Pediatrics and the Canadian Paediatric Society did not recommend the routine use of systemic dexamethasone for the prevention or treatment of chronic lung disease in infants with very low birthweights, because it does not reduce overall mortality and is associated with impaired growth and neurodevelopment delay (317,318).

In an analysis of 595 preterm infants born at 26–32 weeks gestation during a randomized controlled trial for the prevention of lung disease, glucocorticoids given to women at risk of preterm delivery promoted fetal lung maturation, reduced the incidence of respiratory distress syndrome, and reduced neonatal morbidity and mortality (319). Dexamethasone was given as either two doses of 12 mg 24 hours apart or four doses of 6 mg every 6 hours. Mortality was 9.2% after three or more courses, compared with 4.8% after one or two courses. This association was not explained by other factors (maternal or other common preterm morbidities).

The effects of glucocorticoids on uterine activity and preterm labor in high-order multiple gestations have been retrospectively reviewed (SEDA-20, 377) (320). In 15 women with triplet or quadruplet pregnancies, 17 out of 57 courses of betamethasone were associated with episodes of significant contractions requiring tocolytic intervention; 11 of these episodes were associated with cervical change and four resulted in premature delivery. The authors did not recommend the use of glucocorticoids if patients have more than 3.5 contractions per hour.

Prenatal glucocorticoid therapy to enhance fetal lung maturation reduces neonatal morbidity and mortality. However, adverse effects of serial courses of betamethasone on mother and fetus can occur.

Endocrine

Maternal hyperadrenalism occurred after five courses of betamethasone to enhance fetal lung maturation (321).

- A 26-year-old woman was given intravenous salbutamol 0.3 mg/hour for preterm labor, and intramuscular betamethasone 12 mg/day for 2 days. Daily oral tocolysis (salbutamol 2 mg every 6 hours plus nicardipine 50 mg every 12 hours) and betamethasone every week were continued at home for 3 weeks. The mother developed amyotrophy, acne on the face and trunk, moon face, hirsutism with whiskers, and thin skin. Free urinary cortisol was less than 5 micrograms/day (reference range 25–90), plasma cortisol was less than 10 ng/ml (100–200), and the salivary cortisol was less than 0.6 ng/ml (2.3–4.7). One hour after intramuscular tetracosactide 250 micrograms, her plasma cortisol was 102 ng/ml (reference range over 210) and the salivary cortisol was 3.1 ng/ml (13–25), indicating no adrenocortical response. She was given hydrocortisone 20 mg/day, and 2 months later adrenocortical insufficiency persisted, with a plasma cortisol of

152 ng/ml after corticotropin stimulation. One year later, she still required hydrocortisone 10 mg/day.

Hyperadrenalism has never otherwise been reported after the sequential use of glucocorticoids for fetal lung maturation.

A study in 10 women has been conducted to determine whether betamethasone administered at risk of preterm delivery causes adrenal suppression (322). After adrenal stimulation with corticotropin 1 microgram at 24–25 weeks, each woman received two intramuscular doses of betamethasone 12 mg 24 hours apart; 1 week later, another corticotropin test was followed by another two doses of betamethasone; a third corticotropin stimulation test was carried out 1 week later. All the women had normal baseline and stimulated cortisol concentrations during the first corticotropin stimulation test. Mean baseline serum cortisol concentrations fell with each corticotropin stimulation test (from 700 nmol/l (254 micrograms/l) before betamethasone to 120 nmol/l (43 micrograms/l) 1 week after the second course of betamethasone). The mean stimulated cortisol concentrations also fell significantly, from 910 nmol/l (330 micrograms/l) to 326 nmol/l (118 micrograms/l). There was evidence of adrenal suppression in four patients after the first course of betamethasone and in seven patients after the second course. There was no evidence of Addisonian crisis antepartum or intrapartum.

Musculoskeletal

Osteonecrosis of the femoral head can occur with glucocorticoids in nonpregnant individuals, but has not previously been reported in pregnancy (323).

- A 37-year-old white woman was given betamethasone, two doses of 12 mg over a day, at 24 weeks of a twin pregnancy, because of a history of growth restriction in her first pregnancy. At 25 weeks Doppler of the umbilical vessels suggested a reduction in end-diastolic flow in one twin. Betamethasone was prescribed again and was repeated weekly to a total of six courses because of the high risk of preterm delivery. At 30 weeks she complained of pain in the right hip exacerbated by weight bearing, which increased over the following 7 days until standing was impossible. An MRI scan showed avascular necrosis of the femoral head.

Infection risk

The use of betamethasone for the treatment of premature rupture of membranes during pregnancy is associated with an increased prevalence of maternal and neonatal infections. Two reports have described the risk of infections associated with the use of glucocorticoids during pregnancy. Of 374 patients with preterm premature rupture of membranes, 99 received a single course of glucocorticoids, 72 received multiple courses, and 203 were not treated with glucocorticoids (324). Only multiple courses of betamethasone increased the incidence of early-onset neonatal sepsis, chorioamnionitis, and endometritis in mothers. A single course of glucocorticoid was not significantly associated with any maternal or neonatal infectious complications. The incidence of maternal infections in 37 patients who received three or more courses of betamethasone (median 6, range 3–10) because of the risk of preterm delivery has been evaluated, with 70 healthy pregnant women as controls (325). Of those treated with betamethasone, 65% developed infectious diseases compared with 18% of controls. Symptomatic lower urinary tract infections (35 versus 2.7%) and serious bacterial infections (24 versus 0%) were more frequent in treated mothers. Eight of nine serious infections occurred in patients exposed to five or more courses of glucocorticoids.

Singleton pregnancies delivered at 24–34 weeks after antenatal betamethasone exposure have been prospectively analysed, in order to study the incidence of perinatal infection (326). There were 453 patients, 267 of whom took a single course of betamethasone (two doses of 12 mg in 24 hours), and 186 of whom took a multiple course (more than two doses in the 24 hours after the initial course). Multiple courses were significantly associated with early-onset neonatal sepsis (OR = 5.0; 95% CI = 1.0, 23), neonatal death (OR = 2.9; CI = 1.3, 6.9), chorioamnionitis (OR = 10; CI = 2.1, 65), and endometritis (OR = 3.6; CI = 1.7, 8.1). Respiratory distress and intraventricular hemorrhage were similar in the two groups. Although the study was non-randomized the results suggest an increased risk of neonatal infection and death after multiple courses of dexamethasone during pregnancy.

In a retrospective study in 609 mothers and their 713 infants who were treated with 1–12 courses of antenatal glucocorticoids, data from 369 singleton preterm infants born at 34 weeks or later, 210 multiple gestations, and 134 infants delivered at 35 weeks or later were analysed (327). The incidence of respiratory distress syndrome was 45% for single courses and 35% for multiple courses of glucocorticoids (OR = 0.44; 95% CI = 0.25, 0.79). The multiple-course group also had significantly less cases of patent ductus arteriosus (20 versus 13%). The incidences of death before discharge and other neonatal morbidities were similar. The multiple-course group had a significant reduction of 0.46 cm in head circumference at birth when adjusted for gestational age and pre-eclampsia. The two groups had similar birthweights. Infants born at more than 35 weeks, multiple-gestation infants, and infants who were born more than 7 days after the last dose of glucocorticoid had similar outcomes, regardless of the number of courses they had received. Mothers treated with multiple courses compared with a single course had a significantly higher incidence of postpartum endometritis, even though they had a lower incidence of prolonged rupture of membranes (24 versus 33%) and similar cesarean delivery rates. In conclusion, antenatal exposure to multiple courses of glucocorticoids compared with a single course resulted in a significant reduction in the incidence of respiratory distress syndrome in singleton preterm infants delivered within a week of the last glucocorticoid dose. This was associated with a reduction in head circumference at birth and an increased incidence of maternal endometritis. Whether the potential benefits of repeated therapy outweigh the risks will ultimately be determined in randomized controlled trials.

Teratogenicity

Teratogenic effects of glucocorticoids, which have been demonstrated in animal experiments since 1950, have not generally been confirmed in man. The question whether a disease that has had to be treated with glucocorticoids in pregnancy or the glucocorticoid treatment itself may have caused congenital anomalies reported anecdotally usually cannot be answered in any individual case. Dexamethasone, for instance, given in a suppressive dosage, seems to have been therapeutically effective in endocrine abnormal pregnancy with congenital adreno-genital syndrome (328); how is one to distinguish cause and effect here? Cleft lip and palate, seen in animal studies, have not been encountered more often in the offspring of glucocorticoid-treated women than in those of untreated women. In several small series of patients in whom glucocorticoids were used before and during pregnancy, no congenital abnormalities were seen on follow-up, but material on which to base a firm judgement is lacking. Certainly, the evidence to date does not suggest that on teratological grounds one should hesitate to administer glucocorticoids for therapeutic reasons during pregnancy (SEDA-3, 306).

However, first trimester in utero exposure to a glucocorticoid was associated with a small risk of major neonatal malformations, according to the results of a Canadian meta-analysis (329). Six cohort studies and one case-control study were analysed, and the results showed that women who had taken long-term glucocorticoid therapy during pregnancy were more likely to have a baby with a major malformation than women who had not (OR = 2.46; 95% CI = 1.41, 4.29).

Glucocorticoids have been used in cases of hyperemesis gravidarum when standard antiemetics are ineffective. In an observational comparison of women with complicated hyperemesis gravidarum and weight loss, over 5% of pre-pregnant weight treated with ($n = 30$) or without ($n = 25$) glucocorticoids, gestational evolution and singleton birthweights were not different in the two groups (330).

A hydatidiform mole during pregnancy may have been due to the glucocorticoids used in an immunosuppressive regimen (331).

- A 33-year-old woman took immunosuppressive therapy after renal transplantation: ciclosporin (dosage adjusted to achieve blood concentrations of 120–160 ng/ml), azathioprine 1 mg/kg (frequency of administration not stated), and methylprednisolone 40 mg/day from day 1 after transplantation, tapered weekly by 4–8 mg/day. Because of rejection symptoms at weeks 1, 4, and 7, she received three cycles of intravenous methylprednisolone 250 mg/day, each cycle lasting 5–7 days; she also received a bolus dose of methylprednisolone 500 mg on day 0. Pregnancy was diagnosed on day 12 after transplantation (9 weeks after conception). At week 6 after transplantation she had a missed abortion. Curettage was performed and a partial hydatidiform mole was detected. She was discharged at week 10 and immunosuppressive therapy was tapered.

The teratogenic effects of prednisone have been evaluated in a placebo-controlled study in 372 women and a meta-analysis (332). There was no statistical difference in the rate of major anomalies between the glucocorticoid-exposed women and the controls. The meta-analysis included 10 studies (six cohort and four case-control studies), with data from 535 exposed and 50 845 nonexposed women. The odds ratios for major malformations were 1.5 (95% CI = 0.8, 2.6) for the cohort studies and 3.4 (CI = 2.0, 5.7) for the case-control studies. The results suggest that although prednisone does not represent a major teratogenic risk in humans in therapeutic doses, it does increase the risk of oral cleft defects by an order of 3.4-fold.

Fetotoxicity

The effect of prolonged antenatal betamethasone (three or more weekly administrations) has been studied in 414 fetuses (333). Multidose betamethasone was not associated with higher risks of antenatal maternal fever, chorioamnionitis, reduced birthweight, neonatal adrenal suppression, neonatal sepsis, or neonatal death.

The effects of antenatal dexamethasone on birthweight have been studied in 961 infants and matched controls (334). Dexamethasone-treated infants had significantly lower birthweights (after adjustment for week of gestation). The average differences from controls were 12 g at 24–26 weeks, 63 g at 27–29 weeks, 161 g at 30–32 weeks, and 80 g at 33–34 weeks. In the case of preterm rupture of membranes, the data were not conclusive.

Betamethasone, two doses of 12 mg a day apart, in 40 pregnant women (27–34 weeks) caused important changes in fetal physiology (335). Fetal breathing (the number of breathing episodes and the total breathing time in 30 minutes) fell by 83% and fetal limb and trunk movements fell by 53% and 49% respectively. These changes were transient and returned to the range of normality 96 hours after administration. There were no changes in Doppler velocimetry of the umbilical and middle cerebral arteries. Awareness of these effects may prevent unnecessary iatrogenic delivery of preterm infants who present abnormal biophysical profile scores 2 days after glucocorticoid exposure.

Retardation of intrauterine growth by glucocorticoids has been reported not only in animals but also in man. In a 1990 case from France, dwarfism (as well as Cushing's syndrome) was recorded in a child whose mother had received high-dose glucocorticoids during pregnancy.

It has been suggested that the risk of stillbirth may be increased by glucocorticoid treatment; the figures are suggestive, but the possibility that the disorder that led to the use of the glucocorticoid was itself responsible for the less favorable outcome cannot be excluded (336).

Prevention of the respiratory distress syndrome in anticipated prematurity has become a widely accepted (though not uncontroversial) indication for glucocorticoids in late pregnancy, the compound most often used being dexamethasone. The timing of such treatment in late pregnancy seems to be of crucial importance (SEDA-3, 306); the possible adverse effects on the mother and child are still being discussed. The issue has been extensively reviewed (SEDA-17, 445). A meta-analysis of 15 trials, involving 1780 patients treated with glucocorticoids and 1780 controls, has shown a lower risk of the syndrome, and a substantial reduction in neonatal mortality (OR = 0.60; 95% CI = 0.48, 0.76), without a higher risk of infection in the mother or maternal pulmonary edema (SEDA-20, 377) (337). In the mother, labor can be delayed by such glucocorticoid therapy (SEDA-3, 306); the combination of this treatment with sympathomimetic drugs may put the mother at risk of fluid retention with pulmonary edema (SED-12, 990), although it is not clear whether this problem only occurs when both drugs are used.

As far as the child is concerned, there may be only moderate adrenal suppression (338), although in some cases substitution treatment with glucocorticoids can be necessary in such babies; short-term treatment with betamethasone shortly before birth generally does not inhibit the infant's adrenal capacity to react to corticotropin (339). A single case of a leukemoid reaction in a preterm infant has been observed, after the mother was given betamethasone shortly before delivery (SEDA-3, 306).

On the other hand, there are many reports of hypertension (340), and electrocardiographic and other studies have often confirmed the presence of a disproportionately serious and bilateral hypertrophic obstructive cardiomyopathy, which unless it proves fatal is, in general, reversible once the glucocorticoids are withdrawn (SEDA-18, 386). Although the issue is confounded by the possibility that infants with bronchopulmonary dysplasia may be innately hypertensive, there seems no doubt as to the effect.

Most babies treated with glucocorticoids for lung dysplasia also show an appreciable rise in blood urea nitrogen, due almost entirely to an increase in structural protein catabolism (341). Serious gastrointestinal complications can occur. In one typical series of premature neonates treated in this way there were three such instances (perforated duodenal ulcer, perforated gastric ulcer, and upper gastrointestinal hemorrhage, the last two proving fatal) (342); the symptoms are apparently not masked by the glucocorticoid, as one would expect in adults. Treated infants also tend to have a low pH, which is unusual in premature babies (SEDA-18, 445).

Clearly, the duration of such treatment after delivery should be as brief as possible, but there is no reason for such concern as would lead to withholding therapy; one Dutch study with a 10-year follow-up detected no problems with exposed children's intellectual, motor, or social functioning compared with controls (114).

A meta-analysis, including 15 controlled trials and involving more than 1400 women, has shown that antenatal glucocorticoids in women with ruptured membranes may be beneficial in reducing the risks of neonatal death (RR = 0.68; 95% CI = 0.43, 1.07) and respiratory distress syndrome (RR = 0.56; CI = 0.46, 0.70), with no increase in the risk of infection in either the mother (RR = 0.88; CI = 0.61, 1.20) or baby (RR = 1.05; CI = 0.66, 1.68) (343).

A reduction in fetal response to vibroacoustic stimulation (vibroacoustic startle reflex) has been reported during 48 hours after the administration to pregnant women of two doses of betamethasone (12 mg 2 days apart) (344). The authors recommended that this test should not be used to evaluate well-being in fetuses exposed to glucocorticoids.

Susceptibility Factors

Genetic factors

Significant differences in the pharmacokinetics of methylprednisolone have been described in black and white renal transplant patients. Black patients had a slower clearance rate and a lower apparent volume of distribution. They had higher cortisol concentrations throughout the day, with higher nadir concentrations. Some of them had glucocorticoid-associated diabetes, and no white patients did. Further studies are needed to define the differences between the races (SEDA-20, 377) (345).

Age

Children

Inhaled glucocorticoids are recommended as first-line therapy for persistent asthma in children, to reduce both asthma symptoms and inflammatory markers. Treatment should be begun early in the course of the disease, because inhaled glucocorticoids can preserve airway function and prevent airway remodelling and subsequent irreversible airway obstruction (346). Because asthma is a chronic disease requiring long-term treatment, it is very important to balance the safety and efficacy of inhaled glucocorticoids to achieve optimal long-term results. Major safety concerns in children are the potential adverse effects on growth, adrenal function, and bone mass. Overall, the benefits of inhaled glucocorticoids clearly outweigh their potential adverse effects and the risks of poor asthma control. However, high doses of inhaled glucocorticoids in children are still of concern (347). It is of utmost importance to use the lowest effective dose, to limit systemic availability by selecting drugs with high first-pass hepatic inactivation, and to instruct patients on proper inhalation technique. Moreover, the use of adjuvant asthma medications acting by different mechanisms can help to reduce inhaled glucocorticoid dosages (346,347). These add-on therapies include leukotriene modifiers, long-acting beta$_2$-agonists, cromoglicate and nedocromil, and in selected cases theophylline. These agents should be added to, but should not in any case replace, inhaled glucocorticoid therapy (346,347).

The use of postnatal glucocorticoids in very premature infants is controversial; although dexamethasone reduces bronchopulmonary dysplasia, it has been associated with severe adverse effects (348). In 220 infants with a birthweight of 501–1000 g randomized to placebo or dexamethasone (0.15 mg/kg/day for 3 days and tapering over a period of 7 days) the relative risk of death or chronic lung disease compared with controls was 0.9 (95% CI = 0.8–1.1) at 36 weeks of gestational age (304). Infants treated with dexamethasone were less likely to need supplementary oxygen. Dexamethasone was associated with increased risks of hypertension (RR = 7.4; 95% CI = 2.7, 20.2), hyperglycemia (RR = 2.0; 95% CI = 1.1, 3.6), spontaneous gastrointestinal perforation (13 versus 4%), lower weight, and a smaller head circumference.

Elderly people

Prolonged use of glucocorticoids in elderly people can exacerbate diabetes, hypertension, congestive heart failure, and osteoporosis, or cause depression. In a retrospective, controlled study, the risks of high-dose intravenous or oral glucocorticoid therapy were assessed in 55 patients with Crohn's disease who were over the age of 50 years (350). They had a higher risk of developing hypertension, hypokalemia, and changes in mental state.

Hepatic disease

In patients with acute hepatitis and active hepatitis, protein binding of the glucocorticoids will be reduced and peak concentrations of administered glucocorticoids increased. Conversion of prednisone to prednisolone has been reported to be impaired in chronic active liver disease (351). However, although plasma prednisolone concentrations were more predictable after the administration of prednisolone than of prednisone to a group of healthy subjects (352), there was no difference in patients with chronic active hepatitis. There was also impaired elimination of prednisolone in these patients. In a review of the pharmacokinetics of prednisone and prednisolone it was concluded that fear of inadequate conversion of prednisone into prednisolone was not justified (353). Patients with hepatic disease suffer adrenal suppression more readily (91).

Other features of the patient

Menopause

Significant differences in the pharmacokinetics of prednisolone amongst menopausal women have been described (SEDA-21, 419) (354). The postmenopausal women had reduced unbound clearance (30%), reduced total clearance, and an increased half-life. Similar results are seen in the postmenopausal women who took estrogen or estrogen–progestogen therapy.

Protein binding

The association between low serum albumin concentrations and complications of prednisone has been long recognized, and it is an elementary pharmacokinetic principle that concentrations of unbound drug in plasma (the fraction that can reach the tissues) will be increased when binding of a drug to serum albumin is reduced (355).

Systemic lupus erythematosus

In 539 patients with systemic lupus erythematosus, organ damage was associated with glucocorticoid therapy compared with controls (356). Oral prednisone 10 mg/day for 10 years (cumulative dose 36.6 g) was significantly associated with osteoporotic fractures (RR = 2.5; 95% CI = 1.7, 3.7), symptomatic coronary artery disease (RR = 1.7; CI = 1.1, 2.5), and cataracts (RR = 1.7; CI = 1.4, 2.5). Avascular necrosis was associated with high-dose prednisone (at least 60 mg/day for at least 2 months; RR = 1.2; CI = 1.1, 1.4). Intravenous pulses of methylprednisolone (1000 mg for 1–3 days) were associated with a small increase in the risk of osteoporotic fractures (RR = 1.3; CI = 1.0, 1.8).

Drug Administration

Drug contamination

Unregulated Chinese herbal products adulterated with glucocorticoids have been detected (357). Dexamethasone was present in eight of 11 Chinese herbal creams analysed by UK dermatologists. The creams contained dexamethasone in concentrations inappropriate for use on the face or in children (64–1500 micrograms/g). The cream with the highest concentration of dexamethasone was prescribed to treat facial eczema in a 4-month-old baby. In all cases, it had been assumed that the creams did not contain glucocorticoids. The authors were concerned that these patients received both unlabelled and unlicensed topical glucocorticoids. They wrote that "greater regulation and restriction needs to be imposed on herbalists, and continuous monitoring of side effects of these medications is necessary."

Drug dosage regimens

Daily or alternate-day administration

The unwanted effects of the glucocorticoids can be reduced to some extent by altering the dosage routine, for example by giving them on alternate days or giving the total daily dose every morning.

Because of circadian variation in endogenous glucocorticoid secretion, the pituitary–adrenal axis is suppressed more easily in the night than during the day (358). Thus, administration of the total dose as a single dose in the morning is preferable to twice daily dosing or administration in the evening alone.

Alternate-day therapy (giving twice the daily dose on alternate days) can in some cases maintain the therapeutic efficacy of oral glucocorticoids, while reducing their adverse effects (359–361).

Use in fixed combinations

Fixed combinations of oral glucocorticoids with nonsteroidal anti-inflammatory analgesics or broncholytic drugs that have to be given repeatedly during the day are undesirable, since their pattern of administration is determined in part by the demands of the other components; the glucocorticoid is thus likely to be given in such a way that it alters the circadian rhythm of endogenous glucocorticoids.

Pulse or megadose therapy

Extremely large intravenous doses of glucocorticoids given at longer intervals can sometimes be effective when a patient does not respond to conventional high doses. Systemic lupus erythematosus, various rheumatic diseases, and the treatment of renal graft rejection are indications for this type of use (SEDA-6, 331). High doses of glucocorticoids also have an antiemetic effect in patients with cancers.

No adverse effects are to be expected after a single injection of a high dose of a glucocorticoid, but some serious complications have been observed with repeated use, including both infections and the known direct adverse effects of glucocorticoids. Cases of ventricular dysrhythmias and atrial fibrillation have been reported (SEDA-18, 391). With pulse therapy, the nature of the injected glucocorticoid seems to be important; for example, hydrocortisone, which is more rapidly metabolized, seems to be better tolerated than dexamethasone (SEDA-6, 331).

Drug administration route

Most knowledge of the adverse effects of glucocorticoids has been acquired in connection with their use as oral products. However, various other routes of administration have been developed, sometimes specifically in the hope of securing a local therapeutic effect while avoiding systemic adverse reactions. Although experience has shown that the latter cannot be eliminated in this way, they can be diminished in some cases. In other cases, new problems arise. Administration by inhalation is covered in the monograph on inhaled glucocorticoids.

Topical administration to the skin

The percutaneous absorption of high-potency topical glucocorticoids has been documented, but hypothalamic–pituitary–adrenal axis suppression, leading to clinically significant adrenal insufficiency or Cushing's syndrome, is infrequent. Two patients developed adrenal suppression after the unregulated use of betamethasone dipropionate 0.05% ointment (about 80 g/week) or clobetasol 0.05% ointment (up to 100 g/week), obtained without prescription to treat psoriasis (362).

Although glucocorticoids are used to treat eczema, they can sometimes exacerbate it (363).

- A 74-year-old man developed worsening eczema 24 hours after he applied clobetasol (Decloban) to treat chronic eczema of his external ear. Twelve years earlier he had noted exacerbation of a cutaneous lesion after he had applied a topical glucocorticoid. He had also had generalized erythema after an intra-articular injection of paramethasone. Patch tests to a series of glucocorticoids were positive for all drugs except flupametasone, fluocortine, and tixocortol. In addition, intradermal tests were positive to hydrocortisone and prednisolone, despite negative patch tests.

The authors commented that most glucocorticoid-sensitized patients react to several of the same group and less frequently of different groups. No case of hypersensitivity to glucocorticoids of all four classes has previously been reported.

- Chronic lichenified eczema has been attributed to prolonged use of topical methylprednisolone aceponate and budesonide (strength and duration of therapy not stated) in a 26-year-old woman (364). Patch tests were positive for methylprednisolone aceponate and budesonide cream, but negative for all other topical glucocorticoids.

The effects of exposure to topical glucocorticoids during pregnancy have been evaluated in a population-based follow-up study in 363 primigravida exposed to topical glucocorticoids during pregnancy and 9263 controls who received no prescriptions at all (365). The prevalence of malformations was 2.9% among 170 infants exposed to glucocorticoids during the first trimester and 3.6% among the controls. There were no increases in the risks of low birthweight, malformations, or preterm delivery in the offspring of women who were exposed to topical glucocorticoids during pregnancy.

Topical administration to the eye

Glucocorticoids that have been used for local ophthalmic treatment include medrysone, fluorometholone, tetrahydroxytriamcinolone, and clobetasone. Loteprednol etabonate 0.5% increases intraocular pressure less than dexamethasone. Studies on animal models of uveitis and two randomized double-masked trials showed that loteprednol etabonate 0.5% was less potent than dexamethasone, prednisolone acetate 1%, or fluorometholone, which may partly explain the improved toxicity profile of loteprednol etabonate (366).

Clinicians should not prescribe glucocorticoid-containing eye-drops unless they have performed a slit-lamp examination with tonometry, have assurance of appropriate follow-up, and understand the differential diagnosis, evaluation, and treatment. Unless clearly indicated, prescribing volumes larger than 5 ml or providing refillable prescriptions should be avoided. It should be stressed that excessive use of glucocorticoids can result in corneal Herpes infection and mycosis.

Since glucocorticoids reduce the immunological defences of the body to most types of infection, their use in the eyes should be monitored carefully. When long-term use is necessary, even with oral or inhalation therapy, eye examination should be performed every 6 months. The ophthalmological follow-up of patients using topical glucocorticoids should include tonometry at least twice a year, careful slit-lamp examination for early signs of herpetic or fungal keratitis and for changes in the equatorial and posterior subcapsular portions of the lens, examination of pupillary size and lid position, and staining of the cornea to detect possible punctate keratitis. Blood glucose concentrations should be checked if there are symptoms that suggest hyperglycemia.

Sensory systems

Ocular adverse effects of local or systemic administration of glucocorticoids include cataracts, glaucoma, papilledema, pseudotumor cerebri, activation of corneal infections, superficial keratitis, ptosis, pupillary dilatation, conjunctival palpebral petechiae, uveitis, and scleromalacia. Topical ocular application and facial application can cause high glucocorticoid concentrations in the anterior compartment of the eye. Serious visual loss can occur owing to the development of cataract in patients using glucocorticoid creams.

Glucocorticoid creams applied topically to the skin are routinely used in the treatment of many skin disorders, and their use on the face in severe atopic eczema is relatively common. Three patients developed advanced glaucoma while using topical facial glucocorticoids. Two other patients developed ocular hypertension secondary to topical facial glucocorticoids (367).

The use of a combination of a glucocorticoid with an antimicrobial drug is illogical and should generally be avoided because of the possibility of the emergence of resistant bacterial strains. It would be highly preferable if prescriptions for these drugs were issued by ophthalmologists only, at least in those parts of the world where adequate medical services are available.

Three vision-threatening complications have been described due to the indiscriminate use of glucocorticoid-containing eyedrops (368).

- A 31-year-old man noted a blind spot in his right eye. He had worn contact lenses for 10 years to correct his myopia. He had applied Tobradex ointment (tobramycin 0.3% and dexamethasone 0.1%) to each eye every evening for the past 4 years because of irritation due to contact lenses, and continuous refills of this prescription were obtained through an acquaintance who was employed in a pharmacy. With spectacle correction his visual acuity was 20/25 in each eye. The intraocular pressure was 52 mmHg in his right eye and 37 mmHg in his left eye. The optic discs showed glaucomatous cupping in each eye. Automated visual field testing showed superior and inferior arcuate defects typical of glaucoma in both eyes. Slit-lamp biomicroscopy showed mild papillary conjunctivitis bilaterally due to contact lenses. The antibiotic + glucocorticoid ointment was withdrawn and his bilateral glucocorticoid-induced open-angle glaucoma was treated with antiglaucomatous drugs.
- A 15-year-old boy felt a foreign body sensation in his right eye after he had been raking hay. His local physician prescribed a suspension of tobramycin 0.3% + dexamethasone 0.1% tds, but 6 days later referred him for evaluation of a suspected fungal keratitis. He had a corneal epithelial defect with an underlying dense inflammatory infiltrate. Corneal scrapings contained fungal hyphae and *Fusarium* species was identified. Natamycin 5% was administered topically every hour, the infection resolved, and his visual acuity returned to 20/20 despite a dense corneal scar.
- A 56-year-old woman had bilateral primary open-angle glaucoma without visual field loss, which was well controlled with a long-term topical beta-blocker in each eye. She underwent a left dacryocystorhinostomy for nasolacrimal duct obstruction, but developed persistent tearing and irritation of the left eye several months postoperatively. A suspension of tobramycin 0.3% + dexamethasone 0.1% was prescribed, which she continued to use as needed for 6 months. Pain and reduced vision persisted in her left eye. Corrected visual acuity was 20/20 in her right eye and 20/60 in her left eye. The intraocular pressures were 18 mmHg in her right eye and 68 mmHg in her left eye. Automated visual field testing showed a normal field in her right eye, but only a central island and a crescent of temporal visual field in her left eye. External examination showed persistent nasolacrimal duct obstruction on the left side with mild conjunctival injection. The diagnosis was primary open-angle glaucoma in both eyes, which was exacerbated by topically applied glucocorticoids in her left eye. The antibiotic + glucocorticoid suspension was withdrawn, and a topical ocular hypotensive therapeutic regimen was initiated in her left eye.

Susceptibility factors

Local and systemic adverse effects of ophthalmic glucocorticoids occur in children more often, more severely, and more rapidly than in adults, for unknown reasons. It could be that children have relatively immature chamber angles, giving rise to a rapidly increasing intraocular pressure (369).

Glaucoma has been reported after the use of a glucocorticoid ointment in a young boy (369).

- A 6-year-old boy underwent a resection of levator palpebrae superioris for congenital blepharoptosis. Postoperatively, an ointment containing 0.1% dexamethasone and neomycin (Maxitrol) was applied to the operated eyelid three times a day to reduce lid edema. Four days later the surgical correction was satisfactory and there were no symptoms, but the intraocular pressure was raised to 44 mmHg in the operated eye, although normal in the other eye. The glucocorticoid was withdrawn and topical ocular hypotensive agents were prescribed. The intraocular pressure returned to normal the next day, and the antiglaucoma treatments were maintained for 1 week and tapered over the next 2 weeks. Subsequent follow-up confirmed normal intraocular pressure and no glaucomatous damage.

The ocular hypertensive response in this case could have been due to systemic absorption of glucocorticoid through the skin of the eyelid, especially when there was a surgical wound. Alternatively, a sufficient amount of ointment could have seeped over the eyelid margins, causing the rise in intraocular pressure, similar to the application of eye-drops, as has been reported in another child, who also had Cushing's syndrome, a rare result of ophthalmic glucocorticoids (370).

- An 11-year-old boy with iridocyclitis developed Cushing's syndrome, a posterior subcapsular cataract, and increased intraocular pressure in both eyes after the topical administration of prednisolone acetate 1% eyedrops bilaterally for 6 months. The Cushing's syndrome was aggravated when periocular methylprednisolone acetate was started while bilateral posterior subtenon injections of 80 mg of suspension were continued every 6 weeks for 6 months. He had not used systemic glucocorticoids before.

Topical administration to the nose

The local application of glucocorticoids for seasonal or perennial rhinitis often results in systemic adverse effects. The use of nasal sprays containing a glucocorticoid that has specific topical activity (such as beclomethasone dipropionate or flunisolide) seems to reduce the systemic adverse effects, but they can nevertheless occur, even to the extent of suppression of basal adrenal function in children (371). Local adverse effects include *Candida* infection, nasal stinging, epistaxis, throat irritation (372), and, exceptionally, anosmia (373).

Nervous system

Benign intracranial hypertension with nasal glucocorticoids has been reported (374).

- A 13-year-old boy with Crohn's disease in remission, who had taken fluticasone aqueous nasal spray 50 micrograms to each nostril od regularly for 5 days, gave a 10-day history of head and back pain. He had a right sixth nerve palsy with bilateral swelling of his optic discs. An unenhanced computer tomogram was normal and magnetic resonance imaging excluded cavernous sinus thrombosis. The cerebrospinal fluid was clear with no cells, and protein and glucose concentrations were normal.

Although there was no clear temporal relation between the onset of the symptoms and the regular use of fluticasone, the authors proposed that the fluticasone was responsible, because the symptoms resolved after drug withdrawal. The association remains unproven but it does highlight the possibility of an association.

Sensory systems
Nasal budesonide or beclomethasone 100 micrograms bd for 3–9 months had no effect on the eyes in 26 patients who had undergone endoscopic sinus surgery (375). Ophthalmologic examination, tonometry, visual field testing, and biomicroscopic studies showed no evidence of ocular hypertension or posterior subcapsular cataract.

Ear, nose, and throat
The use of intranasal glucocorticoids in the treatment of allergic and vasomotor rhinitis in Sweden has doubled over a period of 5 years, and the number of reported cases of nasal septum perforation increased over the same time (376). The most common risk factor in 32 patients with nasal septum perforation (21 women, 11 men) was glucocorticoid treatment. Information from the Swedish Drug Agency showed that 38 cases of glucocorticoid-induced perforation had been reported over 10 years. The number of adverse effects per million Defined Daily Doses averaged 0.21. The risk of perforation was greatest during the first 12 months of treatment and most cases were in young women.

Endocrine
Aqueous nasal triamcinolone spray 220 or 440 micrograms od for the treatment of allergic rhinitis reportedly had no measurable adverse effects on adrenocortical function in 80 children (aged 6–12 years) in a placebo-controlled, double-blind study (377). Plasma triamcinolone concentrations measured over 6 hours fell rapidly and there was little or no accumulation during 6 weeks.

There have been reports of Cushing's syndrome after prolonged use of intranasal betamethasone 0.1% for chronic catarrh in two boys (378) and from an interaction of nasal fluticasone with ritonavir (379).

- A 30-year-old man who was using an intranasal formulation of fluticasone (therapeutic indication not stated), developed Cushing's syndrome about 5 months after starting ritonavir 600 mg bd, zidovudine, and lamivudine for HIV infection. His plasma cortisol concentrations were undetectable, his corticotrophin was low (under 2 pmol/l), and his 24-hours urinary cortisol excretion was under 30 nmol/l. Further investigations were consistent with secondary adrenal failure or with glucocorticoid use. He admitted to having used a topical glucocorticoid cream for 2 months. However, 6 weeks after he stopped using this cream, his plasma cortisol concentrations were still undetectable. It was then established that he had used nasal fluticasone propionate 200 micrograms/day for about 1 year before starting ritonavir. Ritonavir was replaced by nevirapine, and he continued to use fluticasone nasal spray. Three weeks later, his plasma cortisol concentration had increased to 290 nmol/l. Ritonavir was then added and his plasma cortisol concentration fell rapidly. Ritonavir was stopped again and his cortisol concentration normalized and his Cushingoid facies improved.

The authors thought it likely that inhibition of cytochrome P-450 by ritonavir increased the systemic availability of fluticasone and thus caused Cushing's syndrome in this patient.

Intralesional injection
Intralesional triamcinolone acetonide has been used extensively for the treatment of hypertrophic and keloid scars. Complications are few, usually being local skin color changes, prominent vascular markings, or subcutaneous atrophy. Cushing's syndrome after intralesional administration of triamcinolone acetate has been described in two adults and two children (aged 10 years and 21 months) after treatment of hypertrophic burn scars with intralesional triamcinolone acetonide (SEDA-21, 419) (350). These two children may have had a form of hypersensitivity to triamcinolone acetonide, as Cushing's syndrome was not the result of overdosage.

- Acute anaphylaxis occurred in an 18-year-old man after the third course of intradermal injections of triamcinolone suspension ("Kenalog" 10 mg per treatment) for alopecia areata (380). Subsequent rechallenge with intradermal triamcinolone 1 ml resulted in the same anaphylactic reaction as before and his serum IgE concentration was increased.

Immediate hypersensitivity reactions to paramethasone acetate, causing widespread eruptions, have been described in at least four cases. Delayed allergic reactions are less common.

- A woman had received intralesional paramethasone and other topical glucocorticoids several times for alopecia between the ages of 7 and 18 years (381). When she was 30 she was again treated with intralesional paramethasone for a relapse of alopecia. She developed pruritus after the first intralesional injection and erythema, edema, and vesicles 6–8 hours later. A biopsy showed spongiform lymphocytic folliculitis with spongiosis and exocytosis in the sweat gland ducts and in the pilosebaceous unit. She was treated with triamcinolone cream and her skin lesions resolved. Patch tests were positive for paramethasone, with cross-reactivity to tixocortol pivalate, hydrocortisone, and hydrocortisone butyrate.

Intraspinal injection
Intrathecal
The effects of intrathecal administration, both wanted and unwanted, are still much debated (382). The question as to whether oral glucocorticoid therapy should be preferred to intrathecal injections is raised by the harmful effects that have sometimes occurred after the latter,

although some of these may have been caused by irritative substances in the injection fluid (SEDA-6, 331). The same local glucocorticoid concentrations can probably be attained with fewer problems with oral administration. Epidural injection of glucocorticoids seems to be safer than intrathecal injection, but injection of high doses can cause the same systemic adverse effects as seen with oral treatment. Facial flushing and erythema after lumbar epidural glucocorticoid administration have been reported (SEDA-20, 378) (383).

Glucocorticoids given intrathecally can cause a rise in cerebrospinal fluid protein and carry the risk of arachnoiditis (SED-8, 820). Chemical meningitis has been reported after two intrathecal injections of methylprednisolone acetate (384) and after lumbar facet joint block (SEDA-17, 450). Intraspinal injections of hydrocortisone for multiple sclerosis apparently led in one case to a cauda equina syndrome, with subsequent ulceromutilating acropathy (SEDA-17, 450). Intra-discal injections of triamcinolone acetonide in a number of French cases led to disk or epidural calcification, sometimes symptomless (SEDA-17, 450).

Postlumbar puncture syndrome with abducent nerve palsy followed the use of intrathecal prednisolone for the treatment of low back pain and sciatica (385).

- A 38-year-old woman received intrathecal prednisolone 3 ml (strength not stated) and 1 day later developed a postural headache, nausea, and dizziness. She was treated with intravenous fluids and analgesics. Eight days later she suddenly developed a complete palsy of the right abducent nerve. An MRI brain scan showed contrast meningeal enhancement typical of postlumbar puncture syndrome. She was treated with oral glucocorticoids and blood patching was performed. Her headache began to resolve a week later. Four months later she had almost completely recovered function of her abducent nerve and a repeat MRI scan was normal.

Epidural

The indications, rationale, techniques, alternatives, contraindications, complications, and efficacy of lumbar and caudal epidural glucocorticoid injections have been reviewed (SEDA-21, 420) (386).

Bilateral posterior subcapsular cataracts have been reported after treatment with epidural methylprednisolone for low back pain secondary to degenerative joint disease and disk protrusion (387).

- A 42-year-old man had received 15 epidural injections of methylprednisolone 80 mg over 10 years. About 6 weeks after his last injection, he developed progressively worsening cloudy vision. He had bilateral posterior subcapsular cataracts and subsequently underwent bilateral cataract removal.

The authors commented that it is possible that multiple epidural glucocorticoid injections had contributed to cataract formation. The patient also had several other risk factors for cataracts (cigarette smoking, alcohol consumption, exposure to ultraviolet radiation, low socioeconomic class, and low intake of antioxidant vitamins). However, the role of these other risk factors was speculative.

Symptoms consistent with complex regional pain syndrome have been reported after a cervical epidural glucocorticoid injection (SEDA-22, 451) (388).

Spinal epidural lipomatosis secondary to exogenous administration of glucocorticoids is a rare condition that has been reported almost exclusively in association with systemic treatment. However, local epidural administration has also been implicated (389).

One case of *Staphylococcus aureus* meningitis, a rare complication of epidural analgesia, has been published. The same patient developed a cauda equina syndrome of uncertain etiology, although neural ischemia as a result of meningitis secondary to immunosuppression was possible (SEDA-21, 420) (390). A unique case of transient profound paralysis after epidural glucocorticoid injection (acute paraplegia) has now been reported (SEDA-22, 451) (391). Diplopia associated with the peridural or intrathecal infiltration of prednisolone have not been previously reported (SEDA-22, 451) (392).

Of 31 patients who received 1 ml (40 mg) of methylprednisolone epidurally at the end of microdiscectomy, three developed epidural abscesses (393). These results were compared with a historical series of 400 patients not taking glucocorticoids, who had no deep infection. Although the data were limited, epidural glucocorticoids after discectomy should not be recommended.

Cervical epidural glucocorticoid injection is often used for the treatment of cervical radiculopathy. Subjective patient satisfaction has been reported, but controlled trials have not yet delineated the effectiveness of this procedure. Three cases of severe pain consistent with nerve injury have been reported immediately after cervical epidural glucocorticoid injection, bringing into question the benefit–harm balance of this technique (394).

Intra-articular and periarticular administration

Local injections of glucocorticoids into and around the joints can have a dramatic therapeutic effect, but the catabolic effect can have serious consequences, including adverse effects on joint structure (395) and on local tendons, subcutaneous atrophy, and possibly osteonecrosis. Provided the state of the joint is carefully inspected before any new injection is given, and the interval between the injections is not less than 4 weeks, the risk seems to be small enough to justify treatment in invalidating cases (SEDA-3, 307).

Neuropsychiatric effects of glucocorticoids, like hallucinations, can result from intra-articular administration (SEDA-22, 444) (396).

An acute adrenal crisis occurred in a woman who received an intra-articular glucocorticoid for pseudogout of the knee (397).

- An 87-year-old woman received intra-articular betamethasone (Diprophos) 7 mg on three occasions for painful knee joints over 6 months. Six weeks after the last injection she developed diffuse pain and contractures in the legs, fatigue, nausea, abdominal pain, and weight loss of 6 kg. Both knee joints were tender but there was no effusion. Her serum sodium concentration was 123 mmol/l, serum osmolality 254 mosmol/kg, urine sodium 136 mmol/l, and urinary osmolality

373 mosmol/kg. The syndrome of inappropriate antidiuretic hormone secretion was diagnosed, but despite treatment she remained drowsy and hyponatremic. About a week later, she developed hypotension and symptoms of an acute abdomen. Further investigations showed that her basal cortisol concentration was low (36 nmol/l) but it increased to 481 nmol/l after a short tetracosactide test, consistent with acute adrenal crisis. She recovered rapidly after treatment with oral hydrocortisone, but still required glucocorticoid substitution several months later.

An erythema multiforme-like eruption has been reported after intra-articular triamcinolone in the right knee, with cross-sensitivity to budesonide (398).

- A 70-year-old man had received three intra-articular injections of triamcinolone (dose not stated) into the same knee over 3 months without any allergic reactions. However, 12–24 hours after the last injection he developed pruritus and erythema at the injection site. This eruption was treated with topical budesonide, but within the next few hours, acute eczema developed. The lesions spread to his legs and abdomen, and were erythematous, edematous, and resembled erythema multiforme. He was treated with boric acid solution dressings, emollients, and oral antihistamines. His lesions gradually resolved and did not recur during 8 months of follow-up. A month after the lesions had resolved, he underwent patch testing, which was positive to triamcinolone 1% and budesonide 1% in petrolatum, but negative to other glucocorticoids.

Hiccups have been reported after intra-articular administration (399).

- A 38-year-old man had an intra-articular injection of betamethasone dipropionate (dose not stated) into his right ankle, and the day after had hiccups that lasted for 24 hours and then resolved without treatment. Some months later, because of persistent arthritis, he received a further injection of betamethasone dipropionate into his right ankle. Once again, he had hiccups the following day. On this occasion, the hiccups resolved after 2 weeks, following treatment with levomepromazine.

Anaphylaxis occurred in two women after intra-articular administration of paramethasone plus mepivacaine 2% (400).

- A 44-year-old woman developed generalized pruritus 10 minutes after intra-articular paramethasone and mepivacaine and 30 minutes later developed generalized urticaria, tachycardia, and dyspnea. She received emergency treatment and her condition initially improved. However, her symptoms recurred after 6 hours and she was treated again and then discharged taking oral dexchlorpheniramine. She had a history of allergic contact dermatitis due to nickel sulfate sensitization, and 7 years before had had generalized urticaria and dyspnea after intra-articular administration of a glucocorticoid.
- A 31-year-old woman developed generalized pruritus and urticaria, facial edema, and dyspnea 2 hours after the intra-articular administration of paramethasone and mepivacaine. She was treated with an intramuscular glucocorticoid and antihistamines, with worsening of her symptoms. She received intravenous fluids and dexchlorpheniramine, but her symptoms recurred after 1 hour, when she was given subcutaneous adrenaline, intravenous fluids and dexchlorpheniramine. She was later discharged taking oral diphenhydramine. She had a history of a systemic reaction after the administration of a glucocorticoid and a local anesthetic.

Skin prick tests were positive for isolated paramethasone in both patients, but negative for mepivacaine. There has only been one previous report of anaphylaxis in association with paramethasone.

Osteomyelitis after three glucocorticoid injections for tennis elbow has been reported; the second injection was given 3 months after the first and the third 2 days later (401). This case illustrates the need for vigilance, even after common procedures, and that exacerbation of symptoms after local glucocorticoid injections should prompt the doctor to review the diagnosis and consider the need for further investigation.

Inadvertent intra-arterial injection

Particularly when injecting glucocorticoids locally, for example to relieve arthritis of the wrist, accidental injection into an artery is possible. Severe local ischemia can result (SEDA-17, 450).

Intracapsular injection

The use of implants for augmentation of the breast can lead to capsular contracture. Patients with intractable capsular contracture are treated with intracapsular injection of triamcinolone. Major complications included three cases of major atrophy requiring surgical correction. This problem appeared to have been eliminated by reduction of the dose of triamcinolone from 50 to 25 mg. There was one implant puncture (SEDA-19, 379) (402).

Rectal administration

Systemic absorption of glucocorticoids can occur after rectal administration.

- A 48-year-old woman developed avascular necrosis 9 months after she had completed a 3-month course of hydrocortisone 100 mg retention enemas once or twice daily for ulcerative proctitis (403). An MRI scan showed multiple bony infarcts in her distal femora, proximal tibiae, and posterior proximal right fibular head, extending from the diaphysis to the epiphysis, consistent with avascular necrosis.
- Cushing's syndrome occurred in a 65-year-old woman with ulcerative colitis who received a daily betamethasone enema (404).

The authors of the second report reported the pharmacokinetics of betamethasone after rectal dosing, with plasma concentrations of betamethasone high enough to cause Cushing's syndrome. Suppression of the hypothalamic–pituitary–adrenal axis disappeared after the dosage schedule was changed from daily to three times a week. These findings suggest that a considerable amount of betamethasone is absorbed after rectal dosing.

Occupational exposure

Occupational exposure to glucocorticoids can cause adverse effects. Facial plethora has been found in workers manufacturing synthetic glucocorticoids, some of them having grossly abnormal responses to tetracosactide.

- A 58-year-old woman, who had been involved in the manufacturing of glucocorticoid creams and ointments for over 10 years, developed occupational contact sensitization to topical glucocorticoids (405). Patch tests were positive to hydrocortisone, hydrocortisone butyrate, and tixocortol pivalate. Intradermal tests were positive to hydrocortisone succinate, methylprednisolone, and prednisolone. An oral challenge with betamethasone 0.75 mg, 2.5 mg, and 8 mg on three consecutive days resulted in no adverse reactions.

It has been recommended that all workers manufacturing potent glucocorticoids should be screened regularly for glucocorticoid overdosage and should be moved regularly to units processing other drugs (406).

Drug overdose

High doses of glucocorticoids in patients with cancers can increase the risk of metastases, for example in breast cancer; this has been attributed in some cases to immunosuppression (407). These hormones should therefore only be used in patients with those types of tumors for which they are known to improve the efficacy of the cancer treatment.

A curious reaction to intravenous high-dose dexamethasone, used as an antiemetic agent in cancer chemotherapy or for other purposes, is sudden severe itching, burning, and constrictive pain in the perineal region, which has been described in several published reports (SEDA-11, 336) (408).

Drug–Drug Interactions

Albendazole

Dexamethasone reduced the clearance of albendazole and increased its half-life; plasma concentrations almost doubled (SEDA-22, 450) (409).

Amiodarone

Budesonide for collagenous colitis caused Cushing's syndrome in a patient with chronic renal insufficiency taking amiodarone for paroxysmal atrial fibrillation (410).

- An 81-year-old man with persistent diarrhea was given oral budesonide 9 mg/day, following unsuccessful treatment with mesalazine and prednisone. He was also taking amiodarone 100 mg/day. His diarrhea resolved within 6 weeks, and attempts to reduce the dosage of bzudesonide resulted in recurrent diarrhea. After 11 months he developed Cushing's syndrome, which persisted despite a reduction in dosage to 3 mg/day. His mild diarrhea recurred and the dosage of budesonide was increased to 6 mg/day with worsening of Cushing's syndrome; the dosage was reduced to 3 mg/day. Four weeks later amiodarone was withdrawn. The symptoms of Cushing's syndrome resolved within 4 weeks.

The authors suggested that the development of Cushing's syndrome and its persistence at a low dosage of budesonide was caused by inhibition of the metabolism of budesonide by amiodarone.

Anticoagulants

Intravenous methylprednisolone (1 g/day for 3 days) has been reported to inhibit the metabolism of oral anticoagulants (acenocoumarol and fluindione) in 10 patients, increasing the INR by 8 (range 5–20) (411).

Glucocorticoids can also alter the response to anticoagulants. A raised tolerance to heparin has been reported and a fall in fibrinolytic activity has been seen during glucocorticoid treatment (SED-8, 816). The entire clotting mechanism and particularly the prothrombin time should therefore be checked periodically in patients taking glucocorticoids concomitantly with anticoagulants, particularly if the glucocorticoid dose is changed. In addition there is an increased risk of gastric bleeding in patients taking both glucocorticoids and anticoagulants.

Antifungal azoles

Itraconazole 200 mg/day markedly increased plasma methylprednisolone concentrations and reduced morning plasma cortisol concentrations by over 80% in 10 healthy volunteers (412). The C_{max}, AUC, and half-life of methylprednisolone were increased 1.9, 3.9, and 2.4 times respectively.

Itraconazole 200 mg/day orally for 4 days markedly reduced the clearance and increased the half-life of intravenous methylprednisolone from 2.1 to 4.8 hours in a double-blind, randomized, two-phase, crossover study in nine healthy volunteers (SEDA-23, 430) (413). The volume of distribution was not affected. The mean morning plasma cortisol concentration during the itraconazole phase, measured 24 hours after methylprednisolone, was only 9% of that during the placebo phase (11 versus 117 ng/ml).

The authors of these two reports recommended that care be taken when methylprednisolone is prescribed in combination with itraconazole or other potent inhibitors of CYP3A4.

Itraconazole, given orally increased oral prednisolone concentrations by only 24% (414) but increased intravenous dexamethasone concentrations 3.3-fold and oral dexamethasone 3.7-fold (415).

In another study, ketoconazole was given orally as 200 mg od for 4 days, following a single oral dose of budesonide 3 mg either at the same time as ketoconazole or 12 hours before (416). Ketoconazole increased budesonide concentrations (C_{max} and AUC) 6.8- to 7.6-fold when the two drugs were co-administered; with a 12-hour separation, budesonide concentrations increased only 1.7- to 2.1-fold.

Calcium channel blockers

Methylprednisolone concentrations increased with the co-administration of diltiazem (2.6-fold) and mibefradil (3.8-fold) (417).

Ciclosporin

Glucocorticoids cause additive immunosuppression when they are given with other immunosuppressants, such as ciclosporin (SEDA-22, 451) (418).

Clarithromycin

Clarithromycin inhibits CYP3A4, which is responsible for the metabolic clearance of prednisolone, the biologically active metabolite of prednisone. Clarithromycin (500 mg bd for 2 days) reduced the clearance of methylprednisolone by 65% and significantly increased its plasma concentrations; clarithromycin did not influence the clearance or plasma concentrations of prednisone (419). Acute mania has been reported to be related to inhibition of the metabolic clearance of prednisone by clarithromycin (SEDA-22, 444) (420).

Cyclophosphamide

The effect of prednisone 1 mg/kg on the pharmacokinetics of cyclophosphamide and its initial metabolites 4-hydroxycyclophosphamide and aldophosphamide (the acyclic tautomer of 4-hydroxycyclophosphamide) has been studied between the first and sixth cycles in seven patients (two men) with systemic vasculitis receiving intravenous cyclophosphamide 0.6 g/m^2 as a 1-hour intravenous infusion every 3 weeks for six cycles (421). Prednisone reduced the clearance of cyclophosphamide from 5.8 to 4.0 l/hour, reducing the amount of initial metabolites formed. Although the clinical significance of this interaction is unclear, 4-hydroxycyclophosphamide and aldophosphamide are probably responsible for the cytotoxic activity of cyclophosphamide, and increased cyclophosphamide dosages should be considered in patients taking prednisone.

Diuretics

Glucocorticoids with mineralocorticoid activity potentiate potassium loss when they are given with potassium-wasting diuretics (422).

Grapefruit juice

Methylprednisolone concentrations increased with the co-administration of grapefruit juice (1.75-fold) (423).

Leukotriene receptor antagonists

In a probable pharmacodynamic interaction, severe peripheral edema followed treatment with montelukast and prednisone for asthma (424).

- A 23-year-old man, with a history of asthma, house dust mite allergy, and rhinoconjunctivitis, presented with acute respiratory symptoms. He was given oral cetirizine, inhaled salmeterol, and fluticasone propionate, and oral prednisone 40 mg/day for 1 week and 20 mg/day for 1 week. His asthma recurred when prednisone was withdrawn and he took oral prednisone 60 mg/day for 1 week and 40 mg/day for 1 week. He also took montelukast 10 mg/day. He then developed severe peripheral edema with a gain in weight of 13 kg. Prednisone was withdrawn and his edema resolved. Montelukast was continued.

The author commented that the patient had tolerated prednisone without montelukast and montelukast without prednisone. However, he had severe edema when both drugs were used together. Montelukast may have potentiated glucocorticoid-induced renal tubular sodium and fluid retention. Both have been associated with edema.

Oral contraceptives

Oral contraceptives increased budesonide concentrations by only 22%, but prednisolone concentrations increased by 131%, suggesting a clinically important interaction (425).

Phenobarbital

Phenobarbital increases the metabolism of glucocorticoids, reducing the half-life by some 50% (426).

Phenytoin

Phenytoin increases the metabolism of glucocorticoids, reducing the half-life by some 50% (426).

Rifampicin

Rifampicin and other drugs that induce liver enzymes increase the metabolism of glucocorticoids (427), sufficient to reduce their therapeutic effects, for example in asthma (428).

Salicylates

Glucocorticoids reduce the plasma concentrations of salicylates (429). If they are given with aspirin or other anti-inflammatory drugs, there may be an additive effect on the gastric wall, leading to an increased risk of bleeding and ulceration (430–432).

References

1. Kaiser H. Cortisone derivate in Klinik und Praxis. Stuttgart-New York: Thieme, 1987.
2. Labhart A. Adrenal cortex. In: Labhart A, editor. Clinical Endocrinology. Berlin-Heidelberg-New York: Springer, 1985:373.
3. Medici TC, Ruegsegger P. Does alternate-day cloprednol therapy prevent bone loss? A longitudinal double-blind, controlled clinical study. Clin Pharmacol Ther 1990;48(4):455–66.
4. Iwasaki E, Baba M. [Pharmacokinetics and pharmacodynamics of hydrocortisone in asthmatic children.] Arerugi 1993;42(10):1555–62.
5. Bone RC, Fisher CJ Jr, Clemmer TP, Slotman GJ, Metz CA, Balk RA. A controlled clinical trial of high-dose methylprednisolone in the treatment of severe sepsis and septic shock. N Engl J Med 1987;317(11):653–8.
6. The Veterans Administration Systemic Sepsis Cooperative Study Group. Effect of high-dose glucocorticoid therapy on mortality in patients with clinical signs of systemic sepsis. N Engl J Med 1987;317(11):659–65.
7. Garland JS, Alex CP, Pauly TH, Whitehead VL, Brand J, Winston JF, Samuels DP, McAuliffe TL. A three-day course of dexamethasone therapy to prevent chronic lung

disease in ventilated neonates: a randomized trial. Pediatrics 1999;104(1 Part 1):91–9.
8. Romagnoli C, Zecca E, Vento G, De Carolis MP, Papacci P, Tortorolo G. Early postnatal dexamethasone for the prevention of chronic lung disease in high-risk preterm infants. Intensive Care Med 1999;25(7):717–21.
9. Arias-Camison JM, Lau J, Cole CH, Frantz ID. 3rd. Meta-analysis of dexamethasone therapy started in the first 15 days of life for prevention of chronic lung disease in premature infants. Pediatr Pulmonol 1999;28(3):167–74.
10. Romagnoli C, Zecca E, Vento G, Maggio L, Papacci P, Tortorolo G. Effect on growth of two different dexamethasone courses for preterm infants at risk of chronic lung disease. A randomized trial. Pharmacology 1999;59(5):266–74.
11. Tarnow-Mordi W, Mitra A. Postnatal dexamethasone in preterm infants is potentially lifesaving, but follow up studies are urgently needed. BMJ 1999;319(7222):1385–6.
12. Klein-Gitelman MS, Pachman LM. Intravenous corticosteroids: adverse reactions are more variable than expected in children. J Rheumatol 1998;25(10):1995–2002.
13. Feldweg AM, Leddy JP. Drug interactions affecting the efficacy of corticosteroid therapy. A brief review with an illustrative case. J Clin Rheumatol 1999;5:143–50.
14. Maxwell SR, Moots RJ, Kendall MJ. Corticosteroids: do they damage the cardiovascular system? Postgrad Med J 1994;70(830):863–70.
15. Sato A, Funder JW, Okubo M, Kubota E, Saruta T. Glucocorticoid-induced hypertension in the elderly. Relation to serum calcium and family history of essential hypertension. Am J Hypertens 1995;8(8):823–8.
16. Thedenat B, Leaute-Labreze C, Boralevi F, Roul S, Labbe L, Marliere V, Taieb A. Surveillance tensionnelle des nourrissons traites par corticotherapie generale pour un hemangiome. [Blood pressure monitoring in infants with hemangiomas treated with corticosteroids.] Ann Dermatol Venereol 2002;129(2):183–5.
17. Stewart IM, Marks JSECG. Abnormalities in steroid-treated rheumatoid patients. Lancet 1977;2(8050):1237–8.
18. Baty V, Blain H, Saadi L, Jeandel C, Canton P. Fatal myocardial infarction in an elderly woman with severe ulcerative colitis. what is the role of steroids? Am J Gastroenterol 1998;93(10):2000–1.
19. Machiels JP, Jacques JM, de Meester A. Coronary artery spasm during anaphylaxis. Ann Emerg Med 1996; 27(5):674–5.
20. Sato O, Takagi A, Miyata T, Takayama Y. Aortic aneurysms in patients with autoimmune disorders treated with corticosteroids. Eur J Vasc Endovasc Surg 1995;10(3):366–9.
21. Kotha P, McGreevy MJ, Kotha A, Look M, Weisman MH. Early deaths with thrombolytic therapy for acute myocardial infarction in corticosteroid-dependent rheumatoid arthritis. Clin Cardiol 1998;21(11):853–6.
22. Yunis KA, Bitar FF, Hayek P, Mroueh SM, Mikati M. Transient hypertrophic cardiomyopathy in the newborn following multiple doses of antenatal corticosteroids. Am J Perinatol 1999;16(1):17–21.
23. Gill AW, Warner G, Bull L. Iatrogenic neonatal hypertrophic cardiomyopathy. Pediatr Cardiol 1996; 17(5):335–9.
24. Pokorny JJ, Roth F, Balfour I, Rinehart G. An unusual complication of the treatment of a hemangioma. Ann Plast Surg 2002;48(1):83–7.
25. Kothari SN, Kisken WA. Dexamethasone-induced congestive heart failure in a patient with dilated cardiomyopathy caused by occult pheochromocytoma. Surgery 1998; 123(1):102–5.
26. Kucukosmanoglu O, Karabay A, Ozbarlas N, Noyan A, Anarat A. Marked bradycardia due to pulsed and oral methylprednisolone therapy in a patient with rapidly progressive glomerulonephritis. Nephron 1998;80(4):484.
27. Schult M, Lohmann D, Knitsch W, Kuse ER, Nashan B. Recurrent cardiocirculatory arrest after kidney transplantation related to intravenous methylprednisolone bolus therapy. Transplantation 1999;67(11):1497–8.
28. Brumund MR, Truemper EJ, Lutin WA, Pearson-Shaver AL. Disseminated varicella and staphylococcal pericarditis after topical steroids. J Pediatr 1997; 131(1 Part 1):162–3.
29. Kaiser H. Cortisonderivate in Klink und Praxis, 7th edn. Stuttgart: G.Thieme, 1977.
30. Williamson IJ, Matusiewicz SP, Brown PH, Greening AP, Crompton GK. Frequency of voice problems and cough in patients using pressurized aerosol inhaled steroid preparations. Eur Respir J 1995;8(4):590–2.
31. Lim BS, Choi WY, Choi JW. A case of steroid-induced intractable hiccup. Tuberc Respir Dis 1991;38:304–7.
32. Cersosimo RJ, Brophy MT. Hiccups with high dose dexamethasone administration: a case report. Cancer 1998;82(2):412–14.
33. Ross J, Eledrisi M, Casner P. Persistent hiccups induced by dexamethasone. West J Med 1999;170(1):51–2.
34. Poynter D. Beclomethasone dipropionate aerosol and nasal mucosa. Br J Clin Pharmacol 1977;4(Suppl 3):S295–301.
35. Albucher JF, Vuillemin-Azais C, Manelfe C, Clanet M, Guiraud-Chaumeil B, Chollet F. Cerebral thrombophlebitis in three patients with probable multiple sclerosis. Role of lumbar puncture or intravenous corticosteroid treatment. Cerebrovasc Dis 1999;9(5):298–303.
36. Shinwell ES, Karplus M, Reich D, Weintraub Z, Blazer S, Bader D, Yurman S, Dolfin T, Kogan A, Dollberg S, Arbel E, Goldberg M, Gur I, Naor N, Sirota L, Mogilner S, Zaritsky A, Barak M, Gottfried E. Early postnatal dexamethasone treatment and increased incidence of cerebral palsy. Arch Dis Child Fetal Neonatal Ed 2000;83(3):F177–81.
37. Bentson J, Reza M, Winter J, Wilson G. Steroids and apparent cerebral atrophy on computed tomography scans. J Comput Assist Tomogr 1978;2(1):16–23.
38. Vaughn BV, Ali II, Olivier KN, Lackner RP, Robertson KR, Messenheimer JA, Paradowski LJ, Egan TM. Seizures in lung transplant recipients. Epilepsia 1996;37(12):1175–9.
39. Lorrot M, Bader-Meunier B, Sebire G, Dommergues JP. Hypertension intracranienne benigne: une complication meconnue de la corticotherapie. [Benign intracranial hypertension: an unrecognized complication of corticosteroid therapy.] Arch Pediatr 1999;6(1):40–2.
40. Kalapurakal JA, Silverman CL, Akhtar N, Laske DW, Braitman LE, Boyko OB, Thomas PR. Intracranial meningiomas: factors that influence the development of cerebral edema after stereotactic radiosurgery and radiation therapy. Radiology 1997;204(2):461–5.
41. Laroche F, Chemouilli R, Carlier P. Efficacy of conservative treatment in a patient with spinal cord compression due to corticosteroid-induced epidural lipomatosis. Rev Rheum (English Edn) 1993;30:729–31.
42. Roy-Camille R, Mazel C, Husson JL, Saillant G. Symptomatic spinal epidural lipomatosis induced by a long-term steroid treatment. Review of the literature and report of two additional cases. Spine 1991;16(12):1365–71.
43. Andress HJ, Schurmann M, Heuck A, Schmand J, Lob G. A rare case of osteoporotic spine fracture associated with epidural lipomatosis causing paraplegia following long-term cortisone therapy. Arch Orthop Trauma Surg 2000;120(7–8):484–6.
44. Pinsker MO, Kinzel D, Lumenta CB. Epidural thoracic lipomatosis induced by long-term steroid treatment case illustration. Acta Neurochir (Wien) 1998;140(9):991–2.

45. Parker CT, Jarek MJ, Finger DR. Corticosteroid-associated epidural lipomatosis. J Clin Rheumatol 1999;5:141–2.
46. Donaghy M, Mills KR, Boniface SJ, Simmons J, Wright I, Gregson N, Jacobs J. Pure motor demyelinating neuropathy: deterioration after steroid treatment and improvement with intravenous immunoglobulin. J Neurol Neurosurg Psychiatry 1994;57(7):778–83.
47. Urban RC Jr, Cotlier E. Corticosteroid-induced cataracts. Surv Ophthalmol 1986;31(2):102–10.
48. Kaye LD, Kalenak JW, Price RL, Cunningham R. Ocular implications of long-term prednisone therapy in children. J Pediatr Ophthalmol Strabismus 1993;30(3):142–4.
49. Cumming RG, Mitchell P, Leeder SR. Use of inhaled corticosteroids and the risk of cataracts. N Engl J Med 1997;337(1):8–14.
50. Abramson HA. May corticosteroid cataracts be reversible. J Asthma Res 1977;14(3):vii–viii.
51. Lubkin VL. Steroid cataract – a review and a conclusion. J Asthma Res 1977;14(2):55–9.
52. Forman AR, Loreto JA, Tina LU. Reversibility of corticosteroid-associated cataracts in children with the nephrotic syndrome. Am J Ophthalmol 1977;84(1):75–8.
53. Wingate RJ, Beaumont PE. Intravitreal triamcinolone and elevated intraocular pressure. Aust NZ J Ophthalmol 1999;27(6):431–2.
54. Garbe E, LeLorier J, Boivin JF, Suissa S. Risk of ocular hypertension or open-angle glaucoma in elderly patients on oral glucocorticoids. Lancet 1997;350(9083):979–82.
55. Garbe E, LeLorier J, Boivin JF, Suissa S. Inhaled and nasal glucocorticoids and the risks of ocular hypertension or open-angle glaucoma. JAMA 1997;277(9):722–7.
56. Novack GD. Ocular toxicology. Curr Opin Ophthalmol 1994;5(6):110–14.
57. Opatowsky I, Feldman RM, Gross R, Feldman ST. Intraocular pressure elevation associated with inhalation and nasal corticosteroids. Ophthalmology 1995;102(2):177–9.
58. Kwok AK, Lam DS, Ng JS, Fan DS, Chew SJ, Tso MO. Ocular-hypertensive response to topical steroids in children. Ophthalmology 1997;104(12):2112–16.
59. Gass JD, Little H. Bilateral bullous exudative retinal detachment complicating idiopathic central serous chorioretinopathy during systemic corticosteroid therapy. Ophthalmology 1995;102(5):737–47.
60. Apel A, Campbell I, Rootman DS. Infectious crystalline keratopathy following trabeculectomy and low-dose topical steroids. Cornea 1995;14(3):321–3.
61. Rao GP, O'Brien C, Hicky-Dwyer M, Patterson A. Rapid onset bilateral calcific band keratopathy associated with phosphate-containing steroid eye drops. Eur J Implant Refractive Surg 1995;7:251–2.
62. Ramanathan R, Siassi B, deLemos RA. Severe retinopathy of prematurity in extremely low birth weight infants after short-term dexamethasone therapy. J Perinatol 1995;15(3):178–82.
63. Kushner FH, Olson JC. Retinal hemorrhage as a consequence of epidural steroid injection. Arch Ophthalmol 1995;113(3):309–13.
64. Byers B. Blindness secondary to steroid injections into the nasal turbinates. Arch Ophthalmol 1979;97(1):79–80.
65. Van Dalen JT, Sherman MD. Corticosteroid-induced exophthalmos. Doc Ophthalmol 1989;72(3–4):273–7.
66. Klein JF. Adverse psychiatric effects of systemic glucocorticoid therapy. Am Fam Physician 1992;46(5): 1469–74.
67. Doherty M, Garstin I, McClelland RJ, Rowlands BJ, Collins BJ. A steroid stupor in a surgical ward. Br J Psychiatry 1991;158:125–7.
68. Satel SL. Mental status changes in children receiving glucocorticoids. Review of the literature. Clin Pediatr (Phila) 1990;29(7):383–8.
69. Alpert E, Seigerman C. Steroid withdrawal psychosis in a patient with closed head injury. Arch Phys Med Rehabil 1986;67(10):766–9.
70. Hassanyeh F, Murray RB, Rodgers H. Adrenocortical suppression presenting with agitated depression, morbid jealousy, and a dementia-like state. Br J Psychiatry 1991;159:870–2.
71. Nahon S, Pisanté L, Delas N. A successful switch from prednisone to budesonide for neuropsychiatric adverse effects in a patient with ileal Crohn's disease. Am J Gastroenterol 2001;96(1):1953–4.
72. O'Shea TM, Kothadia JM, Klinepeter KL, Goldstein DJ, Jackson BG, Weaver RG III, Dillard RG. Randomized placebo-controlled trial of a 42-day tapering course of dexamethasone to reduce the duration of ventilator dependency in very low birth weight infants: outcome of study participants at 1-year adjusted age. Pediatrics 1999;104(1 Part 1):15–21.
73. Soliday E, Grey S, Lande MB. Behavioral effects of corticosteroids in steroid–sensitive nephrotic syndrome. Pediatrics 1999;104(4):e51.
74. Kaiser H. Psychische Storungen nach Beclomethasondipropionat-Inhalation? [Mental disorders following beclomethasone dipropionate inhalation?] Med Klin 1978;73(38):1334.
75. Keenan PA, Jacobson MW, Soleymani RM, Mayes MD, Stress ME, Yaldoo DT. The effect on memory of chronic prednisone treatment in patients with systemic disease. Neurology 1996;47(6):1396–402.
76. Oliveri RL, Sibilia G, Valentino P, Russo C, Romeo N, Quattrone A. Pulsed methylprednisolone induces a reversible impairment of memory in patients with relapsing-remitting multiple sclerosis. Acta Neurol Scand 1998;97(6):366–9.
77. Newcomer JW, Selke G, Melson AK, Hershey I, Craft S, Richards K, Alderson AL. Decreased memory performance in healthy humans induced by stress-level cortisol treatment. Arch Gen Psychiatry 1999;56(6):527–33.
78. Aisen PS, Davis KL, Berg JD, Schafer K, Campbell K, Thomas RG, Weiner MF, Farlow MR, Sano M, Grundman M, Thal LJ. A randomized controlled trial of prednisone in Alzheimer's disease. Alzheimer's Dis Cooperative Study. Neurology 2000;54(3):588–93.
79. de Quervain DJ, Roozendaal B, Nitsch RM, McGaugh JL, Hock C. Acute cortisone administration impairs retrieval of long-term declarative memory in humans. Nat Neurosci 2000;3(4):313–14.
80. Moser NJ, Phillips BA, Guthrie G, Barnett G. Effects of dexamethasone on sleep. Pharmacol Toxicol 1996;79(2):100–2.
81. Preda A, Fazeli A, McKay BG, Bowers MB Jr, Mazure CM. Lamotrigine as prophylaxis against steroid-induced mania. J Clin Psychiatry 1999;60(10):708–9.
82. Preda A, Fazeli A, McKay BG, Bowers MB Jr, Mazure CM. Lamotrigine of prophylaxis against steroid-induced mania. J. Clin Psychiatry 1999;60(10):708–9.
83. Brown ES, Suppes T, Khan DA, Carmody TJ 3rd. Mood changes during prednisone bursts in outpatients with asthma. J Clin Psychopharmacol 2002;22(1):55–61.
84. Ilbeigi MS, Davidson ML, Yarmush JM. An unexpected arousal effect of etomidate in a patient on high-dose steroids. Anesthesiology 1998;89(6):1587–9.
85. Kramer TM, Cottingham EM. Risperidone in the treatment of steroid-induced psychosis. J Child Adolesc Psychopharmacol 1999;9(4):315–6.
86. Scheschonka A, Bleich S, Buchwald AB, Ruther E, Wiltfang J. Development of obsessive-compulsive behaviour following cortisone treatment. Pharmacopsychiatry 2002;35(2):72–4.

87. Kamoda T, Nakahara C, Matsui A. A case of empty sella after steroid pulse therapy for nephrotic syndrome. J Rheumatol 1998;25(4):822–3.
88. Rabhan NB. Pituitary-adrenal suppression and Cushing's syndrome after intermittent dexamethasone therapy. Ann Intern Med 1968;69(6):1141–8.
89. Zwaan CM, Odink RJ, Delemarre-van de Waal HA, Dankert-Roelse JE, Bokma JA. Acute adrenal insufficiency after discontinuation of inhaled corticosteroid therapy. Lancet 1992;340(8830):1289–90.
90. Clark DJ, Grove A, Cargill RI, Lipworth BJ. Comparative adrenal suppression with inhaled budesonide and fluticasone propionate in adult asthmatic patients. Thorax 1996;51(3):262–6.
91. Marazzi MG, Agnese G, Gremmo M, Cotellessa M, Garibaldi L. Problemi relativi alla funzionalita surrenalica in corso di terapia cortisonica protratta in soggetti con epatite cronica: nota preliminare. [Problems concerning adrenal function during prolonged corticoid treatment in patients with chronic hepatitis. Preliminary note.] Minerva Pediatr 1978;30(11):937–44.
92. Dutau G, Rochiccioli P. Exploration corticotrope au cours des traitements prolongés par le dipropionate de béclométhasone chez l'enfant. [Corticotropic testing during long-term beclomethasone dipropionate treatment asthmatic children.] Poumon Coeur 1978;34(4):247–53.
93. Sumboonnanonda A, Vongjirad A, Suntornpoch V, Petrarat S. Adrenal function after prednisolone treatment in childhood nephrotic syndrome. J Med Assoc Thai 1994;77(3):126–9.
94. Felner EI, Thompson MT, Ratliff AF, White PC, Dickson BA. Time course of recovery of adrenal function in children treated for leukemia. J Pediatr 2000;137(1):21–4.
95. Reiner M, Galeazzi RL, Studer H. Cushing-Syndrom und Nebennierenrinden-Suppression durch intranasale Anwendung von Dexamethasonpraparaten. [Cushing's syndrome and adrenal suppression by means of intranasal use of dexamethasone preparations.] Schweiz Med Wochenschr 1977;107(49):1836–7.
96. Kay J, Findling JW, Raff H. Epidural triamcinolone suppresses the pituitary–adrenal axis in human subjects. Anesth Analg 1994;79(3):501–5.
97. Boonen S, Van Distel G, Westhovens R, Dequeker J. Steroid myopathy induced by epidural triamcinolone injection. Br J Rheumatol 1995;34(4):385–6.
98. Kobayashi S, Warabi H, Hashimoto H. Hypopituitarism with empty sella after steroid pulse therapy. J Rheumatol 1997;24(1):236–8.
99. Grabner W. Zur induzierten NNR-Insuffizienz bei chirurgischen Eingriffen. [Problems of corticosteroid-induced adrenal insufficiency in surgery.] Fortschr Med 1977;95(30): 1866–8.
100. Mukai T. [Antagonism between parathyroid hormone and glucocorticoids in calcium and phosphorus metabolism.] Nippon Naibunpi Gakkai Zasshi 1965;41(8):950–9.
101. Kahn A, Snapper I, Drucker A. Corticosteroid-induced tetany in latent hypoparathyroidism. Arch Intern Med 1964;114:434–8.
102. Fisher JE, Smith RS, Lagrandeur R, Lorenz RP. Gestational diabetes mellitus in women receiving beta-adrenergics and corticosteroids for threatened preterm delivery. Obstet Gynecol 1997;90(6):880–3.
103. Kim YS, Kim MS, Kim SI, Lim SK, Lee HY, Han DS, Park K. Post-transplantation diabetes is better controlled after conversion from prednisone to deflazacort: a prospective trial in renal transplants. Transpl Int 1997;10(3):197–201.
104. Gurwitz JH, Bohn RL, Glynn RJ, Monane M, Mogun H, Avorn J. Glucocorticoids and the risk for initiation of hypoglycemic therapy. Arch Intern Med 1994;154(1): 97–101.
105. Bagdade JD, Porte D Jr, Bierman EL. Steroid-induced lipemia. A complication of high-dosage corticosteroid therapy. Arch Intern Med 1970;125(1):129–34.
106. Ettinger WH Jr, Hazzard WR. Elevated apolipoprotein-B levels in corticosteroid-treated patients with systemic lupus erythematosus. J Clin Endocrinol Metab 1988;67(3):425–8.
107. Amin SB, Sinkin RA, McDermott MP, Kendig JW. Lipid intolerance in neonates receiving dexamethasone for bronchopulmonary dysplasia. Arch Pediatr Adolesc Med 1999;153(8):795–800.
108. Tiley C, Grimwade D, Findlay M, Treleaven J, Height S, Catalano J, Powles R. Tumour lysis following hydrocortisone prior to a blood product transfusion in T-cell acute lymphoblastic leukaemia. Leuk Lymphoma 1992;8(1–2): 143–6.
109. Lerza R, Botta M, Barsotti B, Schenone E, Mencoboni M, Bogliolo G, Pannacciulli I, Arboscello E. Dexamethazone-induced acute tumor lysis syndrome in a T-cell malignant lymphoma. Leuk Lymphoma 2002;43(5):1129–32.
110. Balli F, Benatti C. Terapia corticosteroidea protratta e metabolismo fosfo-calcico. II. Modificazioni del metabolismo fosfo-calcico in soggetti nefrosici sattoposti a terapia carticosteroidea protratta. [Prolonged corticosteroid therapy and phospho-calcic metabolism. II. Changes of phospho-calcic metabolism in nephrotic subjects subjected to prolonged corticoid therapy.] Minerva Pediatr 1968;20(45): 2315–25.
111. Handa R, Wali JP, Singh RI, Aggarwal P. Corticosteroids precipitating hypocalcemic encephalopathy in hypoparathyroidism. Ann Emerg Med 1995;26(2):241–2.
112. Ravina A, Slezak L, Mirsky N, Bryden NA, Anderson RA. Reversal of corticosteroid-induced diabetes mellitus with supplemental chromium. Diabet Med 1999;16(2):164–7.
113. Schneider J, Burmeister H, Ruiz-Torres A. Langzeitstudien uber die Wirksamkeit der Dauertherapie bei hyperergisch-allergischen Erkrankungen mit Prednisolon. [Longitudinal study about the efficacy of long term prednisolone therapy in hyperergic-allergic diseases.] Verh Dtsch Ges Inn Med 1977;83:1785–8.
114. Schmand B, Neuvel J, Smolders-de Haas H, Hoeks J, Treffers PE, Koppe JG. Psychological development of children who were treated antenatally with corticosteroids to prevent respiratory distress syndrome. Pediatrics 1990;86(1):58–64.
115. Bielawski D, Hiatt IM, Hegyi T. Betamethasone-induced leukaemoid reaction in pre-term infant. Lancet 1978;1(8057):218–19.
116. Craddock CG. Corticosteroid-induced lymphopenia, immunosuppression, and body defense. Ann Intern Med 1978;88(4):564–6.
117. Saxon A, Stevens RH, Ramer SJ, Clements PJ, Yu DT. Glucocorticoids administered in vivo inhibit human suppressor T lymphocyte function and diminish B lymphocyte responsiveness in in vitro immunoglobulin synthesis. J Clin Invest 1978;61(4):922–30.
118. Maeshima E, Yamada Y, Yukawa S. Fever and leucopenia with steroids. Lancet 2000;355(9199):198.
119. Patrassi GM, Sartori MT, Livi U, Casonato A, Danesin C, Vettore S, Girolami A. Impairment of fibrinolytic potential in long-term steroid treatment after heart transplantation. Transplantation 1997;64(11):1610–14.
120. The British Thoracic and Tuberculosis Association. Inhaled corticosteroids compared with oral prednisone in patients starting long-term corticosteroid therapy for asthma. Lancet 1975;2(7933):469–73.

121. Salzman GA, Pyszczynski DR. Oropharyngeal candidiasis in patients treated with beclomethasone dipropionate delivered by metered-dose inhaler alone and with Aerochamber. J Allergy Clin Immunol 1988;81(2):424–8.
122. Linder N, Kuint J, German B, Lubin D, Loewenthal R. Hypertrophy of the tongue associated with inhaled corticosteroid therapy in premature infants. J Pediatr 1995;127(4):651–3.
123. Spiro HM. Is the steroid ulcer a myth? N Engl J Med 1983;309(1):45–7.
124. Messer J, Reitman D, Sacks HS, Smith H Jr, Chalmers TC. Association of adrenocorticosteroid therapy and peptic-ulcer disease. N Engl J Med 1983;309(1):21–4.
125. Conn HO, Poynard T. Corticosteroids and peptic ulcer: meta-analysis of adverse events during steroid therapy. J Intern Med 1994;236(6):619–32.
126. Henry DA, Johnston N, Dobson A, Duggan J. Fatal peptic ulcer complications and the use of non-steroidal antiinflammatory drugs, aspirin, and corticosteroids. BMJ (Clin Res Ed) 1987;295:1227.
127. Suazo-Barahona J, Gallegos J, Carmona-Sanchez R, Martinez R, Robles-Diaz G. Nonsteroidal anti-inflammatory drugs and gastrocolic fistula. J Clin Gastroenterol 1998;26(4):343–5.
128. Shimizu T, Yamashiro Y, Yabuta K. Impaired increase of prostaglandin E2 in gastric juice during steroid therapy in children. J Paediatr Child Health 1994;30(2):169–72.
129. Yamanishi Y, Yamana S, Ishioka S, Yamakido M. Development of ischemic colitis and scleroderma renal crisis following methylprednisolone pulse therapy for progressive systemic sclerosis. Intern Med 1996; 35(7):583–6.
130. Dwarakanath AD, Nash J, Rhodes JM. "Conversion" from ulcerative colitis to Crohn's disease associated with corticosteroid treatment. Gut 1994;35(8):1141–4.
131. Sharma R, Gupta KL, Ammon RH, Gambert SR. Atypical presentation of colon perforation related to corticosteroid use. Geriatrics 1997;52(5):88–90.
132. Candelas G, Jover JA, Fernandez B, Rodriguez-Olaverri JC, Calatayud J. Perforation of the sigmoid colon in a rheumatoid arthritis patient treated with methylprednisolone pulses. Scand J Rheumatol 1998;27(2): 152–3.
133. Weissel M, Hauff W. Fatal liver failure after high-dose glucocorticoid pulse therapy in a patient with severe thyroid eye disease. Thyroid 2000;10(6):521.
134. Nanki T, Koike R, Miyasaka N. Subacute severe steatohepatitis during prednisolone therapy for systemic lupus erythematosis. Am J Gastroenterol 1999;94(11):3379.
135. Dourakis SP, Sevastianos VA, Kaliopi P. Acute severe steatohepatitis related to prednisolone therapy. Am J Gastroenterol 2002;97(4):1074–5.
136. Verrips A, Rotteveel JJ, Lippens R. Dexamethasone-induced hepatomegaly in three children. Pediatr Neurol 1998;19(5):388–91.
137. Hamed I, Lindeman RD, Czerwinski AW. Case report: acute pancreatitis following corticosteroid and azathioprine therapy. Am J Med Sci 1978;276(2):211–19.
138. Di Fazano CS, Messica O, Quennesson S, Quennesson ER, Inaoui R, Vergne P, Bonnet C, Bertin P, Treves R. Two new cases of glucocorticoid-induced pancreatitis. Rev Rhum Engl Ed 1999;66(4):235.
139. Reichert LJ, Koene RA, Wetzels JF. Acute haemodynamic and proteinuric effects of prednisolone in patients with a nephrotic syndrome. Nephrol Dial Transplant 1999;14(1):91–7.
140. Charpin J, Arnaud A, Boutin C, Aubert J, Murisasco A, Gotte G. Long-term corticosteroid therapy and its effect on the kidney. Acta Allergol 1969;24(1):49–56.
141. Gray D, Shepherd H, Daar A, Oliver DO, Morris PJ. Oral versus intravenous high-dose steroid treatment of renal allograft rejection. The big shot or not? Lancet 1978;1(8056):117–18.
142. Toftegaard M, Knudsen F. Massive vasopressin-resistant polyuria induced by dexamethasone. Intensive Care Med 1995;21(3):238–40.
143. Editorial. Nocturia during steroid therapy. BMJ 1970;4(729):193–4.
144. Wendt H. Klinisch-pharmakologische Untersuchungen zur akneinduzierenden Wirkung von Fluorcortinbutylester. [Clinico-pharmacological studies on the acne-inducing action of fluocortin butylester.] Arzneimittelforschung 1977;27(11a):2245–6.
145. Bioulac P, Beylot C. Etude ultrastructurale d'une leucodermie secondaire à une injection intraarticulaire de corticoides. [Ultrastructural study of a leukoderma secondary to an intra-articular injection of corticoides.] Ann Dermatol Venereol 1977;104(12):883–5.
146. Bondy PhK. Disorders of the adrenal cortex. In: Wilson JD and Foster DW editors. Williams' Textbook of Endocrinology, 7th edn. Philadelphia: Saunders, 1985:816.
147. Reinhold K, Schneider L, Hunzelmann N, Krieg T, Scharffetter-Kochanek K. Delayed-type allergy to systemic corticosteroids. Allergy 2000;55(11):1095–6.
148. Shuster S, Raffle EJ, Bottoms E. Skin collagen in rheumatoid arthritis and the effect of corticosteroids. Lancet 1967;2:525.
149. Mathov E, Grad P, Scaglia H. Provocación de hemorrhagias uterinas anormales y hematomas subcutáneos por el uso de la acetonida de la triamcinoona en pacientes alérgicas. [Provocation of uterine hemorrhages and subcutaneous hematomas by the use of triamcinolone acetonide in allergic patients.] Prensa Med Argent 1971;58(16):826–9.
150. Roy A, Leblanc C, Paquette L, Ghezzo H, Cote J, Cartier A, Malo JL. Skin bruising in asthmatic subjects treated with high doses of inhaled steroids: frequency and association with adrenal function. Eur Respir J 1996;9(2):226–31.
151. Korting HC, Unholzer A, Schafer-Korting M, Tausch I, Gassmueller J, Nietsch KH. Different skin thinning potential of equipotent medium-strength glucocorticoids. Skin Pharmacol Appl Skin Physiol 2002;15(2):85–91.
152. Sener O, Caliskaner Z, Yazicioglu K, Karaayvaz M, Ozanguc N. Nonpigmenting solitary fixed drug eruption after skin testing and intra-articular injection of triamcinolone acetonide. Ann Allergy Asthma Immunol 2001;86(3):335–6.
153. Weber F, Barbaud A, Reichert-Penetrat S, Danchin A, Schmutz JL. Unusual clinical presentation in a case of contact dermatitis due to corticosteroids diagnosed by ROAT. Contact Dermatitis 2001;44(2):105–6.
154. Sener O, Caliskaner Z, Yazicioglu K, Karaayvaz M, Ozanguc N. Nonpigmenting solitary fixed drug eruption after skin testing and intra-articular injection of triamcinolone acetonide. Ann Allergy Asthma Immunol 2001;86(3):335–6.
155. Dooms-Goossens A, Andersen KE, Brandao FM, Bruynzeel D, Burrows D, Camarasa J, Ducombs G, Frosch P, Hannuksela M, Lachapelle JM, Lahti A, Menne T, Wahlberg JE, Wilkinson JD. Corticosteroid contact allergy: an EECDRG multicentre study. Contact Dermatitis 1996;35(1):40–4.
156. Quintiliani R. Hypersensitivity and adverse reactions associated with the use of newer intranasal corticosteroids for allergic rhinitis. Curr Ther Res Clin Exp 1996; 57:478–88.
157. Isaksson M, Bruze M, Goossens A, Lepoittevin JP. Patch testing with budesonide in serial dilutions. the significance

of dose, occlusion time and reading time. Contact Dermatitis 1999;40(1):24–31.
158. Murata T, Tanaka M, Dekio I, Tanikawa A, Nishikawa T. Allergic contact dermatitis due to clobetasone butyrate. Contact Dermatitis 2000;42(5):305.
159. O'Hagan AH, Corbett JR. Contact allergy to budesonide in a breath-actuated inhaler. Contact Dermatitis 1999; 41(1):53.
160. Lew DB, Higgins GC, Skinner RB, Snider MD, Myers LK. Adverse reaction to prednisone in a patient with systemic lupus erythematosus. Pediatr Dermatol 1999;16(2):146–50.
161. Garcia-Bravo B, Repiso JB, Camacho F. Systemic contact dermatitis due to deflazacort. Contact Dermatitis 2000;43(6):359–60.
162. Stingeni L, Caraffini S, Assalve D, Lapomarda V, Lisi P. Erythema-multiforme-like contact dermatitis from budesonide. Contact Dermatitis 1996;34(2):154–5.
163. Roujeau JC, Kelly JP, Naldi L, Rzany B, Stern RS, Anderson T, Auquier A, Bastuji-Garin S, Correia O, Locati F, Mockenhaupt M, Paoletti C, Shapiro S, Shear N, Schüpf E, Kaufman DW. Medication use and the risk of Stevens–Johnson syndrome or toxic epidermal necrolysis. N Engl J Med 1995;333(24):1600–7.
164. Ingber A, Trattner A, David M. Hypersensitivity to an oestrogen–progesterone preparation and possible relationship to autoimmune progesterone dermatitis and corticosteroid hypersensitivity. J Dermatol Treat 1999;10:139–40.
165. Picado C, Luengo M. Corticosteroid-induced bone loss. Prevention and management. Drug Saf 1996;15(5):347–59.
166. Wichers M, Springer W, Bidlingmaier F, Klingmuller D. The influence of hydrocortisone substitution on the quality of life and parameters of bone metabolism in patients with secondary hypocortisolism. Clin Endocrinol (Oxf) 1999;50(6):759–65.
167. Krogsgaard MR, Thamsborg G, Lund B. Changes in bone mass during low dose corticosteroid treatment in patients with polymyalgia rheumatica. a double blind, prospective comparison between prednisolone and deflazacort. Ann Rheum Dis 1996;55(2):143–6.
168. Goldstein MF, Fallon JJ Jr, Harning R. Chronic glucocorticoid therapy-induced osteoporosis in patients with obstructive lung disease. Chest 1999;116(6):1733–49.
169. Yosipovitch G, Hoon TS, Leok GC. Suggested rationale for prevention and treatment of glucocorticoid-induced bone loss in dermatologic patients. Arch Dermatol 2001;137(4):477–81.
170. Selby PL, Halsey JP, Adams KR, Klimiuk P, Knight SM, Pal B, Stewart IM, Swinson DR. Corticosteroids do not alter the threshold for vertebral fracture. J Bone Miner Res 2000;15(5):952–6.
171. Zelissen PM, Croughs RJ, van Rijk PP, Raymakers JA. Effect of glucocorticoid replacement therapy on bone mineral density in patients with Addison disease. Ann Intern Med 1994;120(3):207–10.
172. Valero MA, Leon M, Ruiz Valdepenas MP, Larrodera L, Lopez MB, Papapietro K, Jara A, Hawkins F. Bone density and turnover in Addison's disease: effect of glucocorticoid treatment. Bone Miner 1994;26(1):9–17.
173. Heiner JP, Joyce MJ, Carter JR, Makley JT. Atraumatic posterior pelvic ring fractures simulating metastatic disease in patients with metabolic bone disease. Orthopedics 1994;17(3):285–9.
174. Baltzan MA, Suissa S, Bauer DC, Cummings SR. Hip fractures attributable to corticosteroid use. Study Osteoporotic Fractures Group. Lancet 1999;353(9161): 1327.
175. McKenzie R, Reynolds JC, O'Fallon A, Dale J, Deloria M, Blackwelder W, Straus SE. Decreased bone mineral density during low dose glucocorticoid administration in a randomized, placebo controlled trial. J Rheumatol 2000;27(9):2222–6.
176. Walsh LJ, Wong CA, Oborne J, Cooper S, Lewis SA, Pringle M, Hubbard R, Tattersfield AE. Adverse effects of oral corticosteroids in relation to dose in patients with lung disease. Thorax 2001;56(4):279–84.
177. van Everdingen AA, Jacobs JW, Siewertsz Van Reesema DR, Bijlsma JW. Low-dose prednisone therapy for patients with early active rheumatoid arthritis: clinical efficacy, disease-modifying properties, and side effects: a randomized, double-blind, placebo-controlled clinical trial. Ann Intern Med 2002;136(1):1–12.
178. Lukert BP, Adams JS. Calcium and phosphorus homeostasis in man. Effect Corticosteroids. Arch Intern Med 1976;136(11):1249–53.
179. Hahn TJ. Corticosteroid-induced osteopenia. Arch Intern Med 1978;138(Spec No):882–5.
180. Chesney RW, Mazess RB, Hamstra AJ, DeLuca HF, O'Reagan S. Reduction of serum-1, 25-dihydroxyvitamin-D3 in children receiving glucocorticoids. Lancet 1978;2(8100):1123–5.
181. Eastell R. Management of corticosteroid-induced osteoporosis. UK Consensus Group Meeting on Osteoporosis. J Intern Med 1995;237(5):439–47.
182. Goans RE, Weiss GH, Abrams SA, Perez MD, Yergey AL. Calcium tracer kinetics show decreased irreversible flow to bone in glucocorticoid treated patients. Calcif Tissue Int 1995;56(6):533–5.
183. Sasaki N, Kusano E, Ando Y, Yano K, Tsuda E, Asano Y. Glucocorticoid decreases circulating osteoprotegerin (OPG): possible mechanism for glucocorticoid induced osteoporosis. Nephrol Dial Transplant 2001;16(3):479–82.
184. Lespessailles E, Siroux V, Poupon S, Andriambelosoa N, Pothuaud L, Harba R, Benhamou CL. Long-term corticosteroid therapy induces mild changes in trabecular bone texture. J Bone Miner Res 2000;15(4):747–53.
185. Mateo L, Nolla JM, Bonnin MR, Navarro MA, Roig-Escofet D. Sex hormone status and bone mineral density in men with rheumatoid arthritis. J Rheumatol 1995;22(8):1455–60.
186. Harris M, Hauser S, Nguyen TV, Kelly PJ, Rodda C, Morton J, Freezer N, Strauss BJ, Eisman JA, Walker JL. Bone mineral density in prepubertal asthmatics receiving corticosteroid treatment. J Paediatr Child Health 2001;37(1):67–71.
187. Lane NE. An update on glucocorticoid-induced osteoporosis. Rheum Dis Clin North Am 2001;27(1):235–53.
188. Henderson NK, Sambrook PN, Kelly PJ, Macdonald P, Keogh AM, Spratt P, Eisman JA. Bone mineral loss and recovery after cardiac transplantation. Lancet 1995;346(8979):905.
189. Garton MJ, Reid DM. Bone mineral density of the hip and of the anteroposterior and lateral dimensions of the spine in men with rheumatoid arthritis. Effects of low-dose corticosteroids. Arthritis Rheum 1993;36(2):222–8.
190. Saito JK, Davis JW, Wasnich RD, Ross PD. Users of low-dose glucocorticoids have increased bone loss rates: a longitudinal study. Calcif Tissue Int 1995;57(2):115–19.
191. Buckley LM, Leib ES, Cartularo KS, Vacek PM, Cooper SM. Effects of low dose corticosteroids on the bone mineral density of patients with rheumatoid arthritis. J Rheumatol 1995;22(6):1055–9.
192. Fryer JP, Granger DK, Leventhal JR, Gillingham K, Najarian JS, Matas AJ. Steroid-related complications in the cyclosporine era. Clin Transplant 1994;8(3 Part 1): 224–9.
193. Wolpaw T, Deal CL, Fleming-Brooks S, Bartucci MR, Schulak JA, Hricik DE. Factors influencing vertebral bone density after renal transplantation. Transplantation 1994;58(11):1186–9.

194. Yun YS, Kim BJ, Hong SP, Lee TW, Lim CG, Kim MJ. Changes of bone metabolism indices in patients receiving immunosuppressive therapy including low doses of steroids after renal transplantation. Transplant Proc 1996;28(3):1561–4.
195. Saisu T, Sakamoto K, Yamada K, Kashiwabara H, Yokoyama T, Iida S, Harada Y, Ikenoue S, Sakamoto M, Moriya H. High incidence of osteonecrosis of femoral head in patients receiving more than 2 g of intravenous methylprednisolone after renal transplantation. Transplant Proc 1996;28(3):1559–60.
196. Naganathan V, Jones G, Nash P, Nicholson G, Eisman J, Sambrook PN. Vertebral fracture risk with long-term corticosteroid therapy: prevalence and relation to age, bone density, and corticosteroid use. Arch Intern Med 2000;160(19):2917–22.
197. Tattersfield AE, Town GI, Johnell O, Picado C, Aubier M, Braillon P, Karlstrom R. Bone mineral density in subjects with mild asthma randomized to treatment with inhaled corticosteroids or non-corticosteroid treatment for two years. Thorax 2001;56(4):272–8.
198. Sambrook PN. Corticosteroid osteoporosis: practical implications of recent trials. J Bone Miner Res 2000;15(9):1645–9.
199. American College of Rheumatology Task Force on Osteoporosis Guidelines. Recommendations for the prevention and treatment of glucocorticoid-induced osteoporosis. Arthritis Rheum 1996;39(11):1791–801.
200. Bone and Tooth Society. National Osteoporosis Society, Royal College of Physicians. Glucocorticoid-induced Osteoporosis. Guidelines for Prevention and Treatment. London: Royal College of Physicians, 2002.
201. Hart SR, Green B. Osteoporosis prophylaxis during corticosteroid treatment: failure to prescribe. Postgrad Med J 2002;78(918):242–3.
202. Gudbjornsson B, Juliusson UI, Gudjonsson FV. Prevalence of long term steroid treatment and the frequency of decision making to prevent steroid induced osteoporosis in daily clinical practice. Ann Rheum Dis 2002;61(1):32–6.
203. Cino M, Greenberg GR. Bone mineral density in Crohn's disease: a longitudinal study of budesonide, prednisone, and nonsteroid therapy. Am J Gastroenterol 2002; 97(4):915–21.
204. Schwid SR, Goodman AD, Puzas JE, McDermott MP, Mattson DH. Sporadic corticosteroid pulses and osteoporosis in multiple sclerosis. Arch Neurol 1996;53(8):753–7.
205. Lukert BP, Johnson BE, Robinson RG. Estrogen and progesterone replacement therapy reduces glucocorticoid-induced bone loss. J Bone Miner Res 1992;7(9):1063–9.
206. Buckley LM, Leib ES, Cartularo KS, Vacek PM, Cooper SM. Calcium and vitamin D3 supplementation prevents bone loss in the spine secondary to low-dose corticosteroids in patients with rheumatoid arthritis. A randomized, double-blind, placebo-controlled trial. Ann Intern Med 1996;125(12):961–8.
207. Adachi JD, Bensen WG, Bianchi F, Cividino A, Pillersdorf S, Sebaldt RJ, Tugwell P, Gordon M, Steele M, Webber C, Goldsmith CH. Vitamin D and calcium in the prevention of corticosteroid induced osteoporosis: a 3 year followup J Rheumatol 1996;23(6): 995–1000.
208. Talalaj M, Gradowska L, Marcinowska-Suchowierska E, Durlik M, Gaciong Z, Lao M. Efficiency of preventive treatment of glucocorticoid-induced osteoporosis with 25-hydroxyvitamin D3 and calcium in kidney transplant patients. Transplant Proc 1996;28(6):3485–7.
209. Warady BD, Lindsley CB, Robinson FG, Lukert BP. Effects of nutritional supplementation on bone mineral status of children with rheumatic diseases receiving corticosteroid therapy. J Rheumatol 1994;21(3):530–5.
210. Luengo M, Pons F, Martinez de Osaba MJ, Picado C. Prevention of further bone mass loss by nasal calcitonin in patients on long term glucocorticoid therapy for asthma: a two year follow up study. Thorax 1994; 49(11):1099–102.
211. Healey JH, Paget SA, Williams-Russo P, Szatrowski TP, Schneider R, Spiera H, Mitnick H, Ales K, Schwartzberg P. A randomized controlled trial of salmon calcitonin to prevent bone loss in corticosteroid-treated temporal arteritis and polymyalgia rheumatica. Calcif Tissue Int 1996;58(2):73–80.
212. Adachi JD, Bensen WG, Bell MJ, Bianchi FA, Cividino AA, Craig GL, Sturtridge WC, Sebaldt RJ, Steele M, Gordon M, Themeles E, Tugwell P, Roberts R, Gent M. Salmon calcitonin nasal spray in the prevention of corticosteroid-induced osteoporosis. Br J Rheumatol 1997;36(2):255–9.
213. Mulder H, Struys A. Intermittent cyclical etidronate in the prevention of corticosteroid-induced bone loss. Br J Rheumatol 1994;33(4):348–50.
214. Diamond T, McGuigan L, Barbagallo S, Bryant C. Cyclical etidronate plus ergocalciferol prevents glucocorticoid-induced bone loss in postmenopausal women. Am J Med 1995;98(5):459–63.
215. Roux C, Oriente P, Laan R, Hughes RA, Ittner J, Goemaere S, Di Munno O, Pouilles JM, Horlait S, Cortet B. Randomized trial of effect of cyclical etidronate in the prevention of corticosteroid-induced bone loss. Ciblos Study Group. J Clin Endocrinol Metab 1998;83(4):1128–33.
216. Pitt P, Li F, Todd P, Webber D, Pack S, Moniz C. A double blind placebo controlled study to determine the effects of intermittent cyclical etidronate on bone mineral density in patients on long-term oral corticosteroid treatment. Thorax 1998;53(5):351–6.
217. Nordborg E, Schaufelberger C, Andersson R, Bosaeus I, Bengtsson BA. The ineffectiveness of cyclical oral clodronate on bone mineral density in glucocorticoid-treated patients with giant-cell arteritis. J Intern Med 1997;242(5):367–71.
218. Boutsen Y, Jamart J, Esselinckx W, Stoffel M, Devogelaer JP. Primary prevention of glucocorticoid-induced osteoporosis with intermittent intravenous pamidronate: a randomized trial. Calcif Tissue Int 1997;61(4):266–71.
219. Wallach S, Cohen S, Reid DM, Hughes RA, Hosking DJ, Laan RF, Doherty SM, Maricic M, Rosen C, Brown J, Barton I, Chines AA. Effects of risedronate treatment on bone density and vertebral fracture in patients on corticosteroid therapy. Calcif Tissue Int 2000;67(4):277–85.
220. Reid DM, Hughes RA, Laan RF, Sacco-Gibson NA, Wenderoth DH, Adami S, Eusebio RA, Devogelaer JP. Efficacy and safety of daily risedronate in the treatment of corticosteroid-induced osteoporosis in men and women: a randomized trial. European Corticosteroid-Induced Osteoporosis Treatment Study. J Bone Miner Res 2000;15(6):1006–13.
221. Adachi JD, Saag KG, Delmas PD, Liberman UA, Emkey RD, Seeman E, Lane NE, Kaufman JM, Poubelle PE, Hawkins F, Correa-Rotter R, Menkes CJ, Rodriguez-Portales JA, Schnitzer TJ, Block JA, Wing J, McIlwain HH, Westhovens R, Brown J, Melo-Gomes JA, Gruber BL, Yanover MJ, Leite MO, Siminoski KG, Nevitt MC, Sharp JT, Malice MP, Dumortier T, Czachur M, Carofano W, Daifotis A. Two-year effects of alendronate on bone mineral density and vertebral fracture in patients receiving glucocorticoids: a randomized,

double-blind, placebo-controlled extension trial. Arthritis Rheum 2001;44(1):202–11.
222. Rizzoli R, Chevalley T, Slosman DO, Bonjour JP. Sodium monofluorophosphate increases vertebral bone mineral density in patients with corticosteroid-induced osteoporosis. Osteoporos Int 1995;5(1):39–46.
223. Giustina A, Bussi AR, Jacobello C, Wehrenberg WB. Effects of recombinant human growth hormone (GH) on bone and intermediary metabolism in patients receiving chronic glucocorticoid treatment with suppressed endogenous GH response to GH-releasing hormone. J Clin Endocrinol Metab 1995;80(1):122–9.
224. Yonemura K, Kimura M, Miyaji T, Hishida A. Short-term effect of vitamin K administration on prednisolone-induced loss of bone mineral density in patients with chronic glomerulonephritis. Calcif Tissue Int 2000;66(2):123–8.
225. Westeel FP, Mazouz H, Ezaitouni F, Hottelart C, Ivan C, Fardellone P, Brazier M, El Esper I, Petit J, Achard JM, Pruna A, Fournier A. Cyclosporine bone remodeling effect prevents steroid osteopenia after kidney transplantation. Kidney Int 2000;58(4):1788–96.
226. Abe H, Sako H, Okino K, Nakane Y, Kodama M, Park KI, Inoue H, Kim CJ, Tomoyoshi T. Clinical study of aseptic necrosis of bone after renal transplantation. Transplant Proc 1994;26(4):1987.
227. Alarcon GS, Mikhail I, Jaffe KA, Bradley LA, Bailey WC. Hip osteonecrosis secondary to the administration of corticosteroids for feigned bronchial asthma. The clinical spectrum of the factitious disorders. Arthritis Rheum 1994;37(1):139–41.
228. Lausten GS, Lemser T, Jensen PK, Egfjord M. Necrosis of the femoral head after kidney transplantation. Clin Transplant 1998;12(6):572–4.
229. Bauer M, Thabault P, Estok D, Chrinstiansen C, Platt R. Low-dose corticosteroids and avascular necrosis of the hip and knee. Pharmacoepidemiol Drug Saf 2000;9:187–91.
230. McKee MD, Waddell JP, Kudo PA, Schemitsch EH, Richards RR. Osteonecrosis of the femoral head in men following short-course corticosteroid therapy: a report of 15 cases. CMAJ 2001;164(2):205–6.
231. Virik K, Karapetis C, Droufakou S, Harper P. Avascular necrosis of bone: the hidden risk of glucocorticoids used as antiemetics in cancer chemotherapy. Int J Clin Pract 2001;55(5):344–5.
232. Gibson JN, Poyser NL, Morrison WL, Scrimgeour CM, Rennie MJ. Muscle protein synthesis in patients with rheumatoid arthritis: effect of chronic corticosteroid therapy on prostaglandin F2 alpha availability. Eur J Clin Invest 1991;21(4):406–12.
233. Ekstrand A, Schalin-Jantti C, Lofman M, Parkkonen M, Widen E, Franssila-Kallunki A, Saloranta C, Koivisto V, Groop L. The effect of (steroid) immunosuppression on skeletal muscle glycogen metabolism in patients after kidney transplantation. Transplantation 1996;61(6):889–93.
234. Anonymous. Corticosteroid myopathy. Lancet 1970;2:1118.
235. Janssens S, Decramer M. Corticosteroid-induced myopathy and the respiratory muscles. Report of two cases. Chest 1989;95(5):1160–2.
236. Weiner P, Azgad Y, Weiner M. The effect of corticosteroids on inspiratory muscle performance in humans. Chest 1993;104(6):1788–91.
237. Halpern AA, Horowitz BG, Nagel DA. Tendon ruptures associated with corticosteroid therapy. West J Med 1977;127(5):378–82.
238. Pai VS. Rupture of the plantar fascia. J Foot Ankle Surg 1996;35(1):39–40.
239. Motson RW, Glass DN, Smith DA, Daly JR. The effect of short- and long-term corticosteroid treatment on sleep-associated growth hormone secretion. Clin Endocrinol (Oxf) 1978;8(4):315–26.
240. Allen DB, Mullen M, Mullen B. A meta-analysis of the effect of oral and inhaled corticosteroids on growth. J Allergy Clin Immunol 1994;93(6):967–76.
241. Doull IJ, Freezer NJ, Holgate ST. Growth of prepubertal children with mild asthma treated with inhaled beclomethasone dipropionate. Am J Respir Crit Care Med 1995;151(6):1715–19.
242. Whitaker K, Webb J, Barnes J, Barnes ND. Effect of fluticasone on growth in children with asthma. Lancet 1996;348(9019):63–4.
243. Todd G, Dunlop K, McNaboe J, Ryan MF, Carson D, Shields MD. Growth and adrenal suppression in asthmatic children treated with high-dose fluticasone propionate. Lancet 1996;348(9019):27–9.
244. Travis LB, Chesney R, McEnery P, Moel D, Pennisi A, Potter D, Talwalkar YB, Wolff E. Growth and glucocorticoids in children with kidney disease. Kidney Int 1978;14(4):365–8.
245. Rivkees SA, Danon M, Herrin J. Prednisone dose limitation of growth hormone treatment of steroid-induced growth failure. J Pediatr 1994;125(2):322–5.
246. Lai HC, FitzSimmons SC, Allen DB, Kosorok MR, Rosenstein BJ, Campbell PW, Farrell PM. Risk of persistent growth impairment after alternate-day prednisone treatment in children with cystic fibrosis. N Engl J Med 2000;342(12):851–9.
247. Diczfalusy E, Landgren BM. Hormonal changes in the menstrual cycle. In: Diczfalusy D, editor. Regulation of Human Fertility. Copenhagen: Scriptor, 1977:21.
248. Cunningham GR, Goldzieher JW, de la Pena A, Oliver M. The mechanism of ovulation inhibition by triamcinolone acetonide. J Clin Endocrinol Metab 1978;46(1):8–14.
249. Mens JM, Nico de Wolf A, Berkhout BJ, Stam HJ. Disturbance of the menstrual pattern after local injection with triamcinolone acetonide. Ann Rheum Dis 1998;57(11):700.
250. Lopez-Serrano MC, Moreno-Ancillo A, Contreras J, Ortega N, Cabanas R, Barranco P, Munoz-Pereira M. Two cases of specific adverse reactions to systemic corticosteroids. J Invest Allergol Clin Immunol 1996;6(5):324–7.
251. Moreno-Ancillo A, Martin-Munoz F, Martin-Barroso JA, Diaz-Pena JM, Ojeda JA. Anaphylaxis to 6-alpha-methylprednisolone in an eight-year-old child. J Allergy Clin Immunol 1996;97(5):1169–71.
252. van den Berg JS, van Eikema Hommes OR, Wuis EW, Stapel S, van der Valk PG. Anaphylactoid reaction to intravenous methylprednisolone in a patient with multiple sclerosis. J Neurol Neurosurg Psychiatry 1997;63(6):813–14.
253. Figueredo E, Cuesta-Herranz JI, De Las Heras M, Lluch-Bernal M, Umpierrez A, Sastre J. Anaphylaxis to dexamethasone. Allergy 1997;52(8):877.
254. Mace S, Vadas P, Pruzanski W. Anaphylactic shock induced by intraarticular injection of methylprednisolone acetate. J Rheumatol 1997;24(6):1191–4.
255. Hayhurst M, Braude A, Benatar SR. Anaphylactic-like reaction to hydrocortisone. S Afr Med J 1978;53(7):259–60.
256. Srinivasan V, Lanham PR. Acute laryngeal obstruction – reaction to intravenous hydrocortisone? Eur J Anaesthesiol 1997;14(3):342.
257. Vaghjimal A, Rosenstreich D, Hudes G. Fever, rash and worsening of asthma in response to intravenous hydrocortisone. Int J Clin Pract 1999;53(7):567–8.
258. Clear D. Anaphylactoid reaction to methyl prednisolone developing after starting treatment with interferon beta-1b. J Neurol Neurosurg Psychiatry 1999;66(5):690.
259. Schonwald S. Methylprednisolone anaphylaxis. Am J Emerg Med 1999;17(6):583–5.

260. Vanpee D, Gillet JB. Allergic reaction to intravenous methylprednisolone in a woman with asthma. Ann Emerg Med 1998;32(6):754.
261. Polosa R, Prosperini G, Pintaldi L, Rey JP, Colombrita R. Anaphylaxis after prednisone. Allergy 1998;53(3):330–1.
262. Yawalkar N, Hari Y, Helbing A, von Greyerz S, Kappeler A, Baathen LR, Pichler WJ. Elevated serum levels of interleukins 5, 6, and 10 in a patient with drug-induced exanthem caused by systemic corticosteroids. J Am Acad Dermatol 1998;39(5 Part 1):790–3.
263. Heeringa M, Zweers P, de Man RA, de Groot H. Drug Points: Anaphylactic-like reaction associated with oral budesonide. BMJ 2000;321(7266):927.
264. Gomez CM, Higuero NC, Moral de Gregorio A, Quiles MH, Nunez Aceves AB, Lara MJ, Sanchez CS. Urticaria–angioedema by deflazacort. Allergy 2002;57(4):370–1.
265. Staunton H, Stafford F, Leader M, O'Riordain D. Deterioration of giant cell arteritis with corticosteroid therapy. Arch Neurol 2000;57(4):581–4.
266. Schols AM, Wesseling G, Kester AD, de Vries G, Mostert R, Slangen J, Wouters EF. Dose dependent increased mortality risk in COPD patients treated with oral glucocorticoids. Eur Respir J 2001;17(3):337–42.
267. Klaustermeyer WB, Gianos ME, Kurohara ML, Dao HT, Heiner DC. IgG subclass deficiency associated with corticosteroids in obstructive lung disease. Chest 1992;102(4):1137–42.
268. Robinson MJ, Campbell F, Powell P, Sims D, Thornton C. Antibody response to accelerated Hib immunisation in preterm infants receiving dexamethasone for chronic lung disease. Arch Dis Child Fetal Neonatal Ed 1999; 80(1):F69–71.
269. Sprung CL, Caralis PV, Marcial EH, Pierce M, Gelbard MA, Long WM, Duncan RC, Tendler MD, Karpf M. The effects of high-dose corticosteroids in patients with septic shock. A prospective, controlled study. N Engl J Med 1984;311(18):1137–43.
270. Mostafa BE. Fluticasone propionate is associated with severe infection after endoscopic polypectomy. Arch Otolaryngol Head Neck Surg 1996;122(7):729–31.
271. Demitsu T, Kosuge A, Yamada T, Usui K, Katayama H, Yaoita H. Acute generalized exanthematous pustulosis induced by dexamethasone injection. Dermatology 1996;193(1):56–8.
272. Hedderwick SA, Bonilla HF, Bradley SF, Kauffman CA. Opportunistic infections in patients with temporal arteritis treated with corticosteroids. J Am Geriatr Soc 1997;45(3):334–7.
273. Korula J. Tuberculous peritonitis complicating corticosteroid therapy for acute alcoholic hepatitis. Dig Dis Sci 1995;40(10):2119–20.
274. Kim HA, Yoo CD, Baek HJ, Lee EB, Ahn C, Han JS, Kim S, Lee JS, Choe KW, Song YW. *Mycobacterium tuberculosis* infection in a corticosteroid-treated rheumatic disease patient population. Clin Exp Rheumatol 1998;16(1):9–13.
275. di Girolamo C, Pappone N, Melillo E, Rengo C, Giuliano F, Melillo G. Cavitary lung tuberculosis in a rheumatoid arthritis patient treated with low-dose methotrexate and steroid pulse therapy. Br J Rheumatol 1998;37(10):1136–7.
276. Martos A, Podzamczer D, Martinez-Lacasa J, Rufi G, Santin M, Gudiol F. Steroids do not enhance the risk of developing tuberculosis or other AIDS-related diseases in HIV-infected patients treated for *Pneumocystis carinii* pneumonia. AIDS 1995;9(9):1037–41.
277. Bridges MJ, McGarry F. Two cases of *Mycobacterium avium* septic arthritis. Ann Rheum Dis 2002;61(2):186–7.
278. Fernandez-Aviles F, Batlle M, Ribera JM, Matas L, Sabria M, Feliu E. *Legionella* sp pneumonia in patients with hematologic diseases. A study of 10 episodes from a series of 67 cases of pneumonia. Haematologica 1999;84(5):474–5.
279. Rice P, Simmons K, Carr R, Banatvala J. Near fatal chickenpox during prednisolone treatment. BMJ 1994;309(6961):1069–70.
280. Choong K, Zwaigenbaum L, Onyett H. Severe varicella after low dose inhaled corticosteroids. Pediatr Infect Dis J 1995;14(9):809–11.
281. Burnett I. Severe chickenpox during treatment with corticosteroids. Immunoglobulin should be given if steroid dosage was > or = 0.5 mg/kg/day in preceding three months. BMJ 1995;310(6975):327. Erratum in BMJ 1995;310(6978):534.
282. Doherty MJ, Baxter AB, Longstreth WT Jr. Herpes simplex virus encephalitis complicating myxedema coma treated with corticosteroids. Neurology 2001;56(8):1114–5.
283. Pingleton WW, Bone RC, Kerby GR, Ruth WE. Oropharyngeal candidiasis in patients treated with triamcinolone acetonide aerosol. J Allergy Clin Immunol 1977;60(4):254–8.
284. Nenoff P, Horn LC, Mierzwa M, Leonhardt R, Weidenbach H, Lehmann I, Haustein UF. Peracute disseminated fatal *Aspergillus fumigatus* sepsis as a complication of corticoid-treated systemic lupus erythematosus. Mycoses 1995;38(11–12):467–71.
285. Wald A, Leisenring W, van Burik JA, Bowden RA. Epidemiology of *Aspergillus infections* in a large cohort of patients undergoing bone marrow transplantation. J Infect Dis 1997;175(6):1459–66.
286. Machet L, Jan V, Machet MC, Vaillant L, Lorette G. Cutaneous alternariosis: role of corticosteroid-induced cutaneous fragility. Dermatology 1996;193(4):342–4.
287. Fucci JC, Nightengale ML. Primary esophageal histoplasmosis. Am J Gastroenterol 1997;92(3):530–1.
288. Monlun E, de Blay F, Berton C, Gasser B, Jaeger A, Pauli G. Invasive pulmonary aspergillosis with cerebromeningeal involvement after short-term intravenous corticosteroid therapy in a patient with asthma. Respir Med 1997;91(7):435–7.
289. Shetty D, Giri N, Gonzalez CE, Pizzo PA, Walsh TJ. Invasive aspergillosis in human immunodeficiency virus-infected children. Pediatr Infect Dis J 1997;16(2):216–21.
290. Fernandez JM, Sanchez E, Polo FJ, Saez L. Infección pulmonar por *Aspergillus fumigatus* y *Nocardia asteroides* como complicación del tratamiento con glucocorticoides. Med Clin (Barc) 2000;114:358.
291. Carrascosa Porras M, Herreras Martinez R, Corral Mones J, Ares Ares M, Zabaleta Murguiondo M, Ruchel R. Fatal *Aspergillus* myocarditis following short-term corticosteroid therapy for chronic obstructive pulmonary disease. Scand J Infect Dis 2002;34(3):224–7.
292. Vogeser M, Haas A, Ruckdeschel G, von Scheidt W. Steroid-induced invasive aspergillosis with thyroid gland abscess and positive blood cultures. Eur J Clin Microbiol Infect Dis 1998;17(3):215–16.
293. Bower CP, Oxley JD, Campbell CK, Archer CB. Cutaneous *Scedosporium apiospermum* infection in an immunocompromised patient. J Clin Pathol 1999;52(11):846–8.
294. Ioannidou DJ, Stefanidou MP, Maraki SG, Panayiotides JG, Tosca AD. Cutaneous alternariosis in a patient with idiopathic pulmonary fibrosis. Int J Dermatol 2000;39(4):293–5.
295. Pera A, Byun A, Gribar S, Schwartz R, Kumar D, Parimi P. Dexamethasone therapy and *Candida* sepsis in neonates less than 1250 grams. J Perinatol 2002;22(3):204–8.

296. Sen P, Gil C, Estrellas B, Middleton JR. Corticosteroid-induced asthma: a manifestation of limited hyperinfection syndrome due to *Strongyloides stercoralis*. South Med J 1995;88(9):923–7.
297. Mariotta S, Pallone G, Li Bianchi E, Gilardi G, Bisetti A. *Strongyloides stercoralis* hyperinfection in a case of idiopathic pulmonary fibrosis. Panminerva Med 1996;38(1): 45–7.
298. Leung VK, Liew CT, Sung JJ. Fatal strongyloidiasis in a patient with ulcerative colitis after corticosteroid therapy. Am J Gastroenterol 1997;92(8):1383–4.
299. Schipperijn AJM. Flare-up of toxoplasmosis due to corticosteroid therapy in pulmonary sarcoidosis. Ned T Geneesk 1970;114:1710.
300. Cohen SN. Toxoplasmosis in patients receiving immunosuppressive therapy. JAMA 1970;211(4):657–60.
301. Sy ML, Chin TW, Nussbaum E. *Pneumocystis carinii* pneumonia associated with inhaled corticosteroids in an immunocompetent child with asthma. J Pediatr 1995;127(6):1000–2.
302. Bachelez H, Schremmer B, Cadranel J, Mouly F, Sarfati C, Agbalika F, Schlemmer B, Mayaud CM, Dubertret L. Fulminant *Pneumocystis carinii* pneumonia in 4 patients with dermatomyositis. Arch Intern Med 1997;157(13):1501–3.
303. Kanani SR, Knight R. Amoebic dysentery precipitated by corticosteroids. BMJ 1969;3(662):114.
304. Stark AR, Carlo WA, Tyson JE, Papile LA, Wright LL, Shankaran S, Donovan EF, Oh W, Bauer CR, Saha S, Poole WK, Stoll BJ. National Institute of Child Health and Human Development Neonatal Research Network. Adverse effects of early dexamethasone in extremely-low-birth-weight infants. National Institute of Child Health and Human Development Neonatal Research Network. N Engl J Med 2001;344(2):95–101.
305. Lucas A, Coll J, Salinas I, Sanmarti A. Hipertensión intracraneal benigna tras suspensión de corticoterapia en una paciente previaments intervenida por enfermedad de Cushing. [Benign intracranial hypertension following the suspension of corticotherapy in a female patient previously operated on for Cushing's disease.] Med Clin (Barc) 1991;97(12):473.
306. Richards D, Aronson J. The Oxford Handbook of Practical Drug Therapy. Oxford: Oxford University Press, 2004.
307. Morgan J, Lacey JH. Anorexia nervosa and steroid withdrawal. Int J Eat Disord 1996;19(2):213–15.
308. Silverman RA, Newman AJ, LeVine MJ, Kaplan B. Poststeroid panniculitis: a case report. Pediatr Dermatol 1988;5(2):92–3.
309. Le Gall C, Pham S, Vignes S, Garcia G, Nunes H, Fichet D, Simonneau G, Duroux P, Humbert M. Inhaled corticosteroids and Churg–Strauss syndrome: a report of five cases. Eur Respir J 2000;15(5):978–81.
310. Hodgkinson DJ, Williams TJ. Endometrial carcinoma associated with azathioprine and cortisone therapy. A case report. Gynecol Oncol 1977;5(3):308–12.
311. Erban SB, Sokas RK. Kaposi's sarcoma in an elderly man with Wegener's granulomatosis treated with cyclophosphamide and corticosteroids. Arch Intern Med 1988; 148(5):1201–3.
312. Thiagarajan CM, Divakar D, Thomas SJ. Malignancies in renal transplant recipients. Transplant Proc 1998; 30(7):3154–5.
313. Gill PS, Loureiro C, Bernstein-Singer M, Rarick MU, Sattler F, Levine AM. Clinical effect of glucocorticoids on Kaposi sarcoma related to the acquired immunodeficiency syndrome (AIDS). Ann Intern Med 1989; 110(11):937–40.
314. Tebbe B, Mayer-da-Silva A, Garbe C, von Keyserlingk HJ, Orfanos CE. Genetically determined coincidence of Kaposi sarcoma and psoriasis in an HIV-negative patient after prednisolone treatment. Spontaneous regression 8 months after discontinuing therapy. Int J Dermatol 1991;30(2):114–20.
315. Vincent T, Moss K, Colaco B, Venables PJ. Kaposi's sarcoma in two patients following low-dose corticosteroid treatment for rheumatological disease. Rheumatology (Oxford) 2000;39(11):1294–6.
316. Sorensen HT, Mellemkjaer L, Friis S, Olsen JH. Use of systemic corticosteroids and risk of esophageal cancer. Epidemiology 2002;13(2):240–1.
317. Committee on Fetus and Newborn. Postnatal corticosteroids to treat or prevent chronic lung disease in preterm infants. Pediatrics 2002;109(2):330–8.
318. Canadian Paediatric Society and American Academy of Pediatrics. Postnatal corticosteroids to treat or prevent chronic lung disease in preterm infants. Pediatr Child Health 2002;7:20–8.
319. Banks BA, Macones G, Cnaan A, Merrill JD, Ballard PL, Ballard RA; North American TRH Study Group. Multiple courses of antenatal corticosteroids are associated with early severe lung disease in preterm neonates.. J Perinatol 2002;22(2):101–7.
320. Elliott JP, Radin TG. The effect of corticosteroid administration on uterine activity and preterm labor in high-order multiple gestations. Obstet Gynecol 1995;85(2):250–4.
321. Schmitz T, Goffinet F, Barrande G, Cabrol D. Maternal hypercorticism from serial courses of betamethasone. Obstet Gynecol 1999;94(5 Part 2):849.
322. Helal KJ, Gordon MC, Lightner CR, Barth WH Jr Adrenal suppression induced by betamethasone in women at risk for premature delivery. Obstet Gynecol 2000;96(2):287–90.
323. Spencer C, Smith P, Rafla N, Weatherell R. Corticosteroids in pregnancy and osteonecrosis of the femoral head. Obstet Gynecol 1999;94(5 Part 2):848.
324. Vermillion ST, Soper DE, Chasedunn-Roark J. Neonatal sepsis after betamethasone administration to patients with preterm premature rupture of membranes. Am J Obstet Gynecol 1999;181(2):320–7.
325. Rotmensch S, Vishne TH, Celentano C, Dan M, Ben-Rafael Z. Maternal infectious morbidity following multiple courses of betamethasone. J Infect 1999;39(1):49–54.
326. Vermillion ST, Soper DE, Newman RB. Neonatal sepsis and death after multiple courses of antenatal betamethasone therapy. Am J Obstet Gynecol 2000; 183(4):810–14.
327. Abbasi S, Hirsch D, Davis J, Tolosa J, Stouffer N, Debbs R, Gerdes JS. Effect of single versus multiple courses of antenatal corticosteroids on maternal and neonatal outcome. Am J Obstet Gynecol 2000;182(5):1243–9.
328. Stockli A, Keller M. Kongenitales adrenogenitales Syndrom und Schwangerschaft. [Congenital adrenogenital syndrome and pregnancy.] Schweiz Med Wochenschr 1969;99(4):126–8.
329. Beique LC, Friesen MH, Park LY, Diaz-Citrin O, Koren G, Einarson TR. Major malformations associated with corticosteroid exposure during the first trimester: a meta-analysis. Can J Hosp Pharm 1998;51:83.
330. Moran P, Taylor R. Management of hyperemesis gravidarum: the importance of weight loss as a criterion for steroid therapy. QJM 2002;95(3):153–8.
331. Markert UR, Klemm A, Flossmann E, Werner W, Sperschneider H, Funfstuck R. Renal transplantation in early pregnancy with acute graft rejection and development of a hydatidiform mole. Clin Nephrol 1998; 49(6):391–2.

332. Park-Wyllie L, Mazzotta P, Pastuszak A, Moretti ME, Beique L, Hunnisett L, Friesen MH, Jacobson S, Kasapinovic S, Chang D, Diav-Citrin O, Chitayat D, Nulman I, Einarson TR, Koren G. Birth defects after maternal exposure to corticosteroids: prospective cohort study and meta-analysis of epidemiological studies. Teratology 2000;62(6):385–92.
333. Harding JE, Pang J, Knight DB, Liggins GC. Do antenatal corticosteroids help in the setting of preterm rupture of membranes? Am J Obstet Gynecol 2001;184(2):131–9.
334. Bloom SL, Sheffield JS, McIntire DD, Leveno KJ. Antenatal dexamethasone and decreased birth weight. Obstet Gynecol 2001;97(4):485–90.
335. Rotmensch S, Liberati M, Celentano C, Efrat Z, Bar-Hava I, Kovo M, Golan A, Moravski G, Ben-Rafael Z. The effect of betamethasone on fetal biophysical activities and Doppler velocimetry of umbilical and middle cerebral arteries. Acta Obstet Gynecol Scand 1999;78(9):768–73.
336. Warrell DW, Taylor R. Outcome for the foetus of mothers receiving prednisolone during pregnancy. Lancet 1968;1(7534):117–18.
337. Crowley PA. Antenatal corticosteroid therapy: a meta-analysis of the randomized trials, 1972–94. Am J Obstet Gynecol 1995;173(1):322–35.
338. Kairalla AB. Hypothalamic–pituitary–adrenal axis function in premature neonates after extensive prenatal treatment with betamethasone: a case history. Am J Perinatol 1992;9(5–6):428–30.
339. Ohrlander S, Gennser G, Nilsson KO, Eneroth P. ACTH test to neonates after administration of corticosteroids during gestation. Obstet Gynecol 1977;49(6):691–4.
340. Ohlsson A, Calvert SA, Hosking M, Shennan AT. Randomized controlled trial of dexamethasone treatment in very-low-birth-weight infants with ventilator-dependent chronic lung disease. Acta Paediatr 1992; 81(10):751–6.
341. Brownlee KG, Ng PC, Henderson MJ, Smith M, Green JH, Dear PR. Catabolic effect of dexamethasone in the preterm baby. Arch Dis Child 1992;67(1 Spec No):1–4.
342. O'Neil EA, Chwals WJ, O'Shea MD, Turner CS. Dexamethasone treatment during ventilator dependency: possible life threatening gastrointestinal complications. Arch Dis Child 1992;67(1 Spec No):10–1.
343. Harding JE, Pang J, Knight DB, Liggins GC. Do antenatal corticosteroids help in the setting of preterm rupture of membranes? Am J Obstet Gynecol 2001;184(2):131–9.
344. Rotmensch S, Celentano C, Liberati M, Sadan O, Glezerman M. The effect of antenatal steroid administration on the fetal response to vibroacoustic stimulation. Acta Obstet Gynecol Scand 1999;78(10):847–51.
345. Tornatore KM, Biocevich DM, Reed K, Tousley K, Singh JP, Venuto RC. Methylprednisolone pharmacokinetics, cortisol response, and adverse effects in black and white renal transplant recipients. Transplantation 1995;59(5):729–36.
346. Skoner DP. Balancing safety and efficacy in pediatric asthma management. Pediatrics 2002;109(Suppl 2):381–92.
347. Allen DB. Safety of inhaled corticosteroids in children. Pediatr Pulmonol 2002;33(3):208–20.
348. Thebaud B, Lacaze-Masmonteil T, Watterberg K. Postnatal glucocorticoids in very preterm infants: "the good, the bad, and the ugly"? Pediatrics 2001;107(2):413–5.
349. O'Callaghan JW, Brooks PM. Disease-modifying agents and immunosuppressive drugs in the elderly. Clin Rheum Dis 1986;2(1):275–89.
350. Akerkar GA, Peppercorn MA, Hamel MB, Parker RA. Corticosteroid-associated complications in elderly Crohn's disease patients. Am J Gastroenterol 1997;92(3):461–4.
351. Powell LW, Axelsen E. Corticosteroids in liver disease: studies on the biological conversion of prednisone to prednisolone and plasma protein binding. Gut 1972;13(9):690–6.
352. Davis M, Williams R, Chakraborty J, English J, Marks V, Ideo G, Tempini S. Prednisone or prednisolone for the treatment of chronic active hepatitis? A comparison of plasma availability. Br J Clin Pharmacol 1978;5(6):501–5.
353. Frey BM, Frey FJ. Clinical pharmacokinetics of prednisone and prednisolone. Clin Pharmacokinet 1990;19(2):126–46.
354. Harris RZ, Tsunoda SM, Mroczkowski P, Wong H, Benet LZ. The effects of menopause and hormone replacement therapies on prednisolone and erythromycin pharmacokinetics. Clin Pharmacol Ther 1996;59(4):429–35.
355. Lewis GP, Jusko WJ, Graves L, Burke CW. Prednisone side-effects and serum-protein levels. A collaborative study. Lancet 1971;2(7728):778–80.
356. Zonana-Nacach A, Barr SG, Magder LS, Petri M. Damage in systemic lupus erythematosus and its association with corticosteroids. Arthritis Rheum 2000;43(8):1801–8.
357. Keane FM, Munn SE, du Vivier AW, Taylor NF, Higgins EM. Analysis of Chinese herbal creams prescribed for dermatological conditions. BMJ 1999; 318(7183):563–4.
358. Reinberg AE. Chronopharmacology of corticosteroids and ACTH. In: Lammer B, editor. Chronopharmacology. Cellular and Biochemical Interactions. New York and Basel: Marcel Dekker Inc, 1989:137–67.
359. Kimura Y, Fieldston E, Devries-Vandervlugt B, Li S, Imundo L. High dose, alternate day corticosteroids for systemic onset juvenile rheumatoid arthritis. J Rheumatol 2000;27(8):2018–24.
360. Kaiser BA, Polinsky MS, Palmer JA, Dunn S, Mochon M, Flynn JT, Baluarte HJ. Growth after conversion to alternate-day corticosteroids in children with renal transplants: a single-center study. Pediatr Nephrol 1994;8(3):320–5.
361. Blair GP, Light RW. Treatment of chronic obstructive pulmonary disease with corticosteroids. Comparison of daily vs alternate-day therapy. Chest 1984;86(4):524–8.
362. Gilbertson EO, Spellman MC, Piacquadio DJ, Mulford MI. Super potent topical corticosteroid use associated with adrenal suppression: clinical considerations. J Am Acad Dermatol 1998;38(2 Part 2):318–21.
363. Marcos C, Allegue F, Luna I, Gonzalez R. An unusual case of allergic contact dermatitis from corticosteroids. Contact Dermatitis 1999;41(4):237–8.
364. Corazza M, Virgili A. Allergic contact dermatitis from 6alpha-methylprednisolone aceponate and budesonide. Contact Dermatitis 1998;38(6):356–7.
365. Mygind H, Thulstrup AM, Pedersen L, Larsen H. Risk of intrauterine growth retardation, malformations and other birth outcomes in children after topical use of corticosteroid in pregnancy. Acta Obstet Gynecol Scand 2002;81(3):234–9.
366. Whitcup SM, Ferris FL 3rd. New corticosteroids for the treatment of ocular inflammation. Am J Ophthalmol 1999;127(5):597–9.
367. Aggarwal RK, Potamitis T, Chong NH, Guarro M, Shah P, Kheterpal S. Extensive visual loss with topical facial steroids. Eye 1993;7(5):664–6.
368. Baratz KH, Hattenhauer MG. Indiscriminate use of corticosteroid-containing eyedrops. Mayo Clin Proc 1999;74(4):362–6.
369. Chua JK, Fan DS, Leung AT, Lam DS. Accelerated ocular hypertensive response after application of corticosteroid ointment to a child's eyelid. Mayo Clin Proc 2000;75(5):539.
370. Ozerdem U, Levi L, Cheng L, Song MK, Scher C, Freeman WR. Systemic toxicity of topical and periocular

corticosteroid therapy in an 11-year-old male with posterior uveitis. Am J Ophthalmol 2000;130(2):240–1.
371. Priftis K, Everard ML, Milner AD. Unexpected side-effects of inhaled steroids: a case report. Eur J Pediatr 1991;150(6):448–9.
372. Stead RJ, Cooke NJ. Adverse effects of inhaled corticosteroids. BMJ 1989;298(6671):403–4.
373. Whittet HB, Shinkwin C, Freeland AP. Anosmia due to nasal administration of corticosteroid. BMJ 1991;303(6803):651.
374. Bond DW, Charlton CP, Gregson RM. Benign intracranial hypertension secondary to nasal fluticasone propionate. BMJ 2001;322(7291):897.
375. Ozturk F, Yuceturk AV, Kurt E, Unlu HH, Ilker SS. Evaluation of intraocular pressure and cataract formation following the long-term use of nasal corticosteroids. Ear Nose Throat J 1998;77(10):846–51.
376. Cervin A, Andersson M. Intranasal steroids and septum perforation – an overlooked complication? A description of the course of events and a discussion of the causes. Rhinology 1998;36(3):128–32.
377. Nayak AS, Ellis MH, Gross GN, Mendelson LM, Schenkel EJ, Lanier BQ, Simpson B, Mullin ME, Smith JA. The effects of triamcinolone acetonide aqueous nasal spray on adrenocortical function in children with allergic rhinitis J Allergy Clin Immunol 1998;101(2 Part 1): 157–62.
378. Findlay CA, Macdonald JF, Wallace AM, Geddes N, Donaldson MD. Childhood Cushing's syndrome induced by betamethasone nose drops, and repeat prescriptions. BMJ 1998;317(7160):739–40.
379. Hillebrand-Haverkort ME, Prummel MF, ten Veen JH. Ritonavir-induced Cushing's syndrome in a patient treated with nasal fluticasone. AIDS 1999;13(13):1803.
380. Downs AM, Lear JT, Kennedy CT. Anaphylaxis to intradermal triamcinolone acetonide. Arch Dermatol 1998;134(9):1163–4.
381. Miranda-Romero A, Bajo-del Pozo C, Sanchez-Sambucety P, Martinez-Fernandez M, Garcia-Munoz M. Delayed local allergic reaction to intralesional paramethasone acetate. Contact Dermatitis 1998;39(1):31–2.
382. Wilkinson HA. Intrathecal Depo-Medrol: a literature review. Clin J Pain 1992;8(1):49–56.
383. DeSio JM, Kahn CH, Warfield CA. Facial flushing and/or generalized erythema after epidural steroid injection. Anesth Analg 1995;80(3):617–19.
384. Plumb VJ, Dismukes WE. Chemical meningitis related to intrathecal corticosteroid therapy. South Med J 1977;70(10):1241–3.
385. Dumont D, Hariz H, Meynieu P, Salama J, Dreyfus P, Boissier MC. Abducens palsy after an intrathecal glucocorticoid injection. Evidence for a role of intracranial hypotension. Rev Rhum Engl Ed 1998;65(5):352–4.
386. Spaccarelli KC. Lumbar and caudal epidural corticosteroid injections. Mayo Clin Proc 1996;71(2):169–78.
387. Chen YC, Gajraj NM, Clavo A, Joshi GP. Posterior subcapsular cataract formation associated with multiple lumbar epidural corticosteroid injections. Anesth Analg 1998;86(5):1054–5.
388. Siegfried RN. Development of complex regional pain syndrome after a cervical epidural steroid injection. Anesthesiology 1997;86(6):1394–6.
389. Sandberg DI, Lavyne MH. Symptomatic spinal epidural lipomatosis after local epidural corticosteroid injections: case report. Neurosurgery 1999;45(1):162–5.
390. Cooper AB, Sharpe MD. Bacterial meningitis and cauda equina syndrome after epidural steroid injections. Can J Anaesth 1996;43(5 Part 1):471–4.
391. McLain RF, Fry M, Hecht ST. Transient paralysis associated with epidural steroid injection. J Spinal Disord 1997;10(5):441–4.
392. Brocq O, Breuil V, Grisot C, Flory P, Ziegler G, Euller-Ziegler L. Diplopie après infiltrations peridurale et intradurale de prédnisolone. Deux observations. [Diplopia after peridural and intradural infiltrations of prednisolone. 2 cases.] Presse Méd 1997;26(6):271.
393. Lowell TD, Errico TJ, Eskenazi MS. Use of epidural steroids after discectomy may predispose to infection. Spine 2000;25(4):516–19.
394. Field J, Rathmell JP, Stephenson JH, Katz NP. Neuropathic pain following cervical epidural steroid injection. Anesthesiology 2000;93(3):885–8.
395. Sparling M, Malleson P, Wood B, Petty R. Radiographic followup of joints injected with triamcinolone hexacetonide for the management of childhood arthritis. Arthritis Rheum 1990;33(6):821–6.
396. Daragon A, Vittecoq O, Le Loet X. Visual hallucinations induced by intraarticular injection of steroids. J Rheumatol 1997;24(2):411.
397. Wicki J, Droz M, Cirafici L, Vallotton MB. Acute adrenal crisis in a patient treated with intraarticular steroid therapy. J Rheumatol 2000;27(2):510–11.
398. Valsecchi R, Reseghetti A, Leghissa P, Cologni L, Cortinovis R. Erythema-multiforme-like lesions from triamcinolone acetonide. Contact Dermatitis 1998;38(6):362–3.
399. Gutierrez-Urena S, Ramos-Remus C. Persistent hiccups associated with intraarticular corticosteroid injection. J Rheumatol 1999;26(3):760.
400. Montoro J, Valero A, Serra-Baldrich E, Amat P, Lluch M, Malet A. Anaphylaxis to paramethasone with tolerance to other corticosteroids. Allergy 2000;55(2):197–8.
401. Jawed S, Allard SA. Osteomyelitis of the humerus following steroid injections for tennis elbow. Rheumatology (Oxford) 2000;39(8):923–4.
402. Caffee HH. Intracapsular injection of triamcinolone for intractable capsule contracture. Plast Reconstr Surg 1994;94(6):824–8.
403. Braverman DL, Lachmann EA, Nagler W. Avascular necrosis of bilateral knees secondary to corticosteroid enemas. Arch Phys Med Rehabil 1998;79(4):449–52.
404. Tsuruoka S, Sugimoto K, Fujimura A. Drug-induced Cushing syndrome in a patient with ulcerative colitis after betamethasone enema: evaluation of plasma drug concentration. Ther Drug Monit 1998;20(4):387–9.
405. Lauerma AI. Occupational contact sensitization to corticosteroids. Contact Dermatitis 1998;39(6):328–9.
406. Newton RW, Browning MC, Iqbal J, Piercy N, Adamson DG. Adrenocortical suppression in workers manufacturing synthetic glucocorticoids. BMJ 1978; 1(6105):73–4.
407. Nixon DW, Shlaer SM. Fulminant lung metastases from cancer of the breast. Med Pediatr Oncol 1981;9(4):381–5.
408. Klygis LM. Dexamethasone-induced perineal irritation in head injury. Am J Emerg Med 1992;10(3):268.
409. Takayanagui OM, Lanchote VL, Marques MP, Bonato PS. Therapy for neurocysticercosis: pharmacokinetic interaction of albendazole sulfoxide with dexamethasone. Ther Drug Monit 1997;19(1):51–5.
410. Ahle GB, Blum AL, Martinek J, Oneta CM, Dorta G. Cushing's syndrome in an 81-year-old patient treated with budesonide and amiodarone. Eur J Gastroenterol Hepatol 2000;12(9):1041–2.
411. Costedoat-Chalumeau N, Amoura Z, Aymard G, Sevin O, Wechsler B, Du Cacoub PLT, Diquet B, Ankri A, Piette JC. Potentiation of vitamin K antagonists by high-dose intravenous methylprednisolone. Ann Intern Med 2000;132(8):631–5.
412. Varis T, Kaukonen KM, Kivisto KT, Neuvonen PJ. Plasma concentrations and effects of oral methylprednisolone are

considerably increased by itraconazole. Clin Pharmacol Ther 1998;64(4):363–8.
413. Varis T, Kivisto KT, Backman JT, Neuvonen PJ. Itraconazole decreases the clearance and enhances the effects of intravenously administered methylprednisolone in healthy volunteers. Pharmacol Toxicol 1999;85(1):29–32.
414. Varis T, Kivisto KT, Neuvonen PJ. The effect of itraconazole on the pharmacokinetics and pharmacodynamics of oral prednisolone. Eur J Clin Pharmacol 2000; 56(1):57–60.
415. Varis T, Kivisto KT, Backman JT, Neuvonen PJ. The cytochrome P450 3A4 inhibitor itraconazole markedly increases the plasma concentrations of dexamethasone and enhances its adrenal-suppressant effect. Clin Pharmacol Ther 2000;68(5):487–94.
416. Seidegard J. Reduction of the inhibitory effect of ketoconazole on budesonide pharmacokinetics by separation of their time of administration. Clin Pharmacol Ther 2000;68(1):13–17.
417. Varis T, Backman JT, Kivisto KT, Neuvonen PJ. Diltiazem and mibefradil increase the plasma concentrations and greatly enhance the adrenal-suppressant effect of oral methylprednisolone. Clin Pharmacol Ther 2000;67(3):215–21.
418. Quan VA, Saunders BP, Hicks BH, Sladen GE. Cyclosporin treatment for ulcerative colitis complicated by fatal *Pneumocystis carinii* pneumonia. BMJ 1997;314(7077):363–4.
419. Fost DA, Leung DY, Martin RJ, Brown EE, Szefler SJ, Spahn JD. Inhibition of methylprednisolone elimination in the presence of clarithromycin therapy. J Allergy Clin Immunol 1999;103(6):1031–5.
420. Finkenbine R, Gill HS. Case of mania due to prednisone–clarithromycin interaction. Can J Psychiatry 1997;42(7):778.
421. Belfayol-Pisante L, Guillevin L, Tod M, Fauvelle F. Possible influence of prednisone on the pharmacokinetics of cyclophosphamide in systemic vasculitis. Clin Drug Invest 1999;18:225–31.
422. Manchon ND, Bercoff E, Lemarchand P, Chassagne P, Senant J, Bourreille J. Frequence et gravité des interactions médicamenteuses dans une population agée: étude prospective concernant 639 malades. [Incidence and severity of drug interactions in the elderly. a prospective study of 639 patients.] Rev Med Interne 1989;10(6):521–5.
423. Varis T, Kivisto KT, Neuvonen PJ. Grapefruit juice can increase the plasma concentrations of oral methylprednisolone. Eur J Clin Pharmacol 2000;56(6–7):489–93.
424. Geller M. Marked peripheral edema associated with montelukast and prednisone. Ann Intern Med 2000;132(11):924.
425. Seidegard J, Simonsson M, Edsbacker S. Effect of an oral contraceptive on the plasma levels of budesonide and prednisolone and the influence on plasma cortisol. Clin Pharmacol Ther 2000;67(4):373–81.
426. Schönhofer PS. Interaktionen antirheumatisch wirksamer Substanzen. [Interactions of antirheumatic agents.] Internist (Berl) 1979;20(9):433–8.
427. Strayhorn VA, Baciewicz AM, Self TH. Update on rifampin drug interactions III. Arch Intern Med 1997;157(21):2453–8.
428. Dhanoa J, Natu M, Massey S. Worsening of steroid depending bronchial asthma following rifampicin administration. J Assoc Physicians India 1998;46(2):242.
429. Edelman J, Potter JM, Hackett LP. The effect of intra-articular steroids on plasma salicylate concentrations. Br J Clin Pharmacol 1986;21(3):301–7.
430. Nielsen GL, Sorensen HT, Mellemkjoer L, Blot WJ, McLaughlin JK, Tage-Jensen U, Olsen JH. Risk of hospitalization resulting from upper gastrointestinal bleeding among patients taking corticosteroids: a register-based cohort study. Am J Med 2001;111(7):541–5.
431. Garcia Rodriguez LA, Hernandez-Diaz S. The risk of upper gastrointestinal complications associated with non-steroidal anti-inflammatory drugs, glucocorticoids, acetaminophen, and combinations of these agents. Arthritis Res 2001;3(2):98–101.
432. Weil J, Langman MJ, Wainwright P, Lawson DH, Rawlins M, Logan RF, Brown TP, Vessey MP, Murphy M, Colin-Jones DG. Peptic ulcer bleeding: accessory risk factors and interactions with nonsteroidal anti-inflammatory drugs. Gut 2000;46(1):27–31.

Corticosteroids—glucocorticoids, inhaled

See also Corticosteroids—glucocorticoids *and* Inhaler propellants

General Information

Treatment with inhaled glucocorticoids reduces the need for oral glucocorticoids in the treatment of severe asthma. The compounds used for inhalation have high local activity and low systemic availability when delivered to the lung. However, if sufficient amounts of glucocorticoids reach the bronchioles be absorbed, systemic effects will occur. Furthermore, a proportion of the dose intended for inhalation is actually swallowed and is absorbed from the gastrointestinal tract. The consequence is that if sufficiently high doses are used, enough drug will be absorbed from the respiratory and gastrointestinal surfaces to result in systemic effects.

Systemic availability of inhaled glucocorticoids can be reduced in two ways. First, by using esters that reduced local absorption; in the case of beclomethasone the dipropionate is used. Secondly, by using glucocorticoids that are extensively metabolized in the liver after absorption from the gut, such as fluticasone and budesonide. These strategies can be combined: fluticasone is given as the ester fluticasone propionate.

When a patient switches from oral or parenteral therapy to inhalation therapy, the systemic effect is reduced, just as if the dose of systemic glucocorticoid is reduced, and precautions should be taken to avoid withdrawal symptoms.

Systemic availability of inhaled glucocorticoids

The systemic availability of an inhaled glucocorticoid represents the additive and complex combination of pulmonary and gastrointestinal drug absorption. Absorption is influenced by many factors, including delivery device, the use of a spacer, the particle size of the inhaled drug, and the absorption and metabolism of the swallowed drug (1).

In healthy volunteers, high doses of both budesonide and fluticasone were readily absorbed after inhalation from a metered-dose aerosol (2). Fluticasone is extensively metabolized by the liver, so measurable concentrations of parent drug in the systemic circulation reflect efficient absorption across the lung. Lower doses of these inhaled glucocorticoids also result in some systemic absorption, reflected in effects on the hypothalamic–pituitary–adrenal axis (3).

The extent of absorption of inhaled glucocorticoids tends to be less in asthmatic subjects than in healthy volunteers. In a study of fluticasone (500 micrograms via a dry powder device) in asthmatic patients with a wide range of severity, there was a highly significant linear correlation between lung function (expressed as percentage predicted FEV_1) and the absolute magnitude of adrenal suppression (4). In 11 patients with moderately severe asthma (mean FEV_1 54% predicted), who took fluticasone 1000 micrograms/day via a metered-dose inhaler with a spacer, the systemic availability of fluticasone was significantly less (10%) than in 13 healthy controls (21%). The plasma fluticasone concentrations (expressed as AUC) correlated positively with gas transfer (5). In contrast, there was no difference in plasma concentrations of fluticasone and budesonide between 15 mild asthmatics (mean FEV_1 81% predicted) and healthy volunteers after inhalation of 1000 micrograms of either drug with single or repeated dosing (6). Taken together, these studies suggest that patients with severe asthma are protected from the systemic adverse effects of high doses of inhaled glucocorticoids, owing to airways obstruction and reduced lung availability. However, as their lung function improves with continued use of the inhaled glucocorticoids, it is likely that the lung availability of inhaled glucocorticoid will increase. This likely outcome is a compelling argument for reducing the dose of inhaled glucocorticoids to a lowest dose that maintains optimal control of asthma and optimal lung function.

Plasma concentrations have been measured in 13 healthy subjects and eight patients with mild asthma using inhaled fluticasone propionate 1000 micrograms bd via Diskus or pressurized metered-dose inhaler and of budesonide 1000 micrograms bd daily via Turbuhaler for 7 days. Twenty-four-hour plasma cortisol concentrations were determined to assess the systemic activity of fluticasone propionate and budesonide. At steady state, the systemic availability of budesonide via Turbuhaler (39%) was significantly higher than that of fluticasone propionate via Diskus (13%) or inhaler (21%). Fluticasone propionate had a larger distribution volume and slower rates of absorption and clearance. Despite a significantly higher pulmonary availability of budesonide via Turbuhaler, plasma cortisol suppression was less than that of fluticasone propionate via inhaler and similar to that of fluticasone propionate via Diskus. There were no differences between healthy subjects and patients with mild asthma in subgroup analyses. However, this study had some limitations as the doses of fluticasone propionate and budesonide were not equipotent, fluticasone being twice as potent as budesonide (7).

The effects of fluticasone 1500 micrograms/day and budesonide 1600 micrograms/day, both by dry powder inhalation, on three systemic markers (urinary concentrations of total cortisol metabolites, morning serum cortisol, and osteocalcin concentrations) have been investigated in 46 healthy and 31 asthmatic subjects (8). Urinary total cortisol metabolite concentrations represented the most sensitive marker of the systemic effects of inhaled glucocorticoids, and were lower in healthy subjects treated with fluticasone than in asthmatic patients, suggesting greater systemic availability of fluticasone in healthy subjects. A similar correlation was not found for budesonide. Fluticasone impaired the hypothalamic–pituitary–adrenal axis more than budesonide, while budesonide significantly lowered serum osteocalcin concentrations, which reflect osteoblastic activity. The authors suggested that different inhaled glucocorticoids have different effects on the hypothalamic–pituitary–adrenal axis and bone metabolism. This study also had its limitations given that the fluticasone and budesonide doses were not equipotent (9).

The safety and efficacy of fluticasone, beclomethasone dipropionate, and budesonide have been compared in a randomized trial in 133 patients with chronic severe asthma who required at least 1750 micrograms/day of beclomethasone/budesonide (10). The patients were randomized to their regular beclomethasone/budesonide or to fluticasone at about half the dose for 6 months. The patients who used fluticasone had a better safety profile, especially with regard to adrenocortical function and bone turnover, while maintaining asthma control. There were significant increases in morning serum cortisol concentrations, the urine cortisol:creatinine ratio, serum osteocalcin, and the serum (deoxy)-pyridinoline:creatinine ratio only with fluticasone, suggesting less suppression of the hypothalamic–pituitary–adrenal axis. The 2:1 potency ratio for clinical efficacy of fluticasone and budesonide/beclomethasone seems to be maintained even at doses of 2000 micrograms/day or higher.

Since many patients with allergic asthma also have rhinitis, they may be taking both inhaled glucocorticoids for their asthma and intranasal formulations for their hay fever. The total systemic availability of glucocorticoids has been studied after the addition of intranasal therapy in patients already taking inhaled glucocorticoids (11) in 12 moderately severe asthmatic subjects (mean FEV_1 84% predicted), who were randomized in a placebo-controlled, two-way, crossover comparison of inhaled fluticasone (880 micrograms bd) plus intranasal fluticasone (200 micrograms od), inhaled triamcinolone (800 micrograms bd) plus intranasal triamcinolone (220 micrograms od), and respective placebos. Both the inhaled glucocorticoids caused significant suppression of adrenocorticoid activity, although the addition of intranasal formulations did not produce further significant suppression. There were more individual subjects with abnormally low cortisol values when intranasal fluticasone was added. These findings suggest that the dose of intranasal glucocorticoids should be taken into account (particularly if used in the long term) when considering the systemic availability of glucocorticoids used in the treatment of asthma and hay fever.

The concept of the L:T ratio in inhalation therapy is a useful one, where L represents the local or lung availability of an inhaled drug and T the total systemic availability. This ratio will be affected by differences in first-pass metabolism. Another important variable that determines the L:T ratio is the inhalation device. The L:T ratio for budesonide is 0.66–0.85, depending on the method of inhalation (12).

Another way of describing the L:T ratio concept is that of "pulmonary targeting." Drug properties that improve pulmonary targeting include slow absorption from the lungs, low oral systemic availability, and rapid systemic clearance.

Differences in delivery devices can also produce differences in pulmonary targeting by altering the dose of drug deposited in the lungs. Allowing for both drug and inhaler differences, the relative potencies of the commonly used drugs are as follows: fluticasone propionate > budesonide = beclomethasone dipropionate > triamcinolone acetonide = flunisolide. Potency differences can be overcome by giving a larger dose of the less potent drug. However, comparisons between glucocorticoids must measure the systemic effects as well as the lung effect of each dose (13).

Inhalation devices

The importance of the inhalation device has been shown in studies of beclomethasone. Pressurized metered-dose inhalers containing chlorofluorocarbons produce relatively large particles that deposit less than 10% of the delivered dose in the lungs, primarily in the large airways, more than 90% being deposited in the oropharynx. A hydrofluoroalkane beclomethasone multidose aerosol (Qvar 3M Pharmaceuticals) delivers a smaller particle size. More than 50% is deposited in the lungs in animal and mechanical models. This has been confirmed using radiolabelled Qvar in patients with asthma and in healthy volunteers. In these subjects, 50–60% of the dose is deposited throughout the airways and about 30% in the oropharynx. The breath-activated Autohaler provides lung deposition equivalent to an optimally used Qvar inhaler, by automatically delivering drug early in the inhalation. Neither of these devices is improved by the addition of a spacer (14).

Both inhaled and swallowed fractions cause significant systemic activity, the degree of which depends on the inhaler device used. In one study, systemic activity was greater using a dry power inhaler (52%) than a pressurized metered-dose inhaler with a large volume spacer (28%) (15). It was recommended that when high-dose beclomethasone is used, a pressurized metered-dose inhaler with a large volume spacer would help in limiting potential adverse effects.

The systemic availability of inhaled budesonide has been measured in 15 healthy volunteers, using an open crossover design. Each subject was given three treatments, intravenous budesonide 0.5 mg, inhaled budesonide (from a metered-dose inhaler with a Nebuhaler) 1 mg (200 micrograms × 5) plus oral charcoal, and inhaled budesonide 1 mg without oral charcoal. The treatment order was randomized. The mean systemic availability of inhaled budesonide compared with intravenous budesonide was 36% with charcoal and 35% without charcoal, indicating that the absorption of budesonide from the gastrointestinal tract did not contribute to its systemic availability. Pulmonary deposition was 36% with charcoal and 34% without. When the inhaler was used incorrectly, that is, the canister was shaken only before the first of the five inhalations, systemic availability fell by 50%. This shows that the performance of each inhaler is very dependent on proper use (16).

The available studies suggest that fluticasone is more effective than beclomethasone, triamcinolone, or budesonide. However, budesonide delivered by Turbuhaler has equivalent efficacy to fluticasone delivered by metered-dose inhaler or Diskhaler, and is more effective than beclomethasone. When comparative safety is considered, budesonide and triamcinolone delivered by metered-dose inhaler have less systemic activity than fluticasone. Beclomethasone and fluticasone delivered by metered-dose inhaler are equivalent. Budesonide delivered by Turbuhaler has less systemic activity than fluticasone delivered by Diskhaler (17).

The equivalence of inhaled glucocorticoids based on equipotent (cortisol suppression) effects has been studied by the Asthma Clinical Research Network (ACRN). Six different inhaled glucocorticoids and matched placebos (beclomethasone chlorofluorocarbon, budesonide dry powder inhaler, fluticasone dry powder inhaler, fluticasone chlorofluorocarbon metered-dose inhaler, flunisolide chlorofluorocarbon, and triamcinolone chlorofluorocarbon) were compared by measuring their systemic effects (18). Glucocorticoid-naïve patients with asthma ($n = 156$) were enrolled at six centers and a one-week doubling dose design was used for each of the six inhaled glucocorticoids and matched placebos to a total of four doses. The best outcome variable for the reliable assessment of a systemic effect was the 12-hour AUC of the hourly overnight plasma cortisol measurements from 8 p.m. to 8 a.m. Microgram comparisons of the glucocorticoids could only be performed at 10% cortisol suppression, because fluticasone did not cause higher suppression. The following equipotent doses (that is, doses producing equal systemic cortisol suppression) were found: flunisolide 936 micrograms; triamcinolone 787 micrograms; beclomethasone 548 micrograms; fluticasone dry powder: 445 micrograms; budesonide 268 micrograms; and fluticasone metered-dose inhaler 111 micrograms. The ranking of systemic effects was very similar to that found earlier in a large meta-analysis (19).

Dry powder inhaler and pressurized metered-dose inhaler for administration of low-dose budesonide (400 micrograms/day) have been compared (20). Only the dry powder caused suppression of the hypothalamic–pituitary–adrenal axis. As effective inhaled glucocorticoid therapy is expected to cause detectable reductions in the physiological secretion of cortisol (1), low-dose budesonide by pressurized metered-dose inhaler is probably not effective. In another study, budesonide inhalation suspension, developed for nebulization to meet the specific needs of infants and young children, did not cause significant suppression of hypothalamic–pituitary–adrenal axis function (basal plasma cortisol concentrations and corticotropin test) in doses from 0.25 to 1.0 mg (21). However, inhaled fluticasone propionate by pressurized metered-dose inhaler with a spacer in 62 children resulted in abnormal morning cortisol concentrations in 36% (17 using a low dose of 176 micrograms/day; 43 using a high dose, over 880 micrograms/day) (22).

In a randomized, double-blind study, adult asthmatic patients took budesonide 800 micrograms/day over 12 weeks either by Easyhaler ($n = 103$) or by Turbuhaler ($n = 58$) dry powder inhaler. The Easyhaler was equivalent to the Turbuhaler with regard to safety and efficacy, but was more acceptable to the patients (23).

Therapeutic studies

Budesonide

Inhaled budesonide has been studied in the management of moderately severe, acute asthma in children (24). After treatment with nebulized terbutaline, 11 children were randomly allocated to receive one dose of either budesonide 1600 micrograms by Turbuhaler or prednisolone 2 mg/kg. There was no significant difference in the improvement of the pulmonary index score or peak expiratory flow rate. Children treated with budesonide had an earlier clinical response than those given prednisolone. Prednisolone caused a fall in serum cortisol concentration. The authors concluded that children with moderately severe asthma attacks could be effectively treated with a short-term course of inhaled budesonide, starting with a high dose and reducing over the following week.

In 81 patients with acute asthma, mean age 38 years, inhaled budesonide 1600 micrograms bd via Turbuhaler was compared with oral prednisolone (40 mg on day 1, reducing to 5 mg by day 7) in a randomized, double-blind, parallel-group design (25). The mean increase in FEV_1 from baseline to day 7 was 17% with budesonide and 18% with prednisolone. Mean values of morning peak expiratory flow rate increased from day 1 to day 7 by 67 l/second with budesonide and by 57 l/second with prednisolone. There were no statistically significant differences between the groups in either symptoms or the number of doses of rescue medication. The authors concluded that high-dose inhaled budesonide may be a substitute for oral therapy in the treatment of an acute attack of asthma.

The effect of supplementary inhaled budesonide in acute asthma has been evaluated in a randomized, double-blind comparison with standard treatment in 44 children aged 6 months to 18 years with a moderate to severe exacerbation of asthma (26). Prednisone 1 mg/kg orally and nebulized salbutamol (0.15 mg/kg) every 30 minutes for three doses and then every hour for 4 hours were given to all children. In addition, each child was given 2 mg of nebulized budesonide or nebulized isotonic saline. There was a more rapid discharge rate in the budesonide group. There were no adverse effects. The authors concluded that nebulized budesonide may be an effective adjunct to oral prednisone in the management of moderate to severe exacerbations of asthma.

Fluticasone

Inhaled fluticasone 500 micrograms bd from a pressurized metered-dose inhaler for 6 months has been compared with placebo in a randomized, double-blind trial in 280 patients with COPD, aged 50–75 years (27). There was no significant difference in the number of patients who suffered one or more exacerbations. Moderate or severe exacerbations occurred significantly more often with placebo than with fluticasone. Diary-card scores, morning peak expiratory flow rate, clinic FEV_1, FVC, and mid-expiratory flow all improved significantly with fluticasone. Scores for median daily cough and sputum volume were significantly lower with fluticasone than with placebo. At the end of treatment, patients using fluticasone had increased their 6-minute walking distance significantly more than those using placebo. Fluticasone propionate was tolerated, as well as placebo, with few adverse effects and no clinically important effect on mean serum cortisol concentration. The authors suggested that inhaled glucocorticoids may have an important place in the long-term management of patients with COPD.

Local adverse effects

The local adverse effects of inhaled glucocorticoids have been studied in a prospective, cross-sectional, cohort study in 639 asthmatic children using beclomethasone (721 micrograms/day) or budesonide (835 micrograms/day) for at least one month (28). The local adverse effects included cough (40%), thirst (22%), hoarseness (14%), dysphonia (11%), oral candidiasis (11%), perioral dermatitis (2.9%), and tongue hypertrophy (0.1%). A spacer doubled the incidence of coughing.

Potent glucocorticoids in high local doses increase the risk of local infection and even promote atrophy of the bronchial mucosa. The latter effect has not proved clinically important, but there is an increased incidence of oropharyngeal candidiasis. The incidence varies depending on the population studied and the criteria used to make the diagnosis; candidiasis can affect 13–71% of patients, the highest incidence being seen with doses up to 0.8 mg. Candidiasis rarely requires treatment or withdrawal of the drug. Local measures, such as gargling immediately after inhalation of the aerosol, and the use of a large-volume spacer are effective in reducing the incidence of this complication. However, candidiasis can result in dysphonia.

A local myopathy caused by inhaled glucocorticoids can also cause dysphonia. However, patients with asthma have more dysphonia and vocal fold pathology than healthy controls and inhaled glucocorticoids can improve the voice in some patients (SEDA-21, 188).

In some patients, the propellant used in certain aerosols can cause acute bronchoconstriction (SEDA-6, 332).

Organs and Systems

Sensory systems

Cataract

In a population-based cross-sectional study of vision and common eye diseases in 3654 people, 49–97 years of age, inhaled glucocorticoid use was reported by 370 subjects, of whom 164 reported current use and 206 previous use. Subjects who reported using inhaled glucocorticoids had a higher prevalence of nuclear cataracts (OR = 1.5; CI = 1.2, 1.9) and posterior subcapsular cataracts (OR = 1.9; CI = 1.3, 2.8). The highest prevalence (27%) was in patients whose lifetime dose was more than 2000 mg (relative prevalence 5.5) (SEDA-22, 187).

In 3677 patients undergoing cataract extraction over 2 years compared with a matched control group of 21 868 people, the patients were more likely to undergo cataract extraction if they had used inhaled glucocorticoids for more than 3 years (OR = 3.06; CI = 1.53, 6.13). This risk was not significant in patients who used low to medium doses (1000 micrograms/day or less) when the OR was 1.63 (CI = 0.85, 3.13) after 2 years. The OR was higher in patients using average daily doses of beclomethasone dipropionate or budesonide (over 1000 micrograms) (OR = 3.40; CI = 1.49, 7.76) after more than 2 years of treatment (29).

In a nested case-control analysis based on a retrospective, observational, cohort study, 103 289 asthmatic patients using inhaled glucocorticoids were identified from the UK General Practice Database and were compared with 98 527 asthmatic patients with no history of glucocorticoid use (30). There was a slightly increased risk of cataract in those who used inhaled glucocorticoids (RR = 1.3; 95% CI = 1.1, 1.5). The relative risk of cataract was 2.0 in oral glucocorticoid users relative to glucocorticoid non-users (95% CI = 1.5, 2.2). The risk ratio increased with extensive use of inhaled glucocorticoids, but not with moderate use. The association of extensive use with cataract was most pronounced in those aged 70 years and over, and there was no effect in those aged under 40. The increased risk of cataract in patients aged 70 years and over persisted after controlling for cataract risk factors, such as smoking, diabetes mellitus, hypertension, and sex.

In another study, treatment for 2 years with fluticasone propionate (500 micrograms bd) had no significant effect on ophthalmic parameters (glaucoma and posterior subcapsular cataracts) (31). Slit lamp examinations were carried out in 157 asthmatic children treated with inhaled budesonide at a mean daily dose of 504 (range 189–1322) micrograms for 3–6 years (mean 4.4 years). Posterior subcapsular cataract due to budesonide was not detected (32).

Glaucoma

A case-control study compared 9793 patients with open-angle glaucoma or ocular hypertension to 38 325 randomly selected controls (33). There was no association between the use of inhaled or intranasal glucocorticoids and the risk of open-angle glaucoma or ocular hypertension. In patients who were currently using high doses, there was a small but significant increase in risk (OR = 1.44; CI = 1.01, 2.06).

Endocrine

Hypothalamic–pituitary–adrenal axis function provides one of the most sensitive markers of the systemic activity of inhaled glucocorticoids (34), and suppression can be used as a surrogate marker for adverse effects of inhaled glucocorticoids in other tissues.

The different methods of assessing hypothalamic–pituitary–adrenal axis activity in patients using inhaled glucocorticoids have been compared (35). The AUC of serum cortisol concentrations was the most reliable method. There were significant positive correlations between AUC and the 8 a.m. serum and salivary cortisol concentrations. The authors favored the non-invasive method of salivary concentration measurement. However, 24-hour urine collection is not recommended, as it correlated only moderately well. This finding is consistent with the results of other studies. Urinary free-cortisol estimation based on immunoassay after inhaled glucocorticoids may be an unreliable surrogate marker of adrenal suppression, and studies using this method should be interpreted with caution (36).

In a randomized, placebo-controlled study, the activity of the hypothalamic–pituitary–adrenal axis was assessed at baseline and after 21 days by determining 22-hour time-integrated serum cortisol concentrations, 24-hour urinary cortisol (corrected for creatinine), and morning salivary cortisol concentrations in 153 patients with mild to moderate asthma, randomly assigned to either inhaled flunisolide (500 or 1000 micrograms bd), inhaled fluticasone (110, 220, 330, or 440 micrograms bd), oral prednisone (7.5 mg/day), or placebo (19). Flunisolide and fluticasone caused dose-dependent suppression of the hypothalamic–pituitary–adrenal axis, and fluticasone was significantly more potent. However, the lowest fluticasone dose (110 micrograms/day) had no effect. These findings are consistent with those of a previous meta-analysis, which showed that fluticasone caused a greater dose-related suppression of the hypothalamic–pituitary–adrenal axis than other inhaled glucocorticoids (37). Fluticasone is more lipophilic than flunisolide and therefore has a larger volume of distribution and a longer half-life (34), but it is not clear how this might be associated with the larger effect described here.

The effect of fluticasone aqueous nasal spray on the hypothalamic–pituitary–adrenal axis has been compared with that of oral prednisone and placebo, using a 6-hour tetracosactide infusion test in a 4-week, randomized, double-blind, placebo-controlled study in 105 adults with allergic rhinitis randomly assigned to receive fluticasone 200 micrograms od, fluticasone 400 micrograms bd, oral prednisone 7.5 mg od, oral prednisone 15 mg od, or placebo (38). Fluticasone 400 micrograms bd and both doses of prednisone caused a significant reduction in the morning plasma cortisol concentration. The two fluticasone treatments produced no significant change in the hypothalamic–pituitary–adrenal axis response to co-syntropin. This contrasted with oral prednisone 7.5 or 15 mg od, which significantly reduced both plasma cortisol concentrations after co-syntropin and 24-hour urinary cortisol excretion.

A review of the literature from 1 January 1966 to 31 July 1998 identified 27 studies in which the effects of inhaled glucocorticoids on adrenal function were measured. A meta-regression of adrenal suppression in these 27 studies showed that adrenal suppression occurred with high doses of inhaled glucocorticoids (above 1500 micrograms/day; 750 micrograms/day for fluticasone propionate). However, there is a considerable degree of interindividual susceptibility. Meta-analysis showed significantly greater potency for dose-related adrenal suppression with fluticasone propionate compared with beclomethasone dipropionate, budesonide, or triamcinolone acetonide. Prednisolone and fluticasone propionate were approximately equivalent in a dose ratio of 10:1 (19).

Adrenal suppression by inhaled glucocorticoids in children

Inhaled glucocorticoids are being prescribed more and more in younger children at an earlier stage of their disease and for longer periods; children with severe asthma are also treated with larger doses than licensed.

Therefore, considerations of their systemic effects are of importance. Symptomatic adrenal insufficiency has been reported in children after various regimens of inhaled glucocorticoids.

- Four boys 4–8 years old with symptomatic adrenal insufficiency had all used consistent high doses of fluticasone propionate 1000–1500 micrograms/day over extended periods (16 months to 5 years) (39). They presented with acute hypoglycemia secondary to iatrogenic adrenal suppression, with abnormal corticotropin tests, although none had Cushingoid features.
- A 33-year-old man and three children (two girls, one boy, 7–9 years) presented with symptomatic adrenal insufficiency (40). All three children had seizures because of hypoglycemia, and the man had a low blood pressure, nausea, and fatigue. In all cases, corticotropin tests were abnormal, showing adrenal insufficiency. The children had used fluticasone propionate 500–2000 micrograms/day and the man had recently switched from fluticasone propionate 1000–2000 micrograms/day to budesonide dry powder inhaler 800 micrograms/day. Only one of the children had used oral glucocorticoids in the previous year.
- A 21-month-old boy had a hypoglycemia-induced seizure in the setting of adrenal suppression (41). He had been given increasing doses of budesonide up to 2000 micrograms qds and oral glucocorticoids until the age of 15 months.
- A 32-month-old girl developed hypoglycemic seizures (42). She had been given fluticasone propionate 440–880 micrograms/day and up to 5 months before the incident oral glucocorticoids.
- Two girls aged 11 and 16 years, one boy aged 12 years, and one woman aged 54 years developed hypothalamic–pituitary–adrenal axis suppression during treatment with inhaled fluticasone propionate 220–880 micrograms bd for long-term control of asthma; however, two of the patients also took oral prednisone or prednisolone (43). Because of poor growth, an 8-year-old girl's asthma medication was changed from budesonide to fluticasone propionate 250 micrograms/day (44). However, 5 months later she had developed a round face. Her early morning cortisol concentration was less than 30 nmol/l (reference range 140–720) and her growth had been no more than 0.5 cm during the past 5 months. Fluticasone propionate was discontinued. After 1 month, her Cushingoid features had resolved and her fasting morning cortisol concentration was 310 nmol/l.
- A 32-year-old woman's asthma regimen was changed from budesonide to fluticasone propionate 500 micrograms/day and salmeterol (44). Eight months later, she was evaluated because of excessive bodyweight gain; her serum cortisol concentration was 16 nmol/l. Fluticasone propionate was replaced with nedocromil and 1 month later her serum cortisol concentration had normalized.

In addition to these case reports, there has been a survey of symptomatic adrenal suppression associated with inhaled glucocorticoids in the UK (45). Only 24% of the questionnaires were returned (709 responses), and there were 28 cases of symptomatic adrenal suppression reported in children and five in adults (including the 10 cases discussed above). The children presented mostly with hypoglycemia and coma, whereas the adults mainly had lethargy and nausea. No obvious precipitating cause was found in 65% of the cases. In four children, diagnosis was delayed by 3 months to 2 years. All but three patients had been treated with fluticasone propionate alone, but at high daily doses (children 500–2000 micrograms, adults 1000–2000 micrograms). One child had used both fluticasone propionate and budesonide, and one adult and one child used beclomethasone dipropionate.

A series of cases has illustrated the unexpected occurrence of symptomatic adrenal insufficiency in eight asthmatic children using inhaled glucocorticoids (46). The authors concluded that therapeutic doses of inhaled glucocorticoids can provoke paradoxical symptoms of adrenal insufficiency. Very high doses (calculated according to body surface area) may partly explain marked suppression of the hypothalamic–pituitary–adrenal axis. The need to taper inhaled glucocorticoid doses and to recognize the possibility of life-threatening acute adrenal insufficiency is of utmost importance.

In a double-blind, randomized pilot study of the efficacy and adverse effects of inhaled fluticasone in 25 newborn preterm infants who required mechanical ventilation for treatment of respiratory distress syndrome, the infants were randomized to receive inhaled fluticasone 1000 micrograms/day or placebo (47). The hypothalamic–pituitary–adrenal axis was assessed by the response to corticotropin-releasing factor. All basal and post-stimulation plasma corticotropin and serum cortisol concentrations were significantly less with inhaled fluticasone than placebo. Cumulative high-dose inhaled glucocorticoids caused moderately severe suppression of both the pituitary and the adrenal glands. This systemic activity is probably associated with pulmonary vascular absorption that avoids hepatic first-pass metabolism.

Chronic inhalation of beclomethasone dipropionate (up to 1000 micrograms/day) can produce adrenal suppression in some children. This effect is reduced by the attachment of a large volume spacer to the aerosol (SEDA-21, 188). Budesonide inhaled from the Turbuhaler, at doses of 800 or 1600 micrograms/day), did not produce any statistically significant suppression of the hypothalamic–pituitary–adrenal axis compared with placebo. The reduction was significant only after 3200 micrograms/day of budesonide when suppression equivalent to 10 mg/day oral prednisone was seen (48). Fluticasone propionate powder, 500 micrograms bd, given using a Diskhaler, for 104 weeks caused only minimal changes in the hypothalamic–pituitary–adrenal axis (31). Inhaled fluticasone propionate 400 micrograms/day for 8 weeks did not cause adrenal suppression in asthmatic children. In children, the benefit/risk ratio generally decreases at doses above 400 micrograms/day of fluticasone propionate (49). Hypothalamic–pituitary–adrenal axis suppression has been reported with inhaled fluticasone propionate at doses in excess of 1000 micrograms/day (SEDA-21, 188).

Different inhaled glucocorticoids have been compared for their suppressing effects on the hypothalamic–pituitary–adrenal axis (18). In a large meta-analysis, budesonide or beclomethasone dipropionate in doses of over 1500 micrograms/day was associated with adrenal suppression in adults (19). In children, fluticasone propionate 200 micrograms/day or budesonide 400 micrograms/day caused detectable adrenal gland suppression (50). For interpretation of the different studies, it is very important to distinguish between detectable indicators for systemic drug action (that is, reduced morning cortisol) and true suppression of the hypothalamic–pituitary–adrenal axis, as determined by adrenal function tests (standard-dose or low-dose corticotropin test), which are more predictive of possible systemic adverse effects (1).

The fact that fluticasone propionate is involved in the vast majority of the published cases should be discussed further. The systemic concentration of an inhaled glucocorticoid depends on the absorbed fraction of the drug in the gut and in the lung. Swallowed fluticasone propionate is almost completely metabolized in the liver by CYP3A4 (first-pass effect over 99.9%) before reaching the systemic circulation; however, its metabolic clearance can be altered in patients with low CYP3A4 expression and activity (51). Pulmonary absorbed fluticasone propionate is very potent; because of its pronounced lipophilicity, it binds with higher affinity to glucocorticoid receptors and has a larger distribution volume and a longer half-life than other inhaled glucocorticoids (52). These characteristics give it the potential of accumulating with multiple doses.

Other factors that determine the absorbed fraction of inhaled glucocorticoids include the age of the child, as lung deposition of inhaled drugs increases with age (53). Therefore, the minimum effective dose may fall as the child becomes older. Moreover, it is reasonable to hypothesize that systemic absorption will increase once asthma control is established (54). Furthermore, patient adherence and inhaler technique are two factors that can have a large influence on the amount of glucocorticoid inhaled and absorbed.

However, the most important factor is the dose. The safety and efficacy of fluticasone propionate in children in daily doses of 100–200 micrograms have been demonstrated in many studies (55). The doses in the case reports of symptomatic adrenal suppression have to be considered as being excessively high. These reports reflect excessive dosing of inhaled glucocorticoids, and in some cases a residual effect of previous oral glucocorticoid treatment cannot be excluded. The use of excessive doses is empirical and not supported by the literature. All inhaled glucocorticoids have a flat dose–response curve (56). Extensive clinical experience with inhaled glucocorticoids over the past 20 years has suggested that the risk of adrenal insufficiency with inhaled glucocorticoids alone is very low when recommended doses are used (57). To avoid symptomatic adrenal suppression, the lowest effective dose should always be used. Before automatically increasing the dose in refractory patients, the diagnosis should be reconsidered. Furthermore, a reduction in the dosage of inhaled glucocorticoid can also be achieved with the addition of adjuvant therapies, such as leukotriene receptor antagonists and long-acting β_2-adrenoceptor agonists (58).

Monitoring children using inhaled glucocorticoids has been discussed (1). Children using low to moderate doses of inhaled glucocorticoids (up to 200 micrograms of fluticasone propionate or budesonide) do not require routine hypothalamic–pituitary–adrenal axis measurement. In children using consistently higher doses (up to 400 micrograms of fluticasone propionate or budesonide) or using glucocorticoids by other routes, morning plasma cortisol should be monitored periodically because of the increased risk of clinically significant adrenal suppression. If cortisol concentrations are below 276 μmol/l (100 ng/ml), functional testing of the hypothalamic–pituitary–adrenal axis should be considered.

Metabolism

Impaired diabetic control has been reported with high doses of inhaled glucocorticoids.

- A 67-year-old man with asthma and non-insulin-dependent diabetes mellitus, taking glibenclamide 5 mg/day and metformin 1700 mg/day, had glycated hemoglobin concentrations of 7.0–7.3% (59). For asthma, he used nebulized ipratropium bromide 0.5 mg and salbutamol 5 mg qds. He was given inhaled fluticasone propionate 2000 micrograms/day by metered-dose inhaler through a Volumatic spacer device, with beneficial effect. In the third week he developed persistent glycosuria and the dose of fluticasone was reduced stepwise to 500 micrograms/day. He was then rechallenged by increasing his daily dose of fluticasone from 500 to 1000 micrograms. Within a week he had glycosuria, which again resolved on reduction of the dose of fluticasone. His glycated hemoglobin concentration rose to 7.8% after 1000 micrograms/day and to 8.2% after 2000 micrograms/day.
- Deterioration in glucose control occurred in a 64-year-old man with non-insulin-dependent diabetes mellitus (60). High doses of both fluticasone (2000 micrograms/day) and budesonide (2000 micrograms/day) had produced glycosuria despite treatment with glibenclamide and metformin 1700 mg/day. On reducing the dose of budesonide, there was a commensurate fall in glycosylated hemoglobin and glycosuria. There was no glycosuria at a daily maintenance dose of 800 micrograms and the glycosylated hemoglobin fell from 8.2 to 7.2%.

The association between inhaled glucocorticoids and the risk of diabetes mellitus in elderly people (over 65 years) has been investigated in two Canadian studies. In a nested case-control study of the association between current use of inhaled glucocorticoids and the risk of using antidiabetic drugs among 21 645 subjects the risk of diabetes was not statistically significant (61). Moreover, there was no statistically significant increase in risk among users of high-dose beclomethasone compared with non-users. In a retrospective population-based cohort study using administrative databases, the association between oral and inhaled glucocorticoid use and the onset of diabetes mellitus in the elderly was quantified (62). Users of proton pump inhibitors ($n = 53\ 845$) were the controls. Relative to controls, oral glucocorticoid users ($n = 31\ 864$) were more likely to develop diabetes mellitus, but there was no association between the use of inhaled glucocorticoids ($n = 38\ 441$) and diabetes mellitus. These results suggest that the use of inhaled glucocorticoids in elderly people does not significantly increase the risk of diabetes mellitus.

Skin

Reduced skin thickness

Skin thickness (measured with ultrasound) was not significantly different from controls in patients taking low-dose beclomethasone dipropionate (200–800 micrograms/day). There was a reduction in skin thickness of 15–19% in patients using high dose beclomethasone dipropionate (1000–2500 micrograms/day), and 28–33% in patients using long-term oral prednisolone (5–20 mg/day). Bruising occurred in 12% of controls, 33% of patients using low-dose beclomethasone dipropionate, 48% of patients using high-dose beclomethasone dipropionate, and 80% of patients using oral prednisolone (63). Other workers have concluded that patients using beclomethasone dipropionate who report bruising are older (61 versus 52 years), take higher daily doses (1388 versus 1067 micrograms), and have been on treatment longer (55 versus 43 months) (64). The number of bruises seems to be inversely related to the concentration of urinary cortisol (SEDA-21, 188). In children using budesonide (189–1322 micrograms/day) for 3–6 years, there was no increase in bruising (32).

The effect of long-term inhaled glucocorticoids (800–1000 micrograms/day of either budesonide or beclomethasone) on skin collagen synthesis and thickness has been prospectively investigated in 27 consecutive new asthmatic patients (65). Asthma was treated with a moderate dosage of inhaled glucocorticoids. Skin thickness was measured before treatment and at 3 and 6 months using ultrasound on the abdomen and the upper right arm. Suction blisters were induced on the abdominal skin using a disposable suction blister device. Blister fluid was collected and kept frozen for radioimmunoassay of PINP and PIIINP. Skin punch biopsies were taken from the abdominal wall for the determination of skin hydroxyproline. After 1–2 years, 20 subjects attended for a further measurement of skin thickness. Control data were obtained in 14 healthy women who were followed for 6 months. PINP and PIIINP concentrations in blister fluid were followed in eight male volunteers for 1 year. There was no significant change in abdominal skin thickness after 6 months of inhaled glucocorticoids. In the upper arm there was a small, significant reduction from 1.64 to 1.50 mm after 6 months. After 1–2 years the skin thickness in the abdomen and upper arm was unchanged in 14 subjects who had used only inhaled glucocorticoids, but in six patients who had taken supplementary oral glucocorticoids for one to several weeks there was thinning of the skin in the upper arm but not the abdomen. The procollagen propeptides were markedly reduced in blister fluid at 3 and 6 months. There was no significant change in skin collagen expressed as hydroxyproline. Thus, despite evidence of a reduction in collagen synthesis, skin thickness and collagen did not change, possibly because the degradation and turnover of collagen slowed down. However, in the six patients who subsequently used oral glucocorticoids, skin thickness decreased.

Bruising

Since the original observation of the association between high-dose glucocorticoids and purpura and dermal thinning, easy bruising of the skin has become recognized as a systemic adverse effect of inhaled glucocorticoids (63). In a double-blind crossover study 69 asthmatic subjects received either the usual dose of beclomethasone dipropionate or fluticasone (at half the dose of beclomethasone) both for 4 months (66). The frequency and severity of skin bruising were assessed by questionnaire, and the numbers of bruises were assessed by direct examination. The dose of fluticasone was selected on the basis of previous studies that showed that it had comparable efficacy when given in half the dose of beclomethasone. This dose of fluticasone had comparable efficacy with respect to the control of asthma, but there was no skin bruising. These findings suggest that the systemic availability of equieffective doses of fluticasone is less than that of beclomethasone.

Contact allergy

Nasal glucocorticoids and inhaled glucocorticoids can have adverse effects on the nose and mouth, including pruritus, burning, dryness, erythema, edema, dry cough, and odynophagia; less commonly, they can cause eczema and urticaria, particularly on the face. Contact dermatitis to glucocorticoids can be facilitated by impaired epithelial barriers, and has been found in 4.7% of patients receiving topical hydrocortisone (67). Inhaled glucocorticoids can cause hypersensitivity reactions, especially in patients with chronic eczema who have been sensitized to local glucocorticoids.

Tixocortol pivalate is a marker for glucocorticoid contact allergy, as a positive patch test suggests established contact allergy to hydrocortisone, prednisolone, and their derivatives (68). A literature search via Medline from 1966 to May 2000 revealed only one patient hypersensitive to tixocortol pivalate and budesonide in a pilot study in 34 patients (10 with asthma, 13 with rhinitis, 11 with both) (69). From case reports, the prevalence of glucocorticoid-induced contact allergy has been estimated at 2.9–5%.

Based on these observations it has been concluded that patients who use inhaled glucocorticoids and develop unprecedented skin reactions during therapy should be tested for glucocorticoid-related contact allergy (70). Switching from one of the four main glucocorticoid groups to another might prove successful in these cases.

Two cases of perioral dermatitis have been associated with the use of inhaled glucocorticoids (71).

- A 38-year-old woman who had used inhaled beclomethasone daily (dosage not stated) during the winter for the past 5 years for mild asthma, developed a perioral rash with numerous small pustules and papules. She stopped using beclomethasone and was treated with oral erythromycin and topical tretinoin. Her rash resolved within 4 weeks. One year later, she restarted beclomethasone and her rash reappeared after 2 weeks. There was no recurrence of her perioral dermatitis during subsequent treatment with monthly intramuscular injections of betamethasone.
- A 46-year-old woman, who had used inhaled budesonide (dosage not stated) for 8 years for vasomotor rhinitis, developed a recurrent perioral rash, which responded to treatment with oral erythromycin 1 g/day for 6 weeks. One year later, she had a recurrence, which resolved with oral erythromycin. She continued to use inhaled budesonide.

As cross-reactivity within glucocorticoid groups may be clinically relevant, skin patch testing has been proposed in cases of suspected glucocorticoid allergy, to identify the substances that can be safely administered (72). The prevalence of glucocorticoid allergy has been studied by skin patch testing in 30 patients using inhaled or intranasal glucocorticoids (73). Four patients had a positive patch test (three allergic reactions and one irritant reaction). Eight different glucocorticoids were used, but allergic reactions occurred only with budesonide. The authors therefore suggested that budesonide is more likely to cause contact hypersensitivity, but also referred to the possible relevance of allergic or irritant reactions to preservatives.

Contact allergy to glucocorticoids is not rare in patients with atopic dermatitis. In patients with known contact allergy to budesonide, allergic skin reactions can also occur when inhaled forms of the drug are used, as shown by a randomized, double-blind, placebo-controlled study in 15 non-asthmatic patients with budesonide hypersensitivity on patch testing (74). In four of seven patients who used inhaled budesonide, there was reactivation of the 6-week-old patch test sites and they had new distant skin lesions. No flare-up reactions were observed in the other 11 patients (three had used inhaled budesonide and eight placebo for 1 week). None of the patients developed respiratory symptoms; spirometry and peak expiratory flow rates remained normal.

Musculoskeletal

Bone

Studies of the effects of inhaled glucocorticoids have used biochemical markers of bone function and imaging techniques to assess bone mineral density. Some of the biochemical markers are summarized in Table 1. Initial, short-term studies caused concern about the effect of inhaled glucocorticoids on bone metabolism. Beclomethasone dipropionate 2000 micrograms/day reduced serum osteocalcin concentrations at 1 and 2 weeks, and they returned to normal at 1 and 2 weeks after withdrawal. Nebulized budesonide (2000 micrograms bd) produced a similar increase in FEV_1 to oral prednisolone 30 mg/day given over 5 days. Serum osteocalcin was significantly higher: 2.3 (0.9–3.7) ng/ml with budesonide compared with 0.6 (0–1.2) ng/ml with prednisolone. The 24-hour urinary calcium to creatinine ratio was significantly lower in patients treated with nebulized budesonide (SEDA-22, 183). After 4 weeks on beclomethasone dipropionate or budesonide 800 micrograms/day, there were significant but paradoxical changes in osteocalcin and PICP (both markers of bone formation). Osteocalcin concentrations fell, but PICP concentrations rose. Patients on beclomethasone dipropionate 800 micrograms/day followed for 30 months showed no change in markers of resorption (ICTP) or formation (PICP) (SEDA-22, 183).

While biochemical markers of bone metabolism may be sensitive to the effects of glucocorticoids in the short term, the relation between changes in these markers and intermediate measures, such as bone mineral density, and

Table 1 Biochemical markers of bone mineral density

Bone formation	Bone resorption
Blood	*Blood*
Alkaline phosphatase (bone-specific)	Acid phosphatase (acid-resistant)
Osteocalcin	Type I collagen carboxy-terminal telopeptide (ICTP)
Procollagen type I carboxy-terminal propeptide (PICP)	*Urine*
Procollagen type I amino-terminal propeptide (PINP)	Calcium
Procollagen type III amino-terminal propeptide (PIIINP)	Hydroxyproline
	Cross-linked peptides (pyridinium and deoxypyridinoline)

the more important clinical outcomes of fractures, is unknown. In a random stratified sample of 3222 women in the perimenopausal age range (47–56 years), including 119 women with asthma, bone mineral density was measured to determine whether asthma was a risk factor of osteoporosis and to investigate the effect of inhaled glucocorticoids (75). The subjects had predominantly adult-onset asthma, as the age at diagnosis was over 40 years. There were 26 patients who were treated mainly with inhaled glucocorticoids (average daily dose 1000 micrograms). The asthmatic women in this general perimenopausal population had slightly reduced spinal and femoral neck bone mineral density compared with non-asthmatic women. These differences were more prominent in women who were not taking hormone replacement therapy. The reduction in bone mineral density may be due to glucocorticoids, and hormone replacement therapy appears to be protective against bone loss in asthmatics as well as healthy subjects. Cross-sectional studies such as this provide information about association but do not imply causality, for which longitudinal studies are required. Studies of the effects of inhaled glucocorticoids on markers of bone mineral density have provided conflicting data (76).

Effects on bone mineral density

Bone mineral density has been measured in a 3-year prospective study in 109 premenopausal asthmatic women, aged 18–45 years, all of whom used inhaled triamcinolone acetonide (77). They were grouped according to their inhaled glucocorticoid use at base line (no glucocorticoids and triamcinolone less than 800 micrograms/day or more than 800 micrograms/day). Therapy with triamcinolone was associated with a dose-related fall in bone mineral density at the hip overall and the trochanter. There was no effect at the femoral neck or the spine. None of the measured serum or urinary markers of bone turnover predicted the degree of bone loss. The dose-related loss of bone mineral density was suggested to be clinically related to prolonged treatment with inhaled glucocorticoids, and periodic bone mineral density assessment in patients taking high-dose inhaled glucocorticoids was proposed.

The effect of beclomethasone on bone mineral density has been examined over 1 year in 36 premenopausal and early postmenopausal women with asthma using inhaled glucocorticoids (beclomethasone at a mean dose of 542 micrograms/day) compared with 45 healthy matched controls (78). In early postmenopausal asthmatic women using beclomethasone, bone mineral density was significantly lower than in the controls, but not in premenopausal asthmatic women using inhaled beclomethasone. Serum osteocalcin concentrations were lower in the early postmenopausal asthmatic women using inhaled glucocorticoids than in the healthy controls, suggesting reduced bone formation, which leads to more pronounced bone loss. Ovarian hormones were suggested to offset the bone-depleting effects of inhaled beclomethasone in premenopausal women by maintaining or stimulating osteoblastic function.

There were significant reductions in bone mineral density in the lumbar spine and femur in 32 asthmatic women taking long-term inhaled beclomethasone (750–1500 micrograms/day) compared with 26 healthy controls (79). Control subjects and asthmatic patients were matched for age, sex, menopausal status, body-mass index, calcium intake, and physical activity. Loss of bone mass was more pronounced in the postmenopausal women. The authors identified several risk factors for accelerated bone loss in the lumbar spine, including postmenopausal status, low body-mass index, long duration of disease, long-term inhaled glucocorticoid therapy, and higher average daily and cumulative inhaled glucocorticoid doses.

The effects of inhaled budesonide 800 micrograms/day and fluticasone 400 micrograms/day on bone metabolism, morning cortisol concentrations, and clinical parameters have been studied in eight asthmatic patients (80). There were no changes in serum and bone alkaline phosphatase, osteocalcin, carboxyterminal propeptide of type 1 procollagen, and urinary calcium and deoxypyridinoline concentrations over 6 months. The authors concluded that fluticasone is as effective as twice the dose of budesonide in controlling asthmatic symptoms, without adverse effects on bone metabolism.

In a prospective comparison of the changes in bone mineral density in adults with mild asthma, 374 subjects with mild asthma (mean FEV_1 86% predicted; mean age 35 years; 55% women) were randomized to receive inhaled budesonide, inhaled beclomethasone, or non-glucocorticoid treatment (the control group) for 2 years (81). Bone mineral density was measured blind after 6, 12, and 24 months. The median daily doses of budesonide (87 subjects) and beclomethasone (74 subjects) were 389 and 499 micrograms respectively. The mean changes in bone density over 2 years in the budesonide, beclomethasone, and control groups were 0.1, –0.4, and 0.4% in the lumbar spine and –0.9, –0.9, and –0.4% in the neck of the femur. The mean daily dose of inhaled glucocorticoid was related to the reduction in bone mineral density only in the lumbar spine. Low to moderate doses of inhaled glucocorticoids caused little change in bone mineral density over 2 years and provided better asthma control.

In a retrospective cohort comparison of patients using inhaled glucocorticoids or bronchodilators with controls, there was an increased risk of fractures, particularly at the hip and spine, in those using inhaled glucocorticoids. There were no differences in relative fracture risks with different drugs, for example fluticasone, budesonide, beclomethasone (82). In an earlier retrospective study, there was a dose-dependent increase in bone fracture risk with oral glucocorticoids (83).

The effects of inhaled glucocorticoids on bone mineral density (measured using dual X-ray absorptiometry of the spine and hip) and biochemical parameters were followed over 18 months. Mean serum osteocalcin concentrations were significantly lower in patients taking beclomethasone dipropionate or budesonide at doses of 800 micrograms/day and more. However, bone mineral density of the lumbar spine and hip was not affected. The normal advancement of bone mineral density expected in growing children was not affected by inhaled glucocorticoids taken for 7–16 months (SEDA-22, 184).

Treatment with beclomethasone dipropionate 1500 micrograms/day for 6 weeks significantly reduced markers of bone formation (osteocalcin and PICP), whereas fluticasone propionate 750 micrograms/day had no effect. Neither drug affected biochemical markers of bone resorption. There was no significant change in bone density (SEDA-22, 183).

Effects on bone mineral density in children

A cross-sectional study in children (84) showed no significant difference in total and anteroposterior spine bone mineral density between children with asthma treated with long-term budesonide (200–800 micrograms for at least 6 months; $n = 52$) and asthmatic children who had never used inhaled glucocorticoids ($n = 22$). These results are in agreement with those of a larger cross-sectional study of the effects of long-term treatment (3–6 years, mean 4.5 years) with inhaled budesonide on total bone mineral density in children with asthma ($n = 157$). The results provided evidence that long-term treatment with inhaled glucocorticoids in moderate dosages is unlikely to affect bone mineral density adversely in children with asthma (85). However, a study of the association of clinical risk factors and bone density with fractures in 324 prepubertal children, of whom 32 had a fracture, suggested that for total fracture risk bone mineral density may be less important than clinical risk factors (86). In a multivariate model incorporating age, weight, height, breast-feeding history, sports participation, and the use of inhaled glucocorticoids, these factors accounted for 10% of the variability in the risk of fracture. Surprisingly, bone mineral density in the lumbar spine, femoral neck, and total body bone did not differ between those with and without fractures.

In a small cross-sectional study, bone mineral density was studied in 20 prepubertal asthmatic patients treated with moderate to high doses of inhaled glucocorticoids (under 400 micrograms/day beclomethasone or budesonide or over 200 micrograms/day fluticasone) (87). Volumetric trabecular bone mineral density of the lumbar spine and distal radius were measured using dual energy X-ray absorptiometry and were within the reference ranges.

Bone mineral density (measured by dual X-ray absorptiometry) did not change significantly in asthmatic children treated for 3–6 years with a mean daily dose of 504 micrograms (189–1322 micrograms) budesonide (85).

In 23 children, randomized to either fluticasone 100 micrograms bd or beclomethasone 200 micrograms bd for 20 months, there was a significant increase in bone mineral density in the lumbar spine with time, following the normal growth pattern (88).

Comparisons with placebo

More data on the effect of inhaled glucocorticoids on bone mineral density in adults have been generated by the large randomized, multicenter, double-blind, placebo-controlled EUROSCOPE (European Respiratory Society Study on Chronic Obstructive Pulmonary Disease) study of 912 patients with chronic obstructive pulmonary disease randomly assigned to treatment for 3 years with budesonide 800 micrograms/day or placebo (89). There were no significant differences in bone mineral density at L2–4 vertebrae, the femoral neck, trochanter, or Ward's triangle; nor did the fracture rate between budesonide-treated and placebo-treated patients differ. These findings are in contrast to recent data from the Lung Health Study, which showed that triamcinolone 1200 micrograms/day for 4 years was associated with a statistically significant 2% reduction in bone mineral density in the femoral neck compared with placebo (90).

Comparisons of glucocorticoids

In a 12-month, multicenter comparison of fluticasone propionate 250–500 micrograms/day with beclomethasone dipropionate 500–1000 micrograms/day, the two drugs had an equal therapeutic effect. Fluticasone propionate treatment resulted in a higher bone mineral density (assessed at the hip) and higher serum osteocalcin concentrations.

In a prospective randomized comparison of the effects of fluticasone propionate 1000 micrograms/day and budesonide 1600 micrograms/day, over 1 year, bone mineral density measured in the spine was normal at the start of the study and increased slightly with time in both groups, as did serum osteocalcin concentration.

Fluticasone propionate 1000 micrograms/day or beclomethasone dipropionate 2000 micrograms/day taken for 2 years caused no change in biochemical markers of bone metabolism. Bone mineral density, measured by dual X-ray absorptiometry or single-photon absorptiometry, showed no consistent change. However, when bone mineral density was measured using quantitative computed tomography of the lumbar spine, beclomethasone dipropionate was associated with a small fall in bone mineral density, which stabilized by 24 months. It is doubtful that a small fall in bone density seen only on quantitative computed tomography is clinically relevant (SEDA-22, 184).

The efficacy and safety of fluticasone 750 micrograms/day and beclomethasone 1500 micrograms/day delivered by a spacer device have been compared in 30 asthmatic children in a 12-week, randomized, double-blind, crossover study (91). All of the children had persistent asthma requiring 1000–2000 micrograms/day of inhaled glucocorticoids before the trial. There was no significant difference in efficacy, as judged by daytime and nighttime symptom scores and PEFR. There was a minimal reduction in serum cortisol in both groups. Both groups had identical height gain velocities. At the doses used in this trial, the authors were unable to show a safety advantage of fluticasone over beclomethasone, as assessed by cortisol concentrations.

In a 1-year prospective, randomized, open comparison of inhaled fluticasone 500 micrograms bd with budesonide 800 micrograms bd delivered by metered-dose inhaler and large volume spacer, bone mineral density was measured in 29 patients in the lumbar spine and femoral neck (92). Bone mineral density in the spine increased slightly in both groups over the 12 months. Serum osteocalcin concentrations increased from baseline in both treatment groups (fluticasone +17%, budesonide +14%). The percentage change from baseline in bone mineral density of the spine correlated with the increase in serum osteocalcin. Mean serum cortisol concentrations remained in the reference range after both inhaled glucocorticoids.

It can be hypothesized that different glucocorticoids have different systemic effects, and therefore different effects on bone metabolism. An alternative hypothesis is that these effects are dose dependent (58), support for which comes from a population-based case-control study of 16 341 older patients with hip fractures (mean age 79 years) and 29 889 controls; recent use of an inhaled glucocorticoid was associated with a small dose-dependent increase in the risk of hip fracture (93).

Comparisons with other drugs

Bone mineral density was measured after 7.4 months in 49 asthmatic children, 38 of whom took inhaled beclomethasone, average daily dose 276 micrograms, and 11 sodium cromoglicate, average daily dose 30 mg (94). Children who had used beclomethasone had grown as much as those who used sodium cromoglicate. Trabecular and cortical bone mineral density in the proximal forearm and lumbar spine increased to the same extent in both groups.

The effects of fluticasone 50 micrograms bd or sodium cromoglicate 20 mg qds on growth over 12 months have been studied in 122 asthmatic children aged 4–10 years (95). The mean height velocity was 6 cm/year with fluticasone and 6.5 cm/year with sodium cromoglicate. There was no significant treatment difference in the mean 24-hour urinary-free cortisol concentrations at 6 or 12 months. Mean predicted peak expiratory flow rate improved over 1 year in both groups, but to a greater extent with fluticasone. The authors concluded that growth was normal in mildly asthmatic children using fluticasone (50 micrograms bd) for 1 year. Fluticasone was more effective than sodium cromoglicate, with fewer withdrawals and greater improvement in lung function.

Dose relation

Current evidence suggests that the changes in bone mineral density in asthmatic patients who take inhaled glucocorticoids occur within the high therapeutic range of doses. In patients with mild asthma who are well maintained on low doses of inhaled glucocorticoids, the benefits derived from good control of the asthma appear to outweigh any concerns about minor changes in bone mineral density. The picture is less clear in patients with other risk factors, such as estrogen deficiency and advancing years.

No adverse effect on bone has been shown with beclomethasone dipropionate or budesonide at doses less than 1000 micrograms/day or fluticasone propionate less than 500 micrograms/day. Most patients obtain a good therapeutic response at these doses. Higher doses may be required in some patients. Aerosols delivering doses of beclomethasone dipropionate 250 and 500 micrograms, budesonide 400 micrograms and fluticasone propionate 250 and 500 micrograms should be reserved for patients in whom the requirement for a high dose has been demonstrated in an adequate trial of therapy.

In an uncontrolled study, 56 women with asthma taking long-term inhaled glucocorticoids had bone mineral density measurements of the lumbar spine and hip (96). Women who had taken more than three short courses of systemic glucocorticoids per year over the preceding 3 years were excluded. Data on duration of use and dose of inhaled glucocorticoids were obtained from the patients' medical records. Doses of inhaled glucocorticoids were arbitrarily classified as low (under 500 micrograms/day), medium (500–1000 micrograms/day), and high (over 1000 micrograms/day). More than half the women (61%) had reduced bone mineral density at either the hip or lumbar spine. Amongst the postmenopausal women in the study, 17% of those aged under 65 years had osteoporosis compared with 43% of those aged over 65 years. These figures exceeded those from a national sample of estrogen-deficient women, in which 5.7% under the age of 65 and 29% over the age of 65 years had osteoporosis. Bone mineral density loss increased with higher doses of inhaled glucocorticoids, from 5% in the low-dose group to 50% in the high-dose group. Whilst this is a potentially important finding in women at risk of osteoporosis because of the menopause, there are some aspects of the design of the study that limit the applicability of the findings. There was no appropriate age- and ethnicity-matched control group, and the contribution of nasal glucocorticoids was not accurately assessed.

In a large cross-sectional study, patients aged 20–40 years with asthma who had taken inhaled glucocorticoids for a median of 6 years were studied (97). Patients were excluded if they had taken a course of oral or parenteral glucocorticoids in the past 6 months or more than two courses ever, or if they had had more than 10 inhalers of nasal glucocorticoids or more than 10 prescriptions of a dermal glucocorticoid. Computerized records of general practices were used to identify patients for the study. Bone mineral density was measured at the lumbar spine (L2–L4) and the left femur (neck, Ward's triangle, trochanter). The cumulative dose of inhaled glucocorticoid was expressed as a product of the mean daily dose and time (mg days). This information was obtained from a patient questionnaire and validated against general practice computer and paper records. More than half of the patients (119/196) were women and the median cumulative dose of inhaled glucocorticoid was 876 mg (range 88–4380 mg). There was a significant inverse relation between the cumulative dose of inhaled glucocorticoid and bone mineral density at the spine and hip in both men and women. A doubling of cumulative dose was associated with a 0.16 times SD reduction in bone mineral density. Extrapolation from cross-sectional data such as these requires confirmation in longitudinal studies, since bone loss with oral glucocorticoids is more rapid in the first 12–24 months of therapy.

Bone mineral density has been measured at 3-year intervals in 51 patients taking inhaled glucocorticoids for asthma (98). The patients were divided into a high-dose group taking over 800 micrograms/day of beclomethasone or budesonide ($n = 28$, mean dose 983 micrograms/day) and a control group taking no inhaled glucocorticoid or less than 500 micrograms/day ($n = 23$, mean dose 309 micrograms/day). Whilst there were statistically significant reductions in bone markers, such as serum calcium and phosphorus and osteocalcin, over the 3-year period in each group, there was no significant reduction in bone mineral density in either group of asthmatic patients. Although the change in bone mineral density in the high-dose group was small over the 3-year period and not statistically significant, there was a correlation between bone loss and the daily dose of inhaled glucocorticoids. There was no significant correlation between the changes in bone density and either the initial bone density or biomarkers of bone turnover for the level of physical activity. This longitudinal study has shown the unreliability of biomarkers of bone turnover in predicting changes in bone density (and presumably relevant clinical outcomes, such as risk of fracture) and shows the need for measurement of bone mineral density in asthmatic patients who are deemed to be at risk of bone loss. Such patients include those taking oral glucocorticoids, perimenopausal women not taking hormone replacement therapy, and patients who need high doses of inhaled glucocorticoids. Whilst patients in this study did not have significant changes in bone mineral density over 3 years, the effects of higher doses remain uncertain, so it would be prudent to measure bone mineral density in patients who need higher doses.

Time course

The time course of changes in bone mineral density with inhaled glucocorticoids has yet to be determined. Longitudinal studies will be required to determine whether bone loss is most rapid in the first 12–24 months after initiating inhaled glucocorticoid therapy, as is the case with oral glucocorticoids (99) and whether the risk of fracture falls towards baseline after withdrawal of treatment, as was suggested by the GPRD (General Practice Research Database) study (87).

In older women with asthma, who have an increased risk of osteoporosis, there was no significant change in bone mineral density after 1 year of treatment with beclomethasone dipropionate 1000 micrograms/day (100).

Bone mineral density, bone turnover markers, and adrenal glucocorticoid hormones have been measured in 53 patients (34 women, 19 men) with chronic bronchial asthma who took either inhaled beclomethasone or budesonide in doses of at least 1500 micrograms/day for at least 12 months (101). The patients were divided into those who had taken oral glucocorticoids for more than 1 month and those who had not. Bone mineral density was measured at the lumbar spine and the proximal femur. The values were about one standard deviation lower in men and women taking oral glucocorticoids or very high doses of inhaled glucocorticoids. The reduction in bone mineral density was enough to a double the risk of fracture at these sites. There was suppression of both endogenous glucocorticoid and adrenal androgen production in all subjects. Adrenal androgen suppression may increase the susceptibility of postmenopausal women treated with an oral glucocorticoid to bone loss.

Risk of fracture

Although studies in which biochemical markers of bone turnover are measured for periods of 1–2 months do not predict the development of bone thinning, osteoporosis, or fracture, they can be useful in comparing the potential effects on bone of different glucocorticoids. Studies of bone mineral density over longer time periods relate more directly to osteoporosis and fracture risk.

Whilst there have been several studies of the effects of inhaled glucocorticoids on bone mineral density, there are few data on the effects of inhaled glucocorticoids on the risk of fracture. In a retrospective cohort study the risk of fracture was established by examining the General Practice Research Database (GPRD), which is run by the Medicines Control Agency in the UK (87). Users of inhaled glucocorticoids were defined as permanently registered patients aged 18 years or more who received one or more prescriptions for inhaled glucocorticoids during the time from enrolment in the GPRD until the end of data collection. Patients who received a prescription for oral glucocorticoids for a period of 6 months before to 91 days after the last prescription for an inhaled glucocorticoid were excluded. There were two comparison groups: a bronchodilator group, which included adults who received prescriptions for non-systemic glucocorticoids and bronchodilators, and a second control group who received non-systemic glucocorticoids but never inhaled systemic glucocorticoids or bronchodilators. The database included over 440 000 patients and all patients who had fractures were identified from their medical records during the follow-up period, which was 91 days after the last prescription for an inhaled glucocorticoid. The relative rates of non-vertebral, hip, and vertebral fractures during inhaled glucocorticoid treatment compared with controls were 1.15 (95% CI = 1.10, 1.20), 1.22 (CI = 1.04, 1.43), and 1.51 (CI = 1.22, 1.85) respectively. There were no differences between inhaled glucocorticoids and bronchodilators (non-vertebral fracture relative rate = 1). The authors concluded that users of inhaled glucocorticoids may have an increased risk of fracture, particularly at the hip and spine, but that this excess risk may be related more to the underlying respiratory disease than to the inhaled glucocorticoids.

There were no major differences between the three groups in baseline fracture history. About 1% in each cohort recorded a history of non-vertebral fractures in the year before baseline. During the follow-up, the incidence of non-vertebral fractures was 1.4 fractures per 100 persons with inhaled glucocorticoids, 1.4 with bronchodilators, and 1.1 in the control group. Comparing inhaled glucocorticoid users with a control group, there was a dose response for hip and vertebral fractures. For a standardized daily dose of under 300 micrograms/day of budesonide, hip fracture was 0.95, rising to 1.06 at doses of 300–700 micrograms/day and 1.77 at doses of 700 micrograms/day or more. There was no consistent trend in the rate of fractures amongst users of inhaled glucocorticoid compared with bronchodilators.

This is a noteworthy study because it has examined the most important clinical outcome of change in bone mineral density: the risk of fracture. The results point to an increased risk of fracture, especially at the hip and the vertebral bodies, amongst patients who use inhaled glucocorticoids as well as those using bronchodilators, when compared with patients not using these drugs. Fracture risk tended to fall after withdrawal of inhaled glucocorticoids or bronchodilators. These findings suggest that low-dose inhaled glucocorticoids are not associated with an increased risk of fracture and that patients with chronic respiratory disease who use any inhaled therapy are at risk compared with a control population. There were no differences in fracture risk between the various types of bronchodilators, suggesting that the underlying lung disease itself was the basis of risk rather than any particular type of bronchodilator. The authors noted that 1.9% of patients were using doses of budesonide equivalents of over 1500 micrograms/day and that the possibility of a more pronounced increased fracture risk at these high doses cannot be excluded. The age- and sex-specific incidence of fracture in the control group was similar to that of the general population in the GPRD.

Estimates of the important outcome of bone fracture have shown a small increased risk with inhaled glucocorticoids, but this may well be a feature of the disease rather than the therapy, because comparisons with treatment with bronchodilator drugs show no difference between risk factors in patients taking glucocorticoids or bronchodilators.

Prevention of osteoporosis with bisphosphonates

The effect of high-dose inhaled glucocorticoids and antiresorptive therapy with sodium etidronate has been studied for 18 months in 38 Chinese patients (24 men and 14 premenopausal women aged 30–50 years), of whom 28 were asthmatics who had already been treated for at least 12 months with high-dose inhaled glucocorticoids (beclomethasone or budesonide over 1.5 mg/day), and 10 healthy controls (102). The patients were randomly allocated to (1) no supplement, (2) a calcium supplement 1000 mg/day, or (3) cyclical sodium etidronate 400 mg/day for 14 days followed by calcium 1000 mg/day for 76 days. All three groups continued to take inhaled glucocorticoids. Bone mineral density was measured at the lumbar spine and hip. Bone mineral density in the group one patients fell by about 1% over 18 months and rose by about 1.5% in the healthy controls, neither change being significant. In groups 2 and 3 bone mineral density rose significantly at 12 and 18 months by 2 and 3% respectively. Serum osteocalcin concentrations fell significantly in all three groups of asthmatic patients but not in the controls. There were no significant changes in serum alkaline phosphatase or parathyroid hormone. In the patients taking calcium, with or without etidronate, mean serum calcium increased. The authors suggested that calcium supplementation and cyclical etidronate work by reducing bone resorption, and hence reduced bone turnover, rather than by increasing bone formation. This is consistent with the fall in serum osteocalcin.

The efficacy of clodronate in treating glucocorticoid-induced bone loss in asthmatic subjects has been evaluated in a double-blind study in 74 adults (41 women and 33 men, mean age 57 years) with a long history (mean 8.1 years) of oral and inhaled glucocorticoid use, randomized to clodronate 800, 1600, or 2400 mg/day or placebo (103). There was no increase in bone mineral density with placebo or clodronate 800 mg/day, but a significant dose-related increase with clodronate 1600 and 2400 mg/day. The most common adverse effect was gastric irritation in the patients who took the highest dose of clodronate.

Growth

Oral glucocorticoids inhibit growth by blunting pulsatile growth hormone secretion, by decreasing insulin-like growth factor-1 activity, and by directly inhibiting collagen synthesis (104). Although inhalation reduces systemic exposure, concerns have been raised regarding the potential effects on growth and final height in children, especially when inhaled glucocorticoids are used for long periods.

Uninterrupted administration of moderate-dose inhaled glucocorticoids (for example 400 micrograms/day of budesonide equivalents) has been associated with a suppressed growth rate in some children with asthma. Budesonide reduced the growth by 1 and 1.4 cm over 7 and 12 months, respectively (105). Consequently, in the USA, a class label warning for inhaled glucocorticoids about growth retardation in children was introduced in 1998, when the FDA decided to alter the class labeling for all inhaled and nasal glucocorticoids in children, to indicate that the use of recommended doses might be associated with a reduction in growth velocity (19). However, the available studies suggest that in children, the major advantages of adequate asthma control with inhaled glucocorticoids outweigh any potential adverse effects on growth.

However, results from trials in asthmatic children can be flawed by confounding variables. Severe asthma can itself have a negative effect on growth and adversely affect adult height, as with any chronic disease. Even in well-controlled asthma, children typically show retardation in pubertal growth spurt and attain normal adult height later. As growth in children is non-linear over time, trials over short periods are likely to capture short-term effects of inhaled glucocorticoids rather than the long-term outcome. Furthermore, the growth-retarding effect of inhaled glucocorticoids is more pronounced at the start of treatment.

Long-term studies have suggested that a temporary short-term or medium-term reduction in growth velocity is normally compensated for later on, and individuals attain normal adult height (106,107). The effects of inhaled glucocorticoids on growth rate over weeks and months are dose-dependent, and dose-response curves of pulmonary and adverse systemic effects differ widely, so that individual titration of the inhaled glucocorticoid dose according to the severity of the disease is strongly recommended, and the lowest dose of inhaled glucocorticoids that controls the disease should always be preferred. In conclusion, accumulating evidence shows that children with asthma, even when treated with inhaled glucocorticoids for years, attain normal adult height. However, close growth monitoring during inhaled glucocorticoid therapy is recommended, as idiosyncratic responses can occur, probably owing to individual glucocorticoid receptor polymorphism (108).

A two-part review was published in 2002, addressing the difficulties of assessing the effects of asthma therapy on childhood growth and reviewing the published literature based on the authors' recommendations (109,110). In the first part (109), a simple classification system for growth studies was developed:

- comparisons with placebo (type 1 studies);
- comparisons with non-steroidal asthma therapy (type 2 studies);
- comparisons with another inhaled glucocorticoid (type 3 studies);
- comparisons with "real life" asthma therapy (type 4 studies).

In the context of these different study types, the authors also discussed the choice of end-point, key trial design issues, the selection and numbers of subjects in the active and control groups, the duration of assessments, and methods for measuring height and data analysis. They also elaborated specific recommendations regarding study duration, age/sexual maturity of the patients, exclusion criteria for height and growth velocity, permitted therapy during the study, the protocol for height measurement, the numbers of patients for adequate statistical power, and methods for statistical analysis (109).

In the second part, they selected 18 growth studies that included minimal criteria, such as selected control group, measured height by stadiometry, and at least a 12-month duration; they compared the design attributes of these studies with the described recommendations (110). Of the 18 selected studies, 17 were susceptible to one or more important confounding factors; nevertheless, the outcomes of all 18 studies were considered to be consistent. In summary, impaired growth velocity was found with budesonide and beclomethasone dipropionate compared with placebo, non-steroidal treatment, and fluticasone propionate during 1–2 years of therapy, but none of the inhaled glucocorticoids appeared to affect final height (110). Growth in children treated with low-dose fluticasone propionate (up to 200 micrograms/day) for 1 year is similar to growth in those treated with placebo or non-steroidal therapy. Standard pediatric doses of inhaled glucocorticoids (less than 800 micrograms of budesonide and less than 400 micrograms of budesonide or fluticasone) are considered not to affect growth adversely (57,111). The risk of growth suppression depends on the dose, the administration regimen, and the delivery device.

An important confounding factor is the influence of non-adherence to inhaled glucocorticoid treatment (112). Sensitive and reliable measures of adherence should be applied when evaluating long-term effects on height.

The time of dosing can influence the effect of inhaled glucocorticoids on growth suppression in the prepubertal child, since growth hormone secretion is generally confined to nighttime. Therefore, once-daily morning dosing could be advantageous (113).

For clinical practice, the lowest effective dose should be achieved, and all children using inhaled glucocorticoids should have their growth measured every 6 months, as this is a sensitive method of detecting significant systemic effects (57,113).

These results apply to children over 4 years of age; for younger children only assumptions can be entertained and age-specific studies are needed (113).

Dose relation

Lumbar spine bone mineral density has been assessed in 76 prepubertal asthmatics (mean age 7.7 years, 26 girls) using glucocorticoids (114). After stratification for dose and route of administration, the children who used over 800 micrograms/day of inhaled glucocorticoids, with or without intermittent oral glucocorticoids, had a significant lower weight-adjusted bone density than children who used 400–800 micrograms/day of inhaled glucocorticoids (mean difference –0.05 g/cm^2; 95% CI = –0.02, –0.09). Bone mass was similar in children who did not use inhaled glucocorticoids and those who used 400–800 micrograms/day.

The authors of a review concluded, from short-term and intermediate-term growth studies, that there are no clinically significant adverse effects on growth with inhaled glucocorticoids at normal pediatric doses (100–200 micrograms/day budesonide equivalents), but that growth retardation can occur with all inhaled glucocorticoids at higher doses (115). Individual idiosyncratic adverse reactions are rare. Long-term studies and studies that have examined the effect on final adult height have been consistent in showing significantly reduced growth rates during the first months and up to 2 years of treatment with inhaled glucocorticoids. However, children treated with inhaled glucocorticoids attain their predicted adult height to the same extent as their healthy peers. It is important to note that changes in growth rate during the first year of inhaled glucocorticoid treatment cannot be used to predict final adult height.

Growth velocity measured over a 12-month period in prepubertal children with asthma was reduced by prior treatment with inhaled glucocorticoids for an average of 2.7 years. However, measurement of biochemical markers (Table 1) gave conflicting results. Osteocalcin concentrations were reduced, but alkaline phosphatase did not change. PINP and PIIINP were reduced, but PICP increased. ICTP, a marker for collagen I degradation, fell.

Comparisons of glucocorticoids

Fluticasone propionate 400 micrograms/day or budesonide 800 micrograms/day were administered for 20 weeks to children with moderate to severe asthma aged 4–12 years. Fluticasone propionate was superior to budesonide in improving peak expiratory flow and comparable in controlling symptoms. Growth was reduced with budesonide treatment compared with fluticasone propionate treatment mean difference, 6.2 mm (CI = 2.9, 9.6). There was no difference in serum cortisol suppression (116).

Comparisons with other drugs

Beclomethasone dipropionate 400 micrograms/day and salmeterol 50 micrograms bd were compared in asthmatic children treated for 12 months. Beclomethasone dipropionate treatment resulted in better overall asthma control. Over 12 months, linear growth was 3.96 cm/year in the children using beclomethasone dipropionate, compared with 5.40 cm/year in those who used salmeterol and 5.04 cm/year in a placebo group (SEDA-22, 186).

The long-term effects of inhaled glucocorticoids on growth in children have been recently assessed. In the so-called CaAMP Study (117), children aged 5–12 years with mild to moderate asthma were randomized to budesonide 200 micrograms bd (n = 311), nedocromil 8 mg bd (n = 312), or placebo (n = 418). At the end of the 4–6 year treatment period, the mean increase in height in the budesonide group was 1.1 cm less than in the placebo group. The difference between budesonide and placebo in the rate of growth was evident primarily within the first year but did not increase thereafter, and all the groups had similar growth velocity by the end of the treatment period.

Comparisons with oral glucocorticoids

A meta-analysis of 21 studies in which 810 asthmatic children were treated with oral prednisolone (8 trials) and/or beclomethasone dipropionate, dosage range 200–900 micrograms/day (12 trials) has been reported. Significant suppression of growth occurred with oral glucocorticoids but not with beclomethasone dipropionate (118).

Reversibility

Growth data obtained in 50 children who used beclomethasone dipropionate over 7 months suggested that any growth suppression is temporary and that growth velocity recovers during continuing treatment. Growth velocity fell most in the first 6 weeks of treatment, from 0.140 to 0.073 mm/week (0.067 mm/week; 95% CI = 0.015, 0.120). There were similar reductions at 12 and 18 weeks. After this, growth velocity increased to rates seen before treatment began: 0.138 mm/week at 24 weeks and 0.120 mm/week at 30 weeks (119).

Long-term use of beclomethasone dipropionate 400–600 micrograms/day was reported to delay the onset of puberty. However, subsequent catch-up growth was unaffected and subjects reached their normal predicted adult height (120).

Children taking budesonide (mean daily dose 412 micrograms, range 110–877 micrograms) for periods of 3–13 years have been followed to adulthood to determine their final height (107). These 142 budesonide-treated children were compared with 18 control patients with asthma who had never taken inhaled glucocorticoids and 51 healthy siblings of the patients in the budesonide group. These children, who had taken long-term inhaled glucocorticoids, attained normal adult height. There was no evidence of a dose–response relation between the mean daily dose of budesonide, the cumulative dose, or the duration of treatment with budesonide and the difference between the measured and target adult heights.

These studies are important, because several previous reports of growth during a period of 1 year after beginning treatment with inhaled glucocorticoids (in daily doses of about 400 micrograms of budesonide) identified growth retardation of about 1.5 cm. The mechanism for the termination after 1 year of the effects on growth is uncertain.

Immunologic

Hypersensitivity to inhaled glucocorticoids is rare.

- An asthmatic patient using inhaled budesonide and salbutamol developed an acute asthma attack. Despite emergency treatment the patient deteriorated, requiring endotracheal intubation and assisted ventilation, and there was no improvement until the glucocorticoid was withdrawn, after which there was steady improvement. Skin prick tests with prednisolone, sodium hemisuccinate, and 6-methylprednisolone-sodium hemisuccinate were positive. Thirty minutes after intradermal 6-methylprednisolone-sodium hemisuccinate 4 mg, the patient developed a dry cough, dyspnea, and wheezing and a 17% fall in FEV_1.
- A 37-year-old woman who was pregnant developed Churg–Strauss syndrome after withdrawal of her usual high-dose inhaled glucocorticoid therapy (drug not stated) that she had used for 3 years for bronchial asthma (121).

The authors of the second report commented that activated eosinophils and their cytotoxic products, such as eosinophil catatonic protein, may play a part in the pathogenesis of Churg–Strauss syndrome. Measuring serum concentrations of eosinophil catatonic protein may be useful in monitoring disease activity, since concentrations were increased before treatment and normalized afterwards.

Infection risk

Inhaled or topical immunosuppressive and anti-inflammatory glucocorticoids increase the risk of oral candidiasis (122). Patients who harbor oral *Candida* before they use inhaled glucocorticoids may have an increased risk. The location and degree of oral candidiasis seems to be related to dosage, administration frequency, and inhalation technique. Preventive measures include using a spacer, lowering the dosage, and rinsing the mouth after use.

Invasive aspergillosis occurred after high-dose inhaled fluticasone (440 micrograms qds) and zafirlukast 20 mg/day in a 44-year old man with moderately severe asthma; this is the first report of invasive pulmonary aspergillosis associated with an inhaled glucocorticoid (123).

Second-Generation Effects

Teratogenicity

Congenital malformations that may be associated with inhaled budesonide in pregnancy have been evaluated using the Swedish Medical Birth Registry (124). Of 2014 infants whose mothers started to use inhaled budesonide in early pregnancy, 75 (3.7%) had a congenital malformation; the corresponding rate among all infants born in 1995–97 was 3.5%. Five infants had chromosomal anomalies that were unlikely to have been caused by drugs. This study did not identify teratogenic properties of inhaled budesonide.

Drug–Drug Interactions

Itraconazole

Interactions with other drugs can increase plasma concentrations of inhaled glucocorticoids. Itraconazole, a potent inhibitor of CYP3A4, markedly increased plasma concentrations of inhaled budesonide (125).

Ritonavir

Ritonavir, a potent inhibitor of CYP3A4, caused Cushing's syndrome in a patient using fluticasone propionate 1000 micrograms/day (126).

References

1. Allen DB. Sense and sensitivity: assessing inhaled corticosteroid effects on the hypothalamic–pituitary–adrenal axis. Ann Allergy Asthma Immunol 2002; 89(6):537–9.
2. Minto C, Li B, Tattam B, Brown K, Seale JP, Donnelly R. Pharmacokinetics of epimeric budesonide and fluticasone propionate after repeat dose inhalation—intersubject variability in systemic absorption from the lung. Br J Clin Pharmacol 2000;50(2):116–24.
3. Donnelly R, Williams KM, Baker AB, Badcock CA, Day RO, Seale JP. Effects of budesonide and fluticasone on 24-hour plasma cortisol. A dose-response study. Am J Respir Crit Care Med 1997;156(6):1746–51.
4. Weiner P, Berar-Yanay N, Davidovich A, Magadle R. Nocturnal cortisol secretion in asthmatic patients after inhalation of fluticasone propionate. Chest 1999; 116(4):931–4.
5. Brutsche MH, Brutsche IC, Munawar M, Langley SJ, Masterson CM, Daley-Yates PT, Brown R, Custovic A, Woodcock A. Comparison of pharmacokinetics and systemic effects of inhaled fluticasone propionate in patients with asthma and healthy volunteers: a randomised crossover study. Lancet 2000;356(9229):556–61.
6. Lofdahl CG, Thorsson L. No difference between asthmatic patients and healthy subjects in lung uptake of fluticasone propionate. Eur Respir J 1999;14:466S.
7. Harrison TW, Wisniewski A, Honour J, Tattersfield AE. Comparison of the systemic effects of fluticasone propionate and budesonide given by dry powder inhaler in healthy and asthmatic subjects. Thorax 2001;56(3):186–91.
8. Fabbri L, Melara R. Systemic effects of inhaled corticosteroids are milder in asthmatic patients than in normal subjects. Thorax 2001;56(3):165–6.

9. Berend N, Kellett B, Kent N, Sly PD, Bowler S, Burdon J, Dennis C, Gibson P, James A, Jenkins C; Collaborative Study Group of the Australian Lung Foundation. Improved safety with equivalent asthma control in adults with chronic severe asthma on high-dose fluticasone propionate. Respirology 2001;6(3):237–46.
10. Dubus JC, Marguet C, Deschildre A, Mely L, Le Roux P, Brouard J, Huiart L; Reseau de Recherche Clinique en Pneumonologie Pédiatrique. Local side-effects of inhaled corticosteroids in asthmatic children: influence of drug, dose, age, and device. Allergy 2001;56(10):944–8.
11. Wilson AM, Lipworth BJ. 24 hour and fractionated profiles of adrenocortical activity in asthmatic patients receiving inhaled and intranasal corticosteroids. Thorax 1999;54(1):20–6.
12. Borgstrom L. Local versus total systemic bioavailability as a means to compare different inhaled formulations of the same substance. J Aerosol Med 1998;11(1):55–63.
13. Kelly HW. Establishing a therapeutic index for the inhaled corticosteroids. Part I. Pharmacokinetic/pharmacodynamic comparison of the inhaled corticosteroids. J Allergy Clin Immunol 1998;102(4 Pt 2):S36–51.
14. Leach C. Targeting inhaled steroids. Int J Clin Pract Suppl 1998;96:23–7.
15. Trescoli C, Ward MJ. Systemic activity of inhaled and swallowed beclomethasone dipropionate and the effect of different inhaler devices. Postgrad Med J 1998; 74(877):675–7.
16. Thorsson L, Edsbacker S. Lung deposition of budesonide from a pressurized metered-dose inhaler attached to a spacer. Eur Respir J 1998;12(6):1340–5.
17. O'Byrne PM, Pedersen S. Measuring efficacy and safety of different inhaled corticosteroid preparations. J Allergy Clin Immunol 1998;102(6 Pt 1):879–86.
18. Martin RJ, Szefler SJ, Chinchilli VM, Kraft M, Dolovich M, Boushey HA, Cherniack RM, Craig TJ, Drazen JM, Fagan JK, Fahy JV, Fish JE, Ford JG, Israel E, Kunselman SJ, Lazarus SC, Lemanske RF Jr, Peters SP, Sorkness CA. Systemic effect comparisons of six inhaled corticosteroid preparations. Am J Respir Crit Care Med 2002;165(10):1377–83.
19. Lipworth BJ. Systemic adverse effects of inhaled corticosteroid therapy: A systematic review and meta-analysis. Arch Intern Med 1999;159(9):941–55.
20. Goldberg S, Einot T, Algur N, Schwartz S, Greenberg AC, Picard E, Virgilis D, Kerem E. Adrenal suppression in asthmatic children receiving low-dose inhaled budesonide: comparison between dry powder inhaler and pressurized metered-dose inhaler attached to a spacer. Ann Allergy Asthma Immunol 2002;89(6):566–71.
21. Irani AM, Cruz-Rivera M, Fitzpatrick S, Hoag J, Smith JA. Effects of budesonide inhalation suspension on hypothalamic–pituitary–adrenal-axis function in infants and young children with persistent asthma. Ann Allergy Asthma Immunol 2002;88(3):306–12.
22. Eid N, Morton R, Olds B, Clark P, Sheikh S, Looney S. Decreased morning serum cortisol levels in children with asthma treated with inhaled fluticasone propionate. Pediatrics 2002;109(2):217–21.
23. Tukiainen H, Rytila P, Hamalainen KM, Silvasti MS, Keski-Karhu J; Finnish Study Group. Safety, tolerability and acceptability of two dry powder inhalers in the administration of budesonide in steroid-treated asthmatic patients. Respir Med 2002;96(4):221–9.
24. Volovitz B, Bentur L, Finkelstein Y, Mansour Y, Shalitin S, Nussinovitch M, Varsano I. Effectiveness and safety of inhaled corticosteroids in controlling acute asthma attacks in children who were treated in the emergency department: a controlled comparative study with oral prednisolone. J Allergy Clin Immunol 1998;102(4 Pt 1):605–9.
25. Nana A, Youngchaiyud P, Charoenratanakul S, Boe J, Lofdahl CG, Selroos O, Stahl E. High-dose inhaled budesonide may substitute for oral therapy after an acute asthma attack. J Asthma 1998;35(8):647–55.
26. Sung L, Osmond MH, Klassen TP. Randomized, controlled trial of inhaled budesonide as an adjunct to oral prednisone in acute asthma. Acad Emerg Med 1998;5(3):209–13.
27. Paggiaro PL, Dahle R, Bakran I, Frith L, Hollingworth K, Efthimiou J. Multicentre randomised placebo-controlled trial of inhaled fluticasone propionate in patients with chronic obstructive pulmonary disease. International COPD Study Group. Lancet 1998;351(9105):773–80. Erratum in: Lancet 1998;351(9120):1968.
28. Jick SS, Vasilakis-Scaramozza C, Maier WC. The risk of cataract among users of inhaled steroids. Epidemiology 2001;12(2):229–34.
29. Garbe E, Suissa S, LeLorier J. Association of inhaled corticosteroid use with cataract extraction in elderly patients. JAMA 1998;280(6):539–43. Erratum in: JAMA 1998;280(21):1830.
30. Kennedy L, Rusch VW, Strange C, Ginsberg RJ, Sahn SA. Pleurodesis using talc slurry. Chest 1994;106(2):342–6.
31. Li JT, Ford LB, Chervinsky P, Weisberg SC, Kellerman DJ, Faulkner KG, Herje NE, Hamedani A, Harding SM, Shah T. Fluticasone propionate powder and lack of clinically significant effects on hypothalamic–pituitary–adrenal axis and bone mineral density over 2 years in adults with mild asthma. J Allergy Clin Immunol 1999;103(6):1062–8.
32. Agertoft L, Larsen FE, Pedersen S. Posterior subcapsular cataracts, bruises and hoarseness in children with asthma receiving long-term treatment with inhaled budesonide. Eur Respir J 1998;12(1):130–5.
33. Garbe E, LeLorier J, Boivin JF, Suissa S. Inhaled and nasal glucocorticoids and the risks of ocular hypertension or open-angle glaucoma. JAMA 1997;277(9):722–7.
34. Casale TB, Nelson HS, Stricker WE, Raff H, Newman KB. Suppression of hypothalamic–pituitary–adrenal axis activity with inhaled flunisolide and fluticasone propionate in adult asthma patients. Ann Allergy Asthma Immunol 2001;87(5):379–85.
35. Nelson HS, Stricker W, Casale TB, Raff H, Fourre JA, Aron DC, Newman KB. A comparison of methods for assessing hypothalamic–pituitary–adrenal HPA axis activity in asthma patients treated with inhaled corticosteroids. J Clin Pharmacol 2002;42(3):319–26.
36. Fink RS, Pierre LN, Daley-Yates PT, Richards DH, Gibson A, Honour JW. Hypothalamic–pituitary–adrenal axis function after inhaled corticosteroids: unreliability of urinary free cortisol estimation. J Clin Endocrinol Metab 2002;87(10):4541–6.
37. Patel L, Wales JK, Kibirige MS, Massarano AA, Couriel JM, Clayton PE. Symptomatic adrenal insufficiency during inhaled corticosteroid treatment. Arch Dis Child 2001;85(4):330–4.
38. Vargas R, Dockhorn RJ, Findlay SR, Korenblat PE, Field EA, Kral KM. Effect of fluticasone propionate aqueous nasal spray versus oral prednisone on the hypothalamic–pituitary–adrenal axis. J Allergy Clin Immunol 1998;102(2):191–7.
39. Drake AJ, Howells RJ, Shield JP, Prendiville A, Ward PS, Crowne EC. Symptomatic adrenal insufficiency presenting with hypoglycaemia in children with asthma receiving high dose inhaled fluticasone propionate. BMJ 2002;324(7345):1081–2.

40. Todd GR, Acerini CL, Buck JJ, Murphy NP, Ross-Russell R, Warner JT, McCance DR. Acute adrenal crisis in asthmatics treated with high-dose fluticasone propionate. Eur Respir J 2002;19(6):1207–9.
41. Dunlop KA, Carson DJ, Shields MD. Hypoglycemia due to adrenal suppression secondary to high-dose nebulized corticosteroid. Pediatr Pulmonol 2002;34(1):85–6.
42. Kennedy MJ, Carpenter JM, Lozano RA, Castile RG. Impaired recovery of hypothalamic–pituitary–adrenal axis function and hypoglycemic seizures after high-dose inhaled corticosteroid therapy in a toddler. Ann Allergy Asthma Immunol 2002;88(5):523–6.
43. Duplantier JE, Nelson RP Jr, Morelli AR, Good RA, Kornfeld SJ. Hypothalamic–pituitary–adrenal axis suppression associated with the use of inhaled fluticasone propionate. J Allergy Clin Immunol 1998;102(4 Pt 1):699–700.
44. Zimmerman B, Gold M, Wherrett D, Hanna AK. Adrenal suppression in two patients with asthma treated with low doses of the inhaled steroid fluticasone propionate. J Allergy Clin Immunol 1998;101(3):425–6.
45. Todd GR, Acerini CL, Ross-Russell R, Zahra S, Warner JT, McCance D. Survey of adrenal crisis associated with inhaled corticosteroids in the United Kingdom. Arch Dis Child 2002;87(6):457–61.
46. Wilkinson SM, Cartwright PH, English JS. Hydrocortisone: an important cutaneous allergen. Lancet 1991;337(8744):761–2.
47. Ng PC, Fok TF, Wong GW, Lam CW, Lee CH, Wong MY, Lam K, Ma KC. Pituitary–adrenal suppression in preterm, very low birth weight infants after inhaled fluticasone propionate treatment. J Clin Endocrinol Metab 1998;83(7):2390–3.
48. Aaronson D, Kaiser H, Dockhorn R, Findlay S, Korenblat P, Thorsson L, Kallen A. Effects of budesonide by means of the Turbuhaler on the hypothalmic–pituitary–adrenal axis in asthmatic subjects: a dose-response study. J Allergy Clin Immunol 1998;101(3):312–19.
49. Lipworth BJ. Airway and systemic effects of inhaled corticosteroids in asthma: dose response relationship. Pulm Pharmacol 1996;9(1):19–27.
50. Kannisto S, Korppi M, Remes K, Voutilainen R. Adrenal suppression, evaluated by a low dose adrenocorticotropin test, and growth in asthmatic children treated with inhaled steroids. J Clin Endocrinol Metab 2000;85(2):652–7.
51. Shimada T, Yamazaki H, Mimura M, Inui Y, Guengerich FP. Interindividual variations in human liver cytochrome P-450 enzymes involved in the oxidation of drugs, carcinogens and toxic chemicals: studies with liver microsomes of 30 Japanese and 30 Caucasians. J Pharmacol Exp Ther 1994;270(1):414–23.
52. Derendorf H, Hochhaus G, Meibohm B, Mollmann H, Barth J. Pharmacokinetics and pharmacodynamics of inhaled corticosteroids. J Allergy Clin Immunol 1998;101(4 Pt 2):S440–6.
53. Onhoj J, Thorsson L, Bisgaard H. Lung deposition of inhaled drugs increases with age. Am J Respir Crit Care Med 2000;162(5):1819–22.
54. Russell G. Inhaled corticosteroids and adrenal insufficiency. Arch Dis Child 2002;87(6):455–6.
55. Russell G. Fluticasone propionate in children. Respir Med 1994;88(Suppl A):25–9.
56. Bousquet J, Ben-Joseph R, Messonnier M, Alemao E, Gould AL. A meta-analysis of the dose-response relationship of inhaled corticosteroids in adolescents and adults with mild to moderate persistent asthma. Clin Ther 2002;24(1):1–20.
57. Sizonenko PC. Effects of inhaled or nasal glucocorticosteroids on adrenal function and growth. J Pediatr Endocrinol Metab 2002;15(1):5–26.
58. Allen DB. Safety of inhaled corticosteroids in children. Pediatr Pulmonol 2002;33(3):208–20.
59. Faul JL, Tormey W, Tormey V, Burke C. High dose inhaled corticosteroids and dose dependent loss of diabetic control. BMJ 1998;317(7171):1491.
60. Faul JL, Cormican LJ, Tormey VJ, Tormey WP, Burke CM. Deteriorating diabetic control associated with high-dose inhaled budesonide. Eur Respir J 1999; 14(1):242–3.
61. Dendukuri N, Blais L, LeLorier J. Inhaled corticosteroids and the risk of diabetes among the elderly. Br J Clin Pharmacol 2002;54(1):59–64.
62. Blackburn D, Hux J, Mamdani M. Quantification of the risk of corticosteroid-induced diabetes mellitus among the elderly. J Gen Intern Med 2002;17(9):717–20.
63. Capewell S, Reynolds S, Shuttleworth D, Edwards C, Finlay AY. Purpura and dermal thinning associated with high dose inhaled corticosteroids. BMJ 1990;300(6739):1548–51.
64. Mak VH, Melchor R, Spiro SG. Easy bruising as a side-effect of inhaled corticosteroids. Eur Respir J 1992; 5(9):1068–74.
65. Haapasaari K, Rossi O, Risteli J, Oikarinen A. Effects of long-term inhaled corticosteroids on skin collagen synthesis and thickness in asthmatic patients. Eur Respir J 1998;11(1):139–43.
66. Malo JL, Cartier A, Ghezzo H, Mark S, Brown J, Laviolette M, Boulet LP. Skin bruising, adrenal function and markers of bone metabolism in asthmatics using inhaled beclomethasone and fluticasone. Eur Respir J 1999;13(5):993–8.
67. Dooms-Goossens A. Allergy to inhaled corticosteroids: a review. Am J Contact Dermatitis 1995;6:1–3.
68. Isaksson M, Bruze M, Hornblad Y, Svenonius E, Wihl JA. Contact allergy to corticosteroids in asthma/rhinitis patients. Contact Dermatitis 1999;40(6):327–8.
69. Isaksson M. Skin reactions to inhaled corticosteroids. Drug Saf 2001;24(5):369–73.
70. Israel E, Banerjee TR, Garrett MPH, Fitzmaurice GM, Kotlov TV, LaHive K, LeBoff MS. Effects of inhaled glucocorticoids on bone density in premenopausal women. N Engl J Med 2001;345(13):941–7.
71. Shiri J, Amichai B. Perioral dermatitis induced by inhaled corticosteroids. J Dermatol Treat 1998;9:259–60.
72. Ellepola AN, Samaranayake LP. Inhalational and topical steroids, and oral candidosis: a mini review. Oral Dis 2001;7(4):211–16.
73. National Asthma Education Program, National Institutes of Health. Guidelines for the Diagnosis and Management of Asthma. Publication No 91–3042. Bethesda: United States Department of Health and Human Services, 1991.
74. Isaksson M, Bruze M. Allergic contact dermatitis in response to budesonide reactivated by inhalation of the allergen. J Am Acad Dermatol 2002;46(6):880–5.
75. Laatikainen AK, Kroger HP, Tukiainen HO, Honkanen RJ, Saarikoski SV. Bone mineral density in perimenopausal women with asthma: a population-based cross-sectional study. Am J Respir Crit Care Med 1999;159(4 Pt 1):1179–85.
76. Wong CA, Subakumar G, Casey PM. Effects of asthma and asthma therapies on bone mineral density. Curr Opin Pulm Med 2002;8(1):39–44.
77. Fujita K, Kasayama S, Hashimoto J, Nagasaka Y, Nakano N, Morimoto Y, Barnes PJ, Miyatake A. Inhaled corticosteroids reduce bone mineral density in early post-menopausal but not premenopausal asthmatic women. J Bone Miner Res 2001;16(4):782–7.
78. Sivri A, Coplu L. Effect of the long-term use of inhaled corticosteroids on bone mineral density in asthmatic women. Respirology 2001;6(2):131–4.

79. Harmanci E, Colak O, Metintas M, Alatas O, Yurdasiper A. Fluticasone propionate and budesonide do not influence bone metabolism in the long term treatment of asthma. Allergol Immunopathol (Madr) 2001;29(1):22–7.
80. Reilly SM, Hambleton G, Adams JE, Mughal MZ. Bone density in asthmatic children treated with inhaled corticosteroids. Arch Dis Child 2001;84(2):183–4.
81. Tattersfield AE, Town GI, Johnell O, Picado C, Aubier M, Braillon P, Karlstrom R. Bone mineral density in subjects with mild asthma randomised to treatment with inhaled corticosteroids or non-corticosteroid treatment for two years. Thorax 2001;56(4):272–8.
82. Poon E, Fewings JM. Generalized eczematous reaction to budesonide in a nasal spray with cross-reactivity to triamcinolone. Australas J Dermatol 2001;42(1):36–7.
83. Bennett ML, Fountain JM, McCarty MA, Sherertz EF. Contact allergy to corticosteroids in patients using inhaled or intranasal corticosteroids for allergic rhinitis or asthma. Am J Contact Dermat 2001;12(4):193–6.
84. Bahceciler NN, Sezgin G, Nursoy MA, Barlan IB, Basaran MM. Inhaled corticosteroids and bone density of children with asthma. J Asthma 2002;39(2):151–7.
85. Agertoft L, Pedersen S. Bone mineral density in children with asthma receiving long-term treatment with inhaled budesonide. Am J Respir Crit Care Med 1998; 157(1):178–83.
86. Ma DQ, Jones G. Clinical risk factors but not bone density are associated with prevalent fractures in prepubertal children. J Paediatr Child Health 2002;38(5):497–500.
87. van Staa TP, Leufkens HG, Cooper C. Use of inhaled corticosteroids and risk of fractures. J Bone Miner Res 2001;16(3):581–8.
88. Gregson RK, Rao R, Murrills AJ, Taylor PA, Warner JO. Effect of inhaled corticosteroids on bone mineral density in childhood asthma: comparison of fluticasone propionate with beclomethasone dipropionate. Osteoporos Int 1998;8(5):418–22.
89. Johnell O, Pauwels R, Lofdahl CG, Laitinen LA, Postma DS, Pride NB, Ohlsson SV. Bone mineral density in patients with chronic obstructive pulmonary disease treated with budesonide Turbuhaler. Eur Respir J 2002;19(6):1058–63.
90. Lung Health Study Research Group. Effect of inhaled triamcinolone on the decline in pulmonary function in chronic obstructive pulmonary disease. N Engl J Med 2000;343(26):1902–9.
91. Fitzgerald D, Van Asperen P, Mellis C, Honner M, Smith L, Ambler G. Fluticasone propionate 750 micrograms/day versus beclomethasone dipropionate 1500 micrograms/day: comparison of efficacy and adrenal function in paediatric asthma. Thorax 1998;53(8):656–61.
92. Hughes JA, Conry BG, Male SM, Eastell R. One year prospective open study of the effect of high dose inhaled steroids, fluticasone propionate, and budesonide on bone markers and bone mineral density. Thorax 1999;54(3):223–9.
93. Hubbard RB, Smith CJ, Smeeth L, Harrison TW, Tattersfield AE. Inhaled corticosteroids and hip fracture: a population-based case-control study. Am J Respir Crit Care Med 2002;166(12 Pt 1):1563–6.
94. Martinati LC, Bertoldo F, Gasperi E, Fortunati P, Lo Cascio V, Boner AL. Longitudinal evaluation of bone mass in asthmatic children treated with inhaled beclomethasone dipropionate or cromolyn sodium. Allergy 1998;53(7):705–8.
95. Price JF, Russell G, Hindmarsh PC, Weller P, Heaf DP, Williams J. Growth during one year of treatment with fluticasone propionate or sodium cromoglycate in children with asthma. Pediatr Pulmonol 1997;24(3):178–86.
96. Bonala SB, Reddy BM, Silverman BA, Bassett CW, Rao YA, Amara S, Schneider AT. Bone mineral density in women with asthma on long-term inhaled corticosteroid therapy Ann Allergy Asthma Immunol 2000;85(6 Pt 1):495–500.
97. Wong CA, Walsh LJ, Smith CJ, Wisniewski AF, Lewis SA, Hubbard R, Cawte S, Green DJ, Pringle M, Tattersfield AE. Inhaled corticosteroid use and bone-mineral density in patients with asthma. Lancet 2000;355(9213):1399–403.
98. Boulet LP, Milot J, Gagnon L, Poubelle PE, Brown J. Long-term influence of inhaled corticosteroids on bone metabolism and density. Are biological markers predictors of bone loss? Am J Respir Crit Care Med 1999;159(3):838–44.
99. Sambrook P, Birmingham J, Kempler S, Kelly P, Eberl S, Pocock N, Yeates M, Eisman J. Corticosteroid effects on proximal femur bone loss. J Bone Miner Res 1990;5(12):1211–16.
100. Herrala J, Puolijoki H, Impivaara O, Liippo K, Tala E, Nieminen MM. Bone mineral density in asthmatic women on high-dose inhaled beclomethasone dipropionate. Bone 1994;15(6):621–3.
101. Ebeling PR, Erbas B, Hopper JL, Wark JD, Rubinfeld AR. Bone mineral density and bone turnover in asthmatics treated with long-term inhaled or oral glucocorticoids. J Bone Miner Res 1998;13(8):1283–9.
102. Wang WQ, Ip MS, Tsang KW, Lam KS. Antiresorptive therapy in asthmatic patients receiving high-dose inhaled steroids: a prospective study for 18 months. J Allergy Clin Immunol 1998;101(4 Pt 1):445–50.
103. Herrala J, Puolijoki H, Liippo K, Raitio M, Impivaara O, Tala E, Nieminen MM. Clodronate is effective in preventing corticosteroid-induced bone loss among asthmatic patients. Bone 1998;22(5):577–82.
104. Lo Cascio V, Bonucci E, Imbimbo B, Ballanti P, Adami S, Milani S, Tartarotti D, DellaRocca C. Bone loss in response to long-term glucocorticoid therapy. Bone Miner 1990;8(1):39–51.
105. Allen DB. Influence of inhaled corticosteroids on growth: a pediatric endocrinologist's perspective. Acta Paediatr 1998;87(2):123–9.
106. Norjavaara E, Gerhardsson De Verdier M, Lindmark B. Reduced height in swedish men with asthma at the age of conscription for military service. J Pediatr 2000;137(1):25–9.
107. Agertoft L, Pedersen S. Effect of long-term treatment with inhaled budesonide on adult height in children with asthma. N Engl J Med 2000;343(15):1064–9.
108. Brand PL. Inhaled corticosteroids reduce growth. Or do they? Eur Respir J 2001;17(2):287–94.
109. Price J, Hindmarsh P, Hughes S, Effthimiou J. Evaluating the effects of asthma therapy on childhood growth: principles of study design. Eur Respir J 2002;19(6):1167–78.
110. Price J, Hindmarsh P, Hughes S, Efthimiou J. Evaluating the effects of asthma therapy on childhood growth: what can be learnt from the published literature? Eur Respir J 2002;19(6):1179–93.
111. Wolthers OD. Growth problems in children with asthma. Horm Res 2002;57(Suppl 2):83–7.
112. Wolthers OD, Allen DB. Inhaled corticosteroids, growth, and compliance. N Engl J Med 2002;347(15):1210–11.
113. Allen DB. Inhaled corticosteroid therapy for asthma in preschool children: growth issues. Pediatrics 2002; 109(Suppl 2):373–80.
114. Pedersen S. Do inhaled corticosteroids inhibit growth in children? Am J Respir Crit Care Med 2001;164(4):521–35.
115. Thorsson L, Edsbacker S, Kallen A, Lofdahl CG. Pharmacokinetics and systemic activity of fluticasone via Diskus and pMDI, and of budesonide via Turbuhaler. Br J Clin Pharmacol 2001;52(5):529–38.

116. Ferguson AC, Spier S, Manjra A, Versteegh FG, Mark S, Zhang P. Efficacy and safety of high-dose inhaled steroids in children with asthma: a comparison of fluticasone propionate with budesonide. J Pediatr 1999;134(4):422–7.
117. The Childhood Asthma Management Program Research Group. Long-term effects of budesonide or nedocromil in children with asthma. N Engl J Med 2000;343(15):1054–63.
118. Allen DB, Mullen M, Mullen B. A meta-analysis of the effect of oral and inhaled corticosteroids on growth. J Allergy Clin Immunol 1994;93(6):967–76.
119. Doull IJ, Campbell MJ, Holgate ST. Duration of growth suppressive effects of regular inhaled corticosteroids. Arch Dis Child 1998;78(2):172–3.
120. Balfour-Lynn L. Growth and childhood asthma. Arch Dis Child 1986;61(11):1049–55.
121. Priori R, Tomassini M, Magrini L, Conti F, Valesini G. Churg–Strauss syndrome during pregnancy after steroid withdrawal. Lancet 1998;352(9140):1599–600.
122. Sears MR, Taylor DR. The beta 2-agonist controversy. Observations, explanations and relationship to asthma epidemiology. Drug Saf 1994;11(4):259–83.
123. Leav BA, Fanburg B, Hadley S. Invasive pulmonary aspergillosis associated with high-dose inhaled fluticasone. N Engl J Med 2000;343(8):586.
124. Kallen B, Rydhstroem H, Aberg A. Congenital malformations after the use of inhaled budesonide in early pregnancy. Obstet Gynecol 1999;93(3):392–5.
125. Raaska K, Niemi M, Neuvonen M, Neuvonen PJ, Kivisto KT. Plasma concentrations of inhaled budesonide and its effects on plasma cortisol are increased by the cytochrome P4503A4 inhibitor itraconazole. Clin Pharmacol Ther 2002;72(4):362–9.
126. Clevenbergh P, Corcostegui M, Gerard D, Hieronimus S, Mondain V, Chichmanian RM, Sadoul JL, Dellamonica P. Iatrogenic Cushing's syndrome in an HIV-infected patient treated with inhaled corticosteroids (fluticasone propionate) and low dose ritonavir enhanced PI containing regimen. J Infect 2002;44(3):194–5.

Corticosteroids—glucocorticoids, topical

See also Glucocorticosteroids

The local adverse effects of topical glucocorticoids (1,2) are listed in Table 1. They include transient local erythema, calcinosis cutis, cramps (due to injection of crystals into a vessel), amaurosis (a dubious report), depigmentation, skin atrophy, and skin necrosis (3,4). The systemic adverse effects of topical glucocorticoids (5–8), which are those to be expected from systemic use, are also listed in Table 1.

Table 1 Local adverse effects of topical glucocorticoids

Effects on the pilosebaceous unit
Perioral dermatitis (SEDA-5, 151)
Steroid rosacea or rosacea-like dermatitis; cannot be differentiated from perioral dermatitis and can be identical
Steroid acne
Exacerbation of pre-existing rosacea
Hypertrichosis of the face

Atrophic changes
Cigarette-paper wrinkling of the skin
Telangiectasia (SEDA-6, 153)
Petechiae, ecchymoses
Striae rubrae distensae, mainly in the inguinal and axillary region (occlusion effect)
Susceptibility of the skin to minor trauma
Fragile skin in surgery
Delayed wound healing
Worsening of existing ulceration
Photosensitivity of atrophic skin

Effects on the immune system
Aggravation of pre-existing folliculitis
Development of extensive, but unrecognized dermatophytic infections ("tinea incognito")
Perpetuation of masked infections with *Candida albicans*
Conversion of scabies into the Norwegian type
Widespread lesions of molluscum contagiosum
"Galloping" impetigo
(Possibly) exacerbation or dissemination of viral skin infections
Generalized pustular psoriasis
Generalized urticaria
Spreading of malignant skin lesions
Suppression of pruritus
Allergic contact dermatitis* (SEDA-15, 139)

Ocular effects
Ocular hypertension
Open-angle glaucoma (9)
Uveitis
Posterior subcapsular cataracts (9)

Nasal effects
Nasal septal perforation (steroid aerosols)

Skin lesions
Acne
Hirsutism
Ecchymoses
Milia
Granuloma gluteale infantum
Pseudocicatrices stellaires spontanées
Eczema craquelatum after withdrawal
Elastoidosis cutanée nodulaire à cystes et à comedones Favre-Raacouchot
Erythrosis interfollicularis colli
Cutis punctata linearis colli or "stippled skin"

Effects on skin color
Hypopigmentation
Hyperpigmentation
Striae

Miscellaneous effects
Tachyphylaxis to the vasoconstrictor effect of topical glucocorticoids

Systemic adverse effects of topical administration
Cushing's syndrome
Suppression of the hypothalamic–pituitary–adrenal axis
Growth retardation (SEDA-6, 151)
Hyperglycemia
Benign intracranial hypertension after withdrawal
Subcapsular cataract
Pancreatitis
Bony avascular necrosis (9)
Psychiatric symptoms
Fluid retention
Hypertension (SEDA-7, 167)

*Cross-allergy between glucocorticoids is infrequent (10–12).

References

1. De Groot AC, Weyland JW, Nater JP. Unwanted Effects of Cosmetics and Drugs used in Dermatology. 3rd ed. Amsterdam: Elsevier, 1994.
2. Miller JA, Munro DD. Topical corticosteroids: clinical pharmacology and therapeutic use Drugs 1980;19(2): 119–34.
3. Rimbaud P, Meynadier J, Guilhou JJ, Meynadier J. Complications dermatologiques locales secondaires aux injections cortisonées. [Local dermatological complications secondary to corticosteroid injections.] Nouv Presse Méd 1974;3(11):665–8.
4. Davy A, Guillerot E, Boyer C. A propas d'un accident iatrogène consecutif à une injection de corticoïdes au cou de pied. [An iatrogenic complication subsequent to an injection of corticoids into the instep.] Phlebologie 1986;39(3):527–37.
5. Walsh P, Aeling JL, Huff L, Weston WL. Hypothalamus–pituitary–adrenal axis suppression by superpotent topical steroids. J Am Acad Dermatol 1993;29(3):501–3.
6. Dhein S. Cushing-Syndrom nach externer Glukokortikoid-Applikation bei psoriasis. [Cushing syndrome following external glucocorticoid administration in psoriasis.] Z Hautkr 1986;61(3):161–6.
7. Lawlor F, Ramabala K. Iatrogenic Cushing's syndrome—a cautionary tale. Clin Exp Dermatol 1984;9(3):286–9.
8. Olsen EA, Cornell RC. Topical clobetasol-17-propionate: review of its clinical efficacy and safety. J Am Acad Dermatol 1986;15(2 Pt 1):246–55.
9. McLean CJ, Lobo RF, Brazier DJ. Cataracts, glaucoma, and femoral avascular necrosis caused by topical corticosteroid ointment. Lancet 1995;345(8945):330.
10. Isaksson M, Dooms-Goossens AN. Contact allergens—what's new? Corticosteroids. Clin Dermatol 1997; 15(4):527–31.
11. Dooms-Goossens A. Allergy to inhaled corticosteroids: a review. Am J Contact Dermatitis 1995;6:1–3.
12. Whitmore SE. Delayed systemic allergic reactions to corticosteroids. Contact Dermatitis 1995;32(4):193–8.

Corticosteroids—mineralocorticoids

General Information

Aldosterone is the principal physiological salt-retaining mineralocorticoid, but it is unsuitable for routine medical use since it is rapidly inactivated when given orally. Desoxycorticosterone (DCA, DOCA, desoxycortone) was used for a long time, but it had to be taken sublingually (or implanted or injected) to avoid inactivation during passage through the liver. Overdosage of desoxycorticosterone, leading to hypertensive encephalopathy and permanent brain damage, has been described (SED-8, 820).

The approximate potency of various mineralocorticoids relative to cortisone is shown in Table 1.

Fludrocortisone is the compound that is most often used at present for long-term mineralocorticoid treatment. The dose of fludrocortisone needed in chronic adrenocortical insufficiency varies very widely, from 0.05 to 1.0 mg/day. In salt-losing forms of the congenital adrenogenital syndrome up to 0.2 mg/day may be needed. In doses appropriate to the individual's needs, adverse reactions to the glucocorticoid effects of fludrocortisone rarely prove problematic; the main problem is to adjust the dosage (as well as salt intake) to these needs, since the adverse effects that can be experienced mainly reflect relative overdosage; if high doses are to be used, meticulous monitoring is required.

Table 1 Approximate potency of various mineralocorticoids relative to cortisone

Compound	Route of administration	Mineralocorticoid effect	Glucocorticoid effect
Cortisone	Oral	1	1
Desoxycorticosterone	Sublingual	50	Negligible
Fludrocortisone	Oral	150	10–20
Aldosterone	Injected	500	None

Organs and Systems

Cardiovascular

Edema, hypertension, and cardiac hypertrophy can occur with fludrocortisone (1). Hypertension is the most common reason for reducing the dosage.

Fluid retention due to mineralocorticoid effects can cause cardiac failure (1).

- Congestive heart failure occurred in a 47-year-old woman after she had taken fludrocortisone 100 micrograms/day for 2 weeks for Addison's disease (2). Ten months later, fludrocortisone 25 micrograms/day was restarted, and the dosage was increased to 100 micrograms/day over 2 months. At follow-up after 4 months she was well, without fluid retention or electrolyte abnormalities.

Electrolyte balance

Hypokalemia due to fludrocortisone can cause muscle weakness (3).

Drug–Drug Interactions

Phenytoin

In two patients with adrenal insufficiency, phenytoin increased fludrocortisone dosage requirements (4).

Potassium-sparing diuretics

Potassium-sparing diuretics, such as prorenoate and spironolactone, can prevent the potassium-losing effects of fludrocortisone (5).

References

1. Hussain RM, McIntosh SJ, Lawson J, Kenny RA. Fludrocortisone in the treatment of hypotensive disorders in the elderly. Heart 1996;76(6):507–9.

2. Bhattacharyya A, Tymms DJ. Heart failure with fludrocortisone in Addison's disease. J R Soc Med 1998;91(8):433–4.
3. Rivera VM. Fludrocortisone acetate and muscular weakness. JAMA 1973;225:993.
4. Keilholz U, Guthrie GP Jr. Adverse effect of phenytoin on mineralocorticoid replacement with fludrocortisone in adrenal insufficiency. Am J Med Sci 1986;291(4):280–3.
5. Ramsay LE, Shelton JR, Tidd MJ. The pharmacodynamics of single doses of prorenoate potasssium and spironolactone in fludrocortisone treated normal subjects. Br J Clin Pharmacol 1976;3(3):475–82.

Corticotrophins (corticotropin and tetracosactide)

General Information

The adrenocorticotrophic hormone ACTH (corticotropin) stimulates the adrenal cortex to secrete the glucocorticoids hydrocortisone (cortisol) and corticosterone, the mineralocorticoid aldosterone, and a number of weakly androgenic substances, as well as a small amount of testosterone. Aldosterone synthesis is also regulated by renin and angiotensin.

This monograph should be read in conjunction with the monograph on glucocorticoids. It is not always clear which adverse effects are specific to corticotrophins and which simply result from the secretion of the glucocorticoids that they induce; conversely, almost any adverse effect associated with glucocorticoids can in principle also occur with corticotrophins.

Structures and nomenclature

Natural ACTH (corticotropin) is a polypeptide consisting of 39 amino acids. Its hormonal activity is related to the first 24 amino acids in a sequence that is found in both animal and human pituitary glands. The differing sequences of the remaining 15 amino acids in animals can lead to antibody formation and hence to allergic reactions when animal hormones are injected into humans. From 1970 onwards, therefore, even highly purified corticotropin preparations of animal origin were largely displaced by the so-called "synthetic ACTH" or "synthetic corticotropin," better known by its generic name of tetracosactide (rINN), which contains only the first 24 amino acids, hence avoiding much of the antigenicity of the complete molecule. Collectively, corticotropin and tetracosactide are known as the corticotrophins.

Since the development of tetracosactide, other modifications to the corticotropin molecule have been made, and some clinical work has been done with products containing fewer than 24 amino acids, for example 1–18. However, none has proved more usable than tetracosactide. The replacement of some naturally occurring amino acids by others may intensify or prolong the effect of the polypeptide.

Production and elimination

Fluctuations in the rates of secretion of glucocorticoids from the adrenal cortex are determined by variations in the rate of release of corticotropin from the anterior pituitary, and this in turn is controlled by the hypothalamic corticotropin-releasing hormone (CRH). Since release of CRH is affected by circulating glucocorticoid concentrations, a negative-feedback control operates to keep the system in balance. It follows from this that if glucocorticoids are administered exogenously they will operate through this feedback to suppress adrenal function.

The mode of inactivation and excretion of corticotropin is still almost completely unknown; its biological half-life has been variously assessed as several minutes or several hours.

Uses

Corticotrophins can be used diagnostically to investigate adrenocortical insufficiency. Corticotropin has also been used therapeutically in most of the conditions for which systemic glucocorticoids are indicated, although such use is now fairly limited. However, corticotropin is used in certain neurological disorders, such as infantile spasms and multiple sclerosis. The main indications for corticotropin and tetracosactide are thus diagnostic rather than therapeutic; for the latter purpose they are being increasingly replaced by CRH.

General adverse effects

Corticotrophins share all the adverse effects of glucocorticoids, including impaired immunity, but they do not depress adrenocortical function. In addition, the melanocyte-stimulating hormone (MSH) sequence in the corticotropin molecule can result in hyperpigmentation, and induction of androgen secretion can lead to virilization. Corticotrophins also have additional unwanted effects of their own, such as myoclonic encephalopathy and adrenal hemorrhage. Hypersensitivity reactions occur occasionally, but have become less frequent since older preparations of animal origin were phased out. Tumor-inducing effects have not been observed.

Organs and Systems

Cardiovascular

Corticotropin has been reported to cause enlargement of cardiac tumors in tuberous sclerosis (1).

- A female infant with tuberous sclerosis had multiple large cardiac tumors in the left and right ventricles. Corticotropin was given (dose not stated; once a day for 2 weeks, tapering over 3 months) at 4 months for infantile spasms. At 6 months a heart murmur was detected. Echocardiography showed pronounced enlargement of the tumors in both ventricles and a small tumor extending from the upper portion of the interventricular septum into the left ventricular outflow tract. An electrocardiogram showed 2–3 mm ST segment depression in leads I, aVL, and V4-6. Gated single photon emission CT showed low perfusion at the lateral and inferior regions of the left ventricle, indicating myocardial ischemia.

Corticotropin was withdrawn and 3 months later the patient was asymptomatic. An echocardiogram showed that the tumors had reduced in size, and there was concomitant improvement in the electrocardiogram.

There is a risk of myocardial hypertrophy in children on prolonged treatment with ACTH (2), an effect that could reflect increased androgen secretion and thus be more likely to occur than with glucocorticoids.

Hypertension, with or without simultaneous hypertrophic myopathy, is a common feature of adrenal stimulation that seems to be common with depot tetracosactide but not simple tetracosactide (3). During treatment for infantile spasms, hypertension occurred more often in those treated with high doses (SEDA-19, 374) (4), and changes in cardiac function, such as left ventricular shortening fraction, can occur early and sometimes before systolic hypertension (SEDA-19, 374) (5).

Respiratory

Corticotropin and to a lesser extent tetracosactide can cause asthma in sensitive subjects (6). The question as to whether tetracosactide or glucocorticoids should be preferred for the treatment of chronic asthmatic bronchitis has been discussed mainly with respect to adverse effects, particularly adverse endocrine effects and effects on growth. An earlier belief that corticotropin might be more effective in children has not been confirmed.

Nervous system

In 138 Japanese patients with West syndrome treated with low-dose tetracosactide, the initial effects on seizures and long-term outcome were not related to dose (daily dose 0.005–0.032 mg/kg, 0.2–1.28 IU/kg; total dose 0.1–0.87 mg/kg, 4–35 IU/kg) (7). There were moderate or severe adverse effects in 30% of the patients. There was slight loss of brain volume on CT/MRI scans in 64% of the patients, moderate loss in 23%, and severe loss in 4%. The severity of adverse effects correlated with the total dose of corticotropin, and the severity of brain volume loss due to corticotropin correlated well with the daily and total doses. The authors recommended a reduction in the dose of corticotropin in order to avoid serious adverse effects.

Brain shrinkage has been described as a possible adverse effect of corticotropin treatment of infantile spasms, and this has been confirmed using magnetic resonance imaging (SEDA-20, 368) (8,9). Changes in midline structures (volume reductions in the pons, corpus callosum, and cerebellum) seem to show that the beneficial effect of corticotropin in infantile spasms could be due to a direct effect on the brainstem. Cerebral shrinkage and subdural hematoma occurred after the administration of high doses of corticotropin for West syndrome (total dose 4.5–6.75 mg) and subdural hematoma occurred in two children (aged 2 and 5 months) during the administration of low doses of tetracosactide (0.01 mg/kg/day; total dose 0.24–0.26 mg) (10).

Drowsiness, hypotonia, and irritability were observed in 37% of infants given corticotropin in a randomized comparison of corticotropin with vigabatrin in the treatment of infantile spasms (SEDA-22, 442) (11).

Myoclonic encephalopathy appears to be a specific, if rare, complication of corticotropin, not seen with the glucocorticoids (12).

Sensory systems

Bilateral subcapsular cataracts and glaucoma have been reported as possible risks (13), but they presumably reflect glucocorticoid effects.

Bilateral macular degeneration has been described with tetracosactide (13), but presumably reflects glucocorticoid effects.

Central serous retinopathy has been linked to the therapeutic use of corticotrophins or glucocorticoids or to endogenous corticotropin hypersecretion. Bilateral central serous retinopathy has been reported in a woman treated with tetracosactide intramuscularly (SEDA-22, 442) (14).

Psychological, psychiatric

Mood changes continue to be reported in association with corticotropin (15). Emotional instability or psychotic tendencies can be aggravated, while euphoria, insomnia, and personality changes such as hypomania and depression can be precipitated, sometimes even with psychotic manifestations. Although it seems reasonable to assume that one is dealing here mainly with an effect of the glucocorticoids secreted in response to corticotropin, it should be recalled that segments of the corticotropin molecule themselves have effects on brain function and could conceivably play a role.

Endocrine

Corticotropin can promote the development of a more or less pronounced Cushingoid state. Corticotropin also increases the metabolic clearance rate of cortisol, aldosterone, and desoxycorticosterone (SEDA-1, 282).

Prolonged stimulation by corticotropin leads to adrenocortical cell hyperplasia and an increase in the size and weight of the adrenal glands; massive enlargement can be demonstrated by computerized tomography as well as clinical examination (16).

Acute adrenal hemorrhage, either unilateral (17) or bilateral (18), has been observed repeatedly after corticotropin administration, and causes an acute abdominal crisis. Although it is usually seen in children, hemorrhage can also occur in adults (SEDA-17, 451).

Even a single dose of corticotropin can cause inhibition of thyrotrophic hormone secretion (19), although the effect is brief. Conversely, thyroid hormones increase the sensitivity of adrenocortical cells in vitro to corticotropin (20) and hyperthyroidism increases sensitivity to corticotropin (21,22).

Corticotropin suppresses the growth hormone response to hypoglycemia (23).

Androgen secretion due to corticotropin can cause virilization in women (24).

Fluid balance

Corticotropin affects mineral and fluid balance in varying degrees, as would be expected from its effect on mineralocorticoid secretion.

Hematologic

Marked leukocytosis has been described, despite the absence of infection, in a patient treated with tetracosactide (SED-12, 980); the effect may well have been due to glucocorticoid secretion rather than to tetracosactide itself.

Gastrointestinal

A relative indication for corticotropin is the occasional gastrointestinal intolerance that occurs with oral glucocorticoids. In these cases, however, only the local effects of the glucocorticoids can be avoided, and not their systemic effects on the gastrointestinal tract (25).

Urinary tract

Renal calcinosis can develop as a result of hypercalciuria and is a major concern in the treatment of infantile spasms with corticotropin. In 16 infants, corticotropin, often associated with anticonvulsants, results in increased urinary excretion of calcium and phosphate, with increased parathormone serum concentrations and in some cases generalized aminoaciduria (26). This makes it imperative that the dose of corticotropin and the duration of treatment be kept to the minimum required to ensure efficacy. In one case in which calcified stones were removed surgically, recurrence was apparently prevented, despite the presence of a Cushingoid state, by long-term chlorothiazide (27).

Skin

Allergic skin reactions, for example urticaria, can occur. Since the first 13 amino acids in the corticotropin peptide are the same as in MSH, treatment with corticotropin can occasionally cause hyperpigmentation. The shorter peptide chain in tetracosactide can even cause rather more pronounced melanocyte-stimulatory effects. Long-term treatment with depot tetracosactide has itself caused melanoderma (SED-12, 980) and, in one series of 41 patients, there was hyperpigmentation in 3 of them (SEDA-1, 281).

Immunologic

Although the incidence of severe allergic reactions to natural corticotropin of animal origin fell as progressively purer products were introduced, the problem remained for a small minority of patients. Exact figures are difficult to cite, but hypersensitivity reactions have sometimes even been described in patients with no history of corticotropin treatment, presumably sensitized by other animal material. Hypersensitivity to corticotropin generally causes only dizziness, nausea and vomiting, or cutaneous hypersensitivity reactions, but in several instances shock with circulatory failure has been observed (28). In a number of patients who were allergic to porcine corticotropin, no such problems were observed when tetracosactide was given. This suggests that the absence of most of the antigenic part of the original molecule reduces the risk of hypersensitivity reactions. However, the smaller synthetic molecule can still stimulate the formation of antibodies in some individuals (SEDA-12, 979) (29).

However, allergic reactions and anaphylactic shock have been observed during treatment with tetracosactide and have even proved fatal. Local reactions have even been seen after the administration of small doses for intracutaneous testing. In the early years of tetracosactide use, the frequency of local and general reactions to a long-acting acetylated tetracosactide was estimated at as little as one in 30 000 (SED-12, 979), but it is doubtful whether this figure can be supported today, unless one interprets it as referring only to major calamities. Indeed, subclinical immune reactions to both natural and tetracosactide appear to be fairly common during long-term treatment of patients with asthma, with an incidence of intradermal reactions of about 50%, a prevalence of IgE antibodies that is significantly higher than in controls, and a high incidence of low-titer agglutinating antibodies to corticotropin. The antibodies can result in a gradual loss of effect.

Infection risk

Pneumonia due to *Pneumocystis jiroveci* (formerly *Pneumocystis carinii*) has been attributed to high-dose corticotropin (30).

- An infant girl was given corticotropin 80 U/day for infantile spasms. After 5 weeks she became increasingly lethargic, with reduced oral intake, cough, an increased respiratory rate (50 breaths/minute), and a fever of 38.6°C. Investigations were consistent with pneumonia and she was given intravenous ceftriaxone. She initially improved, but 36 hours later her respiratory distress worsened and she required intubation and mechanical ventilation. The diagnosis of *P. jiroveci* pneumonia was confirmed and she was given intravenous co-trimoxazole and glucocorticoids. Her respiratory distress resolved and she was extubated 10 days later. Immunological testing after the withdrawal of corticotropin did not show any abnormalities that could have predisposed her to *P. jiroveci* pneumonia.

The authors commented that a transient immunodeficiency related to corticotrophin may have predisposed to the development of *P. jiroveci* pneumonia.

Long-Term Effects

Drug withdrawal

Relative adrenocortical insufficiency can follow withdrawal of corticotropin treatment (presumably because the cortex has adapted itself to a constant high level of stimulation) and can persist for some months. Glucocorticoid substitution has to be provided during this period. The risk of this effect can be reduced by keeping the dose of corticotropin as low as possible.

Second-Generation Effects

Pregnancy

There are no firm data on the use of corticotropin in pregnancy; both glucocorticoid and androgenic effects might be expected to affect the fetus.

Susceptibility Factors

Age

Although it has been stated in reviews that treatment with corticotropin inhibits growth much less than glucocorticoid treatment does, the growth hormone response to stimuli is reduced, and since growth hormone secretion is impaired during corticotropin treatment, claims for the greater safety of this therapy in children with asthma must be treated with reservations.

Other features of the patient

Susceptibility factors for adverse effects are as for glucocorticoids. In addition, patients with a known allergic tendency should preferably not receive these substances, unless sufficient supervision is possible to cope with unexpected allergic reactions, at least until tolerance has been demonstrated.

Drug–Drug Interactions

Coumarin anticoagulants

In 10 of 14 patients taking dicoumarol or phenindione who also took corticotropin for 4–9 days, there was a small increase in the effects of the anticoagulants (31). One patient taking ethyl biscoumacetate developed bleeding after taking corticotropin 20 mg/day for 3 days (32). However, in contrast, reduced efficacy of ethyl biscoumacetate has been described (33).

References

1. Hiraishi S, Iwanami N, Ogawa N. Images in cardiology. Enlargement of cardiac rhabdomyoma and myocardial ischaemia during corticotropin treatment for infantile spasm. Heart 2000;84(2):170.
2. Lang D, Muhler E, Kupferschmid C, Tacke E, von Bernuth G. Cardiac hypertrophy secondary to ACTH treatment in children. Eur J Pediatr 1984;142(2):121–5.
3. Kusse MC, van Nieuwenhuizen O, van Huffelen AC, van der Mey W, Thijssen JH, van Ree JM. The effect of non-depot ACTH(1–24) on infantile spasms. Dev Med Child Neurol 1993;35(12):1067–73.
4. Hrachovy RA, Frost JD Jr, Glaze DG. High-dose, long-duration versus low-dose, short-duration corticotropin therapy for infantile spasms. J Pediatr 1994;124(5 Pt 1):803–6.
5. Starc TJ, Bierman FZ, Pavlakis SG, Challenger ME, De Vivo DC, Gersony WM. Cardiac size and function during adrenocorticotropic hormone-induced systolic systemic hypertension in infants. Am J Cardiol 1994;73(1):57–64.
6. Grabner W. Zur induzierten NNR-Insuffizienz. (Problems of corticosteroid-induced adrenal insufficiency in surgery.) Fortschr Med 1977;95(30):1866–8.
7. Ito M, Aiba H, Hashimoto K, Kuroki S, Tomiwa K, Okuno T, Hattori H, Go T, Sejima H, Dejima S, Ikeda H, Yoshioka M, Kanazawa O, Kawamitsu T, Ochi J, Miki N, Noma H, Oguro K, Ozaki N, Tamamoto A, Matsubara T, Miyajima T, Fujii T, Konishi Y, Okuno T, Hojo H. Low-dose ACTH therapy for West syndrome: initial effects and long-term outcome. Neurology 2002;58(1):110–14.
8. Konishi Y, Yasujima M, Kuriyama M, Konishi K, Hayakawa K, Fujii Y, Ishii Y, Sudo M. Magnetic resonance imaging in infantile spasms: effects of hormonal therapy. Epilepsia 1992;33(2):304–9.
9. Konishi Y, Hayakawa K, Kuriyama M, Saito M, Fujii Y, Sudo M. Effects of ACTH on brain midline structures in infants with infantile spasms. Pediatr Neurol 1995;13(2):134–6.
10. Ito M, Miyajima T, Fujii T, Okuno T. Subdural hematoma during low-dose ACTH therapy in patients with West syndrome. Neurology 2000;54(12):2346–7.
11. Vigevano F, Cilio MR. Vigabatrin versus ACTH as first-line treatment for infantile spasms: a randomized, prospective study. Epilepsia 1997;38(12):1270–4.
12. Rutgers AW, Links TP, le Coultre R, Begeer JH. Behavioural disturbances after effective ACTH-treatment of the dancing-eyes syndrome. Dev Med Child Neurol 1988;30(3):408–9.
13. Williamson J, Dalakos TG. Posterior subcapsular cataracts and macular lesions after long-term corticotrophin therapy. Br J Ophthalmol 1967;51(12):839–42.
14. Zamir E. Central serous retinopathy associated with adrenocorticotrophic hormone therapy. A case report and a hypothesis. Graefes Arch Clin Exp Ophthalmol 1997;235(6):339–44.
15. Minden SL, Orav J, Schildkraut JJ. Hypomanic reactions to ACTH and prednisone treatment for multiple sclerosis. Neurology 1988;38(10):1631–4.
16. Liebling MS, Starc TJ, McAlister WH, Ruzal-Shapiro CB, Abramson SJ, Berdon WE. ACTH induced adrenal enlargement in infants treated for infantile spasms and acute cerebellar encephalopathy. Pediatr Radiol 1993;23(6):454–6.
17. Levin TL, Morton E. Adrenal hemorrhage complicating ACTH therapy in Crohn's disease. Pediatr Radiol 1993;23(6):457–8.
18. Dunlap SK, Meiselman MS, Breuer RI, Panella JS, Ficho TW, Reid SE Jr. Bilateral adrenal hemorrhage as a complication of intravenous ACTH infusion in two patients with inflammatory bowel disease. Am J Gastroenterol 1989;84(10):1310–12.
19. Prummel MF, Brokken LJ, Wiersinga WM. Ultra short-loop feedback control of thyrotropin secretion. Thyroid 2004;14(10):825–9.
20. Simonian MH. ACTH and thyroid hormone regulation of 3 beta-hydroxysteroid dehydrogenase activity in human fetal adrenocortical cells. J Steroid Biochem 1986; 25(6):1001–6.
21. Jasani MK. Anti-inflammatory steroids: mode of action in rheumatoid arthritis and homograft reaction. In: Born GVR, Farah A, Herken H, Welch AD, editors. Handbook of Experimental Pharmacology. Berlin–Heidelberg–New York: Springer-Verlag, 1979:589.
22. Labhart A, Martz G. Fundamentals of hormone treatment of nonendocrine disorders. In: Labhart A, editor. Clinical Endocrinology. Berlin–Heidelberg–New York: Springer-Verlag, 1986:1067.
23. McGregor VP, Banarer S, Cryer PE. Elevated endogenous cortisol reduces autonomic neuroendocrine and symptom responses to subsequent hypoglycemia. Am J Physiol Endocrinol Metab 2002;282(4):E770–7.
24. Garren LD, Gill GN, Masui H, Walton GM. On the mechanism of action of ACTH. Recent Prog Horm Res 1971;27:433–78.
25. Mathies H. Probleme der symptomatischen Therapie rheumatischer Erkrankungen mit Glukokortikoiden und nichtsteroidalen Antirheumatika. [Problems in symptomatic therapy of rheumatic diseases with glucocorticoids and nonsteroidal anti-rheumatic agents.] Internist (Berl) 1979;20(9):414–25.
26. Riikonen R, Simell O, Jaaskelainen J, Rapola J, Perheentupa J. Disturbed calcium and phosphate homeostasis during treatment with ACTH of infantile spasms. Arch Dis Child 1986;61(7):671–6.

27. Katzir Z, Shvil Y, Landau EH, Popovtzer MM. Thiazide therapy for ACTH-induced hypercalciuria and nephrolithiasis. Acta Paediatr 1992;81(3):277–9.
28. Riikonen R, Simell O, Dunkel L, Santavuori P, Perheentupa J. Hormonal background of the hypertension and fluid derangements associated with adrenocorticotrophic hormone treatment of infants. Eur J Pediatr 1989;148(8):737–41.
29. Glass D, Nuki G, Daly JR. Development of antibodies during long-term therapy with corticotrophin in rheumatoid arthritis. II. Zinc tetracosactrin (Depot Synacthen). Ann Rheum Dis 1971;30(6):593–6.
30. Dunagan DP, Rubin BK, Fasano MB. *Pneumocystis carinii* pneumonia in a child receiving ACTH for infantile spasms. Pediatr Pulmonol 1999;27(4):286–9.
31. Hellem AJ, Solem JH. The influence of ACTH on prothrombin–proconvertin values in blood during treatment with dicumarol and phenylindanedione. Acta Med Scand 1954;150(5):389–93.
32. Van Cauwenberge H, Jaques LB. Haemorrhagic effect of ACTH with anticoagulants. Can Med Assoc J 1958; 79(7):536–40.
33. Chatterjea JB, Salomon L. Antagonistic effect of A.C.T.H. and cortisone on the anticoagulant activity of ethyl biscoumacetate. BMJ 1954;4891:790–2.

Corynebacterium parvum

General Information

Inactivated *Corynebacterium parvum* has been tried as an adjuvant in patients with cancer and in the treatment of malignant pleural effusions. Fever and chills were frequent, with sustained fever and chest or abdominal pain in several patients (1,2).

References

1. Ludwig Lung Cancer Study Group. Adverse effect of intrapleural *Corynebacterium parvum* as adjuvant therapy in resected stage I and II non-small cell carcinoma of the lung. J Thorac Cardiovasc Surg 1985;89(6):842–7.
2. Foresti V. Intrapleural *Corynebacterium parvum* for recurrent malignant pleural effusions. Respiration 1995;62(1):21–6.

Coumarin

General Information

The plant lactone coumarin (not to be confused with coumarin anticoagulants) is a constituent of some plants, including:

- *Alyxia lucida*
- *Dalea tuberculata*
- *Dipteryx odorata*
- *Dipteryx oppositofolia*
- *Levisticum officinale*
- *Melilotus officinalis*
- *Scabiosa comosa.*

Organs and Systems

Hematologic

Coumarin is devoid of anticoagulant activity, but the molding of sweet clover can give it hemorrhagic potential by transforming coumarin to the anticoagulant dicoumarol. This transformation could explain a case of abnormal clotting function and mild bleeding after the drinking of an herbal tea prepared from tonka beans, sweet clover, and several other ingredients. Unfortunately, this possibility was not investigated, as the reporting physician was not aware of the exact phytochemistry and pharmacology of coumarin-yielding plants.

Liver

Coumarin has hepatotoxic potential in man, when taken in daily doses of 25–100 mg (1). Bile-duct carcinomas have been reported to occur in rats fed coumarin, but the correctness of this diagnosis has been seriously criticized.

Reference

1. Cox D, O'Kennedy R, Thornes RD. The rarity of liver toxicity in patients treated with coumarin (1,2-benzopyrone). Hum Toxicol 1989;8(6):501–6.

Coumarin anticoagulants

General Information

The coumarins were first discovered in Wisconsin, when bleeding in cattle was found to be due to the consumption of bruised sweet clover in the 1920s (1). The causative agent, dicoumarol, was isolated in 1940, and a range of related compounds was then synthesized, the most popular of which proved to be warfarin (named after the Wisconsin Alumni Research Foundation). Other coumarins that have been used are acenocoumarol (nicoumalone), bishydroxycoumarin, dicoumarol, ethyl biscoumacetate, and phenprocoumon.

The coumarins act as competitive inhibitors of vitamin K epoxide reductase, which is responsible for regenerating reduced vitamin K from vitamin K epoxide after it has been consumed as a co-factor in the synthesis of coagulation factors II, VII, IX, and X.

Uses

The main use of the coumarins is in the treatment and prevention of thromboembolic disease, including deep vein thrombosis, pulmonary embolism, and cerebral embolism from cardiac and other sources.

Protein C, another vitamin K-dependent serine protease zymogen in plasma, is a regulatory protein that, when activated, limits the activity of two activated procoagulant co-factors, factors Va and VIIIa. Heterozygotes for hereditary isolated protein C deficiency tend to develop a thrombotic disease which has been successfully treated with long-term coumarins (2,3). Apparently, the balance between the activities of protein C and the procoagulant factors (II, VII, IX, and X), which is disturbed in protein C-deficient patients, is restored during long-term treatment with coumarins.

Non-anticoagulant uses

Warfarin reduces calcium deposition in spontaneously degenerated bioprosthetic valves (4).

Both direct and indirect antitumor actions of anticoagulants have been postulated on the basis of experimental findings in animals (5). Warfarin given alone or in combination with cytostatic drugs reduces the size of fibrosarcomas in animals (5,6) and of osteosarcomas in man (7), and consequently prolongs survival times in both. The Cooperative Studies Program of the Veterans Administration Medical Research Service suggests that, among patients with various tumors, those with small-cell carcinoma of the lung had a significantly longer survival (about 4 years instead of 2) when warfarin was added to standard treatment (8). There were no differences in survival between warfarin-treated and control groups for advanced non-small-cell lung cancers, colorectal, head and neck, and prostate cancers (9). However, the contention that cancer morbidity and/or mortality is reduced in anticoagulated patients is not substantiated by the results of a retrospective study of 378 patients who had been taking anticoagulants for about 10 years on average (10).

It has been suggested that warfarin may have a specific effect on tumor-cell growth via the inhibition of protein synthesis (11). Another explanation of the effect of the drug is a reduction in the co-adherence of tumor cells, which renders them more vulnerable to the actions of defence mechanisms. The reduction in co-adherence is thought to be caused by an inhibitory action of anticoagulants on the fibrin network that is vital for tumor cell growth. This hypothesis, which is supported by dose dependence of the inhibitory effect of both heparin and warfarin (12), has been studied in a controlled randomized trial of the use of streptokinase after surgery for tumors of the large bowel (6).

Supercoumarins

Resistance to warfarin emerged soon after its original use as a poison for rodents. Second-generation anticoagulants, termed "superwarfarins," were subsequently developed and are sold as rodenticides for pest control. These include agents such as brodifacoum and difenacoum, which typically have much longer half-lives than warfarin. There have been several published case reports of accidental or intentional poisoning due to these drugs (13,14), which can result in prolonged coagulopathy (15,16).

In 10 762 children aged 6 years and under who unintentionally took single doses of brodifacoum, there were no deaths or major adverse effects, although 67 reported evidence of coagulopathy (17). There were minor and moderate adverse effects in 38 and 54 children, respectively. About half of the children received some form of gastrointestinal decontamination, which had no effect on the distribution of outcomes but caused adverse effects in 42 patients.

Ingestion of a small amount of a superwarfarin does not require specific therapy (18,19). However, if the coagulopathy due to a superwarfarin is severe, large doses of vitamin K may be required (15). Recombinant activated factor VII has been successfully used to treat superwarfarin poisoning (20).

When cases of unexplained acquired coagulopathy and selective deficiency of vitamin K-dependent clotting factors occur in patients in the absence of liver disease or inhibitors, physicians should consider the possibility of superwarfarin poisoning as a cause.

General adverse effects

The major adverse effect of the coumarins is hemorrhage and, exceptionally, hemorrhagic skin necrosis. Administration during pregnancy can cause an embryopathy. Allergic reactions are extremely rare. Tumor-inducing effects have not been reported.

Organs and Systems

Cardiovascular

Vasodilatory effects on the coronary arteries, peripheral veins, and capillaries, with purple toes as one of the most obvious consequences (21,22), have been reported. Sensations of cold may be due to increased loss of body heat caused by peripheral vasodilatation (23).

Cholesterol embolization, which promptly improves after the drug is withdrawn (24), may explain the purple-toe phenomenon.

Nervous system

Apart from cerebral hemorrhage, coumarins have no direct adverse effects on the nervous system.

Endocrine

An antithyroid effect of bishydroxycoumarin has been suspected (25).

Metabolism

Dicoumarol has been reported to have a uricosuric effect (26).

Hematologic

Hemorrhage

Bleeding is the major complication of coumarin anticoagulants. The annual incidence of major bleeding among 4060 patients in the AFFIRM trial, who were followed for an average of 3.5 years, was about 2% per year (27).

Dose-dependency

The intensity and stability of treatment, in addition to the beneficial effect of the coumarins, determine the rate and severity of bleeding complications. The average annual frequencies of fatal, major, and major and minor bleeding during warfarin therapy were 0.6, 3.0, and 9.6% respectively (28). The relationship between the intensity of anticoagulant therapy and the risk of bleeding is very strong, both in patients with deep vein thrombosis tissue and in those with mechanical heart valves. In randomized trials for these indications, the incidence of major bleeding in patients randomly assessed to less intense warfarin therapy (targeted INR 2.0–3.0) has been less than half the incidence found in patients randomly assigned to more intense anticoagulation (INR more than 3) (29). The bleeding risk increases dramatically when the INR is higher than 4.0 (30), especially the risk of intracranial hemorrhage. Less intense warfarin therapy has been used in patients with non-rheumatic atrial fibrillation, with only a very slight increase in major bleeding compared with placebo. In such patients, an INR of 2.5 (range 2.0–3.0) minimizes both hemorrhage and thromboembolism (31).

Time-dependency

Although bleeding can occur at any time, if the effective dose of drug increases, whether because of a change in dose or an interaction, most studies have reported higher frequencies of bleeding soon after the start of treatment. In one study the incidence of major bleeding fell from 3.0% per month during the first month of outpatient warfarin therapy to 0.8% per month during the rest of the first year of therapy and to 0.3% per month thereafter (32). Increased variation in anticoagulant effect, as reflected by time-dependent variation in the INR is associated with an increased frequency of hemorrhage independent of the mean INR (33,34).

Susceptibility factors

Important susceptibility factors include age, endogenous coagulation defects, thrombocytopenia, hypertension, cerebrovascular disease, thyroid disease, renal insufficiency, liver disease, tumors, cerebrovascular disease, alcoholism, a history of gastrointestinal bleeding (peptic ulcer disease alone without past bleeding is not associated with an increased risk of bleeding), and an inability to adhere to the regimen.

Management

The management of coumarin toxicity depends on the INR and whether there is bleeding.

- INR more than 0.5 over the target but under 5.0: reduce the dose
- INR 5.0–8.0: withhold the drug and restart once the INR is below 5.0
- INR over 8.0 and no bleeding: withhold the drug and restart once the INR is below 5.0
- INR over 8.0 with bleeding: withhold the drug and give vitamin K_1 (phytomenadione) 0.5 mg intravenously or 5 mg orally
- INR over 8.0 with life-threatening hemorrhage: withhold the drug and give a prothrombin complex concentrate (such as Beriplex-P/N or Prothromplex-T) 50 U/kg (35); if this is not available, give fresh frozen plasma 15 ml/kg.

If rapid and complete reversal is required (for example before a procedure such as a liver biopsy), vitamin K_1 (phytomenadione) 5–10 mg can be given slowly (1 mg/minute).

Other effects

Blood and plasma viscosity fall by 5–10% during the administration of coumarins in healthy volunteers and in patients with coronary artery disease (36). This may also explain, at least partly, the antianginal effect of coumarins. The mechanism might be related to changes in the protein composition of the plasma.

A reversible increase in white cell count has been reported with long-term use of acenocoumarol (37).

Hemolytic anemia thought to be related to warfarin has been reported (38).

Gastrointestinal

Gastrointestinal complications due to coumarins are limited to hemorrhage.

Liver

Only a few cases of hepatic injury have been documented in patients taking coumarins. In some of them, rechallenge caused a relapse (39). The usual presentation was with a cholestatic illness, beginning about 10 days after the coumarin anticoagulant was started, sometimes associated with eosinophilia. In Switzerland, oral anticoagulants were involved in only 11 of 674 reports of drug-induced liver disease collected during 1981–95. Seven cases were due to phenprocoumon and three to acenocoumarol. The severity ranged from asymptomatic rises in liver enzymes to cholestatic hepatitis. The interval between administration and onset of symptoms varied from 2 days to several weeks or months (40).

Subacute liver failure necessitating orthotopic liver transplantation has been reported with phenprocoumon (41).

- A 39-year-old woman developed idiopathic thrombosis of the posterior tibial vein. Oral contraceptives and resistance to activated protein C were identified as risk factors. After initial treatment with intravenous heparin, she was given phenprocoumon and the oral contraceptive was withdrawn. After 4 months she developed subacute liver failure and phenprocoumon was withdrawn immediately. Autoimmune disease, viral hepatitis, toxic causes, and Budd–Chiari syndrome were excluded. Despite symptomatic treatment, she deteriorated further and orthotopic liver transplantation was performed. Histopathology of the explanted liver further excluded ischemic liver cell necrosis and Budd–Chiari syndrome.

Urinary tract

In one case, multisystem abnormalities, including renal insufficiency, were caused by cholesterol embolization. Withdrawal of the anticoagulant resulted in dramatically improved renal function (24).

Skin

Maculopapular rashes with cross-sensitivity between coumarin derivates have been reported (42). Non-pruritic purpuric skin eruptions, histologically presenting as vasculitis and reappearing on rechallenge with warfarin or acenocoumarol, have been described (43).

Skin necrosis

Skin necrosis is a rare but serious complication of oral anticoagulation, seen typically during induction of therapy and occurring in about 0.01–0.1% of patients (44). It is conceivable that this condition is more common than is generally recognized, because many formes frustes can occur, presenting as painful cellulitis without hemorrhagic necrosis. Severe skin necrosis in a patient taking an oral anticoagulant was first described in 1943, but not documented in a series of patients until 11 years later (45). The morbidity of this complication is high and, despite treatment, about 50% of patients ultimately require surgical intervention and in some cases skin grafting.

There is convincing evidence that skin necrosis occurs exclusively in patients with excessively severe initial coumarin-induced hypocoagulability (46). As a rule, excessive doses have been given, resulting in severe and rapid reductions in the concentrations of factor VII and protein C (47,48).

Time-course

Familiarity with the clinical and histological pictures is essential, because the earliest signs and symptoms must be recognized if necrosis is to be prevented. The lesion does not usually occur before the second day of treatment or after the second week of treatment has started; most commonly it appears between the third and fifth day (49,50). There are occasionally exceptions to this rule; warfarin-induced skin necrosis can occur several days after discontinuation of warfarin (51) and some cases have been reported during long-term treatment (52,53). However, as a general rule, when skin necrosis occurs after 10 days of warfarin therapy, another cause must be sought.

Presentation

The lesion often appears symmetrically or at a pair of unrelated sites, with a predilection for parts of the body rich in fatty tissue, such as the breasts, abdomen, buttocks, thighs, and calves (54). Feet and toes are seldom affected, male genitalia only rarely (45,55,56), and the vagina and uterus very exceptionally (57).

The lesion begins with an evanescent, painful, slightly raised, more or less clearly demarcated erythematous patch. Histological examination at this stage reveals slight round-cell perivascular infiltration of the corium, edema, and swelling of the capillary endothelium, particularly at the cutis/subcutis boundary (the dermovascular loop), with fibrin thrombi in the small venules. Patches of necrotic fatty tissue, slight polymorphonuclear perivascular infiltration, and patchy interstitial edema as well as bleeding are present at this stage. Very soon, petechiae appear and become confluent within 24 hours, forming purple ecchymotic lesions surrounded by a sharply defined zone of hyperemia. During the next 24 hours, thrombotic occlusion of the veins causes infarction with necrosis of the skin, subcutaneous fat, and sometimes also of deeper anatomical structures. Hemorrhagic blisters characterize the onset of irreversible necrosis of the skin. Laboratory investigation may reveal diffuse intravascular coagulation and even hemolytic anemia (58).

Mechanism

The pathogenesis is still not completely elucidated, but data suggest that transient protein C deficiency may be causative.

Hemorrhagic skin necrosis has been described with all coumarins and indanediones. During the initial phase of oral anticoagulant treatment with these agents, the plasma concentration of protein C falls rapidly in parallel with factor VII. The half-lives of protein C and factor VII are much shorter than those of factors II, IX, and X, and during this initial phase of oral anticoagulation, there is therefore a striking imbalance between procoagulant factors (factors IX, X, and II) and anticoagulant vitamin K-dependent factors (protein C).

Susceptibility factors

Probably because of the sites of predilection, women account for about 80% of cases (49).

Patients with hereditary protein C deficiency (59,60) or acquired functional protein C deficiency (61) are particularly susceptible to the development of hemorrhagic skin necrosis. However, skin necrosis has also been reported in patients with deficiency of protein S (a co-factor for protein C), in patients at high thrombogenic risk linked to a constitutional antithrombin III deficit, and in patients with antiphospholipid antibodies associated with systemic lupus erythematosus (62,63).

Prevention

Prevention of coumarin-induced skin necrosis can be achieved by avoiding initial overshooting of the coumarin effect. A primary cautious initial dosage is mandatory (60), especially in elderly people, who require a smaller dose than younger age groups (one-third less on average) (64). Secondly, adequate patient surveillance is essential. The development of full-blown skin necrosis can usually be prevented by the administration, at the first signs of a developing lesion, of vitamin K_1 (46). If the lesions progress, the oral anticoagulant should preferably be withdrawn.

Prevention of recurrence of coumarin necrosis in patients with protein C deficiency, if treatment is necessary, could consist of transient simultaneous infusion of fresh frozen plasma (leading to a constant concentration of protein C) and heparin both before and at the first time of administration of an oral anticoagulant, associated or not with protein C concentrate (65,66).

Musculoskeletal

Preliminary results that suggested coumarin-associated reduction in bone density have not been confirmed. In a study from the Osteoporotic Fractures Research Group, 6201 postmenopausal women who were either users ($n = 149$) or non-users of warfarin were assessed for fractures and bone mineral density. Over 2 years, the two groups had similar age-adjusted heel and hip bone mineral density measurements. During an average of 3.5 years, non-traumatic, non-vertebral fractures occurred in 10% of warfarin users and 9.3% of non-users (67).

However, bones that fracture during oral anticoagulant therapy require more time to form adequate amounts of callus. This may be explained by an anticoagulant-induced increase in the size of fracture hematoma. However, the observation that warfarin inhibits calcification inside artificial hearts implanted in calves adds to the body of evidence indicating that coumarin depresses not only coagulation factors, but also other (Gla)-containing proteins, for example osteocalcin, a shortage of which may also delay skeletal calcification (68). Osteocalcin is a non-collagenous bone matrix protein containing gamma-carboxyglutamic acid, the synthesis of which is vitamin K-dependent. During oral anticoagulation with phenprocoumon, osteocalcin concentrations were lower than in control subjects, whereas the proportion of non-carboxylated osteocalcin was significantly higher than in healthy subjects (69). Since osteocalcin concentrations reflect bone formation, but not bone resorption activity, the reduced serum total osteocalcin concentrations during oral anticoagulation do not necessarily imply that bone loss occurs in these patients. However, reduced bone formation and impaired gamma-carboxylation of osteocalcin in patients treated with phenprocoumon can be clinically important in circumstances such as fracture healing or when there is pre-existing bone disease. It has been suggested that vitamin D regulates the synthesis of vitamin K-dependent bone protein, but no significant effect of the duration of phenprocoumon therapy on parathormone and vitamin D concentrations has been observed (69).

Immunologic

Skin-test reactivity, that is induration and tissue factor generation by monocytes, is reduced by therapeutic doses of oral anticoagulants, but lymphocyte transformation activity is not. This constitutes the rationale for the use of oral anticoagulants in the treatment of immune diseases characterized by fibrin deposition, such as allograft rejection and lupus nephritis (70).

Second-Generation Effects

Pregnancy

Antithrombotic treatment during pregnancy carries a well-established and substantial risk for both mother and fetus (71). The mother has an increased chance of abortion and of perinatal bleeding complications.

Contraceptive counselling must be given to all women who need anticoagulants. Recommendations for the use of anticoagulants during pregnancy have been reassessed in various publications (72–75). In cases of previous venous thrombosis and/or pulmonary embolism, two reasonable approaches are possible. One can either use low-dose heparin throughout pregnancy followed by an oral anticoagulant postpartum for 4–6 weeks, or one can choose to initiate clinical surveillance combined with periodic venous non-invasive tests followed by an oral anticoagulant postpartum for 4–6 weeks. If venous thrombosis occurs, heparin should be used until term, withdrawn immediately before delivery, and then both heparin and an oral anticoagulant can be started postpartum. When pregnancy is planned in patients who are taking long-term oral anticoagulants, the physician should either replace the oral anticoagulant with heparin before conception is attempted, or perform frequent pregnancy tests and substitute oral anticoagulant for heparin when pregnancy is achieved.

In patients with artificial heart valves, management in pregnancy is problematic, because the efficacy of heparin has not been established. Two approaches have been recommended. One can use heparin in a therapeutic dosage throughout pregnancy or use heparin until the 13th week, followed by an oral anticoagulant until the middle of the third trimester, and then heparin until delivery.

Teratogenicity

Vitamin K antagonists, including hydroxycoumarin derivatives and indan-1,3-dione-derived drugs, can be teratogenic and can also induce bleeding in the fetus (71,72,76–79). Adverse fetal outcomes occur in about one-third of pregnancies after either oral anticoagulants or heparin (77). This surprisingly high figure, which is often quoted, should be tempered by the consideration that these data are largely (if not exclusively) derived from women with heart valves taking relatively large doses of warfarin in order to maintain the INR at around 4. Some have suggested that the risk of fetal embryopathy is lower in women taking lower doses for prophylaxis or treatment of deep venous thrombosis (80).

The pattern of teratogenicity of congeners of the vitamin K antagonist group is generally known as warfarin embryopathy, also referred to as the fetal-warfarin syndrome and Conradi–Hünermann syndrome, although the latter term also covers an identical hereditary disorder. The pattern is now considered to represent a specific group of malformations occurring in some fetuses exposed to a vitamin K antagonist during the first trimester, with a critical period during the sixth to twelfth weeks of gestation. The minimal criteria for the diagnosis include either nasal hypoplasia or stippled epiphyses. In severe cases the forehead is bossed and the nose is sunken, with deep grooves between the alae nasi and the tip of the nose; other skeletal deformities can also be present. Half the affected children have upper airway obstruction, secondary to underdeveloped cartilage. Radiography shows stippling (caused by abnormal focal calcification of the epiphyseal regions), preferentially in the axial skeleton, for example the proximal femur, and in the calcanei. Children with milder defects can show catch-up growth, and stippling can disappear after the first year of life; however, in severe cases the nose remains small and sunken. It is questionable whether mental retardation is part of the syndrome, since it has only been observed in cases of exposure for at least two trimesters.

The belief that the incidence of the overt syndrome is of the order of 5% seems to have been confirmed by a review of 186 studies: among 1325 pregnant women who took anticoagulant drugs, 970 were allocated to warfarin and the incidence of warfarin embryopathy was 4.6% (81). However, in a prospective survey of 72 pregnant women with cardiac valve prostheses, the incidence of coumarin embryopathy was 25% in the 12 pregnancies in which heparin was not substituted for acenocoumarol until after the 7th week, and 30% in the 37 pregnancies in which acenocoumarol was given throughout pregnancy. There were no signs of coumarin embryopathy when acenocoumarol was withdrawn from the sixth to the twelfth weeks of gestation and the women were treated instead with heparin (82).

Oral anticoagulation may cause warfarin embryopathy by inhibiting post-translational carboxylation of proteins needed in the normal ossification process. Intensity of treatment appears to be of importance, since there were no cases of warfarin embryopathy in 44 consecutive children of 42 mothers exposed in the first trimester, but who had prothrombin times prolonged by 40–60% (83,84). Experiments in rats in which highly intensive long-term anticoagulant therapy produced excessive mineralization disorders favor this causal relation (85).

Another possible adverse reaction is the occurrence of central nervous system anomalies in fetuses exposed to vitamin K antagonists at any time during pregnancy. The anomalies may result from fetal intracerebral hemorrhage with scarring. There are two patterns: one consists of dorsal midline dysplasia, expressed as agenesis of the corpus callosum, Dandy-Walker malformation, midline cerebral atrophy, or possible encephalocele; the other consists of ventral midline dysplasia, characterized by optic atrophy. The patients are never completely normal on follow-up, and the resulting personal and social burdens are considerable. According to a review (81), there were central nervous system anomalies in 26 (2.7%) of 970 pregnancies in which warfarin was used. Neonates can also have hemorrhagic complications if a pregnant mother takes an oral anticoagulant near term. The neonatal liver is immature, and concentrations of vitamin K-dependent coagulation factors are low. Although maternal warfarin concentrations are in the therapeutic range, bleeding can occur in neonates. Warfarin in particular should be avoided beyond 36 weeks of gestation (86).

Other consequences of oral anticoagulation during pregnancy are spontaneous abortion, stillbirth, and premature birth (87).

Lactation

In contrast to heparin, coumarins are secreted into the breast milk, but it has long been known that prothrombin activity in the plasma of neonates whose mothers take coumarins is not significantly reduced (88–90) and that warfarin does not have anticoagulant effects in breast-fed infants when given to nursing mothers (89,91). These conclusions are subject to the reservation that in some of the studies the dose of anticoagulant was low (89). Acenocoumarol-treated breastfeeding mothers can as a rule safely breastfeed their infants (92,93); nevertheless, it is prudent to check the infant's prothrombin time in such cases.

There are differences between infants in their sensitivity to coumarins. Some experts therefore recommended weekly oral administration of 1 mg of vitamin K_1 to the child if the mother is taking a coumarin and breastfeeding (94).

Susceptibility Factors

Genetic factors

There is a strong association between CYP2C9 variant alleles and warfarin dosage requirements (95), and the CYP2C9*2 and CYP2C9*3 variant alleles, which are associated with reduced enzyme activity, have been associated with significant reductions in mean warfarin dosage requirements (96). The possession of a variant allele may also be associated with an increased risk of adverse effects (97). The CYP2C9 genotype is also relevant to acenocoumarol (98). Other polymorphisms, such as those that affect CYP3A4 or CYP1A2, may also be important (96). The molecular basis of warfarin resistance is unclear but could be due to unusually high CYP2C9 activity (pharmacokinetic resistance) or to abnormal activity of vitamin K epoxide reductase (pharmacodynamic resistance) (96).

There is also a rare ala-10 mutation in the propeptide of factor IX, which leads to an increased risk of bleeding when starting anticoagulation with coumarin anticoagulants (99,100).

Age

Age is generally considered as an important susceptibility factor for bleeding during oral anticoagulant treatment (101). The frequency of bleeding was higher in elderly patients in four of five cohort studies of warfarin-related bleeding, published over a 10-year period (29,33). In one study (30), age was the only significant independent risk factor for subdural hemorrhage, apart from the intensity of anticoagulation, whereas age was only of borderline significance for intracerebral hemorrhage. Various explanations could account for the effect of age: co-medication, co-morbidity, increased sensitivity to warfarin, and impaired vascular integrity. Elderly patients, especially those with moderate hypertension, cerebral thrombosis, or a latent gastrointestinal ulcer, should be supervised closely (102).

Other features of the patient

Susceptibility factors for bleeding with oral anticoagulants, apart from age, include (29):

- endogenous coagulation defects
- thrombocytopenia
- hypertension
- cerebrovascular disease
- thyroid disease
- renal insufficiency
- liver disease
- tumors
- cerebrovascular disease
- alcoholism
- a history of gastrointestinal bleeding (peptic ulcer disease alone without past bleeding is not associated with an increased risk of bleeding)
- an inability to adhere to the regimen.

Patients with hypothyroidism and hyperthyroidism should all be carefully monitored because the response is greatly reduced in hypothyroidism and greatly enhanced in hyperthyroidism (103). The increased warfarin sensitivity is said to be related to increased degradation of clotting factors. When the thyroid disease is treated, the susceptibility of these patients to coumarins gradually normalizes.

Since vitamin K is one of the vitamins whose absorption is significantly affected by diarrhea, a raised INR and bleeding can occur during episodes of diarrhea (104). Therefore, patients who have diarrhea or reduced food intake should have their INR evaluated more often and their anticoagulant doses adjusted appropriately.

For oral anticoagulant prophylaxis, the overall number of bleeding patients with organic lesions exceeds 50%. Most have prothrombin times within the usual target range. It is therefore clear that all cases of major (or recurrent mild) internal hemorrhagic complications should be investigated for possible underlying organic disease. In one study, patients with hemorrhagic complications, despite a prothrombin time within the target range, were more likely to have an underlying pathological lesion as a direct cause of bleeding than patients whose bleeding occurred when the prothrombin time was above the target range (105).

Drug–Drug Interactions

General

Commonly prescribed drugs can potentiate or antagonize the anticoagulant effect of coumarin drugs in several ways:

- by interfering with the absorption of the drug
- by inhibiting intestinal bacterial production and absorption of vitamin K_2
- by inhibiting the absorption of vitamin K_1 present in food
- by altering the binding of the coumarins to plasma proteins
- by altering the metabolism of the drug by liver microsomes.

Competition for metabolic pathways (for example cytochrome P_{450} isozymes) could lead to an increase in the anticoagulant effect, and/or the pharmacological effects of a drug whose active metabolites are produced by the same metabolic pathway. Hence, any patient taking an oral anticoagulant who has another drug added to or withdrawn from the regimen must have prothrombin time carefully monitored to avoid important changes in the intensity of treatment.

The information on interactions given in Table 1 is mainly based on well-documented prospective studies and, in a few instances, on anecdotal reports. A given interaction may hold for one but not for another coumarin congener.

Alcohol

Alcoholics can drink ethanol in amounts large enough (200 g) to inhibit warfarin clearance as an acute effect. However, daily consumption of ethanol for a period of 3 weeks in the form of wine taken with meals in moderate amounts (28 g/day) or even in liberal amounts (56 g/day) had no effect on the hypoprothrombinemia induced by warfarin (256).

Although long-term alcohol can induce some cytochrome P_{450} isozymes, such as CYP1A1, CYP1A2 (257), CYP2B1, and CYP2E1 (258), these effects are not relevant to the coumarins, which are mostly metabolized by CYP2C9.

A report of ethanol potentiation of aspirin-induced prolongation of bleeding time (259) is of importance, in view of a putative increase, due to alcohol intake, of the hemorrhagic risk accompanying outpatient oral anticoagulation.

Co-amoxiclav

In a case-control study in 300 previously stable outpatients taking phenprocoumon or acenocoumarol with INR values of 6.0 or more and 302 matched controls with INR values within the target range, potentially interacting drugs were predominantly antibacterial drugs (260). A course of co-amoxiclav was associated with a small increase in risk (OR = 2.4; 95% CI = 1.0, 5.5). Of 87 potentially interacting drugs, 45 were not used during the 4-week study and only 15 drugs were used by at least 10 patients. The authors concluded that unless no therapeutic alternative is available, co-amoxiclav should be avoided in patients taking coumarins. If no therapeutic alternative is available, increased monitoring of INR values is warranted to prevent overanticoagulation and potential bleeding complications.

Co-trimoxazole

In a case-control study in 300 previously stable outpatients taking phenprocoumon or acenocoumarol, with INR values of 6 or more, and 302 matched controls with INR values within the target range, potentially interacting drugs were predominantly antibacterial drugs (260). A course of co-trimoxazole was associated with a large increase in the risk of excess anticoagulation (adjusted OR = 24; 95% CI = 2.8, 209). Of 87 potentially interacting drugs 45 were not used during the 4-week study and only 15 drugs were used by at least 10 patients. The authors concluded that unless no therapeutic alternative is available, co-trimoxazole should be avoided in patients taking coumarins. If no therapeutic alternative is available, increased monitoring of INR values is warranted to prevent overanticoagulation and potential bleeding complications.

Danshen

- Potentiation of the effect of warfarin by danshen (the root of *Salvia miltiorrhiza*), a widely used traditional Chinese herbal medicine, particularly for cardiovascular complaints, has been described in a 62-year-old man with a mechanical mitral valve prosthesis (159).

Fluoroquinolones

A series of cases of coagulopathy due to an interaction of warfarin with ciprofloxacin has been extracted from the FDA's Spontaneous Reporting System database, including all cases reported from 1987 to 1997, combined with two of the author's own cases (261). Soon after the introduction of ciprofloxacin in 1987, hemorrhagic events from hypoprothrombinemia were reported in patients taking warfarin. However, several prospective studies of combining ciprofloxacin and other fluoroquinolones with warfarin failed to show a significant change in INR (Table 2). Although it is impossible to estimate the frequency of the ciprofloxacin/warfarin interaction from these or other descriptive data, it can be concluded that potentiation of anticoagulant effect by ciprofloxacin occurs most often in older patients and those taking multiple medications.

Methylprednisolone

Potentiation of the effects of vitamin K antagonists by high-dose intravenous methylprednisolone has been prospectively studied in 10 consecutive patients and 5 controls after the observation of a sharp increase in the International Normalized Ratio (INR) in a patient taking oral anticoagulation after concomitant administration of methylprednisolone (1 g/day for 3 days) (262). The mean INR was 2.8 (range 2.0–3.8) at baseline and increased to 8.0 (5.3–20). The maximum increase in INR occurred after a mean of 93 (29–156) hours. The coumarins taken by these patients were fluindione in eight and acenocoumarol in two. The prothrombin time in the controls

Table 1 Important drug–drug interactions with coumarin anticoagulants

Drug	Effect on anticoagulant response	Mechanism	Comment
Acetylsalicylic acid and other salicylates	Potentiation (106,107) (at doses over 1.5 g/day) even with topical application (108)	Unknown	Avoid concurrent use: can also impair platelet aggregation and cause peptic erosion and ulceration
Allopurinol	Potentiation (109)	Inhibition of microsomal enzymes (110)	Adjust dosage
Aminoglutethimide	Reduction possible (111)	Unknown	Adjust dosage
Aminoglycoside antibiotics	Potentiation possible (112)	Reduced availability of vitamin K (113)	Monitor INR
Amiodarone	Potentiation (114–117)	Reduced warfarin and acenocoumarol clearances (114,117)	Adjust dosage
Anabolic steroids and androgens (C17-alkylated)	Potentiation (118)	Unknown	Adjust dosage
Antacids containing magnesium	Potentiation possible (119) (only documented for dicoumarol)	Increased absorption (119)	Of no practical importance
Azapropazone	Potentiation (120)	Displacement from binding sites on plasma proteins (121); inhibition of metabolism causes peptic ulceration	Avoid concurrent use
Azathioprine	Reduction (122,123)	Unknown	
Azithromycin	Potentiation (124)	Inhibition of microsomal enzymes possible	Monitor INR or avoid concurrent use
Barbiturates	Reduction (125)	Induction of microsomal enzymes (126)	Adjust dosage
Benziodarone	Potentiation (127)	Unknown	Adjust dosage
Bezafibrate	Potentiation (128,129)	Unknown	Adjust dosage
Carbamazepine	Reduction (130,131)	Induction of microsomal enzymes (131)	Adjust dosage
Carbimazole	Reduction (132)	Decreased catabolism of vitamin K-dependent clotting	Adjust dosage
Cetirizine	Potentiation (133)	Unknown	Anecdotal
Cephalosporins	Potentiation possible (134,135)	Inhibition of hepatic vitamin K metabolism (136)	Monitor INR
Chloral hydrate and related compounds	Minor potentiation during initial phase of anticoagulation therapy, not during maintenance therapy (108,137)	Displacement from binding sites on plasma proteins	Usually of no practical importance
Chloramphenicol	Potentiation (138,139) even with ocular administration (140)	Unknown	Adjust dosage Monitor INR
Chlortalidone	Pseudoreduction	Hemoconcentration (141)	No practical importance
Colestyramine	Reduction (142,143)	Reduced absorption and interruption of enterohepatic circulation (142,143)	Adjust dosage: separate dosage of these two drugs by a long time interval
Cimetidine	Potentiation (144); not documented for phenprocoumon (145)	Stereoselective inhibition of warfarin metabolism (146)	Adjust dosage
Ciprofloxacin	Potentiation possible (147,148)	Unknown	Monitor INR
Cisapride	Potentiation (149)	Inhibition of microsomal enzymes possible	Monitor INR
Clarithromycin	Potentiation (150–152)	Inhibition of microsomal enzymes possible	Monitor INR or avoid concurrent use
Clofibrate	Potentiation (153)	Unknown	Adjust dosage
Co-trimoxazole	Potentiation (154,155)	Unknown	Adjust dosage
Cyclophosphamide	Reduction possible (156)	Unknown	Anecdotal
Ciclosporin	Reduction possible (157)	Unknown	Adjust dosage
Danazol	Potentiation (158)		
Danshen	Potentiation (159)	Unknown	Anecdotal
Dicloxacillin	Reduction (160)	Unknown	Monitor INR
Diflunisal	Potentiation possible (161)	Can impair platelet aggregation and cause peptic ulceration	Avoid concurrent use

Drug	Effect on anticoagulant response	Mechanism	Comment
Disulfiram	Potentiation (162,163)	Inhibition of microsomal enzymes (162)	Adjust dosage
Erythromycin	Potentiation possible (164,165)	Reduced warfarin clearance (166)	Monitor INR
Etacrynic acid	Potentiation possible (167)	Unknown	Anecdotal
Fenofibrate	Potentiation (168)	Displacement from binding sites on plasma proteins	Adjust dosage Monitor INR
Floctafenine	Minor potentiation (169)	Unknown	Monitor INR
Fluconazole	Potentiation possible (170–172)	Unknown	Monitor INR
Fluorouracil	Potentiation possible (173)	Unknown	Monitor INR
Fluoxetine	Potentiation (174)	Unknown	Adjust dosage or avoid concurrent use
Flurbiprofen	Potentiation possible (175,176)	Unknown	Monitor INR
Fluvastatin	Potentiation possible (177)	Unknown	Monitor INR
Furosemide	Reduction (178)	Hemoconcentration	Monitor INR
Ginseng	Reduction (179)	Unknown	Anecdotal
Glucagon	Potentiation (180)	Unknown	Avoid concurrent use
Glucocorticoids	Ambiguous (181,182)		No practical importance
Glutethimide	Reduction (183)	Induction of microsomal enzymes (183)	Adjust dosage
Griseofulvin	Reduction (184)	Unknown	Adjust dosage
Haloperidol	Reduction possible (185)	Unknown	Anecdotal
Indometacin	Potentiation possible (186)	Unknown	Monitor INR
Isoniazid	Potentiation possible (187)	Unknown	Anecdotal
Itraconazole	Potentiation possible (188)	Unknown	Monitor INR
Ketoconazole	Potentiation possible (189)	Unknown	Monitor INR
Lovastatin	Potentiation possible (190)	Unknown	Monitor INR
Mefenamic acid	Potentiation possible (191)	Fibrinolysis	No clinical importance
Mercaptopurine	Reduction (192)	Unknown	Adjust dosage
Mesalazine	Reduction (193,194)	Unknown	Monitor INR
Metronidazole	Potentiation (195)	Stereoselective inhibition of metabolism (warfarin) (195)	Adjust dosage
Miconazole	Potentiation possible (196–198) even with topical application (197,199,200)	Inhibition of metabolism (201)	Avoid concurrent use or contraindicated
Nafcillin	Reduction possible (202,203)	Unknown	Anecdotal
Nalidixic acid	Potentiation possible (204,205)	Unknown	Anecdotal
Norfloxacin	Potentiation (147)	Unknown	Monitor INR
Nutritional formulations	Reduction (206)	Increased availability of vitamin K (206)	Adjust dosage
Ofloxacin	Potentiation (207)	Unknown	Monitor INR
Omeprazole	Potentiation (208)	Unknown	Monitor INR
Oral contraceptives	Ambiguous (209,210)	Unknown	No practical importance
Paracetamol	Potentiation during long-term administration (211,212)	Unknown	Use paracetamol for limited periods Monitor INR
Phenylbutazone	Potentiation (213)	Displacement from binding sites on plasma proteins; stereoselective inhibition of metabolism (warfarin); causes peptic ulceration (214,215)	Avoid concurrent use
Phenytoin	Reduction (216); warfarin may give potentiation (217,218)	Unknown	Adjust dosage
Piracetam	Potentiation possible (219)	Unknown	Anecdotal
Piroxicam	Potentiation (220)	Unknown	Monitor INR
Pravastatin	Potentiation (221)	Unknown	Monitor INR
Proguanil	Potentiation (222)	Unknown	Monitor INR
Propafenone	Potentiation (223)	Unknown	Monitor INR
Propranolol	Potentiation (224)	Inhibition of metabolism	Monitor INR
Quinidine	Potentiation possible (225,226)	Pharmacodynamic interaction	Monitor INR

Continued

Table 1 Continued

Drug	Effect on anticoagulant response	Mechanism	Comment
Ranitidine	Possible potentiation at high dosages (227)	Unknown	Monitor INR if high dosage
Rifampicin	Reduction (228)	Induction of microsomal enzymes (229,230)	Adjust dosage
Ritonavir	Reduction (231)	Unknown	Monitor INR
Saquinavir	Potentiation (232)	Inhibition of microsomal enzymes	Monitor INR
Simvastatin	Potentiation (233,234)	Unknown	Adjust dosage Monitor INR
Spironolactone	Pseudoreduction (235)	Hemoconcentration	No practical importance
Sucralfate	Reduction possible (236,237)		Anecdotal
Sulfinpyrazone	Potentiation possible (238–241) (not documented with phenprocoumon) (240)	Inhibition of microsomal enzymes (242)	Adjust dosage
Sulfonamides	Potentiation possible (243,244)	Unknown	Anecdotal
Sulindac	Potentiation possible (245,246)	Unknown	Monitor INR
Tamoxifen	Potentiation possible (247,248)	Unknown	Adjust dosage
Tetracyclines	Potentiation possible (139,154)	Reduced availability of vitamin K (113)	Monitor INR
Thiouracils	Reduction	Reduced catabolism of vitamin K-dependent clotting factors	Adjust dosage
Thyroid hormones	Potentiation (148,249)	Increased catabolism of vitamin K-dependent clotting factors (132)	Adjust dosage
Tramadol	Potentiation possible (250,251)	Inhibition of microsomal enzymes	Monitor INR
Ubidecarone	Reduction (252)	Unknown	Adjust dosage
Vitamin E	Potentiation possible (253)	Unknown	Anecdotal
Zafirlukast	Potentiation possible (254)	Unknown	Monitor INR
Zileuton (255)	Potentiation	Unknown	Adjust dosage Monitor INR

Table 2 Prospective interaction studies of fluoroquinolones with warfarin

Study design	N	Source of subjects	Drug	Coagulation effect	Reference
Single arm	9	Warfarin clinic	Ciprofloxacin	None	(264)
Single arm	16	Warfarin clinic	Ciprofloxacin	*R*-warfarin	(265)
Placebo-controlled[a]	36	Warfarin clinic	Ciprofloxacin	*R*-warfarin	(266)
Randomized crossover[b]	6	Healthy volunteers	Enoxacin	*R*-warfarin	(267)
Randomized crossover[c]	10	Healthy volunteers	Ofloxacin	None	(268)
Single arm	7	Healthy volunteers	Ofloxacin	None	(269)
Single arm	10	Healthy volunteers	Temafloxacin	None	(270)

[a]Randomized, double-blind, placebo-controlled study
[b]Randomized, double-blind, placebo-controlled, multicenter study
[c]Randomized, two-way, crossover study

remained stable. A similar rise in INR was described in two patients with multiple sclerosis taking warfarin (263).

The mechanism of the interaction of methylprednisolone with oral anticoagulants has not been elucidated, but it might be due to inhibition of anticoagulant catabolism. In the three patients in whom the authors assayed fluindione concentrations, these increased in parallel with the INR. The administration of high-dose methylprednisolone to patients taking oral anticoagulants is not rare; daily monitoring of INR or even reducing the anticoagulant dose before administering methylprednisolone is advised.

Miconazole

Interactions between coumarins and miconazole have been reported, although the mechanism of the interaction is not known. There have been two separate reports of potentiation of the anticoagulant effect of acenocoumarol by non-systemic administration of miconazole. Three patients taking long-term acenocoumarol who used miconazole gel for oral candidiasis had significant rises in INR (197). In two other patients vaginal miconazole potentiated the anticoagulant effect of acenocoumarol (198).

NSAIDs

The COX-2 selective non-steroidal anti-inflammatory drug celecoxib did not alter the pharmacokinetics or the hypoprothrombinemic effect of warfarin in 24 healthy subjects (30). However, there have been at least two reports of increased INR in patients taking stable warfarin therapy and celecoxib (31,101).

Another COX-2-selective non-steroidal anti-inflammatory drug, rofecoxib, increased plasma concentrations of the biologically less active isomer, $R(+)$ warfarin, which accounted for an approximately 8% increase in INR at steady state in healthy volunteers (33).

Standard monitoring of INR in patients taking warfarin should be performed when therapy with celecoxib or rofecoxib is begun or changed.

Paracetamol

In a prospective, case-control study, designed to determine causes of INRs over 6.0 in an outpatient anticoagulant unit, there was a clear dose-dependent association between the use of paracetamol (acetaminophen) and having an INR greater than 6.0 (212). The authors studied 93 patients with INRs over 6.0 (cases) and 196 patients with INRs of 1.7–3.3 (controls) during warfarin therapy. The likelihood of an INR greater than 6.0 increased from an odds ratio of 3.5 for doses of 2275–4549 mg per week, to 6.9 for doses of 4550–9099 mg per week, to a 10-fold increase at a dose of over 9100 mg per week.

Paracetamol also potentiates the effects of acenocoumarol (211) and although a study with phenprocoumon showed no interaction (271), the study was too small and not well designed to detect an effect of the sort that has been shown in case-control studies.

Ribavirin

Inhibition of the effect of warfarin by ribavirin has been described.

- In a 61-year-old man, who was taking long-term warfarin after a heart valve replacement, the dose of warfarin had to be increased by 40% after the introduction of ribavirin for chronic hepatitis C; the inhibition of the effect of warfarin was reproduced on rechallenge (272).

The mechanism of this effect was not clear.

Ritonavir

Inhibition of the effect of acenocoumarol by ritonavir has been described.

- A 46-year-old man with two prosthetic heart valves taking acenocoumarol started to take ritonavir 600 mg/day. Despite a progressive increase in the dose of acenocoumarol to three times the original dose, it was impossible to achieve a therapeutic INR, and the ritonavir was withdrawn (273).

The authors proposed that ritonavir had induced CYP1A2, CYP1A4, and CYP2C9/19 activity, leading to increased metabolism, at least of acenocoumarol. However, this effect was the opposite of what was expected, since ritonavir is a potent inhibitor of most hepatic isoenzymes.

Salicylates

Salicylates can interact with warfarin in different ways. They displace warfarin from albumin binding sites, and this can result in a transient increase in anticoagulant activity, which is usually clinically unimportant. They can also cause peptic ulceration and reduce platelet aggregation, making bleeding more likely and slower to stop when it occurs.

There was a rise in INR from 2.8 to 12 when a topical pain-relieving gel containing methylsalicylate was applied to the knees of a 22-year-old white woman taking stable warfarin anticoagulation (274).

Other similar cases have been reported (275).

Food–Drug Interactions

Cranberry juice

Cranberry juice has been reported to enhance the action of warfarin (276).

- After a chest infection, a man in his 70s had a poor appetite for 2 weeks and ate next to nothing, taking only cranberry juice as well as his regular drugs (digoxin, phenytoin, and warfarin) (277). Six weeks later his international normalised ratio was over 50, having previously been stable. He died of gastrointestinal and pericardial haemorrhage. He had not taken any over-the-counter preparations or herbal medicines, and he had been taking his drugs correctly.

The Committee on Safety of Medicines has received several other reports through the yellow card reporting scheme about a possible interaction between warfarin and cranberry juice. In one case, this effect was suggested to have been due to contamination with salicylic acid, which displaces warfarin from protein binding sites (278).

Smoking

Cigarette smoking altered the clearance and apparent volume of distribution of warfarin, although the net effect on anticoagulant activity was negligible both in volunteers (279) and patients (280).

Monitoring Therapy

There are no clear guidelines about how often the INR should be measured in patients taking coumarins. However, it should be done quite frequently at the start of therapy when the risk of bleeding is higher (32). Monitoring anticoagulant therapy is greatly improved by the use of anticoagulation clinics or anticoagulation management services in which the management is conducted by registered nurses, pharmacists, or physicians using dosage adjustment protocols developed by experts in the field (281).

References

1. Duxbury BM, Poller L. The oral anticoagulant saga: past, present, and future. Clin Appl Thromb Hemost 2001;7(4):269–75.

2. Griffin JH, Evatt B, Zimmerman TS, Kleiss AJ, Wideman C. Deficiency of protein C in congenital thrombotic disease. J Clin Invest 1981;68(5):1370–3.
3. Marlar RA, Kleiss AJ, Griffin JH. Mechanism of action of human activated protein C, a thrombin-dependent anticoagulant enzyme. Blood 1982;59(5):1067–72.
4. Stein PD, Riddle JM, Kemp SR, Lee MW, Lewis JW, Magilligan DJ Jr. Effect of warfarin on calcification of spontaneously degenerated porcine bioprosthetic valves. J Thorac Cardiovasc Surg 1985;90(1):119–25.
5. Hilgard P, Schulte H, Wetzig G, Schmitt G, Schmidt CG. Oral anticoagulation in the treatment of a spontaneously metastasising murine tumour (3LL). Br J Cancer 1977;35(1):78–86.
6. Thornes RD. Adjuvant therapy of cancer via the cellular immune mechanism or fibrin by induced fibrinolysis and oral anticoagulants. Cancer 1975;35(1):91–7.
7. Hoover HC Jr, Ketcham AS, Millar RC, Gralnick HR. Osteosarcoma: improved survival with anticoagulation and amputation. Cancer 1978;41(6):2475–80.
8. Zacharski LR, Henderson WG, Rickles FR, Forman WB, Cornell CJ Jr, Forcier RJ, Edwards R, Headley E, Kim SH, O'Donnell JR, O'Dell R, Tornyos K, Kwaan HC. Effect of warfarin on survival in small cell carcinoma of the lung. Veterans Administration Study No. 75. JAMA 1981;245(8):831–5.
9. Zacharski LR, Henderson WG, Rickles FR, Forman WB, Cornell CJ Jr, Forcier RJ, Edwards RL, Headley E, Kim SH, O'Donnell JF, et al. Effect of warfarin anticoagulation on survival in carcinoma of the lung, colon, head and neck, and prostate. Final report of VA Cooperative Study #75. Cancer 1984;53(10):2046–52.
10. Annegers JF, Zacharski LR. Cancer morbidity and mortality in previously anticoagulated patients. Thromb Res 1980;18(3–4):399–403.
11. Hilgard P, Maat B. Mechanism of lung tumour colony reduction caused by coumarin anticoagulation. Eur J Cancer 1979;15(2):183–7.
12. Lione A, Bosmann HB. The inhibitory effect of heparin and warfarin treatments on the intravascular survival of B16 melanoma cells in syngeneic C57 mice. Cell Biol Int Rep 1978;2(1):81–6.
13. Poovalingam V, Kenoyer DG, Mahomed R, Rapiti N, Bassa F, Govender P. Superwarfarin poisoning—a report of 4 cases. S Afr Med J 2002;92(11):874–6.
14. Sharma P, Bentley P. Of rats and men: superwarfarin toxicity. Lancet 2005;365(9459):552–3.
15. Tsutaoka BT, Miller M, Fung SM, Patel MM, Olson KR. Superwarfarin and glass ingestion with prolonged coagulopathy requiring high-dose vitamin K1 therapy. Pharmacotherapy 2003;23(9):1186–9.
16. Sarin S, Mukhtar H, Mirza MA. Prolonged coagulopathy related to superwarfarin overdose. Ann Intern Med 2005;142(2):156.
17. Shepherd G, Klein-Schwartz W, Anderson BD. Acute, unintentional pediatric brodifacoum ingestions. Pediatr Emerg Care 2002;18(3):174–8.
18. Mullins ME, Brands CL, Daya MR. Unintentional pediatric superwarfarin exposures: do we really need a prothrombin time? Pediatrics 2000;105(2):402–4.
19. Ingels M, Lai C, Tai W, Manning BH, Rangan C, Williams SR, Manoguerra AS, Albertson T, Clark RF. A prospective study of acute, unintentional, pediatric superwarfarin ingestions managed without decontamination. Ann Emerg Med 2002;40(1):73–8.
20. Zupancic-Salek S, Kovacevic-Metelko J, Radman I. Successful reversal of anticoagulant effect of superwarfarin poisoning with recombinant activated factor VII. Blood Coagul Fibrinolysis 2005;16(4):239–44.
21. Akle CA, Joiner CL. Purple toe syndrome. J R Soc Med 1981;74(3):219.
22. Feder W, Auerbach R. "Purple toes": an uncommon sequela of oral coumarin drug therapy. Ann Intern Med 1961;55:911–17.
23. Burton JL, Pennock P. Anticoagulants and "feeling cold". Lancet 1979;1(8116):608.
24. Bruns FJ, Segel DP, Adler S. Control of cholesterol embolization by discontinuation of anticoagulant therapy. Am J Med Sci 1978;275(1):105–8.
25. Walters MB. The relationship between thyroid function and anticoagulant thrapy. Am J Cardiol 1963;11:112–14.
26. Christensen F. Uricosuric effect of dicoumarol. Acta Med Scand 1964;175:461–8.
27. DiMarco JP, Flaker G, Waldo AL, Corley SD, Greene HL, Safford RE, Rosenfeld LE, Mitrani G, Nemeth M; AFFIRM Investigators. Factors affecting bleeding risk during anticoagulant therapy in patients with atrial fibrillation: observations from the Atrial Fibrillation Follow-up Investigation of Rhythm Management (AFFIRM) study. Am Heart J 2005;149(4):650–6.
28. Landefeld CS, Beyth RJ. Anticoagulant-related bleeding: clinical epidemiology, prediction, and prevention. Am J Med 1993;95(3):315–28.
29. Levine MN, Raskob G, Landefeld S, Kearon C. Hemorrhagic complications of anticoagulant treatment. Chest 1998;114(5 Suppl):S511–23.
30. Hylek EM, Singer DE. Risk factors for intracranial hemorrhage in outpatients taking warfarin. Ann Intern Med 1994;120(11):897–902.
31. Hylek EM, Skates SJ, Sheehan MA, Singer DE. An analysis of the lowest effective intensity of prophylactic anticoagulation for patients with nonrheumatic atrial fibrillation. N Engl J Med 1996;335(8):540–6.
32. Landefeld CS, Goldman L. Major bleeding in outpatients treated with warfarin: incidence and prediction by factors known at the start of outpatient therapy. Am J Med 1989;87:153.
33. Fihn SD, McDonell M, Martin D, Henikoff J, Vermes D, Kent D, White RH. Risk factors for complications of chronic anticoagulation. A multicenter study. Warfarin Optimized Outpatient Follow-up Study Group. Ann Intern Med 1993;118(7):511–20.
34. The Stroke Prevention in Atrial Fibrillation Investigators. Bleeding during antithrombotic therapy in patients with atrial fibrillation. Arch Intern Med 1996;156(4):409–16.
35. Makris M, Greaves M, Phillips WS, Kitchen S, Rosendaal FR, Preston EF. Emergency oral anticoagulant reversal: the relative efficacy of infusions of fresh frozen plasma and clotting factor concentrate on correction of the coagulopathy. Thromb Haemost 1997;77(3):477–80.
36. Mayer GA. Blood viscosity and oral anticoagulant therapy. Am J Clin Pathol 1976;65(3):402–6.
37. Herrmann KS, Kreuzer H. Beobachtung einer Acenocoumarol induzierten Granulocytose. [Observation of acenocoumarol-induced granulocytosis.] Klin Wochenschr 1988;66(14):639–42.
38. Dybedal I, Lamvik J. Warfarin as a probable cause of haemolytic anaemia. Thromb Haemost 1990;63(1):143.
39. Adler E, Benjamin SB, Zimmerman HJ. Cholestatic hepatic injury related to warfarin exposure. Arch Intern Med 1986;146(9):1837–9.
40. Ciorciaro C, Hartmann K, Stoller R, Kuhn M. Leberschäden durch Coumarin-antikoagulantien: Erfahrungen der IKS und der SANZ. [Liver injury caused by coumarin anticoagulants: experience of the IKS (Intercanton Monitoring Station) and the SANZ (Swiss Center for Drug Monitoring).] Schweiz Med Wochenschr 1996;126(49):2109–13.

41. Mix H, Wagner S, Boker K, Gloger S, Oldhafer KJ, Behrend M, Flemming P, Manns MP. Subacute liver failure induced by phenprocoumon treatment. Digestion 1999;60(6):579–82.
42. Kruis-de Vries MH, Stricker BH, Coenraads PJ, Nater JP. Maculopapular rash due to coumarin derivatives. Dermatologica 1989;178(2):109–11.
43. Susano R, Garcia A, Altadill A, Ferro J. Hypersensitivity vasculitis related to nicoumalone. BMJ 1993;306(6883):973.
44. Cole MS, Minifee PK, Wolma FJ. Coumarin necrosis–a review of the literature. Surgery 1988;103(3):271–7.
45. Verhagen H. Local haemorrhage and necrosis of the skin and underlying tissues, during anti-coagulant therapy with dicumarol or dicumacyl. Acta Med Scand 1954;148(6):453–67.
46. van Amstel WJ, Boekhout-Mussert MJ, Loeliger EA. Successful prevention of coumarin-induced hemorrhagic skin necrosis by timely administration of vitamin K_1. Blut 1978;36(2):89–93.
47. Loeliger EA, Paul LC, Van Brummelen P, Bieger R. Is coumarin-induced haemorrhagic necrosis of the skin the result of hypoproconvertinaemic bleeding in non-specifically inflamed skin patches? Neth J Med 1975;18(1):12–16.
48. Horn JR, Danziger LH, Davis RJ. Warfarin-induced skin necrosis: report of four cases. Am J Hosp Pharm 1981;38(11):1763–8.
49. Eby CS. Warfarin-induced skin necrosis. Hematol Oncol Clin North Am 1993;7(6):1291–300.
50. Gelwix TJ, Beeson MS. Warfarin-induced skin necrosis. Am J Emerg Med 1998;16(5):541–3.
51. Wynn SS, Jin DK, Essex DW. Warfarin-induced skin necrosis occurring four days after discontinuation of warfarin. Haemostasis 1997;27(5):246–50.
52. Goldberg SL, Orthner CL, Yalisove BL, Elgart ML, Kessler CM. Skin necrosis following prolonged administration of coumarin in a patient with inherited protein S deficiency. Am J Hematol 1991;38(1):64–6.
53. Sternberg ML, Pettyjohn FS. Warfarin sodium-induced skin necrosis. Ann Emerg Med 1995;26(1):94–7.
54. Torngren S, Somell A. Warfarin skin necrosis of the breast. Acta Chir Scand 1982;148(5):471–2.
55. Barkley C, Badalament RA, Metz EN, Nesbitt J, Drago JR. Coumarin necrosis of the penis. J Urol 1989;141(4):946–8.
56. Kandrotas RJ, Deterding J. Genital necrosis secondary to warfarin therapy. Pharmacotherapy 1988;8(6):351–4.
57. Haefeli H. Uterusnekrose bei Cumarin-Therapie. Fortschr Geburtslilfe Gynekol 1969;39:49.
58. DiCato M-A, Ellman L. Letter: Coumadin-induced necrosis of breast, disseminated intravascular coagulation, and hemolytic anemia. Ann Intern Med 1975;83(2):233–4.
59. Broekmans AW, Bertina RM, Loeliger EA, Hofmann V, Klingemann HG. Protein C and the development of skin necrosis during anticoagulant therapy. Thromb Haemost 1983;49(3):251.
60. Samama M, Horellou MH, Soria J, Conard J, Nicolas G. Successful progressive anticoagulation in a severe protein C deficiency and previous skin necrosis at the initiation of oral anticoagulant treatment. Thromb Haemost 1984;51(1):132–3.
61. Teepe RG, Broekmans AW, Vermeer BJ, Nienhuis AM, Loeliger EA. Recurrent coumarin-induced skin necrosis in a patient with an acquired functional protein C deficiency. Arch Dermatol 1986;122(12):1408–12.
62. Comp PC, Elrod JP, Karzenski S. Warfarin-induced skin necrosis. Semin Thromb Hemost 1990;16(4):293–8.
63. Wattiaux MJ, Herve R, Robert A, Cabane J, Housset B. Imbert JC. Coumarin-induced skin necrosis associated with acquired protein S deficiency and antiphospholipid antibody syndrome. Arthritis Rheum 1994;37(7):1096–100.
64. Shepherd AM, Hewick DS, Moreland TA, Stevenson IH. Age as a determinant of sensitivity to warfarin. Br J Clin Pharmacol 1977;4(3):315–20.
65. Lewandowski K, Zawilska K. Protein C concentrate in the treatment of warfarin-induced skin necrosis in the protein C deficiency. Thromb Haemost 1994;71(3):395.
66. Zauber NP, Stark MW. Successful warfarin anticoagulation despite protein C deficiency and a history of warfarin necrosis. Ann Intern Med 1986;104(5):659–60.
67. Jamal SA, Browner WS, Bauer DC, Cummings SR. Warfarin use and risk for osteoporosis in elderly women. Study of Osteoporotic Fractures Research Group. Ann Intern Med 1998;128(10):829–32.
68. Pierce WS, Donachy JH, Rosenberg G, Baier RE. Calcification inside artificial hearts: inhibition by warfarin-sodium. Science 1980;208(4444):601–3.
69. Pietschmann P, Woloszczuk W, Panzer S, Kyrle P, Smolen J. Decreased serum osteocalcin levels in phenprocoumon-treated patients. J Clin Endocrinol Metab 1988;66(5):1071–4.
70. Edwards RL, Rickles FR. Delayed hypersensitivity in man: effects of systemic anticoagulation. Science 1978;200(4341):541–3.
71. Hirsh J, Cade JF, Gallus AS. Anticoagulants in pregnancy: a review of indications and complications. Am Heart J 1972;83(3):301–5.
72. Ginsberg JS, Hirsh J. Use of antithrombotic agents during pregnancy. Chest 1998;114(Suppl 5):S524–30.
73. Ginsberg JS, Hirsh J. Use of antithrombotic agents during pregnancy. Chest 1992;102(Suppl 4):S385–90.
74. Ginsberg JS, Hirsh J. Use of antithrombotic agents during pregnancy. Chest 1995;108(Suppl 4):S305–11.
75. Greer IA. Thrombosis in pregnancy: maternal and fetal issues. Lancet 1999;353(9160):1258–65.
76. Ginsberg JS, Hirsh J. Optimum use of anticoagulants in pregnancy. Drugs 1988;36(4):505–12.
77. Hall JG, Pauli RM, Wilson KM. Maternal and fetal sequelae of anticoagulation during pregnancy. Am J Med 1980;68(1):122–40.
78. Stevenson RE, Burton OM, Ferlauto GJ, Taylor HA. Hazards of oral anticoagulants during pregnancy. JAMA 1980;243(15):1549–51.
79. Wellesley D, Moore I, Heard M, Keeton B. Two cases of warfarin embryopathy: a re-emergence of this condition? Br J Obstet Gynaecol 1998;105(7):805–6.
80. Vitale N, De Feo M, De Santo LS, Pollice A, Tedesco N, Cotrufo M. Dose-dependent fetal complications of warfarin in pregnant women with mechanical heart valves. J Am Coll Cardiol 1999;33(6):1637–41.
81. Ginsberg JS, Hirsh J. Use of anticoagulants during pregnancy. Chest 1989;95(Suppl 2):S156–60.
82. Iturbe-Alessio I, Fonseca MC, Mutchinik O, Santos MA, Zajarias A, Salazar E. Risks of anticoagulant therapy in pregnant women with artificial heart valves. N Engl J Med 1986;315(22):1390–3.
83. Kort HI, Cassel GA. An appraisal of warfarin therapy during pregnancy. S Afr Med J 1981;60(15):578–9.
84. Olwin JH, Koppel JL. Anticoagulant therapy during pregnancy. A new approach. Obstet Gynecol 1969;34(6):847–52.
85. Price PA, Williamson MK, Haba T, Dell RB, Jee WS. Excessive mineralization with growth plate closure in rats on chronic warfarin treatment. Proc Natl Acad Sci USA 1982;79(24):7734–8.
86. Bates SM, Ginsberg JS. Anticoagulants in pregnancy: fetal defects. London: Bailliere Tindall, 1997:479.
87. Chong MK, Harvey D, de Swiet M. Follow-up study of children whose mothers were treated with warfarin during pregnancy. Br J Obstet Gynaecol 1984;91(11):1070–3.

88. Ludwig H. Antikoagulantien in der Schwangerschaft und im Wochenbett. [Anticoagulants in pregnancy and puerperium.] Geburtshilfe Frauenheilkd 1970;30(4):337–47.
89. Orme ML, Lewis PJ, de Swiet M, Serlin MJ, Sibeon R, Baty JD, Breckenridge AM. May mothers given warfarin breast-feed their infants? BMJ 1977;1(6076):1564–5.
90. De Swiet M, Lewis PJ. Excretion of anticoagulants in human milk. N Engl J Med 1977;297(26):1471.
91. McKenna R, Cole ER, Vasan U. Is warfarin sodium contraindicated in the lactating mother? J Pediatr 1983;103(2):325–7.
92. Houwert-de Jong M, Gerards LJ, Tetteroo-Tempelman CA, de Wolff FA. May mothers taking acenocoumarol breast feed their infants? Eur J Clin Pharmacol 1981;21(1):61–4.
93. Fondevila CG, Meschengieser S, Blanco A, Penalva L, Lazzari MA. Effect of acenocoumarine on the breast-fed infant. Thromb Res 1989;56(1):29–36.
94. Eckstein HB, Jack B. Breast-feeding and anticoagulant therapy. Lancet 1970;1(7648):672–3.
95. Aithal GP, Day CP, Kesteven PJ, Daly AK. Association of polymorphisms in the cytochrome P450 CYP2C9 with warfarin dose requirement and risk of bleeding complications. Lancet 1999;353(9154):717–19.
96. Daly AK, Aithal GP. Genetic regulation of warfarin metabolism and response. Semin Vasc Med 2003;3(3):231–8.
97. Oldenburg J, Kriz K, Wuillemin WA, Maly FE, von Felten A, Siegemund A, Keeling DM, Baker P, Chu K, Konkle BA, Lammle B, Albert T; Study Group on Hereditary Warfarin Sensitivity. Genetic predisposition to bleeding during oral anticoagulant therapy: evidence for common founder mutations (FIXVal-10 and FIXThr-10) and an independent CpG hotspot mutation (FIXThr-10). Thromb Haemost 2001;85(3):454–7.
98. Visser LE, van Vliet M, van Schaik RH, Kasbergen AA, De Smet PA, Vulto AG, Hofman A, van Duijn CM, Stricker BH. The risk of overanticoagulation in patients with cytochrome P450 CYP2C9*2 or CYP2C9*3 alleles on acenocoumarol or phenprocoumon. Pharmacogenetics 2004;14(1):27–33.
99. Chu K, Wu SM, Stanley T, Stafford DW, High KA. A mutation in the propeptide of Factor IX leads to warfarin sensitivity by a novel mechanism. J Clin Invest 1996;98(7):1619–25.
100. Baker P, Clarke K, Giangrande P, Keeling D. Ala-10 mutations in the factor IX propeptide and haemorrhage in a patient treated with warfarin. Br J Haematol 2000;108(3):663.
101. Beyth RJ, Shorr RI. Epidemiology of adverse drug reactions in the elderly by drug class. Drugs Aging 1999;14(3):231–9.
102. Launbjerg J, Egeblad H, Heaf J, Nielsen NH, Fugleholm AM, Ladefoged K. Bleeding complications to oral anticoagulant therapy: multivariate analysis of 1010 treatment years in 551 outpatients. J Intern Med 1991;229(4):351–5.
103. Self TH, Straughn AB, Weisburst MR. Effect of hyperthyroidism on hypoprothrombinemic response to warfarin. Am J Hosp Pharm 1976;33(4):387–9.
104. Smith JK, Aljazairi A, Fuller SH. INR elevation associated with diarrhea in a patient receiving warfarin. Ann Pharmacother 1999;33(3):301–4.
105. Landefeld CS, Rosenblatt MW, Goldman L. Bleeding in outpatients treated with warfarin: relation to the prothrombin time and important remediable lesions. Am J Med 1989;87(2):153–9.
106. Watson RM, Pierson RN Jr. Effect of anticoagulant therapy upon aspirin-induced gastrointestinal bleeding. Circulation 1961;24:613–16.
107. Chesebro JH, Fuster V, Elveback LR, McGoon DC, Pluth JR, Puga FJ, Wallace RB, Danielson GK, Orszulak TA, Piehler JM, Schaff HV. Trial of combined warfarin plus dipyridamole or aspirin therapy in prosthetic heart valve replacement: danger of aspirin compared with dipyridamole. Am J Cardiol 1983;51(9):1537–41.
108. Boston Collaborative Drug Surveillance Program, Boston Universtiy Medical Center. Interaction between chloral hydrate and warfarin. N Engl J Med 1972;286(2):53–5.
109. Jahnchen E, Meinertz I, Gilfrich HJ. Interaction of allopurinol with phenprocoumon in man. Klin Wochenschr 1977;55(15):759–61.
110. Vesell ES, Passananti GT, Greene FE. Impairment of drug metabolism in man by allopurinol and nortriptyline. N Engl J Med 1970;283(27):1484–8.
111. Bruning PF. Personal communication, Antoni van Leeuwenhoekhuis. Het Nederlands Kanker Instituut, Amsterdam, 1983.
112. Udall JA. Human sources and absorption of vitamin K in relation to anticoagulation stability. JAMA 1965;194(2):127–9.
113. O'Reilly RA, Aggeler PM. Determinants of the response to oral anticoagulant drugs in man. Pharmacol Rev 1970;22(1):35–96.
114. Caraco Y, Chajek-Shaul T. The incidence and clinical significance of amiodarone and acenocoumarol interaction. Thromb Haemost 1989;62(3):906–8.
115. Hamer A, Peter T, Mandel WJ, Scheinman MM, Weiss D. The potentiation of warfarin anticoagulation by amiodarone. Circulation 1982;65(5):1025–9.
116. Martinowitz U, Rabinovich J, Goldfarb D, Many A, Bank H. Interaction between warfarin sodium and amiodarone. N Engl J Med 1981;304(11):671–2.
117. Watt AH, Stephens MR, Buss DC, Routledge PA. Amiodarone reduces plasma warfarin clearance in man. Br J Clin Pharmacol 1985;20(6):707–9.
118. Pyerele K, Kekki M. Decreased anticoagulant tolerance during methandrostenolone therapy. Scand J Clin Lab Invest 1963;15:367–74.
119. Ambre JJ, Fischer LJ. Effect of coadministration of aluminum and magnesium hydroxides on absorption of anticoagulants in man. Clin Pharmacol Ther 1973;14(2):231–7.
120. Green AE, Hort JF, Korn HE, Leach H. Potentiation of warfarin by azapropazone. BMJ 1977;1(6075):1532.
121. McElnay JC, D'Arcy PF. Interaction between azapropazone and warfarin. Experientia 1978;34(10):1320–1.
122. Rivier G, Khamashta MA, Hughes GR. Warfarin and azathioprine: a drug interaction does exist. Am J Med 1993;95(3):342.
123. Singleton JD, Conyers L. Warfarin and azathioprine: an important drug interaction. Am J Med 1992;92(2):217.
124. Woldtvedt BR, Cahoon CL, Bradley LA, Miller SJ. Possible increased anticoagulation effect of warfarin induced by azithromycin. Ann Pharmacother 1998;32(2):269–70.
125. Robinson DS, MacDonald MG. The effect of phenobarbital administration on the control of coagulation achieved during warfarin therapy in man. J Pharmacol Exp Ther 1966;153:250.
126. Levy G, O'Reilly RA, Aggeler PM, Keech GM. Parmacokinetic analysis of the effect of barbiturate on the anticoagulant action of warfarin in man. Clin Pharmacol Ther 1970;11(3):372–7.
127. Pyorala K, Ikkala E, Siltanen P. Benziodarone (Amplivix) and anticoagulant therapy. Acta Med Scand 1963;173:385–9.
128. Blum A, Seligmann H, Livneh A, Ezra D. Severe gastrointestinal bleeding induced by a probable hydroxycoumarin-bezafibrate interaction. Isr J Med Sci 1992;28(1):47–9.
129. Beringer TR. Warfarin potentiation with bezafibrate. Postgrad Med J 1997;73(864):657–8.
130. Denbow CE, Fraser HS. Clinically significant hemorrhage due to warfarin-carbamazepine interaction. South Med J 1990;83(8):981.

131. Hansen JM, Siersbaek-Nielsen K, Skovsted L. Carbamazepine-induced acceleration of diphenylhydantoin and warfarin metabolism in man. Clin Pharmacol Ther 1971;12(3):539–43.
132. Loeliger EA, Van der Esch B, Mattern MJ, Hemker HC. The biological disappearance rate of prothrombin, factors VII, IX and X from plasma in hypothyroidism, hyperthuroidism, and during fever. Thromb Diath Haemorrh 1964;10:267–77.
133. Berod T, Mathiot I. Probable interaction between cetirizine and acenocoumarol. Ann Pharmacother 1997;31(1):122.
134. Rymer W, Greenlaw CW. Hypoprothrombinemia associated with cefamandole. Drug Intell Clin Pharm 1980;14:780.
135. Parker SW, Baxter J, Beam TR Jr. Cefoperazone-induced coagulopathy. Lancet 1984;1(8384):1016.
136. Bechtold H, Andrassy K, Jahnchen E, Koderisch J, Koderisch H, Weilemann LS, Sonntag HG, Ritz E. Evidence for impaired hepatic vitamin K_1 metabolism in patients treated with N-methyl-thiotetrazole cephalosporins. Thromb Haemost 1984;51(3):358–61.
137. Udall JA. Warfarin interactions with chloral hydrate and glutethimide. Curr Ther Res Clin Exp 1975;17(1):67–74.
138. Christensen LK, Skovsted L. Inhibition of drug metabolism by chloramphenicol. Lancet 1969;2(7635):1397–9.
139. Magid E. Tolerance to anticoagulants during antibiotic therapy. Scand J Clin Lab Invest 1962;14:565.
140. Leone R, Ghiotto E, Conforti A, Velo G. Potential interaction between warfarin and ocular chloramphenicol. Ann Pharmacother 1999;33(1):114.
141. O'Reilly RA, Sahud MA, Aggeler PM. Impact of aspirin and chlorthalidone on the pharmacodynamics of oral anticoagulant drugs in man. Ann NY Acad Sci 1971;179:173–86.
142. Robinson DS, Benjamin DM, McCormack JJ. Interaction of warfarin and nonsystemic gastrointestinal drugs. Clin Pharmacol Ther 1971;12(3):491–5.
143. Meinertz T, Gilfrich HJ, Groth U, Jonen HG, Jahnchen E. Interruption of the enterohepatic circulation of phenprocoumon by cholestyramine. Clin Pharmacol Ther 1977;21(6):731–5.
144. Serlin MJ, Sibeon RG, Mossman S, Breckenridge AM, Williams JR, Atwood JL, Willoughby JM. Cimetidine: interaction with oral anticoagulants in man. Lancet 1979;2(8138):317–19.
145. Harenberg J, Zimmermann R, Staiger C, de Vries JX, Walter E, Weber E. Lack of effect of cimetidine on action of phenprocoumon. Eur J Clin Pharmacol 1982;23(4):365–7.
146. Toon S, Hopkins KJ, Garstang FM, Rowland M. Comparative effects of ranitidine and cimetidine on warfarin in man. Br J Clin Pharmacol 1986;21:P565.
147. Jolson HM, Tanner LA, Green L, Grasela TH Jr. Adverse reaction reporting of interaction between warfarin and fluoroquinolones. Arch Intern Med 1991;151(5):1003–4.
148. Costigan DC, Freedman MH, Ehrlich RM. Potentiation of oral anticoagulant effect by L-thyroxine. Clin Pediatr (Phila) 1984;23(3):172–4.
149. Raburn M. Hypoprothrombinemia induced by warfarin sodium and cisapride. Am J Health Syst Pharm 1997;54(3):320–1.
150. Grau E, Real E, Pastor E. Interaction between clarithromycin and oral anticoagulants. Ann Pharmacother 1996;30(12):1495–6.
151. Sanchez B, Muruzabal MJ, Peralta G, et al. Clarithromycin oral anticoagulants interaction: report of five cases. Clin Drug Invest 1997;13:220–2.
152. Oberg KC. Delayed elevation of international normalized ratio with concurrent clarithromycin and warfarin therapy. Pharmacotherapy 1998;18(2):386–91.
153. O'Reilly RA, Sahud MA, Robinson AJ. Studies on the interaction of warfarin and clofibrate in man. Thromb Diath Haemorrh 1972;27(2):309–18.
154. O'Donnell D. Antibiotic-induced potentiation of oral anticoagulant agents. Med J Aust 1989;150(3):163–4.
155. O'Reilly RA, Motley CH. Racemic warfarin and trimethoprim–sulfamethoxazole interaction in humans. Ann Intern Med 1979;91(1):34–6.
156. Tashima CK. Cyclophosphamide effect on coumarin anticoagulation. South Med J 1979;72(5):633–4.
157. Snyder DS. Interaction between cyclosporine and warfarin. Ann Intern Med 1988;108(2):311.
158. Meeks ML, Mahaffey KW, Katz MD. Danazol increases the anticoagulant effect of warfarin. Ann Pharmacother 1992;26(5):641–2.
159. Izzat MB, Yim AP, El-Zufari MH. A taste of Chinese medicine! Ann Thorac Surg 1998;66(3):941–2.
160. Mailloux AT, Gidal BE, Sorkness CA. Potential interaction between warfarin and dicloxacillin. Ann Pharmacother 1996;30(12):1402–7.
161. Serlin MJ, Mossman S, Sibeon RG, Tempero KF, Breckenridge AM. Interaction between diflunisal and warfarin. Clin Pharmacol Ther 1980;28(4):493–8.
162. O'Reilly RA. Interaction of sodium warfarin and disulfiram (antabuse) in man. Ann Intern Med 1973;78(1):73–6.
163. O'Reilly RA. Dynamic interaction between disulfiram and separated enantiomorphs of racemic warfarin. Clin Pharmacol Ther 1981;29(3):332–6.
164. Bartle WR. Possible warfarin–erythromycin interaction. Arch Intern Med 1980;140(7):985–7.
165. Grau E, Fontcuberta J, Felez J. Erythromycin-oral anticoagulants interaction. Arch Intern Med 1986;146(8):1639.
166. Bachmann K, Schwartz JI, Forney R Jr, Frogameni A, Jauregui LE. The effect of erythromycin on the disposition kinetics of warfarin. Pharmacology 1984;28(3):171–6.
167. Petrick RJ, Kronacher N, Alcena V. Interaction between warfarin and ethacrynic acid. JAMA 1975;231(8):843–4.
168. Ascah KJ, Rock GA, Wells PS. Interaction between fenofibrate and warfarin. Ann Pharmacother 1998;32(7–8):765–8.
169. Boeijinga JK, van de Broeke RN, Jochemsen R, Breimer DD, Hoogslag MA, Jeletich-Bastiaanse A. De invloed van floctafenine (Idalon) op antistollingsbehandeling met coumarinderivaten. [The effect of floctafenine (Idalon) on anticoagulant treatment with coumarin derivatives.] Ned Tijdschr Geneeskd 1981;125(47):1931–5.
170. Seaton TL, Celum CL, Black DJ. Possible potentiation of warfarin by fluconazole. DICP 1990;24(12):1177–8.
171. Baciewicz AM, Menke JJ, Bokar JA, Baud EB. Fluconazole–warfarin interaction. Ann Pharmacother 1994;28(9):1111.
172. Gericke KR. Possible interaction between warfarin and fluconazole. Pharmacotherapy 1993;13(5):508–9.
173. Brown MC. Multisite mucous membrane bleeding due to a possible interaction between warfarin and 5-fluorouracil. Pharmacotherapy 1997;17(3):631–3.
174. Dent LA, Orrock MW. Warfarin–fluoxetine and diazepam–fluoxetine interaction. Pharmacotherapy 1997; 17(1):170–2.
175. Marbet GA, Duckert F, Walter M, Six P, Airenne H. Interaction study between phenprocoumon and flurbiprofen. Curr Med Res Opin 1977;5(1):26–31.
176. Stricker BH, Delhez JL. Interactions between flurbiprofen and coumarins. BMJ (Clin Res Ed) 1982;285(6344):812–13.
177. Trilli LE, Kelley CL, Aspinall SL, Kroner BA. Potential interaction between warfarin and fluvastatin. Ann Pharmacother 1996;30(12):1399–402.
178. Laizure SC, Madlock L, Cyr M, Self T. Decreased hypoprothrombinemic effect of warfarin associated with furosemide. Ther Drug Monit 1997;19(3):361–3.

179. Janetzky K, Morreale AP. Probable interaction between warfarin and ginseng. Am J Health Syst Pharm 1997;54(6):692–3.
180. Koch-Weser J. Potentiation by glucagon of the hypoprothrombinemic action of warfarin. Ann Intern Med 1970;72(3):331–5.
181. Chatterjea JB, Salomon L. Antagonistic effect of A.C.T.H. and cortisone on the anticoagulant activity of ethyl biscoumacetate. BMJ 1954;4891:790–2.
182. Hellem AJ, Solem JH. The influence of ACTH on prothrombin-proconvertin values in blood during treatment with dicumarol and phenylindanedione. Acta Med Scand 1954;150(5):389–93.
183. MacDonald MG, Robinson DS, Sylwester D, Jaffe JJ. The effects of phenobarbital, chloral betaine, and glutethimide administration on warfarin plasma levels and hypoprothrombinemic responese in man. Clin Pharmacol Ther 1969;10(1):80–4.
184. Cullen SI, Catalano PM. Griseofulvin–warfarin antagonism. JAMA 1967;199(8):582–3.
185. Oakley DP, Lautch H. Haloperidol and anticoagulant treatment. Lancet 1963;41:1231.
186. Chan TY, Lui SF, Chung SY, Luk S, Critchley JA. Adverse interaction between warfarin and indomethacin. Drug Saf 1994;10(3):267–9.
187. Rosenthal AR, Self TH, Baker ED, Linden RA. Interaction of isoniazid and warfarin. JAMA 1977;238(20):2177.
188. Yeh J, Soo SC, Summerton C, Richardson C. Potentiation of action of warfarin by itraconazole. BMJ 1990;301(6753):669.
189. Smith AG. Potentiation of oral anticoagulants by ketoconazole. BMJ (Clin Res Ed) 1984;288(6412):188–9.
190. Ahmad S. Lovastatin. Warfarin interaction. Arch Intern Med 1990;150(11):2407.
191. Holmes EL. Experimental observations on flufenamic, mefenamic, and meclofenamic acids. IV. Toleration by normal human subjects. Ann Phys Med 1966;(Suppl):36–49.
192. Spiers AS, Mibashan RS. Letter: Increased warfarin requirement during mercaptopurine therapy: a new drug interaction. Lancet 1974;2(7874):221–2.
193. Self TH. Interaction of warfarin and aminosalicylic acid. JAMA 1973;223(11):1285.
194. Marinella MA. Mesalamine and warfarin therapy resulting in decreased warfarin effect. Ann Pharmacother 1998;32(7–8):841–2.
195. O'Reilly RA. The stereoselective interaction of warfarin and metronidazole in man. N Engl J Med 1976;295(7):354–7.
196. Watson PG, Lochan RG, Redding VJ. Drug interactions with coumarin derivative anticoagulants. BMJ (Clin Res Ed) 1982;285(6347):1045–6.
197. Ortin M, Olalla JI, Muruzabal MJ, Peralta FG, Gutierrez MA. Miconazole oral gel enhances acenocoumarol anticoagulant activity: a report of three cases. Ann Pharmacother 1999;33(2):175–7.
198. Lansdorp D, Bressers HP, Dekens-Konter JA, Meyboom RH. Potentiation of acenocoumarol during vaginal administration of miconazole. Br J Clin Pharmacol 1999;47(2):225–6.
199. Colquhoun MC, Daly M, Stewart P, Beeley L. Interaction between warfarin and miconazole oral gel. Lancet 1987;1(8534):695–6.
200. Marotel C, Cerisay D, Vasseur P, Rouvier B, Chabanne JP. Potentialisation des effets de l'acenocoumarol par le gel buccal de miconazole. [Potentiation of the effects of acenocoumarol by a buccal gel of miconazole.] Presse Méd 1986;15(33):1684–5.
201. O'Reilly RA, Goulart DA, Kunze KL, Neal J, Gibaldi M, Eddy AC, Trager WF. Mechanisms of the stereoselective interaction between miconazole and racemic warfarin in human subjects. Clin Pharmacol Ther 1992;51(6):656–67.
202. Qureshi GD, Reinders TP, Somori GJ, Evans HJ. Warfarin resistance with nafcillin therapy. Ann Intern Med 1984;100(4):527–9.
203. Taylor AT, Pritchard DC, Goldstein AO, Fletcher JL Jr. Continuation of warfarin–nafcillin interaction during dicloxacillin therapy. J Fam Pract 1994;39(2):182–5.
204. Hoffbrand BI. Interaction of nalidixic acid and warfarin. BMJ 1974;2(920):666.
205. Leor J, Levartowsky D, Sharon C. Interaction between nalidixic acid and warfarin. Ann Intern Med 1987;107(4):601.
206. Lee M, Schwartz RN, Sharifi R. Warfarin resistance and vitamin K. Ann Intern Med 1981;94(1):140–1.
207. Baciewicz AM, Ashar BH, Locke TW. Interaction of ofloxacin and warfarin. Ann Intern Med 1993;119(12):1223.
208. Ahmad S. Omeprazole–warfarin interaction. South Med J 1991;84(5):674–5.
209. de Teresa E, Vera A, Ortigosa J, Pulpon LA, Arus AP, de Artaza M. Interaction between anticoagulants and contraceptives: an unsuspected finding. BMJ 1979;2(6200):1260–1.
210. Monig H, Baese C, Heidemann HT, Ohnhaus EE, Schulte HM. Effect of oral contraceptive steroids on the pharmacokinetics of phenprocoumon. Br J Clin Pharmacol 1990;30(1):115–18.
211. Bagheri H, Bernhard NB, Montastruc JL. Potentiation of the acenocoumarol anticoagulant effect by acetaminophen. Ann Pharmacother 1999;33(4):506.
212. Hylek EM, Heiman H, Skates SJ, Sheehan MA, Singer DE. Acetaminophen and other risk factors for excessive warfarin anticoagulation. JAMA 1998;279(9):657–62.
213. Aggeler PM, O'Reilly RA, Leong L, Kowitz PE. Potentiation of anticoagulant effect of warfarin by phenylbutazone. N Engl J Med 1967;276(9):496–501.
214. Lewis RJ, Trager WF, Chan KK, Breckenridge A, Orme M, Roland M, Schary W. Warfarin. Stereochemical aspects of its metabolism and the interaction with phenylbutazone. J Clin Invest 1974;53(6):1607–17.
215. O'Reilly RA, Goulart DA. Comparative interaction of sulfinpyrazone and phenylbutazone with racemic warfarin: alteration in vivo of free fraction of plasma warfarin. J Pharmacol Exp Ther 1981;219(3):691–4.
216. Hansen JM, Siersbaek-Nielsen K, Kristensen M, Skovsted L, Christensen LK. Effect of diphenylhydantoin on the metabolism of dicoumarol in man. Acta Med Scand 1971;189(1–2):15–19.
217. Nappi JM. Warfarin and phenytoin interaction. Ann Intern Med 1979;90(5):852.
218. Levine M, Sheppard I. Biphasic interaction of phenytoin warfarin interaction. Postgrad Med J 1991;67:98.
219. Pan HY, Ng RP. The effect of Nootropil in a patient on warfarin. Eur J Clin Pharmacol 1983;24(5):711.
220. Rhodes RS, Rhodes PJ, Klein C, Sintek CD. A warfarin–piroxicam drug interaction. Drug Intell Clin Pharm 1985;19(7–8):556–8.
221. Trenque T, Choisy H, Germain ML. Pravastatin: interaction with oral anticoagulant? BMJ 1996;312(7035):886.
222. Jassal SV. Warfarin potentiated by proguanil. BMJ 1991;303(6805):789.
223. Kates RE, Yee YG, Kirsten EB. Interaction between warfarin and propafenone in healthy volunteer subjects. Clin Pharmacol Ther 1987;42(3):305–11.
224. Scott AK, Park BK, Breckenridge AM. Interaction between warfarin and propranolol. Br J Clin Pharmacol 1984;17(5):559–64.
225. Koch-Weser J. Quinidine-induced hypoprothrombinemic hemorrhage in patients on chronic warfarin therapy. Ann Intern Med 1968;68(3):511–17.

226. Trenk D, Mohrke W, Warth L, Jahnchen E. Determination of the interaction of 3S-hydroxy-10,11-dihydroquinidine on the pharmacokinetics and pharmacodynamics of warfarin. Arzneimittelforschung 1993;43(8):836–41.
227. Baciewicz AM, Morgan PJ. Ranitidine-warfarin interaction. Ann Intern Med 1990;112(1):76–7.
228. O'Reilly RA. Interaction of chronic daily warfarin therapy and rifampin. Ann Intern Med 1975;83(4):506–8.
229. O'Reilly RA. Interaction of sodium warfarin and rifampin. Studies in man. Ann Intern Med 1974;81(3):337–40.
230. Heimark LD, Gibaldi M, Trager WF, O'Reilly RA, Goulart DA. The mechanism of the warfarin–rifampin drug interaction in humans. Clin Pharmacol Ther 1987;42(4):388–94.
231. Knoell KR, Young TM, Cousins ES. Potential interaction involving warfarin and ritonavir. Ann Pharmacother 1998;32(12):1299–302.
232. Darlington MR. Hypoprothrombinemia during concomitant therapy with warfarin and saquinavir. Ann Pharmacother 1997;31(5):647.
233. Grau E, Perella M, Pastor E. Simvastatin–oral anticoagulant interaction. Lancet 1996;347(8998):405–6.
234. Risc IR. Bilateral subdural hematoma caused by simvastatin during warfarin treatment. Case report. Acta Neurol Scandinavica 1997;96:339.
235. O'Reilly RA. Spironolactone and warfarin interaction. Clin Pharmacol Ther 1980;27(2):198–201.
236. Braverman SE, Marino MT. Sucralfate—warfarin interaction. Drug Intell Clin Pharm 1988;22(11):913.
237. Mungall D, Talbert RL, Phillips C, Jaffe D, Ludden TM. Sucralfate and warfarin. Ann Intern Med 1983;98(4):557.
238. Michot F, Holt NF, Fontanilles F. Uber die Beeinflussung der gerinnungshemmenden Wirkung von Acenocoumarol durch Sulfinpyrazon. [The effect of sulfinpyrazone on the coagulation-inhibiting action of acenocoumarol.] Schweiz Med Wochenschr 1981; 111(8):255–60.
239. Nenci GG, Agnelli G, Berrettini M. Biphasic sulphinpyrazone–warfarin interaction. BMJ (Clin Res Ed) 1981;282(6273):1361–2.
240. O'Reilly RA. Phenylbutazone and sulfinpyrazone interaction with oral anticoagulant phenprocoumon. Arch Intern Med 1982;142(9):1634–7.
241. Toon S, Low LK, Gibaldi M, Trager WF, O'Reilly RA, Motley CH, Goulart DA. The warfarin–sulfinpyrazone interaction: stereochemical considerations. Clin Pharmacol Ther 1986;39(1):15–24.
242. Walter E, Staiger C, de Vries J, Zimmermann R, Weber E. Induction of drug metabolizing enzymes by sulfinpyrazone. Eur J Clin Pharmacol 1981;19(5):353–8.
243. Self TH, Evans W, Ferguson T. Interaction of sulfisoxazole and warfarin. Circulation 1975;52(3):528.
244. Sioris LJ, Weibert RT, Pentel PR. Potentiation of warfarin anticoagulation by sulfisoxazole. Arch Intern Med 1980;140(4):546–7.
245. Carter SA. Potential effect of sulindac on response of prothrombin-time to oral anticoagulants. Lancet 1979; 2(8144):698–9.
246. Loftin JP, Vesell ES. Interaction between sulindac and warfarin: different results in normal subjects and in an unusual patient with a potassium-losing renal tubular defect. J Clin Pharmacol 1979;19(11–12):733–42.
247. Lodwick R, McConkey B, Brown AM. Life threatening interaction between tamoxifen and warfarin. BMJ (Clin Res Ed) 1987;295(6606):1141.
248. Gustovic P, Baldin B, Tricoire MJ, Chichmanian RM. Interaction tamoxifene–acenocoumarol. Une interaction potentiellement dangereuse. [Tamoxifen–acenocoumarol interaction. A potentially dangerous interaction.] Therapie 1994;49(1):55–6.
249. Owens JC, Neely WB, Owen WR. Effect of sodium dextrothyroxine in patients receiving anticoagulants. N Engl J Med 1962;266:76–9.
250. Scher ML, Huntington NH, Vitillo JA. Potential interaction between tramadol and warfarin. Ann Pharmacother 1997;31(5):646–7.
251. Sabbe JR, Sims PJ, Sims MH. Tramadol-warfarin interaction. Pharmacotherapy 1998;18(4):871–3.
252. Spigset O. Reduced effect of warfarin caused by ubidecarenone. Lancet 1994;344(8933):1372–3.
253. Corrigan JJ Jr, Marcus FI. Coagulopathy associated with vitamin E ingestion. JAMA 1974;230(9):1300–1.
254. Morkunas A, Graeme K. Zafirlukast warfarin drug interaction with gastrointestinal bleeding. J Toxicol 1997;35:501.
255. Awni WM, Hussein Z, Granneman GR, Patterson KJ, Dube LM, Cavanaugh JH. Pharmacodynamic and stereoselective pharmacokinetic interactions between zileuton and warfarin in humans. Clin Pharmacokinet 1995;29(Suppl 2):67–76.
256. O'Reilly RA. Lack of effect of mealtime wine on the hypoprothrombinemia of oral anticoagulants. Am J Med Sci 1979;277(2):189–94.
257. Kukongviriyapan V, Senggunprai L, Prawan A, Gaysornsiri D, Kukongviriyapan U, Aiemsa-Ard J. Salivary caffeine metabolic ratio in alcohol-dependent subjects. Eur J Clin Pharmacol 2004;60(2):103–7.
258. Badger TM, Huang J, Ronis M, Lumpkin CK. Induction of cytochrome P450 2E1 during chronic ethanol exposure occurs via transcription of the CYP 2E1 gene when blood alcohol concentrations are high. Biochem Biophys Res Commun 1993;190(3):780–5.
259. Deykin D, Janson P, McMahon L. Ethanol potentiation of aspirin-induced prolongation of the bleeding time. N Engl J Med 1982;306(14):852–4.
260. Penning-van Beest FJ, van Meegen E, Rosendaal FR, Stricker BH. Drug interactions as a cause of overanticoagulation on phenprocoumon or acenocoumarol predominantly concern antibacterial drugs. Clin Pharmacol Ther 2001;69(6):451–7.
261. Ellis RJ, Mayo MS, Bodensteiner DM. Ciprofloxacin–warfarin coagulopathy: a case series. Am J Hematol 2000;63(1):28–31.
262. Leizorovicz A, Haugh MC, Chapuis FR, Samama MM, Boissel JP. Low molecular weight heparin in prevention of perioperative thrombosis. BMJ 1992;305(6859):913–20.
263. Nurmohamed MT, Rosendaal FR, Buller HR, Dekker E, Hommes DW, Vandenbroucke JP, Briet E. Low-molecular-weight heparin versus standard heparin in general and orthopaedic surgery: a meta-analysis. Lancet 1992;340(8812):152–6.
264. Rindone JP, Kelley CL, Jones WN, Garewal HS. Hypoprothrombinemic effect of warfarin not influenced by ciprofloxacin. Clin Pharm 1991;10(2):136–8.
265. Bianco TM, Bussey HI, Farnett LE, Linn WD, Roush MK, Wong YW. Potential warfarin–ciprofloxacin interaction in patients receiving long-term anticoagulation. Pharmacotherapy 1992;12(6):435–9.
266. Israel DS, Stotka J, Rock W, Sintek CD, Kamada AK, Klein C, Swaim WR, Pluhar RE, Toscano JP, Lettieri JT, Heller AH, Polk RE. Effect of ciprofloxacin on the pharmacokinetics and pharmacodynamics of warfarin. Clin Infect Dis 1996;22(2):251–6.
267. Toon S, Hopkins KJ, Garstang FM, Aarons L, Sedman A, Rowland M. Enoxacin-warfarin interaction: pharmacokinetic and stereochemical aspects. Clin Pharmacol Ther 1987;42(1):33–41.

268. Rocci ML Jr, Vlasses PH, Distlerath LM, Gregg MH, Wheeler SC, Zing W, Bjornsson TD. Norfloxacin does not alter warfarin's disposition or anticoagulant effect. J Clin Pharmacol 1990;30(8):728–32.
269. Verho M, Malerczyk V, Rosenkranz B, Grotsch H. Absence of interaction between ofloxacin and phenprocoumon. Curr Med Res Opin 1987;10(7):474–9.
270. Wyld P, Nimmo W, Millar W, Coles S, Abbott S. The lack of potentiation of the anticoagulant effect of warfarin when administered concurrently with temafloxacin, 1991.
271. Gadisseur AP, Van Der Meer FJ, Rosendaal FR. Sustained intake of paracetamol (acetaminophen) during oral anticoagulant therapy with coumarins does not cause clinically important INR changes: a randomized double-blind clinical trial. J Thromb Haemost 2003;1(4):714–17.
272. Schulman S. Inhibition of warfarin activity by ribavirin. Ann Pharmacother 2002;36(1):72–4.
273. Llibre JM, Romeu J, Lopez E, Sirera G. Severe interaction between ritonavir and acenocoumarol. Ann Pharmacother 2002;36(4):621–3.
274. Leizorovicz A, Simonneau G, Decousus H, Boissel JP. Comparison of efficacy and safety of low molecular weight heparins and unfractionated heparin in initial treatment of deep venous thrombosis: a meta-analysis. BMJ 1994;309(6950):299–304.
275. Ramanathan M. Warfarin—topical salicylate interactions: case reports. Med J Malaysia 1995;50(3):278–9.
276. Grant P. Warfarin and cranberry juice: an interaction? J Heart Valve Dis 2004;13(1):25–6.
277. Suvarna R, Pirmohamed M, Henderson L. Possible interaction between warfarin and cranberry juice. BMJ 2003;327(7429):1454.
278. Isele H. Todliche Blutung unter Warfarin plus Preiselbeersaft. Liegt's an der Salizylsaure? [Fatal bleeding under warfarin plus cranberry juice. Is it due to salicylic acid?] MMW Fortschr Med 2004;146(11):13.
279. Bachmann K, Shapiro R, Fulton R, Carroll FT, Sullivan TJ. Smoking and warfarin disposition. Clin Pharmacol Ther 1979;25(3):309–15.
280. Weiner B, Faraci PA, Fayad R, Swanson L. Warfarin dosage following prosthetic valve replacement: effect of smoking history. Drug Intell Clin Pharm 1984; 18(11):904–6.
281. Ansell JE, Buttaro ML, Thomas OV, Knowlton CH. Consensus guidelines for coordinated outpatient oral anticoagulation therapy management. Anticoagulation Guidelines Task Force. Ann Pharmacother 1997;31(5):604–15.

COX-2 inhibitors

See also Individual agents

General Information

The cyclo-oxygenase (COX) that is responsible for prostaglandin synthesis exists in two isoforms, COX-1 and COX-2, which differ in their structure, regulation, expression, and function. COX-1 is expressed normally in a constant amount in almost all body tissues and produces prostaglandins important for the maintenance of normal homeostasis. In particular, among other important functions, they help to protect the gastrointestinal mucosa against ulceration and regulate renal function and platelet activity. COX-1 appears to be largely unaffected by inflammatory stimuli. In contrast, the COX-2 isoform is constitutively expressed only in the brain, in bone (associated with osteoblast activity), in the female reproductive tract (associated with both the ovulatory cycle and implantation of fertilized ova), and in the kidney, where it may play an important role in regulating renal function. In many other cells COX-2 is expressed at very low levels or is undetectable, but it is readily induced by inflammatory cytokines, mitogens, and endotoxins. Therefore, prostaglandins generated by COX-2 mediate pain and inflammation in many tissues and probably also have a role in renal, brain, and reproductive physiology, and in tissue repair (1–4).

Traditional NSAIDs inhibit both COX-1 and COX-2, providing benefit at sites of inflammation, but at the cost of potential adverse effects related to COX-1 inhibition, particularly in areas such as the gastrointestinal mucosa, platelets, and the kidney. The development of a drug that inhibits only COX-2 would offer the promise of relieving pain and inflammation without some, if not all, of these adverse effects. However, the concept that selective inhibition of COX-2 is only a positive event and inhibition of COX-1 a bad one may be simplistic, as it is flawed by many experimental data that have also implicated COX-2 as an integral component in the maintenance of physiological homeostasis (3). In particular, COX-2 may reduce inflammation by generating anti-inflammatory prostanoids (5); COX-2, like COX-1, may be present in normal gastric mucosa (6,7) and can play a physiological role there in defense mechanisms (8,9), and there is evidence that prostaglandins derived from COX-2 may be important in the healing of gastric ulcers (9–12). Furthermore, COX-2 inhibition alone may be insufficient to resolve inflammation and pain (13), suggesting that COX-1 inhibition may play a role in reducing inflammation as well (14). Although the relevance of these experimental observations to the possible beneficial role of COX-2 activity is uncertain, they cannot be simply dismissed.

Nearly all of the traditional NSAIDs are predominantly COX-1-selective. In fact, only two of them, meloxicam and nimesulide (1,2), have been shown to have some COX-2 selectivity in humans. Two other NSAIDs, etodolac and nabumetone, may be COX-2 preferential inhibitors, but the evidence is less convincing than for meloxicam or nimesulide. Unfortunately, despite their wide use, clinical and epidemiological evidence that supports the claim of better tolerability of these preferential inhibitors with respect to other NSAIDs, is scanty and even controversial (1,4). Furthermore, for both meloxicam and nimesulide there are data consistent with reduced COX-2 selectivity at high doses, those usually used in clinical practice. These considerations have prompted research for more selective COX-2 inhibitors, and three compounds, celecoxib, parecoxib, and rofecoxib, have become available. These compounds are much more selective than previous preferential inhibitors and they have no effect on COX-1 (COX-1 sparing drugs) over the whole range of doses used and concentrations achieved in clinical use. In particular, they have been shown in humans to spare gastric COX-1 to a much greater extent than traditional NSAIDs.

Is there convincing evidence that COX-2-selective NSAIDs offer a distinct therapeutic advantage over non-selective ones? To prove the usefulness of these compounds, clinical studies should show:

- whether the COX-2 selective inhibitors are as effective as older NSAIDs in the relief of pain and/or inflammation;
- whether in the effective dosage range there is evidence of less damage to the mucosa of the upper gastrointestinal tract than with conventional NSAIDs;
- whether there are any effects on platelet in effective doses;
- whether unexpected adverse drug reactions compromise the safety of these compounds.

As far as the last of these criteria is concerned, the finding that rofecoxib increases the risk of cardiovascular disease (heart attacks and strokes) during long-term therapy has led to a reappraisal of the role of the COX-2 inhibitors. Furthermore, both rofecoxib and valdecoxib have been withdrawn by their manufacturers, the former because of its adverse cardiovascular effects and the latter because of an increased risk of cardiovascular events after coronary artery bypass surgery and reports of potentially fatal skin reactions.

Clinical studies

Both celecoxib and rofecoxib have been evaluated in large randomized trials lasting from weeks to 1 year, for the relief of the signs and symptoms of osteoarthritis or rheumatoid arthritis in adults (1,15–21). In all of these studies both compounds have been shown to be more effective than placebo and at least as effective as traditional NSAIDs (that is ibuprofen, diclofenac, nabumetone, naproxen). However, there is less information about their efficacy as analgesics. A few randomized, double-blind trials have shown that both compounds are more effective than placebo; rofecoxib was as effective as non-selective NSAIDs (ibuprofen, naproxen) in relieving the pain of osteoarthritis or after dental surgery, but celecoxib was less effective (22–26). Rofecoxib was also analgesic in patients with primary dysmenorrhea (27). However, there are no published data on the usefulness of COX-2-selective NSAIDs in other types of acute pain, such as that related to acute gout, migraine, cancer, or biliary or ureteric colic.

General adverse effects

Although the scientific literature has been flooded by articles and reviews on the use of selective COX-2 inhibitors (coxibs), the safe prescribing and use of these compounds is controversial (28–31).

COX-2 selectivity may be a double-edged sword. Because the cardiovascular risk outweighs the gastrointestinal risk in adults with rheumatoid arthritis or osteoarthritis, the harm would outweigh the benefits in most clinical settings. This means that the total number of serious adverse events would be increased by COX-2-selective NSAIDs compared with non-selective NSAIDs. COX-2 selectivity, which is an appealing theoretical concept, might be a clinical failure (30).

Much information on celecoxib and rofecoxib has come from two large pivotal randomized clinical trials, the Celecoxib Long-term Arthritis Safety Study (CLASS) and Vioxx Gastrointestinal Outcomes Research (VIGOR) studies, in which the efficacy and safety of the two coxibs and various non-selective NSAIDs were compared (32,33).

Summary

The COX-2-selective inhibitors are as efficacious as traditional NSAIDs in treating inflammation and pain due to osteoarticular diseases. However, there are questions to be addressed before COX-2-selective inhibitors can be considered to be definitely safer than traditional NSAIDs (4). Among these questions the most important relate to the possibility that COX-2 inhibitors may cause complicated ulceration in some subgroup of patients and may retard ulcer healing in others. Therefore, whether the COX-2 inhibitors in place of non-selective NSAIDs will prove to be cost-effective by reducing ulcer-related morbidity remains to be demonstrated. Moreover, it is likely that such drugs can cause the same renal problems as traditional NSAIDs do. Finally, the effect of COX-2 inhibitors on the incidence of vascular disease will need strict scrutiny, since vascular disease is a commoner cause of death than ulcer perforation or bleeding and since some of them clearly increase the long-term risk of heart attacks and strokes. Only their continuing use and postmarketing surveillance studies will demonstrate their strengths and weaknesses with respect to non-selective NSAIDs.

Organs and Systems

Cardiovascular

Prothrombotic effects

COX-2 inhibitors inhibit the synthesis of prostacyclin in the vascular wall but not platelet thromboxane production. They could therefore theoretically increase the risk of cardiovascular events by shifting the hemostatic balance toward a prothrombotic state. However, it is not clear that theory has much impact on reality.

Information about this topic comes from the two large studies, CLASS and VIGOR, from a pooled cardiovascular safety analysis using individual patient data derived from all rofecoxib phase IIb to V trials conducted by the manufacturer that lasted at least 2 weeks, and from the adverse events reporting system in the USA (34). As a result of these and other studies the COX-2 inhibitors, rofecoxib and valdecoxib, have been voluntarily withdrawn from the market by their manufacturers, and other COX-2 inhibitors are under scrutiny.

In VIGOR, rofecoxib 50 mg/day was associated with a higher rate of non-fatal myocardial infarction (0.4%) than the non-selective COX-2 inhibitor naproxen 500 mg bd (0.1%) (RR = 0.2; CI = 0.1, 0.7) (33). In CLASS there was no difference in the rates of myocardial infarction in patients taking celecoxib (0.5%) and those taking ibuprofen or diclofenac (0.4%). However, the protocols of the two studies differed substantially with respect to the use of aspirin. In VIGOR, the patients were not allowed to take aspirin or any other antiplatelet drug, while in

CLASS one-fifth of the patients took aspirin. A re-analysis of CLASS for cardiovascular thromboembolic events, including myocardial infarction, stroke, cardiovascular deaths, and peripheral events, showed no significant increase with celecoxib versus NSAIDs (35).

The results of VIGOR might be explained by a significant prothrombotic effect of rofecoxib and/or an antithrombotic effect of naproxen, which may have a significant antiplatelet effect. To clarify this, the annualized myocardial infarction rates in both VIGOR and CLASS were compared with those found in placebo-treated patients with similar cardiac risk factors enrolled in three meta-analyses of four aspirin primary prevention trials (34,36). The analysis showed 0.24 and 0.30% increases over placebo in cardiovascular events for rofecoxib and celecoxib respectively, suggesting a prothrombotic potential of both COX-2 inhibitors. However, these results have been heavily criticized (37–43), because of many potential pitfalls in the comparisons of patient populations in different trials. The results from a recently reported pooled analysis of individual patient data combined across rofecoxib phase IIb to phase V trials seem to be more reliable (44). Cardiovascular events were assessed across 23 studies. Comparisons were made between patients taking rofecoxib and those taking placebo, naproxen, or other non-selective NSAIDs (diclofenac, ibuprofen, and nabumetone). The major outcome measure was the combined end-point used by the Anti-platelet Trialist Collaboration, which includes cardiovascular death, hemorrhagic death, death of unknown cause, non-fatal myocardial infarction, and non-fatal stroke. More than 28 000 patients, representing more than 14 000 patient-years at risk, were analysed. The relative risk for an end-point was 0.84 (95% CI = 0.51, 1.38) when comparing rofecoxib with placebo; 0.79 (95% CI = 0.40, 1.55) when comparing rofecoxib with non-selective NSAIDs; and 1.69 (95% CI = 1.07, 2.69) when comparing rofecoxib with naproxen. These data provide no evidence for an excess of cardiovascular events for rofecoxib relative to either placebo or the non-selective NSAIDs that were studied. Instead, the difference between rofecoxib and naproxen showed that naproxen was associated with a reduced risk of cardiovascular events.

The cardiovascular results in VIGOR may have occurred simply by chance, given the low number of events, or because naproxen may have a cardioprotective effect similar to that of aspirin, or because rofecoxib 50 mg/day could have prothrombotic effects, especially in the absence of concomitant COX-1 inhibition in patients at increased risk of cardiovascular thromboembolic events. Because there was no untreated group in VIGOR, we do not know whether this finding suggests a protective effect of naproxen or a harmful effect of rofecoxib. All three explanations are plausible, and they are not mutually exclusive.

It has been suggested that the increase in thrombotic cardiovascular events in rofecoxib-treated patients probably represents the antiplatelet effect of naproxen (34,45,46). Naproxen has a long pharmacodynamic half-life and inhibits platelet aggregation by 88% for up to 8 hours (47).

In VIGOR (30,33), the incidence of confirmed thrombotic cardiovascular events was 0.6% higher with rofecoxib than with naproxen (RR = 2.4; 95% CI = 3.9, 4.0).

Some data may help to answer the important question of whether the relative difference in the incidence of myocardial infarction in VIGOR was due to a harmful effect of rofecoxib or a beneficial effect of naproxen. Although contrasting data have been published (48), the hypothesis that naproxen has a cardioprotective effect has gained wider support (49). Only one of the four most recently published studies negated a potential cardioprotective effect of naproxen.

However, an analysis of FDA data suggested an increase in serious cardiac events with celecoxib (30). The incidence of serious cardiac adverse events (myocardial infarction, combined anginal events, and atrial dysrhythmias) was 0.6% higher with celecoxib than with other NSAIDs (RR = 1.55; CI = 1.04, 2.30). The reasons for these inconsistencies are not clear.

In an 11-year observational study in new users of non-selective, non-aspirin NSAIDs ($n = 181\ 441$) and an equal number of non-users there was no evidence of a protective effect of naproxen (50). During 532 634 person-years of follow-up there were 6382 cases of serious coronary heart disease (11.9 per 1000 person-years). Multivariate-adjusted rate ratios for current and former use of non-aspirin NSAIDs were 1.05 (95% CI = 0.97, 1.14) and 1.02 (0.97, 1.08) respectively. Rate ratios for ibuprofen, naproxen, and other NSAIDs were 1.15 (1.02, 1.28), 0.95 (0.82, 1.09), and 1.03 (0.92, 1.16) respectively. There was no protection in long-term users with uninterrupted use; the rate ratio among current users with more than 60 days of continuous use was 1.05 (0.91, 1.21). When naproxen was directly compared with ibuprofen, the rate ratio in current users was 0.83 (0.69, 0.98). This study therefore seems to have shown no cardioprotective effect of naproxen. However, the study had a number of important limitations, including: lack of information about some important confounders (smoking, obesity), possible exposure misclassification, and lack of information about over-the-counter use of aspirin.

Opposite evidence has emerged from three case-control studies from the USA, Canada, and the UK, which showed that the rates of myocardial infarction in patients taking naproxen were lower than in patients not taking any NSAIDs (51,52) and those taking other NSAIDs (53).

In the first study, 4425 patients hospitalized with acute myocardial infarction who used NSAIDs were compared with 17 700 controls in a large health-care database in the USA (51). Multivariate models were constructed to control for potential confounders. A quarter of the cases and controls had also filled a prescription for an NSAID in the 6 months before the study. Overall, the NSAID users had the same risk of acute myocardial infarction as non-users, but naproxen users had a significantly lower risk of acute myocardial infarction compared with those who were not taking NSAIDs (adjusted OR = 0.84; 95% CI = 0.72, 0.98). The cardioprotective effect of naproxen was very modest compared with aspirin (a 44% reduction in the risk of acute myocardial infarction in the Physician Health Study (54)).

The second study was a case-control study sponsored by Merck & Co (the manufacturers of celecoxib), in which the risk of acute thromboembolic cardiovascular events among 16 937 patients aged 40–75 years with rheumatoid arthritis using naproxen was examined using the British General Practice Research Database (52). Each patient with a first thromboembolic event (n = 809: 435 myocardial infarctions, 347 strokes, 27 sudden deaths) was matched with four controls. The results suggested that patients with rheumatoid arthritis who currently use naproxen have a significantly lower risk of thromboembolic events relative to those who have not used naproxen in the past year (RR = 0.61; 0.39, 0.94). However, the risk was not lower with previous use of naproxen, suggesting that any effect of naproxen is likely to be short-lived. Moreover, the significantly lower risk of myocardial infarction with current naproxen was not found when myocardial infractions were analysed separately (RR = 0.57; 0.3, 1.06). There was no protective effect for thromboembolic events with current use of non-naproxen NSAIDs.

The third study was also sponsored by Merck & Co and was designed to examine the association between the use of naproxen and other non-selective NSAIDs and hospitalization for acute myocardial infarction (53). In a database of 14 163 patients aged 65 years or older who were hospitalized for acute myocardial infarction and an equal number of age-matched controls, concurrent exposure to naproxen had a protective effect against myocardial infarction compared with the other non-selective non-aspirin NSAIDs (RR = 0.79; CI = 0.63, 0.99). This effect was present only with concurrent naproxen exposure and was stronger in long-term users. However, this study also had several limitations: some important risk factors, such as smoking and obesity, could not be assessed, patients who died of myocardial infarction before reaching the hospital were not included, and there was uncertainty about concurrent use of over-the-counter drugs, especially aspirin.

In conclusion, although these three studies suggest that patients who take naproxen have a lower incidence of myocardial infarction than those who take other NSAIDs or who do not take NSAIDs, the data do not provide definitive evidence that naproxen is cardioprotective. The data therefore raise a cautionary flag about the risk of severe cardiovascular events with COX-2 inhibitors and again call for more studies.

Hypertension

The shift in hemostatic balance toward a prothrombotic state might not be the only mechanism by which COX-2 inhibitors could increase the risk of cardiovascular adverse effects. In fact, non-selective NSAIDs can raise blood pressure and antagonize the hypotensive effect of antihypertensive medications to an extent that may increase hypertension-related morbidity (55,56). The problem is clinically relevant, as arthritis and hypertension are common co-morbid conditions in elderly people, requiring concurrent therapy.

Information on the effect of COX-2-selective inhibitors on arterial blood pressure is scanty. In VIGOR, more patients developed hypertension with rofecoxib than naproxen. For rofecoxib, the mean increase in blood pressure was 4.6/1.7 mmHg compared with a 1.0/0.1 mmHg increase with naproxen (34). Previous work has shown that a 2 mmHg reduction in diastolic blood pressure can result in about a 40% reduction in the rate of stroke and a 25% reduction in the rate of myocardial infarction (57). The effect of celecoxib on blood pressure was evaluated in a post hoc analysis using the safety database generated during the celecoxib clinical development program in more than 13 000 subjects (58). The incidence of hypertension after celecoxib was greater than that after placebo but similar to that after non-selective NSAIDs. Hypertension and exacerbation of pre-existing hypertension occurred, respectively, in 0.8 and 0.6% of patients. Furthermore, there was no evidence of interactions between celecoxib and other antihypertensive drugs.

The safety profiles of celecoxib (200 mg/day) and rofecoxib (25 mg/day) have recently been compared in a 6-week, randomized, parallel-group, double-blind trial in 810 patients with osteoarthritis aged 65 years or over taking antihypertensive drugs (59). The primary endpoints were edema and changes in systolic and diastolic blood pressures, measured at baseline and after 1, 2, and 6 weeks. Systolic blood pressure rose significantly in 17% of rofecoxib-treated patients (n = 399) compared with 11% of celecoxib-treated patients (n = 411), a statistically significant difference, at any time in the study. Diastolic blood pressure rose in 2.3% of rofecoxib-treated patients compared with 1.5% of celecoxib-treated patients, a non-significant difference. At week 6, the change from baseline in mean systolic blood pressure was +2.6 mmHg for rofecoxib compared with –0.5 mmHg for celecoxib, a highly significant difference. Nearly twice as many rofecoxib-treated than celecoxib-treated patients had edema. Despite some limitations, this study provides some evidence that COX-2-selective inhibitors may differ in their ability to alter arterial blood pressure.

Cardiac dysrhythmias

There have been reports of celecoxib-associated torsade de pointes in three patients who had never had any complaints before celecoxib administration; the dysrhythmia did not recur after the drug was withdrawn (60). However, all three patients had cardiac abnormalities that might have predisposed them to the development of torsade de pointes, and the follow-up period was too short to evaluate possible spontaneous recurrence. The hypothesis that celecoxib is dysrhythmogenic requires confirmation.

Respiratory

Most people tolerate aspirin well, but not patients with asthma, of whom there is a subgroup in whom aspirin precipitates asthmatic attacks (61,62). This is a distinct clinical syndrome, called aspirin-induced asthma, which affects about 10% of adults with asthma (63). Aspirin-induced asthma is usually accompanied by naso-ocular symptoms and can be triggered not only by aspirin, but by several NSAIDs, a fact that makes immunological cross-reactivity most unlikely. The propensity of an NSAID to precipitate an attack of asthma is probably related to inhibition of COX (63). There is evidence that potent inhibitors of COX-1 (such as ibuprofen, indometacin, and naproxen) are more likely to precipitate bronchoconstriction than NSAIDs that inhibit COX-2 preferentially (such as meloxicam and nimesulide) (64,65). A widely accepted hypothesis is that in patients with asthma and aspirin intolerance, NSAID-induced COX inhibition results in increased products from the 5-lipoxygenase pathway, the leukotrienes, which are both potent bronchoconstrictors and also inducers of mucous hypersecretion and airway edema. The leukotrienes implicated in aspirin intolerance are cysteinyl leukotrienes (61,63), but leukotriene release is probably not the only pathogenic mechanism.

The hypothesis that in aspirin-induced asthma the attacks are triggered by inhibition of COX-1 and not COX-2 has been tested in three small studies, two of which were double-blind and placebo-controlled (66–68). In the first study (66) 12 patients with aspirin-induced asthma were challenged with increasing doses of rofecoxib (1.25–25 mg/day for 5 days); no patients had any adverse symptoms, and biochemical markers that reflect intolerance to aspirin in asthma (urinary leukotriene E4 and 9α-11β-PGF-2) were unchanged.

In the second study, 60 aspirin-sensitive asthmatics were challenged with oral rofecoxib (12.5 and 25 mg/day for 2 days) (67). There were no signs or symptoms of asthma in any patient and no reductions in FEV_1.

In the third study, 27 patients with stable chronic asthma in whom inhalation of lysine aspirin caused a 20% fall in FEV_1 were challenged with increasing doses of oral celecoxib (from 10 to 200 mg/day); they do not develop bronchoconstriction or other extrapulmonary reactions (68).

So, is the safety of COX-2 inhibitors in patients with aspirin-induced asthma sufficiently well documented? Avoidance of NSAIDs is crucial in patients with asthma who have aspirin sensitivity, and hitherto two alternative analgesic options have been available: paracetamol and non-acetylated salicylates. Paracetamol is a generally safe substitute; however, it is a weak COX inhibitor and, albeit very rarely, patients who are sensitive to aspirin have an adverse reaction to high-dose paracetamol (69). Choline magnesium salicylate and salicylic acid are also weak COX inhibitors and should therefore be used with care in these patients. The results of the above-mentioned studies suggest that rofecoxib and celecoxib can be taken safely by patients with aspirin-induced asthma. However, this conclusion must be treated with caution, as only a few patients were studied and this does not exclude COX-2 inhibitors from participating in other types of reactions, including immune recognition after prior treatment.

Nervous system

Aseptic meningitis is a rare complication of NSAID therapy. Five serious cases of aseptic meningitis associated with rofecoxib have been reported (70).

- A 55-year-old woman who had taken rofecoxib for 1 month reported numbness and tingling on the left side of the tongue and left hand (71). The association between paresthesia and rofecoxib was supported by the time-course of the reaction and resolution after withdrawal.

Because this patient was using other medications (paroxetine, zolpidem, and sumatriptan), which can have a similar effect, this report requires confirmation.

Hematologic

Platelets have only the COX-1 isoform for generating thromboxane to precipitate platelet aggregation. Therefore, selective COX-2 inhibitors have no effect on platelet aggregation or bleeding time (3,72). On the other hand, COX-2 plays a role in the production of endothelial PGI2. In vitro studies have shown that COX-2 expression is up-regulated in endothelial cells by laminar shear stress (73). Furthermore, selective COX-2 inhibitors reduce systemic PGI-2 production in healthy volunteers (74). The clinical implications of these observations are unknown. In theory, COX-2 selective NSAIDs might increase the risk of thromboembolic cardiovascular events because of preferential inhibition of endothelial prostacyclin synthesis without corresponding inhibition of platelet thromboxane synthesis, but no reliable data are available on the occurrence of cardiovascular events in patients treated with COX-2 selective or non-selective NSAIDs.

Gastrointestinal

Gastric damage

Evidence that the COX-2 selective agents cause less damage to the gastrointestinal mucosa than traditional NSAIDs is still limited. Gastrointestinal tolerability has been evaluated by measuring the frequency and severity of gastrointestinal adverse effects during randomized comparative efficacy trials, by performing microbleeding or endoscopic studies, and by evaluating the incidence of severe ulcer complications. Evidence from efficacy trials suggests an incidence of unwanted gastrointestinal effects (dyspepsia, epigastric abdominal pain, nausea, or diarrhea) similar to that caused by the traditional NSAIDs (1,15–17,20,75). The withdrawal rate from clinical trials because of unwanted effects (gastrointestinal or as a whole) was also similar, the only exception being one study in which fewer patients with rheumatoid arthritis stopped taking celecoxib than stopped taking diclofenac (16). However, the clinical importance of the frequency and severity of symptoms is uncertain. In fact, it is well known that symptoms do not necessarily predict the presence of mucosal damage, and it is still unclear if patients who have dyspeptic symptoms associated with NSAIDs are at greater or lesser risk of serious gastrointestinal complications (SEDA-15, 92) (SEDA-17, 103), the crucial question in evaluating these drugs.

In endoscopic comparisons of the new compounds with placebo or older NSAIDs, in both healthy volunteers and patients with rheumatoid arthritis or osteoarthritis, endoscopically observed lesions (erosions, ulcers) in the stomach and duodenum were undoubtedly fewer with the two COX-2-selective compounds than with non-selective NSAIDs (16,75–78) and were similar to those found with placebo (1).

However, the clinical significance of endoscopically detected erosions and ulcers is debatable (SEDA-14, 79) (SEDA-20, 97), as there is much controversy about whether endoscopic ulcers are surrogates for clinical outcomes such as perforation, obstruction, and gastrointestinal bleeding (78). Thus, although endoscopic studies are an important step in the evaluation of COX-2-selective inhibitors, large-scale, prospective, randomized outcome studies are necessary before we can definitively determine if these drugs will indeed represent significantly safer alternatives to the older NSAIDs. Unfortunately, these prospective comparative complication trials are difficult to perform, as the absolute rate of serious gastrointestinal complications (perforation, obstruction, and bleeding) is low (about 2% per year) (78) and so a large number of patients must be studied.

Suggestions for improved gastrointestinal safety of COX-2-selective inhibitors have come from two studies, which addressed the problem of sample size by pooling published and unpublished randomized, double-blind trials of varying design and duration, comparing celecoxib, rofecoxib, non-selective NSAIDs (diclofenac, ibuprofen, nabumetone), and placebo in patients with osteoarthritis and/or rheumatoid arthritis.

In the first study the results of eight studies were pooled (79). The sample size of 5435 patients was large enough to detect even small differences in rates of complicated ulcers (perforation, symptomatic ulcers, and bleeding ulcers). Over 12 months complicated ulcers occurred at a rate of 1.33 per 100 patient-years with rofecoxib and 2.60 per 100 patient-years with non-selective NSAIDs. The analysis of confirmed upper gastrointestinal perforations, symptomatic ulcers, and upper gastrointestinal bleeding showed a relative risk (RR) with rofecoxib versus NSAIDs of 0.51 (95% CI = 0.26, 1.00). The difference between rofecoxib and the usual NSAIDs in the incidence of perforation, symptomatic ulcers, and bleeding ulcers became statistically significant as early as 6 weeks and remained so up to 12 months. However, this study has some limitations: first, it was not a prospective analysis or a properly conducted meta-analysis; secondly, there were only enough patient-years of exposure to compare rofecoxib with pooled traditional NSAIDs rather than individual drugs; thirdly, the confidence intervals were wide and compatible with no difference between the two treatment groups; fourthly, the time to exposure with any selective drug or placebo was too short to give a good prediction of actual complication rates with typical use.

In the second analysis, data from 14 studies of the efficacy of celecoxib in osteoarthritis or rheumatoid arthritis in 11 007 patients were pooled (80,81). Gastrointestinal complications (bleeding, obstruction, or perforation) occurred in 0.2% of the patients per year of exposure to celecoxib and in 1.7% per year of exposure to traditional NSAIDs. The absolute risk reduction was 1.5% (CI = 0.4, 2.6). This study, too, had some limitations. In fact, ulcer complication was not the specified end-point of the studies that were pooled, and about 15% of celecoxib-treated patients took a dose below that indicated for arthritis.

Assuming that a COX-2-selective inhibitor will prevent complicated ulcers in 50% of patients, it has been calculated that the NNT for avoiding one complicated ulcer each year in low-risk patients with rheumatoid arthritis (that is with a 0.4% risk of ulcer complications) is 500. On the other hand, in patients at higher risk (that is a 5% risk for ulcer complications) the NNT is 40 (82). It is therefore of paramount importance that studies currently under way confirm the same benefit from COX-2-selective agents in patients with a high risk of ulcer complications (that is aged 75 years or older, with a prior history of ulcer and gastrointestinal tract bleeding, taking low-dose aspirin for cardiovascular disease).

Two large trials have addressed the efficacy of COX-2 selective inhibitors and the associated risk of gastrointestinal complications: the CLASS and the VIGOR trial (32,33).

The CLASS consisted of two separate studies, in which celecoxib was compared with ibuprofen and diclofenac; the results obtained from the two traditional NSAIDs were pooled for analysis. Overall, 3987 patients with osteoarthritis and rheumatoid arthritis took celecoxib (400 mg bd), 1985 patients took ibuprofen (800 mg tds), and 1996 took diclofenac (75 mg bd). The study lasted 13 months, but only the data from 6 months of follow-up were published initially.

There was no statistically significant difference between the two groups in the incidence of the primary end-point of complicated ulcers (upper gastrointestinal bleeding, ulcer perforation, gastric outlet obstruction); the annualized incidence of complicated ulcers in patients taking celecoxib was 0.76% (11 events per 1441 patient-years) versus an incidence of 1.45% (20 events per 1384 patient-years) in patients taking the non-selective NSAIDs, a non-significant difference. However, for the composite end-point of upper gastrointestinal ulcer complications plus symptomatic gastroduodenal ulcers, celecoxib was significantly better tolerated than traditional NSAIDs; the annualized incidence was 2.08% (30 events per 1441 patient-years) with celecoxib versus 3.54% (49 events per 1384 patient-years) for patients taking traditional NSAIDs, significantly different.

The lack of difference in the rate of ulcer complications between the two treatments appeared to be a function of the higher-than-expected rate of complicated ulcers in those taking celecoxib compared with previous studies (81). Further analysis showed that this increase in complications was likely to be attributable to concurrent low-dose aspirin; the annualized incidence of upper gastrointestinal tract ulcer complications and of symptomatic gastroduodenal ulcers in patients not taking low-dose aspirin was significantly lower with celecoxib than with non-selective NSAIDs (0.44% or 5 events per 1143 patient-years versus 1.27% or 14 events per 1101 patient-years respectively). In patients taking aspirin, the annualized incidence of upper gastrointestinal complications and symptomatic ulcers were not significantly different (4.7% or 14 events per 298 patient-years in patients taking celecoxib versus 6.0% or 17 events per 283 patient-years in those taking traditional NSAIDs).

Moreover, the overall incidence of gastrointestinal symptoms in patients taking celecoxib was only slightly lower than that of patients taking the traditional NSAIDs, as was the rate of withdrawal due to gastrointestinal intolerance in both users and non-users of low-dose aspirin.

This subgroup analysis shows what might be called "competing co-morbidity"; that is, in the subgoup of patients taking aspirin as prophylaxis against ischemic heart disease, the gastrointestinal safety advantage of celecoxib over traditional NSAIDs was almost totally wiped out by the use of aspirin (83).

Despite that, the authors of CLASS concluded by stating that celecoxib caused fewer symptomatic ulcers and ulcer complications than ibuprofen or diclofenac at 6 months.

However, these conclusions were not only contradicted by the published data (32), but were also called into question by subsequent information on the trial available to the FDA (84,85). As was first described on the FDA website, the published account of CLASS differed from the original protocol in many respects (in primary outcomes, statistical analysis, and trial duration). In particular, the published article represented selective reporting of the combined analysis of only the first 6 months of two separate protocols of longer duration: the first a 12-month comparison of celecoxib with diclofenac and the other a 16-month comparison of celecoxib with ibuprofen. The unpublished data show that by week 65 celecoxib was associated with a similar number of ulcer complications as diclofenac and ibuprofen and that the relative risks of both complicated ulcers and all serious gastrointestinal adverse events were higher at 12–16 months than they were at 6 months, suggesting an increased risk of serious adverse events with celecoxib long-term therapy.

Serious criticism was therefore aimed at the authors on the grounds of design, data analysis, and misleading presentation of the results. They were charged with having published and circulated overoptimistic short-term pooled data from different protocols, and of omitting disappointing long-term data. They replied to these criticisms, but their explanations were not considered to be convincing (86–88). Furthermore, Pharmacia, the manufacturers of celecoxib, continue to present inappropriately pooled short-term results from different protocols performed in different continents with different comparator drugs for the SUCCESS 1 trial, the successor to CLASS (86–88).

In the VIGOR study, 8076 patients with rheumatoid arthritis were randomly assigned to receive rofecoxib 50 mg/day or naproxen 500 mg bd. The primary end-point was a confirmed clinical upper gastrointestinal event (gastroduodenal perforation or obstruction, upper gastrointestinal bleeding, and symptomatic gastroduodenal ulcer).

Overall, confirmed upper gastrointestinal events occurred in 177 patients, 56 with rofecoxib ($n = 4047$), and 121 in those taking naproxen ($n = 4029$). In 53 of these patients (16 taking rofecoxib and 37 taking naproxen) the event was complicated. That means that during a median follow-up of 9.0 months, there were 2.1 confirmed gastrointestinal events per 100 patient-years with rofecoxib compared with 4.5 per 100 patient-years with naproxen (RR = 0.5; 95% CI = 0.2, 0.8). The respective rates of complicated ulcers (perforation, obstruction, and bleeding) were 0.6 per 100 patient-years and 1.4 per 100 patient-years (RR = 0.4; 95% CI = 0.2, 0.8).

It is also worth noting that the most common adverse events that led to withdrawal of treatment, excluding the primary gastrointestinal end-points, were dyspepsia, abdominal pain, epigastric discomfort, nausea, and heartburn and that significantly fewer patients discontinued treatment as a result of any one of these five upper gastrointestinal symptoms in the rofecoxib group (3.5%) than in the naproxen group (4.9%).

Problems have also occurred in interpreting the results of VIGOR (33). There were significantly fewer upper gastrointestinal adverse events with rofecoxib compared with naproxen, but an unexpected substantial excess of serious cardiovascular events, making the overall safety of rofecoxib uncertain. When the complete data from VIGOR were presented and all serious adverse events were included (not just gastrointestinal events) the patients who took naproxen had fewer overall serious events: 9.3% of the patients who took rofecoxib had a serious adverse event, compared with 7.8% of those who took naproxen (RR = 0.81; 95% CI = 0.62, 0.97).

The reasons for the discrepancy between celecoxib and rofecoxib in the frequency of upper gastrointestinal complications are not clear, but some hypotheses have been proposed. First, aspirin was used concomitantly with celecoxib (20% of patients) in CLASS but not in VIGOR, increasing the risk of gastrointestinal damage. Secondly, diclofenac (which has greater COX-2 selectivity than naproxen) was used as a comparator in CLASS. Thirdly, the dosages of celecoxib were too high and at the doses studied in CLASS celecoxib might not have had true selectivity for COX-2. Finally, the selectivity of celecoxib for COX-2 is probably lower than that of rofecoxib. Therefore, given major differences in study design and data analysis between the two trials, a valid comparison of the two coxibs is not possible from these data alone; a head-to-head comparison in a large outcome study is needed (89).

Two recently published articles have helped to clarify this point: a systematic review of randomized clinical trials on the upper gastrointestinal safety of celecoxib (90) and a population-based retrospective cohort comparison of the rate of upper gastrointestinal hemorrhages in over 40 000 NSAID-naïve elderly users of non-selective NSAIDs, celecoxib, or rofecoxib with the rate in 100 000 patients who had not been exposed to NSAIDs (91).

In the systematic review, all published and unpublished randomized clinical trials that compared at least 12 weeks of celecoxib treatment with placebo or a traditional NSAID (diclofenac, ibuprofen, naproxen) were analysed. Nine of 17 trials fulfilled the inclusion criteria (a total of 15 187 patients). Withdrawals because of drug-related gastrointestinal adverse effects, ulcers detected at endoscopy, and complicated ulcers were used as measures of gastrointestinal tolerability. Compared with those taking non-selective NSAIDs, the patients who took celecoxib had a lower rate of withdrawals because of adverse gastrointestinal effects at 12 weeks (3.2 versus 6.2%), but there was no significant difference between celecoxib and NSAIDs in the incidence of withdrawals for all adverse events. The incidence of ulcers detected at routine endoscopy at 12 weeks was also lower in patients who took celecoxib compared with those who took non-selective NSAIDs (6.2 versus 23%). In four trials that provided information on the incidence of ulcers detected by endoscopy according to whether or not patients were taking concomitant aspirin up to 325 mg/day, the benefit provided by celecoxib was greater in patients not taking aspirin. The incidences of ulcers were as follows:

- celecoxib alone 6.2%;
- celecoxib + aspirin 12%;
- non-selective NSAID alone 25%;
- non-selective NSAID + aspirin 26%.

However, these results must be treated with great caution, as the total number of patients who took prophylactic aspirin was small (150 taking celecoxib and 140 taking non-selective NSAIDs) and the largest number of patients came from a single trial (CLASS).

The same warning applies to evaluation of the incidence of complicated ulcers (bleeds, perforation, and obstructions). The incidence of these serious events with celecoxib was 2.7% (11 events) versus 5% (20 events) in patients taking diclofenac or ibuprofen, a non-significant difference.

This meta-analysis has provided further evidence that celecoxib has better upper gastrointestinal tolerability that some traditional NSAIDs when withdrawal from trials due to drug-related adverse effects or ulceration detected during routine endoscopy are used as measures of tolerability. However, not all ulcers detected by endoscopy progress to a serious event, and many probably heal spontaneously; the clinical relevance of this measure is therefore controversial. On the other hand, there is a consensus that ulcer complications, the prime cause of concern with NSAIDs, should be the primary end-point of outcome studies aimed at evaluating the gastrointestinal toxicity of NSAIDs. Unfortunately, this consensus is counterbalanced by the problems of doing such studies, as they need to be very large to achieve even marginal power and there are also problems in evaluating the clinical outcomes (89).

Another study that deserves attention was an observational study of upper gastrointestinal hemorrhage in over 40 000 elderly patients taking COX-2-selective drugs (celecoxib, rofecoxib) or non-selective NSAIDs with and without misoprostol, compared with 100 000 non-NSAID users (91). Of about 1.3 million potential subjects aged 65 years and over, 364 686 (28%) were given an NSAID during the study period (about 1 year). From the total elderly population, the authors identified 5391 users of non-selective NSAIDs, 5087 users of diclofenac plus misoprostol, 14 583 users of rofecoxib, 18 908 users of celecoxib, and 100 000 controls. Most of the users of non-selective NSAIDs were taking naproxen (32%), ibuprofen (23%), or diclofenac (20%). During over 55 000 person-years of follow-up, there were 187 hospitalizations for upper gastrointestinal hemorrhage. Relative to the non-users, there was a significantly greater risk of upper gastrointestinal hemorrhage in the patients who took non-selective NSAIDs (adjusted risk ratio 4.0; 95% CI = 2.3, 6.9), diclofenac plus misoprostol (3.0; 1.7, 5.6), or rofecoxib (1.9; 1.3, 2.6), but not celecoxib (1.0; 0.7, 1.6). There were also significant differences in the risks of upper gastrointestinal hemorrhage. Relative to celecoxib users, there was a higher risk of hospitalization for upper gastrointestinal hemorrhage, not only among users of non-selective NSAIDs and diclofenac plus misoprostol but also among users of rofecoxib.

This study has provided further evidence that the risk of upper gastrointestinal hemorrhage with COX-2 inhibitors is significantly lower than with conventional NSAIDs, whether or not they are taken with misoprostol. The apparently greater risk of gastrointestinal hemorrhage with rofecoxib than with celecoxib needs confirmation, as the study had some limitations, of which the most important were the low absolute number of events in the study group and the retrospective design.

What are the implications of these data on the use of the coxibs? Overall they suggest that COX-2 selective inhibitors are less likely to cause upper gastrointestinal damage than some traditional NSAIDs. This advantage is measured by a lower number of events that represent a composite end-point of gastrointestinal toxicity, such as endoscopically detected symptomatic ulcers and serious ulcer complications (perforation, obstruction, bleeding). However, this may not be true in all patients, especially in those who simultaneously take aspirin. This question is of major clinical importance, as many patients with osteoarthritis or rheumatoid arthritis use low-dose aspirin for cardiovascular prophylaxis. We do not know whether gastrointestinal safety is preserved with the use of such combinations, nor whether a proton pump inhibitor should be added in this situation. Furthermore, the data on which of the coxibs has better gastrointestinal tolerability are inconclusive. Large outcome studies will be necessary to solve these questions.

A final consideration is worthwhile. To focus attention only on gastrointestinal events may provide an incomplete picture of the benefit/harm profile of the COX-2 inhibitors. Meta-analysis of mortality and morbidity outcomes from CLASS and VIGOR has suggested that total mortality was higher with coxibs than with non-selective NSAIDs, although the difference was not statistically significant (30). Moreover, if one takes into account the incidence of serious adverse events (including death, admission to hospital, and any life-threatening event or events leading to serious disability) as a combined measure of harm, the incidence was significantly higher with COX-2 selective compounds than with other NSAIDs, and complicated gastrointestinal ulcers accounted for only a small proportion of total serious adverse events. Non-gastrointestinal serious adverse events call for more attention.

Two other aspects of gastrointestinal toxicity have yet to be studied. First, the use of COX-2 inhibitors in patients with inflammatory bowel disease, in whom it is likely that COX-2 activity is upregulated (92) and in whom traditional NSAIDs may exacerbate the disease. Experimental colitis has been induced both in COX-2-deficient mice and in rats treated with COX-2-selective inhibitors (93). However, in healthy volunteers, rofecoxib did not alter intestinal permeability, in contrast to indometacin, which increased it (94). Studies in patients with inflammatory bowel disease are necessary before considering COX-2 selective inhibitors to be safe in these patients (95).

Secondly, a possible beneficial role of COX-2 on the stomach should also be taken into account. In mice, COX-2 is expressed at the borders of gastric ulcers and has been implicated as a critical factor in promoting repair (11). Whether these experimental data have any clinical relevance is unknown, but this issue raises the possibility that individuals with pre-existing peptic ulcers who take COX-2 selective drugs may be at risk of delayed ulcer healing and potential complications. This issue may be of particular concern in patients with ulcers due to *Helicobacter pylori* infection.

In conclusion, clinical trials have shown that COX-2-selective NSAIDs seem to be less toxic to the gastrointestinal mucosa than traditional ones. However, life-threatening ulcer complications have been reported in patients taking both celecoxib (81,96,97) and rofecoxib (79). The FDA and other regulatory authorities require that drug information sheets for celecoxib and rofecoxib carry gastrointestinal ulcer warnings similar to those for older NSAIDs.

Large bowel damage

Little is known about the effects of COX-2 inhibitors on the colon, although animal evidence suggests that they can worsen or precipitate acute colitis. Features similar to those seen in cases of ischemic colitis have been reported in a patient taking rofecoxib (98).

- A 52-year-old woman with a colostomy for a tumor of the sigmoid colon developed low back pain that radiated to the legs. A bone scan showed no evidence of tumor. She was given rofecoxib 25 mg/day and 4 days later noticed bloody diarrhea from the colostomy. At colonoscopy a large portion of the transverse colon was seen to be hemorrhagic, with nodularity, a superficial exudate, and mucosal edema, with a well-demarcated transition to normal areas. Despite extensive investigations, no plausible cause of the bloody diarrhea and colitis were found, except the possible involvement of rofecoxib. She stopped taking it and was given intravenous fluids. After 4 days the colostomy stopped oozing blood; colonoscopy showed no evidence of hemorrhage and the mucosa was regenerative. Bleeding did not recur.

Pancreas

Two case reports have suggested a potential association between the sulfonamide group in celecoxib and the development of acute pancreatitis (99,100). The cause of acute pancreatitis in patients taking celecoxib is speculative, but sulfonamides are known to cause pancreatitis, and one of these patients reported an allergy to sulfa medication. Thus, the reaction might have been allergic in nature.

Urinary tract

Kidneys

Renal dysfunction after therapy with COX-2 inhibitors is not unexpected. COX-2 is expressed in the normal human kidney, especially in endothelial and smooth muscle cells of the vasculature and glomerular epithelial cells. Angiotensin II and endothelin induce and upregulate COX-2 and prostaglandin synthesis. Furthermore, it seems reasonable to hypothesize that intrarenal dependence on COX-2-synthesized prostaglandins increases in heart failure, liver failure, volume depletion, and chronic renal disease (101). It is thought that in healthy kidneys COX-2 plays an important role in the balance of water and electrolytes, and its activity is upregulated in patients with reduced left ventricular filling pressure, to help maximize renal blood flow.

As experience with COX-2-selective inhibitors accumulates, it appears that the pattern of nephrotoxicity is similar to that of traditional NSAIDs (102,103). Non-selective NSAIDs can cause hemodynamically mediated acute renal insufficiency in predisposed patients and can cause sodium and water retention, causing peripheral edema and hypertension. Efficacy trials have shown a similar incidence of pedal edema, renal adverse effects, and hypertension with COX-2 selective and non-selective NSAIDs (18,75).

- A 43-year-old woman with rheumatoid arthritis developed dizziness having taken celecoxib 200 mg/day for 2 weeks. At the start of treatment she had normal renal function (104). Her serum creatinine was 670 μmol/l (7.4 mg/dl) and blood urea nitrogen 30 mmol/l (90 mg/dl). Creatinine clearance was 16 ml/minute. Urinalysis was normal and casts were not present. Urinary chemical analysis showed a sodium concentration of 18 mmol/l, a fractional excretion of sodium of 0.3, and a renal failure index of 0.493, consistent with prerenal acute renal insufficiency. Celecoxib was withdrawn. Although her renal function then improved, her serum creatinine was still abnormal (4.7 mg/dl) 1 month later.

In a randomized comparison of celecoxib and diclofenac plus omeprazole, renal adverse events, including hypertension, peripheral edema, and renal insufficiency, were common and similar in the two groups (105). They occurred in the 24% of the patients who took celecoxib and in 31% of those who took diclofenac plus omeprazole. Among patients with renal impairment at baseline, 51% of those who took celecoxib and 41% of those who took diclofenac plus omeprazole had renal adverse events. Careful monitoring of renal function in patients taking COX-2 inhibitors or traditional NSAIDs is mandatory, especially in high-risk subjects (for example those with pre-existing renal disease, diabetes, or heart failure).

Two studies in healthy volunteers have shown that the effects of COX-2 inhibitors on renal function are similar to those of traditional non-selective NSAIDs (106,107). The first was a short-term crossover study on renal function in healthy elderly subjects treated with rofecoxib and naproxen. Although there was a greater fall in glomerular filtration rate with naproxen, reductions in the urinary excretion of sodium, prostaglandin E-2, and 6-keto-prostaglandin F-1α were similar with the two compounds (106). In the second study in elderly people taking a low-salt diet, rofecoxib and indometacin significantly lowered the glomerular filtration to a similar extent (107).

However, these data are limited and must be interpreted with caution, since NSAIDs have significant toxic effects on the kidney only in patients at risk (that is those with volume depletion, heart failure, cirrhosis, intrinsic renal disease, and hypercalcemia), in whom the secretion of vasodilator prostaglandins is increased in an attempt to counteract the effect of increased renal vasoconstrictors, such as angiotensin II.

The incidence of adverse effects related to renal function in CLASS and VIGOR was low and similar (0.9% with celecoxib and 1.2% with rofecoxib). The incidence of increased creatinine and urea nitrogen concentrations was slightly lower in patients taking celecoxib than in those taking ibuprofen or diclofenac. Similar results have been documented in two other clinical trials. The first compared celecoxib with diclofenac in long-term management of rheumatoid arthritis in 430 patients (16). There were only small increases in serum creatinine concentration (from 93 μmol/l at baseline to 96 μmol/l at the final visit) and serum urea concentration (from 6.0 to 6.4 mmol/l). There was a similar increase in patients taking diclofenac. The second trial, in 1149 patients, compared celecoxib with naproxen; serum creatinine concentrations were not affected by either celecoxib or naproxen (75). However, data from these clinical trials must be interpreted with caution, as patients at major risk of renal adverse events were likely to be excluded.

In contrast, published case reports and case series have provided more insight into the potential nephrotoxicity associated with COX-2-selective inhibitors. Taken together, these case reports suggest that COX-2 inhibitors, like non-selective NSAIDs, produce similar and consistent renal adverse effects in patients with one or more risk factors that induce prostaglandin-dependent renal function (that is patients with renal and cardiovascular disease and taking a number of culprit medications, such as diuretics and ACE inhibitors). Acute renal insufficiency, disturbances in volume status (edema, heart failure), metabolic acidosis, hyperkalemia, and hyponatremia have been commonly described. The duration of treatment with COX-2 inhibitors before the development of clinically recognized renal impairment ranged from a few days to 3–4 weeks. Withdrawal of COX-2 inhibitors and supportive therapy most often resulted in resolution of renal dysfunction, but in some patients hemodialysis was required (102,108–112).

The renal safety of rofecoxib and celecoxib has been studied using the database of spontaneous reports of adverse drug reactions in the WHO Monitoring Center in Uppsala (113). Disproportionality in the association between COX-2 selective inhibitors and renal-related adverse drug reactions was evaluated using a Bayesian confidence propagation neural network method, in which a statistical parameter (the information component: IC) was calculated for each drug-reaction combination. In this method an IC value significantly greater than 0 implies that the association of a drug-reaction pair is stronger than background; the higher the IC value, the more the combination stands out from the background. As with non-selective NSAIDs, both COX-2 selective inhibitors were associated with renal-related adverse drug reactions. IC values were significantly different for the following comparisons: water retention, abnormal renal function, renal insufficiency, cardiac failure, and hypertension. However, the adverse renal impact of rofecoxib was significantly greater than that of celecoxib. Renal-related events for rofecoxib were two- to four-fold higher than for celecoxib and the severity of these reported adverse reactions was also more serious. Studies based on spontaneous reports have many limitations and their results must therefore be confirmed by additional epidemiological studies that can provide more accurate information on incidence rates and risk factors.

Rare reports of acute reversible renal impairment have been recorded in patients with predisposing factors (109).

Whether selective COX-2 inhibitors can cause the other types of renal toxicity that are associated with non-selective NSAIDs (that is acute interstitial nephritis, nephrotic syndrome with or without renal insufficiency) is not known.

Bladder

The use of NSAIDs to treat and prevent bladder spasms has been documented in clinical trials (114) and their role in relaxing bladder smooth muscle has experimental support (115). Three elderly patients who used rofecoxib or celecoxib developed acute but reversible urinary retention (116). Each had co-morbidities likely to cause bladder dysfunction, and the administration of a COX-2 inhibitor may have caused further relaxation of the detrusor muscle, resulting in urinary retention.

Skin

There have been reports of maculopapular rash (117) and severe erythema multiforme (toxic epidermal necrolysis) (118) with celecoxib. Three patients developed erythema multiforme while taking rofecoxib (119). All were well documented, and oral rechallenge with rofecoxib, positive in two of them, confirmed the role of rofecoxib in the pathogenesis of this adverse reaction.

- Swelling and wrinkling of the palms soon after exposure to water occurred in an 18-year-old-woman taking rofecoxib for mixed connective tissue disease (120). The swelling followed exposure for 1 to a few minutes to water at any temperature. The swelling developed rapidly and was accompanied by symptoms of mild pain and discomfort. Over the following 2 hours, the palms would return to normal. Because of the temporal correlation with the use of rofecoxib, it was withdrawn, and 3 weeks later her symptoms had almost completely resolved.

The authors speculated that this phenomenon might have been due to increased salt content of the skin caused by the rofecoxib, resulting in increased water-binding capacity of keratin.

Musculoskeletal

An in vitro experiment on cartilage explants from patients with osteoarthritis showed upregulation of COX-2 activity, which may be linked to cartilage repair (121). If this is true, long-term use of COX-2 inhibitor NSAIDs could have harmful effect on joints. Preliminary data suggest that these drugs are efficacious in osteoarthritis, at least in the short term.

Reproductive system

Many reproductive processes (ovulation, fertilization, implantation, decidualization, and parturition) depend on prostaglandin ligand–receptor interactions. It is therefore not surprising that selective COX-2 inhibition has a negative local effect on ovulation, resulting in delayed follicular rupture and infertility, without affecting peripheral hormonal cyclicity (122,123).

There have been several case reports that non-selective NSAIDs (diclofenac, naproxen, piroxicam) can cause infertility, attributed to "luteinized unruptured ovarian follicles" syndrome (124–126). Now the syndrome has been documented in a double-blind, randomized, placebo-controlled study, in which women were assessed over two menstrual cycles while taking rofecoxib (123). Women who are trying to become pregnant should avoid taking any NSAIDs if possible, and those who need one for a chronic rheumatic disorder should be aware of possible infertility; in such cases further investigation is not required, as withdrawal of the drug restores fertility.

Immunologic

There is considerable difficulty and controversy in identifying and classifying allergic reactions to NSAIDs, for many reasons (127). First, the difficulty in making a definite diagnosis in patients who have these reactions without provocative challenge with the suspected drug and other NSAIDs. Secondly, reactions are characterized by a large spectrum of target organ responses to NSAIDs, and the same drug can cause different types of reactions in different organs in the same or different individuals. Thirdly, a patient can have a similar reaction to a structurally different NSAID. Finally, reports of these reactions include different, often imprecise, terms, making interpretation difficult. It is worth evaluating the safety of new coxibs in patients who cannot tolerate non-selective NSAIDs.

Anaphylaxis due to celecoxib has been described (SEDA 26, 121). Life-threatening anaphylaxis, with urticaria, angioedema, and bronchospasm, has also been described 30 minutes after a dose of celecoxib for arthritis of the hip (128).

Allergic vasculitis has been reported in association with various NSAIDs, and has been attributed to celecoxib (129,130), including one case with a fatal outcome (131).

Whether allergic reactions to celecoxib occur more often in patients who report a previous reaction to sulfonamides, and should therefore be contraindicated in such patients, is still unknown (132).

Angioedema has been attributed to rofecoxib (SEDA-26, 121).

- A 60-year-old man developed angioedema after taking two doses of rofecoxib 12.5 mg 18 and 12 hours before (133). Despite intensive treatment he developed pulmonary hemorrhagic edema and died a day later. He had fibrotic lung disease, which may have predisposed him to the lethal event.

The tolerability of rofecoxib in patients with cutaneous allergic and pseudoallergic adverse reactions to non-selective NSAIDs has been confirmed in a study in 139 patients with NSAID-induced adverse reactions: 60 with urticaria alone (43%), 34 with angioedema (25%), 34 with angioedema plus urticaria (2.9%), and 2 with Stevens–Johnson syndrome (1.4%) (134). They all underwent a single-blind, placebo-controlled oral challenge with increasing doses of rofecoxib, and 138 of them tolerated it without adverse reactions. Only one had mild urticaria on the arms. Rofecoxib may be a useful alternative in patients with NSAID hypersensitivity.

Anaphylaxis

Among the anaphylactic reactions to NSAIDs that result in different types of reaction (urticaria, angioedema, asthma, or hypotension), there have been very few reports of anaphylactic shock. However, anaphylaxis has been described in patients taking celecoxib (135,136) or rofecoxib (137). Rofecoxib caused anaphylaxis in a patient who had had a similar reaction to diclofenac, suggesting that COX-2 inhibitors may be not safe in all individuals who have adverse reactions to non-selective COX inhibitors. It also suggests that different mechanisms may be involved in patients with asthma and in those with anaphylactoid reactions to NSAIDs.

Sulfonamide-like allergic adverse reactions

Concerns that COX-2 inhibitors may be associated with an increased risk of allergic reactions in patients with a history of sulfonamide hypersensitivity arise from the molecular structures of these compounds (SEDA-24, 119) (138).

A sulfur component is necessary for the receptor binding of both celecoxib and rofecoxib, but their structures differ and they have different potentials for causing allergic reactions. Consequently, celecoxib is thought to be contraindicated in patients with a history of allergy to sulfonamides. The available data on the immunological tolerability profile of celecoxib and rofecoxib are scanty but merit attention.

Sulfonamide-like adverse drug reactions seem to occur more frequently with celecoxib than with rofecoxib, according to a report from Sweden (139). The investigators identified a profile of 19 typical sulfonamide-like adverse reactions from published papers and the WHO Adverse Drug Reactions database from 1968 to 2000, and compared this profile with reported adverse drug reactions associated with celecoxib and rofecoxib. The WHO database contained 11 514 reports about celecoxib describing 21 292 suspected adverse drug reactions and 10 200 reports about rofecoxib describing 18 585 suspected drug reactions. The relative reporting rate of sulfonamide-like adverse drug reactions was almost twice as high for celecoxib as for rofecoxib (RR = 1.8; 95% CI = 1.6, 1.9) for all reports and for reports that listed a COX-2 inhibitor as the only suspected drug. The reporting rate for 15 of the 19 sulfonamide-like adverse drug reactions was higher for celecoxib than for rofecoxib, with significant differences for rash (RR = 2.3; CI = 2.0, 2.6), urticaria (RR = 2.0; CI = 1.6, 24), Stevens–Johnson syndrome (RR = 3.6; CI = 1.4, 12), and photosensitivity (RR = 2.4; CI = 1.5, 4.0). Fatal adverse drug reactions fitting the typical sulfonamide profile also occurred more often with celecoxib than with rofecoxib (1.8; CI = 0.9, 4.0).

Even though serious sulfonamide reactions are rare, their clinical impact warrants close monitoring as more data become available, and physicians should be aware of possible sulfonamide allergy when prescribing COX-2 inhibitors, in particular celecoxib.

There have been single case reports of sulfonamide-like allergic reactions in patients taking celecoxib; in two cases sulfonamide allergy was ignored and was discovered only after an adverse reaction to celecoxib (140) or rofecoxib (141) had occurred.

Urticaria and angioedema

Of 110 patients with a history of urticaria and angioedema triggered by one or more non-selective NSAIDs, who were submitted to 184 single-blind, placebo-controlled oral challenges with the suspected NSAID, patients with a positive challenge underwent further oral challenge with various COX-2 inhibitors (celecoxib and rofecoxib, and also nimesulide and meloxicam, which are relatively selective COX-2 inhibitors) (142). The maximal challenge doses were celecoxib 200 mg, rofecoxib 25 mg, meloxicam 15 mg, and nimesulide 100 mg. Reactions (expressed as a percentage of tested patients with a positive test) varied among the COX-2 inhibitors: 33% (10/30) for celecoxib, 21% (16/75) for nimesulide, 17% (8/46) for meloxicam, and 3% (1/33) for rofecoxib. This suggests that the degree of cross-reactivity of COX-2 inhibitors was related to the degree of in vitro COX-1 inhibition, since meloxicam, nimesulide, and celecoxib inhibit COX-1 to a similar extent (143). The results also suggested that the most selective COX-2 inhibitor (rofecoxib) might be relatively safe in a patient with NSAID-induced urticaria/angioedema.

In another study, 34 patients with a history of urticaria and/or angioedema after ingestion of at least two chemically unrelated non-selective NSAIDs, 22 of whom also had chronic urticaria, all underwent a single-blind, placebo-controlled oral tolerance test with rofecoxib (12 and 25 mg 1 hour apart) (144). Rofecoxib caused urticaria and/or angioedema in 6/34 patients (18%), with no difference between patients with or without a history of chronic urticaria.

There was even better tolerability of rofecoxib in another study in 33 patients with documented urticaria/angioedema after ingestion of two different NSAIDs (145). The patients underwent provocative tests with increasing doses of rofecoxib (from 6.25 to 25 mg); at the end of the challenge all tolerated rofecoxib 25 mg.

Other single case reports have supported the evidence of better tolerability of COX-2-selective inhibitors (in particular rofecoxib) in patients with a history of urticaria/angioedema (64,146). However, contrasting data have shown cross-reactivity of celecoxib with other NSAIDs and between celecoxib and rofecoxib (147).

Why are COX-2-selective drugs better tolerated? The mechanisms underlying intolerance to chemically unrelated NSAIDs are unknown, but it has been hypothesized that intolerant patients may have exaggerated sensitivity to the effects of leukotrienes, which are more active than histamine in inducing wheal and flare reactions. Blockade of both COX-1 and COX-2 by non-selective NSAIDs increases the production of leukotrienes by the lipoxygenase pathway, whereas COX-2-selective agents do not increase the production of LTB_4 or cysteinyl LTS. However, this may not be the only pathogenic mechanism, as some drugs probably trigger histamine release from mast cells and basophils non-specifically, and others may trigger immunological cross-reactivity. Overall, the above-mentioned studies and clinical experience suggest that urticaria and angioedema can occur with COX-2 inhibitors, albeit with a lower frequency than with non-selective NSAIDs.

Second-Generation Effects

Fetotoxicity

A single case report supports the hypothesis that a COX-2-selective NSAID might have the efficacy of indometacin as a tocolytic agent without its adverse effects in the fetus (148).

Drug–Drug Interactions

Lithium

A possible interaction of rofecoxib with lithium has been reported (149).

- A 73-year-old man with manic-depressive illness, who had taken lithium for 40 years, underwent coronary bypass surgery and was given long-term warfarin. He developed signs of lithium intoxication (confusion, irritability, tremor, and gait disturbance) after having taken rofecoxib 12.5 mg/day for 9 days for arthritis. Rofecoxib had been chosen in order to avoid a possible drug interaction with warfarin. Lithium and rofecoxib were withdrawn and the signs resolved within 1 week. His serum lithium concentration was 1.5 mmol/l and his serum creatinine 1430 μmol/l.

Both lithium and rofecoxib have been associated with nephrotoxicity, and it is likely that lithium intoxication was caused by concomitant administration of rofecoxib, causing a reversible reduction in renal function.

Propofol

A single perioperative dose of parecoxib did not alter the disposition or the clinical effects of a bolus of propofol (150).

Sex hormones

Rofecoxib did not cause any clinically important changes in ethinylestradiol and norethindrone pharmacokinetics in 18 subjects (151).

References

1. Feldman M, McMahon AT. Do cyclooxygenase-2 inhibitors provide benefits similar to those of traditional nonsteroidal anti-inflammatory drugs, with less gastrointestinal toxicity? Ann Intern Med 2000;132(2):134–43.
2. Hawkey CJ. COX-2 inhibitors. Lancet 1999;353(9149): 307–14.
3. Crofford LJ, Lipsky PE, Brooks P, Abramson SB, Simon LS, van de Putte LB. Basic biology and clinical application of specific cyclooxygenase-2 inhibitors. Arthritis Rheum 2000;43(1):4–13.
4. Brooks P, Emery P, Evans JF, Fenner H, Hawkey CJ, Patrono C, Smolen J, Breedveld F, Day R, Dougados M, Ehrich EW, Gijon-Banos J, Kvien TK, Van Rijswijk MH, Warner T, Zeidler H. Interpreting the clinical significance of the differential inhibition of cyclooxygenase-1 and cyclooxygenase-2. Rheumatology (Oxford) 1999;38(8):779–88.
5. Gilroy DW, Colville-Nash PR, Willis D, Chivers J, Paul-Clark MJ, Willoughby DA. Inducible cyclooxygenase may

have anti-inflammatory properties. Nat Med 1999; 5(6):698–701.
6. Zimmermann KC, Sarbia M, Schror K, Weber AA. Constitutive cyclooxygenase-2 expression in healthy human and rabbit gastric mucosa. Mol Pharmacol 1998;54(3):536–40.
7. Iseki S. Immunocytochemical localization of cyclooxygenase-1 and cyclooxygenase-2 in the rat stomach. Histochem J 1995;27(4):323–8.
8. Robert A, Nezamis JE, Lancaster C, Davis JP, Field SO, Hanchar AJ. Mild irritants prevent gastric necrosis through "adaptive cytoprotection" mediated by prostaglandins. Am J Physiol 1983;245(1):G113–21.
9. Gretzer B, Ehrlich K, Maricic N, Lambrecht N, Respondek M, Peskar BM. Selective cyclo-oxygenase-2 inhibitors and their influence on the protective effect of a mild irritant in the rat stomach. Br J Pharmacol 1998;123(5):927–35.
10. Schmassmann A. Mechanisms of ulcer healing and effects of nonsteroidal anti-inflammatory drugs. Am J Med 1998;104(3A):S43–51.
11. Mizuno H, Sakamoto C, Matsuda K, Wada K, Uchida T, Noguchi H, Akamatsu T, Kasuga M. Induction of cyclooxygenase 2 in gastric mucosal lesions and its inhibition by the specific antagonist delays healing in mice. Gastroenterology 1997;112(2):387–97.
12. Takahashi S, Shigeta J, Inoue H, Tanabe T, Okabe S. Localization of cyclooxygenase-2 and regulation of its mRNA expression in gastric ulcers in rats. Am J Physiol 1998;275(5 Pt 1):G1137–45.
13. Seibert K, Zhang Y, Leahy K, Hauser S, Masferrer J, Perkins W, Lee L, Isakson P. Pharmacological and biochemical demonstration of the role of cyclooxygenase 2 in inflammation and pain. Proc Natl Acad Sci USA 1994;91(25):12013–17.
14. Wallace JL, Bak A, McKnight W, Asfaha S, Sharkey KA, MacNaughton WK. Cyclooxygenase 1 contributes to inflammatory responses in rats and mice: implications for gastrointestinal toxicity. Gastroenterology 1998;115(1): 101–9.
15. Bensen WG, Fiechtner JJ, McMillen JI, Zhao WW, Yu SS, Woods EM, Hubbard RC, Isakson PC, Verburg KM, Geis GS. Treatment of osteoarthritis with celecoxib, a cyclooxygenase-2 inhibitor: a randomized controlled trial. Mayo Clin Proc 1999;74(11):1095–105.
16. Emery P, Zeidler H, Kvien TK, Guslandi M, Naudin R, Stead H, Verburg KM, Isakson PC, Hubbard RC, Geis GS. Celecoxib versus diclofenac in long-term management of rheumatoid arthritis: randomised double-blind comparison. Lancet 1999;354(9196):2106–11.
17. Zhao SZ, McMillen JI, Markenson JA, Dedhiya SD, Zhao WW, Osterhaus JT, Yu SS. Evaluation of the functional status aspects of health-related quality of life of patients with osteoarthritis treated with celecoxib. Pharmacotherapy 1999;19(11):1269–78.
18. Schnitzer TJ, Truitt K, Fleischmann R, Dalgin P, Block J, Zeng Q, Bolognese J, Seidenberg B, Ehrich EW. The safety profile, tolerability, and effective dose range of rofecoxib in the treatment of rheumatoid arthritis. Phase II Rofecoxib Rheumatoid Arthritis Study Group. Clin Ther 1999;21(10):1688–702.
19. Ehrich EW, Schnitzer TJ, McIlwain H, Levy R, Wolfe F, Weisman M, Zeng Q, Morrison B, Bolognese J, Seidenberg B, Gertz BJ. Effect of specific COX-2 inhibition in osteoarthritis of the knee: a 6 week double blind, placebo controlled pilot study of rofecoxib. Rofecoxib Osteoarthritis Pilot Study Group. J Rheumatol 1999;26(11):2438–47.
20. Day R, Morrison B, Luza A, Castaneda O, Strusberg A, Nahir M, Helgetveit KB, Kress B, Daniels B, Bolognese J, Krupa D, Seidenberg B, Ehrich E. A randomized trial of the efficacy and tolerability of the COX-2 inhibitor rofecoxib vs ibuprofen in patients with osteoarthritis. Rofecoxib/Ibuprofen Comparator Study Group. Arch Intern Med 2000;160(12):1781–7.
21. Cannon GW, Caldwell JR, Holt P, McLean B, Seidenberg B, Bolognese J, Ehrich E, Mukhopadhyay S, Daniels B. Rofecoxib, a specific inhibitor of cyclooxygenase 2, with clinical efficacy comparable with that of diclofenac sodium: results of a one-year, randomized, clinical trial in patients with osteoarthritis of the knee and hip. Rofecoxib Phase III Protocol 035 Study Group. Arthritis Rheum 2000;43(5):978–87.
22. Anonymous. Celecoxib for arthritis. Med Lett Drugs Ther 1999;41(1045):11–12.
23. Anonymous. Rofecoxib for osteoarthritis and pain. Med Lett Drugs Ther 1999;41(1056):59–61.
24. Morrison BW, Christensen S, Yuan W, Brown J, Amlani S, Seidenberg B. Analgesic efficacy of the cyclooxygenase-2-specific inhibitor rofecoxib in post-dental surgery pain: a randomized, controlled trial. Clin Ther 1999;21(6):943–53.
25. Malmstrom K, Daniels S, Kotey P, Seidenberg BC, Desjardins PJ. Comparison of rofecoxib and celecoxib, two cyclooxygenase-2 inhibitors, in postoperative dental pain: a randomized, placebo- and active-comparator-controlled clinical trial. Clin Ther 1999;21(10):1653–63.
26. Ehrich EW, Dallob A, De Lepeleire I, Van Hecken A, Riendeau D, Yuan W, Porras A, Wittreich J, Seibold JR, De Schepper P, Mehlisch DR, Gertz BJ. Characterization of rofecoxib as a cyclooxygenase-2 isoform inhibitor and demonstration of analgesia in the dental pain model. Clin Pharmacol Ther 1999;65(3):336–47.
27. Morrison BW, Daniels SE, Kotey P, Cantu N, Seidenberg B. Rofecoxib, a specific cyclooxygenase-2 inhibitor, in primary dysmenorrhea: a randomized controlled trial. Obstet Gynecol 1999;94(4):504–8.
28. Juni P, Rutjes AW, Dieppe PA. Are selective COX 2 inhibitors superior to traditional non steroidal anti-inflammatory drugs? BMJ 2002;324(7349):1287–8.
29. Jones R. Efficacy and safety of COX 2 inhibitors. BMJ 2002;325(7365):607–8.
30. Wright JM. The double-edged sword of COX-2 selective NSAIDs. CMAJ 2002;167(10):1131–7.
31. McCormack JP, Rangno R. Digging for data from the COX-2 trials. CMAJ 2002;166(13):1649–50.
32. Silverstein FE, Faich G, Goldstein JL, Simon LS, Pincus T, Whelton A, Makuch R, Eisen G, Agrawal NM, Stenson WF, Burr AM, Zhao WW, Kent JD, Lefkowith JB, Verburg KM, Geis GS. Gastrointestinal toxicity with celecoxib vs nonsteroidal anti-inflammatory drugs for osteoarthritis and rheumatoid arthritis: the CLASS study: a randomized controlled trial. Celecoxib Long-term Arthritis Safety Study. JAMA 2000;284(10): 1247–55.
33. Bombardier C, Laine L, Reicin A, Shapiro D, Burgos-Vargas R, Davis B, Day R, Ferraz MB, Hawkey CJ, Hochberg MC, Kvien TK, Schnitzer TJ; VIGOR Study Group. Comparison of upper gastrointestinal toxicity of rofecoxib and naproxen in patients with rheumatoid arthritis. N Engl J Med 2000;343(21):1520–8.
34. Mukherjee D, Nissen SE, Topol EJ. Risk of cardiovascular events associated with selective COX-2 inhibitors. JAMA 2001;286(8):954–9.
35. White WB, Faich G, Whelton A, Maurath C, Ridge NJ, Verburg KM, Geis GS, Lefkowith JB. Comparison of thromboembolic events in patients treated with celecoxib, a cyclooxygenase-2 specific inhibitor, versus ibuprofen or diclofenac. Am J Cardiol 2002;89(4):425–30.
36. Sanmuganathan PS, Ghahramani P, Jackson PR, Wallis EJ, Ramsay LE. Aspirin for primary prevention of

coronary heart disease: safety and absolute benefit related to coronary risk derived from meta-analysis of randomised trials. Heart 2001;85(3):265–71.
37. Fleming M. Cardiovascular events and COX-2 inhibitors. JAMA 2001;286(22):2808.
38. Burnakis TG. Cardiovascular events and COX-2 inhibitors. JAMA 2001;286(22):2808.
39. Konstam MA, Demopoulos LA. Cardiovascular events and COX-2 inhibitors. JAMA 2001;286(22):2809.
40. Grant KD. Cardiovascular events and COX-2 inhibitors. JAMA 2001;286(22):2809.
41. Haldey EJ, Pappagallo M. Cardiovascular events and COX-2 inhibitors. JAMA 2001;286(22):2809–10.
42. McGeer PL, McGeer EG, Yasojima K. Cardiovascular events and COX-2 inhibitors. JAMA 2001;286(22):2810.
43. White WB, Whelton A. Cardiovascular events and COX-2 inhibitors. JAMA 2001;286(22):2811–12.
44. Konstam MA, Weir MR, Reicin A, Shapiro D, Sperling RS, Barr E, Gertz BJ. Cardiovascular thrombotic events in controlled, clinical trials of rofecoxib. Circulation 2001;104(19):2280–8.
45. FitzGerald GA, Cheng Y, Austin S. COX-2 inhibitors and the cardiovascular system. Clin Exp Rheumatol 2001; 19(6 Suppl 25):S31–6.
46. Wooltorton E. What's all the fuss? Safety concerns about COX-2 inhibitors rofecoxib (Vioxx) and celecoxib (Celebrex). CMAJ 2002;166(13):1692–3.
47. Van Hecken A, Schwartz JI, Depre M, De Lepeleire I, Dallob A, Tanaka W, Wynants K, Buntinx A, Arnout J, Wong PH, Ebel DL, Gertz BJ, De Schepper PJ. Comparative inhibitory activity of rofecoxib, meloxicam, diclofenac, ibuprofen, and naproxen on COX-2 versus COX-1 in healthy volunteers. J Clin Pharmacol 2000;40(10):1109–20.
48. Cleland JG. No reduction in cardiovascular risk with NSAIDs-including aspirin? Lancet 2002;359(9301):92–3.
49. Dalen JE. Selective COX-2 Inhibitors, NSAIDs, aspirin, and myocardial infarction. Arch Intern Med 2002; 162(10):1091–2.
50. Ray WA, Stein CM, Hall K, Daugherty JR, Griffin MR. Non-steroidal anti-inflammatory drugs and risk of serious coronary heart disease: an observational cohort study. Lancet 2002;359(9301):118–23.
51. Solomon DH, Glynn RJ, Levin R, Avorn J. Nonsteroidal anti-inflammatory drug use and acute myocardial infarction. Arch Intern Med 2002;162(10):1099–104.
52. Watson DJ, Rhodes T, Cai B, Guess HA. Lower risk of thromboembolic cardiovascular events with naproxen among patients with rheumatoid arthritis. Arch Intern Med 2002;162(10):1105–10.
53. Rahme E, Pilote L, LeLorier J. Association between naproxen use and protection against acute myocardial infarction. Arch Intern Med 2002;162(10):1111–15.
54. Steering Committee of the Physicians' Health Study Research Group. Final report on the aspirin component of the ongoing Physicians' Health Study. N Engl J Med 1989;321(3):129–35.
55. Johnson AG, Nguyen TV, Day RO. Do nonsteroidal anti-inflammatory drugs affect blood pressure? A meta-analysis. Ann Intern Med 1994;121(4):289–300.
56. Whelton A. Renal and related cardiovascular effects of conventional and COX-2-specific NSAIDs and non-NSAID analgesics. Am J Ther 2000;7(2):63–74.
57. Collins R, Peto R, MacMahon S, Hebert P, Fiebach NH, Eberlein KA, Godwin J, Qizilbash N, Taylor JO, Hennekens CH. Blood pressure, stroke, and coronary heart disease. Part 2. Short-term reductions in blood pressure: overview of randomised drug trials in their epidemiological context. Lancet 1990;335(8693):827–38.
58. Whelton A, Maurath CJ, Verburg KM, Geis GS. Renal safety and tolerability of celecoxib, a novel cyclooxygenase-2 inhibitor. Am J Ther 2000;7(3):159–75.
59. Whelton A, Fort JG, Puma JA, Normandin D, Bello AE, Verburg KM; SUCCESS VI Study Group. Cyclooxygenase-2-specific inhibitors and cardiorenal function: a randomized, controlled trial of celecoxib and rofecoxib in older hypertensive osteoarthritis patients. Am J Ther 2001;8(2):85–95.
60. Pathak A, Boveda S, Defaye P, Mansourati J, Mallaret M, Thebault L, Galinier M, Blanc JJ, Montastruc JL. Celecoxib-associated torsade de pointes. Ann Pharmacother 2002;36(7–8):1290–1.
61. Levy S, Volans G. The use of analgesics in patients with asthma. Drug Saf 2001;24(11):829–41.
62. Szczeklik A, Nizankowska E, Duplaga M. Natural history of aspirin-induced asthma. AIANE Investigators. European Network on Aspirin-Induced Asthma. Eur Respir J 2000;16(3):432–6.
63. Szczeklik A, Stevenson DD. Aspirin-induced asthma: advances in pathogenesis and management. J Allergy Clin Immunol 1999;104(1):5–13.
64. Kosnik M, Music E, Matjaz F, Suskovic S. Relative safety of meloxicam in NSAID-intolerant patients. Allergy 1998;53(12):1231–3.
65. Bianco S, Robuschi M, Petrigni G, Scuri M, Pieroni MG, Refini RM, Vaghi A, Sestini PS. Efficacy and tolerability of nimesulide in asthmatic patients intolerant to aspirin. Drugs 1993;46(Suppl 1):115–20.
66. Szczeklik A, Nizankowska E, Bochenek G, Nagraba K, Mejza F, Swierczynska M. Safety of a specific COX-2 inhibitor in aspirin-induced asthma. Clin Exp Allergy 2001;31(2):219–25.
67. Stevenson DD, Simon RA. Lack of cross-reactivity between rofecoxib and aspirin in aspirin-sensitive patients with asthma. J Allergy Clin Immunol 2001;108(1):47–51.
68. Dahlen B, Szczeklik A, Murray JJ; Celecoxib in Aspirin-Intolerant Asthma Study Group. Celecoxib in patients with asthma and aspirin intolerance. N Engl J Med 2001;344(2):142.
69. Settipane RA, Stevenson DD. Cross sensitivity with acetaminophen in aspirin-sensitive subjects with asthma. J Allergy Clin Immunol 1989;84(1):26–33.
70. Bonnel RA, Villalba ML, Karwoski CB, Beitz J. Aseptic meningitis associated with rofecoxib. Arch Intern Med 2002;162(6):713–15.
71. Daugherty KK, Gora-Harper ML. Idiopathic paresthesia reaction associated with rofecoxib. Ann Pharmacother 2002;36(2):264–6.
72. Simon LS, Lanza FL, Lipsky PE, Hubbard RC, Talwalker S, Schwartz BD, Isakson PC, Geis GS. Preliminary study of the safety and efficacy of SC-58635, a novel cyclooxygenase 2 inhibitor: efficacy and safety in two placebo-controlled trials in osteoarthritis and rheumatoid arthritis, and studies of gastrointestinal and platelet effects. Arthritis Rheum 1998;41(9):1591–602.
73. Topper JN, Cai J, Falb D, Gimbrone MA Jr. Identification of vascular endothelial genes differentially responsive to fluid mechanical stimuli: cyclooxygenase-2, manganese superoxide dismutase, and endothelial cell nitric oxide synthase are selectively up-regulated by steady laminar shear stress. Proc Natl Acad Sci USA 1996;93(19):10417–22.
74. McAdam BF, Catella-Lawson F, Mardini IA, Kapoor S, Lawson JA, Fitzgerald GA. Systemic biosynthesis of prostacyclin by cyclooxygenase (COX)-2: the human

pharmacology of a selective inhibitor of COX-2. Proc Natl Acad Sci USA 1999;96(1):272–7.
75. Simon LS, Weaver AL, Graham DY, Kivitz AJ, Lipsky PE, Hubbard RC, Isakson PC, Verburg KM, Yu SS, Zhao WW, Geis GS. Anti-inflammatory and upper gastrointestinal effects of celecoxib in rheumatoid arthritis: a randomized controlled trial. JAMA 1999;282(20):1921–8.
76. Lanza FL, Rack MF, Simon TJ, Quan H, Bolognese JA, Hoover ME, Wilson FR, Harper SE. Specific inhibition of cyclooxygenase-2 with MK-0966 is associated with less gastroduodenal damage than either aspirin or ibuprofen. Aliment Pharmacol Ther 1999;13(6):761–7.
77. Laine L, Harper S, Simon T, Bath R, Johanson J, Schwartz H, Stern S, Quan H, Bolognese J. A randomized trial comparing the effect of rofecoxib, a cyclooxygenase 2-specific inhibitor, with that of ibuprofen on the gastroduodenal mucosa of patients with osteoarthritis. Rofecoxib Osteoarthritis Endoscopy Study Group. Gastroenterology 1999;117(4):776–83.
78. Wolfe MM, Lichtenstein DR, Singh G. Gastrointestinal toxicity of nonsteroidal antiinflammatory drugs. N Engl J Med 1999;340(24):1888–99.
79. Langman MJ, Jensen DM, Watson DJ, Harper SE, Zhao PL, Quan H, Bolognese JA, Simon TJ. Adverse upper gastrointestinal effects of rofecoxib compared with NSAIDs. JAMA 1999;282(20):1929–33.
80. Goldstein JL, Agrawal NM, Silverstein F, Kaiser J, Burr AM, Verburg KM, et al. Celecoxib is associated with a significantly lower incidence of clinically significant upper gastrointestinal (UGI) events in osteoarthritis (OA) and rheumatoid arthritis (RA) patients as compared to NSAIDs. Gastroenterology 1999;116:A174.
81. Goldstein JL, Silverstein FE, Agrawal NM, Hubbard RC, Kaiser J, Maurath CJ, Verburg KM, Geis GS. Reduced risk of upper gastrointestinal ulcer complications with celecoxib, a novel COX-2 inhibitor. Am J Gastroenterol 2000;95(7):1681–90.
82. Peterson WL, Cryer B. COX-1-sparing NSAIDs—is the enthusiasm justified? JAMA 1999;282(20):1961–3.
83. Boers M. NSAIDS and selective COX-2 inhibitors: competition between gastroprotection and cardioprotection. Lancet 2001;357(9264):1222–3.
84. Hrachovec JB, Mora M. Reporting of 6-month vs 12-month data in a clinical trial of celecoxib. JAMA 2001; 286(19):2398.
85. Wright JM, Perry TL, Bassett KL, Chambers GK. Reporting of 6-month vs 12-month data in a clinical trial of celecoxib. JAMA 2001;286(19):2398–400.
86. Geis GS. CLASS clarification: reaffirms the medical importance of the analyses and results. BMJ USA 2002;2:522–3.
87. Juni P, Rutjes AWS, Dieppe P. Pharmacia addresses June 1 editorial regarding CLASS study: authors' response. BMJ 2002;324:1287–8.
88. Budenholzer BR, Geis GS, Mamdani M, Juurlink DN, Anderson GM, Stover RR, Juni P, Rutjes AW, Dieppe PA. Are selective COX 2 inhibitors superior to traditional NSAIDs? BMJ 2002;325:161.
89. Hawkey CJ. Outcomes studies of drug induced ulcer complications: do we need them and how should they be done? BMJ 2000;321(7256):291–3.
90. Deeks JJ, Smith LA, Bradley MD. Efficacy, tolerability, and upper gastrointestinal safety of celecoxib for treatment of osteoarthritis and rheumatoid arthritis: systematic review of randomised controlled trials. BMJ 2002;325(7365):619.
91. Mamdani M, Rochon PA, Juurlink DN, Kopp A, Anderson GM, Naglie G, Austin PC, Laupacis A. Observational study of upper gastrointestinal haemorrhage in elderly patients given selective cyclo-oxygenase-2 inhibitors or conventional non-steroidal anti-inflammatory drugs. BMJ 2002;325(7365):624.
92. Hendel J, Nielsen OH. Expression of cyclooxygenase-2 mRNA in active inflammatory bowel disease. Am J Gastroenterol 1997;92(7):1170–3.
93. Reuter BK, Asfaha S, Buret A, Sharkey KA, Wallace JL. Exacerbation of inflammation-associated colonic injury in rat through inhibition of cyclooxygenase-2. J Clin Invest 1996;98(9):2076–85.
94. Sigthorsson G, Crane R, Simon T, Hoover M, Quan H, Bolognese J, Bjarnason I. COX-2 inhibition with rofecoxib does not increase intestinal permeability in healthy subjects: a double blind crossover study comparing rofecoxib with placebo and indomethacin. Gut 2000;47(4):527–32.
95. Bjarnason I, Thjodleifsson B. Gastrointestinal toxicity of non-steroidal anti-inflammatory drugs: the effect of nimesulide compared with naproxen on the human gastrointestinal tract. Rheumatology (Oxford) 1999;38(Suppl 1):24–32.
96. Reuben SS, Steinberg R. Gastric perforation associated with the use of celecoxib. Anesthesiology 1999;91(5):1548–9.
97. Mohammed S, Croom DW 2nd. Gastropathy due to celecoxib, a cyclooxygenase-2 inhibitor. N Engl J Med 1999;340(25):2005–6.
98. Freitas J, Farricha V, Nascimento I, Borralho P, Parames A. Rofecoxib: a possible cause of acute colitis. J Clin Gastroenterol 2002;34(4):451–3.
99. Godino J, Butani RC, Wong PWK, Murphy FT. Acute drug-induced pancreatitis associated with celecoxib. J Clin Rheumatol 1999;5:305–7.
100. Carrillo-Jimenez R, Nurnberger M. Celecoxib-induced acute pancreatitis and hepatitis: a case report. Arch Intern Med 2000;160(4):553–4.
101. Dunn MJ. Are COX-2 selective inhibitors nephrotoxic? Am J Kidney Dis 2000;35(5):976–7.
102. Perazella MA, Tray K. Selective cyclooxygenase-2 inhibitors: a pattern of nephrotoxicity similar to traditional non-steroidal anti-inflammatory drugs. Am J Med 2001; 111(1):64–7.
103. Noroian G, Clive D. Cyclo-oxygenase-2 inhibitors and the kidney: a case for caution. Drug Saf 2002;25(3):165–72.
104. Alkhuja S, Menkel RA, Alwarshetty M, Ibrahimbacha AM. Celecoxib-induced nonoliguric acute renal failure. Ann Pharmacother 2002;36(1):52–4.
105. Chan FK, Hung LC, Suen BY, Wu JC, Lee KC, Leung VK, Hui AJ, To KF, Leung WK, Wong VW, Chung SC, Sung JJ. Celecoxib versus diclofenac and omeprazole in reducing the risk of recurrent ulcer bleeding in patients with arthritis. N Engl J Med 2002;347(26):2104–10.
106. Whelton A, Schulman G, Wallemark C, Drower EJ, Isakson PC, Verburg KM, Geis GS. Effects of celecoxib and naproxen on renal function in the elderly. Arch Intern Med 2000;160(10):1465–70.
107. Swan SK, Rudy DW, Lasseter KC, Ryan CF, Buechel KL, Lambrecht LJ, Pinto MB, Dilzer SC, Obrda O, Sundblad KJ, Gumbs CP, Ebel DL, Quan H, Larson PJ, Schwartz JI, Musliner TA, Gertz BJ, Brater DC, Yao SL. Effect of cyclooxygenase-2 inhibition on renal function in elderly persons receiving a low-salt diet. A randomized, controlled trial. Ann Intern Med 2000;133(1):1–9.
108. Boyd IW, Mathew TH, Thomas MC. COX-2 inhibitors and renal failure: the triple whammy revisited. Med J Aust 2000;173(5):274.
109. Perazella MA, Eras J. Are selective COX-2 inhibitors nephrotoxic? Am J Kidney Dis 2000;35(5):937–40.
110. Pfister AK, Crisalli RJ, Carter WH. Cyclooxygenase-2 inhibition and renal function. Ann Intern Med 2001;134(11):1077.

111. Graham MG. Acute renal failure related to high-dose celecoxib. Ann Intern Med 2001;135(1):69–70.
112. Wolf G, Porth J, Stahl RA. Acute renal failure associated with rofecoxib. Ann Intern Med 2000;133(5):394.
113. Zhao SZ, Reynolds MW, Lejkowith J, Whelton A, Arellano FM. A comparison of renal-related adverse drug reactions between rofecoxib and celecoxib, based on the World Health Organization/Uppsala Monitoring Centre safety database. Clin Ther 2001; 23(9):1478–91.
114. Park JM, Houck CS, Sethna NF, Sullivan LJ, Atala A, Borer JG, Cilento BG, Diamond DA, Peters CA, Retik AB, Bauer SB. Ketorolac suppresses postoperative bladder spasms after pediatric ureteral reimplantation. Anesth Analg 2000;91(1):11–15.
115. Park JM, Schnermann JB, Briggs JP. Cyclooxygenase-2. A key regulator of bladder prostaglandin formation. Adv Exp Med Biol 1999;462:171–81.
116. Gruenenfelder J, McGuire EJ, Faerber GJ. Acute urinary retention associated with the use of cyclooxygenase-2 inhibitors. J Urol 2002;168(3):1106.
117. Verbeiren S, Morant C, Charlanne H, Ajebbar K, Caron J, Modiano P. Toxidermie au célécoxib (Cerebrex®) avec test epicutané positif. [Celecoxib induced toxiderma with positive patch-test.] Ann Dermatol Venereol 2002;129(2):203–5.
118. Berger P, Dwyer D, Corallo CE. Toxic epidermal necrolysis after celecoxib therapy. Pharmacotherapy 2002; 22(9):1193–5.
119. Sarkar R, Kaur C, Kanwar AJ. Erythema multiforme due to rofecoxib. Dermatology 2002;204(4):304–5.
120. Carder KR, Weston WL. Rofecoxib-induced instant aquagenic wrinkling of the palms. Pediatr Dermatol 2002;19(4):353–5.
121. Amin AR, Attur M, Patel RN, Thakker GD, Marshall PJ, Rediske J, Stuchin SA, Patel IR, Abramson SB. Superinduction of cyclooxygenase-2 activity in human osteoarthritis-affected cartilage. Influence of nitric oxide. J Clin Invest 1997;99(6):1231–7.
122. Norman RJ. Reproductive consequences of COX-2 inhibition. Lancet 2001;358(9290):1287–8.
123. Pall M, Friden BE, Brannstrom M. Induction of delayed follicular rupture in the human by the selective COX-2 inhibitor rofecoxib: a randomized double-blind study. Hum Reprod 2001;16(7):1323–8.
124. Smith G, Roberts R, Hall C, Nuki G. Reversible ovulatory failure associated with the development of luteinized unruptured follicles in women with inflammatory arthritis taking non-steroidal anti-inflammatory drugs. Br J Rheumatol 1996;35(5):458–62.
125. Akil M, Amos RS, Stewart P. Infertility may sometimes be associated with NSAID consumption. Br J Rheumatol 1996;35(1):76–8.
126. Mendonca LL, Khamashta MA, Nelson-Piercy C, Hunt BJ, Hughes GR. Non-steroidal anti-inflammatory drugs as a possible cause for reversible infertility. Rheumatology (Oxford) 2000;39(8):880–2.
127. Stevenson DD, Sanchez-Borges M, Szczeklik A. Classification of allergic and pseudoallergic reactions to drugs that inhibit cyclooxygenase enzymes. Ann Allergy Asthma Immunol 2001;87(3):177–80.
128. Grob M, Pichler WJ, Wuthrich B. Anaphylaxis to celecoxib. Allergy 2002;57(3):264–5.
129. Skowron F, Berard F, Bernard N, Balme B, Perrot H. Cutaneous vasculitis related to celecoxib. Dermatology 2002;204(4):305.
130. Jordan KM, Edwards CJ, Arden NK. Allergic vasculitis associated with celecoxib. Rheumatology (Oxford) 2002;41(12):1453–5.
131. Schneider F, Meziani F, Chartier C, Alt M, Jaeger A. Fatal allergic vasculitis associated with celecoxib. Lancet 2002;359(9309):852–3.
132. Wiholm BE, Shear NH, Knowles S, Shapiro L. Should celecoxib be contraindicated in patients who are allergic to sulfonamides? Drug Saf 2002;25(4):297–9.
133. Kumar NP, Wild G, Ramasamy KA, Snape J. Fatal haemorrhagic pulmonary oedema and associated angioedema after the ingestion of rofecoxib. Postgrad Med J 2002;78(921):439–40.
134. Nettis E, Di PR, Ferrannini A, Tursi A. Tolerability of rofecoxib in patients with cutaneous adverse reactions to nonsteroidal anti-inflammatory drugs. Ann Allergy Asthma Immunol 2002;88(3):331–4.
135. Levy MB, Fink JN. Anaphylaxis to celecoxib. Ann Allergy Asthma Immunol 2001;87(1):72–3.
136. Habki R, Vermeulen C, Bachmeyer C, Charoud A, Mofredj A. Choc anaphylactique au célécoxib. [Anaphylactic shock induced by celecoxib.] Ann Med Interne (Paris) 2001;152(5):355.
137. Schellenberg RR, Isserow SH. Anaphylactoid reaction to a cyclooxygenase-2 inhibitor in a patient who had a reaction to a cyclooxygenase-1 inhibitor. N Engl J Med 2001;345(25):1856.
138. Knowles S, Shapiro L, Shear NH. Should celecoxib be contraindicated in patients who are allergic to sulfonamides? Revisiting the meaning of "sulfa" allergy. Drug Saf 2001;24(4):239–47.
139. Wiholm BE. Identification of sulfonamide-like adverse drug reactions to celecoxib in the World Health Organization database. Curr Med Res Opin 2001;17(3):210–16.
140. Anonymous. COX-2 inhibitor-induced rash. Consultant 2001;41:1338.
141. Kaur C, Sarkar R, Kanwar AJ. Fixed drug eruption to rofecoxib with cross-reactivity to sulfonamides. Dermatology 2001;203(4):351.
142. Sanchez Borges M, Capriles-Hulett A, Caballero-Fonseca F, Perez CR. Tolerability to new COX-2 inhibitors in NSAID-sensitive patients with cutaneous reactions. Ann Allergy Asthma Immunol 2001;87(3):201–4.
143. Warner TD, Giuliano F, Vojnovic I, Bukasa A, Mitchell JA, Vane JR. Nonsteroid drug selectivities for cyclo-oxygenase-1 rather than cyclo-oxygenase-2 are associated with human gastrointestinal toxicity: a full in vitro analysis. Proc Natl Acad Sci USA 1999;96(13):7563–8.
144. Asero R. Tolerability of rofecoxib. Allergy 2001; 56(9):916–17.
145. Berges-Gimeno MP, Camacho-Garrido E, Garcia-Rodriguez RM, Alfaya T, Martin Garcia C, Hinojosa M. Rofecoxib safe in NSAID hypersensitivity. Allergy 2001;56(10):1017–18.
146. Enrique E, Cistero-Bahima A, San Miguel-Moncin MM, Alonso R. Rofecoxib should be tried in NSAID hypersensitivity. Allergy 2000;55(11):1090.
147. Kelkar PS, Butterfield JH, Teaford HG. Urticaria and angioedema from cyclooxygenase-2 inhibitors. J Rheumatol 2001;28(11):2553–4.
148. Sawdy R, Slater D, Fisk N, Edmonds DK, Bennett P. Use of a cyclo-oxygenase type-2-selective non-steroidal anti-inflammatory agent to prevent preterm delivery. Lancet 1997;350(9073):265–6.
149. Lundmark J, Gunnarsson T, Bengtsson F. A possible interaction between lithium and rofecoxib. Br J Clin Pharmacol 2002;53(4):403–4.
150. Ibrahim A, Park S, Feldman J, Karim A, Kharasch ED. Effects of parecoxib, a parenteral COX-2-specific inhibitor, on the pharmacokinetics and pharmacodynamics of propofol. Anesthesiology 2002;96(1):88–95.
151. Schwartz JI, Wong PH, Porras AG, Ebel DL, Hunt TR, Gertz BJ. Effect of rofecoxib on the pharmacokinetics of chronically administered oral contraceptives in healthy female volunteers. J Clin Pharmacol 2002;42(2):215–21.

Cremophor

General Information

Cremophor is a non-ionic solubilizer and emulsifier that is made by reacting ethylene oxide with castor oil (1). It is a pale yellow oily liquid consisting of a mixture of components, primarily polyethylene glycol conjugates. Fatty acid esters of polyethyleneglycol are also present, as well as hydrophilic polyethylene glycols and ethoxylated glycerol. It is present in intravenous formulations of the anticancer drugs teniposide and paclitaxel. The paclitaxel formulation consists of 6 mg/ml in 50% ethanol and 50% Cremophor. Thus, a patient receiving paclitaxel in the widely used dose of 175 mg/m^2 will also receive about 14 ml/m^2 of Cremophor.

Anaphylactoid reactions can occur after the intravenous administration of Cremophor (SEDA-22, 526) when it is used as a diluent of alfadolone/afaxolone (SED-11, 211) (2), ciclosporin (3), paclitaxel (4), propanidid (SED-11, 211) (5,6), teniposide (7), and vitamin K (8,9). Cardiorespiratory arrest after intravenous miconazole has been attributed to the histamine-releasing properties of Cremophor (10).

In a study of the effects of Cremophor after 74 cycles of doxorubicin in Cremophor in 39 patients, there were no major hypersensitivity reactions to Cremophor, and no patients had their infusion discontinued or modified (11). Adverse effects that were considered to be potentially related to Cremophor were cutaneous (pruritus, flushing, or rashes), hypotension or dizziness, and headache. Because of the subjective nature of some of these symptoms, they were classified as grade 1 (mild and not requiring treatment or interfering with function), grade 2 (moderate, causing some impairment of function but not requiring hospitalization), or grade 3 (severe, requiring hospitalization or causing significant interference with function). No grade 2 or 3 toxicity was recorded at the first three doses. One patient at level 4A had grade 2 dizziness, one patient at level 5 had grade 2 rash, one patient at level 5 had grade 3 headache and grade 3 pruritus, and one patient at level 6 had grade 3 hypotension and grade 3 rash. In no patient did these symptoms occur with doxorubicin alone, confirming their relation to Cremophor. These symptoms began several hours to days after Cremophor and persisted for 1–2 weeks, with the exception of the patient at level 5, whose pruritus gradually resolved over 3 months after discontinuing Cremophor.

Organs and Systems

Hematologic

The hematological toxicity of Cremophor has been evaluated after 74 cycles of doxorubicin in Cremophor in 39 patients (11). The principal effect was neutropenia. The incidence of grade 4 neutropenia increased with increasing doses of Cremophor from 1 to 60 ml/m^2. Grade 4 neutropenia occurred in zero of three patients at 1 ml/m^2, one of four patients at 7.5 ml/m^2, four of six patients at 15 ml/m^2, and 11 of 16 patients at 30 ml/m^2. When the dose of doxorubicin was reduced, grade 4 neutropenia occurred in one of six patients at 45 ml/m^2 and two of four patients at 60 ml/m^2. Febrile neutropenia occurred in one patient at 15 ml/m^2, three patients at 30 ml/m^2, one patient at 45 ml/m^2, and one patient at 60 ml/m^2. There was one death from neutropenic sepsis at 30 ml/m^2.

References

1. Anonymous. Cremophor EL. BASF Technical Leaflet MEF 1986;074e.
2. Anonymous. Glaxo discontinues Althesin. Scrip 1984;882:17.
3. Volcheck GW, Van Dellen RG. Anaphylaxis to intravenous cyclosporine and tolerance to oral cyclosporine: case report and review. Ann Allergy Asthma Immunol 1998;80(2):159–63.
4. Rowinsky EK, Eisenhauer EA, Chaudhry V, Arbuck SG, Donehower RC. Clinical toxicities encountered with paclitaxel (Taxol). Semin Oncol 1993;20(4 Suppl 3):1–15.
5. Baraka A, Sfeir S. Anaphylactic cardiac arrest in a parturient. Response of the newborn. JAMA 1980;243(17):1745–6.
6. Dye D, Watkins J. Suspected anaphylactic reaction to Cremophor EL. BMJ 1980;280(6228):1353.
7. Weiss RB. Hypersensitivity reactions. Semin Oncol 1992;19(5):458–77.
8. Martin JC. Anaphylactoid reactions and vitamin K. Med J Aust 1991;155(11–12):851.
9. Leo MA, Kim C, Lowe N, Lieber CS. Interaction of ethanol with beta-carotene: delayed blood clearance and enhanced hepatotoxicity. Hepatology 1992;15(5):883–91.
10. Drouhet E, Dupont B. Evolution of antifungal agents: past, present, and future Rev Infect Dis 1987;9(Suppl 1): S4–14.
11. Millward MJ, Webster LK, Rischin D, Stokes KH, Toner GC, Bishop JF, Olver IN, Linahan BM, Linsenmeyer ME, Woodcock DM. Phase I trial of cremophor EL with bolus doxorubicin. Clin Cancer Res 1998;4(10):2321–9.

Cromoglicate sodium

General Information

Cromoglicate disodium salt (cromoglicate sodium) is available as a powder for inhalation. Each capsule contains 20 mg. The usual dose is 1 capsule inhaled four times daily. It is also dispensed in a multidose-pressurized aerosol delivering 1 or 5 mg per actuation. A 1.0% nebulizer solution (20 mg dissolved in 2 ml of distilled water) is also available. It is nebulized over 15 minutes and has the same effect as 20 mg given as a powder (1). Cromoglicate is taken regularly in chronic asthma and when it is effective it improves symptoms and lung function and reduces the need for bronchodilators. It has a steroid-sparing effect and should be tried before inhaled steroids are used, especially in children. It is a prophylactic drug and is not effective in acute asthma.

A liquid form is also available for use in rhinitis and ocular conditions. When applied topically to the eye cromoglicate is effective in the treatment of vernal keratoconjunctivitis (vernal catarrh, spring catarrh), allergic conjunctivitis, and hay fever.

Cromoglicate inhibits mast-cell degranulation and histamine release induced by phospholipase A2, but does not interfere with the interaction of antigen and reaginic antibodies. Evidence is accumulating that it has an important stabilizing action on leukocytes, apart from mast cells, such as neutrophils, eosinophils, and monocytes, and that it also affects nerve reflexes in the lung (2).

The overall incidence of adverse effects was about 2% when using inhaled cromoglicate (3). Most of the observed adverse effects are mild and transient and do not require withdrawal of therapy. Adverse effects such as laryngeal edema, swollen parotid glands, bronchospasm, joint swelling, nausea, cough, headache, nasal congestion, rash, and urticaria have been reported in only one in 10 000 patients (SEDA-12, 142). The American Academy of Allergy and Immunology reported two 10-year safety reports involving 424 and 85 patients. These emphasized the safety of long-term treatment with cromoglicate. The only serious adverse effects were three cases of pulmonary infiltration and eosinophilia (SEDA-6, 171). In another series of 375 patients, only eight experienced adverse reactions; these included dermatitis with pruritus, myositis, and gastroenteritis (SEDA-4, 120).

While no systemic or severe adverse reactions have been attributed to ocular cromoglicate even after as long as 8 months of therapy, transient local stinging and burning have been reported in 13–77% of patients who used the original formulation of this drug, which contained 2-phenylethyl alcohol as a preservative. These effects regressed during continued treatment and can vary greatly depending on both the individual and the underlying disease. Ocular cromoglicate without 2-phenylethyl alcohol has been reported to be more effective than formulations that contain this preservative; stinging, leading to increased lacrimation, dilutes the drug and reduces the time for which it is retained in the conjunctival sac. The desired topical effects of cromoglicate are therefore reduced if it is formulated with 2-phenylethyl alcohol.

Organs and Systems

Cardiovascular

- A woman developed peripheral eosinophilia and pericarditis with cardiac tamponade after using cromoglicate (SEDA-4, 120). Cellular and humoral sensitivity to cromoglicate were demonstrated and she recovered following pericardiocentesis.

Respiratory

Initial bronchospasm, seen in some patients, is thought to be due to the irritant effect of the dry powder. This can be prevented by prior inhalation of a $beta_2$-adrenoceptor agonist. In one case, a severe asthmatic reaction occurred and was thought to be reflexogenic in origin (SEDA-4, 120). Inhalation of nebulized cromoglicate by asthmatic children causes a reduction in forced mid-expiratory flow rate equivalent to that seen with distilled water (SEDA-17, 205). Bronchospasm and breathlessness as a result of hypersensitivity are rare, but do occur.

Rarely, a hypersensitivity reaction can cause bronchospasm or aggravation of existing asthma and a progressive fall in FEV_1, resulting in dyspnea (4).

Three cases of pulmonary infiltration with eosinophilia were reported among a total of 509 patients treated with cromoglicate (SEDA-6, 171).

- A 7-year-old asthmatic child, sensitive to timothy grass, used inhaled cromoglicate for 1 week and developed cyanosis, hypotension, and cardiopulmonary arrest. IgE involvement was demonstrated by passive transfer of the patient's serum to the mother (5).

Ear, nose, throat

Intranasal use of cromoglicate can cause sneezing and nasal congestion. There is nasal irritation in 35% of patients, swollen sore eyes in 17%, and a sore throat in 21%. The sensitive nasal mucosa can be susceptible to irritation by any nasal spray (6).

Nervous system

Most investigators have referred to headaches, but no clear relation to cromoglicate has been seen in any study. Dizziness has been reported, but may be connected with hyperventilation during the inhalation of the powder.

Sensory systems

The irritant effect of cromoglicate can cause lacrimation and inflammatory changes in the eye.

An allergic reaction to cromoglicate eye drops has been reported. After application of the eye-drops intense itching, burning, redness, and severe swelling of both conjunctivae developed immediately. Skin prick tests and conjunctival provocation with pure cromoglicate were positive. Circulating IgE-specific antibodies to cromoglicate were demonstrated by RAST (7).

Gastrointestinal

Nausea can occur. Esophagitis following inhalation of cromoglicate has been reported. It was much improved by prophylactic antacids given before each inhalation (SEDA-5, 169). In a patient with lactose intolerance, cromoglicate disodium capsules with lactose produced nausea, bloating, and flatulence. Lactose-free formulations produced no such symptoms (SEDA-13, 135).

Liver

Minor abnormalities of liver function have been described when cromoglicate is used orally for ulcerative colitis (8).

- A 45-year-old woman developed liver disease, vasculitis, and peripheral eosinophilia (SEDA-4, 120). Liver biopsy showed inflammatory changes with infiltration of eosinophils. Withdrawal of the drug markedly improved the symptoms.

Skin

Skin reactions including dermatitis with pruritus have been reported in patients using cromoglicate. Urticaria or maculopapular rashes occur rarely.

Musculoskeletal

Bone mineral density was measured after 7.4 months in 49 asthmatic children, 38 of whom took inhaled beclomethasone, average daily dose 276 μg, and 11 sodium cromoglicate, average daily dose 30 mg. Children who had used beclomethasone had grown as much as those who used sodium cromoglicate. Trabecular and cortical bone mineral density in the proximal forearm and lumbar spine increased to the same extent in both groups.

The effects of fluticasone 50 μg bd or cromoglicate 20 mg qds on growth over 12 months have been studied in 122 asthmatic children aged 4–10 years (9). The mean height velocity was 6 cm/year with fluticasone and 6.5 cm/year with sodium cromoglicate. There was no significant treatment difference in the mean 24-hour urinary free cortisol concentrations at 6 or 12 months. Mean predicted peak expiratory flow rate improved over 1 year in both groups, but to a greater extent with fluticasone. Fluticasone was more effective than sodium cromoglicate, with fewer withdrawals and greater improvement in lung function.

Immunologic

Immunological reactions to cromoglicate can involve the pericardium, the lung, the eye, the nasal mucosa, the skin, the joints, and the liver. Rarely, a hypersensitivity reaction can cause fever (4). A survey of the world literature up to 1982 found 13 cases of facial rash, urticaria, and/or generalized dermatitis, and one of nasal congestion. In 19 patients there was bronchospasm and/or pulmonary edema, eventually culminating in shock. Four cases of eosinophilic or granulomatous pulmonary infiltration, one of liver disease and vasculitis, one of pericarditis, and three of polymyositis were reported.

IgE and/or specifically reactive lymphocytes do not mediate many of the adverse reactions to cromoglicate, which mimic allergic processes of the immediate or delayed type. These reactions fulfilled the criteria that characterize pseudo-allergic reactions (3,10). There is a much higher incidence of such adverse reactions when cromoglicate is used orally in the treatment of food allergy, as high as 29% of cases treated (3,10).

The US Food and Drug Administration has issued a report (SEDA-7, 1) on a suspected case of cromoglicate-induced lupus-like syndrome. Treatment with cromoglicate for 6 months resulted in arthritis, positive LE cells, and a positive antinuclear factor. After withdrawal of cromoglicate, the signs and symptoms regressed. Although this does not prove cause and effect, the report suggests a similarity between lupus-like syndrome and some of the adverse reactions that were listed earlier in the US data sheet (SEDA-3, 48).

Second-Generation Effects

Teratogenicity

Cromoglicate probably does not reach the fetus after inhalation, as systemic blood concentrations are extremely low (11). Animal testing did not show any teratogenic effects.

A critical review of drug therapy for allergic rhinitis during pregnancy has been published (12). Mast cell stabilizers are not teratogenic and can be considered as excellent first-line choices to treat allergic conjunctivitis and rhinitis. However, any recommendation should be accompanied by informed consent.

Drug Administration

Drug administration route

No systemic or severe adverse reactions have been attributed to ocular sodium cromoglicate, even after as long as 8 months of therapy. However, transient local stinging and burning were reported in 13–77% of patients who used the original formulation of this drug, which contained 2-phenylethyl alcohol as a preservative. These effects regressed during continued treatment and varied greatly depending on the individual and the underlying disease. Ocular sodium cromoglicate without 2-phenylethyl alcohol has been reported to be more effective; stinging, leading to increased lacrimation, dilutes the drug and reduces the time it is retained in the conjunctival sac. The desired topical effects of sodium cromoglicate are therefore reduced if it is formulated with 2-phenylethyl alcohol.

References

1. Marks MB. Nebulized cromolyn sodium: efficacy and safety. Immunol Allergy Pract 1984;6:130–4.
2. Garland LG. Pharmacology of prophylactic anti-asthma drugs. In: Page CP, Barnes PJ, editors. Pharmacology of Asthma. Berlin: Springer-Verlag, 1991:261–90.
3. Kallos P, Kallos L. Pseudo-allergic reactions due to sodium cromoglycate. In: Dukor P, Kallos P, Schlumberger HD, West GB, editors. Pseudo-allergic Reactions. Involvement of Drugs and Chemicals. Basel: Karger, 1982:122–32.
4. Repo UK, Nieminen P. Pulmonary infiltrates with eosinophilia and urinary symptoms during disodium cromoglycate treatment. A case report. Scand J Respir Dis 1976;57(1):1–4.
5. Brown LA, Kaplan RA, Benjamin PA, Hoffman LS, Shearer WT. Immunoglobulin E-mediated anaphylaxis with inhaled cromolyn sodium. J Allergy Clin Immunol 1981;68(6):416–20.
6. Brown HM, Engler C, English JR. A comparative trial of flunisolide and sodium cromoglycate nasal sprays in the treatment of seasonal allergic rhinitis. Clin Allergy 1981;11(2):169–73.
7. Valdivieso R, Subiza J, Varela-Losada S, Subiza JL, Narganes MJ, Cabrera M, Serrano L. Severe allergic conjunctivitis and chemosis caused by disodium cromoglycate. J Investig Allergol Clin Immunol 1998;8(1):58–60.
8. Mani V, Lloyd G, Green FH, Fox H, Turnberg LA. Treatment of ulcerative colitis with oral disodium cromoglycate. A double-blind controlled trial. Lancet 1976;1(7957):439–41.

9. Price JF, Russell G, Hindmarsh PC, Weller P, Heaf DP, Williams J. Growth during one year of treatment with fluticasone propionate or sodium cromoglycate in children with asthma. Pediatr Pulmonol 1997;24(3):178–86.
10. Sheffer AL, Rocklin RE, Goetzl EJ. Immunologic components of hypersensitivity reactions to cromolyn sodium. N Engl J Med 1975;293(24):1220–4.
11. Walker SR, Evans ME, Richards AJ, Paterson JW. The fate of (14 C)disodium cromoglycate in man. J Pharm Pharmacol 1972;24(7):525–31.
12. Mazzotta P, Loebstein R, Koren G. Treating allergic rhinitis in pregnancy. Safety considerations. Drug Saf 1999;20(4):361–75.

Crotetamide

General Information

Crotetamide is a mixture in equal parts by weight of cropropamide and crotethamide. It has similar actions to doxapram hydrochloride and has been used as a respiratory stimulant in man as well as illicitly in racehorses. When crotetamide was given intravenously, the incidence of adverse effects was 25% (1–3).

Organs and Systems

Nervous system

Flushing, paresthesia, headache, restlessness, muscle twitching, tremor, and dyspnea have been ascribed to crotetamide. Convulsions have been reported but are rare.

References

1. Merck & Co. The Merck Index. 1960.
2. Entretiens de Physiopathologie Respiratoire, Nancy 21–23. Septembre, 1962. Place des analeptiques en pathologie respiratoire. [The role of analeptic agents in respiratory pathology.] Presse Méd 1963;71:1336.
3. New and Non-Official Drugs. 1964.

Crystalloids

General Information

Potassium and sodium salts are given intravenously in solutions to replace body fluids and electrolytes. Adverse effects are rare and usually limited to the effects of overtransfusion.

Microwave heating of crystalloid fluids has been recommended as a method of correcting hypothermia during resuscitation. Severe full-thickness burns and venous thrombosis occurred after infusion of over-heated crystalloid fluid in the management of a ruptured aortic aneurysm in a 75-year-old man (1). Measuring the temperature of the fluid before starting the infusion is necessary to avoid this complication.

Organs and Systems

Nervous system

Central pontine myelinolysis has been reported in patients given intravenous saline (2). Pontine and extrapontine myelinolysis are generally considered to be linked with rapid correction of severe hyponatremia, for example in the treatment of hyponatremia in patients with so-called hyperosmolar non-ketoacidotic hyperglycemia reference. Neurological deterioration is likely to result. It is not certain what rate of sodium repletion is safe. The best data available suggest that correction should not exceed 12 mmol/l per day, although more rapid correction may be safe. The duration of treatment also seems to be important: 12 mmol/l per day may be excessive if continued for more than 2 or 3 days.

Accurate control of the serum sodium is a major difficulty in the setting of severe hyponatremia. The administration of an amount of hypertonic saline calculated to raise the sodium to mildly hyponatremic concentrations can result in serum sodium in the normonatremic or even hypernatremic range. The serum sodium should not be allowed to raise more that 12 mmol/l over the first 24 hours, and even less over each subsequent 24-hour period. It is clear that an amount of saline calculated to raise the serum sodium by a given amount affects individuals differently. This makes frequent monitoring of serum sodium mandatory.

Gastrointestinal

Gastric and upper small bowel necrosis have been described after oral ingestion of massive amounts of concentrated saline (1 kg of sodium chloride in 660 ml of water) as an emetic.

Second-Generation Effects

Pregnancy

The value of intravenous crystalloid administration in preventing hypotension developing during spinal anesthesia in parturition has been questioned (3). Moreover, the association between increasing crystalloid volume and reducing postpartum colloid osmotic pressure raises concerns about the risks of maternal and fetal pulmonary edema. In a comparative study of the dose–response effects of crystalloid fluids before spinal anesthesia, all groups had a fall in mean arterial blood pressure and systemic vascular resistance index, measured using non-invasive thoracic impedance monitoring (3). The extent of the fall did not differ according to the volume given. There were no differences in neonatal colloid osmotic pressure with varying preload. No apparent benefit is to be gained in healthy parturients by giving crystalloid in volumes up to 30 ml/kg.

References

1. Sieunarine K, White GH. Full-thickness burn and venous thrombosis following intravenous infusion of microwave-heated crystalloid fluids. Burns 1996;22(7):568–9.
2. Laureno R, Karp BI. Pontine and extrapontine myelinolysis following rapid correction of hyponatraemia. Lancet 1988;1(8600):1439–41.

3. Park GE, Hauch MA, Curlin F, Datta S, Bader AM. The effects of varying volumes of crystalloid administration before cesarean delivery on maternal hemodynamics and colloid osmotic pressure. Anesth Analg 1996; 83(2):299–303.

Cucurbitaceae

See also Herbal medicines

General Information

The genera in the family of Cucurbitaceae (Table 1) include cucumbers, gourds, and melons.

Bryonia alba

Bryonia alba (white bryony) contains toxic triterpenoids called cucurbitacins.

Adverse effects

Cucurbitacins are drastic laxatives and emetics and can cause the symptoms of food poisoning (1).

Citrullus colocynthis

The dried pulp of the fruit of *Citrullus colocynthis* (colocynth) is a drastic laxative, which contains toxic cucurbitacins.

Table 1 The genera of Cucurbitaceae

Apodanthera (apodanthera)
Benincasa (benincasa)
Brandegea (starvine)
Bryonia (bryony)
Cayaponia (melonleaf)
Citrullus (watermelon)
Coccinia (coccinia)
Ctenolepis (ctenolepis)
Cucumis (melon)
Cucumeropsis (cucumeropsis)
Cucurbita (gourd)
Cyclanthera (cyclanthera)
Doyerea (doyeria)
Ecballium (squirting cucumber)
Echinocystis (echinocystis)
Echinopepon (balsam apple)
Fevillea (fevillea)
Hodgsonia (hodgsonia)
Ibervillea (globeberry)
Lagenaria (lagenaria)
Luffa (luffa)
Marah (manroot)
Melothria (melothria)
Momordica (momordica)
Psiguria (pygmymelon)
Sechium (sechium)
Sicana (sicana)
Sicyos (burr cucumber)
Sicyosperma (sicyosperma)
Telfairia (telfairia)
Thladiantha (thladiantha)
Trichosanthes (trichosanthes)
Tumamoca (tumamoca)

Adverse effects

A man experienced vomiting, colicky pain, and bloody diarrhea after self-medication with *C. colocynthis* (2). Hemorrhagic colitis secondary to ingestion of colocynth has been reported (2). In three cases of toxic acute colitis 8–12 hours after ingestion of colocynth for ritual purposes, the prominent clinical feature was dysenteric diarrhea; colonoscopic changes included congestion and hyperemia of the mucosa with abundant exudates but no ulceration or pseudopolyp formation; there was rapid recovery within 3–6 days, with normal endoscopy at day 14 (3).

Ecballium elaterium

Ecballium elaterium (squirting cucumber) contains toxic cucurbitacins, which are violent purgatives. It is used in the Mediterranean as a purgative and in treating sinusitis.

Adverse effects

Intranasal use of *E. elaterium* has been associated with Quincke's edema (4) and with fatal cardiac and renal failure (5).

A report from a poisons unit in Israel included 13 patients who had used the juice of the squirting cucumber, either orally or topically, for unreported reasons (6). They subsequently had edema of the pharynx, dyspnea, drooling, dysphagia, vomiting, and conjunctivitis. With symptomatic treatment they recovered within a few days.

In a retrospective chart analysis in a Greek ENT department 42 patients with allergic reactions to *E. elaterium*, including upper airway edema, were identified (7). Treatment with glucocorticoids and antihistamines resulted in full recovery in all cases.

Momordica charantia

Oral formulations of *Momordica charantia* (karela fruit, bitter melon) have hypoglycemic activity in non-insulin dependent diabetes mellitus (8,9), and can interfere with conventional treatment with diet and chlorpropamide (10). In 15 patients aged 52–65 years a soft extract of *M. charantia* plus half doses of metformin or glibenclamide or both in combination caused hypoglycemia greater than that caused by full doses during treatment for 7 days (11). Subcutaneous injection of a principle obtained from the fruit may lower blood glucose concentrations in juvenile diabetes.

Adverse effects

Metabolism

M. charantia can cause hypoglycemic coma and convulsions in children (12).

Drug interactions

M. charantia inhibits P glycoprotein in vitro and drug interactions can therefore be expected (13).

Sechium edule

The tuber of *Sechium edule* (chayote) is valued as a potent diuretic by Latin American populations. Its use as a decoction by a pregnant woman suffering from pedal edema may have been the cause of a severe case of hypokalemia (14).

References

1. Kirschman JC, Suber RL. Recent food poisonings from cucurbitacin in traditionally bred squash. Food Chem Toxicol 1989;27(8):555–6.
2. Al Faraj S. Haemorrhagic colitis induced by *Citrullus colocynthis*. Ann Trop Med Parasitol 1995;89(6):695–6.
3. Goldfain D, Lavergne A, Galian A, Chauveinc L, Prudhomme F. Peculiar acute toxic colitis after ingestion of colocynth: a clinicopathological study of three cases. Gut 1989;30(10):1412–18.
4. Plouvier B, Trotin F, Deram R, De Coninck P, Baclet JL. Concombre d'ane (*Ecbalium elaterium*) une cause peu banale d'oedème de Quincke. [Squirting cucumber (*Ecbalium elaterium*), an uncommon cause of Quincke's edema.] Nouv Presse Méd 1981;10(31):2590.
5. Vlachos P, Kanitsakis NN, Kokonas N. Fatal cardiac and renal failure due to *Ecbalium elaterium* (squirting cucumber). J Toxicol Clin Toxicol 1994;32(6):737–8.
6. Raikhlin-Eisenkraft B, Bentur Y. *Ecbalium elaterium* (squirting cucumber)—remedy or poison? J Toxicol Clin Toxicol 2000;38(3):305–8.
7. Kloutsos G, Balatsouras DG, Kaberos AC, Kandiloros D, Ferekidis E, Economou C. Upper airway edema resulting from use of *Ecballium elaterium*. Laryngoscope 2001;111(9):1652–5.
8. Welihinda J, Karunanayake EH, Sheriff MH, Jayasinghe KS. Effect of *Momordica charantia* on the glucose tolerance in maturity onset diabetes. J Ethnopharmacol 1986;17(3):277–82.
9. Leatherdale BA, Panesar RK, Singh G, Atkins TW, Bailey CJ, Bignell AH. Improvement in glucose tolerance due to *Momordica charantia* (karela). BMJ (Clin Res Ed) 1981;282(6279):1823–4.
10. Aslam M, Stockley IH. Interaction between curry ingredient (karela) and drug (chlorpropamide). Lancet 1979;1(8116):607.
11. Tongia A, Tongia SK, Dave M. Phytochemical determination and extraction of *Momordica charantia* fruit and its hypoglycemic potentiation of oral hypoglycemic drugs in diabetes mellitus (NIDDM). Indian J Physiol Pharmacol 2004;48(2):241–4.
12. Basch E, Gabardi S, Ulbricht C. Bitter melon (*Momordica charantia*): a review of efficacy and safety. Am J Health Syst Pharm 2003;60(4):356–9.
13. Limtrakul P, Khantamat O, Pintha K. Inhibition of P-glycoprotein activity and reversal of cancer multidrug resistance by *Momordica charantia* extract. Cancer Chemother Pharmacol 2004;54(6):525–30.
14. Jensen LP, Lai AR. Chayote (*Sechium edule*) causing hypokalemia in pregnancy. Am J Obstet Gynecol 1986;155(5):1048–9.

Cuprammonium cellulose

General Information

Cuprammonium cellulose is a constituent of some dialysis membranes (1).

Organs and Systems

Immunologic

Anaphylaxis as an adverse effect of hemodialysis has been analysed from records of about 260 000 courses of dialysis treatment, at three centers. There were 21 severe reactions over the 10.5-year period of the survey, all highly suggestive of anaphylaxis (2). Reactions occurred within minutes of initiating dialysis and were characterized by cardiopulmonary, mucocutaneous, and/or gastrointestinal tract symptoms. Four respiratory arrests occurred and there was one death. When the individual histories and treatments were analysed, there was strong evidence that hollow-fiber dialysers made of cuprammonium cellulose were responsible. No obvious factors could be found to identify predisposed patients; suboptimal rinsing of the cuprammonium cellulose hollow-fiber dialysers before use may have been responsible for some of the reactions. Repeated dialysis anaphylaxis in one patient has been reported (3).

References

1. Bowry SK. Dialysis membranes today. Int J Artif Organs 2002;25(5):447–60.
2. Daugirdas JT, Ing TS, Roxe DM, Ivanovich PT, Krumlovsky F, Popli S, McLaughlin MM. Severe anaphylactoid reactions to cuprammonium cellulose hemodialyzers. Arch Intern Med 1985;145(3):489–94.
3. Wenzel-Seifert K, Sharma AM, Keller F. Repeated dialysis anaphylaxia. Nephrol Dial Transplant 1990;5(9):821–4.

Cupressaceae

See also Herbal medicines

General Information

The genera in the family of Cupressaceae (Table 1) include cedar, cypress, and juniper.

Juniperus communis

Extracts of *Juniperus communis* and other species are used in cosmetics, as hair conditioners, and in fragrances (1). The volatile oil distilled from the berries of *Juniperus communis* (juniper) can act as a gastrointestinal irritant. It is said that excessive doses can cause renal damage, and use during pregnancy is discouraged because of a fear that this might also stimulate the uterus.

Table 1 The genera of Cupressaceae

Callitris (cypress pine)
Calocedrus (incense cedar)
Chamaecyparis (cedar)
Cupressus (cypress)
Cupressocyparis
Juniperus (juniper)
Platycladus (platycladus)
Tetraclinis (tetraclinis)
Thuja (red cedar)

Reference

1. Anonymous. Final report on the safety assessment of *Juniperus communis* extract, *Juniperus oxycedrus* extract, *Juniperus oxycedrus* tar, *Juniperus phoenicea* extract, and *Juniperus virginiana* extract. Int J Toxicol 2001; 20(Suppl 2):41–56.

Cyanoacrylates

General Information

Cyanoacrylate (Histoacryl) is a tissue adhesive used in duraplasty. The sites at which it is used should be carefully chosen. Cyanoacrylates are also in use for embolization of arteriovenous malformations in the brain. The risk of this procedure is the creation of pulmonary emboli after acrylate glue injection, particularly when delivery systems without flow arrest are used in high-flow vascular brain lesions. Techniques using acetic acid to delay polymerization time and "sandwich" techniques, in which glue is pushed with dextrose, appear to be more likely to cause this complication (1).

Organs and Systems

Immunologic

Infection can develop in the frontal area and at the lateral base of the skull after the use of cyanoacrylates, even after a symptom-free interval of several years; the lesions can be characterized by infected granular nodules, chronic sinusitis, or otogenic meningitis (2).

References

1. Pelz DM, Lownie SP, Fox AJ, Hutton LC. Symptomatic pulmonary complications from liquid acrylate embolization of brain arteriovenous malformations. AJNR Am J Neuroradiol 1995;16(1):19–26.
2. Chilla R. Histoacryl-induzierte Spatkomplikationen nach Duraplastiken an der Fronto- und Otobasis. [Late histoacryl-induced complications of dura surgery in the frontal and lateral base of the skull.] HNO 1987;35(6):250–1.

Cycadaceae

See also Herbal medicines

General Information

The family of Cycadaceae contains the single genus *Cycas*.

Cycas circinalis

The seeds of *Cycas circinalis* (false sago palm, queen sago) contain the non-protein amino acid beta-*N*-methylamino-L-alanine, which is similar to the neurotoxic amino acid beta-*N*-oxalylamino-L-alanine. Monkeys fed this amino acid develop a syndrome that closely resembles the disease that is known by the Chamorros of Guam as lytico-bodig, a complex of amyotrophic lateral sclerosis parkinsonism dementia that occurs in Guam, where the seeds of *C. circinalis* are a traditional staple of the indigenous diet (1). Consumption of flying foxes may also generate sufficiently high cumulative doses of *Cycas* neurotoxins, since the flying foxes forage on cycad seeds (2). The risk may be increased by the use of poultices prepared from cycad seeds as a topical cure for skin lesions in Eastern Irian Jaya (New Guinea), Indonesia.

Adverse effects

In a retrospective chart review at the Poison Control Center in Taiwan from 1990 to 2001 there were 21 cases of *Cycas* seed poisoning (3). The patients had taken 1–30 seeds for cosmetic use (5%), as edible food (70%), or for health promotion (10%), cancer prevention (10%), and gastrointestinal discomfort (5%). All had eaten the seeds after washing and cooking them. The time from ingestion to the onset of symptoms ranged from 30 minutes to 7 hours (mean 2.8 hours). All the patients except one presented with gastrointestinal disturbances, and 90% sought medical care at the emergency department. Severe vomiting was the most striking symptom. There was no respiratory depression. Within 24 hours all had recovered. Six patients had blood cyanide or thiocyanate concentrations measured, and although they were higher than normal, they did not reach the toxic range.

References

1. Spencer PS, Nunn PB, Hugon J, Ludolph A, Roy DN. Motorneurone disease on Guam: possible role of a food neurotoxin. Lancet 1986;1(8487):965.
2. Cox PA, Sacks OW. Cycad neurotoxins, consumption of flying foxes, and ALS-PDC disease in Guam. Neurology 2002;58(6):956–9.
3. Chang SS, Chan YL, Wu ML, Deng JF, Chiu T, Chen JC, Wang FL, Tseng CP. Acute *Cycas* seed poisoning in Taiwan. J Toxicol Clin Toxicol 2004;42(1):49–54.

Cyclandelate

General Information

The spasmolytic action of cyclandelate, an ester of mandelic acid, was described as early as 1959, but only in later years have its properties been more fully investigated. It appears to act as a calcium channel blocker in smooth muscle and platelets, this effect being partly due to inhibition of phosphodiesterases. It also produces increased deformability of erythrocytes, the mechanism of which is so far unknown, although phosphodiesterase inhibition may again be responsible. Cyclandelate also reduces the activity of the rate-limiting enzyme in the biosynthesis of cholesterol (HMG-CoA), and its "antidiabetic" properties may be due to inhibition of aldose reductase.

Cyclandelate is mainly given to elderly patients with mild to moderate cognitive impairment; it is also used in the prophylaxis of migraine. Its efficacy is not impressive (SEDA-21, 215) (1).

Major adverse effects have not been reported with dosages of 1.6 g/day. Gastrointestinal upset, flushing, and tingling are rare and minor complaints. Even elderly patients apparently tolerate 3.2 g/day without problems (SEDA-9, 189).

Reference

1. Diener HC, Krupp P, Schmitt T, Steitz G, Milde K, Freytag S. Cyclandelate in the prophylaxis of migraine: a placebo-controlled study. Cephalalgia 2001;21(1):66–70.

Cyclazocine

General Information

Cyclazocine is an agonist at OP_2 (κ) opioid receptors and it is its affinity for these receptors that is thought to account for disruption of the normal sleep pattern, urination, and sustained arousal that it causes (1). Visual disturbances and racing thoughts have also been reported and are subject to tolerance (2).

Long-Term Effects

Drug withdrawal

Abrupt withdrawal resulted in a classical withdrawal syndrome, but without drug-seeking behavior (2). Adverse effects could be minimized by gradual increments in daily dosage over 3 weeks.

References

1. Pickworth WB, Neidert GL, Kay DC. Cyclazocine-induced sleep disruptions in nondependent addicts. Prog Neuropsychopharmacol Biol Psychiatry 1986;10(1):77–85.
2. Resnick RB, Schuyten-Resnick E, Washton AM. Narcotic antagonists in the treatment of opioid dependence: review and commentary. Compr Psychiatry 1979;20(2): 116–25.

Cyclizine

See also Antihistamines

General Information

Cyclizine is a first-generation antihistamine, a piperazine derivative, with sedative and antimuscarinic activity, although its sedative effects are not marked.

Organs and Systems

Nervous system

Four cases of dystonic reactions caused by single doses of cyclizine have been reported (1–4).

Long-Term Effects

Drug abuse

Abuse of cyclizine in teenagers has been described (5).

References

1. King H, Corry P, Wauchob T, Barclay P. Probable dystonic reaction after a single dose of cyclizine in a patient with a history of encephalitis. Anaesthesia 2003;58(3):257–60.
2. Dagg LE, Wrathall DW. Dystonic reactions to cyclizine. Anaesthesia 2003;58(7):724.
3. Sewell A, Nixon M. Dystonic reaction to cyclizine. Anaesthesia 2003;58(9):928.
4. Michailidou M, Peck T. Dystonic reaction to cyclizine. Anaesthesia 2004;59(4):413–14.
5. Bassett KE, Schunk JE, Crouch BI. Cyclizine abuse by teenagers in Utah. Am J Emerg Med 1996;14(5):472–4.

Cyclobenzaprine

General Information

Cyclobenzaprine is a centrally acting skeletal-muscle relaxant, claimed to be effective in providing relief of muscle spasm, pain and tenderness, and in reducing the limitations imposed thereby on normal daily activities. The recommended total oral daily dose is 10–30 mg (1). It is structurally similar to the tricyclic antidepressants and adverse effects similar to those seen with the tricyclic antidepressants are therefore to be expected.

The most common adverse effects of cyclobenzaprine are somnolence, dry mucous membranes, dizziness, and confusion. Less commonly, tachycardia, dysarthria, disorientation, and hallucinations have been reported (2).

Organs and Systems

Cardiovascular

Cyclobenzaprine can occasionally cause marked arteriolar spasm due to increased adrenergic tone, precipitating Raynaud's syndrome (SEDA-6, 132).

Psychological, psychiatric

Rarely, manic psychosis can be activated in patients with bipolar affective disorders (3).

First-onset paranoid psychosis has also been reported (4).

- A 36-year-old woman with no past psychiatric problems took 23 tablets of cyclobenzaprine (10 mg each) over 6 weeks to ease back pain resulting from a back injury. She developed insomnia, reduced appetite, poor concentration, irritability, disorganized thoughts, persecutory delusions, and auditory hallucinations. Cyclobenzaprine was withdrawn and a course of loxapine was started, leading to rapid and complete resolution of her agitation and psychotic symptoms within 72 hours. Loxapine was subsequently quickly withdrawn with no ill effects and she recovered fully.

The authors thought that this psychotic episode was related to cyclobenzaprine, in view of the temporal relation of the symptoms to the administration of cyclobenzaprine and their rapid resolution after withdrawal.

Drug Administration

Drug overdose

Common effects of cyclobenzaprine overdose were lethargy, agitation, sinus tachycardia, and both hypertension and hypotension (5).

References

1. Azoury FJ. Double-blind comparison of Parafon Forte and Flexeril in the treatment of acute musculoskeletal disorders. Curr Ther Res 1979;26:189.
2. Nibbelink DW, Strickland SC. Cyclobenzaprine (Flexeril) Report of a postmarketing surveillance program. Curr Ther Res 1980;28:894.
3. Beeber AR, Manring JM Jr. Psychosis following cyclobenzaprine use. J Clin Psychiatry 1983;44(4):151–2.
4. O'Neil BA, Knudson GA, Bhaskara SM. First episode psychosis following cyclobenzaprine use. Can J Psychiatry 2000;45(8):763–4.
5. Spiller HA, Winter ML, Mann KV, Borys DJ, Muir S, Krenzelok EP. Five-year multicenter retrospective review of cyclobenzaprine toxicity. J Emerg Med 1995;13(6):781–5.

Cyclofenil

General Information

Cyclofenil is a weak non-steroidal estrogen related to diethylstilbestrol. For a number of years it was used for inducing ovulation, but has lost favor; more recently there have been studies of its possible effects in Raynaud's phenomenon secondary to scleroderma (1).

Up to 2% of patients taking cyclofenil complain of nausea, vomiting, hot flushes, or headache. Mild abdominal pain has been reported in up to 18%, ovarian enlargement without cysts in 3%, and galactorrhea in 4%. There have been a few case reports of hemolytic anemia (SED-12, 1034) (2).

Organs and Systems

Liver

Cyclofenil can cause reversible mild cholestatic jaundice. The authors of a review of 30 patients with hepatic reactions to cyclofenil concluded that liver derangement due to cyclofenil is probably related to metabolic hypersusceptibility rather than to a direct toxic effect (3). There is a surprising lack of such reports from countries where cyclofenil was widely used: in France, at least, the number of cases of hepatitis occurring is known to have been much greater than that reported in print, and the drug was abandoned in that country in 1988.

References

1. Pope J, Fenlon D, Thompson A, Shea B, Furst D, Wells G, Silman A. Cyclofenil for Raynaud's phenomenon in progressive systemic sclerosis. Cochrane Database Syst Rev 2000;(2):CD000955.
2. Wollheim FA, Ljunggren HO, Blom-Bulow B. Hemolytic anemia during cyclofenil treatment of scleroderma. Acta Med Scand 1981;210(5):429–30.
3. Olsson R, Tyllstrom J, Zettergren L. Hepatic reactions to cyclofenil. Gut 1983;24(3):260–3.

Cyclopentolate hydrochloride

General Information

Cyclopentolate is an anticholinergic drug used as a mydriatic.

Organs and Systems

Skin

Contact urticaria has been reported with cyclopentolate (1).

- A 72-year-old man, with a history of adverse reactions to sulfonamides, had erythema, edema, itching, burning of the eye, and an urticarial rash on his right cheek after the administration of several drugs to his right eye. Patch testing was performed and the cyclopentolate hydrochloride patch showed erythema after 15 minutes and an itching wheal after 30 minutes. No immediate or delayed reaction was observed with any of the other eye-drops. Patch tests with cyclopentolate hydrochloride in eight healthy volunteers were negative.

Reference

1. Munoz-Bellido FJ, Beltran A, Bellido J. Contact urticaria due to cyclopentolate hydrochloride. Allergy 2000;55(2): 198–9.

Cyclophosphamide

General Information

Cyclophosphamide is an alkylating nitrogen mustard derivative mainly used in oncology patients (1) or in conditioning regimens for bone marrow transplantation. Its immunosuppressant properties have been used in organ transplantation and more often in chronic inflammatory disorders or autoimmune diseases.

Observational studies

Cyclophosphamide has been investigated in a wide range of diseases, but results in aplastic anemia and idiopathic pulmonary fibrosis have been disappointing. In a low dose (2 mg/kg/day), it produced minimal efficacy in 19 patients with idiopathic pulmonary fibrosis who had failed to respond to a glucocorticoid or who had had adverse effects (2). Moreover, 13 patients had cyclophosphamide-induced adverse effects, which required drug withdrawal in 9. The most frequent were severe gastrointestinal effects, leukopenia, and skin rashes. In another study, high-dose cyclophosphamide plus ciclosporin (50 mg/kg/day for 4 days) was compared with antithymocyte globulin plus ciclosporin in patients with severe aplastic anemia, but the trial was prematurely stopped after only 31 patients had been enrolled because of three early deaths in patients taking cyclophosphamide (3). Subsequent analysis showed excess morbidity and mortality in patients taking cyclophosphamide, with six proven or suspected cases of systemic fungal infection (including the three deaths) compared with no cases in the other group, but no significant difference in the hematological response rates between the groups. In addition, the durations of hospital stay, neutropenia, and antibacterial treatment were longer with cyclophosphamide. Based on these results, the authors concluded that cyclophosphamide should not be used in aplastic anemia.

General adverse effects

Common adverse effects observed at low doses of cyclophosphamide are similar to, but less frequent than, those observed in oncology patients. They include gastrointestinal disturbances (mostly nausea), hematological toxicity (mostly leukopenia), alopecia, and infectious complications (4,5).

Organs and Systems

Cardiovascular

Cardiac toxicity can be observed at high doses of cyclophosphamide (usually over 1.5 g/m^2/day), and acute myocardial necrosis or severe cardiac failure have been anecdotally reported after smaller dosages (SEDA-21, 386).

High-dose cyclophosphamide (120–200 mg/kg) can cause lethal cardiotoxicity, and severe congestive heart failure can develop 1–10 days after the first dose. Severe congestive heart failure is accompanied by electrocardiographic findings of diffuse voltage loss, cardiomegaly, pulmonary vascular congestion, and pleural and pericardial effusions. Pathological findings include hemorrhagic myocardial necrosis, thickening of the left ventricular wall, and fibrinous pericarditis.

Of 80 patients who received cyclophosphamide 50 mg/kg/day for 4 days in preparation for bone marrow grafting 17% had symptoms consistent with cyclophosphamide cardiotoxicity (6). Six died from congestive heart failure. Older patients were at greatest risk of developing cardiotoxicity.

In six patients who developed heart failure after high-dose conditioning therapy before stem cell transplantation, cyclophosphamide was suspected, despite the possible involvement of four drugs (7). The authors suggested monitoring high-risk patients.

Corrected QT dispersion was a predictor of acute heart failure after high-dose cyclophosphamide chemotherapy (5.6 g/m^2 over 4 days) in 19 patients (8).

Respiratory

Cyclophosphamide-induced pneumonitis has been described in 29 cases (9). Considering the widespread use of this drug over many years, this is a rare adverse effect. It does not clearly correlate with dosage (SED-8, 1112) (SED-13, 1122). From a review of 12 case reports and a retrospective analysis of six other patients (including four with Wegener's granulomatosis), in whom cyclophosphamide was thought to be the only causative factor, two distinct clinical patterns of pneumonitis with different prognoses were identified (10). Early-onset pneumonitis ($n = 8$) occurred acutely within 1–8 months of treatment, and complete recovery was noted after cyclophosphamide withdrawal and prednisone treatment. In contrast, late-onset pneumonitis ($n = 10$) developed insidiously over several months (eventually after cyclophosphamide withdrawal) in patients maintained taking low daily doses for months to years. These patients had progressive pulmonary fibrosis unresponsive to glucocorticoid therapy, and six died of respiratory failure. Radiological pleural thickening may be an early sign of late-onset lung toxicity.

Nervous system

Progressive multifocal leukoencephalopathy is sometimes associated with Wegener's granulomatosis, but one case occurred in a patient who was taking low-dose cyclophosphamide, with subsequent significant improvement on withdrawal of the drug (SEDA-19, 347).

Sensory systems

Blurred vision is sometimes reported after high intravenous doses of cyclophosphamide, and there has been one report of transient myopia that recurred after each monthly intravenous pulse (11).

Endocrine

Even low-dose intravenous cyclophosphamide can cause a syndrome that resembles inappropriate secretion of antidiuretic hormone, with severe hyponatremia and symptoms of water intoxication (SEDA-19, 347) (SEDA-21, 386). A direct effect on the renal tubules is likely, but no other nephrotoxic effects have been documented.

Hematologic

Leukopenia, and less commonly thrombocytopenia or anemia, due to cyclophosphamide are typically dose-related in the therapeutic range. Cyclophosphamide-induced anemia has led to retinopathy presenting as striated hemorrhage of the retina (12).

Relative eosinophilia and increased interleukin-4 secretion were found in one study, suggesting that an immune deviation toward a type-2 T helper cell (Th2) response can occur (13). The clinical relevance of these findings as regards hypersensitivity reactions is unknown.

The idea that the degree of leukocyte suppression can be used to predict the success of adjuvant chemotherapy has been applied to combined treatment with cyclophosphamide, methotrexate, and 5-fluorouracil for breast cancer; the lower the nadir leukocyte count, the greater the incidence of metastatic disease-free survival (14).

Mouth and teeth

Unilateral necrosis of the tongue has been attributed to cyclophosphamide (15).

- A 62-year-old woman with invasive ductal carcinoma of the breast was treated with epirubicin and cyclophosphamide. She rapidly developed swelling and necrosis of the tongue and consequent airway obstruction necessitating tracheostomy. After excision of the necrosis, the swelling of the tongue and the airway obstruction resolved.

Because of the temporal connection between the necrosis and the chemotherapy, the authors suspected an adverse effect, although they could not exclude a paraneoplastic pathogenesis.

Gastrointestinal

Nausea and vomiting are infrequent with daily low-dose cyclophosphamide (4).

Two-thirds of patients treated with cyclophosphamide orally for 4 months plus intravenous 5-fluorouracil and methotrexate for breast cancer developed Barrett's epithelium (16), perhaps as a result of esophagitis, rather than through mucosal re-epithelialization by undifferentiated stem cells (17).

Toxic megacolon occurred after five cycles of epirubicin 70 mg/m^2, 5-fluorouracil 500 mg/m^2, and oral cyclophosphamide 75 mg/m^2 for 14 days (18). The clinical presentation included a raised erythrocyte sedimentation rate and a colonic diameter of greater than 9 cm; the outcome can be fatal.

Liver

Cyclophosphamide-induced, dose-related liver damage is probably caused as a result of impaired clearance of its metabolite acrolein (19). This causes raised serum transaminases (20) and can be aggravated by prior exposure to azathioprine.

Acute reversible cytolytic or cholestatic jaundice can also occur after low-dose cyclophosphamide in adults and children (SED-13, 1122) (SEDA-19, 347) (SEDA-20, 342) (SEDA-21, 386). Acute liver failure required liver transplantation in one patient (21). Although glucocorticoids were given concomitantly in most of these patients, no data are available to indicate a possibly increased hepatotoxic potential of this drug combination.

Hepatic veno-occlusive disease was attributed to low-dose cyclophosphamide in a 2-year-old child, and in repeated episodes of serum transaminase fluctuations in a patient with hepatitis C virus infection (SEDA-19, 347).

Late hepatotoxicity has also been reported with low-dose cyclophosphamide (22).

- A 67-year-old man with Sjögren's syndrome took cyclophosphamide for 2 years, a cumulative dose of 40.5 g. He then developed severe progressive jaundice due to acute hepatocellular injury. Gallstones and acute viral hepatitis were excluded, and only anti-smooth muscle antibodies were weakly positive. Liver histology showed marked ballooning of the hepatocytes and cell loss, cytoplasmic and canalicular cholestasis, and infiltration of the portal tract with inflammatory cells. Complete resolution occurred 6 weeks after cyclophosphamide withdrawal.

The authors emphasized this was the first case suggesting a cumulative hepatotoxic effect of low-dose cyclophosphamide. Previous rare cases of low-dose cyclophosphamide-induced acute hepatitis have usually occurred within the first 2 months.

Urinary tract

Hemorrhagic cystitis and bladder cancer are well-known complications of cyclophosphamide. The damage to the urinary bladder epithelium is caused by acrolein, a metabolite of cyclophosphamide that is excreted in the urine. In bone marrow transplant recipients, prior administration of busulfan, which itself causes hemorrhagic cystitis, can increase this risk (23). Mesna (2-mercaptoethane sodium sulfonate) is used to prevent this adverse effect. It is excreted by the kidney, and it binds and detoxifies acrolein in the urine; mesna also prevents the breakdown of acrolein precursors. Intravesical prostaglandin E_2 has been suggested as an alternative treatment (23).

The incidence of cystitis and/or dysuria was only 8% in 531 women with breast cancer who were given oral cyclophosphamide 60 mg/m^2/day for 1 year; the majority of cases were only grade 1 (24).

Upper renal tract disorders with ureteric reflux and bilateral hydronephrosis has been briefly reported in a patient with a history of cyclophosphamide-induced cystitis (SEDA-22, 410–411).

In 155 patients with Wegener's granulomatosis, of whom 142 took daily oral cyclophosphamide, the most frequent long-term cyclophosphamide-related adverse effects were cystitis despite mesna therapy (12%) and myelodysplasia (8%) (25). Patients who took a cumulative dose of over 100 g had a two-fold greater risk of cystitis and/or myelodysplasia than patients who took under 100 g. The authors emphasized that cyclophosphamide therapy should be as short as possible, with mesna and close surveillance in order to reduce treatment-associated morbidity.

Cyclophosphamide was thought to have favored the development of emphysematous cystitis in a 73-year-old man (26).

Skin

High doses of cyclophosphamide can cause the erythrodysesthesia syndrome, that is erythema of the hands and feet (27).

Stevens–Johnson syndrome developed in two patients, including one with positive rechallenge (SEDA-20, 342).

Five of thirty-two patients treated with the alternating drug regimen CAMBO-VIP (cyclophosphamide, doxorubicin, methotrexate, bleomycin, vincristine, etoposide, ifosfamide, and prednisolone) for non-Hodgkin's lymphoma developed blisters under the thickened skin of the palms and/or soles, followed by desquamation (28).

Discrete cutaneous hyperpigmentation occurred in two patients after high-dose chemotherapy with cyclophosphamide, etoposide, and carboplatin (29).

Hair

Alopecia occurs in patients taking cyclophosphamide, but it is less common and less severe in patients taking low doses. Mild to moderate alopecia was observed in 17% of patients with Wegener's granulomatosis (4).

Nails

Beau's lines (transverse ridging of the nails) developed after multiple drug therapy for Hodgkin's disease, including cyclophosphamide (30).

Reproductive system

In autoimmune diseases cyclophosphamide can cause menstrual disorders (oligomenorrhea or sustained amenorrhea) and ultimately sterility or premature menopause. This has been particularly exemplified in lupus erythematosus, and several studies have shown a high prevalence of menstrual disorders or premature ovarian failure in cyclophosphamide-treated patients, or a significantly higher incidence of both complications compared with other immunosuppressive regimens or healthy controls (31–33).

Of 17 adult men who had been treated before puberty for sarcoma with high-dose pulse cyclophosphamide (median dose 20.5 m/m^2) as part of regimens containing vincristine, dactinomycin, and cyclophosphamide, with or without doxorubicin, 10 had azoospermia, five had oligospermia, and only two had normal sperm counts (34). The authors concluded that a previous suggestion that puberty acts as a protection to infertility was not borne out and that the risk of infertility was proportional to the cumulative dose of cyclophosphamide.

Susceptibility factors have been investigated in a large retrospective study of 274 patients aged under 45 years, of whom 70 had received cyclophosphamide, 84 azathioprine but not cyclophosphamide, and 88 either no drug or hydroxychloroquine alone (35). The overall incidence of ovarian failure, defined as sustained amenorrhea for at least 12 months and documented by reduced estradiol concentrations, was 26, 1, and 0% respectively. The mean delay to onset of the first missed menses was 4.4 months. A higher age at the start of treatment and cumulative dose were independent risk factors for cyclophosphamide-induced ovarian failure. The incidences were 14, 28, and 50% in patients aged under 30 years, 30–39 years, and over 40 years respectively, and 4, 26, 31, 70% for cumulative doses of under 10, 10–20, 20–30, and over 40 g, respectively.

Immunologic

Type I hypersensitivity

Anaphylactic reactions have very rarely occurred after intravenous cyclophosphamide (SED-8, 1126) (SEDA-17, 522) (36), and positive skin tests to the parent drug and/or 4-hydroxycyclophosphamide were found in several well-documented case reports (SEDA-19, 347). Although other mechanisms could be considered, a possible IgE antibody-mediated reaction was substantiated by the positivity of immediate skin tests to cyclophosphamide metabolites in five patients, and the recurrence of symptoms following intravenous or oral rechallenge in several of them (37).

Cyclophosphamide reportedly caused a type I hypersensitivity reaction in a patient with systemic lupus erythematosus (38).

- A 17-year-old Chinese girl with systemic lupus erythematosus developed acute angioedema over the neck, chest, and larynx, and required mechanical ventilation. She had received two previous courses of cyclophosphamide without incident. She developed urticaria 30 minutes after an infusion of cyclophosphamide, without angioedema, stridor, wheezing, or hypotension. Skin prick testing with cyclophosphamide was negative. Four weeks later, 15 minutes after the start of an infusion of cyclophosphamide, she developed generalized urticaria. Further infusions were given with diphenhydramine premedication.

In the absence of drug-induced angioedema or anaphylaxis, monthly therapy with cyclophosphamide can be continued with antihistamine premedication in patients who have allergic reactions.

Infection risk

Owing to its effects on cellular and humoral immune responses, and independently of leukopenia, cyclophosphamide can induce more frequent and more severe infectious complications (SED-13, 1123) (SEDA-20, 343). Older age and total cumulative dose are possible susceptibility factors for severe infectious episodes. More specifically, an increased risk of severe, life-threatening *Pneumocystis jiroveci* pneumonia has been identified, particularly in patients with lymphopenia (39,40). There was also a 10- to 20-fold increase in *Herpes zoster* infections (41,42). Fatal aspergillosis and disseminated cryptococcosis have been sometimes reported (SEDA-20, 343) (43). Infections were mostly reported in patients who were also taking glucocorticoids, and a synergistic effect with glucocorticoids is likely to be relevant in causation (41,44); all the same, there is direct evidence that cyclophosphamide itself is involved. Its role was investigated in a retrospective study of 100 patients with systemic lupus erythematosus: 45% developed serious bacterial infections (58%), opportunistic infections (24%), or *H. zoster* infections (18%), compared with 12% in 43 patients taking high-dose glucocorticoids alone (45). Infections were more frequent with sequential intravenous and oral cyclophosphamide (68%) than with intravenous cyclophosphamide (39%) or oral cyclophosphamide (40%), and leukopenia was an additional risk factor. Other investigators have similarly adduced evidence of more frequent infections, particularly *P. jiroveci* pneumonia, in patients receiving cyclophosphamide plus glucocorticoids daily rather than alternate-day glucocorticoids (41).

- A 72-year-old man with autoimmune thrombocytopenia had taken prednisone (30 mg/day) for 1 year, when he was found to have systemic lupus erythematosus (46). Prednisone was continued and he started to take chloroquine (250 mg/day) and monthly cyclophosphamide (0.75 g/m^2). Three weeks after the first bolus of cyclophosphamide, he complained of fever and dyspnea, and chest X-rays showed bilateral pulmonary infiltrates. Despite prompt medical management, he died 5 days after admission with cytomegalovirus-induced interstitial pneumonia.

In addition to cyclophosphamide, this patient had several susceptibility factors for fatal infection, namely age (older than 50 years) and a low leukocyte nadir (2900×10^6/l) after treatment with cyclophosphamide and prednisone.

Long-Term Effects

Tumorigenicity

Although tumor induction has mostly been documented in patients treated for cancer, long-term cyclophosphamide treatment for non-neoplastic conditions can also increase the incidence of certain neoplasms. Whether this oncogenic effect is a consequence of drug-induced chromosomal aberrations rather than immunosuppression is unclear. An increased incidence of bladder cancers, skin cancers, and myeloproliferative disorders was found in a 20-year follow-up study of 119 patients with rheumatoid arthritis, and a high dose of cyclophosphamide (mean total dose of 80 g) was the main susceptibility factor (47).

In another study in patients with Wegener's granulomatosis there was an 11-fold increase in the incidence of lymphomas compared with the general population (41). In contrast, previous exposure to cyclophosphamide did not appear to be associated with a significantly higher risk of cancer in patients with systemic lupus erythematosus, but the number of cases was very low (48).

Myelodysplastic syndromes

Cyclophosphamide can cause myelodysplastic syndromes, particularly after prolonged treatment. The type of myelodysplastic syndromes and cytogenetic abnormalities that developed after treatment with alkylating agents for rheumatic diseases have been described in eight patients (mean age 57 years), of whom seven had taken oral cyclophosphamide and one chlorambucil (49). The mean cumulative dose of cyclophosphamide was 118 g for a mean cumulative duration of 4.4 years, and the myelodysplastic syndrome was diagnosed 0–4 years (mean 2.4 years) after the end of treatment. Concomitant immunosuppressive drugs were given in four of seven cyclophosphamide-treated patients. Cytogenetic abnormalities of chromosome 5 and/or 7, which are characteristic of treatment-related myelodysplastic syndromes, were found in all patients. Only two patients were still alive at the time of the report, and the outcome was remarkably poor in patients with chromosome 5 deletion. This study suggested that a high cumulative dose of cyclophosphamide is a risk factor for hematological malignancies, and that patients require long-term surveillance.

Urinary tract tumors

Squamous cell carcinoma of the bladder has been reported 4 years after pulsed cyclophosphamide therapy (50). However, the authors noted that other susceptibility factors, such as bladder diverticula and human papilloma virus infection, occurred in the intervening period and they speculated on the cumulative risk.

- A 72-year old woman who received 1400 mg cyclophosphamide over 2 weeks for Wegener's granulomatosis had gross hematuria and dysuria (51). Cystoscopy was normal, but there was marked irregularity of the mucosa of the upper ureteric mucosa, the renal pelvis, and the renal calyces on retrograde ureteropyelography. Nephroscopy showed a gray necrotic uroepithelium with dystrophic calcification.

The risk of bladder cancer persists for as long as 20 years after cyclophosphamide withdrawal. In a retrospective analysis, half of the 145 patients on long-term treatment for Wegener's granulomatosis had microscopic or gross hematuria, among whom 70% had cystoscopic features compatible with cyclophosphamide-induced bladder injury (52). Seven patients (5%) developed bladder cancer, a 31-fold higher incidence than in the general population. As previous episodes of hematuria were found in all seven patients and the drug was the only significant risk factor for bladder cancer, prompt cystoscopy should be done in any patient who develops gross hematuria, even after treatment withdrawal. Another study showed an excess in the incidence of bladder cancer in patients with multiple sclerosis who received cyclophosphamide and who also had an indwelling catheter (53).

Renal adenocarcinoma has been reported in a 50-year-old man after 3 years of cyclophosphamide treatment for hepatic sarcoidosis (54).

Other tumors

It has been suggested that cyclophosphamide can contribute to the risk of cervical dysplasia. In a retrospective study of 110 patients with systemic lupus erythematosus, cervical dysplasia was significantly more frequent in patients who had received intravenous cyclophosphamide (10 of 61) than in a control group who did not receive cyclophosphamide (two of 49) (55). In addition, cervical pathology worsened during cyclophosphamide therapy in all four patients with pre-existing cervical dysplasia, and one patient developed in situ cervical carcinoma.

- A 54-year-old man with polyarteritis nodosa developed hepatic angiosarcoma after taking cyclophosphamide for 13 years (56). Although this may have been coincidental, the authors found two other published reports of this very rare tumor in patients taking long-term cyclophosphamide.

To determine the frequency and types of malignancies that occur in children with end-stage renal insufficiency who required renal replacement therapy, data from 249 patients were analysed retrospectively (57). There were 22 malignancies in 21 patients; skin cancers accounted for 59% and non-Hodgkin's lymphomas for 23%. At 25 years after first renal replacement therapy, the probability of developing a malignancy was 17%. The incidence of cancers overall was 10-fold higher than in the general population. For cancers other than melanoma and non-Hodgkin's lymphoma, the standardized risks were 222 and 46 respectively. The use of more than 20 mg/kg cyclophosphamide was associated with an increased risk of malignancy. Six patients died as a result of their malignancy, accounting for 9.5% of overall mortality. The long-term risk of certain malignancies is significantly increased in children who have undergone renal replacement therapy, especially after treatment with cyclophosphamide.

Second-Generation Effects

Fertility

Cyclophosphamide, or testicular and cranial irradiation, in the treatment of childhood malignancies can lead to small testicular size and decreased sperm production in adulthood (58). Of 17 adult male survivors of childhood sarcomas treated before puberty with high-dose cyclophosphamide, only two had normal sperm counts, 10 had azoospermia, and five had oligospermia (34). The two patients with normal sperm counts had taken the lowest doses of cyclophosphamide.

Gonadal toxicity has been documented in both men and women receiving cyclophosphamide (4). In men, the incidence of transient or permanent oligospermia/azoospermia is 50–90%, and in prepubertal patients spermatogenesis will more readily return to normal than adults. In one study, testosterone prophylaxis given at the same time as cyclophosphamide reduced the incidence of disorders of spermatogenesis and accelerated spermatogenesis recovery after cyclophosphamide discontinuation, but few patients were evaluable (59).

Of 23 men treated with either cyclophosphamide or non-alkylating agent combinations, there was a dose-related disturbance of gonadotrophin secretion in the cyclophosphamide group (60). The chances of maintaining normal gonadal function after combined treatment of Hodgkin's disease are significantly greater among girls than boys at 9-year follow-up (61). Pre- and post-pubescent boys were affected by six cycles of MOPP, whether or not pelvic radiation was administered; on the other hand, in girls similarly treated, ovarian function was directly affected by the number of courses of chemotherapy and the ovarian radiation dose (62). In a study of male gonadal function at 9 years follow-up after regimens containing cyclophosphamide, mechlorethamine, vincristine, or procarbazine, there was azoospermia, whereas regimens containing dactinomycin and vinblastine did not have a toxic effect on spermatogenesis (63). Testicular volume and sperm count in 18 patients, 1–3 years after chemotherapy, showed that all those who had received chemotherapy that did not include cisplatin had normal testicular size and sperm counts, whereas of seven who had received cisplatin, six had small testes and azoospermia and one was oligozoospermic with normal-sized testes (64).

The risk of ovarian failure and infertility has been studied in 84 women with an underlying inflammatory disease receiving intravenous cyclophosphamide (65). The incidence of sustained amenorrhea was 22% and was independent of the underlying inflammatory disease. After treatment with cyclophosphamide following bone marrow transplantation, ovarian function can occasionally recover, resulting in a successful pregnancy up to 7 years after treatment (66). No specific factors correlated with recovery of normal ovarian function. However, recovery was rare if the patient had undergone concurrent total body irradiation (67).

Pregnancy

Cyclophosphamide crosses the placenta and reaches an amniotic fluid concentration of 25%. Six pregnancies occurred in women taking cyclophosphamide; three had induced abortions, one had a spontaneous abortion, and two had normal pregnancies. After withdrawal of cyclophosphamide, 16 women became pregnant; three had induced abortions for severe morphological anomalies, three had spontaneous miscarriages, and 10 delivered healthy infants. Contraception during intravenous cyclophosphamide therapy is recommended, and after withdrawal, pregnancy is possible, with a favourable outcome in two-thirds of cases.

Teratogenicity

The FDA has classified cyclophosphamide as a pregnancy risk factor D drug: it is teratogenic in animals, but population studies have not conclusively shown teratogenicity in humans. However, in a study of in utero first-trimester exposure to four doses of cyclophosphamide 20 mg/kg it was concluded that cyclophosphamide is a human teratogen, that there is a distinct embryopathic phenotype, and that there are serious doubts about the safety of cyclophosphamide in pregnancy (68). The congenital malformation rate has been estimated at 10–44% (69).

Reported congenital abnormalities are many and include facial and palate defects, skin and skeletal anomalies, and visceral malformations. Based on one case and a review of six previous reports of malformations after in utero exposure to cyclophosphamide in the first trimester, a distinct embryopathy due to cyclophosphamide has been suggested (68). The proposed phenotype included growth deficiency, developmental delay, craniosynostosis, blepharophimosis, flat nasal bridge, abnormal ears, and distal limb defects; chromosomes were normal.

In one case of first-trimester exposure to cyclophosphamide in a woman pregnant with twins, the male twin was born with multiple congenital abnormalities and developed papillary thyroid cancer at 11 years of age and stage III neuroblastoma at 14 years of age; the female twin was unaffected (70).

Most cases have been reported in patients with cancer who were also exposed to other antineoplastic drugs or to irradiation. The potential for congenital abnormalities in the offspring of men treated with cyclophosphamide is yet unknown.

Fetotoxicity

The effects of second- or third-trimester exposure to cyclophosphamide are poorly documented, although normal children have been described (71). However, in other cases growth retardation and neutropenia have been reported (72).

Drug Administration

Drug dosage regimens

In inflammatory or autoimmune diseases, both daily oral and cyclic pulse intravenous cyclophosphamide regimens are used, but it is unclear whether one route of administration should be preferred to another. The cumulative dose obtained in those given an intravenous pulse regimen is consistently lower than in those given daily oral administration, and the incidence of bladder cancer or infection is expected to be lower in the former. However, the choice of the maintenance regimen remains a dilemma as regards efficacy and toxicity (73). For example, in one study in 50 patients with Wegener's granulomatosis there was a similar overall incidence of adverse effects in patients treated with prednisone plus oral cyclophosphamide compared with those who received prednisone plus intravenous pulse cyclophosphamide (74). Patients in the oral group had a higher incidence of severe or fatal infectious complications, but a lower incidence of cumulative relapse rates at 4.5 years.

In 47 patients intravenous pulsed cyclophosphamide was as effective as daily oral cyclophosphamide, but caused fewer adverse effects (75). The patients were randomized to receive monthly intravenous pulses of cyclophosphamide (0.75 g/m^2, $n = 22$) or daily oral cyclophosphamide (2 mg/kg/day, $n = 25$) for at least 1 year. Both groups received glucocorticoids. Whereas efficacy end-points did not show significant differences between the two groups, leukopenia (18 versus 60%) and severe infections (14% with no deaths versus 40% with three deaths) were significantly less frequent with intravenous pulsed cyclophosphamide. As a result, the probability of freedom from adverse effects (no deaths, severe infections, leukopenia, or thrombocytopenia) over a 12-month period was only about 25% in the oral group, compared with 70% in the intravenous group. In addition, and based on the findings of a significantly lower serum follicle-stimulating hormone concentration at 3 and 6 months and a 57% reduction in the total dose in the intravenous pulse group, the intravenous pulse regimen was expected to produce fewer adverse gonadal effects and a reduced risk of malignancies.

Drug–Drug Interactions

Cisplatin

A 4-year follow-up of comparison of a combination of cyclophosphamide with either 50 mg/m^2 or 100 mg/m^2 of cisplatin in ovarian cancer has been reported (76). Peripheral neuropathy was dose-limiting and persistent. Ten of thirty-one patients had significant toxicity in the high-dose group compared with one of 24 in the low-dose group.

Fluconazole

Cyclophosphamide is a prodrug that requires cytochrome P_{450}-dependent hepatic activation to produce alkylating species and several inactive by-products. However, very few metabolic interactions involving cyclophosphamide have been reported. In a retrospective study of 22 children treated with cyclophosphamide for cancer or bone marrow transplantation, cyclophosphamide clearance was significantly lower in nine patients taking fluconazole compared with 13 patients not taking it (77). In vitro studies in human liver microsomes confirmed that the rate of 4-hydroxylation of cyclophosphamide was inhibited by fluconazole.

Prednisolone

Daily prednisolone significantly reduced the total clearance of cyclophosphamide and the peak concentration and AUC of 4-hydroxycyclophosphamide (78). It is not known whether this interaction has clinical consequences.

References

1. Fraiser LH, Kanekal S, Kehrer JP. Cyclophosphamide toxicity. Characterising and avoiding the problem. Drugs 1991;42(5):781–95.
2. Zisman DA, Lynch JP 3rd, Toews GB, Kazerooni EA, Flint A, Martinez FJ. Cyclophosphamide in the treatment of idiopathic pulmonary fibrosis: a prospective study in patients who failed to respond to corticosteroids. Chest 2000;117(6):1619–26.
3. Tisdale JF, Dunn DE, Geller N, Plante M, Nunez O, Dunbar CE, Barrett AJ, Walsh TJ, Rosenfeld SJ, Young NS. High-dose cyclophosphamide in severe aplastic anaemia: a randomised trial. Lancet 2000;356(9241):1554–9.
4. Langford CA. Complications of cyclophosphamide therapy. Eur Arch Otorhinolaryngol 1997;254(2):65–72.
5. Omdal R, Husby G, Koldingsnes W. Intravenous and oral cyclophosphamide pulse therapy in rheumatic diseases: side effects and complications. Clin Exp Rheumatol 1993;11(3):283–8.
6. Goldberg MA, Antin JH, Guinan EC, Rappeport JM. Cyclophosphamide cardiotoxicity: an analysis of dosing as a risk factor. Blood 1986;68(5):1114–18.
7. Mugitani A, Yamane T, Park K, Im T, Tatsumi N, Tatsumi Y. Cardiac complications after high-dose chemotherapy with peripheral blood stem cell transplantation. J Jpn Soc Cancer Ther 1996;31:255–62.
8. Nakamae H, Tsumura K, Hino M, Hayashi T, Tatsumi N. QT dispersion as a predictor of acute heart failure after high-dose cyclophosphamide. Lancet 2000;355(9206):805–6.
9. Glatt E, Henke M, Sigmund G, Costabel U. Cyclophosphamid-induzierte Pneumonitis. [Cyclophosphamide-induced pneumonitis.] Rofo 1988;148(5):545–9.
10. Malik SW, Myers JL, DeRemee RA, Specks U. Lung toxicity associated with cyclophosphamide use. Two distinct patterns. Am J Respir Crit Care Med 1996; 154(6 Pt 1):1851–6.
11. Arranz JA, Jimenez R, Alvarez-Mon M. Cyclophosphamide-induced myopia. Ann Intern Med 1992;116(1):92–3.
12. Kadoya K, Suda Y, Tonaki M, et al. Two cases of anemic retinopathy. Folia Ophthalmol Jpn 1989;40:148.

13. Smith DR, Balashov KE, Hafler DA, Khoury SJ, Weiner HL. Immune deviation following pulse cyclophosphamide/methylprednisolone treatment of multiple sclerosis: increased interleukin-4 production and associated eosinophilia. Ann Neurol 1997;42(3):313–18.
14. Poikonen P, Saarto T, Lundin J, Joensuu H, Blomqvist C. Leucocyte nadir as a marker for chemotherapy efficacy in node-positive breast cancer treated with adjuvant CMF. Br J Cancer 1999;80(11):1763–6.
15. Buch RS, Schmidt M, Reichert TE. Akute Nekrose der Zunge unter Epirubicin-Cyclophosphamid-Therapie bei einem invasiv duktalen Mammakarzinom. [Acute tongue necrosis provoked by epirubicin–cyclophosphamide treatment for invasive ductal breast cancer.] Mund Kiefer Gesichtschir 2003;7(3):175–9.
16. Spechler S. Columnar-lined (Barrett's) esophagus. Curr Opin Gastroenterol 1991;7:557–61.
17. Mullai N, Sivarajan KM, Shiomoto G. Barrett esophagus. Ann Intern Med 1991;114(10):913.
18. de Gara CJ, Gagic N, Arnold A, Seaton T. Toxic megacolon associated with anticancer chemotherapy. Can J Surg 1991;34(4):339–41.
19. Honjo I, Suou T, Hirayama C. Hepatotoxicity of cyclophosphamide in man: pharmacokinetic analysis. Res Commun Chem Pathol Pharmacol 1988;61(2):149–65.
20. Shaunak S, Munro JM, Weinbren K, Walport MJ, Cox TM. Cyclophosphamide-induced liver necrosis: a possible interaction with azathioprine. Q J Med 1988;67(252): 309–17.
21. Gustafsson LL, Eriksson LS, Dahl ML, Eleborg L, Ericzon BG, Nyberg A. Cyclophosphamide-induced acute liver failure requiring transplantation in a patient with genetically deficient debrisoquine metabolism: a causal relationship? J Intern Med 1996;240(5):311–14.
22. Mok CC, Wong WM, Shek TW, Ho CT, Lau CS, Lai CL. Cumulative hepatotoxicity induced by continuous low-dose cyclophosphamide therapy. Am J Gastroenterol 2000;95(3):845–6.
23. Thomas AE, Patterson J, Prentice HG, Brenner MK, Ganczakowski M, Hancock JF, Pattinson JK, Blacklock HA, Hopewell JP. Haemorrhagic cystitis in bone marrow transplantation patients: possible increased risk associated with prior busulphan therapy. Bone Marrow Transplant 1987;1(4):347–55.
24. Budd GT, Green S, O'Bryan RM, Martino S, Abeloff MD, Rinehart JJ, Hahn R, Harris J, Tormey D, O'Sullivan J, et al. Short-course FAC-M versus 1 year of CMFVP in node-positive, hormone receptor-negative breast cancer: an intergroup study. J Clin Oncol 1995;13(4):831–9.
25. Reinhold-Keller E, Beuge N, Latza U, de Groot K, Rudert H, Nolle B, Heller M, Gross WL. An interdisciplinary approach to the care of patients with Wegener's granulomatosis: long-term outcome in 155 patients. Arthritis Rheum 2000;43(5):1021–32.
26. Abuzarad H, Gadallah MF, Rabb H, Vermess M, Ramirez G. Emphysematous cystitis: possible side-effect of cyclophosphamide therapy. Clin Nephrol 1998;50(6):394–6.
27. Matsuyama JR, Kwok KK. A variant of the chemotherapy-associated erythrodysesthesia syndrome related to high-dose cyclophosphamide. DICP 1989;23(10):776,778–9.
28. Hirano M, Okamoto M, Maruyama F, Ezaki K, Shimizu K, Ino T, Matsui T, Sobue R, Shinkai K, Miyazaki H, et al. Alternating non-cross-resistant chemotherapy for non-Hodgkin's lymphoma of intermediate-grade and high-grade malignancy. A pilot study. Cancer 1992;69(3):772–7.
29. Singal R, Tunnessen WW Jr, Wiley JM, Hood AF. Discrete pigmentation after chemotherapy. Pediatr Dermatol 1991;8(3):231–5.
30. Requena L. Chemotherapy-induced transverse ridging of the nails. Cutis 1991;48(2):129–30.
31. Wang CL, Wang F, Bosco JJ. Ovarian failure in oral cyclophosphamide treatment for systemic lupus erythematosus. Lupus 1995;4(1):11–14.
32. Gonzalez-Crespo MR, Gomez-Reino JJ, Merino R, Ciruelo E, Gomez-Reino FJ, Muley R, Garcia-Consuegra J, Pinillos V, Rodriguez-Valverde V. Menstrual disorders in girls with systemic lupus erythematosus treated with cyclophosphamide. Br J Rheumatol 1995;34(8):737–41.
33. McDermott EM, Powell RJ. Incidence of ovarian failure in systemic lupus erythematosus after treatment with pulse cyclophosphamide. Ann Rheum Dis 1996;55(4):224–9.
34. Kenney LB, Laufer MR, Grant FD, Grier H, Diller L. High risk of infertility and long term gonadal damage in males treated with high dose cyclophosphamide for sarcoma during childhood. Cancer 2001;91(3):613–21.
35. Mok CC, Lau CS, Wong RW. Risk factors for ovarian failure in patients with systemic lupus erythematosus receiving cyclophosphamide therapy. Arthritis Rheum 1998;41(5):831–7.
36. Salles G, Vial T, Archimbaud E. Anaphylactoid reaction with bronchospasm following intravenous cyclophosphamide administration. Ann Hematol 1991;62(2–3):74–5.
37. Popescu N, Sheehan M, Kouides P, Loughner JE, Condemi JJ, Looney RJ, Leddy JP. Allergic reactions to cyclophosphamide: delayed clinical expression associated with positive immediate skin tests to drug metabolites in five patients. J Allerg Clin Immunol 1995;95:288.
38. Thong BY, Leong KP, Thumboo J, Koh ET, Tang CY. Cyclophosphamide type I hypersensitivity in systemic lupus erythematosus. Lupus 2002;11(2):127–9.
39. Jarrousse B, Guillevin L, Bindi P, Hachulla E, Leclerc P, Gilson B, Remy P, Rossert J, Jacquot C, Gilson B. Increased risk of *Pneumocystis carinii* pneumonia in patients with Wegener's granulomatosis. Clin Exp Rheumatol 1993;11(6):615–21.
40. Porges AJ, Beattie SL, Ritchlin C, Kimberly RP, Christian CL. Patients with systemic lupus erythematosus at risk for *Pneumocystis carinii* pneumonia. J Rheumatol 1992;19(8):1191–4.
41. Hoffman GS, Kerr GS, Leavitt RY, Hallahan CW, Lebovics RS, Travis WD, Rottem M, Fauci AS. Wegener granulomatosis: an analysis of 158 patients. Ann Intern Med 1992;116(6):488–98.
42. Kahl LE. *Herpes zoster* infections in systemic lupus erythematosus: risk factors and outcome. J Rheumatol 1994;21(1):84–6.
43. Kattwinkel N, Cook L, Agnello V. Overwhelming fatal infection in a young woman after intravenous cyclophosphamide therapy for lupus nephritis. J Rheumatol 1991;18(1):79–81.
44. Bradley JD, Brandt KD, Katz BP. Infectious complications of cyclophosphamide treatment for vasculitis. Arthritis Rheum 1989;32(1):45–53.
45. Pryor BD, Bologna SG, Kahl LE. Risk factors for serious infection during treatment with cyclophosphamide and high-dose corticosteroids for systemic lupus erythematosus. Arthritis Rheum 1996;39(9):1475–82.
46. Garcia-Porrua C, Gonzalez-Gay MA, Perez de Llano LA, Alvarez-Ferreira J. Fatal interstitial pneumonia due to cytomegalovirus following cyclophosphamide treatment in a patient with systemic lupus erythematosus. Scand J Rheumatol 1998;27(6):465–6.
47. Radis C, Kwoh C, Morgan M, et al. Risk of malignancy in cyclophosphamide treated patients with rheumatoid arthritis: a 20-year follow-up study. Arthr Rheum 1993;36(Suppl):R19.

48. Pettersson T, Pukkala E, Teppo L, Friman C. Increased risk of cancer in patients with systemic lupus erythematosus. Ann Rheum Dis 1992;51(4):437–9.
49. McCarthy CJ, Sheldon S, Ross CW, McCune WJ. Cytogenetic abnormalities and therapy-related myelodysplastic syndromes in rheumatic disease. Arthritis Rheum 1998;41(8):1493–6.
50. Wang JS, Hsieh SP, Jiaan BP, Tseng HH. Human papillomavirus in cyclophosphamide and diverticulum-associated squamous cell carcinoma of urinary bladder: a case report. Zhonghua Yi Xue Za Zhi (Taipei) 1996;57(4):305–9.
51. Aviles RJ, Vlahakis SA, Elkin PL. Cyclophosphamide-associated uroepithelial toxicity. Ann Intern Med 1999;131(7):549.
52. Talar-Williams C, Hijazi YM, Walther MM, Linehan WM, Hallahan CW, Lubensky I, Kerr GS, Hoffman GS, Fauci AS, Sneller MC. Cyclophosphamide-induced cystitis and bladder cancer in patients with Wegener granulomatosis. Ann Intern Med 1996;124(5):477–84.
53. De Ridder D, van Poppel H, Demonty L, D'Hooghe B, Gonsette R, Carton H, Baert L. Bladder cancer in patients with multiple sclerosis treated with cyclophosphamide. J Urol 1998;159(6):1881–4.
54. Das D, Smith A, Warnes TW. Hepatic sarcoidosis and renal carcinoma. J Clin Gastroenterol 1999;28(1):61–3.
55. Bateman H, Yazici Y, Leff L, Peterson M, Paget SA. Increased cervical dysplasia in intravenous cyclophosphamide-treated patients with SLE: a preliminary study. Lupus 2000;9(7):542–4.
56. Rosenthal AK, Klausmeier M, Cronin ME, McLaughlin JK. Hepatic angiosarcoma occurring after cyclophosphamide therapy: case report and review of the literature. Am J Clin Oncol 2000;23(6):581–3.
57. Coutinho HM, Groothoff JW, Offringa M, Gruppen MP, Heymans HS. De novo malignancy after paediatric renal replacement therapy. Arch Dis Child 2001;85(6): 478–83.
58. Siimes MA, Rautonen J. Small testicles with impaired production of sperm in adult male survivors of childhood malignancies. Cancer 1990;65(6):1303–6.
59. Masala A, Faedda R, Alagna S, Satta A, Chiarelli G, Rovasio PP, Ivaldi R, Taras MS, Lai E, Bartoli E. Use of testosterone to prevent cyclophosphamide-induced azoospermia. Ann Intern Med 1997;126(4):292–5.
60. Hoorweg-Nijman JJ, Delemarre-van de Waal HA, de Waal FC, Behrendt H. Cyclophosphamide-induced disturbance of gonadotropin secretion manifesting testicular damage. Acta Endocrinol (Copenh) 1992;126(2):143–8.
61. Jackson DV Jr, Craig JB, Spurr CL, White DR, Muss HB, Cruz JM, Richards F, Powell BL. Vincristine infusion with CHOP-CCNU in diffuse large-cell lymphoma. Cancer Invest 1990;8(1):7–12.
62. Ortin TT, Shostak CA, Donaldson SS. Gonadal status and reproductive function following treatment for Hodgkin's disease in childhood: the Stanford experience. Int J Radiat Oncol Biol Phys 1990;19(4):873–80.
63. Aubier F, Flamant F, Brauner R, Caillaud JM, Chaussain JM, Lemerle J. Male gonadal function after chemotherapy for solid tumors in childhood. J Clin Oncol 1989;7(3):304–9.
64. Siimes MA, Elomaa I, Koskimies A. Testicular function after chemotherapy for osteosarcoma. Eur J Cancer 1990;26(9):973–5.
65. Huong du L, Amoura Z, Duhaut P, Sbai A, Costedoat N, Wechsler B, Piette JC. Risk of ovarian failure and fertility after intravenous cyclophosphamide. A study in 84 patients. J Rheumatol 2002;29(12):2571–6.
66. Sanders JE, Buckner CD, Amos D, Levy W, Appelbaum FR, Doney K, Storb R, Sullivan KM, Witherspoon RP, Thomas ED. Ovarian function following marrow transplantation for aplastic anemia or leukemia. J Clin Oncol 1988;6(5):813–18.
67. Gradishar WJ, Schilsky RL. Effects of cancer treatment on the reproductive system. Crit Rev Oncol Hematol 1988;8(2):153–71.
68. Enns GM, Roeder E, Chan RT, Ali-Khan Catts Z, Cox VA, Golabi M. Apparent cyclophosphamide (Cytoxan) embryopathy: a distinct phenotype? Am J Med Genet 1999;86(3):237–41.
69. Roubenoff R, Hoyt J, Petri M, Hochberg MC, Hellmann DB. Effects of antiinflammatory and immunosuppressive drugs on pregnancy and fertility. Semin Arthritis Rheum 1988;18(2):88–110.
70. Zemlickis D, Lishner M, Erlich R, Koren G. Teratogenicity and carcinogenicity in a twin exposed in utero to cyclophosphamide. Teratog Carcinog Mutagen 1993;13(3):139–43.
71. Peretz B, Peretz T. The effect of chemotherapy in pregnant women on the teeth of offspring. Pediatr Dent 2003; 25(6):601–4.
72. Kerr JR. Neonatal effects of breast cancer chemotherapy administered during pregnancy. Pharmacotherapy 2005;25(3):438–41.
73. Werth VP. Pulse intravenous cyclophosphamide for treatment of autoimmune blistering disease. Is there an advantage over oral routes? Arch Dermatol 1997;133(2): 229–30.
74. Guillevin L, Cordier JF, Lhote F, Cohen P, Jarrousse B, Royer I, Lesavre P, Jacquot C, Bindi P, Bielefeld P, Desson JF, Detree F, Dubois A, Hachulla E, Hoen B, Jacomy D, Seigneuric C, Lauque D, Stern M, Longy-Boursier M. A prospective, multicenter, randomized trial comparing steroids and pulse cyclophosphamide versus steroids and oral cyclophosphamide in the treatment of generalized Wegener's granulomatosis. Arthritis Rheum 1997;40(12):2187–98.
75. Haubitz M, Schellong S, Gobel U, Schurek HJ, Schaumann D, Koch KM, Brunkhorst R. Intravenous pulse administration of cyclophosphamide versus daily oral treatment in patients with antineutrophil cytoplasmic antibody-associated vasculitis and renal involvement: a prospective, randomized study. Arthritis Rheum 1998;41(10):1835–44.
76. Kaye SB, Paul J, Cassidy J, Lewis CR, Duncan ID, Gordon HK, Kitchener HC, Cruickshank DJ, Atkinson RJ, Soukop M, Rankin EM, Davis JA, Reed NS, Crawford SM, MacLean A, Parkin D, Sarkar TK, Kennedy J, Symonds RP. Mature results of a randomized trial of two doses of cisplatin for the treatment of ovarian cancer. Scottish Gynecology Cancer Trials Group. J Clin Oncol 1996;14(7):2113–19.
77. Yule SM, Walker D, Cole M, McSorley L, Cholerton S, Daly AK, Pearson AD, Boddy AV. The effect of fluconazole on cyclophosphamide metabolism in children. Drug Metab Dispos 1999;27(3):417–21.
78. Belfayol-Pisante L, Guillevin L, Tod M, Fauvelle F. Possible influence of prednisone on the pharmacokinetics of cyclophosphamide in systemic vasculitis. Clin Drug Invest 1999;18:225–31.

Cyclopropane

See also General anesthetics

General Information

Cyclopropane is an inhalational anesthetic gas. Its minimum alveolar concentration (MAC) is 9.2%. Because of the risk of explosion, it is usually administered by closed circuit (1).

Organs and Systems

Cardiovascular

Cardiac dysrhythmias, which can be ventricular, can complicate the use of cyclopropane (2), and the risk is increased in patients who have also been given catecholamines (3).

Nervous system

Delirium can occur in patients given cyclopropane (4).

Gastrointestinal

Nausea and vomiting are fairly frequent after recovery from cyclopropane anesthesia (5,6).

Liver

Liver dysfunction due to cyclopropane, as judged by effects on indocyanine green clearance, has been reported (7).

Urinary tract

Cyclopropane has an antidiuretic effect that is partly reversed by alcohol (8).

Body temperature

There has been a report of malignant hyperthermia in a patient who was given cyclopropane during cesarean section (9), consistent with the in vitro effect of cyclopropane on caffeine-induced muscle contraction (10).

References

1. Jansen U, Moller-Petersen J, Pedersen S. Eksplosionsdod fald under cyklopropan–anaestesi. [A fatal case after explosion during cyclopropane anesthesia.] Ugeskr Laeger 1979;141(49):3375.
2. Hansen DD, Fernandes A, Skovsted P, Berry P. Cyclopropane anaesthesia for renal transplantation. Report of 100 cases. Br J Anaesth 1972;44(6):584–9.
3. Wong KC. Sympathomimetic drugs. In: Smith NT, Miller RD, Corbascio AN, editors. Drug Interactions in Anesthesia. Philadelphia: Lea & Febiger, 1981:66.
4. Denson JS. Cyclopropane. Int Anesthesiol Clin 1963;21:1005–32.
5. Gold MI. Postanesthetic vomiting in the recovery room. Br J Anaesth 1969;41(2):143–9.
6. Kenny GN. Risk factors for postoperative nausea and vomiting. Anaesthesia 1994;49(Suppl):6–10.
7. Abdel Salam AR, Drummond GB, Bauld HW, Scott DB. Clearance of indocyanine green as an index of liver function during cyclopropane anaesthesia and induced hypotension. Br J Anaesth 1976;48(3):231–8.
8. Deutsch S, Pierce EC Jr, Vandam LD. Cyclopropane effects on renal function in normal man. Anesthesiology 1967;28(3):547–58.
9. Lips FJ, Newland M, Dutton G. Malignant hyperthermia triggered by cyclopropane during cesarean section. Anesthesiology 1982;56(2):144–6.
10. Reed SB, Strobel GE Jr. An in-vitro model of malignant hyperthermia: differential effects of inhalation anesthetics on caffeine-induced muscle contractures. Anesthesiology 1978;48(4):254–9.

Cycloserine

See also Antituberculosis drugs

General Information

Cycloserine is an aminoisoxazolidone that shows no cross-resistance with other tuberculostatic agents (1). Because of its high toxicity, it should only be used when microorganisms are resistant to other drugs (relapse or primary resistance). It is usually given orally.

Organs and Systems

Nervous system

Cycloserine can cause headache, somnolence, and tremor (2). In mice, L-cycloserine protects against auditory-invoked seizures by binding to pyridoxal phosphate in the presence of zinc ions (3). The addition of a fluoroquinolone can increase the risk of nervous system effects (4).

Psychological, psychiatric

Cycloserine can cause altered mood, cognitive deterioration, dysarthria, confusion, and even psychotic crises (2).

Susceptibility Factors

Renal disease

Cycloserine accumulates to toxic concentrations in patients with renal insufficiency (5).

References

1. Peloquin CA. Pharmacology of the antimycobacterial drugs. Med Clin North Am 1933;77(6):1253–62.
2. Mitchell RS, Lester W. Clinical experience with cycloserine in the treatment of tuberculosis. Scand J Respir Dis Suppl 1970;71:94–108.
3. Chung SH, Johnson MS, Gronenborn AM. L-cycloserine: a potent anticonvulsant. Epilepsia 1984;25(3):353–62.
4. Berning SE. The role of fluoroquinolones in tuberculosis today. Drugs 2001;61(1):9–18.
5. Wareska W, Klott M, Izdebska-Makosa Z. Wydalenie cykloseryny w przypadkach schorze'n nerkowych. [Excretion of cycloserine in cases of kidney diseases.] Gruzlica 1963;31:664–8.

Cyproheptadine

See also Antihistamines

General Information

Cyproheptadine is a first-generation antihistamine with antiserotoninergic effects (SEDA-12, 142). It has been used because of its appetite-stimulating capacity.

Drowsiness and other adverse effects common to the first-generation antihistamines are common.

Organs and Systems

Psychological, psychiatric

A central anticholinergic syndrome with psychotic symptoms in a 9-year-old boy on therapeutic doses has also been described (1).

Cyproheptadine (6 mg/day) was considered to be the most likely cause of aggressive behaviour in a 5-year-old boy (2).

Long-Term Effects

Drug dependence

A case of cyproheptadine dependence has been reported (SEDA-12, 142).

Drug Administration

Drug overdose

Cyproheptadine caused a reversible toxic psychosis in a patient with renal impairment and low body weight after an incidental overdose of 24 mg within 24 hours (SEDA-2, 150).

References

1. Watemberg NM, Roth KS, Alehan FK, Epstein CE. Central anticholinergic syndrome on therapeutic doses of cyproheptadine. Pediatrics 1999;103(1):158–60.
2. Strayhorn JM Jr. Case study: cyproheptadine and aggression in a five-year-old boy. J Am Acad Child Adolesc Psychiatry 1998;37(6):668–70.

Cytarabine

See also Cytostatic and immunosuppressant drugs

General Information

Cytarabine is a pyrimidine nucleoside that is used to treat acute myelogenous leukemia and lymphocytic leukemias. It is activated intracellularly by deoxycytidine kinase to phosphorylated nucleotides that interfere with DNA synthesis in the S phase of the cell, and is rapidly deaminated intracellularly to the inactive metabolite uracil arabinoside.

Organs and Systems

Respiratory

Two cases of respiratory failure occurred during induction chemotherapy for acute myelomonocytic leukemia with cytarabine and all-*trans*-retinoic acid (1). The authors attributed this to a manifestation of the retinoic acid syndrome. Both patients developed acute respiratory failure with widespread pulmonary infiltrates about 60 hours after starting chemotherapy. Both were managed successfully using high-dose dexamethasone and ventilation.

Nervous system

Central nervous system disturbances, especially impaired cerebellar function, limit doses of cytarabine, and age is an important predictive factor. Of 418 patients who received 36–48 g/m^2 only 35 (8%) had severe cerebellar toxicity, which was irreversible or fatal in 4 (1%) (2). Patients over 50 years of age were significantly more likely to develop cerebellar problems than younger patients (26/137, 19%, compared with 9/281, 3%); a second course did not increase the incidence, implying that it is the individual rather than the cumulative dose that is important.

The cerebellar syndrome is the most common complication of high-dose cytarabine therapy. In a study of the cerebellar syndrome caused by cytarabine (3), in which it was found in seven of 30 patients treated, symptoms of toxicity appeared between the third and seventh days of chemotherapy, manifesting first as lethargy and confusion (3). Within the next 24 hours there were signs of cerebellar dysfunction, including dysarthria, ataxia, tremor, nystagmus, and dysmetria. In most patients in whom neurotoxicity developed, liver function worsened during chemotherapy. Abnormal liver function at the start of therapy and the development of neurotoxicity appear to be linked. The symptoms of neurotoxicity resolved within 4–49 days.

Aseptic meningitis can also occur in patients given cytarabine (4,5), and signs of cerebellar dysfunction after the administration of cytarabine 24 g/m^2 have been reported in association with aseptic meningitis (6).

Sensory systems

Keratoconjunctivitis is a complication of cytarabine therapy, with a reported incidence of 30–100% and commonly associated with high doses (3 g/m^2). Corneal and conjunctival toxicity have been described after therapy for 4 days with 235 mg (100 mg/m^2) daily (7).

Gastrointestinal

The addition of cytarabine 10 mg/m^2/day subcutaneously for 10 days to interferon monotherapy more than doubled the incidence of gastrointestinal toxicity in the treatment of chronic myeloid leukemia in 139 patients (8).

Skin

Acute, painful, swollen, and self-limiting erythema of the hands and soles has been reported after induction therapy for acute myeloid leukemia and attributed to cytarabine (9).

Immunologic

A hypersensitivity reaction has been ascribed to cytarabine (10).

Drug Administration

Drug administration route

The safe intrathecal administration of a long-acting formulation of cytarabine has been reported (11).

Drug–Drug Interactions

Daunorubicin

Hepatotoxicity, with either hyperbilirubinemia or increased alkaline phosphatase activity, occurred in five of 14 patients in a trial of cytarabine 200 mg/m^2/day for 9 days by continuous infusion and daunorubicin 70 mg/m^2/day for 3 days (12).

References

1. Lester WA, Hull DR, Fegan CD, Morris TC. Respiratory failure during induction chemotherapy for acute myelomonocytic leukaemia (FAB M4Eo) with ara-C and all-trans retinoic acid. Br J Haematol 2000;109(4):847–50.
2. Herzig RH, Hines JD, Herzig GP, Wolff SN, Cassileth PA, Lazarus HM, Adelstein DJ, Brown RA, Coccia PF, Strandjord S, et al. Cerebellar toxicity with high-dose cytosine arabinoside. J Clin Oncol 1987;5(6):927–32.
3. Nand S, Messmore HL Jr, Patel R, Fisher SG, Fisher RI. Neurotoxicity associated with systemic high-dose cytosine arabinoside. J Clin Oncol 1986;4(4):571–5.
4. Pease CL, Horton TM, McClain KL, Kaplan SL. Aseptic meningitis in a child after systemic treatment with high dose cytarabine. Pediatr Infect Dis J 2001;20(1):87–9.
5. van den Berg H, van der Flier M, van de Wetering MD. Cytarabine-induced aseptic meningitis. Leukemia 2001;15(4):697–9.
6. Thordarson H, Talstad I. Acute meningitis and cerebellar dysfunction complicating high-dose cytosine arabinoside therapy. Acta Med Scand 1986;220(5):493–5.
7. Thaler J, Hilbe W. Comparative analysis of two consecutive phase II studies with IFN-alpha and IFN-alpha + ara-C in untreated chronic-phase CML patients. Austrian CML Study Group Bone Marrow Transplant 1996;17(Suppl 3):S25–8.
8. Shall L, Lucas GS, Whittaker JA, Holt PJ. Painful red hands: a side-effect of leukaemia therapy. Br J Dermatol 1988;119(2):249–53.
9. Barletta JP, Fanous MM, Margo CE. Corneal and conjunctival toxicity with low-dose cytosine arabinoside. Am J Ophthalmol 1992;113(5):587–8.
10. Williams SF, Larson RA. Hypersensitivity reaction to high-dose cytarabine. Br J Haematol 1989;73(2):274–5.
11. Jaeckle KA, Phuphanich S, Bent MJ, Aiken R, Batchelor T, Campbell T, Fulton D, Gilbert M, Heros D, Rogers L, O'Day SJ, Akerley W, Allen J, Baidas S, Gertler SZ, Greenberg HS, LaFollette S, Lesser G, Mason W, Recht L, Wong E, Chamberlain MC, Cohn A, Glantz MJ, Gutheil JC, Maria B, Moots P, New P, Russell C, Shapiro W, Swinnen L, Howell SB. Intrathecal treatment of neoplastic meningitis due to breast cancer with a slow-release formulation of cytarabine. Br J Cancer 2001;84(2):157–63.
12. Kouides PA, Rowe JM. A dose intensive regimen of cytosine arabinoside and daunorubicin for chronic myelogenous leukemia in blast crisis. Leuk Res 1995;19(10):763–70.

Cytostatic and immunosuppressant drugs

See also Individual agents *and* Alkylating cytostatic agents

General Information

Cytostatic drugs generally have both anticancer and immunosuppressive properties, while immunosuppressant drugs have more specific immunosuppressive effects, although this is a somewhat arbitrary distinction. The following list of drugs is based on the classification used in the *British National Formulary*. Monoclonal antibodies and corticosteroids are not included in this list.

A. Cytostatic drugs

1. Alkylating drugs
   Nitrosoureas: carmustine (BCNU), lomustine (CCNU), nimustine (ACNU), streptozocin.
   N-lost derivatives: chlormethine (mechlorethamine, mustine, nitrogen mustard), cyclophosphamide, estramustine.
   Others: busulfan, chlorambucil, dacarbazine, ifosfamide, melphalan, mitobronitol, mitomycin, procarbazine, thiotepa, temozolomide, treosulfan.
2. Antimetabolites
   Folic acid antagonists: methotrexate, raltitrexed.
   Purine derivatives: cladribine (2-chlorodeoxyadenosine), fludarabine, mercaptopurine, pentostatin (deoxycoformycin), tioguanine.
   Pyrimidine derivatives: capecitabine, cytarabine, fluorouracil (SEDA-23, 476), gemcitabine, tegafur.
3. Cytostatic antibiotics
   Anthracyclines (SEDA-25, 533): aclarubicin, daunorubicin, doxorubicin, epirubicin, idarubicin.
   Others: acivicin, amsacrine, bleomycin, dactinomycin (actinomycin D), mitoxantrone.
4. Photodynamic drugs: porfimer, temoporfin.
5. Platinum compounds (SEDA-26, 490): carboplatin, cisplatin, oxaliplatin.
6. Taxanes: docetaxel, paclitaxel (SEDA-21, 463).
7. Topoisomerase inhibitors (SEDA-27, 477)
   Inhibitors of topoisomerase type 1: irinotecan, topotecan.
   Inhibitors of topoisomerase type 2: etoposide, teniposide.
8. Vinca alkaloids (SEDA-28, 538): vinblastine, vincristine, vindesine, vinorelbine.
9. Others: bexarotene, bortezomib, colaspase and crisantaspase (asparaginases), hydroxycarbamide (hydroxyurea).

B. Immunosuppressant drugs

1. Antiproliferative immunosuppressants: azathioprine, mycophenolate mofetil.

2. Calcineurin inhibitors: ciclosporin, everolimus, pimecrolimus, sirolimus, tacrolimus, temsirolimus.

General adverse effects

There are several types of adverse effects that the cytostatic drugs have in common. These include hyperuricemia (as a result of tumor lysis syndrome), bone marrow suppression, oral mucositis, gastrointestinal discomfort, and alopecia. These are dealt with under the relevant headings below.

Individual drugs also have specific adverse effects. However, one of the difficulties in attributing adverse effects to individual cytostatic and immunosuppressant drugs is the common use of multidrug or multi-intervention studies. A good example of this is the Phase I Study of Foscan-Mediated Photodynamic Therapy and Surgery in Patients with Mesothelioma, in which the authors could not separate the adverse effects, which included local effects, cardiotoxicity, and hepatotoxicity, according to causative drug or procedure (1).

Extravasation of cytostatic drugs

Extravasation is leakage of intravenous drugs from a vein into the surrounding tissues. This can cause local pain accompanied by burning or stinging, erythema, swelling, and tenderness. Not all cytostatic drugs are harmful to the tissues after extravasation. The different types of drugs are classified in Table 1.

The management of extravasation of cytostatic drugs has been reviewed (2–5) and guidelines have been suggested (http://www.ucht.n-i.nhs.uk/pubinfo/Extravasation_of_intravenous_drugs).

Local extravasation

- Stop administering the drug and explain to the patient that extravasation may have occurred.
- Put on gloves and goggles.
- Leave the cannula in place.
- Attach a 20 ml syringe and try to withdraw residual drug.
- Give specific antidotes for specific cytostatic drugs (Table 2).
- Remove the cannula.
- Do not apply pressure, which increases the area of extravasation.
- Apply a thermal pack (for vesicant, exfoliant, and irritant drugs only) (Table 2).
- Raise the limb for 48 hours for vesicant drugs.
- Review vesicant extravasation in 24 hours.
- Consult a plastic surgeon if necessary.

Extravasation from a central venous catheter

If the patient complains of altered sensation, pain, burning, or swelling at the central venous catheter site or in the ipsilateral chest, or if there is a change in intravenous flow rate, extravasation may have occurred.

- Stop administering the drug and explain to the patient that extravasation may have occurred.
- Put on gloves and goggles.
- Attach a 20 ml syringe and try to withdraw residual drug from the line.
- If the reason for extravasation is needle dislodgement, and if aspiration through the needle was unsuccessful, remove the needle and try to aspirate subcutaneously in the pocket and surrounding tissues.
- Give specific antidotes for specific cytostatic drugs (Table 2).
- If a needle is still in situ it should be removed after instillation of the antidote; the antidote can also be injected into the surrounding tissues if needed.
- Do not apply pressure, which increases the area of extravasation.
- Apply a thermal pack (for vesicant, exfoliant, and irritant drugs only) (Table 2).

Table 1 Classification of cytostatic drugs according to their ability to cause tissue damage after extravasation (from http://www.ucht.n-i.nhs.uk/pubinfo/Extravasation_of_intravenous_drugs)

Vesicants[a]	Exfoliants[b]	Irritants[c]	Inflammatory agents[d]	Neutral agents[e]
Amsacrine	Aclarubicin	Carboplatin	Etoposide phosphate	Asparaginase
Chlormethine	Carmustine	Daunorubicin liposomal	Fluorouracil	Bleomycin
Dactinomycin	Cisplatin	Doxorubicin liposomal	Methotrexate	Cladribine
Daunorubicin	Dacarbazine	Etoposide	Raltitrexed	Cyclophosphamide
Doxorubicin	Docetaxel	Irinotecan		Cytarabine
Epirubicin	Floxuridine	Teniposide		Fludarabine
Idarubicin	Mitoxantrone			Gemcitabine
Mitomycin	Oxaliplatin			Ifosfamide
Streptozocin	Paclitaxel			Interleukin-2
Vinca alkaloids	Topotecan			Melphalan
	Treosulfan			Pentostatin
				Thiotepa
				Interferon alfa

[a]Vesicants cause pain, inflammation, and blistering of the skin and underlying tissues, leading to tissue death and necrosis
[b]Exfoliants cause inflammation and shedding of the skin, but are less likely to cause tissue death
[c]Irritants cause inflammation and irritation, but rarely cause tissue damage
[d]Inflammatory agents cause mild to moderate inflammation and flare in local tissues
[e]Neutral agents do not cause inflammation or tissue damage

Table 2 Specific antidotes for cytostatic drugs after extravasation

Drug	Antidote	Instructions	Comments
Anthracyclines	Dimethylsulfoxide Dexrazoxane	Apply dimethylsulfoxide 99% topically Give intravenous dexrazoxane 1000 mg/m^2 on days 1 and 2 and 500 mg/m^2 on day 3; most effective if the first dose is given within 6 hours	Apply a cold pack for 15 minutes, four times a day. Inspect after 24 hours and 7 days. If there are signs of erythema or ulceration after 7 days, discuss with a plastic surgeon
Chlormethine	Sodium thiosulfate	Dilute 0.6 ml of sodium thiosulfate 50% with 9.4 ml of water for injection. Inject 4 ml through the cannula, then remove the cannula. Infiltrate with 0.2 ml subcutaneously over and around the affected area	Apply a cold pack for 15 minutes, four times a day. Inspect after 24 hours and 7 days. If there are signs of erythema or ulceration after 7 days, discuss with a plastic surgeon
Cisplatin[a,b]	Sodium thiosulfate	Dilute 0.6 ml of sodium thiosulfate 50% with 9.4 ml of water for injection. Inject 4 ml through the cannula, then remove the cannula. Infiltrate with 0.2 ml subcutaneously over and around the affected area	Apply a warm pack for 15 minutes, four times a day. Inspect after 24 hours and 7 days. If there are signs of erythema or ulceration after 7 days, discuss with a plastic surgeon
Vinca alkaloids	Hyaluronidase	Mix 1500 units of hyaluronidase with 1 ml of sodium chloride 0.9% for injection. Inject 0.5 ml through the cannula. Remove the cannula. Infiltrate with 0.2 ml subcutaneously over and around the affected area	Apply a warm pack for 15 minutes, four times a day. Inspect after 24 hours and 7 days. If there are signs of erythema or ulceration after 7 days, discuss with a plastic surgeon

[a]High concentration only
[b]Sodium thiosulfate should only be used if a large volume (greater than 20 ml) of concentrated cisplatin (that is a concentration over 0.5 mg/ml) has extravasated

- Review vesicant extravasation in 24 hours.
- Extravasation in the deep part of a central venous catheter will require referral to a plastic surgeon.

Review articles

Some review articles on the adverse effects of cytostatic drugs and related topics are listed in Table 3.

Organs and Systems

Nervous system

Neurological symptoms occur in more than 20% of patients with cancer and can be increased by cytostatic drugs. Acute and late neurotoxic syndromes involve a number of cytostatic agents (Table 4).

The late nervous system effects in survivors 7 years after treatment for childhood acute lymphoblastic leukemia include impaired concentration, attention, and memory (32).

The late effect of chemotherapy and radiotherapy for nervous system lymphoma has been studied in 15 patients; 10 had severe symptomatic diffuse changes in the white matter within 8 months of completing treatment (33).

Endocrine

Combined cytostatic drug therapy for Hodgkin's disease in childhood often results in abnormal endocrine function, particularly increases in follicle-stimulating hormone, prolactin, and thyroid-stimulating hormone (34).

Metabolism

Hyperglycemia was reported in 21 of 56 patients who received weekly paclitaxel with oral estramustine and carboplatin (4-weekly); under 10% required pharmacological intervention (35). There was mild hyperphosphatemia in 24.

There was fasting hypoglycemia in 19 of 35 children with acute lymphoblastic leukemia receiving maintenance therapy of daily oral mercaptopurine and weekly oral methotrexate; all the children improved on withdrawal of chemotherapy and 10 of 15 normalized (36).

There have been cases of acute tumor lysis syndrome in patients with melanoma (37) and light-chain amyloidosis (38). The authors reviewed the incidence of acute tumor lysis syndrome in these diseases, which are less typically associated with it.

Hematologic

The authors of a study in 101 patients concluded that in addition to the dose of chemotherapy and the administration of hemopoietic growth factors, poor performance status and a high concentration of soluble p75-R-TNF can predict the occurrence of chemotherapy-induced myelosuppression in lymphoma (39).

In 43 patients, raised plasma concentrations of FLT3-L (an fms-like tyrosine kinase) in patients who had previously received chemotherapy predicted the stage of recovery of the bone-marrow compartment (40). FLT3-L seems to identify the likelihood that the patient will have severe thrombocytopenia if additional cytostatic therapy is given. Knowledge of bone-marrow activity

Table 3 Some review articles in cytostatic drug therapy

	Topic	Reference
Adverse effects	The relation between a drug's adverse effects spectrum and its pharmacological action	(6)
	Adverse effects profiles of individual drugs	(7)
	Prognostic factors	(8)
	Anemia	(9)
	Nausea and vomiting	(10)
	The relation between toxicity and efficacy	(11,12)
Treatment of specific cancers	Colorectal cancers	(13)
	Lymphomas	(14)
	Melanoma	(15)
	Metastatic breast cancer	(16)
	Prostate cancer	(17)
	Soft tissue sarcomas	(18)
	Testicular carcinoma, non-seminomatous	(19)
Administration	The relation between a drug's adverse effects spectrum and its dosage regimen	(20–22)
	Effects of dosage regimens in combined therapy	(23,24,25)
	Effects of the route of administration	(26,27)
	Dose-finding techniques	(28)
	Preventing dose-limiting adverse effects in patients with nasopharyngeal carcinoma	(96)
	Oral versus intravenous therapy in small cell lung cancer	(29)
Susceptibility factors	Effects of sex	(30)
	The expression and prognostic significance of P glycoprotein in adult solid tumors	(31)

should permit more aggressive therapy, by establishing the earliest possible time for dosing with any cytostatic agent for which myelosuppression is the dose-limiting toxic effect.

Mouth and teeth

Cytostatic drugs can cause oral mucositis, which characteristically affects the whole buccal mucosa (41). It is caused by damage to the oropharyngeal epithelium which has a rapid turnover. The oral mucosa can also be affected by infection. Susceptibility factors include age, nutritional status, tumor type, oral hygiene, and neutrophil count.

Oral mucositis causes pain, interferes with nutrition, and can lead to systemic infection and other complications that increase morbidity and mortality (42). Interventions that have been used to prevent oral mucositis or reduce its severity and sequelae include meticulous pretransplantation and continuing mouth care, calcium phosphate solution, treatment with near-infrared light and lower-energy laser light, interleukin-11, sucralfate, oral glutamine, rinsing with granulocyte-macrophage colony-stimulating factor, tretinoin, keratinocyte growth factor, and amifostine. However, very few interventions have been shown to be effective compared with placebo.

Table 4 Neurotoxic effects of cytostatic drugs

Drug	Neurotoxicity
Asparaginase	Acute encephalopathy
Bortezomib	Peripheral neuropathy
Busulfan	Seizures
Carmustine	Brain damage in conventional doses when combined with radiation
Chlorambucil	Disorientation, cognitive dysfunction
Chlormethine	Rare encephalopathy following high doses
Cisplatin	Peripheral neuropathy, deafness, cerebral cortical blindness, seizures
Cytarabine	Cerebellar ataxia in high doses
Fluorouracil	Cerebellar ataxia in high doses
Ifosfamide	Mild memory disturbances
Methotrexate	Acute meningitis; acute fatal cerebral dysfunction; chronic leukoencephalopathy
Oxaliplatin	Acute and chronic sensory neuropathy
Taxanes	Peripheral neuropathy
Vinblastine	Jaw pain, myopathy, inappropriate ADH secretion
Vincristine	Peripheral neuropathy, abdominal pain, constipation
Vindesine	Overdose or accidental intrathecal injection is usually fatal
Vinorelbine	Sensorimotor distal symmetrical axonal neuropathy

In a retrospective analysis over 13 years of cytostatic therapy for various conditions, six doses of etoposide each of 250 mg/m^2 caused grade 4 mucositis and 50% of patients who received epirubicin 120 mg/m^2 developed grade 2 or 3 mucositis (43). Severe stomatitis complicated epirubicin 1250 mg/m^2 (44).

A scoring system for mucositis has been proposed and validated (45) and multivariate analysis has been used to identify contributory factors (46). A diagnosis of leukemia, the use of total body irradiation or allogenic transplantation in treatment, or delayed neutrophil recovery were associated with an increased incidence of oral mucositis.

It has been proposed that a change in serum diamine oxidase activity is a very sensitive surrogate for early signs of upper gastrointestinal tract mucositis (47).

Gastrointestinal

Nausea and vomiting are common adverse effects of cytostatic drugs (48). They can be acute (occurring within 24 hours of therapy), delayed (persisting for 6–7 days after therapy), or anticipatory (occurring before chemotherapy) (49). Their treatment has been reviewed (50,51).

Diarrhea can also occur (52) and is particularly problematic with some drugs, such as irinotecan (53). Its management has been reviewed (54).

In a retrospective analysis over 13 years of cytostatic therapy for various conditions there were 12 cases in which chemotherapy had caused gastrointestinal perforation (43). Six doses of etoposide each of 250 mg/m^2 induced an advanced stage (grade 4) of mucositis. Fifty percent of patients receiving epirubicin 120 mg/m^2

developed grade 2 or 3 mucositis. Severe stomatitis complicated epirubicin 1250 mg/m^2 (44).

Increased intestinal permeability has been shown in children receiving low-dose methotrexate therapy (44).

Liver

Of 54 patients with non-small-cell lung cancers treated with a combination of gemcitabine 1000 mg/m^2 on days 1 and 8 and paclitaxel 200 mg/m^2 on day 1, six had abnormal but significantly raised transaminases (55). The authors believed that this was drug-induced, but could not rule out underlying liver disease.

Urinary tract

Hemolytic-uremic syndrome in association with thrombotic thrombocytopenic purpura has been reported in a patient receiving pentostatin (deoxycoformycin) after exposure to only 15 mg/m^2 given over 3 days (56).

Skin

There has been a report of six cases of a variant of the palmar-plantar erythrodysesthesia syndrome (hand-foot syndrome), in which patients who had previously reported the syndrome developed it again when they were treated with completely different chemotherapeutic drugs (57). The recall syndrome was of mild to moderate intensity, less severe than the primary syndrome, and self-limiting in all cases.

Four cases of hyperkeratotic seborrheic warts appearing over a 2-year period, 25 years after the patients had been started on azathioprine 2.5 mg/kg, have been reported (58).

Calciphylaxis is a rare, often fatal disease, characterized clinically by progressive cutaneous necrosis and ulceration and histologically by vascular calcification and thrombosis. It has been described in association with end-stage renal disease and hyperparathyroidism.

- A 64-year-old woman who 3 months before had finished a course of cyclophosphamide, doxorubicin, and fluorouracil chemotherapy for breast carcinoma developed calciphylaxis (59). She had no renal disease and had normal renal function and parathyroid hormone concentrations.

The authors speculated that the cause may have been chemotherapy-induced functional deficiency of protein C and protein S.

Musculoskeletal

Bone mineral density has been used to help predict which children who have had chemotherapy may subsequently develop osteoporosis (60).

Reproductive system

Gynecomastia is frequent in men with testicular tumors that produce large amounts of human chorionic gonadotrophin (HCG), and its appearance after completion of chemotherapy may indicate residual or recurrent disease. However, not uncommonly, gynecomastia is a harmless, although troubling, late adverse effect of chemotherapy. In 16 patients who developed gynecomastia 2–9 months after treatment, and who were in complete remission, estradiol concentrations were raised; follicle-stimulating hormone (FSH) produced a higher estradiol/testosterone ratio than similarly treated patients without gynecomastia (61). It is likely that this was due to increased secretion of testicular estrogen in response to a compensatory increase in pituitary gonadotrophins after cytostatic damage to Leydig cells and spermatogenesis.

The gonadal effects of MOPP (mechlorethamine + Oncovin (vincristine) + procarbazine + prednisone/prednisolone) and MVPP (mustine + vinblastine + procarbazine + prednisone/prednisolone) in patients with Hodgkin's disease have been described (SEDA-11, 397) (SEDA-11, 403). Similar studies have been conducted in patients treated with ABVD (adriamycin + bleomycin + vinblastine + dacarbazine) and COPP (cyclophosphamide + vincristine + procarbazine + prednisone) (62). The results suggested that all men have irreversible sterility with preservation of normal Leydig cell function after COPP, which is more spermatotoxic than MOPP and much more so than ABVD. Ovarian failure was age-related after COPP, occurring in 86% of those over 24 years of age at the time of therapy, compared with 28% in women patients less than 24 years old. In contrast to men, sterility in women was always associated with ovarian endocrine failure requiring estrogen replacement. Pregnancies and normal births did occur: 14 women became pregnant and five healthy children were born. It has been proposed that analogues of gonadotropin-releasing hormone preserve gonadal function during the administration of anticancer drugs to premenopausal women.

Infection risk

Infections are major causes of morbidity and mortality in the period after transplantation, whichever immunosuppressive regimen is used, in particular bacterial infections and viral infections (cytomegalovirus, *Herpes simplex* virus, Epstein–Barr virus), but also protozoal and fungal infections (63–65). Based on an analysis of medical and autopsy records, infections were the cause of death in 70% of transplant patients, with bacteria (50%) or fungi (29%) as the most common pathogens (66).

Long-Term Effects

Mutagenicity

An increased incidence of gene aberration is to be expected in the offspring of men being treated at the time of conception with chemotherapy for testicular tumors (67). Various drug regimens for Hodgkin's disease and high-grade non-Hodgkin's lymphoma produce different patterns of changes in sister chromatid exchange frequency, and the changes may reflect the potential of the drugs concerned to induce second malignancies (68).

Tumorigenicity

Malignant tumors have been documented with increasing frequency over the last 35 years as a long-term complication of cytostatic and immunosuppressant therapy.

Alkylating agents have been implicated in the causation of secondary tumors, including acute myeloid leukemia, myelodysplastic syndromes (69), solid tumors (70,71), Hodgkin's disease (72,73), ovarian cancer (74,75), and gastric cancer (69). Survival from the time of diagnosis of secondary malignancies is usually very short (69).

Risks in patients with Hodgkin's disease

The actuarial risks of developing secondary malignancies and/or myelodysplastic syndrome at 5, 10, and 15 years after treatment for Hodgkin's disease have been calculated (76).

In a multicenter, case-control study, the incidence of acute myeloid leukemia in treated Hodgkin's disease was 64 times higher than in the general population, the risk being greater in men. There was also a significant association between the development of acute myeloid leukemia in those patients and the use of extensive radiotherapy, vincristine + procarbazine, splenectomy, and the dose of chlormethine (73). The problem is thought to be the result of chromosomal aberrations developing in patients treated with alkylating agents (77), although there is no general agreement about this (75).

Among 679 patients receiving chemotherapy for advanced Hodgkin's disease, there were four deaths due to secondary malignancies (78). There were 75 deaths in all during 3 years, of which the vast majority were related to disseminated Hodgkin's disease.

The increased incidence of breast cancer after treatment of Hodgkin's disease may be related to supradiaphragmatic irradiation, but the risk was higher in patients with ovarian cancer, which is consistent with a common predisposition to breast and ovarian cancer. However, cytostatic drugs may have contributed to the risk.

Risks in patients with leukemias

The nucleoside analogues fludarabine, pentostatin, and cladribine have not traditionally been associated with secondary malignancies. Long-term follow-up for 5–7.5 years of 2014 patients who had received these agents for chronic lymphoid leukemia and hairy cell leukemia has been reviewed (79). Of 111 malignancies that were detected, the three most common were lymphoma ($n = 25$), prostate cancer ($n = 19$), and lung cancer ($n = 15$). While these incidences suggested significant additional risks beyond those in the normal population, the authors could not conclude beyond a reasonable doubt that the increased risks were greater than expected.

Chemotherapy-related myelodysplastic syndrome has been reported in association with adult T cell leukemia (80).

Risks in patients with Wilms' tumor

The National Wilms' Tumor Study Group has reported the incidence of second malignant neoplasms in 5278 patients treated over 22 years (81). There were 43 second malignant neoplasms, whereas only five were expected. Fifteen years after the diagnosis of Wilms' tumor, the cumulative incidence of a second malignant neoplasm was 1.6% and increasing steadily. Abdominal irradiation, given as part of the initial therapy, increased the risk, and doxorubicin potentiated the radiation effect. Among 234 patients who received doxorubicin and over 35 Gy of abdominal radiation, eight second malignant neoplasms were observed, whereas only 0.22 were expected. Treatment for relapse further increased the risk by a factor of 4–5.

Risks in patients with other tumors

Lymphoblastic leukemia has been described after treatment of a malignant germ cell tumor; it was suggested that this was related to the etoposide component of the treatment, and that development of secondary leukemia after etoposide may not be confined to the myeloid cell lineage (82).

A large international collaborative study by cancer registries has published the incidence of second malignancies following testicular cancer, ovarian cancer, and Hodgkin's disease (83): 3157 second cancers were observed among 133 411 patients diagnosed between 1945 and 1984. Patients with Hodgkin's disease were at particular risk, having an 80% excess of cancers. It confirms the high incidence of this complication noted in other reports involving smaller numbers of patients (84,85).

Other conclusions deriving from the international collaborative study (83) include the following:

- patients with testicular cancer had a 30% greater probability of developing cancers than the general population, and those with ovarian cancer 20%;
- leukemia, previously linked to alkylating agents, occurred in excess after testicular cancer, ovarian cancer, and Hodgkin's disease (relative risk 6.1), as did non-Hodgkin's lymphoma (relative risk 1.8) (the latter particularly after Hodgkin's disease);
- other cancers with significant excesses were lung cancer following Hodgkin's disease (relative risk 1.9), breast cancer following Hodgkin's disease (relative risk 1.4), and bladder cancer following ovarian cancer and Hodgkin's disease (relative risks 1.7 and 2.2 in women, respectively);
- a marked excess in incidence of secondary malignancies was found in the salivary gland, thyroid, bone, and connective tissue (there was a smaller excess for colorectal cancers following ovarian cancer).

It is likely that there is a casual relation between treatment of a first malignancy and development of a second. Alkylating agents are strongly implicated in the pathogenesis of the leukemias. Non-Hodgkin's lymphoma occurred after a 10-year latency in patients with ovarian cancer, suggesting a possible radiation effect, but early in patients with testicular tumors or Hodgkin's disease, possibly related to the immunosuppressive effect of cytostatic drugs. The excess of bladder cancers in patients with Hodgkin's disease and ovarian cancer may be related to radiotherapy (subdiaphragmatic in the former), and/or cyclophosphamide, which is widely used in the treatment of both and is a human bladder carcinogen.

Risks in transplant recipients

Although the risk of secondary malignancy clearly outweighs that of under-treatment in transplant patients, increasing periods of survival extend the importance of this problem and the need for close monitoring. Considerable amounts of data are accumulating based on multicenter or single-center experience, but they reflect the use of various immunosuppressive regimens and prophylactic antiviral treatments, and use different approaches to the calculation of risk incidence. Estimates of risk therefore vary widely between studies and no direct comparison is as a rule possible. However, updated data from the Cincinnati Transplant Tumor Registry, published in 1993, have helped to define comprehensively the characteristics of neoplasms observed in organ transplant recipients (86). Skin and lip cancers were the most common, and non-Hodgkin's lymphomas represent the majority of lymphoproliferative disorders with an incidence some 30- to 50-fold higher than in controls. An excess of Kaposi's sarcomas, carcinomas of the vulva and perineum, hepatobiliary tumors, and various sarcomas is also reported. By contrast, the incidence of common neoplasms encountered in the general population is not increased. In renal transplant patients, the actuarial cumulative risk of cancer is 14–18% at 10 years and 40–50% at 20 years (87,88). Skin cancers accounted for about half of the cases.

There is controversy about which factors (duration of treatment, total dosage, the degree of immunosuppression, or the type of immunosuppressive regimen) are the most relevant to determining risk. Partial or complete regression of lymphoproliferative disorders and Kaposi's sarcomas after reduction of immunosuppressive therapy argues strongly for the role of the degree of immunosuppression (86). The incidence of cancer was also significantly higher in renal transplant patients receiving triple therapy regimens compared with double therapy (89). Similarly, aggressive immunosuppressive therapy may account for the higher incidence of lymphomas in cardiac versus renal allograft patients. In a large, multicenter study involving more than 52 000 kidney or heart transplant patients between 1983 and 1991, the rate of non-Hodgkin's lymphomas in the first year after transplantation was 0.2% in kidney recipients and 1.2% in heart recipients, and fell substantially thereafter (90). Initial immunosuppression with azathioprine and ciclosporin, and prophylactic treatment with antilymphocyte antibodies or muromonab was associated with a significantly increased incidence of non-Hodgkin's lymphomas compared with other immunosuppressive regimens, which confirmed the major role of the degree of immunosuppression. Other studies have confirmed that immunosuppression per se rather than a single agent is responsible for the increased risk of cancer (SEDA-20, 340). Finally, the most striking difference between conventional and modern immunosuppressive regimens, including ciclosporin, was the average time to the appearance of tumors, in particular skin cancers and lymphomas, which was shorter in ciclosporin-treated patients (91,92).

The risk of malignant disease in renal transplant recipients increases with time after the transplant. The commonest cancers in this setting are squamous carcinoma of the skin and lip, in situ carcinoma of the cervix, and non-Hodgkin's lymphoma. An increased incidence of hepatocellular carcinoma has been reported (93). In Australia and New Zealand tumors of the urogenital tract, especially of the kidney and bladder, are the commonest non-cutaneous tumors encountered in renal transplant recipients (94). Severe metaplastic and dysplastic changes, suggestive of premalignancy, have been found in the lining epithelium of collecting ducts and tubules of cadaveric renal transplants in two patients receiving azathioprine and prednisolone (95).

Second-Generation Effects

Fertility

A reduced chance of paternity has been reported in 67% of patients who had been treated with MOPP/ABVD for Hodgkin's disease. This included oligospermia, asthenozoospermia, and/or teratozoospermia. The recovery of spermatogenesis was documented in only 40% (97).

Teratogenicity

The outcomes of pregnancies after the use of immunosuppressive drugs, in particular in renal transplant patients, have been reported, and hundreds of pregnancies have been analysed (98). The largest experience is that derived from the National Transplantation Pregnancy Registry, which has been built up in the USA since 1991 (99). This registry has accumulated data on more than 900 pregnancies, of which 83% followed kidney transplantation. Overall, the immunosuppressive regimens commonly used in transplant patients (that is azathioprine-based or ciclosporin-based programmes) do not appear to increase the overall risk of congenital malformations or to produce a specific pattern of malformation. There was no difference in the rate of malformations when comparing ciclosporin to other immunosuppressive regimens or to the baseline risk of malformations (100,101). Ectopic pregnancies and miscarriages seemed to occur at a similar rate as in the general population. The most common complications were frequent prematurity and more frequent intrauterine growth retardation with low birth weight. Susceptibility factors associated with adverse pregnancy outcomes included a short interval between transplantation and pregnancy (less than 1–2 years), graft dysfunction before or during pregnancy, and hypertension (102). Possible long-term effects of in utero exposure to immunosuppressive drugs are still seldom investigated. There is no evidence that physical and mental development or renal function are altered in children. In one study, there were changes in T lymphocyte development in seven children born to mothers who had taken azathioprine or ciclosporin, but immune function assays were normal, suggesting that fetal immune system development is not affected (103).

References

1. Friedberg JS, Mick R, Stevenson J, Metz J, Zhu T, Buyske J, Sterman DH, Pass HI, Glatstein E, Hahn SM. A phase I study of Foscan-mediated photodynamic therapy and surgery in patients with mesothelioma. Ann Thorac Surg 2003;75(3):952–9.
2. Dorr RT. Antidotes to vesicant chemotherapy extravasations. Blood Rev 1990;4(1):41–60.

3. Nogler-Semenitz E, Mader I, Furst-Weger P, Terkola R, Wassertheurer S, Giovanoli P, Mader RM. Paravasation von Zytostatika. [Extravasation of cytotoxic agents.] Wien Klin Wochenschr 2004;116(9–10):289–95.
4. Rauh J, Pluntke S, Muller Ch. Paravenose Zytostatikainjektion: Prophylaxe und Sofortmassnahmen im Notfall. [Treatment of perivascular extravasation of cytostatic agents.] MMW Fortschr Med 2004; 146(31–32):23–24, 26–7.
5. Jordan K, Grothe W, Schmoll HJ. Paravasation von Zytostatika: Prävention und Therapie. [Extravasation of chemotherapeutic agents: prevention and therapy.] Dtsch Med Wochenschr 2005;130(1–2):33–7.
6. Booser DJ, Hortobagyi GN. Anthracycline antibiotics in cancer therapy. Focus on drug resistance. Drugs 1994;47(2):223–58.
7. Safra T, Groshen S, Jeffers S, Tsao-Wei DD, Zhou L, Muderspach L, Roman L, Morrow CP, Burnett A, Muggia FM. Treatment of patients with ovarian carcinoma with pegylated liposomal doxorubicin: analysis of toxicities and predictors of outcome. Cancer 2001;91(1):90–100.
8. Freyer G, Rougier P, Bugat R, Droz JP, Marty M, Bleiberg H, Mignard D, Awad L, Herait P, Culine S, Trillet-Lenoir V. Prognostic factors for tumour response, progression-free survival and toxicity in metastatic colorectal cancer patients given irinotecan (CPT-11) as second-line chemotherapy after 5FU failure. CPT-11 F205, F220, F221 and V222 study groups. Br J Cancer 2000;83(4):431–7.
9. Barrett-Lee PJ, Bailey NP, O'Brien ME, Wager E. Large-scale UK audit of blood transfusion requirements and anaemia in patients receiving cytotoxic chemotherapy. Br J Cancer 2000;82(1):93–7.
10. Tsavaris N, Kosmas C, Mylonakis N, Bacoyiannis C, Kalergis G, Vadiaka M, Boulamatsis D, Iakovidis V, Kosmidis P. Parameters that influence the outcome of nausea and emesis in cisplatin based chemotherapy. Anticancer Res 2000;20(6C):4777–83.
11. Jodrell DI, Stewart M, Aird R, Knowles G, Bowman A, Wall L, Cummings J, McLean C. 5-fluorouracil steady state pharmacokinetics and outcome in patients receiving protracted venous infusion for advanced colorectal cancer. Br J Cancer 2001;84(5):600–3.
12. Mayers C, Panzarella T, Tannock IF. Analysis of the prognostic effects of inclusion in a clinical trial and of myelosuppression on survival after adjuvant chemotherapy for breast carcinoma. Cancer 2001;91(12):2246–57.
13. Lavery IC, Lopez-Kostner F, Pelley RJ, Fine RM. Treatment of colon and rectal cancer. Surg Clin North Am 2000;80(2):535–69.
14. Carrion JR, Garcia Arroyo FR, Salinas P. Infusional chemotherapy (EPOCH) in patients with refractory or relapsed lymphoma. Am J Clin Oncol 1995;18(1):44–6.
15. Reeves ME, Coit DG. Melanoma. A multidisciplinary approach for the general surgeon. Surg Clin North Am 2000;80(2):581–601.
16. Hayes DF, Henderson IC, Shapiro CL. Treatment of metastatic breast cancer: present and future prospects. Semin Oncol 1995;22(2 Suppl 5):5–21.
17. Klein EA. Hormone therapy for prostate cancer: a topical perspective. Urology 1996;47(Suppl 1A):3–12.
18. Demetri GD, Elias AD. Results of single-agent and combination chemotherapy for advanced soft tissue sarcomas. Implications for decision making in the clinic. Hematol Oncol Clin North Am 1995;9(4):765–85.
19. Kennedy BJ, Torkelson J, Fraley EE. Optimal number of chemotherapy courses in advanced nonseminomatous testicular carcinoma. Am J Clin Oncol 1995;18(6):463–8.
20. Cure H, Chevalier V, Pezet D, Bousquet J, Focan C, Levi F, Garufi C, Chipponi J, Chollet P. Phase II trial of chronomodulated infusion of 5-fluorouracil and folinic acid in metastatic colorectal cancer. Anticancer Res 2000;20(6C):4649–53.
21. Hartmann JT, Kanz L, Bokemeyer C. Phase II study of continuous 120-hour-infusion of mitomycin C as salvage chemotherapy in patients with progressive or rapidly recurrent gastrointestinal adenocarcinoma. Anticancer Res 2000;20(2B):1177–82.
22. Bogliolo G, Pannacciulli I, Desalvo L, Barsotti B, Lerza R, Mencoboni M, Arboscello E. Advanced colorectal cancer: quality of life and toxicity in patients after weekly 24-hour continuous infusions of biomodulated 5-fluorouracil. Anticancer Res 2000;20(1B):501–4.
23. Cardoso F, Ferreira Filho AF, Crown J, Dolci S, Paesmans M, Riva A, Di Leo A, Piccart MJ. Doxorubicin followed by docetaxel versus docetaxel followed by doxorubicin in the adjuvant treatment of node positive breast cancer: results of a feasibility study. Anticancer Res 2001;21(1B):789–95.
24. Spielmann M, Tubiana-Hulin M, Namer M, Mansouri H, Bougnoux P, Tubiana-Mathieu N, Lotz V, Eymard JC. Sequential or alternating administration of docetaxel (Taxotere) combined with FEC in metastatic breast cancer: a randomised phase II trial. Br J Cancer 2002;86(5):692–7.
25. Gelderblom H, Mross K, ten Tije AJ, Behringer D, Mielke S, van Zomeren DM, Verweij J, Sparreboom A. Comparative pharmacokinetics of unbound paclitaxel during 1- and 3-hour infusions. J Clin Oncol 2002;20(2):574–81.
26. Vogl TJ, Engelmann K, Mack MG, Straub R, Zangos S, Eichler K, Hochmuth K, Orenberg E. CT-guided intratumoural administration of cisplatin/epinephrine gel for treatment of malignant liver tumours. Br J Cancer 2002;86(4):524–9.
27. Kovacs AF, Obitz P, Wagner M. Monocomponent chemoembolization in oral and oropharyngeal cancer using an aqueous crystal suspension of cisplatin. Br J Cancer 2002;86(2):196–202.
28. Miller VA, Rigas JR, Francis PA, Grant SC, Pisters KM, Venkatraman ES, Woolley K, Heelan RT, Kris MG. Phase II trial of a 75-mg/m2 dose of docetaxel with prednisone premedication for patients with advanced non-small cell lung cancer. Cancer 1995;75(4):968–72.
29. Miller AA, Herndon JE 2nd, Hollis DR, Ellerton J, Langleben A, Richards F 2nd, Green MR. Schedule dependency of 21-day oral versus 3-day intravenous etoposide in combination with intravenous cisplatin in extensive-stage small-cell lung cancer: a randomized phase III study of the Cancer and Leukemia Group B. J Clin Oncol 1995;13(8):1871–9.
30. Sloan JA, Goldberg RM, Sargent DJ, Vargas-Chanes D, Nair S, Cha SS, Novotny PJ, Poon MA, O'Connell MJ, Loprinzi CL. Women experience greater toxicity with fluorouracil-based chemotherapy for colorectal cancer. J Clin Oncol 2002;20(6):1491–8.
31. Leighton JC Jr, Goldstein LJ. P-glycoprotein in adult solid tumors. Expression and prognostic significance. Hematol Oncol Clin North Am 1995;9(2):251–73.
32. Langer T, Martus P, Ottensmeier H, Hertzberg H, Beck JD, Meier W. CNS late-effects after ALL therapy in childhood. Part III. Neuropsychological performance in long-term survivors of childhood ALL: impairments of concentration, attention, and memory. Med Pediatr Oncol 2002;38(5): 320–8.
33. Herrlinger U, Schabet M, Brugger W, Kortmann RD, Kanz L, Bamberg M, Dichgans J, Weller M. Primary central nervous system lymphoma 1991–1997: outcome and late adverse effects after combined modality treatment. Cancer 2001;91(1):130–5.
34. Perrone L, Sinisi AA, Tullio M, et al. Endocrine function in subjects treated for childhood Hodgkin's disease. J Pediatr Endocrinol 1989;3:175.

35. Kelly WK, Curley T, Slovin S, Heller G, McCaffrey J, Bajorin D, Ciolino A, Regan K, Schwartz M, Kantoff P, George D, Oh W, Smith M, Kaufman D, Small EJ, Schwartz L, Larson S, Tong W, Scher H. Paclitaxel, estramustine phosphate, and carboplatin in patients with advanced prostate cancer. J Clin Oncol 2001;19(1):44–53.
36. Halonen P, Salo MK, Makipernaa A. Fasting hypoglycemia is common during maintenance therapy for childhood acute lymphoblastic leukemia. J Pediatr 2001;138(3):428–31.
37. Castro MP, VanAuken J, Spencer-Cisek P, Legha S, Sponzo RW. Acute tumor lysis syndrome associated with concurrent biochemotherapy of metastatic melanoma: a case report and review of the literature. Cancer 1999;85(5):1055–9.
38. Akasheh MS, Chang CP, Vesole DH. Acute tumour lysis syndrome: a case in AL amyloidosis. Br J Haematol 1999;107(2):387.
39. Voog E, Bienvenu J, Warzocha K, Moullet I, Dumontet C, Thieblemont C, Monneret G, Gutowski MC, Coiffier B, Salles G. Factors that predict chemotherapy-induced myelosuppression in lymphoma patients: role of the tumor necrosis factor ligand-receptor system. J Clin Oncol 2000;18(2):325–31.
40. Blumenthal RD, Lew W, Juweid M, Alisauskas R, Ying Z, Goldenberg DM. Plasma FLT3-L levels predict bone marrow recovery from myelosuppressive therapy. Cancer 2000;88(2):333–43.
41. Amadio P, Ferrau F, Priolo D, Toscano G, Colina P, Mare M, Zavettieri M, La Torre F, Mesiti M, Maisano R. Prevenzione e trattamento della mucosite da chemioterapici antiblastici. [Prevention and treatment of mucositis from cytotoxic chemotherapy.] Clin Ter 2002;153(2):127–34.
42. Gabriel DA, Shea T, Olajida O, Serody JS, Comeau T. The effect of oral mucositis on morbidity and mortality in bone marrow transplant. Semin Oncol 2003;30(6 Suppl 18):76–83.
43. Ricci JL, Turnbull AD. Spontaneous gastroduodenal perforation in cancer patients receiving cytotoxic therapy. J Surg Oncol 1989;41(4):219–21.
44. Vorobiof DA, Falkson G. Phase II study of high-dose 4′-epidoxorubicin in the treatment of advanced gastrointestinal cancer. Eur J Cancer Clin Oncol 1989; 25(3):563–4.
45. Sonis ST, Eilers JP, Epstein JB, LeVeque FG, Liggett WH Jr, Mulagha MT, Peterson DE, Rose AH, Schubert MM, Spijkervet FK, Wittes JP. Validation of a new scoring system for the assessment of clinical trial research of oral mucositis induced by radiation or chemotherapy. Mucositis Study Group. Cancer 1999;85(10):2103–13.
46. Rapoport AP, Miller Watelet LF, Linder T, Eberly S, Raubertas RF, Lipp J, Duerst R, Abboud CN, Constine L, Andrews J, Etter MA, Spear L, Powley E, Packman CH, Rowe JM, Schwertschlag U, Bedrosian C, Liesveld JL. Analysis of factors that correlate with mucositis in recipients of autologous and allogeneic stem-cell transplants. J Clin Oncol 1999;17(8):2446–53.
47. Tsujikawa T, Uda K, Ihara T, Inoue T, Andoh A, Fujiyama Y, Bamba T. Changes in serum diamine oxidase activity during chemotherapy in patients with hematological malignancies. Cancer Lett 1999;147(1–2):195–8.
48. Freeman AJ, Cullen MH. Advances in the management of cytotoxic drug-induced nausea and vomiting. J Clin Pharm Ther 1991;16(6):411–21.
49. Schnell FM. Chemotherapy-induced nausea and vomiting: the importance of acute antiemetic control. Oncologist 2003;8(2):187–98.
50. de Wit R, van Alphen MM. Nieuwe ontwikkelingen in de behandeling van misselijkheid en braken door chemotherapie. [New developments in the treatment of nausea and vomiting caused by chemotherapy.] Ned Tijdschr Geneeskd 2003;147(15):690–4.
51. Tonato M, Clark-Snow RA, Osoba D, Del Favero A, Ballatori E, Borjeson S. Emesis induced by low or minimal emetic risk chemotherapy. Support Care Cancer 2005;13(2):109–11.
52. Arnold RJ, Gabrail N, Raut M, Kim R, Sung JC, Zhou Y. Clinical implications of chemotherapy-induced diarrhea in patients with cancer. J Support Oncol 2005;3(3):227–32.
53. Kobayashi K. [Chemotherapy-induced diarrhea.] Gan To Kagaku Ryoho 2003;30(6):765–71.
54. O'Brien BE, Kaklamani VG, Benson AB 3rd. The assessment and management of cancer treatment-related diarrhea. Clin Colorectal Cancer 2005;4(6):375–81.
55. Douillard JY, Lerouge D, Monnier A, Bennouna J, Haller AM, Sun XS, Assouline D, Grau B, Riviere A. Combined paclitaxel and gemcitabine as first-line treatment in metastatic non-small cell lung cancer: a multicentre phase II study. Br J Cancer 2001;84(9):1179–84.
56. Leach JW, Pham T, Diamandidis D, George JN. Thrombotic thrombocytopenic purpura–hemolytic uremic syndrome (TTP–HUS) following treatment with deoxycoformycin in a patient with cutaneous T cell lymphoma (Sézary syndrome): A case report. Am J Hematol 1999;61(4):268–70.
57. Hui YF, Giles FJ, Cortes JE. Chemotherapy-induced palmar–plantar erythrodysesthesia syndrome—recall following different chemotherapy agents. Invest New Drugs 2002;20(1):49–53.
58. Moens C, Moens P, Philippart G. Azathioprine and warts. Ann Rheum Dis 1990;49(4):269.
59. Goyal S, Huhn KM, Provost TT. Calciphylaxis in a patient without renal failure or elevated parathyroid hormone: possible aetiological role of chemotherapy. Br J Dermatol 2000;143(5):1087–90.
60. Arikoski P, Komulainen J, Riikonen P, Jurvelin JS, Voutilainen R, Kroger H. Reduced bone density at completion of chemotherapy for a malignancy. Arch Dis Child 1999;80(2):143–8.
61. Saeter G, Fossa SD, Norman N. Gynaecomastia following cytotoxic therapy for testicular cancer. Br J Urol 1987;59(4):348–52.
62. Kreuser ED, Xiros N, Hetzel WD, Heimpel H. Reproductive and endocrine gonadal capacity in patients treated with COPP chemotherapy for Hodgkin's disease. J Cancer Res Clin Oncol 1987;113(3):260–6.
63. Garcia VD, Keitel E, Almeida P, Santos AF, Becker M, Goldani JC. Morbidity after renal transplantation: role of bacterial infection. Transplant Proc 1995;27(2):1825–6.
64. Wade JJ, Rolando N, Hayllar K, Philpott-Howard J, Casewell MW, Williams R. Bacterial and fungal infections after liver transplantation: an analysis of 284 patients. Hepatology 1995;21(5):1328–36.
65. Singh N, Yu VL. Infections in organ transplant recipients. Curr Opin Infect Dis 1996;9:223–9.
66. Reis MA, Costa RS, Ferraz AS. Causes of death in renal transplant recipients: a study of 102 autopsies from 1968 to 1991. J R Soc Med 1995;88(1):24–7.
67. Schubert J, Tolkendorf E, Held HJ, et al. Can the genetic risk be evaluated for offspring of testicular cancer patients exposed to chemotherapy treatment? Aktuel Urol 1989;20:199.
68. Brown T, Dawson AA, Bennett B, Moore NR. The effects of four drug regimens on sister chromatid exchange frequency in patients with lymphomas. Cancer Genet Cytogenet 1988;36(1):89–102.
69. Bennett JM, Moloney WC, Greene MH, Boice JD Jr. Acute myeloid leukemia and other myelopathic disorders following treatment with alkylating agents. Hematol Pathol 1987;1(2):99–104.
70. Pedersen-Bjergaard J, Ersbal J, Hansen V, et al. Blasenkarzinom nach Cyclophosphamid-Langzeittherapie. Aktuel Urol 1988;19:275.

71. O'Keane JC. Carcinoma of the urinary bladder after treatment with cyclophosphamide. N Engl J Med 1988;319(13):871.
72. Mahe M, Raffi F, Rojouan J, et al. Cancers secondaires après maladie de Hodgkin. Semin Hop Paris 1988;64:3013.
73. van der Velden JW, van Putten WL, Guinee VF, Pfeiffer R, van Leeuwen FE, van der Linden EA, Vardomskaya I, Lane W, Durand M, Lagarde C, et al. Subsequent development of acute non-lymphocytic leukemia in patients treated for Hodgkin's disease. Int J Cancer 1988;42(2):252–5.
74. Guyotat D, Coiffier B, Campos L, Archimbaud E, Treille D, Ehrsam A, Fiere D. Acute leukaemia following high-dose chemoradiotherapy with bone marrow rescue for ovarian teratoma. Acta Haematol 1988;80(1):52–3.
75. Einhorn N, Eklund G, Lambert B. Solid tumours and chromosome aberrations as late side effects of melphalan therapy in ovarian carcinoma. Acta Oncol 1988; 27(3):215–19.
76. Hoppe RT. Secondary leukemia and myelodysplastic syndrome after treatment for Hodgkin's disease. Leukemia 1992;6(Suppl 4):155–7.
77. Genuardi M, Zollino M, Serra A, Leone G, Mancini R, Mango G, Neri G. Long-term cytogenetic effects of antineoplastic treatment in relation to secondary leukemia. Cancer Genet Cytogenet 1988;33(2):201–11.
78. Hancock BW, Gregory WM, Cullen MH, Hudson GV, Burton A, Selby P, Maclennan KA, Jack A, Bessell EM, Smith P, Linch DC; British National Lymphoma Investigation; Central Lymphoma Group. ChlVPP alternating with PABlOE is superior to PABlOE alone in the initial treatment of advanced Hodgkin's disease: results of a British National Lymphoma Investigation/Central Lymphoma Group randomized controlled trial. Br J Cancer 2001;84(10):1293–300.
79. Cheson BD, Vena DA, Barrett J, Freidlin B. Second malignancies as a consequence of nucleoside analogue therapy for chronic lymphoid leukemias. J Clin Oncol 1999;17(8):2454–60.
80. Kawabata H, Utsunomiya A, Hanada S, Makino T, Takatsuka Y, Takeuchi S, Suzuki S, Suzumiya J, Ohshima K, Horiike S. Myelodysplastic syndrome in a patient with adult T cell leukaemia. Br J Haematol 1999;106(3):702–5.
81. Breslow NE, Takashima JR, Whitton JA, Moksness J, D'Angio GJ, Green DM. Second malignant neoplasms following treatment for Wilms' tumor: a report from the National Wilms' Tumor Study Group. J Clin Oncol 1995;13(8):1851–9.
82. Bokemeyer C, Freund M, Schmoll HJ, Rieder H, Fonatsch C. Secondary lymphoblastic leukemia following treatment of a malignant germ cell tumour. Ann Oncol 1992;3(9):772.
83. Kaldor JM, Day NE, Band P, Choi NW, Clarke EA, Coleman MP, Hakama M, Koch M, Langmark F, Neal FE, et al. Second malignancies following testicular cancer, ovarian cancer and Hodgkin's disease: an international collaborative study among cancer registries. Int J Cancer 1987;39(5):571–85.
84. Pedersen-Bjergaard J, Specht L, Larsen SO, Ersboll J, Struck J, Hansen MM, Hansen HH, Nissen NI. Risk of therapy-related leukaemia and preleukaemia after Hodgkin's disease. Relation to age, cumulative dose of alkylating agents, and time from chemotherapy. Lancet 1987;2(8550):83–8.
85. Blayney DW, Longo DL, Young RC, Greene MH, Hubbard SM, Postal MG, Duffey PL, DeVita VT Jr. Decreasing risk of leukemia with prolonged follow-up after chemotherapy and radiotherapy for Hodgkin's disease. N Engl J Med 1987;316(12):710–14.
86. Penn I. Tumors after renal and cardiac transplantation. Hematol Oncol Clin North Am 1993;7(2):431–45.
87. Gaya SB, Rees AJ, Lechler RI, Williams G, Mason PD. Malignant disease in patients with long-term renal transplants. Transplantation 1995;59(12):1705–9.
88. London NJ, Farmery SM, Will EJ, Davison AM, Lodge JP. Risk of neoplasia in renal transplant patients. Lancet 1995;346(8972):403–16.
89. Kehinde EO, Petermann A, Morgan JD, Butt ZA, Donnelly PK, Veitch PS, Bell PR. Triple therapy and incidence of de novo cancer in renal transplant recipients. Br J Surg 1994;81(7):985–6.
90. Opelz G, Henderson R. Incidence of non-Hodgkin lymphoma in kidney and heart transplant recipients. Lancet 1993;342(8886–8887):1514–6.
91. Gruber SA, Gillingham K, Sothern RB, Stephanian E, Matas AJ, Dunn DL. De novo cancer in cyclosporine-treated and non-cyclosporine-treated adult primary renal allograft recipients. Clin Transplant 1994;8(4):388–95.
92. Hiesse C, Kriaa F, Rieu P, Larue JR, Benoit G, Bellamy J, Blanchet P, Charpentier B. Incidence and type of malignancies occurring after renal transplantation in conventionally and cyclosporine-treated recipients: analysis of a 20-year period in 1600 patients. Transplant Proc 1995;27(1):972–4.
93. Gruber S, Dehner LP, Simmons RL. De novo hepatocellular carcinoma without chronic liver disease but with 17 years of azathioprine immunosuppression. Transplantation 1987;43(4):597–600.
94. Mittal BV, Cotton RE. Severely atypical changes in renal epithelium in biopsy and graft nephrectomy specimens in two cases of cadaver renal transplantation. Histopathology 1987;11(8):833–41.
95. Kelly G, Scheibner A, Murray E, Sheil R, Tiller D, Horvath J. T6+ and HLA-DR+ cell numbers in epidermis of immunosuppressed renal transplant recipients. J Cutan Pathol 1987;14(4):202–6.
96. Schwarz LR. Elimination of dose limiting toxicities of cisplatin, 5-fluorouracil, and leucovorin using a weekly 24-hour infusion schedule for the treatment of patients with nasopharyngeal carcinoma. Cancer 1996;78(3):566–7.
97. Viviani S, Ragni G, Santoro A, Perotti L, Caccamo E, Negretti E, Valagussa P, Bonadonna G. Testicular dysfunction in Hodgkin's disease before and after treatment. Eur J Cancer 1991;27(11):1389–92.
98. Ramsey-Goldman R, Schilling E. Immunosuppressive drug use during pregnancy. Rheum Dis Clin North Am 1997;23(1):149–67.
99. Armenti VT, Moritz MJ, Davison JM. Drug safety issues in pregnancy following transplantation and immunosuppression: effects and outcomes. Drug Saf 1998;19(3):219–32.
100. Armenti VT, Ahlswede KM, Ahlswede BA, Jarrell BE, Moritz MJ, Burke JF. National Transplantation Pregnancy Registry—outcomes of 154 pregnancies in cyclosporine-treated female kidney transplant recipients. Transplantation 1994;57(4):502–6.
101. Cararach V, Carmona F, Monleon FJ, Andreu J. Pregnancy after renal transplantation: 25 years experience in Spain. Br J Obstet Gynaecol 1993;100(2):122–5.
102. Armenti VT, Ahlswede BA, Moritz MJ, Jarrell BE. National Transplantation Pregnancy Registry: analysis of pregnancy outcomes of female kidney recipients with relation to time interval from transplant to conception. Transplant Proc 1993;25(1 Pt 2):1036–7.
103. Pilarski LM, Yacyshyn BR, Lazarovits AI. Analysis of peripheral blood lymphocyte populations and immune function from children exposed to cyclosporine or to azathioprine in utero. Transplantation 1994;57(1):133–44.

D

Dabequine

General Information

Dabequine is a 4-aminoquinoline derivative, the adverse reaction pattern of which is unknown. The WHO Scientific Group's report concerning this drug dates from 1984 and there seems to be little or no later information on it in humans.

Dacarbazine and temozolomide

See also Cytostatic and immunosuppressant drugs

General Information

Dacarbazine is converted to an active metabolite that is thought to be an alkylating agent. It has been used to treat metastatic melanoma and, in combination regimens, soft-tissue sarcomas and Hodgkin's disease.

Temozolomide is structurally related to dacarbazine and is thought to act via the same active metabolite. It has been used to treat malignant gliomas and malignant melanoma.

Organs and Systems

Hematologic

- Temozolomide-related myelodysplastic syndrome has been reported in a 44-year-old woman with recurrent anaplastic astrocytoma in association with a cytogenetic deletion in chromosome 3 (1).

Liver

Hepatotoxicity has been reported with single-dose dacarbazine (2,3), presenting as acute liver necrosis with hepatic venous thrombosis, which can be fatal.

- Severe hepatic insufficiency in a 69-year-old man after two courses of dacarbazine, 250 mg/m^2/day for 5 days, was successfully treated with intravenous hydrocortisone 300 mg/m^2/day (4).

Fatal hepatotoxicity has also been associated with dacarbazine 500 mg/day for 5 days (5). The cause of this effect is unclear; an allergic hepatic vasculitis with thrombosis is possible.

Skin

Phototoxic reactions occurred in 10 patients with malignant melanoma when they were given dacarbazine (6). In five patients who were tested there was increased sensitivity to ultraviolet A; patch-testing in six showed no type IV allergies. In five patients oral temozolomide did not cause phototoxicity.

References

1. Su YW, Chang MC, Chiang MF, Hsieh RK. Treatment-related myelodysplastic syndrome after temozolomide for recurrent high-grade glioma. J Neurooncol 2005;71(3):315–18.
2. Ceci G, Bella M, Melissari M, Gabrielli M, Bocchi P, Cocconi G. Fatal hepatic vascular toxicity of DTIC. Is it really a rare event? Cancer 1988;61(10):1988–91.
3. Lejeune FJ, Macher, E, Kleeberg U, Rumke P, Prade M, Thomas D, Sucin S. An assessment of DTIC vs levamisole or placebo in treatment of high risk stage I patients after surgical removal of a primary melanoma of the skin: a phase III adjuvant study. EORTC protocol 18761. Eur J Cancer Clin Oncol 1988;24(Suppl 2):581–90.
4. Herishanu Y, Lishner M, Kitay-Cohen Y. The role of glucocorticoids in the treatment of fulminant hepatitis induced by dacarbazine. Anticancer Drugs 2002;13(2):177–9.
5. McClay E, Lusch CJ, Mastrangelo MJ. Allergy-induced hepatic toxicity associated with dacarbazine. Cancer Treat Rep 1987;71(2):219–20.
6. Treudler R, Georgieva J, Geilen CC, Orfanos CE. Dacarbazine but not temozolomide induces phototoxic dermatitis in patients with malignant melanoma. J Am Acad Dermatol 2004;50(5):783–5.

Daclizumab

See also Monoclonal antibodies

General Information

Daclizumab, a humanized antibody directed against the alfa chain of the interleukin-2 receptor, has been used for initial immunosuppression in transplant patients. In a phase III trial in 275 patients who received ciclosporin, glucocorticoids, and daclizumab or placebo, there were no specific adverse effects associated with daclizumab (1). In particular, the cytokine-release syndrome did not occur, and there was no difference in the incidence of fungal or cytomegalovirus infections between the two groups.

Organs and Systems

Immunologic

The efficacy of daclizumab in acute and chronic glucocorticoid-refractory graft-versus-host disease has been studied in 16 patients, of whom nine responded (2). However 14 developed infectious complications during treatment, with a high incidence of cytomegalovirus reactivation; there were three infection-related deaths.

References

1. Charpentier B, Thervet E. Placebo-controlled study of a humanized anti-TAC monoclonal antibody in dual therapy for prevention of acute rejection after renal transplantation. Transplant Proc 1998;30(4):1331–2.
2. Willenbacher W, Basara N, Blau IW, Fauser AA, Kiehl MG. Treatment of steroid refractory acute and chronic graft-versus-host disease with daclizumab. Br J Haematol 2001;112(3):820–3.

Dactinomycin

See also Cytostatic and immunosuppressant drugs

General Information

Dactinomycin is used to treat cancers in children, in particular Wilms' tumor. It has similar adverse effects to doxorubicin.

Organs and Systems

Respiratory

Dactinomycin increases the pulmonary toxic effects of radiation by an estimated 30%, and reduces the radiation tolerance of the lung by at least 20% (1).

Liver

Several cases of hepatotoxicity have been reported in children receiving dactinomycin for Wilms' tumor (2–5). The hepatotoxicity of dactinomycin is dose- and schedule-related; mild hepatotoxicity is described in up to 12% of patients (6).

Five of 40 patients, who received a pulsed regimen of 60 μg/kg of dactinomycin every 3 weeks up to and including week 15, developed severe hepatotoxicity, with sharp rises in liver function test values, ascites, and liver enlargement. One child with complicating factors died and the others recovered. All five had possible contributing factors, such as repeated anesthesia (3).

References

1. Cohen IJ, Loven D, Schoenfeld T, Sandbank J, Kaplinsky C, Yaniv Y, Jaber L, Zaizov R. Dactinomycin potentiation of radiation pneumonitis: a forgotten interaction. Pediatr Hematol Oncol 1991;8(2):187–92.
2. Green DM, Finklestein JZ, Norkool P, D'Angio GJ. Severe hepatic toxicity after treatment with single-dose dactinomycin and vincristine. A report of the National Wilms' Tumor Study. Cancer 1988;62(2):270–3.
3. D'Angio GJ. Hepatotoxicity with actinomycin D. Lancet 1987;2(8550):104.
4. Pritchard J, Raine J, Wallendszus K. Hepatotoxicity of actinomycin-D. Lancet 1989;1(8630):168.
5. White L, Tobias V, Hughes DW. Actinomycin D-induced hepatotoxicity. Pediatr Hematol Oncol 1989;6(1):53–7.
6. D'Angio GJ. Hepatotoxicity and actinomycin D. Lancet 1990;335(8700):1290.

Danaparoid sodium

General Information

Danaparoid is a low molecular heparinoid consisting of a mixture of sulfated glycosaminoglycans (heparan, dermatan, and chondroitin sulfates). It has an antithrombotic effect via antithrombin III-mediated inhibition of factor Xa and to a lesser extent through inhibition of factor IIa. The ratio of antifactor Xa to antifactor IIa is over 20.

Danaparoid is as effective as heparins in inhibiting the formation of thrombi. Its major advantage over low molecular weight heparins is its low rate of cross-reactivity with heparin-associated antibodies from patients with heparin-induced thrombocytopenia (1). It is therefore indicated in patients with heparin-associated thrombocytopenia who require further anticoagulation after withdrawal of heparin. However, it should not be used if there is in vitro cross-reactivity between heparin and danaparoid. Cross-reactivity is uncommon but can result in thrombotic complications, as reported in a case with a fatal outcome (2).

Organs and Systems

Hematologic

Severe bleeding is uncommon with danaparoid but was 3.1% in one series (3).

Immunologic

Delayed hypersensitivity reactions have been reported in patients given danaparoid (4).

References

1. Wilde MI, Markham A. Danaparoid. A review of its pharmacology and clinical use in the management of heparin-induced thrombocytopenia. Drugs 1997;54(6):903–24.
2. Tardy B, Tardy-Poncet B, Viallon A, Piot M, Mazet E. Fatal danaparoid-sodium induced thrombocytopenia and arterial thromboses. Thromb Haemost 1998;80(3):530.
3. Magnani HN. Orgaran (danaparoid sodium) use in the syndrome of heparin-induced thrombocytopenia. Platelets 1997;8:74.
4. Koch P, Munssinger T, Rupp-John C, Uhl K. Delayed-type hypersensitivity skin reactions caused by subcutaneous unfractionated and low-molecular-weight heparins: tolerance of a new recombinant hirudin. J Am Acad Dermatol 2000;42(4):612–19.

Dantrolene

General Information

Dantrolene, a hydantoin derivative, is well established in clinical practice, being of greatest value for the reduction of clonus and involuntary muscle spasms (1,2). The recommended oral doses for the treatment of spastic conditions are 75–400 mg/day.

Dantrolene (1,2) is the agent of choice for treatment of malignant hyperthermia and greatly reduces the mortality to under 10% if given in time (3) together with general supportive measures.

Dantrolene differs from the centrally acting muscle relaxants in that its site of action is beyond the muscle cell membrane. It interferes with the excitation–contraction coupling mechanism of striated muscle, presumably by inhibition of calcium release from the sarcoplasmic reticulum.

The most common adverse reactions, seen in up to 75% of patients, are weakness, fatigue, drowsiness, and dizziness. Nausea, vomiting, and diarrhea or constipation are also common, but all these adverse reactions tend to disappear as treatment continues. In general, by adjusting the dose a satisfactory effect can be achieved with acceptable adverse effects.

Rare, but occasionally very serious, adverse effects include hepatotoxicity, respiratory depression, seizures, pleuropericardial reaction, and lymphocytic lymphoma (SEDA-5, 137).

Organs and Systems

Respiratory

Muscle weakness associated with the oral prophylactic use of dantrolene in a patient with compromised respiratory function is reported to have exacerbated postoperative respiratory depression to such an extent that artificial ventilation was required (SEDA-14, 114) (4).

Pleuropericardial reactions, with sterile effusions and eosinophilia, have also rarely been reported in patients taking 225–400 mg/day for 3 months to 4 years (5). There is no proof of a causal relation, but the chemically related nitrofurantoin has also been associated with pulmonary reactions. Patients taking dantrolene should be screened periodically.

Nervous system

Numbness of the hands and feet has been reported (6); long-term use of the structurally related phenytoin has been incriminated in causing polyneuropathy.

Exacerbation or precipitation of seizures has been reported in children with cerebral palsy taking long-term treatment with high doses of dantrolene (4–12 mg/kg) (7).

Sensory systems

Deafness occurred after 5 days' treatment with dantrolene 25 mg/day in a patient who was also taking long-term baclofen and diazepam (8). This may have been coincidental, but the authors suggested that dantrolene may have caused the effect by interfering with the release of calcium from the sarcoplasmic reticulum. It is therefore interesting that one hypothesis that explains the ototoxicity of aminoglycoside antibiotics involves disturbance of calcium ion binding and phosphorylation processes (SED-11, 549).

Hematologic

Fatal lymphocytic lymphoma has been described during high-dose dantrolene therapy (600 mg/day over 3 years) (9). Although the association was only circumstantial, another hydantoin derivative, phenytoin, is known to cause pseudolymphoma.

Liver

Hepatotoxicity from dantrolene consists mainly of minor liver function disturbances (in 1% of patients), with symptoms in 0.35–0.5% and fatal hepatitis in 0.3% (10,11). The risk of severe liver damage is greater with doses above 300–400 mg/day, with prolonged treatment (more than 60 days), in women and in patients older than 35 years.

Reproductive system

Dantrolene may have contributed to uterine atony, with resulting excessive hemorrhage when given prophylactically after a cesarean section (12).

Drug–Drug Interactions

Calcium channel blockers

The combination of dantrolene with calcium channel blockers, such as verapamil, can result in severe cardiovascular depression and hyperkalemia (SEDA-12, 113) (13,14), so that extreme care is required.

Metoclopramide

The absorption of oral dantrolene can be significantly increased by metoclopramide (15). As the risk of hepatotoxicity has been related to the dosage of dantrolene, increased clinical surveillance is necessary to avoid toxicity of dantrolene during concurrent treatment with metoclopramide.

References

1. Britt BA. Dantrolene. Can Anaesth Soc J 1984;31(1):61–75.
2. Ward A, Chaffman MO, Sorkin EM. Dantrolene. A review of its pharmacodynamic and pharmacokinetic properties and therapeutic use in malignant hyperthermia, the neuroleptic malignant syndrome and an update of its use in muscle spasticity. Drugs 1986;32(2):130–68.
3. Kolb ME, Horne ML, Martz R. Dantrolene in human malignant hyperthermia. Anesthesiology 1982;56(4):254–62.
4. Hara Y, Kato A, Horikawa H, Kato Y, Ichiyanagi K. [Postoperative respiratory depression thought to be due to oral dantrolene pretreatment in a malignant hyperthermia-susceptible patient.] Masui 1988;37(4):483–7.
5. Petusevsky ML, Faling LJ, Rocklin RE, Snider GL, Merliss AD, Moses JM, Dorman SA. Pleuropericardial reaction to treatment with dantrolene. JAMA 1979;242(25):2772–4.
6. Luisto M, Moller K, Nuutila A, Palo J. Dantrolene sodium in chronic spasticity of varying etiology. A double-blind study. Acta Neurol Scand 1982;65(4):355–62.
7. Denhoff E, Feldman S, Smith MG, Litchman H, Holden W. Treatment of spastic cerebral-palsied children with sodium dantrolene. Dev Med Child Neurol 1975;17(6):736–42.
8. Pace-Balzan A, Ramsden RT. Sudden bilateral sensorineural hearing loss during treatment with dantrolene sodium (Dantrium). J Laryngol Otol 1988;102(1):57–8.
9. Wan HH, Tucker JS. Dantrolene and lymphocytic lymphoma. Postgrad Med J 1980;56(654):261–2.
10. Utili R, Boitnott JK, Zimmerman HJ. Dantrolene-associated hepatic injury. Incidence and character. Gastroenterology 1977;72(4 Pt 1):610–16.
11. Pinder RM, Brogden RN, Speight TM, Avery GS. Dantrolene sodium: a review of its pharmacological properties and therapeutic efficacy in spasticity. Drugs 1977;13(1):3–23.
12. Weingarten AE, Korsh JI, Neuman GG, Stern SB. Postpartum uterine atony after intravenous dantrolene. Anesth Analg 1987;66(3):269–70.

13. Saltzman LS, Kates RA, Corke BC, Norfleet EA, Heath KR. Hyperkalemia and cardiovascular collapse after verapamil and dantrolene administration in swine. Anesth Analg 1984;63(5):473–8.
14. Rubin AS, Zablocki AD. Hyperkalemia, verapamil, and dantrolene. Anesthesiology 1987;66(2):246–9.
15. Gilman TM, Segal JL, Brunnemann SR. Metoclopramide increases the bioavailability of dantrolene in spinal cord injury. J Clin Pharmacol 1996;36(1):64–71.

Dapsone and analogues

General Information

Dapsone is 4,4-diaminodiphenylsulfone (DDS, avlosulfone, disulfone) (SEDA-17, 352). It is a bacteriostatic antileprosy drug with a sulfonamide-like structure. The dosage should be 50–100 mg/day in adults (1). In children aged 3–5 years, the dosage should be reduced according to weight to, for example, 25 mg/day (2).

Studies of patients with borderline leprosy have suggested that dapsone has mild immunosuppressive effects (SEDA-18, 30). Thus, it has been given with some success to patients with dermatitis herpetiformis, subcorneal pustular dermatosis, bullous dermatoses, relapsing polychondritis, thrombocytopenic purpura (3), giant cell arteritis (4), rheumatoid arthritis, and systemic lupus erythematosus (5).

Dapsone is an alternative drug for *Pneumocystis jiroveci* pneumonia prophylaxis in individuals who cannot tolerate co-trimoxazole, and although this has become less of a problem since the advent of highly active antiretroviral drug therapy in countries able to afford these regimens, further data on the toxicity of dapsone in children are welcome. In a multicenter study from the USA daily and weekly dapsone regimens have been compared in 94 HIV-infected children, monitoring hematological and liver toxicity and the incidence of skin rashes, *P. jiroveci* pneumonia, or death (6). They concluded that the weekly regimen produced less hematological toxicity, but that this advantage was offset by a trend toward higher breakthrough rates of *P. jiroveci* pneumonia.

Dapsone analogues

The sulfone acedapsone (rINN) (4,4′-diacetyldiaminodiphenylsulfone, DADDS) is the diacetyl derivative of dapsone with a long half-life (7). However, its plasma concentrations are much lower than those of dapsone and it could enhance the emergence of resistant strains of *Mycobacterium leprae*. Its adverse effects are similar to those of dapsone, which it can replace if gastrointestinal symptoms become severe. It is available in an enteric-coated formulation, given in a dosage of 330 mg/day.

General adverse effects

The adverse effects of dapsone have been comprehensively reviewed (8). The most common untoward effect is hemolysis of varying degree; it is usually mild, except in patients with glucose-6-phosphate dehydrogenase (G6PD) deficiency. Methemoglobinemia and Heinz body formation also occur and methemoglobinemia can be a problem at doses over 200 mg/day. Agranulocytosis is rare but potentially fatal. Mild gastrointestinal complaints and neurological effects of dapsone are not uncommon. Under 0.5% of the patients taking prolonged dapsone therapy develop the dapsone syndrome (SEDA-16, 347). Other rare adverse effects include peripheral neuropathy, psychosis, hepatitis, nephritic syndrome, and renal papillary necrosis. Hypoalbuminemia has been seen after prolonged dapsone therapy of dermatitis herpetiformis (9). Erythema nodosum leprosum may be due to an immune complex mechanism; the antigen is provided by the bacteria and their degeneration products, possibly as a kind of Jarisch–Herxheimer reaction (10). Anaphylactic shock and tachycardia are rare. Rashes, serious cutaneous reactions, and erythema nodosum may have an immunological basis. Tumor-inducing effects have not been reported.

In France, dapsone is available in combination with ferrous oxalate as Disulone (Aventis), and in 1983–98, 249 adverse reactions were reported to French pharmacovigilance centers, mainly blood dyscrasias (often neutropenia and agranulocytosis, rarely hemolysis and anemia) (11). Five patients died; three of them had septicemia secondary to agranulocytosis. There were 29 cases of dapsone syndrome, 39 skin reactions, 27 cases of liver damage, and 27 cases of neurological and psychiatric adverse effects. Patients taking dapsone need to be under close medical supervision for early recognition of adverse reactions.

Organs and Systems

Cardiovascular

Signs of heart failure with edema, ascites, and severe hypoalbuminemia have been described in the treatment of dermatitis herpetiformis with dapsone (9).

Respiratory

Two cases of pulmonary eosinophilia attributed to dapsone were reported in 1998. Four cases had previously been reported, in which the fixed combination of dapsone and pyrimethamine (a malaria prophylactic) had been implicated, but only one previous report had implicated dapsone alone.

- A French woman with chronic urticaria (12) and an Indian man with lepromatous leprosy (13) developed fever, wheezing, and breathlessness. Both had peripheral eosinophilia and chest X-rays showed infiltrates. The woman's symptoms began 2 weeks after she started to take dapsone but recurred a few hours after a subsequent rechallenge. The man's symptoms occurred a few hours after each daily dose. Symptoms in both cases resolved within a few days of stopping dapsone.

Nervous system

Dapsone-induced neuropathy is not common (14), in spite of its widespread use in a variety of unrelated disorders. It has not been reported in patients with leprosy, but it would be easy to miss, since worsening neuropathy would readily be attributed to the underlying disease.

Neuropathy has not been reported in patients with leprosy taking the usually recommended dosage of 100 mg/day. Isolated cases of dapsone-induced peripheral neuropathy, including motor and minor sensory defects, have been published (15,16). The clinical characteristics include a motor neuropathy affecting the extremities with onset within 5 years after the start of dapsone therapy in doses of over 300 mg/day. Complete recovery from the neuropathy almost always occurs after the dose is reduced or the drug is withdrawn.

Infection with *M. leprae* affects the peripheral nerves and the dermis, causing an accumulation of macrophages and other immune cells at the infected site (17).

Sensory systems

Ocular toxicity is rare with dapsone. Reduced visual acuity has been described after overdosage (18).

Psychological, psychiatric

Dapsone-induced psychosis has rarely been reported (SEDA-15, 331) (19).

Hematologic

The most common adverse effect of dapsone therapy is hemolysis (SEDA-15, 331). In varying degrees, it develops in nearly all patients taking dapsone in dosages of 200–300 mg/day. Even with the usual dose of 100 mg/day in normal persons and 50 mg/day in patients with G6PD deficiency, there can be some degree of hemolysis (20,21). Red cell survival can be reduced by dapsone, depending on the dose of the sulfone and its oxidizing activity, but hemolytic anemia generally does not occur without a preexisting disorder of the erythrocytes or bone marrow. The hemolysis can be so severe that manifestations of hypoxia become striking (20).

- Mild hemolytic anemia occurred in a breast-fed infant and his mother, who had continuously been taking 100–150 mg/day; dapsone and its metabolite, monoacetyldapsone, were identified in the infant's serum (SEDA-8, 290).

Dapsone is an oxidant and can trigger methemoglobinemia and delayed sulfhemoglobinemia (SEDA-8, 289) (22). Methemoglobinemia remains subclinical in most cases. However, it can be accurately inferred by a discrepancy between the oxygen saturation measured by pulse oximetry and the concentration of oxygen in the arterial blood (22). Methemoglobinemia at concentrations over 10% produces a visible lavender-colored cyanosis, and concentrations over 35% result in weakness and shortness of breath. Methemoglobinemia can be minimized by the administration of an antioxidant, such as vitamin C or vitamin E (23). Methemoglobinemia disappears after withdrawal of dapsone (SEDA-10, 273).

- A patient who had been taking dapsone inappropriately instead of an antispasmodic that had been prescribed for a spinal condition, because of incorrect labeling in a pharmacy, developed methemoglobinemia (24). Methylene blue was given intravenously and may have contributed to the severe hemolysis that followed.

Agranulocytosis is a rare complication of dapsone treatment (25).

Liver

Jaundice and hepatitis can occur as part of the sulfone syndrome with dapsone (26). Previous liver damage can predispose to serious hepatic or other adverse effects.

Urinary tract

Renal insufficiency can be associated with severe hemolysis due to dapsone (27).

Skin

Pruritus and various forms of rash can occur with dapsone. In 17 cases of dapsone syndrome, the symptoms developed on average 27 days after the start of treatment. The skin lesions took the form of erythematous papules and plaques ($n = 13$), eczematous lesions ($n = 4$), and associated bullous lesions ($n = 2$) (28). The other manifestations were: fever ($n = 16$), pruritus ($n = 15$), lymphadenopathy ($n = 14$), hepatomegaly ($n = 10$), icterus and oral erosions ($n = 5$ each), photosensitivity ($n = 4$), and splenomegaly ($n = 2$).

Serious cutaneous reactions, such as exfoliative dermatitis, toxic epidermal necrolysis, and erythema multiforme bullosum are extremely rare. Erythema nodosum leprosum has been described during dapsone therapy, mostly in the lepromatous type of leprosy (10). If erythema nodosum develops before the start of therapy, the drug should be withheld until the reaction has disappeared. Severe erythema nodosum can be controlled by short-term glucocorticoid therapy. Desensitization to dapsone in patients with hypersensitivity reactions has been proposed (29).

Immunologic

The sulfones occasionally exacerbate lepromatous leprosy, the so-called sulfone syndrome or dapsone syndrome, which resembles acute infectious mononucleosis (SEDA-16, 347) (30), and can develop 3–6 weeks after the start of treatment in malnourished patients. It appears to be an allergic reaction. It includes fever, malaise, pruritus, exfoliative dermatitis, photosensitivity, polyarthritis (31), jaundice and even hepatic necrosis, hepatosplenomegaly, lymphadenopathy, methemoglobinemia, and anemia. The syndrome is accompanied by the formation of atypical T lymphocytes with markedly increased spontaneous thymidine uptake (SEDA-8, 289). The full syndrome is probably rare, but it is important to recognize its partial expression (5,32,33). It has been suggested that it has become more common since the introduction of multidrug therapy (34), especially with rifampicin plus dapsone. The syndrome usually resolves rapidly after withdrawal of dapsone and with glucocorticoid treatment (for example prednisolone 30–60 mg/day). However, it can also end in a fatal allergic reaction (SEDA-12, 259).

Anaphylactic shock and tachycardia are among the most severe allergic reactions to dapsone (34).

Second-Generation Effects

Pregnancy

The use of antileprosy drugs during pregnancy depends upon the severity of the disease and the relative need for treatment. Even though untoward effects on the fetus have not been reported, treatment of leprosy during pregnancy probably predisposes to erythema nodosum leprosum; if this occurs during pregnancy, clofazimine is considered the best drug available (35).

Lactation

Dapsone passes into the breast milk, with a milk to plasma AUC ratio of 0.22:0.45 (36). Assuming a daily milk ingestion of 1 liter by the infant, the maximum percentage of the maternal dose in milk was 14% over 9 days. Usually no adverse effects are noted in the newborn, unless there is G6PD deficiency.

Susceptibility Factors

Genetic factors

Glucose-6-phosphate dehydrogenase deficiency is a risk factor for hemolytic anemia (37–39).

To what extent phenotype (fast versus slow acetylators) affects the metabolism of dapsone is controversial. Since dapsone is acetylated in the liver, an effect might be anticipated (SEDA-4, 217) (40), but has not been demonstrated.

Hepatic disease

Previous liver damage predisposes to adverse effects during dapsone therapy (41).

Other features of the patient

Malnutrition predisposes to adverse effects during dapsone therapy (42).

Drug Administration

Drug administration route

Aqueous or oily suspensions of dapsone for intramuscular injection can be used to ensure adherence and to prevent resistance due to irregular drug intake. The therapeutic efficacy of intramuscular formulations lasts 3–4 weeks (43).

Drug overdose

Several reports of accidental poisoning with dapsone in children have appeared since the early 1980s. Two reports (44,45) have emphasized the persistence of the problem, although the number of childhood cases has fallen over the years. Poisoning with dapsone results in cyanosis due to methemoglobinemia, vomiting, mental confusion, tachycardia, and dyspnea. It has been suggested that treatment with multiple doses of activated charcoal may be sufficient for less severely poisoned children (methemoglobin concentration below 30%) and that a single dose of methylthioninium chloride (methylene blue) should be given to those with higher concentrations (45).

Drug–Drug Interactions

Clofazimine

In 28 patients with lepromatous leprosy, clofazimine did not influence the urinary excretion of dapsone, except in one case (46).

Rifamycins

When rifampicin was given, dapsone blood concentrations were lowered and urinary excretion was increased during the first 2 days; however, blood concentrations remained in the therapeutic range (47).

References

1. Garg SK, Kumar B, Bakaya V, Lal R, Shukla VK, Kaur S. Plasma dapsone and its metabolite monoacetyldapsone levels in leprotic patients. Int J Clin Pharmacol Ther Toxicol 1988;26(11):552–4.
2. Thangaraj RH, Yawalkar SJ. Leprosy for Medical Practitioners and Paramedical Workers. 2nd ed. Basel: Ciba-Geigy, 1987.
3. Godeau B, Oksenhendler E, Bierling P. Dapsone for autoimmune thrombocytopenic purpura. Am J Hematol 1993;44(1):70–2.
4. Liozon F, Vidal E, Barrier JH. Dapsone in giant cell arteritis treatment. Eur J Intern Med 1993;4:207.
5. Kraus A, Jakez J, Palacios A. Dapsone induced sulfone syndrome and systemic lupus exacerbation. J Rheumatol 1992;19(1):178–80.
6. McIntosh K, Cooper E, Xu J, Mirochnick M, Lindsey J, Jacobus D, Mofenson L, Yogev R, Spector SA, Sullivan JL, Sacks H, Kovacs A, Nachman S, Sleasman J, Bonagura V, McNamara J. Toxicity and efficacy of daily vs. weekly dapsone for prevention of *Pneumocystis carinii* pneumonia in children infected with human immunodeficiency virus. ACTG 179 Study Team. AIDS Clinical Trials Group. Pediatr Infect Dis J 1999;18(5):432–9.
7. George J, Balakrishnan S. Blood dapsone levels in leprosy patients treated with acedapsone. Indian J Lepr 1986;58(3):401–6.
8. Zhu YI, Stiller MJ. Dapsone and sulfones in dermatology: overview and update. J Am Acad Dermatol 2001;45(3):420–34.
9. Cowan RE, Wright JT. Dapsone and severe hypoalbuminaemia in dermatitis herpetiformis. Br J Dermatol 1981;104(2):201–4.
10. Somorin AO. Erythema nodosum leprosum in Nigeria. Int J Dermatol 1975;14(9):664–6.
11. Benedetti-Bardet C, Guy C, Boudignat O, Regnier-Zerbib A, Ollagnier M. Centres Regionaux de Pharmacovigilance. Effets indésirables de la Disulone: résultants de l'enquête française de pharmacovigilance. [Adverse effects of Disulone; results of the France pharmacovigilance inquiry. Regional Centers of Pharmacovigilance.] Therapie 2001;56(3):295–9.
12. Jaffuel D, Lebel B, Hillaire-Buys D, Pene J, Godard P, Michel FB, Blayac JP, Bousquet J, Demolyi P. Eosinophilic pneumonia induced by dapsone. BMJ 1998;317(7152):181.
13. Arunthathi S, Raju S. Dapsone-induced pulmonary eosinophilia without cutaneous allergic manifestations—an unusual encounter—a case report. Acta Leprol 1998;11(2):3–5.
14. Saqueton AC, Lorincz AL, Vick NA, Hamer RD. Dapsone and peripheral motor neuropathy. Arch Dermatol 1969;100(2):214–7.

15. Waldinger TP, Siegle RJ, Weber W, Voorhees JJ. Dapsone-induced peripheral neuropathy. Case report and review. Arch Dermatol 1984;120(3):356–9.
16. Ahrens EM, Meckler RJ, Callen JP. Dapsone-induced peripheral neuropathy. Int J Dermatol 1986;25(5):314–16.
17. Kaplan G, Cohn ZA. The immunobiology of leprosy. Int Rev Exp Pathol 1986;28:45–78.
18. Alexander TA, Raju R, Kuriakose T, Cherian AM. Presumed DDS ocular toxicity. Indian J Ophthalmol 1989;37(3):150–1.
19. Balkrishna, Bhatia MS. Dapsone induced psychosis. J Indian Med Assoc 1989;87(5):120–1.
20. Mandell GL, Sande MA. Antimicrobial agents: drugs used in the chemotherapy of tuberculosis and leprosy. In: Goodman Gilman A, Rall TW, Nies AS, Taylor P, editors. Goodman and Gilman's The Pharmacological Basis of Therapeutics.8th ed. Chapter 49. New York: Pergamon Press, 1990:1146 .
21. Byrd SR, Gelber RH. Effect of dapsone on haemoglobin concentration in patients with leprosy. Lepr Rev 1991;62(2):171–8.
22. Trillo RA Jr, Aukburg S. Dapsone-induced methemoglobinemia and pulse oximetry. Anesthesiology 1992;77(3):594–6.
23. Prussick R, Ali MA, Rosenthal D, Guyatt G. The protective effect of vitamin E on the hemolysis associated with dapsone treatment in patients with dermatitis herpetiformis. Arch Dermatol 1992;128(2):210–13.
24. Southgate HJ, Masterson R. Lessons to be learned: a case study approach: prolonged methaemoglobinaemia due to inadvertent dapsone poisoning; treatment with methylene blue and exchange transfusion. J R Soc Health 1999;119(1):52–5.
25. Braude AL, Davis Ch E, Fierer J. Infectious Diseases and Medical Microbiology. 2nd ed. Philadelphia: WB Saunders, 1966:1171.
26. Tomecki KJ, Catalano CJ. Dapsone hypersensitivity. The sulfone syndrome revisited. Arch Dermatol 1981;117(1):38–9.
27. Chugh KS, Singhal PC, Sharma BK, Mahakur AC, Pal Y, Datta BN, Das KC. Acute renal failure due to intravascular hemolysis in the North Indian patients. Am J Med Sci 1977;274(2):139–46.
28. Kumar RH, Kumar MV, Thappa DM. Dapsone syndrome—a five year retrospective analysis. Indian J Lepr 1998;70(3):271–6.
29. Browne SG. Desensitization for dapsone dermatitis. BMJ 1963;5358:664–6.
30. Chan HL, Lee KO. Tonsillar membrane in the DDS (dapsone) syndrome. Int J Dermatol 1991;30(3):216–17.
31. Pavithran K. Dapsone syndrome with polyarthritis: a case report. Indian J Lepr 1990;62(2):230–2.
32. Johnson DA, Cattau EL Jr, Kuritsky JN, Zimmerman HJ. Liver involvement in the sulfone syndrome. Arch Intern Med 1986;146(5):875–7.
33. Mohle-Boetani J, Akula SK, Holodniy M, Katzenstein D, Garcia G. The sulfone syndrome in a patient receiving dapsone prophylaxis for *Pneumocystis carinii* pneumonia. West J Med 1992;156(3):303–6.
34. Richardus JH, Smith TC. Increased incidence in leprosy of hypersensitivity reactions to dapsone after introduction of multidrug therapy. Lepr Rev 1989;60(4):267–73.
35. Duncan ME, Pearson JM. The association of pregnancy and leprosy—III. Erythema nodosum leprosum in pregnancy and lactation. Lepr Rev 1984;55(2):129–42.
36. Edstein MD, Veenendaal JR, Newman K, Hyslop R. Excretion of chloroquine, dapsone and pyrimethamine in human milk. Br J Clin Pharmacol 1986;22(6):733–5.
37. Editorial. Adverse reactions to dapsone. Lancet 1981;2(8239):184–5.
38. Menezes S, Rege VL, Sehgal VN. Dapsone haemolysis in leprosy. A preliminary report. Lepr India 1981;53(1):63–9.
39. Halmekoski J, Mattila MJ, Mustakallio KK. Metabolism and haemolytic effect of dapsone and its metabolites in man. Med Biol 1978;56(4):216–21.
40. Peters JH, Gordon GR, Levy L, Strokan MA, Jacobson RR, Enna CD, Kirchheimer WF. Metabolic disposition of dapsone in patients with dapsone-resistant leprosy. Am J Trop Med Hyg 1974;23(2):222–30.
41. Goette DK. Dapsone-induced hepatic changes. Arch Dermatol 1977;113(11):1616–17.
42. Gawkrodger DJ, Ferguson A, Barnetson RS. Nutritional status in patients with dermatitis herpetiformis. Am J Clin Nutr 1988;48(2):355–60.
43. Modderman ES, Huikeshoven H, Zuidema J, Leiker DL, Merkus FW. Intramuscular injection of dapsone in therapy for leprosy: a new approach. Int J Clin Pharmacol Ther Toxicol 1982;20(2):51–6.
44. Carrazza MZ, Carrazza FR, Oga S. Clinical and laboratory parameters in dapsone acute intoxication. Rev Saude Publica 2000;34(4):396–401.
45. Bucaretchi F, Miglioli L, Baracat EC, Madureira PR, Capitani EM, Vieira RJ. Exposicao aguda a dapsona e metemoglobinemia em criancas: tratamento com doses multiplas de carvao ativado. [Acute dapsone exposure and methemoglobinemia in children: treatment with multiple doses of activated charcoal with or without the administration of methylene blue.] J Pediatr (Rio J) 2000;76(4):290–4.
46. Grabosz JA, Wheate HW. Effect of clofazimine on the urinary excretion of DDS (dapsone). Int J Lepr Other Mycobact Dis 1975;43(1):61–2.
47. Balakrishnan, Seshadri PS. Drug interactions—the influence of rifampicin and clofazimine on the urinary excretion of DDS. Lepr India 1981;53(1):17–22.

Daptomycin

General Information

Daptomycin is a novel lipopeptide antibiotic, an inhibitor of lipoteichoic acid synthesis, with potent bactericidal activity against most clinically important Gram-positive bacteria, including resistant strains (1,2).

When daptomycin 4 mg/kg was given intravenously to seven healthy men the mean peak concentrations in plasma and inflammatory fluid were 78 and 28 μg/ml respectively; the mean half-lives were 7.7 and 13 hours respectively; the overall penetration of total drug into the inflammatory fluid was 68% and the mean urinary recovery over 24 hours was 60% (3).

Organs and Systems

Musculoskeletal

Daptomycin may have adverse effects on skeletal muscle, since it increases serum creatine kinase activity. To find the dosing regimen that has the least effects on skeletal muscle, dogs were given repeated intravenous daptomycin every 24 hours or every 8 hours for 20 days (4). The results suggested that adverse effects on skeletal muscle are primarily related to dosing frequency but not peak plasma concentrations, and once-daily administration appeared to minimize the potential for daptomycin-related skeletal-muscle effects, possibly by allowing more time between doses for repair of subclinical effects.

Long-Term Effects

Drug tolerance

The activity of daptomycin against both vancomycin-sensitive and vancomycin-resistant *Enterococcus faecalis* was greater than that of quinupristin + dalfopristin (5). Daptomycin was as active as quinupristin + dalfopristin but more active than linezolid. At concentrations four times the MIC, daptomycin and vancomycin achieved 99.9% killing of methicillin-resistant *Staphylococcus aureus* after 8 hours, which was greater than the killing seen with linezolid and quinupristin + dalfopristin. However, the antibacterial activity of daptomycin strongly depended on the calcium concentration of the medium.

References

1. Stephenson J. Researchers describe latest strategies to combat antibiotic-resistant microbes. JAMA 2001;285(18):2317–18.
2. Anonymous. Daptomycin. Cidecin, Dapcin, LY 146032. Drugs R D 2002;3(1):33–9.
3. Wise R, Gee T, Andrews JM, Dvorchik B, Marshall G. Pharmacokinetics and inflammatory fluid penetration of intravenous daptomycin in volunteers. Antimicrob Agents Chemother 2002;46(1):31–3.
4. Oleson FB Jr, Berman CL, Kirkpatrick JB, Regan KS, Lai JJ, Tally FP. Once-daily dosing in dogs optimizes daptomycin safety. Antimicrob Agents Chemother 2000;44(11):2948–53.
5. Rybak MJ, Hershberger E, Moldovan T, Grucz RG. In vitro activities of daptomycin, vancomycin, linezolid, and quinupristin–dalfopristin against staphylococci and enterococci, including vancomycin-intermediate and -resistant strains. Antimicrob Agents Chemother 2000;44(4):1062–6.

Decamethonium

See also Neuromuscular blocking drugs

General Information

Decamethonium, a depolarizing neuromuscular blocker, is little used nowadays. A dose of 3 mg provides adequate relaxation for intra-abdominal surgery for about 15 minutes, supplements being required at intervals of 10–30 minutes. It is not as rapid in onset of action as suxamethonium. It is not hydrolysed by plasma cholinesterase, but is eliminated by the kidneys (1).

Tachyphylaxis occurs and a phase II block develops readily (2). In high doses, muscarinic actions can be seen and histamine release can occur.

Organs and Systems

Cardiovascular

Cardiovascular effects are less frequent than with suxamethonium; a reduction in heart rate sometimes occurs after a second dose.

Nervous system

Fasciculation occurs, with similar consequences to those described with suxamethonium.

Myotonia has been precipitated by decamethonium in patients with myotonia congenita and dystrophia myotonica (3).

Susceptibility Factors

Decamethonium depends on renal excretion for the termination of its effects and is therefore contraindicated in renal insufficiency (1).

The action of decamethonium is prolonged by hypothermia (4).

Drug–Drug Interactions

Hexafluorenium and decamethonium are antagonistic. Potentiation of decamethonium block has been reported with ketamine, and can occur with neostigmine.

References

1. Prescott LF. Mechanisms of renal excretion of drugs (with special reference to drugs used by anaesthetists). Br J Anaesth 1972;44(3):246–51.
2. Hughes R, Al-Azawi S, Payne JP. Tachyphylaxis after repeated dosage of decamethonium in anaesthetized man. Br J Clin Pharmacol 1982;13(3):355–9.
3. Orndahl G, Stenberg K. Myotonic human musculature: stimulation with depolarizing agents. Mechanical registration of the effects of succinyldicholine, succinylmonocholine and decamethonium. Acta Med Scand 1962;172(Suppl 389):3–29.
4. England AJ, Wu X, Richards KM, Redai I, Feldman SA. The influence of cold on the recovery of three neuromuscular blocking agents in man. Anaesthesia 1996;51(3):236–40.

Deferiprone

General Information

Deferiprone is an alpha-ketohydroxypyridine compound with metal-chelating properties (1). It is absorbed within minutes after oral administration and reaches maximum blood concentrations within 1 hour. It has a half-life of 1–2 hours, and is almost completely undetectable in blood within 5–7 hours after a single dose. Deferiprone is mostly metabolized to a glucuronide conjugate that reaches maximum blood concentrations within 1.0–1.5 hours. Deferiprone, its iron complex, and its glucuronide conjugate are detectable in the urine, and in most instances the total amount of all three accounts for almost 100% of the

Table 1 Metal stability constants of deferiprone, deferoxamine, and diethylenetriaminepentaacetic acid (DTPA)

Ion	Deferiprone	Deferoxamine	DTPA
Fe^{3+}	35.0	30.6	28.6
Cu^{2+}	19.6	14.0	21.0
Zn^{2+}	13.5	11.1	18.4
Ni^{2+}	12.1	10.0	20.2
Co^{3+}	11.7	11.0	19.0

dose. Deferiprone is not excreted in the feces. However, there is much interindividual variation in its metabolism. The order of metal binding by deferiprone at pH 7.4 is iron > copper > aluminium > zinc (1) (see Table 1).

Deferiprone has a concentration-dependent affinity for iron, with a higher binding constant than deferoxamine or diethylenetriaminepentaacetic acid (DTPA). However, it takes three molecules of deferiprone to bind one molecule of iron, whereas deferoxamine binds iron in a 1:1 ratio. For this reason, deferiprone must be present in very high concentrations, close to toxic concentrations, to be effective (2). Deferiprone dissociates from iron when its concentration in body fluids falls to the concentration achieved just a few hours after oral administration (3). Deferiprone is effective in excreting iron in iron storage diseases and aluminium in patients on hemodialysis (1).

Iron chelation treatment has dramatically improved the prognosis of patients with beta-thalassemia (4). Parenteral deferoxamine reduces tissue iron stores, prevents iron-induced organ damage, and reduces morbidity and mortality. However, the burden of prolonged subcutaneous portable pump infusions, adverse reactions, patient non-compliance, and high cost are limiting factors, which have stimulated the development of orally active compounds. Combinations of chemically different types of chelators, which have different iron-carrying capacities and access different iron compartments, may work synergistically and result in increased efficacy, whereas lower doses of individual drugs may be less toxic (5). Examples are parenteral deferoxamine with oral deferiprone or 2,3-dihydroxybenzoic acid (2,3-DHB), or oral deferiprone with oral *N,N′-bis*(2-hydroxybenzyl)ethylenediamine-*N,N′*-diacetic acid (HDEB). Iron bound to a "shuttle," an oral agent that mobilizes tissue iron, is exchanged in the blood stream with a "sink," such as parenteral deferoxamine, and excreted via the kidneys, while the shuttle is reused. Combinations of different iron chelators can enhance iron excretion, target specific iron compartments, minimize adverse effects, increase treatment options, improve adherence to therapy, and facilitate individualization of therapy. Increasing understanding of the kinetics of iron metabolism, iron overload, and the complexity of chelation should further improve therapeutic strategies.

Observational studies

Since the controversy about the safety of deferiprone (SEDA-18, 250), its position as a therapeutic agent has been clarified (1). In the absence of iron storage, deferoxamine is undoubtedly toxic. However, it has been accepted, in spite of serious toxicity, because of the great need of an effective iron chelator for oral use (SEDA-18, 250). In this context, two studies are important, because they cast doubt on the efficacy of deferiprone (6,7). In the first, a long-term study in 51 transfusion-dependent iron-overloaded patients, 19 withdrew because of adverse events: arthropathy (stiffness, crepitus, effusion; $n=5$), gastrointestinal symptoms (severe nausea, anorexia, vomiting; $n=5$), granulocytopenia ($n=3$), renal insufficiency ($n=1$), and tachycardia ($n=1$) (6). In the second study, in 26 patients who continued to use the drug, there was generally no satisfactory reduction in iron stores. On the other hand, deferiprone caused fewer adverse effects and was more effective in patients who were previously well-chelated and had lower initial ferritin concentrations. Also, in the long run deferiprone did not adequately control the body iron burden. In addition, in this study the alarming suspicion was raised that deferiprone can paradoxically worsen hepatic fibrosis in patients with thalassemia major, based on hepatic biopsies in 19 patients (7).

In contrast, studies in Italy and the USA have reached more positive conclusions. Of 187 patients with thalassemia who were unable or unwilling to use deferoxamine, 162 completed 1 year of treatment with deferiprone (75 mg/kg/day) (8). One patient developed agranulocytosis and another nine had various degrees of neutropenia (altogether 5%). Other reasons for withdrawal were nausea and vomiting ($n=4$; total frequency 24% of patients), thrombocytopenia below 100×10^9/l ($n=2$), and a fall in serum alanine transaminase ($n=2$). Arthralgia developed in 11 patients (6%). In 29 patients who had not adhered well to deferoxamine and who took deferiprone (70 mg/kg/day) with a minimum follow-up of 1 year, adverse effects were pain in the knees in three patients, reversible neutropenia in one, and gastric intolerance in one (9). A repeat liver biopsy in 20 patients showed a reduction in the grade of liver siderosis and of iron content in seven. Worsening of hepatic fibrosis was not mentioned.

In 11 Greek patients who took deferiprone 75–100 mg/kg/day for 6 months, there were no serious adverse events of any kind (10).

In a Lebanese study in 17 patients, mainly with thalassemia major, there were no serious adverse reactions to deferiprone 50–75 mg/kg/day (11). Joint pain, stiffness, or swelling occurred in six patients; the symptoms were severe in two and mild in four patients. Seven patients had nausea, especially in the first month of treatment, and two had a reduced appetite. Headache developed in four patients. Mouth ulcers, sore throat, bitter taste, and fatigue occurred in single cases. In one patient there was a weakly positive ANF after 6 months. There were no cases of granulocytopenia and in none of the patients did adverse effects require drug withdrawal. The authors suggested that environmental or hereditary factors might have influenced the results.

In a large-scale program for the controlled use of deferiprone, established in 1997 by the Italian Ministry of Health, 86 centers collected information about 532 patients (12). In 187 patients, 269 events led to interruption of treatment, often transient. Permanent withdrawal because of adverse events occurred in 47 patients (8.9%). Reasons for withdrawal of treatment in 64 patients included non-compliance ($n = 30$), a serum ferritin concentration above 4000 ng/ml ($n = 14$), and a ferritin concentration below 500 ng/ml ($n = 3$). The most common adverse events were mild to severe granulocytopenia (4.3%), arthralgia (3.9%), gastrointestinal discomfort (3.2%), including nausea, vomiting, and abdominal pain, and transient increases in alanine transaminase activity (2.8%); however, the alanine transaminase results were not clearly presented in the report. Adverse events that were not established as adverse effects were urticaria, erythema, dermatitis, fever, flu-like symptoms, and "infectious episodes"; the authors did not comment on these.

Comparative studies

Deferiprone and deferoxamine have been compared in Lebanese patients, mainly with thalassemia major, of whom 17 used oral deferiprone 75 mg/kg/day and 40 received subcutaneous deferoxamine 20–50 mg/kg/day on 5 days a week; the patients were followed for 2 years (13). All those who took deferiprone did so because deferoxamine had not been suitable, due to either non-compliance or adverse reactions. One of those taking deferiprone withdrew for unknown reasons (and was excluded from the study). Deferiprone was commonly associated with orange discoloration of the urine. Six patients complained of joint pains, mainly in large joints (moderate to severe in two and mild in four), not requiring drug withdrawal. Seven patients reported nausea, four had headaches, two rashes, and two fatigue. Abdominal discomfort, mouth ulcers, and sore throat each occurred in one patient. Although two patients had transient falls in neutrophil count (to 1.3×10^9 and 1.44×10^9/l), presumably secondary to a viral infection, there were no cases of agranulocytosis.

Organs and Systems

Cardiovascular

Since circulating deferiprone-iron complexes can easily dissociate, deferiprone can redistribute iron in the body (14). Although this might theoretically lead to the precipitation or aggravation of heart failure (14), no such cases have as yet been reported.

Sensory systems

Eight patients with deferoxamine-related hearing loss were switched to deferiprone (dose not specified). In five there was deterioration in hearing (15).

Metal metabolism

Zinc deficiency was detected in 12 out of 84 patients, but withdrawal of deferoxamine was not needed (16). In another study, zinc excretion was moderately increased in three of 16 patients, and two had reduced serum zinc concentrations (17). None had clinical signs of zinc deficiency.

Hematologic

Agranulocytosis is a major limitation to the use of deferiprone and has an estimated frequency of 1.6% (16–21). Moderate leukopenia is more common.

Oxidation of deferiprone with hypochlorous acid, the major oxidant of neutrophil leukocytes, results in the formation of a chemically reactive species, consistent with the quinone metabolite of deferiprone. Deferiprone-related agranulocytosis presumably results from a T cell-mediated immunological reaction, induced by a reactive metabolite of deferiprone (18). In one case agranulocytosis and systemic vasculitis (with arthritis, palpable purpura of the legs, erythema of the palms and soles, and desquamation of the skin over the distal phalanges) occurred in association with deferiprone (22).

In 51 children with thalassemia studied in the All India Institute of Medical Sciences some degree of granulocytopenia developed in 12, 7 of whom were taking a low dose (50 mg/kg/day) and 5 a high dose (75 mg/kg/day) (23). Four had neutrophil counts well below 1×10^9/l; one developed a serious infection. Deferiprone was restarted in nine of the 12, leading to a relapse of granulocytopenia after 5 months in only one. The mechanism may be different for moderate and severe granulocytopenia. The authors suggested that the high prevalence of granulocytopenia in the Indian study could have been secondary to conditions such as poor transfusion schedules, poor nutritional status, higher serum ferritin concentrations, or genetic factors. In another study, five of 13 patients were re-challenged and granulocytopenia recurred (18).

In a large-scale program for the controlled use of deferiprone, established in 1997 by the Italian Ministry of Health, 86 centers collected information about 532 patients (12). Agranulocytosis developed in five patients, three of whom had previously had transient episodes of granulocytopenia, while using deferiprone; deferiprone was permanently withdrawn and all five recovered. There were episodes of less profound neutropenia in 18 other patients. In eight patients with neutropenia deferiprone was restarted; in one case agranulocytosis recurred and in three there was a relapse of less severe neutropenia; in the other four patients rechallenge was uneventful. Granulocytopenia occurred predominantly in patients with an intact spleen and in the younger age group (under 18 years); however, splenectomy was more frequent in the older patients. The risk of agranulocytosis is higher during the first months of exposure and probably falls with time.

In a patient with sickle cell anemia there was an increase in the frequency of sickle cell crises during the use of deferiprone (17).

Gastrointestinal

Nausea, occasionally with vomiting, occurred in six out of 20 children taking deferiprone (21). In another study, in 38 patients with transfusional iron overload, three withdrew because of severe nausea and another three had mild gastrointestinal complaints (17). The daily doses were 3–6 g (50–100 mg/kg).

Liver

In 84 patients receiving deferiprone, there were transient increases in liver enzymes in 44%, but persistent liver dysfunction leading to withdrawal occurred in only one (16).

Deferiprone paradoxically worsened hepatic fibrosis in patients with thalassemia major, based on hepatic biopsies in 19 patients (7). On the other hand, in another study of 20 liver biopsies, worsening of hepatic fibrosis was not mentioned (9).

In view of the suspicion that deferiprone can cause hepatic fibrosis, experience at the Sydney Children's Hospital in Australia has been reviewed, encompassing two liver biopsies in 14 patients taking deferiprone and 22 receiving deferoxamine (SEDA-23, 240) (24). The liver iron concentrations in the two groups, both at initial biopsy and subsequent biopsy, were not significantly different. Fibrosis progressed in five of 14 deferiprone users and in eight of 22 deferoxamine users. Progression greater than 1 unit occurred in four of 14 deferiprone users and two of 22 deferoxamine users. In those with positive hepatitis C serology, fibrosis showed progression in one of three patients using deferiprone and two of nine deferoxamine users; these findings were not significantly different. Pericellular fibrosis and Councilman bodies were seen in some patients: four of 11 deferiprone users and one of 20 deferoxamine users, a significant difference. However, errors in the presentation of the data hindered interpretation of the findings.

A further study has provided some reassurance. Three pathologists evaluated 112 coded liver biopsies obtained from 56 patients before and after deferiprone treatment (median duration 3.5 years). They found no evidence that deferiprone had worsened hepatic fibrosis (25). In view of the history of this problem, it is worth noting that "The International Safety Monitoring Committee that commissioned this study [was] an independent body of scientists," and that "The members of the Safety Monitoring Committee and the authors [had] no financial interest in the development of deferiprone."

Skin

In 38 patients with transfusional iron overload, deferiprone had to be withdrawn in one case because of a rash (17). Another patient developed a systemic vasculitis with arthritis, palpable purpura of the legs, erythema of the palms and soles, and desquamation over the distal phalanges. This patient had also had agranulocytosis in association with deferiprone (22).

Musculoskeletal

Deferoxamine commonly causes arthropathy of the knees, hips, shoulders, wrists, and fingers (1,17,26–32). Symptoms range from pain to inflammation and restriction of movement. Knee radiographs in one patient showed thalassemic changes, joint effusions, and minor degenerative changes in the patellofemoral joint. Magnetic resonance imaging confirmed effusions, with no evidence of synovial hypertrophy or cartilage abnormalities. The synovial fluid was a sterile transudate without inflammatory cells and low concentrations of deferiprone uncomplexed to iron. Arthroscopy showed mild synovial hypertrophy and hyperplasia, with iron staining. Synovial biopsy showed mild synovial lining cell proliferation and extensive iron deposition, without evidence of an inflammatory or allergic reaction. Since circulating deferiprone-iron complexes can easily dissociate, iron redistribution might play a role in the development of arthropathy (14). High concentrations of iron relative to deferiprone were detected in synovial fluid, suggesting that iron is shifted by deferiprone from body stores to the joints and that incomplete complexation may result in the formation of catalytic iron.

A joint effusion developed in one of 14 children using deferiprone (24).

Immunologic

A few observations have suggested that deferiprone can cause a lupus-like syndrome, with antinuclear and antihistone antibodies (33,34), but this suspicion is still unproven (29,35).

Infection risk

- An 82-year-old woman with a myelodysplastic syndrome died of *Escherichia coli* septicemia after 5 months of treatment with deferiprone (17). There was no granulocytopenia.

Death

The preliminary results of adding deferiprone to conventional treatment in order to reduce mortality from acute *Plasmodium falciparum* malaria suggest benefit (36). In 24 patients who were given deferiprone there were two deaths, compared with four in the control group of 21 patients. One patient who was given deferiprone died of unexplained pneumonia.

Second-Generation Effects

Fetotoxicity

Deferiprone inhibits intracellular ribonucleotide reductase, a rate-limiting enzyme in DNA synthesis, and in animal experiments it is toxic to proliferating tissues, especially the bone marrow. It has a pattern of adverse effects similar to those of cytotoxic drugs and is teratogenic and embryotoxic in animals (14,37).

References

1. Kontoghiorghes GJ. New concepts of iron and aluminium chelation therapy with oral L1 (deferiprone) and other chelators. A review. Analyst 1995;120(3):845–51.
2. Nathan DG. An orally active iron chelator. N Engl J Med 1995;332(14):953–4.
3. Nathan DG. Deferiprone in iron overload. N Engl J Med 1995;333:599.
4. Kontoghiorghes GJ. Clinical use, therapeutic aspects and future potential of deferiprone in thalassemia and other conditions of iron and other metal toxicity. Drugs Today (Barc) 2001;37(1):23–35.
5. Giardina PJ, Grady RW. Chelation therapy in beta-thalassemia: an optimistic update. Semin Hematol 2001;38(4):360–6.
6. Hoffbrand AV, Al-Refaie F, Davis B, Siritanakatkul N, Jackson BF, Cochrane J, Prescott E, Wonke B. Long-term trial of deferiprone in 51 transfusion-dependent iron overloaded patients. Blood 1998;91(1):295–300.

7. Olivieri NF, Brittenham GM, McLaren CE, Templeton DM, Cameron RG, McClelland RA, Burt AD, Fleming KA. Long-term safety and effectiveness of iron-chelation therapy with deferiprone for thalassemia major. N Engl J Med 1998;339(7):417–23.
8. Cohen A, Galanello R, Piga A, Vullo C, Tricta F. A multi-center safety trial of the oral iron chelator deferiprone. Ann NY Acad Sci 1998;850:223–6.
9. Mazza P, Amurri B, Lazzari G, Masi C, Palazzo G, Spartera MA, Giua R, Sebastio AM, Suma V, De Marco S, Semeraro F, Moscogiuri R. Oral iron chelating therapy. A single center interim report on deferiprone (L1) in thalassemia. Haematologica 1998;83(6):496–501.
10. Rombos Y, Tzanetea R, Konstantopoulos K, Simitzis S, Zervas C, Kyriaki P, Kavouklis M, Aessopos A, Sakellaropoulos N, Karagiorga M, Kalotychou V, Loukopoulos D. Chelation therapy in patients with thalassemia using the orally active iron chelator deferiprone (L1). Haematologica 2000;85(2):115–17.
11. Taher A, Chamoun FM, Koussa S, Saad MA, Khoriaty AI, Neeman R, Mourad FH. Efficacy and side effects of deferiprone (L1) in thalassemia patients not compliant with desferrioxamine. Acta Haematol 1999;101(4):173–7.
12. Ceci A, Baiardi P, Felisi M, Cappellini MD, Carnelli V, De Sanctis V, Galanello R, Maggio A, Masera G, Piga A, Schettini F, Stefano I, Tricta F. The safety and effectiveness of deferiprone in a large-scale, 3-year study in Italian patients. Br J Haematol 2002;118(1):330–6.
13. Taher A, Sheikh-Taha M, Koussa S, Inati A, Neeman R, Mourad F. Comparison between deferoxamine and deferiprone (L1) in iron-loaded thalassemia patients. Eur J Haematol 2001;67(1):30–4.
14. Berdoukas V, Bentley P, Frost H, Schnebli HP. Toxicity of oral iron chelator L1. Lancet 1993;341(8852):1088.
15. Chiodo AA, Alberti PW, Sher GD, Francombe WH, Tyler B. Desferrioxamine ototoxicity in an adult transfusion-dependent population. J Otolaryngol 1997;26(2):116–22.
16. Al-Refaie FN, Hershko C, Hoffbrand AV, Kosaryan M, Olivieri NF, Tondury P, Wonke B. Results of long-term deferiprone (L1) therapy: a report by the International Study Group on Oral Iron Chelators. Br J Haematol 1995;91(1):224–9.
17. Kersten MJ, Lange R, Smeets ME, Vreugdenhil G, Roozendaal KJ, Lameijer W, Goudsmit R. Long-term treatment of transfusional iron overload with the oral iron chelator deferiprone (L1): a Dutch multicenter trial. Ann Hematol 1996;73(5):247–52.
18. Loebstein R, Diav-Citrin O, Atanackovic G, Olivieri NF, Koren G. Deferiprone-induced agranulocytosis. A critical review of five rechallenged cases. Clin Drug Invest 1997;13:345–9.
19. al-Refaie FN, Veys PA, Wilkes S, Wonke B, Hoffbrand AV. Agranulocytosis in a patient with thalassaemia major during treatment with the oral iron chelator, 1,2-dimethyl-3-hydroxypyrid-4-one. Acta Haematol 1993;89(2):86–90.
20. al-Refaie FN, Wonke B, Hoffbrand AV. Deferiprone-associated myelotoxicity Eur J Haematol 1994;53(5):298–301.
21. Adhikari D, Roy TB, Biswas A, Chakraborty ML, Bhattacharya B, Maitra TK, Basu AK, Chandra S. Efficacy and safety of oral iron chelating agent deferiprone in beta-thalassemia and hemoglobin E-beta thalassemia. Indian Pediatr 1995;32(8):855–61.
22. Castriota-Scanderbeg A, Sacco M. Agranulocytosis, arthritis and systemic vasculitis in a patient receiving the oral iron chelator L1 (deferiprone). Br J Haematol 1997;96(2):254–5.
23. Pati HP, Choudhry VP. Deferiprone (L1) associated neutropenia in beta thalassemia major: an Indian experience. Eur J Haematol 1999;63(4):267–8.
24. Berdoukas V, Bohane T, Eagle C, Lindeman R, DeSilva K, Tobias V, Painter D, Fraser I. The Sydney Children's Hospital experience with the oral iron chelator deferiprone (L1). Transfus Sci 2000;23(3):239–40.
25. Wanless IR, Sweeney G, Dhillon AP, Guido M, Piga A, Galanello R, Gamberini MR, Schwartz E, Cohen AR. Lack of progressive hepatic fibrosis during long-term therapy with deferiprone in subjects with transfusion-dependent beta-thalassemia. Blood 2002;100(5):1566–9.
26. Olivieri NF, Brittenham GM, Matsui D, Berkovitch M, Blendis LM, Cameron RG, McClelland RA, Liu PP, Templeton DM, Koren G. Iron-chelation therapy with oral deferipronein patients with thalassemia major. N Engl J Med 1995;332(14):918–22.
27. Bartlett AN, Hoffbrand AV, Kontoghiorghes GJ. Long-term trial with the oral iron chelator 1,2-dimethyl-3-hydroxypyrid-4-one (L1). II. Clinical observations. Br J Haematol 1990;76(2):301–4.
28. Agarwal MB, Viswanathan C, Ramanathan J, Massil DE, Shah S, Gupte SS, Vasandani D, Puniyani RR. Oral iron chelation with L1. Lancet 1990;335(8689):601.
29. Olivieri NF, Matsui D, Liu PP, Blendis L, Cameron R, McClelland RA, Templeton DM, Koren G. Oral iron chelation with 1,2-dimethyl-3-hydroxypyrid-4-one (L1) in iron loaded thalassemia patients. Bone Marrow Transplant 1993;12(Suppl 1):9–11.
30. Berkovitch M, Laxer RM, Inman R, Koren G, Pritzker KP, Fritzler MJ, Olivieri NF. Arthropathy in thalassaemia patients receiving deferiprone. Lancet 1994;343 (8911):1471–2.
31. al-Refaie FN, Wonke B, Hoffbrand AV. Arthropathy in thalassaemia patients receiving deferiprone. Lancet 1994;344(8917):262–3.
32. Olivieri NF. Arthropathy in thalassaemia patients receiving deferiprone. Lancet 1994;344(8917):263.
33. Mehta J, Singhal S, Revankar R, Walvalkar A, Chablani A, Mehta BC. Fatal systemic lupus erythematosus in patient taking oral iron chelator L1. Lancet 1991;337(8736):298.
34. Mehta J, Singhal S, Mehta BC. Oral iron chelator L1 and autoimmunity. Blood 1993;81(7):1970–1.
35. Al-Refaie FN, Hoffbrand AV, Nortey P, Wonke B, Wickens DG. Oral iron chelator L1 and autoimmunity. Blood 1993;81(7):1971–2.
36. Mohanty D, Ghosh K, Pathare AV, Karnad D. Deferiprone (L1) as an adjuvant therapy for *Plasmodium falciparum* malaria. Indian J Med Res 2002;115:17–21.
37. Hershko C. Development of oral iron chelator L1. Lancet 1993;341(8852):1088–9.

Deferoxamine

General Information

Deferoxamine is a polyhydroxamine acid with specific affinity for iron and, less strongly, aluminium. It is a naturally occurring siderophore produced by *Streptomyces pilosus*.

Uses

Deferoxamine is used in the treatment of acute iron poisoning and in iron storage diseases, notably beta-thalassemia (1). The usual regimen is 40 mg/kg/day as a subcutaneous infusion over 10–12 hours, starting at an early age (3 years). During erythrocyte transfusion, deferoxamine 300 mg/kg can be given intravenously over 24 hours. Vitamin C 100 mg/day can also be given orally to facilitate mobilization of stored iron. With such a regimen the duration and quality of life in thalassemia can be greatly improved (2,3). Another indication for deferoxamine is aluminium storage in patients on hemodialysis.

Iron chelation treatment has dramatically improved the prognosis of patients with beta-thalassemia (4). Parenteral deferoxamine reduces tissue iron stores, prevents iron-induced organ damage, and reduces morbidity and mortality. However, the burden of prolonged subcutaneous portable pump infusions, adverse reactions, patient non-compliance, and high cost are limiting factors, which have stimulated the development of orally active compounds. Combinations of chemically different types of chelators, which have different iron-carrying capacities and access different iron compartments, may work synergistically and result in increased efficacy, whereas lower doses of individual drugs may be less toxic (5). Examples are parenteral deferoxamine with oral deferiprone or 2,3-dihydroxybenzoic acid (2,3-DHB), or oral deferiprone with oral *N,N'*-*bis*(2-hydroxybenzyl)ethylenediamine-*N,N'*-diacetic acid (HDEB). Iron bound to a "shuttle," an oral agent that mobilizes tissue iron, is exchanged in the blood stream with a "sink," such as parenteral deferoxamine, and excreted via the kidneys, while the shuttle is reused. Combinations of different iron chelators can enhance iron excretion, target specific iron compartments, minimize adverse effects, increase treatment options, improve adherence to therapy, and facilitate individualization of therapy. Increasing understanding of the kinetics of iron metabolism, iron overload, and the complexity of chelation should further improve therapeutic strategies.

Comparative studies

Deferiprone and deferoxamine have been compared in Lebanese patients, mainly with thalassemia major, of whom 17 used oral deferiprone, 75 mg/kg/day for 2 years, and 40 received subcutaneous deferoxamine 20–50 mg/kg/day on 5 days a week (6). Those who received deferoxamine had done so for 4–24 years and were followed for 2 years. Infusion site reactions occurred in 34 patients, including pain, tenderness, itching, burning, erythema, swelling, induration, and lipodystrophy. Five patients had disturbances of vision and hearing, three had growth retardation. Six patients had increased heart rates, four had dizziness, and one had leg cramps.

General adverse effects

Deferoxamine is only used parenterally. It is more toxic when used in patients with a low iron burden. After subcutaneous infusion many patients have some local irritation and swelling. Rapid intravenous injection can be followed by flushing, wheals, tachycardia, hypotension, acute adult respiratory distress, and renal insufficiency; shock or convulsions can also occur. Headache, blurred vision, dysuria, diarrhea, and leg or hand cramps have been reported. Intramuscular injection can be painful. Hypersensitivity reactions occasionally occur, with rash, fever, and edema; anaphylactic shock has been encountered (SEDA-7, 262) (7,8). As a test dose in patients with aluminium storage disease, a low dose (500 mg in 100 ml of 0.9% saline) is usually effective and safe (9). At the higher doses used in treatment, nausea, itching, dizziness, or more serious reactions can occur. When deferoxamine is given early in childhood, osteopathy and growth impairment can occur.

Withholding iron is an important protection strategy of the body against microbial and neoplastic cells, and cellular iron depletion plays a prominent role in cell-mediated immune defence (10). The use of deferoxamine is associated with an increased risk of life-threatening opportunistic infections, notably yersiniosis and mucormycosis; such infections can affect various organ systems and pose diagnostic problems. Hypersensitivity reactions can occur but are infrequent. Rare cases of anaphylactic shock, thrombocytopenia, and bone marrow failure have been described. Tumor-inducing effects have not been reported. Deferoxamine is teratogenic in animals.

Organs and Systems

Cardiovascular

Although rarely described, hypotension can be a significant problem in patients receiving deferoxamine, especially when it is given too rapidly by intravenous injection (11); it is possibly due to histamine release (12). Dose reduction alleviates the hypotension. Anaphylactic shock has only rarely been reported (SEDA-7, 262).

In a single report, soft-tissue swelling around the elbow and localized mild pitting edema were thought to have been induced by deferoxamine (13). Although the clinical features suggested a deep-vein thrombosis, this was ruled out by a phlebogram.

In iron storage disease, ascorbic acid should be given only after adequate serum concentrations of deferoxamine have been attained, in order to prevent serious cardiac arrhythmia (14). Opportunistic fungal infections associated with deferoxamine may also involve the heart muscle and usually have a fatal outcome (15–17).

There was severe phlebitis in cancer patients receiving deferoxamine (50 mg/kg/day by intravenous infusion over 72 hours) and iron sorbitol citrate in an attempt to enhance doxorubicin activity (18). Dilution of the drug in large volumes of saline did not prevent this adverse effect.

Respiratory

Deferoxamine by continuous infusion can cause life-threatening acute adult respiratory distress syndrome, with respiratory failure, hypoxia, pulmonary edema, low pulmonary compliance, and a reduced pulmonary capillary wedge pressure (19,20). Respiratory distress can start 32–72 hours after the infusion. Lung biopsy shows diffuse abnormalities with alveolar damage, interstitial fibrosis, and inflammatory infiltration with lymphocytes, eosinophils, mast cells, and some erythrocytes. It is therefore recommended that deferoxamine should not be given as a continuous infusion for more than 24 hours (21). Although the mechanism is unknown, it has been suggested that deferoxamine causes lung damage by paradoxically increasing the production of free radicals, as a result of extended exposure of the lungs to ferrioxamine (21). However, others have emphasized that pulmonary endothelial cells are sensitive to macrophage-generated oxidants, and have proposed that in chelating, intracellular iron deferoxamine may acutely reduce the synthesis of catalase and heme, and that readily available extracellular heme subsequently enters cells, is broken down, and releases iron in the presence of low concentrations of catalase, which catalyses oxidant damage (22).

- In one patient, pulmonary symptoms occurred after 7 days of continuous deferoxamine infusion (dyspnea, tachypnea, tachycardia, pleuritic chest pain, and fever) and were diagnosed as pulmonary microemboli (23).

Respiratory distress and interstitial infiltrates have also been reported in children receiving deferoxamine for iron poisoning or refractory cancers (24,25).

Lung damage was attributed to high doses of deferoxamine in 17 patients with beta-thalassemia major who were given 33 courses by continuous intravenous infusion of 10 days duration in doses up to 10 mg/kg/hour (26). Respiratory dysfunction developed in two girls given the highest doses (aged 11 and 15 years). The symptoms were dyspnea, tachypnea, tachycardia, and low-grade fever. Arterial blood gas measurements showed hypoxemia and hypercapnia. Chest X-rays showed bilateral interstitial infiltrates. In one patient, mechanical ventilation was needed for 2 weeks and it took 8 months before pulmonary function returned to normal. In both patients deferoxamine was reintroduced later on without relapse.

The lungs can also be involved in deferoxamine-associated infections, such as systemic mucormycosis, which often runs a fatal course (16,17,27,28).

- Pneumonia during treatment with high doses of deferoxamine (2–2.5 g by continuous infusion) in a patient with thalassemia major was found to be caused by *Pneumocystis jiroveci* (29).

Nervous system

The use of deferoxamine to reduce aluminium overload in hemodialysis patients can exacerbate aluminium encephalopathy and precipitate dialysis dementia (30–34). Confusion, disorientation, agitation, aggression, abnormal behavior, speech arrest, myoclonus, hallucinations, and seizures can occur. Some patients are very sensitive to this effect, and a test dose of deferoxamine is advisable in order to ascertain whether aluminium is excessively mobilized (35).

Deferoxamine can modify the electroencephalogram, with progressive slowing and bilateral paroxysms (36).

Nausea and vomiting often develop in patients with rheumatoid arthritis after 4–12 days of treatment with deferoxamine, presumably as a result of chelation of iron from the central nervous system (37). Two patients who took the phenothiazine derivative prochlorperazine during treatment of rheumatoid arthritis with deferoxamine lost consciousness for 48–72 hours, possibly because this combination of drugs removed essential iron from the nervous system (38).

Headache, loss of vision, disturbed consciousness, and various other neurological symptoms can be alarming signs of deferoxamine-associated systemic mucormycosis with cerebral involvement, a condition that is usually fatal (15–17).

Sensorimotor neurotoxicity, with paresthesia, areflexia, reduced vibration and position sense, muscle weakness of the arms, and concomitant disturbances of vision and hearing, has been described in two thalassemia patients during the intravenous administration of high dosages of deferoxamine (120 mg/kg/day) (28).

Neurophysiological evaluation of 40 patients with beta-thalassemia major showed abnormal findings in brainstem-evoked potentials: auditory (25%), visual (15%), and somatosensory (7.5%); some had abnormal nerve conduction velocity (25%) and 15% had involvement of multiple neural pathways (39). Subclinical involvement of the auditory pathway was statistically associated with a higher mean daily dose of deferoxamine and a longer duration of treatment. Abnormalities of the somatosensory pathways were related to old age, a long duration of deferoxamine use, and low serum copper concentrations. Multiple neural pathway involvement was related to the duration of treatment. However, deferoxamine is only partly responsible for the subclinical abnormalities of neural pathways often found in patients with beta-thalassemia major.

Sensory systems

The reported frequency of sensorineural toxicity of deferoxamine varies. Some degree of visual and auditory toxicity can occur in about one-third of patients (40), and impairment of vision and hearing can occur simultaneously (41).

- A 25-year-old woman with beta-thalassemia, who had received subcutaneous deferoxamine 2 g/day (50 mg/kg) for 7 days a week for 3 years, developed visual loss. Her best-corrected visual acuity was 20/60 bilaterally. Automated perimetry showed bilateral central scotomata, and a Farnsworth Panel D-15 test showed an irregular pattern of errors. There were no lens opacities, and fundoscopy and fluorescein angiography were normal. Audiometry showed a bilateral high-frequency sensorineural deficit. Two days after withdrawal of deferoxamine and oral administration of zinc sulfate 20 mg/day, the central scotomata disappeared and her color vision and audiographic abnormalities reversed completely. The serum ferritin concentration was 656 ng/ml.

Since the serum ferritin concentration was relatively low, the original dose of deferoxamine may have been too high. Although zinc concentrations were not measured before treatment, the rapid and complete improvement in 48 hours after starting zinc sulfate suggested that deferoxamine-induced zinc deficiency may also have played a role.

Eyes

In aluminium-overloaded dialysis patients, acute visual impairment can occur after only the first or second intravenous test dose of 40 mg/kg deferoxamine (42–44). Visual symptoms are of retinal origin and include impairment of color vision, night blindness, and reduced visual acuity; serious and persistent visual loss can occur

(42,45–48). Color blindness is of the tritan type, involving the blue–yellow axis (49). A light- and electron-microscopic study showed loss of microvilli from the apical surface, patchy depigmentation, vacuolation of the cytoplasm, swelling and calcification of mitochondria, and thickening of Bruch's membrane (50). Optic neuritis and pigmentary retinal degeneration can develop (51–55).

In one prospective study in 17 patients with hemolytic anemia (aged 5–25 years) lens opacities were found in 41%, changes in the retinal pigment epithelium in 35%, tortuosity of retinal vessels in 24%, dilatation and sheathing of retinal vessels in 18%, defects in color vision in 29%, and abnormal dark adaptation in 18% (56). In many other studies much lower frequencies were found. Perhaps retinal injury is related to the depletion of metals such as zinc, copper, and/or iron (57). On the other hand, ocular and auditory disturbances are not infrequent in patients with thalassemia, iron storage diseases (58,59), or uremia (45), and may be coincidental in patients receiving deferoxamine (60).

The sensorineural toxicity of deferoxamine is much more pronounced in patients without iron storage disease (for example rheumatoid arthritis). Ocular toxicity was also apparent in cancer patients receiving deferoxamine and iron sorbitol citrate in an attempt to enhance doxorubicin activity (18). Careful estimation of the necessary doses of deferoxamine and regular ophthalmological monitoring can often prevent serious injury. Visual evoked potentials can be used to monitor patients receiving high doses of deferoxamine (61). It is of great diagnostic and prognostic importance to keep in mind that a sudden loss of vision or other neurological events in a patient receiving deferoxamine can also be the first sign of life-threatening cerebral mucormycosis (62).

Cataract has been observed in animals, but even after prolonged use of deferoxamine it has only rarely been reported in humans (63,64).

- Two patients with transfusion-related hemochromatosis, who received deferoxamine 9 g/week and 10 g/month to a total dose of 39 g, and one with hemodialysis-related aluminium storage, who received 9 g/week, experienced gradual loss of visual acuity (65). There was pigmentary mottling near the maculae and electroretinography was abnormal in the two patients studied.

Acute loss of visual acuity has been described after a single test dose of deferoxamine (66).

- A 58-year-old patient with proliferative glomerulonephritis suddenly suffered loss of visual acuity (320/200 in both eyes) and disturbance of color vision 2 hours after hemodialysis, during which deferoxamine 10 mg/kg had been given to test for aluminium storage. Computerized campimetry showed bilateral central scotomata. Recovery was good but slow: within 3 months visual acuity had increased to 20/30, but bilateral pigmentary macular changes persisted.

In a study in China, electroretinographic responses and dark adaptation visual thresholds showed subtle but significant retinal dysfunction in elderly chronically transfused patients with thalassemia receiving deferoxamine (67). The authors concluded that the findings suggested that iron accumulation and not deferoxamine toxicity played a major role in these patients.

Ears

Ototoxicity due to deferoxamine ranges from a subclinically abnormal audiogram, through mid- to high-frequency neurosensorial hearing loss of the cochlear type, to acute deafness (SED-12, 552) (46). The ototoxic effects of deferoxamine have been studied in 70 adult transfusion-dependent patients (40). Characteristically there was high-frequency sensorineural hearing loss; tinnitus was less frequent. In five of eight patients with deferoxamine-related hearing loss who were switched to deferiprone there was a deterioration of hearing (40).

There are two risk factors: a high total cumulative deferoxamine dose and a low serum ferritin concentration. In order to prevent deferoxamine ototoxicity, a therapeutic index has been proposed, defined as the daily dose of deferoxamine (in mg/kg/day) divided by the serum ferritin concentration (ng/ml) (SED-12, 552) (68). A therapeutic index of 0.027 is considered to be associated with a low risk of deterioration of hearing. Regular audiometric follow-up, with special attention to the frequencies of 3 and 6 kHz, can help to detect and prevent permanent hearing loss.

Of 75 adults with thalassemia major (age range 17–32 years) 50 had normal audiography (69). Of the other 25, 13 had a sensorineural deficit of 35 dB or less, with high frequency losses, and two had a deficit of 35–75 dB. There was no association between hearing loss and age, ferritin concentration, or therapeutic index. The authors concluded that their findings were not different from those in a healthy population of the same age and were not suggestive of an ototoxic effect of deferoxamine.

In an Iranian study, the incidence of sensorineural hearing impairment in 128 patients taking deferoxamine was assessed by otological examination and pure tone audiometry (70). Patients who received deferoxamine subcutaneously every other day were compared with those who received it for 6 days a week. In both groups the average daily dose was the same, 21–39 mg/kg/day, since the alternate-day group received double doses. Of the patients in the once-a-day group there was hearing loss at a frequency of 8000 Hz in the right ear in 28% and in the left ear in 23%. In the alternate-day group, hearing loss was more common: 45% and 42% respectively. It appears that the maximum plasma deferoxamine concentration is a determinant of sensorineural toxicity. There was no relation between ototoxicity and either the serum ferritin concentration (which was meticulously controlled) or the duration of deferoxamine treatment.

Mineral balance

The administration of deferoxamine to dialysis patients in order to chelate aluminium is often associated with asymptomatic hypocalcemia, which can in turn aggravate hyperparathyroidism (12). Deferoxamine-induced hypocalcemia can be corrected with supplements of vitamin D and calcium carbonate.

- In an 8-month-old child the administration of deferoxamine for chelation of aluminium, which had accumulated as a result of total parenteral nutrition, caused sustained hypocalcemia without concomitant hypercalciuria (71).

Presumably, the reduced calcium concentrations in this case reflected bone regeneration following the disappearance of aluminium from the bone.

Hematologic

Deferoxamine has a strong depressant effect on proliferation of bone marrow cultures in vitro (72). On the other hand, deferoxamine improves hemopoiesis in patients with anemia, for example in rheumatoid arthritis, hemolysis, or myelodysplastic syndromes, and reduces transfusion dependency (73–78). The mechanism is unknown, but increased erythropoietin responsiveness secondary to iron chelation may play a role (77).

In 11 hemodialysis patients who also received recombinant human erythropoietin for anemia secondary to renal failure, deferoxamine increased the proliferation of erythroid precursor cells and had a synergistic in vivo effect on erythropoietin (79,80).

When used in patients without iron overload, deferoxamine can cause iron deficiency (12). In 20 patients, there were falls in ferritin concentrations in six, requiring withdrawal of deferoxamine and parenteral administration of iron dextran (12). Monitoring ferritin concentrations is therefore recommended in patients receiving deferoxamine for aluminium overload. On the other hand, the administration of deferoxamine (500 mg/day by subcutaneous infusion) improves chronic anemia in patients with rheumatoid arthritis (77). This effect is thought to be achieved through increased erythropoietin responsiveness, secondary to iron chelation. Iron chelation with deferoxamine also improves hemopoiesis in patients with myelodysplastic syndromes and can reduce transfusion dependency (78). Exactly how deferoxamine works in these patients remains to be explained.

There have been rare reports of thrombocytopenia and aplastic anemia with pancytopenia, attributed to deferoxamine (81,82). Deferoxamine can accumulate in renal insufficiency if repeated doses are given, and it has been advised that platelet counts should be monitored in such patients (81).

Gastrointestinal

Gastrointestinal upsets are frequent after parenteral administration of deferoxamine (12). In addition to nausea, vomiting, and abdominal cramps, passage of black stools can occur, perhaps because of increased stool iron content. Nausea, anorexia, and vomiting often occur when deferoxamine is used in rheumatoid arthritis or Alzheimer's disease (32,83).

Urinary tract

The iron–deferoxamine complex gives the urine a reddish-brown color.

In 27 patients with thalassemia, subcutaneous deferoxamine caused a clinically significant reduction in renal glomerular filtration rate in 40% and a mild reduction in another 40% (84). In all cases of severe reductions the glomerular filtration rate tended to return to baseline on withdrawal of deferoxamine. There was also a significant increase in urine volume during deferoxamine therapy.

Deferoxamine has occasionally been reported to cause renal insufficiency (85,86) and adequate hydration and repeated measurements of renal function are recommended in patients receiving intravenous deferoxamine. Perhaps the inability to reabsorb sodium and to concentrate urine during administration of deferoxamine is due to a diuretic effect of ferrioxamine (87).

Skin

Subcutaneous deferoxamine often causes local irritation, pruritus, and swelling of the skin at infusion sites (11,88–90). Dilution of the deferoxamine solution reduces the frequency, and the addition of 1–2 mg hydrocortisone to the solution can alleviate the problem. Occasionally, severe local reactions with fever occur, leading to withdrawal (89). Disfiguring lumps can develop and can serve as foci for bacterial infection. Proper needle placement in deep subcutaneous sites and rotation of sites around the lower abdomen, thighs, buttocks, and arms usually allow sufficient time for one area to heal before it is used again.

Rapid intravenous infusion of deferoxamine (more than 25 mg/kg over 30 minutes) can cause vertigo, hypotension, diffuse erythema, and generalized pruritus (11). Such reactions reverse on withdrawal of the infusion, although occasionally a fluid bolus and/or an antihistamine may be needed to reverse the symptoms more rapidly. This reaction is considered to be due to histamine release and not to be immunological in nature; patients can be safely treated later at a lower rate of infusion.

- An edematous, erythematous, itchy rash developed on the legs of a 62-year-old woman within 48 hours after infusion of deferoxamine (91).
- Porphyria cutanea tarda-like skin lesions on the dorsum of the hands and forearms, worsening with sun exposure, has been described in association with penicillamine (12).

In another study, deferoxamine was used successfully as a treatment for hemodialysis-related porphyria cutanea tarda (92).

Skin lesions imitating vasculitis or cutaneous infarction can be the first manifestation of life-threatening mucormycosis (93,94).

Musculoskeletal

Bone dysplasia

In children, deferoxamine can cause bone dysplasia, especially when it is started at a young age (95–100). Injury to the metaphyseal growth plate cartilage affects the development of tubular bones and vertebrae. The lesions are reminiscent of scurvy, but the mechanism is uncertain. Perhaps a combination of mechanisms is involved, of which the most relevant seem to be defective function of iron-dependent enzymes and chelation of other metals, such as zinc, copper, and aluminium. Deferoxamine-induced bone dysplasia can cause reduced body height and spinal deformities. Metaphyseal changes can be detected at an early stage by serial radiography. When they are found, the nightly dose of deferoxamine should be reduced to the lowest dose that results in a negative iron balance, and growth rate should be carefully observed.

The issue of deferoxamine osteochondropathy is even more complex, because thalassemia itself is also associated with growth impairment and body disproportionality with truncal shortening, whether puberty is induced or spontaneous (101).

Presentation

Of 476 patients in a multicenter study 40% had a short trunk and 18% short stature; in 14% there was disproportion between the upper and lower body segments (102). Spinal growth deficit starts early in infancy and is progressive. Deferoxamine-induced bone dysplasia has been identified as a contributing factor, in addition to thalassemia, hypogonadism, and siderosis. In addition to a short trunk, platyspondylosis and signs of bone dysplasia are characteristic features of bone lesions due to deferoxamine (102). The same group studied three children with beta-thalassemia (one girl aged 7 and two boys aged 6 and 12) (103). The ages of first exposure to deferoxamine were 2.5, 2, and 1.5 years and the mean daily doses were 48, 49, and 55 mg/kg/day respectively (route not stated). All three had short stature, a short trunk, and reduced growth velocity. One had protrusion of the sternum and another had genu valgum. Radiographs of the spine and long bones showed various degrees of osteopenia, platyspondylosis, cupped metaphysis of the distal femur, and pseudocystic cavities with sclerotic borders at distal and proximal metaphyses of the tibia. A reduction in the dosage of deferoxamine was followed by improvement in the bone lesions and growth velocity but not height. The authors concluded that in all children receiving deferoxamine, regular radiological and growth evaluation is needed, in order to limit bone dysplasia and short stature.

Another patient had pain and swelling at the anterior ends of the eighth and ninth ribs (104). This patient had been treated with subcutaneous deferoxamine since the age of 3 years with 37–66 mg/kg/day for 6 days a week. Radiologically there were rickets-like "rosary" lesions of the costochondral junctions. The pain disappeared within a few days after withdrawal of deferoxamine and reappeared after readministration. The mechanism underlying rickets-like changes due to deferoxamine is not known.

In a long-term evaluation of 29 patients with transfusion-dependent thalassemia major there were deferoxamine-induced skeletal changes in 15 patients: metaphyseal and spinal changes in five and spinal changes alone in 10 (105). After a reduction in the dosage of deferoxamine, the metaphyseal changes regressed in two but progressed in three, whereas the spinal changes were unchanged or progressed. Two patients required surgical intervention for marked valgus knee deformities. Of a further 21 patients with growth retardation and skeletal dysplasia, secondary to deferoxamine, four underwent surgery to correct genu valgum (106). Bone histology showed abnormal chondrocytes, alteration of staining pattern of cartilage, irregular columnar cartilage, and lacunae in the cartilaginous tissue. Bone microfractures were sometimes present. Bone microstructure showed varying degrees of impaired mineralization and the hardness of bone tissue was reduced. Bone apatite was quantitatively reduced.

Two Chinese studies in 35 consecutive patients with thalassemia on a hypertransfusion scheme plus chelation therapy have confirmed that deferoxamine-induced bone dysplasia was associated with height reduction and occurred at doses below 50 mg/kg/day (107,108).

In the first study, the patients had radiography of the left hand for bone age determination, and 12 had deferoxamine-induced long bone dysplasia (107). There was irregularity at the physeal–metaphyseal junction of the distal ulna (the site most frequently affected) and radius; metaphyseal sclerosis was also common, especially of the ulna, but also of the radius, metacarpals, and phalanges. Radiolucent lesions occasionally accompanied metaphyseal sclerosis. In six patients with relatively mild lesions, the dysplastic changes had been missed or not mentioned.

In another study, probably in the same 35 patients, coronal T1-weighted MRI scanning of the femur was performed, and in 11 patients also of the patella (108). In the distal but not proximal femurs of 11 of the 35 patients the following abnormalities were seen (in decreasing frequency): blurred physeal–metaphyseal junction, distal metaphyseal areas of hyperintensity, physeal widening, metadiaphyseal lesions, and (in only two) patellar lesions. Patients with MRI evidence of bone dysplasia had a significantly greater reduction in height than patients without.

Of 180 thalassemic patients receiving chelation therapy with subcutaneous deferoxamine, five had deferoxamine-induced serious rickets-like lesions of the long bones; two more had vertebral compression without long bone involvement (109). A microstructural analysis was made of tibia biopsy specimens taken in six patients during orthopaedic surgery and a biopsy of the iliac crest in one. With microradiography and X-ray diffraction there was irregular and reduced mineralization in all seven patients, compared with autopsy bone tissue. Apparently the osteochondrodystrophic lesions in deferoxamine osteopathy are areas with poor mineralization. The bone tissue does not reach maturity, and reduced microhardness leads to an increased risk of microfractures.

In a separate study, apparently in the same seven patients, the histological findings were presented (110). All the bone specimens showed a similar pathological pattern, with irregular columnar cartilage, lacunae in the cartilaginous tissue, abnormal chondrocytes, and impaired mineralization. Microfractures were common and were a likely explanation for the pain experienced by the patients.

Of 41 patients in Hong Kong with transfusion-dependent homozygous beta-thalassemia, who received subcutaneous infusion of deferoxamine in doses not exceeding 50 mg/kg/day, 16 had radiographic evidence of deferoxamine-induced bone dysplasia (111). All 16 had metaphyseal sclerosis of long bones (arms, hands, legs, and/or ribs); three had irregular sclerosis at the costochondral junction; one had platyspondyly. There was osteoporosis (unrelated to deferoxamine), as indicated by thinning of the metacarpal cortex, in 17 patients, eight with and nine without deferoxamine dysplasia. Two patients had evidence of medullary expansion; however, they were from mainland China and had had irregular blood transfusions and no chelation therapy, and it was unrelated to deferoxamine.

Diagnosis
The use of sonography as a cheap and easy tool in the assessment of deferoxamine-induced bone dysplasia of the knee has been studied in 32 patients with thalassemia major (112). Characteristic lesions were notching at the metaphyseal corner, a blurred or irregular peripheral juxtaphyseal–metaphyseal contour, and widening of the peripheral juxtaphyseal–metaphyseal echogenic interface. There were 14 true positive results, 10 true negative, 7 false negative, and 1 false positive. Thus, sonography is specific but not sensitive in the diagnosis of deferoxamine-induced dysplasia. Because of its high specificity, low cost, and non-invasiveness, sonography may have a role in the longitudinal monitoring of deferoxamine-induced bone dysplasia.

Mechanism
The mechanism underlying the effect of deferoxamine on bone formation has not been identified. In one study in 21 thalassemic patients with growth retardation and skeletal dysplasia secondary to deferoxamine, there were reduced concentrations of growth hormone in 72% of patients with bone dysplasia, compared with 41% of patients without (106). Four patients with growth hormone deficiency were treated with human recombinant growth hormone. Growth velocity doubled in two patients and one patient had a partial response; the fourth patient did not respond. There was a fall in growth velocity after 1 year of treatment with growth hormone in the partial responder and in one of the responders.

Management
The following strategy may be helpful in preventing bone dysplasia during treatment with deferoxamine (105,106):

- Chelation therapy should be started after the age of 3 years and when iron accumulation has become established.
- The dosage of deferoxamine should be established on the basis of iron balance and dose–response curves.
- Deferoxamine dosages above 50 mg/kg/day subcutaneously should be avoided.
- The deferoxamine dosage should be reduced if serum ferritin values are consistently below 1500–1000 ng/ml, or if the patient has reduced growth velocity.
- It is important to detect bone changes as early as possible, since a timely reduction in deferoxamine dosage or a switch to deferiprone can prevent serious skeletal injury.

A change from deferoxamine to deferiprone led to general improvement in a 14-year-old boy with deferoxamine-induced osteochondropathy (113). Unfortunately, the patient's sitting height had deteriorated, illustrating the irreversibility of platyspondylosis.

Sexual function

Repeated monilial vaginitis was reported in patients receiving deferoxamine for dialysis-related aluminium overload (12).

Immunologic

Generalized hypersensitivity reactions and anaphylactic shock can occur but are infrequent. Hypersensitivity reactions to deferoxamine may require permanent withdrawal, worsening the prognosis in thalassemia. However, successful desensitization has been achieved in three patients with previous deferoxamine hypersensitivity, enabling continued administration of deferoxamine (8,114,115).

Infection risk
In many species, from mammals to microbes, iron is essential, and the extremely low free iron content of the blood is an important antimicrobial factor. Many microorganisms do not produce siderophores and are entirely dependent on the iron content of their direct environment; usually their inability to produce siderophores is associated with low infectivity. In the case of increased availability of iron, for example in iron storage diseases, patients may have increased susceptibility to infectious diseases (116–118). Furthermore, iron impairs granulocyte function (119,120) and monocytic function (94). An abundance of publications has shown that the use of deferoxamine in iron storage disease, dialysis patients, or acute iron poisoning (121) can promote the development of infections, notably with microorganisms that are iron-dependent and are known to be otherwise only slightly infective (SED-12, 553) (122–126). Besides providing iron to these microorganisms by acting as a siderophore, deferoxamine can deplete the pool of iron available to the macrophage cytotoxic system (127), and adversely influence the immune system (29,35).

Yersinia enterocolitica or *Yersinia pseudotuberculosis*, *Pneumocystis jiroveci* (29), *Staphylococcus aureus* (128), *Cunninghamella bertholletiae* (127), and *Rhizopus* spp. have been involved. The diagnosis of these spontaneously rare infections may be even more difficult, because the deferoxamine-associated form can have an unusual and atypical course.

Mucormycosis
Many reports of fatal cases of mucormycosis have underlined the danger of acquiring disseminated fungal infection in patients receiving deferoxamine (15–17,93,94,129–135). Boelaert and co-workers of the International Registry of Mucormycosis in Dialysis Patients (Algemeen Ziekenhuis Sint Jan, B-8000 Brugge, Belgium) collected data on a total of 62 cases of mucormycosis, of which 59 were studied in detail (136); 78% of these patients were receiving deferoxamine. The infection presented as disseminated mucormycosis in 44%, rhinocerebral in 31%, and other forms in 25%, and ran a fatal course in 52 patients (86%). The fungus (cultured in only 36%) was always *Rhizopus* (in spite of the fact that human mucormycosis can be caused by various other fungal genera (for example *Mucor*, *Absida*, and *Cunninghamella*). The finding that the species was *R. microsporus* in all identified cases is at variance with the usual predominance of *R. oryzae* in patients with diabetes mellitus. Patients using deferoxamine who present with fever, sinusitis, dry cough, hemoptysis (28), acute loss of vision (62), or neurological symptoms should undergo evaluation for mucormycosis.

Occasionally, such conditions can start with skin lesions imitating vasculitis (93) or cutaneous infarction (94), or present with cavernous sinus or carotid arterial thrombosis (131). Although mucormycosis often has a fatal course, it can have a favorable prognosis if diagnosed early and treated aggressively with surgery and antifungal drugs (28). Many patients have several risk factors for mucormycosis in addition to deferoxamine (for example hemochromatosis, diabetes mellitus, splenectomy, immune suppression) and the contribution of deferoxamine can be difficult to prove or quantify in individual cases.

Yersinia enterocolitica

Infections with *Y. enterocolitica*, a Gram-negative aerobic and facultatively anaerobic, non-spore-forming bacterium, can occur in immunocompromized patients, and enteritis and lymphadenopathy are characteristic. However, in deferoxamine-treated patients septicemia predominates, and peritonitis and intestinal perforation (123) have been reported; the fatality rate is high (119,121,126,137–143). In all patients receiving deferoxamine, children and adults, the appearance of fever and other non-specific signs of infection should be a reason to think of yersiniosis. Children with acute iron poisoning are also at risk. In view of the severity of *Yersinia* sepsis, the prophylactic use of antibiotics has been advised whenever deferoxamine is administered to children from areas with a high incidence of yersiniosis (121). There have been single case reports of neck abscess (*Salmonella choleraesuis*) and of osteomyelitis of the ilium (*S. aureus*) during the use of deferoxamine (144,145). In the latter case bacterial contamination was considered to have occurred during insertion of the needle or during the preparation or infusion of the deferoxamine solution.

Long-Term Effects

Tumorigenicity

Deferoxamine is used experimentally in a variety of diseases, including Kaposi's sarcoma, and in vitro tests have suggested that it inhibits the growth of sarcoma-derived cells (146). Unfortunately, the intralesional injection of deferoxamine led to paradoxical exacerbation of Kaposi's sarcoma of the skin and the development of numerous sarcomatous papules in the area of injection, whereas there were no changes in untreated lesions (147).

Second-Generation Effects

Teratogenicity

Deferoxamine is teratogenic in animals, but experience in humans is not so far suggestive of deferoxamine-related malformations (148–150).

Susceptibility Factors

Age

The administration of high subcutaneous doses of deferoxamine to young children with thalassemia before iron overload has been established and is associated with a significant reduction in mean body length (151,152). Impairment of growth is associated with a rickets-like syndrome and joint stiffness. Metabolic studies have shown reduced hair and leukocyte zinc concentrations and leukocyte alkaline phosphatase activity. Retardation of growth may be related to chelation of trace elements (for example zinc), to a direct toxic effect of unchelated deferoxamine by inhibiting critical iron-dependent enzymes, or to both. It is advised that in thalassemia major, treatment with deferoxamine be started only after iron accumulation is established, that is at around 3 years of age, after 20–30 blood transfusions, when ferritin concentrations are in the range 800–1000 ng/ml. Deferoxamine doses should be established on the basis of studies of iron balance and dose–response curves, and longitudinal growth monitoring is warranted.

Children are also susceptible to opportunistic infection, notably *Y. enterocolitica* sepsis (142). In 10 children receiving intravenous deferoxamine (25 mg/kg) there were unexpected infections in four; three had episodes of fever and *S. aureus* in blood cultures, and one had *Y. enterocolitica* sepsis (128). Because of the possibility of septicemic dissemination secondary to digestive *Y. enterocolitica* infection, the occurrence of febrile diarrhea in a child with thalassemia is a reason for immediate withdrawal of deferoxamine and the administration of antimicrobial therapy (co-trimoxazole) (142).

Other features of the patient

A possible relation has been suggested between toxicity and the ratio of metabolite B of deferoxamine to unmetabolized deferoxamine (SEDA-18, 250) and there is a relation between regular deferoxamine treatment in respect to the degree of iron overload, as defined by the therapeutic index, that is the daily dose of deferoxamine in mg/kg/day divided by the serum ferritin concentration in ng/ml (SED-13, 621), and the ratio of metabolite B to total deferoxamine (deferoxamine plus ferrioxamine) in the plasma or urine (153). This is consistent with the hypothesis that metabolite B of deferoxamine, which is a product of the intercellular metabolism of iron-free but not iron-bound deferoxamine, inversely reflects the availability of iron in the plasma compartment. In patients who receive a high amount of chelation (measured as mean daily dose of deferoxamine in mg/kg) in relation to iron stores (as reflected by serum ferritin in ng/ml), the proportion of iron-free deferoxamine that is available for metabolism is greater. Therefore, the proportion of metabolite B is higher in the urine or blood of patients who are relatively well chelated. These findings suggest that the ratio of metabolite B/ferrioxamine, expressed either as plasma AUCs or urine concentrations, reflects the availability of chelatable iron, and hence the risk from excess deferoxamine administration at the time the measurement is taken, but that there is unlikely to be an inherent qualitative difference in deferoxamine metabolism in at-risk patients. Further study is needed to determine whether this is of value in identifying patients with increased risk of adverse effects prospectively.

Drug Administration

Drug administration route

Intravenous deferoxamine can be indicated in gross iron overload, serious cardiomyopathy, or intolerance of or non-adherence to subcutaneous administration. The results of continuous 24-hour deferoxamine infusion via indwelling intravenous catheters in 17 patients (25 intravenous lines) have been presented (154). The doses of deferoxamine were calculated with reference to the serum ferritin concentration, with a view to maintaining the therapeutic index (mean daily dose in mg/kg divided by the serum ferritin concentration in ng/ml) below 0.025. The usual regimen was 6 or 7 days of continuous treatment. Only eight patients received mean daily deferoxamine doses exceeding 50 mg/kg at any time. The mean number of catheter days per patient was 697 and the median follow-up was 54 months (the longest study reported to date). The main catheter-related complications were infection (1.15 events per 1000 catheter days) and thromboembolism (0.48 events per 1000 catheter days). There were 10 episodes of bacteremic infection (with a variety of species) and 11 of port or exit-site infections (mainly coagulase-negative staphylococci). Line thrombosis occurred in four instances, pulmonary embolism in two, superior vena cava thrombosis in one, and internal jugular thrombosis in one. Since deferoxamine is a risk factor for acquiring bacterial and fungal infections (SED-14, 717), it is noteworthy that the observed rate of infection was similar to that in other patient groups. During this study, audiometric abnormalities were not observed. Only one of the 17 patients, while the therapeutic index was briefly exceeded (mean daily dose of deferoxamine 80 mg/kg), had manifestations of deferoxamine toxicity, with visual field and acuity defects (retinopathy). In this patient full resolution occurred over 9 months after dosage reduction.

The local tolerability of subcutaneous bolus injections of deferoxamine has been studied in 27 patients; deferoxamine was given 12-hourly into the abdominal wall on 5 days per week (30 mg/kg/day) (155). The patients had iron overload due to multiple transfusions and were treated for a mean period of 20 months. All had mild transient painless swelling during injection, disappearing within 10–15 minutes. Two also had pain at the injection site, with redness in one case.

Drug–Drug Interactions

Artemisinin derivatives

Co-administration of artemisinin derivatives, such as artesunate, with deferoxamine can be useful in patients with cerebral malaria, because of the combination of rapid parasite clearance by the former and central nervous system protection by the latter. Artesunate has been studied alone and in combination with deferoxamine in a single-blind comparison (156). Adverse effects were generally mild and there were no differences between the two regimens.

Ascorbic acid

There is a complex interaction between ascorbic acid, iron, and deferoxamine (157). Ascorbic acid appears to be essential for the mobilization of stored iron into a labile pool, available for chelation therapy. As a result, the administration of deferoxamine to patients with ascorbic acid deficiency will have a limited effect. On the other hand, ascorbic acid increases the toxic effects of iron, especially on the heart. In order to prevent serious cardiac dysrhythmias, ascorbic acid should only be given after deferoxamine infusion has been started and adequate serum concentrations of deferoxamine have been reached (SEDA-8, 239) (158). Ascorbic acid reduces ferric to ferrous iron, and it is the reduced iron that is responsible for the generation of highly reactive free radicals, causing tissue injury (157). Ascorbic acid up to 2 g/day stimulates deferoxamine-mediated urinary iron excretion, probably without adverse cardiac results (159). However, a report of the precipitation of cardiomyopathy with a dose of 1 g/day of ascorbic acid in a patient with hemochromatosis not receiving deferoxamine provides reason for caution in this respect (160). Interestingly, this patient later had a rapid beneficial response to deferoxamine on the heart, even before significant iron chelation could have been established. Presumably deferoxamine detoxifies iron by the inhibition of Fe^{2+}-induced hydroxyl radical generation and lipid peroxidation.

Methotrexate

In 21 children the liberation of "catalytic iron" in acute myeloid leukemia appeared to aggravate the adverse effects of high-dose methotrexate chemotherapy (161). This finding suggests that the toxicity of chemotherapy might be reduced by the co-administration of iron chelators.

Prochlorperazine

The combination of prochlorperazine and deferoxamine can cause loss of consciousness (38).

Interference with Diagnostic Tests

Iron-binding capacity

In the presence of deferoxamine, misinterpretation of the measurement of the iron-binding capacity can occur (125).

Radioactive ^{67}gallium scanning

Experience in a patient with a cerebral hemorrhage showed that chelation of gallium by deferoxamine can interfere with the diagnostic value of a ^{67}Ga scan (162).

References

1. Pauschinger U, Janssen G, Gobel U. Homozygote-beta-Thalassämie. Erhähte Morbidität bei inkonsequenter Therapie im Kindes-oder Jugendalter. Monatsschr Kinderheilkd 1996;144:1068–72.
2. Pekrun A, Fleckenstein W, Schroter W. Homozygote-beta-Thalassämie. Erfolgreiche Therapie mit Deferoxamin und Hochtransfusionsregime. Monatsschr Kinderheilkd 1996;144:699–701.

3. Giardina PJ, Ehlers KH, Grady RW, Lesser ML, New MI, Hilgartner MW. Progress in the management of thalassemia: over a decade and a half of experience with subcutaneous desferrioxamine. Bone Marrow Transplant 1997;19(Suppl 2):9–10.
4. Kontoghiorghes GJ. Clinical use, therapeutic aspects and future potential of deferiprone in thalassemia and other conditions of iron and other metal toxicity. Drugs Today (Barc) 2001;37(1):23–35.
5. Giardina PJ, Grady RW. Chelation therapy in beta-thalassemia: an optimistic update. Semin Hematol 2001;38(4):360–6.
6. Taher A, Sheikh-Taha M, Koussa S, Inati A, Neeman R, Mourad F. Comparison between deferoxamine and deferiprone (L1) in iron-loaded thalassemia patients. Eur J Haematol 2001;67(1):30–4.
7. Athanasion A, Shepp MA, Necheles TF. Anaphylactic reaction to desferrioxamine. Lancet 1977;2(8038):616.
8. Miller KB, Rosenwasser LJ, Bessette JA, Beer DJ, Rocklin RE. Rapid desensitisation for desferrioxamine anaphylactic reaction. Lancet 1981;1(8228):1059.
9. Janssen MJ, van Boven WP. Efficacy of low-dose desferrioxamine for the estimation of aluminium overload in haemodialysis patients. Pharm World Sci 1996;18(5):187–91.
10. Weinberg ED. Development of clinical methods of iron deprivation for suppression of neoplastic and infectious diseases. Cancer Invest 1999;17(7):507–13.
11. Fosburg MT, Nathan DG. Treatment of Cooley's anemia. Blood 1990;76(3):435–44.
12. McCarthy JT, Milliner DS, Johnson WJ. Clinical experience with desferrioxamine in dialysis patients with aluminium toxicity. Q J Med 1990;74(275):257–76.
13. Jacobs P, Wood L, Bird AR, Ultmann JE. Pseudo deep-vein thrombosis following desferrioxamine infusion: a previously unreported adverse reaction? Lancet 1990;336(8718):815.
14. Stephens AD. Cystinuria and its treatment: 25 years experience at St. Bartholomew's Hospital. J Inherit Metab Dis 1989;12(2):197–209.
15. Hamdy NA, Andrew SM, Shortland JR, Boletis J, Raftery AT, Kanis JA, Brown CB. Fatal cardiac zygomycosis in a renal transplant patient treated with desferrioxamine. Nephrol Dial Transplant 1989;4(10):911–13.
16. Daly AL, Velazquez LA, Bradley SF, Kauffman CA. Mucormycosis: association with deferoxamine therapy. Am J Med 1989;87(4):468–71.
17. Arizono K, Fukui H, Miura H, Hayano K, Otsuka Y, Tajiri M. [A case report of rhinocerebral mucormycosis in hemodialysis patient receiving deferoxamine.] Nippon Jinzo Gakkai Shi 1989;31(1):99–103.
18. Voest EE, Neijt JP, Keunen JE, Dekker AW, van Asbeck BS, Nortier JW, Ros FE, Marx JJ. Phase I study using desferrioxamine and iron sorbitol citrate in an attempt to modulate the iron status of tumor cells to enhance doxorubicin activity. Cancer Chemother Pharmacol 1993;31(5):357–62.
19. Freedman MH, Grisaru D, Olivieri N, MacLusky I, Thorner PS. Pulmonary syndrome in patients with thalassemia major receiving intravenous deferoxamine infusions. Am J Dis Child 1990;144(5):565–9.
20. Castriota Scanderbeg A, Izzi GC, Butturini A, Benaglia G. Pulmonary syndrome and intravenous high-dose desferrioxamine. Lancet 1990;336(8729):1511.
21. Tenenbein M, Kowalski S, Sienko A, Bowden DH, Adamson IY. Pulmonary toxic effects of continuous desferrioxamine administration in acute iron poisoning. Lancet 1992;339(8795):699–701.
22. Weitman SD, Buchanan GR, Kamen BA. Pulmonary toxicity of deferoxamine in children with advanced cancer. J Natl Cancer Inst 1991;83(24):1834–5.
23. Cianciulli P. Pulmonary embolism and intravenous high-dose desferrioxamine. Haematologica 1992;77(4):368–9.
24. Helson L, Helson C, Braverman S, Deb G, Donfrancesco A. Desferrioxamine in acute iron poisoning. Lancet 1992;339(8809):1602–3.
25. Anderson KJ, Rivers RP. Desferrioxamine in acute iron poisoning. Lancet 1992;339(8809):1602.
26. Rego EM, Neto EB, Simoes BP, Zago MA. Dose-dependent pulmonary syndrome in patients with thalassemia major receiving intravenous deferoxamine. Am J Hematol 1998;58(4):340–1.
27. Kubota N, Miyazawa K, Shoji N, Sumi M, Nakajima A, Kimura Y, Oshiro H, Ebihara Y, Ohyashiki K. A massive intraventricular thrombosis by disseminated mucormycosis in a patient with myelodysplastic syndrome during deferoxamine therapy. Haematologica 2003;88(11):EIM13.
28. Venkattaramanabalaji GV, Foster D, Greene JN, Muro-Cacho CA, Sandin RL, Saez R, Robinson LA. Mucormycosis associated with deferoxamine therapy after allogeneic bone marrow transplantation. Cancer Control 1997;4(2):168–71.
29. Kouides PA, Slapak CA, Rosenwasser LJ, Miller KB. *Pneumocystis carinii* pneumonia as a complication of desferrioxamine therapy. Br J Haematol 1988;70(3):383–4.
30. Ogborn MR, Dorcas VC, Crocker JF. Deferoxamine and aluminum clearance in pediatric hemodialysis patients. Pediatr Nephrol 1991;5(1):62–4.
31. Sherrard DJ, Walker JV, Boykin JL. Precipitation of dialysis dementia by deferoxamine treatment of aluminum-related bone disease. Am J Kidney Dis 1988;12(2):126–30.
32. McCauley J, Sorkin MI. Exacerbation of aluminium encephalopathy after treatment with desferrioxamine. Nephrol Dial Transplant 1989;4(2):110–14.
33. Lillevang ST, Pedersen FB. Exacerbation of aluminium encephalopathy after treatment with desferrioxamine. Nephrol Dial Transplant 1989;4(7):676.
34. Olivieri NF, Matsui D, Liu PP, Blendis L, Cameron R, McClelland RA, Templeton DM, Koren G. Oral iron chelation with 1,2-dimethyl-3-hydroxypyrid-4-one (L1) in iron loaded thalassemia patients. Bone Marrow Transplant 1993;12(Suppl 1):9–11.
35. Weinberg K. Novel uses of deferoxamine. Am J Pediatr Hematol Oncol 1990;12(1):9–13.
36. Brancaccio D, Avanzini G, Padovese P, Gallieni M, Franceschetti S, Panzica F, Anelli A, Colantonio G, Martinelli D, Bugiani O. Desferrioxamine infusion can modify EEG tracing in haemodialysed patients. Nephrol Dial Transplant 1991;6(4):264–8.
37. Polson RJ, Jawed A, Bomford A, Berry H, Williams R. Treatment of rheumatoid arthritis with desferrioxamine: relation between stores of iron before treatment and side effects. BMJ (Clin Res Ed) 1985;291(6493):448.
38. Blake DR, Winyard P, Lunec J, Williams A, Good PA, Crewes SJ, Gutteridge JM, Rowley D, Halliwell B, Cornish A, et al Cerebral and ocular toxicity induced by desferrioxamine. Q J Med 1985;56(219):345–55.
39. Zafeiriou DI, Kousi AA, Tsantali CT, Kontopoulos EE, Augoustidou-Savvopoulou PA, Tsoubaris PD, Athanasiou MA. Neurophysiologic evaluation of long-term desferrioxamine therapy in beta-thalassemia patients. Pediatr Neurol 1998;18(5):420–4.
40. Chiodo AA, Alberti PW, Sher GD, Francombe WH, Tyler B. Desferrioxamine ototoxicity in an adult transfusion-dependent population. J Otolaryngol 1997; 26(2):116–22.
41. Pinna A, Corda L, Carta F. Rapid recovery with oral zinc sulphate in deferoxamine-induced presumed optic

neuropathy and hearing loss. J Neuroophthalmol 2001;21(1):32–3.
42. Yaqoob M, Ahmad R, Roberts N, Helliwell T. Low-dose desferrioxamine test for the diagnosis of aluminium-related bone disease in patients on regular haemodialysis. Nephrol Dial Transplant 1991;6(7):484–6.
43. Rivera CF, Fontan MP, Cabanas M, Moncalian J, Arrojo F, Valdes F. Toxicidad ocular irreversible tras administratión de una dosis aislada de desferroxiamina en hemodiálisis. Nefrologia 1990;10:431–4.
44. Ravelli M, Scaroni P, Mombelloni S, Movilli E, Feller P, Apostoli P, De Maria G, Valotti C, Sciuto G, Maiorca R. Acute visual disorders in patients on regular dialysis given desferrioxamine as a test. Nephrol Dial Transplant 1990;5(11):945–9.
45. Hamed LM, Winward KE, Glaser JS, Schatz NJ. Optic neuropathy in uremia. Am J Ophthalmol 1989;108(1):30–5.
46. Cases A, Kelly J, Sabater F, Torras A, Grino MC, Lopez-Pedret J, Revert L. Ocular and auditory toxicity in hemodialyzed patients receiving desferrioxamine. Nephron 1990;56(1):19–23.
47. Bournerias F, Monnier N, Dufier JL, Reveillaud RJ. Toxicité oculaire sévère de la desferrioxamine chez l'hémodialysé. [Severe ocular toxicity of desferrioxamine in the hemodialyzed patient.] Nephrologie 1987;8(1):27–9.
48. Bene C, Manzler A, Bene D, Kranias G. Irreversible ocular toxicity from single "challenge" dose of deferoxamine. Clin Nephrol 1989;31(1):45–8.
49. Cases A, Kelly J, Sabater J, Campistol JM, Torras A, Montoliu J, Lopez I, Revert L. Acute visual and auditory neurotoxicity in patients with end-stage renal disease receiving desferrioxamine. Clin Nephrol 1988;29(4):176–8.
50. Rahi AH, Hungerford JL, Ahmed AI. Ocular toxicity of desferrioxamine: light microscopic histochemical and ultrastructural findings. Br J Ophthalmol 1986;70(5):373–81.
51. Lakhanpal V, Schocket SS, Jiji R. Deferoxamine (Desferal)-induced toxic retinal pigmentary degeneration and presumed optic neuropathy. Ophthalmology 1984;91(5):443–51.
52. Blake DR, Winyard P, Lunec J, Williams A, Good PA, Crewes SJ, Gutteridge JM, Rowley D, Halliwell B, Cornish A, et al. Cerebral and ocular toxicity induced by desferrioxamine. QJ Med 1985;56(219):345–55.
53. Borgna-Pignatti C, De Stefano P, Broglia AM. Visual loss in patient on high-dose subcutaneous desferrioxamine. Lancet 1984;1(8378):681.
54. Sanchez Dalmau BF, Vela Payan MD. Retinopatía por desferroxiamina. [Retinopathy caused by desferrioxamine.] Med Clin (Barc) 1996;107(16):636.
55. Albalate M, Velasco L, Ortiz A, Monzu B, Casado S, Caramelo C. High risk of retinal damage by desferrioxamine in dialysis patients. Nephron 1996;73(4):726–7.
56. Dennerlein JA, Lang GE, Stahnke K, Kleihauer E, Lang GK. Okulare Befunde bei Desferaltherapie. [Ocular findings in Desferal therapy.] Ophthalmologe 1995;92(1):38–42.
57. De Virgiliis S, Congia M, Turco MP, Frau F, Dessi C, Argiolu F, Sorcinelli R, Sitzia A, Cao A. Depletion of trace elements acute ocular toxicity induced by desferrioxamine in patients with thalassaemia. Arch Dis Child 1988;63(3):250–5.
58. Barratt PS, Toogood IR. Hearing loss attributed to desferrioxamine in patients with beta-thalassaemia major. Med J Aust 1987;147(4):177–9.
59. Gelmi C, Borgna-Pignatti C, Franchin S, Tacchini M, Trimarchi F. Electroretinographic and visual-evoked potential abnormalities in patients with beta-thalassemia major. Ophthalmologica 1988;196(1):29–34.
60. Rinaldi M, Della Corte M, Ruocco V, D'Onofrio C, Zanotta G, Romano A. Ocular involvement correlated with age in patients affected by major and intermedia beta-thalassemia treated or not with desferrioxamine. Metab Pediatr Syst Ophthalmol 1993;16(1–2):23–5.
61. Marciani MG, Cianciulli P, Stefani N, Stefanini F, Peroni L, Sabbadini M, Maschio M, Trua G, Papa G. Toxic effects of high-dose deferoxamine treatment in patients with iron overload: an electrophysiological study of cerebral and visual function. Haematologica 1991;76(2):131–4.
62. Murray MF, Galetta SL, Raps EC, Kenyon L, Brennan PJ. Deferoxamine-associated mucormycosis in a non-dialysis patient. Infect Dis Clin Pract 1996;5:395–7.
63. Caballero LG. Toxicidad auditiva, visual y neurologica de la desferroxamina. [Auditory, visual and neurologic toxicity of deferoxamine.] Rev Med Chil 1989;117(5):557–61.
64. Bloomfield SE, Markenson AL, Miller DR, Peterson CM. Lens opacities in thalassemia. J Pediatr Ophthalmol Strabismus 1978;15(3):154–6.
65. Szwarcberg J, Mack G, Flament J. Toxicité oculaire de la deféroxamine. [Ocular toxicity of deferoxamine: description and analysis of three observations.] J Fr Ophtalmol 2002;25(6):609–14.
66. Sanchez Rodriguez A, Martin Oterino JA, Fidalgo Fernandez MA. Unusual toxicity of deferoxamine. Ann Pharmacother 1999;33(4):505–6.
67. Jiang C, Hansen RM, Gee BE, Kurth SS, Fulton AB. Rod and rod mediated function in patients with beta-thalassemia major. Doc Ophthalmol 1998–99;96(4):333–45.
68. Sacco M, Meleleo D, Tricarico N, Greco Miani A, Serra E, Parlatore L. Valutazione dell' ototossicita della desferrioxamina in pazienti talasemici. [Evaluation of desferrioxamine ototoxicity in thalassemic patients. Follow-up over a 5-year period and results.] Minerva Pediatr 1994;46(5):225–30.
69. Ambrosetti U, Donde E, Piatti G, Cappellini MD. Audiological evaluation in adult beta-thalassemia major patients under regular chelation treatment. Pharmacol Res 2000;42(5):485–7.
70. Karimi M, Asadi-Pooya AA, Khademi B, Asadi-Pooya K, Yarmohammadi H. Evaluation of the incidence of sensorineural hearing loss in beta-thalassemia major patients under regular chelation therapy with desferrioxamine. Acta Haematol 2002;108(2):79–83.
71. Klein GL, Snodgrass WR, Griffin MP, Miller NL, Alfrey AC. Hypocalcemia complicating deferoxamine therapy in an infant with parenteral nutrition-associated aluminum overload: evidence for a role of aluminum in the bone disease of infants. J Pediatr Gastroenterol Nutr 1989;9(3):400–3.
72. Nocka KH, Pelus LM. Cell cycle specific effects of deferoxamine on human and murine hematopoietic progenitor cells. Cancer Res 1988;48(13):3571–5.
73. Praga M, Andres A, de la Serna J, Ruilope LM, Nieto J, Estenoz J, Millet VG, Arnaiz F, Rodicio JL. Improvement of anaemia with desferrioxamine in haemodialysis patients. Nephrol Dial Transplant 1987;2(4):243–7.
74. Swartz R, Dombrouski J, Burnatowska-Hledin M, Mayor G. Microcytic anemia in dialysis patients: reversible marker of aluminum toxicity. Am J Kidney Dis 1987;9(3):217–23.
75. Felipe C, Rivera M, Orofino L, Matesanz R, Ortuno J. Effect of desferrioxamine on anaemia of haemodialysis patients. Nephrol Dial Transplant 1988;3(1):105–6.
76. Cuvelier R, Deceuninck P. Desferrioxamine improves anaemia in haemodialysis patients without aluminum or iron overload. Nephrol Dial Transplant 1988;3(1):104.
77. Salvarani C, Baricchi R, Lasagni D, Boiardi L, Piccinini R, Brunati C, Macchioni P, Portioli I. Effects

of desferrioxamine therapy on chronic disease anemia associated with rheumatoid arthritis. Rheumatol Int 1996;16(2):45–8.
78. Jensen PD, Heickendorff L, Pedersen B, Bendix-Hansen K, Jensen FT, Christensen T, Boesen AM, Ellegaard J. The effect of iron chelation on haemopoiesis in MDS patients with transfusional iron overload. Br J Haematol 1996;94(2):288–99.
79. Aucella F, Scalzulli P, Musto P, Prencipe M, Valente GL, Vigilante M, Carotenuto M, Stallone C. Synergic effect of desferoxamine (DFO) and recombinant erythropoietin on erythroid precursors proliferation in chronic renal failure. G Ital Nefrol 1998;15:241–7.
80. Aucella F, Vigilante M, Scalzulli P, Musto P, Prencipe M, Valente GL, Carotenuto M, Stallone C. Synergistic effect of desferrioxamine and recombinant erythropoietin on erythroid precursor proliferation in chronic renal failure. Nephrol Dial Transplant 1999;14(5):1171–5.
81. Walker JA, Sherman RA, Eisinger RP. Thrombocytopenia associated with intravenous desferrioxamine. Am J Kidney Dis 1985;6(4):254–6.
82. Sofroniadou K, Drossou M, Foundoulaki L, Konstantopoulos K, Kyriakoy D, Zervas J. Acute bone marrow aplasia associated with intravenous administration of deferoxamine (desferrioxamine). Drug Saf 1990;5(2):152–4.
83. Kruck TP, Fisher EA, McLachlan DR. A predictor for side effects in patients with Alzheimer's disease treated with deferoxamine mesylate. Clin Pharmacol Ther 1993;53(1):30–7.
84. Koren G, Kochavi-Atiya Y, Bentur Y, Olivieri NF. The effects of subcutaneous deferoxamine administration on renal function in thalassemia major. Int J Hematol 1991;54(5):371–5.
85. Batey R, Scott J, Jain S, Sherlock S. Acute renal insufficiency occurring during intravenous desferrioxamine therapy. Scand J Haematol 1979;22(3):277–9.
86. Koren G, Bentur Y, Strong D, Harvey E, Klein J, Baumal R, Spielberg SP, Freedman MH. Acute changes in renal function associated with deferoxamine therapy. Am J Dis Child 1989;143(9):1077–80.
87. Koren G, Bentur Y, Li Volti S, et al Comments. Am J Dis Child 1990;144:1096–70.
88. Giardini C, Galimberti M, Lucarelli G, Polchi P, Angelucci E, Baronciani D, Gaziev D, Erer B, Ripalti M, Rapa S, Muretto P. Desferrioxamine therapy of secondary hemochromatosis after BMT for thalassemia. Bone Marrow Transplant 1997;19(Suppl 2):119–22.
89. Giardini C, Galimberti M, Lucarelli G, Polchi P, Angelucci E, Baronciani D, Gaziev D, Erer B, La Nasa G, Barbanti I, Muretto P. Desferrioxamine therapy accelerates clearance of iron deposits after bone marrow transplantation for thalassaemia. Br J Haematol 1995;89(4):868–73.
90. Brittenham GM, Griffith PM, Nienhuis AW, McLaren CE, Young NS, Tucker EE, Allen CJ, Farrell DE, Harris JW. Efficacy of deferoxamine in preventing complications of iron overload in patients with thalassemia major. N Engl J Med 1994;331(9):567–73.
91. Venencie PY, Rain B, Blanc A, Tertian G. Toxidermie la déferoxamine (Desféral). [Deferoxamine (Desferal) dermatitis.] Ann Dermatol Venereol 1988;115(11):1174.
92. Praga M, Enriquez de Salamanca R, Andres A, Nieto J, Oliet A, Perpina J, Morales JM. Treatment of hemodialysis-related porphyria cutanea tarda with deferoxamine. N Engl J Med 1987;316(9):547–8.
93. Sombolos K, Kalekou H, Barboutis K, Tzarou V. Fatal phycomycosis in a hemodialyzed patient receiving deferoxamine. Nephron 1988;49(2):169–70.
94. Sane A, Manzi S, Perfect J, Herzberg AJ, Moore JO. Deferoxamine treatment as a risk factor for zygomycete infection. J Infect Dis 1989;159(1):151–2.
95. Brill PW, Winchester P, Giardina PJ, Cunningham-Rundles S. Deferoxamine-induced bone dysplasia in patients with thalassemia major. Am J Roentgenol 1991;156(3):561–5.
96. Orzincolo C, Castaldi G, De Sanctis V, Scutellari PN, Ciaccio C, Vullo C. Lesioni scheletriche simil-rachitiche e/o scorbutiche nella beta-talassemia major. [Rickets-and/or scurvy-like bone lesions in beta-thalassemia major.] Radiol Med (Torino) 1990;80(6):823–9.
97. Orzincolo C, Scutellari PN, Castaldi G. Growth plate injury of the long bones in treated beta-thalassemia. Skeletal Radiol 1992;21(1):39–44.
98. Olivieri NF, Koren G, Harris J, Khattak S, Freedman MH, Templeton DM, Bailey JD, Reilly BJ. Growth failure and bony changes induced by deferoxamine. Am J Pediatr Hematol Oncol 1992;14(1):48–56.
99. Hartkamp MJ, Babyn PS, Olivieri F. Spinal deformities in deferoxamine-treated homozygous beta-thalassemia major patients. Pediatr Radiol 1993;23(7):525–8.
100. Miller TT, Caldwell G, Kaye JJ, Arkin S, Burke S, Brill PW. MR imaging of deferoxamine-induced bone dysplasia in an 8-year-old female with thalassemia major. Pediatr Radiol 1993;23(7):523–4.
101. Filosa A, Di Maio S, Baron I, Esposito G, Galati MG. Final height and body disproportion in thalassaemic boys and girls with spontaneous or induced puberty. Acta Paediatr 2000;89(11):1295–301.
102. Caruso-Nicoletti M, De Sanctis V, Capra M, Cardinale G, Cuccia L, Di Gregorio F, Filosa A, Galati MC, Lauriola A, Malizia R, Mangiagli A, Massolo F, Mastrangelo C, Meo A, Messina MF, Ponzi G, Raiola G, Ruggiero L, Tamborino G, Saviano A. Short stature and body proportion in thalassaemia. J Pediatr Endocrinol Metab 1998;11(Suppl 3):811–16.
103. Caruso-Nicoletti M, Di Bella D, Pizzarelli G, Leonardi C, Sciuto C, Coco M, Di Gregorio F. Growth failure and bone lesions due to desferrioxamine in thalassaemic patients. J Pediatr Endocrinol Metab 1998;11(Suppl 3):957–60.
104. Lauriola AL, Tangerini A, Lodi A, Gamberini MR, Testa MR, Orzincolo C, De Sanctis V, Vullo C. Rachitic rosary in a well chelated thalassaemic patient with primary amenorrhea (patient report). J Pediatr Endocrinol Metab 1998;11(Suppl 3):979–80.
105. Naselli A, Vignolo M, Di Battista E, Garzia P, Forni GL, Traverso T, Aicardi G. Long-term follow-up of skeletal dysplasia in thalassaemia major. J Pediatr Endocrinol Metab 1998;11(Suppl 3):817–25.
106. De Sanctis V, Stea S, Savarino L, Scialpi V, Traina GC, Chiarelli GM, Sprocati M, Govoni R, Pezzoli D, Gamberini R, Rigolin F. Growth hormone secretion and bone histomorphometric study in thalassaemic patients with acquired skeletal dysplasia secondary to desferrioxamine. J Pediatr Endocrinol Metab 1998;11(Suppl 3):827–33.
107. Chan Y, Li C, Chu WC, Pang L, Cheng JC, Chik KW. Deferoxamine-induced bone dysplasia in the distal femur and patella of pediatric patients and young adults: MR imaging appearance. Am J Roentgenol 2000;175(6):1561–6.
108. Chan YL, Li CK, Pang LM, Chik KW. Desferrioxamine-induced long bone changes in thalassaemic patients—radiographic features, prevalence and relations with growth. Clin Radiol 2000;55(8):610–14.
109. de Sanctis V, Savarino L, Stea S, Cervellati M, Ciapetti G, Tassinari L, Pizzoferrato A. Microstructural analysis of severe bone lesions in seven thalassemic patients treated with deferoxamine. Calcif Tissue Int 2000;67(2):128–33.

110. de Sanctis V, Stea S, Savarino L, Granchi D, Visentin M, Sprocati M, Govoni R, Pizzoferrato A. Osteochondrodystrophic lesions in chelated thalassemic patients: an histological analysis. Calcif Tissue Int 2000;67(2):134–40.
111. Chan YL, Pang LM, Chik KW, Cheng JC, Li CK. Patterns of bone diseases in transfusion-dependent homozygous thalassaemia major: predominance of osteoporosis and desferrioxamine-induced bone dysplasia. Pediatr Radiol 2002;32(7):492–7.
112. Chan YL, Chu CW, Chik KW, Pang LM, Shing MK, Li CK. Deferoxamine-induced dysplasia of the knee: sonographic features and diagnostic performance compared with magnetic resonance imaging. J Ultrasound Med 2001;20(7):723–8.
113. Mangiagli A, De Sanctis V, Campisi S, Di Silvestro G, Urso L. Treatment with deferiprone (L1) in a thalassemic patient with bone lesions due to desferrioxamine. J Pediatr Endocrinol Metab 2000;13(6):677–80.
114. Cianciulli P, Sorrentino F, Maffei L, Amadori S. Continuous low-dose subcutaneous desferrioxamine (DFO) to prevent allergic manifestations in patients with iron overload. Ann Hematol 1996;73(6):279–81.
115. Bousquet J, Navarro M, Robert G, Aye P, Michel FB. Rapid desensitisation for desferrioxamine anaphylactoid reaction. Lancet 1983;2(8354):859–60.
116. Seifert A, von Herrath D, Schaefer K. Iron overload, but not treatment with desferrioxamine favours the development of septicemia in patients on maintenance hemodialysis. Q J Med 1987;65(248):1015–24.
117. Chiu HY, Flynn DM, Hoffbrand AV, Politis D. Infection with *Yersinia enterocolitica* in patients with iron overload. BMJ (Clin Res Ed) 1986;292(6513):97.
118. Mofenson HC, Caraccio TR, Sharieff N. Iron sepsis: *Yersinia enterocolitica* septicemia possibly caused by an overdose of iron. N Engl J Med 1987;316(17):1092–3.
119. Waterlot Y, Cantinieaux B, Hariga-Muller C, De Maertelaere-Laurent E, Vanherweghem JL, Fondu P. Impaired phagocytic activity of neutrophils in patients receiving haemodialysis: the critical role of iron overload. BMJ (Clin Res Ed) 1985;291(6494):501–4.
120. Emami A, Fagundus DM. Granulocyte dysfunction in patients with iron overload. Br J Haematol 1990;74(4):546–7.
121. Hadjiminas JM. Yersiniosis in acutely iron-loaded children treated with desferrioxamine. J Antimicrob Chemother 1988;21(5):680–1.
122. Abcarian PW, Demas BE. Systemic *Yersinia enterocolitica* infection associated with iron overload and deferoxamine therapy. Am J Roentgenol 1991;157(4):773–5.
123. Mazzoleni G, deSa D, Gately J, Riddell RH. *Yersinia enterocolitica* infection with ileal perforation associated with iron overload and deferoxamine therapy. Dig Dis Sci 1991;36(8):1154–60.
124. Nouel O, Voisin PM, Vaucel J, Dartois-Hoguin M, Le Bris M. Association d'une septicémie à *Yersinia enterocolitica*, d'une hémochromatose idiopathique et d'un traitement par deferoxamine. [*Yersinia enterocolitica* septicemia associated with idiopathic hemochromatosis and deferoxamine therapy. A case.] Presse Méd 1991;20(31):1494–6.
125. Pierron H, Gillet R, Perrimond H, Broudeur JC, Soudry G. Yersiniose et dyshémoglobinose. Á propos de 4 observations. [*Yersinia* infection and hemoglobin disorder.Apropos of 4 cases.] Pediatrie 1990;45(6):379–82.
126. Kaneko T, Abe F, Ito M, Hotchi M, Yamada K, Okada Y. Intestinal mucormycosis in a hemodialysis patient treated with desferrioxamine. Acta Pathol Jpn 1991;41(7):561–6.
127. Rex JH, Ginsberg AM, Fries LF, Pass HI, Kwon-Chung KJ. *Cunninghamella bertholletiae* infection associated with deferoxamine therapy. Rev Infect Dis 1988;10(6):1187–94.
128. Eijgenraam FJ, Donckerwolcke RA. Treatment of iron overload in children and adolescents on chronic haemodialysis. Eur J Pediatr 1990;149(5):359–62.
129. Goodill JJ, Abuelo JG. Mucormycosis—a new risk of deferoxamine therapy in dialysis patients with aluminum or iron overload? N Engl J Med 1987;317(1):54.
130. Boelaert JR, van Roost GF, Vergauwe PL, Verbanck JJ, de Vroey C, Segaert MF. The role of desferrioxamine in dialysis-associated mucormycosis: report of three cases and review of the literature. Clin Nephrol 1988;29(5):261–6.
131. Van Johnson E, Kline LB, Julian BA, Garcia JH. Bilateral cavernous sinus thrombosis due to mucormycosis. Arch Ophthalmol 1988;106(8):1089–92.
132. Veis JH, Contiguglia R, Klein M, Mishell J, Alfrey AC, Shapiro JI. Mucormycosis in deferoxamine-treated patients on dialysis. Ann Intern Med 1987;107(2):258.
133. Anonymous. Mucormycosis induced by deferoxamine mesylate. Information on Adverse Reactions to Drugs. Japan: Pharmaceutical Affairs Bureau, Ministry of Health and Welfare, February 1988.
134. Boelaert JR, Fenves AZ, Coburn JW. Mucormycosis among patients on dialysis. N Engl J Med 1989;321(3):190–1.
135. Nakamura M, Weil WB Jr, Kaufman DB. Fatal fungal peritonitis in an adolescent on continuous ambulatory peritoneal dialysis: association with deferoxamine. Pediatr Nephrol 1989;3(1):80–2.
136. Slade MP, McNab AA. Fatal mucormycosis therapy associated with deferoxamine. Am J Ophthalmol 1991;112(5):594–5.
137. Boyce N, Wood C, Holdsworth S, Thomson NM, Atkins RC. Life-threatening sepsis complicating heavy metal chelation therapy with desferrioxamine. Aust NZ J Med 1985;15(5):654–5.
138. Melby K, Slordahl S, Gutteberg TJ, Nordbo SA. Septicaemia due to *Yersinia enterocolitica* after oral overdoses of iron. BMJ (Clin Res Ed) 1982;285(6340):467–8.
139. Robins-Browne RM, Prpic JK. Desferrioxamine and systemic yersiniosis. Lancet 1983;2(8363):1372.
140. Waterlot Y, Vanherweghem JL. Desferrioxamine en hémodialyse á l'origine d'une septicémie *Yersinia enterocolitica.* [Desferrioxamine in hemodialysis as the cause of *Yersinia enterocolitica* septicemia.] Presse Méd 1985;14(12):699.
141. Gallant T, Freedman MH, Vellend H, Francombe WH. *Yersinia sepsis* in patients with iron overload treated with deferoxamine. N Engl J Med 1986;314(25):1643.
142. Chirio R, Collignon A, Sabbah L, Lestradet H, Torlotin JC. Infections á *Yersinia enterocolitica* et thalassémie majeure chez l'enfant. [*Yersinia enterocolitica* infections and thalassemia major in children.] Ann Pediatr (Paris) 1989;36(5):308–14.
143. Masters AP, Hopkinson RB. *Yersinia enterocolitica* septicaemia. Intensive Care Med 1988;14(5):585–7.
144. Behr MA, McDonald J. *Salmonella* neck abscess in a patient with beta-thalassemia major: case report and review. Clin Infect Dis 1996;23(2):404–5.
145. McLean TW, Kurth S, Gee B. Pelvic osteomyelitis in a sickle-cell patient receiving deferoxamine. Am J Hematol 1996;53(4):284–5.
146. Simonart T, Degraef C, Andrei G, Mosselmans R, Hermans P, Van Vooren JP, Noel JC, Boelaert JR, Snoeck R, Heenen M. Iron chelators inhibit the growth and induce the apoptosis of Kaposi's sarcoma cells and of their putative endothelial precursors. J Invest Dermatol 2000;115(5):893–900.
147. Simonart T, Boelaert JR, Van Vooren JP. Enhancement of classic Kaposi's sarcoma growth after intralesional injections of desferrioxamine. Dermatology 2002;204(4):290–2.

148. McElhatton PR, Roberts JC, Sullivan FM. The consequences of iron overdose and its treatment with desferrioxamine in pregnancy. Hum Exp Toxicol 1991;10(4):251–9.
149. Briggs GG, Freeman RK, Yaffe SJ. Drugs in Pregnancy and Lactation. 2nd ed. Baltimore: Williams and Wilkins, 1986;121.
150. Tampakoudis P, Tantanassis T, Lazaridis E, Tsatalas K, Mantalenakis S. Akzidentelle Desferoxaminmedikation in der Früschwangerschaft bei homozygoter Beta-Thalassämie; Literaturübersicht. [Accidental desferoxamine medication during early pregnancy with homozygous beta-thalassaemia; review of the literature.] Geburtshilfe Frauenheilkd 1996;56:680–3.
151. De Virgiliis S, Congia M, Frau F, Argiolu F, Diana G, Cucca F, Varsi A, Sanna G, Podda G, Fodde M, et al Deferoxamine-induced growth retardation in patients with thalassemia major. J Pediatr 1988;113(4):661–9.
152. Piga A, Luzzatto L, Capalbo P, Gambotto S, Tricta F, Gabutti V. High-dose desferrioxamine as a cause of growth failure in thalassemic patients. Eur J Haematol 1988;40(4):380–1.
153. Porter JB, Faherty A, Stallibrass L, Brookman L, Hassan I, Howes C. A trial to investigate the relationship between DFO pharmacokinetics and metabolism and DFO-related toxicity. Ann NY Acad Sci 1998;850:483–7.
154. Davis BA, Porter JB. Long-term outcome of continuous 24-hour deferoxamine infusion via indwelling intravenous catheters in high-risk beta-thalassemia. Blood 2000;95(4):1229–36.
155. Franchini M, Gandini G, de Gironcoli M, Vassanelli A, Borgna-Pignatti C, Aprili G. Safety and efficacy of subcutaneous bolus injection of deferoxamine in adult patients with iron overload. Blood 2000;95(9):2776–9.
156. Looareesuwan S, Wilairatana P, Vannaphan S, Gordeuk VR, Taylor TE, Meshnick SR, Brittenham GM. Co-administration of desferrioxamine B with artesunate in malaria: an assessment of safety and tolerance. Ann Trop Med Parasitol 1996;90(5):551–4.
157. Roeser HP. The role of ascorbic acid in the turnover of storage iron. Semin Hematol 1983;20(2):91–100.
158. Nienhuis AW. Vitamin C and iron. N Engl J Med 1981;304(3):170–1.
159. Van der Weyden MB. Vitamin C, desferrioxamine and iron loading anemias. Aust NZ J Med 1984;14(5):593–5.
160. Rowbotham B, Roeser HP. Iron overload associated with congenital pyruvate kinase deficiency and high dose ascorbic acid ingestion. Aust NZ J Med 1984;14(5):667–9.
161. Carmine TC, Evans P, Bruchelt G, Evans R, Handgretinger R, Niethammer D, Halliwell B. Presence of iron catalytic for free radical reactions in patients undergoing chemotherapy: implications for therapeutic management. Cancer Lett 1995;94(2):219–26.
162. Baker DL, Manno CS. Rapid excretion of gallium-67 isotope in an iron-overloaded patient receiving high-dose intravenous deferoxamine. Am J Hematol 1988;29(4):230–2.

Defibrotide

General Information

Defibrotide is a polydeoxyribonucleotide extracted from mammalian organ. Its antithrombotic activity is partly ascribed to enhancement of eicosanoid metabolism, in particular increased release of prostacyclin, with ensuing vasodilatation and inhibition of platelet aggregation. An additional mechanism is activation of the fibrinolytic system, primarily increased activation of tissue plasminogen in the vessel wall.

The antithrombotic potential of defibrotide has been reported in patients with hepatic veno-occlusive disease after stem cell transplantation. In a randomized, placebo-controlled trial in 310 patients with claudication there was significant improvement in walking distance with defibrotide, but no difference in efficacy between the two doses of the drug tested (800 and 1200 mg/day) (1). Twenty patients stopped taking the drug because of cardiovascular events, the preset endpoints of the study. Seven others stopped because of adverse drug reactions, mainly gastrointestinal intolerance and skin reactions. They were equally distributed among the placebo and the two defibrotide groups.

Reference

1. Violi F, Marubini E, Coccheri S, Nenci GG. Improvement of walking distance by defibrotide in patients with intermittent claudication—results of a randomized, placebo-controlled study (the DICLIS study). Defibrotide Intermittent CLaudication Italian Study. Thromb Haemost 2000;83(5):672–7.

Delavirdine

See also Non-nucleoside reverse transcriptase inhibitors (NNRTIs)

General Information

Delavirdine is a non-nucleoside reverse transcriptase inhibitor, which is dosed three times daily. No food restrictions apply. It is metabolized mainly by CYP3A, and so interactions with other drugs that use this metabolic pathway can occur.

Organs and Systems

Skin

The most frequent adverse effect of delavirdine is a rash, which usually occurs during the first 3 months of therapy in up to 50% of individuals. It is usually mild and resolves spontaneously in most patients or can be treated successfully with a short course of antihistamines. Interruption of treatment is required in less than 4% of patients (1,2).

Immunologic

Severe hypersensitivity reactions, including anaphylaxis, can occur and may necessitate drug withdrawal (3).

Drug–Drug Interactions

Antacids

Antacids interfere with the absorption of delavirdine and should therefore not be given concomitantly (4).

Administration of antacids and buffered formulations of didanosine should be separated from that of delavirdine by at least 1 hour.

Didanosine

Didanosine interferes with the absorption of delavirdine and should therefore not be given concomitantly (5).

Enzyme inducers

Concomitant use of inducers of cytochrome P450, such as rifampicin, rifabutin, phenytoin, phenobarbital, or carbamazepine, should be avoided, since they significantly reduce delavirdine plasma concentrations (4).

HIV protease inhibitors

By inhibiting their metabolism, ritonavir potentiates the actions of other protease inhibitors. The addition of delavirdine instead of another NNRTI in three patients taking protease inhibitors plus ritonavir further increased the exposure to the protease inhibitors (6). Combining delavirdine with indinavir removes the food restrictions during indinavir administration (4). The superior virological response observed in antiretroviral regimens containing delavirdine and protease inhibitors has been attributed in part to the pharmacokinetic interaction.

Statins

- Rhabdomyolysis with acute renal insufficiency has been reported in a 63-year-old man who was taking atorvastatin 20 mg/day and delavirdine 400 mg 8-hourly (7).

The authors suggested that delavirdine had inhibited the metabolism of atorvastatin by inhibiting CYP3A4.

References

1. Been-Tiktak AM, Boucher CA, Brun-Vezinet F, Joly V, Mulder JW, Jost J, Cooper DA, Moroni M, Gatell JM, Staszewski S, Colebunders R, Stewart GJ, Hawkins DA, Johnson MA, Parkin JM, Kennedy DH, Hoy JF, Borleffs JC. Efficacy and safety of combination therapy with delavirdine and zidovudine: a European/Australian phase II trial. Int J Antimicrob Agents 1999;11(1):13–21.
2. Friedland GH, Pollard R, Griffith B, Hughes M, Morse G, Bassett R, Freimuth W, Demeter L, Connick E, Nevin T, Hirsch M, Fischl M. Efficacy and safety of delavirdine mesylate with zidovudine and didanosine compared with two-drug combinations of these agents in persons with HIV disease with CD4 counts of 100 to 500 cells/mm^3 (ACTG 261). ACTG 261 Team. J Acquir Immune Defic Syndr 1999;21(4):281–92.
3. Mills G, Morgan J, Hales G, Smith D. Acute hypersensitivity with delavirdine. Antivir Ther 1999;4(1):51.
4. Tran JQ, Gerber JG, Kerr BM. Delavirdine: clinical pharmacokinetics and drug interactions. Clin Pharmacokinet 2001;40(3):207–26.
5. Morse GD, Fischl MA, Shelton MJ, Cox SR, Driver M, DeRemer M, Freimuth WW. Single-dose pharmacokinetics of delavirdine mesylate and didanosine in patients with human immunodeficiency virus infection. Antimicrob Agents Chemother 1997;41(1):169–74.
6. Harris M, Alexander C, O'Shaughnessy M, Montaner JS. Delavirdine increases drug exposure of ritonavir-boosted protease inhibitors. AIDS 2002;16(5):798–9.
7. Castro JG, Gutierrez L. Rhabdomyolysis with acute renal failure probably related to the interaction of atorvastatin and delavirdine. Am J Med 2002;112(6):505.

Desflurane

See also General anesthetics

General Information

Desflurane is identical in structure to isoflurane, except that it is halogenated completely with fluorine instead of fluorine and chlorine. Desflurane is a volatile anesthetic that combines low blood gas solubility with moderate potency and high volatility. Its pharmacology has been reviewed (1,2).

Compared with volatile anesthetics in current use, desflurane has the advantages of being practically inert and of having a low blood-gas partition coefficient (0.4), making its onset and offset of action rapid. Its disadvantages include its low boiling point (close to room temperature) and the fact that it requires a specially heated vaporizer for delivery. It is also irritating to airways, precluding its use for induction of anesthesia and making the safety of mask anesthesia questionable. It also has excitatory effects on the sympathetic nervous system, causing tachycardia and mydriasis, which can make it difficult to judge the adequacy of anesthetic depth.

When desflurane is used with the proper equipment, alveolar concentrations can be adjusted more rapidly and precisely during administration, and recovery is quicker in both the short and long term than with other agents (3).

In a prospective, randomized study of 120 patients undergoing day-surgery, desflurane and sevoflurane were associated with shorter times to awakening, extubation, and orientation than propofol by infusion (4). Average times to awakening at the end of anesthesia were 5, 5, and 8 minutes respectively.

Organs and Systems

Cardiovascular

Desflurane increases the heart rate and reduces both mean arterial pressure and systemic vascular resistance while maintaining cardiac output (5,6). In high concentrations it can cause transient activation of the sympathetic nervous system, predisposing to hypertension and dysrhythmias (7).

Despite some coronary vasodilatation in dogs, there is no evidence of coronary steal in man. Desflurane may benefit elderly patients by allowing more rapid recovery from anesthesia (8).

Respiratory

Desflurane is a mild respiratory irritant (6). Moderate to severe laryngospasm and moderate to severe coughing occurred often (50% of cases) during induction of anesthesia with desflurane in 206 children aged 1 month to 12 years; the authors concluded that the high incidence of these airway complications during induction limit the use of desflurane in children, but that anesthesia could be safely maintained with desflurane after induction with another anesthetic (9).

Nervous system

Increasing doses of desflurane caused no demonstrable fall in cerebral blood flow. Consequently, it can be advocated for patients undergoing neurosurgical procedures (10).

Neuromuscular function

Depression of neuromuscular function occurred 10 minutes after the introduction of desflurane 1.3% in a 32-year-old man who had previously received midazolam, fentanyl, and thiopental for induction. On withdrawal his neuromuscular function returned to baseline (11).

Liver

Poorly metabolized gases are generally safer than those that undergo extensive metabolism. Desflurane is poorly metabolized, and appeared to have no toxic effects on the liver and kidneys in 13 young men (12).

However, a case of severe hepatotoxicity after desflurane anesthesia has been reported (13).

- An obese 37-year-old woman with a past history of allergy to penicillin, nickel, and cobalt, and unexplained mild hepatitis 6 weeks after halothane anesthesia 9 years before, was given an anesthetic including etomidate, alcuronium, metamizole, piritramizide, fentanyl, nitrous oxide, and desflurane. Ten days later she developed the symptoms and signs of hepatitis, an eosinophilia, and raised hepatic enzymes, including alanine transaminase 1776 IU/l, aspartate transaminase 1258 IU/l, gamma-glutamyl transpeptidase 48 IU/l, and bilirubin 503 μmol/l. After exclusion of common causes of hepatitis, a liver biopsy confirmed acute hepatitis. There were increased titers of antitrifluoroacetylated IgG antibodies, which peaked at 0.159 on day 25 postoperatively. She eventually recovered.

This patient had multiple risk factors for anesthesia-induced hepatitis, including obesity, middle age, female sex, a history of drug allergies, and multiple exposures to fluorinated anesthetic agents. Desflurane has a very low rate of hepatic oxidative metabolism (0.02 versus 20% for halothane), and is considered to be one of the safest volatile agents as far as hepatotoxicity is concerned. Nevertheless, this case shows that it can cause severe hepatotoxicity.

Urinary tract

The effects of sevoflurane, isoflurane, and desflurane on macroscopic renal structure have been studied in 24 patients undergoing nephrectomy (14). All the anesthetics were administered using a fresh gas flow of 1 l/minute and a sodium hydroxide absorber and had an average duration of 3 hours. No injury to nephrons was observed by pathologists blinded to which anesthetic agent had been used. Postoperative creatinine concentrations and urine volumes did not differ significantly between the groups.

Body temperature

- Malignant hyperthermia has been described in a 10-year-old boy who received thiopental and suxamethonium for induction of anesthesia, followed by desflurane for maintenance of anesthesia (15).

The role of suxamethonium must also be considered in this case.

Susceptibility Factors

Age

In old people, the MAC of desflurane, with or without nitrous oxide, was less than that in patients aged 18–65 years. Doses of desflurane must therefore be reduced in older people, as with all other inhalation agents (16).

Drug–Drug Interactions

Adrenaline

Adrenaline used during anesthesia can cause ventricular dysrhythmias. The threshold dose of adrenaline for dysrhythmias is reduced by halothane, but not by desflurane; the dose of adrenaline required to produce dysrhythmias in 50% of patients was three times that needed when anesthesia was with halothane (17).

Fentanyl

The MAC of desflurane was significantly reduced 25 minutes after a single dose of fentanyl (18).

Propofol

Desflurane-based anesthesia, with and without prophylactic ondansetron, to reduce the incidence of postoperative nausea and vomiting, has been compared with a propofol infusion in 90 women of ASA grades 1 and 2 undergoing outpatient gynecological laparoscopic surgery (19). The incidence of postoperative nausea and vomiting was 80% with desflurane alone, 40% with desflurane plus ondansetron, and 20% with propofol. Postoperative antiemetic requirements were larger and times-to-home readiness longer with desflurane alone, but sedation and analgesic requirements were similar. The high incidence of postoperative nausea and vomiting suggests that routine antiemetic prophylaxis should be considered in outpatients receiving desflurane-based anesthesia.

Rocuronium

Both desflurane and sevoflurane significantly increase the neuromuscular blocking effects of rocuronium compared with isoflurane or propofol (20,21).

References

1. Westrin P. Intravenous and inhalational anaesthetic agents. Baillière's Clin Anaesthesiol 1996;10:687–715.
2. Anonymous. Sevoflurane and desflurane: comparison with older inhalational anaesthetics. Drugs Ther Perspect 1996;7:1–5.
3. Eger EI 2nd. Desflurane animal and human pharmacology: aspects of kinetics, safety, and MAC. Anesth Analg 1992;75(Suppl 4):S3–9.
4. Song D, Joshi GP, White PF. Fast-track eligibility after ambulatory anesthesia: a comparison of desflurane, sevoflurane, and propofol. Anesth Analg 1998;86(2):267–73.
5. Rodig G, Wild K, Behr R, Hobbhahn J. Effects of desflurane and isoflurane on systemic vascular resistance during hypothermic cardiopulmonary bypass. J Cardiothorac Vasc Anesth 1997;11(1):54–7.
6. Warltier DC, Pagel PS. Cardiovascular and respiratory actions of desflurane: is desflurane different from isoflurane? Anesth Analg 1992;75(Suppl 4):S17–31.
7. Bunting HE, Kelly MC, Milligan KR. Effect of nebulized lignocaine on airway irritation and haemodynamic changes during induction of anaesthesia with desflurane. Br J Anaesth 1995;75(5):631–3.
8. Bennett JA, Lingaraju N, Horrow JC, McElrath T, Keykhah MM. Elderly patients recover more rapidly from desflurane than from isoflurane anesthesia. J Clin Anesth 1992;4(5):378–81.
9. Zwass MS, Fisher DM, Welborn LG, Cote CJ, Davis PJ, Dinner M, Hannallah RS, Liu LM, Sarner J, McGill WA, et al Induction and maintenance characteristics of anesthesia with desflurane and nitrous oxide in infants and children. Anesthesiology 1992;76(3):373–8.
10. Ornstein E, Young WL, Fleischer LH, Ostapkovich N. Desflurane and isoflurane have similar effects on cerebral blood flow in patients with intracranial mass lesions. Anesthesiology 1993;79(3):498–502.
11. Kelly RE, Lien CA, Savarese JJ, Belmont MR, Hartman GS, Russo JR, Hollmann C. Depression of neuromuscular function in a patient during desflurane anesthesia. Anesth Analg 1993;76(4):868–71.
12. Weiskopf RB, Eger EI 2nd, Ionescu P, Yasuda N, Cahalan MK, Freire B, Peterson N, Lockhart SH, Rampil IJ, Laster M. Desflurane does not produce hepatic or renal injury in human volunteers. Anesth Analg 1992;74(4):570–4.
13. Berghaus TM, Baron A, Geier A, Lamerz R, Paumgartner G, Conzen P. Hepatotoxicity following desflurane anesthesia. Hepatology 1999;29(2):613–14.
14. Annila P, Rorarius M, Reinikainen P, Oikkonen M, Baer G. Effect of pre-treatment with intravenous atropine or glycopyrrolate on cardiac arrhythmias during halothane anaesthesia for adenoidectomy in children. Br J Anaesth 1998;80(6):756–60.
15. Fu ES, Scharf JE, Mangar D, Miller WD. Malignant hyperthermia involving the administration of desflurane. Can J Anaesth 1996;43(7):687–90.
16. Gold MI, Abello D, Herrington C. Minimum alveolar concentration of desflurane in patients older than 65 yr. Anesthesiology 1993;79(4):710–14.
17. Moore MA, Weiskopf RB, Eger EI 2nd, Wilson C, Lu G. Arrhythmogenic doses of epinephrine are similar during desflurane or isoflurane nesthesia in humans. Anesthesiology 1993;79(5):943–7.
18. Sebel PS, Glass PS, Fletcher JE, Murphy MR, Gallagher C, Quill T. Reduction of the MAC of desflurane with fentanyl. Anesthesiology 1992;76(1):52–9.
19. Eriksson H, Korttila K. Recovery profile after desflurane with or without ondansetron compared with propofol in patients undergoing outpatient gynecological laparoscopy. Anesth Analg 1996;82(3):533–8.
20. Lowry DW, Mirakhur RK, Carrol MT. Time course of action of rocuronium during sevoflurane, isoflurane or i.v. anaesthesia. Br J Anaesth 1998;80:544.
21. Wulf H, Ledowski T, Linstedt U, Proppe D, Sitzlack D. Neuromuscular blocking effects of rocuronium during desflurane, isoflurane, and sevoflurane anaesthesia. Can J Anaesth 1998;45(6):526–32.

Desloratadine

See also Antihistamines

General Information

Desloratadine is the primary metabolite of loratadine, with superior H_1 receptor binding, potent antihistaminic activity compared with the parent compound, and proven efficacy in allergic disease (1). It is effective and well tolerated in seasonal allergic rhinitis, including relief of nasal congestion (2–4).

In a randomized, open, four-way, crossover study in 20 healthy men desloratadine was given as single doses (5, 7.5, 10, and 20 mg) in four different treatment periods with 14 days between each dose. The C_{max} for all doses occurred at 4 hours after administration, with a half-life of 21–24 hours. There were no dose-related differences in drug absorption rate, and even the 20 mg dose was well tolerated (5). The systemic availability of desloratadine was unaffected by food in healthy adult volunteers (6).

Organs and Systems

Cardiovascular

In a large, multicenter, double-blind, placebo-controlled, parallel-group study of the efficacy and tolerability of desloratadine in 346 patients with seasonal allergic rhinitis, the symptoms improved significantly and there was no significant effect on the QT_c interval (7).

In a multicenter, randomized, double-blind, placebo-controlled study in 190 patients, desloratadine was effective in the treatment of moderate to severe chronic idiopathic urticaria, with no adverse electrocardiographic effects (8).

In healthy volunteers, 12 men and 12 women, there was no prolongation of the QT_c interval after co-administration of desloratadine with erythromycin (9).

Nervous system

Desloratadine appears to be minimally sedative, given that several studies, published in abstract, have shown no impairment in terms of wakefulness or psychomotor performance (10–12). Moreover, in a study in which desloratadine was effective and well tolerated in patients with seasonal allergic rhinitis there were no clinically significant sedative effects (7).

Psychological, psychiatric

The results of several studies suggest that desloratadine has minimal or no effects on cognitive functions and psychomotor performance (13–15).

Susceptibility Factors

Genetic factors

The effect of race on desloratadine pharmacokinetics at steady state has been examined (16). The authors concluded that no dosage adjustments for desloratadine were required.

Age

The effect of age on desloratadine pharmacokinetics at steady state has been examined (17). The authors concluded that no dosage adjustments for desloratadine were required.

Sex

The effect of sex on desloratadine pharmacokinetics at steady state has been examined (16). The authors concluded that no dosage adjustments for desloratadine were required.

Drug–Drug Interactions

Azithromycin

The effect of co-administration of azithromycin on plasma concentrations of desloratadine has been examined in a randomized third-party-blind, placebo-controlled, parallel-group study in 90 healthy volunteers (18). An initial loading dose of azithromycin (500 mg) was given on day 3, followed by 250 mg od for 4 days. Concomitant azithromycin had little effect (<15%) on either the C_{max} or AUC of desloratadine, and there were no statistically significant increases in the PR, QT, QT_c interval, QRS complex duration, or ventricular rate after administration of desloratadine with or without azithromycin.

Erythromycin

There was no clinically relevant interaction between desloratadine and erythromycin (9).

Fluoxetine

Co-administration of desloratadine with fluoxetine did not result in clinically relevant changes in the pharmacokinetics of either drug in 54 healthy volunteers (19).

Grapefruit juice

In an unblinded, randomized, single-dose, crossover study in 24 healthy adults, grapefruit juice had no effect on the systemic availability of oral desloratadine (20). There were no clinically significant electrocardiographic changes after co-administration of grapefruit juice with desloratadine compared with desloratadine alone.

Ketoconazole

The electrocardiographic safety of desloratadine in combination with the CYP3A4 inhibitor ketoconazole has been assessed in a randomized, two-way, crossover, third-party-blind, multiple-dose, placebo-controlled study over 10 days in 24 healthy volunteers (21). Compared with desloratadine alone there were no significant or clinically important changes in QT_c, QT, PR, or QRS intervals when desloratadine (7.5 mg/day, that is 50% higher than the recommended dose) was co-administered with ketoconazole (200 mg bd). There was a 1.3-fold increase in desloratadine C_{max} when it was co-administered with ketoconazole, but this was judged not to be clinically important. The authors concluded that co-administration of desloratadine with ketoconazole has no clinically relevant electrocardiographic or pharmacodynamic implications. There was no clinically relevant interaction between desloratadine and ketoconazole (21).

References

1. McClellan K, Jarvis B. Desloratadine. Drugs 2001; 61(6):789–96.
2. Horak F, Stubner UP, Zieglmayer R, Ing D, Harris AG. Effect of desloratadine versus placebo on nasal airflow and subjective measures of nasal obstruction in subjects with grass pollen-induced allergic rhinitis in an allergen-exposure unit. J Allergy Clin Immunol 2002;109(6):956–61.
3. Bachert C, Virchow CJ Jr, Plenker A. Desloratadine in the treatment of seasonal allergic rhinitis: results of a large observational study. Clin Drug Invest 2002;22:43–52.
4. Wilson AM, Haggart K, Sims EJ, Lipworth BJ. Effects of fexofenadine and desloratadine on subjective and objective measures of nasal congestion in seasonal allergic rhinitis. Clin Exp Allergy 2002;32(10):1504–9.
5. Gupta S, Banfield C, Affrime M, Marco A, Cayen M, Herron J, Padhi D. Desloratadine demonstrates dose proportionality in healthy adults after single doses. Clin Pharmacokinet 2002;41(Suppl 1):1–6.
6. Gupta S, Banfield C, Affrime M, Marbury T, Padhi D, Glue P. Oral bioavailability of desloratadine is unaffected by food. Clin Pharmacokinet 2002;41(Suppl 1):7–12.
7. Meltzer EO, Prenner BM, Nayak A; The Desloratadine Study Group. Efficacy and tolerability of once-daily 5 mg desloratadine, an H_1-receptor antagonist, in patients with seasonal allergic rhinitis: assessment during the spring and fall allergy seasons. Clin Drug Invest 2001;21:25–32.
8. Ring J, Hein R, Gauger A, Bronsky E, Miller B, Breneman D, Conneley M, Corren J, Ceuppens J, Fierlbeck G, Friday G, Goldberg P, Graft D, Holst T, Honsinger R, Hornmark A-M, Kaiser H, Kaplan R, Kempers S, Lockey R, Miller SD, Nayak A, Nayak N, Pariser D, Prenner B, Ruzicka T, Stewart GE II, Thompson M, Wein M. Once-daily desloratadine improves the signs and symptoms of chronic idiopathic urticaria: a randomized, double-blind, placebo-controlled study. Int J Dermatol 2001;40(1):72–6.
9. Banfield C, Hunt T, Reyderman L, Statkevich P, Padhi D, Affrime M. Lack of clinically relevant interaction between desloratadine and erythromycin. Clin Pharmacokinet 2002;41(Suppl 1):29–35.
10. Scharf MB, Kay GC, Rikken G, Danzig MR, Staudinger H. Desloratadine has no effect on wakefulness or psychomotor performance. Allergy 2000;55(Suppl 63):Abstract 280.

11. Vuurman E, Ramaekers JG, Rikken G, De Halleux F. Desloratadine does not impair actual driving performance: a three way crossover comparison with diphenhydramine and placebo. Allergy 2000;55(Suppl 63):Abstract 263.
12. Valk PJL, Van Roon DB, Simons M, Rikken G, Lether IC, Staudinger H. No impairment of flying ability with desloratadine use in healthy volunteers under conditions of simulated cabin pressure. Allergy 2001;56(Suppl 68):Abstract 229.
13. Wilken JA, Kane RL, Ellis AK, Rafeiro E, Briscoe MP, Sullivan CL, Day JH. A comparison of the effect of diphenhydramine and desloratadine on vigilance and cognitive function during treatment of ragweed-induced allergic rhinitis. Ann Allergy Asthma Immunol 2003;91(4):375–85.
14. Nicholson AN, Handford AD, Turner C, Stone BM. Studies on performance and sleepiness with the H_1-antihistamine, desloratadine. Aviat Space Environ Med 2003;74(8):809–15.
15. Valk PJ, Van Roon DB, Simons RM, Rikken G. Desloratadine shows no effect on performance during 6 h at 8,000 ft simulated cabin altitude. Aviat Space Environ Med 2004;75(5):433–8.
16. Affrime M, Banfield C, Gupta S, Cohen A, Boutros T, Thonoor M, Cayen M. Effect of race and sex on single and multiple dose pharmacokinetics of desloratadine. Clin Pharmacokinet 2002;41(Suppl 1):21–8.
17. Affrime M, Gupta S, Banfield C, Cohen A. A pharmacokinetic profile of desloratadine in healthy adults, including elderly. Clin Pharmacokinet 2002;41(Suppl 1):13–19.
18. Gupta S, Banfield C, Kantesaria B, Marino M, Clement R, Affrime M, Batra V. Pharmacokinetic and safety profile of desloratadine and fexofenadine when coadministered with azithromycin: a randomized, placebo-controlled, parallel-group study. Clin Ther 2001;23(3):451–66.
19. Gupta S, Banfield C, Kantesaria B, Flannery B, Herron J. Pharmacokinetics/pharmacodynamics of desloratadine and fluoxetine in healthy volunteers. J Clin Pharmacol 2004;44(11):1252–9.
20. Banfield C, Gupta S, Marino M, Lim J, Affrime M. Grapefruit juice reduces the oral bioavailability of fexofenadine but not desloratadine. Clin Pharmacokinet 2002;41(4):311–18.
21. Banfield C, Herron J, Keung A, Padhi D, Affrime M. Desloratadine has no clinically relevant electrocardiographic or pharmacodynamic interactions with ketoconazole. Clin Pharmacokinet 2002;41(Suppl 1):37–44.

Desmopressin

See also Vasopressin and analogues

General Information

Desmopressin (*N*-deamino-8-D-arginine vasopressin, dDAVP) is a longer acting analogue of vasopressin. It has very little vasoactive effect but is antidiuretic by an action on vasopressin V_2 receptors in the renal tubule and is used to treat central diabetes insipidus and nocturnal enuresis.

At higher doses desmopressin also has significant hematological effects and can significantly boost concentrations of factor VIII and von Willebrand factor (VWF) in the blood. Desmopressin is therefore a valuable agent for the treatment of mild and moderate hemophilia A (congenital or acquired) and type 1 von Willebrand disease, in which the VWF protein structure is normal but the plasma concentration is reduced (1). By contrast with conventional coagulation factor concentrates, desmopressin is cheap and is free from the risk of transmission of viral infections, which have proved such a problem in the past. It is also very useful in the treatment of carriers of hemophilia A, many of whom have significant reductions in the baseline concentration of factor VIII. By contrast, desmopressin has no effect on the concentration of factor IX, and is thus of no value in hemophilia B (Christmas disease). It is also of little value in type 2 (abnormal VWF structure) von Willebrand's disease, which accounts for about 15–20% of all cases. The administration of desmopressin to patients with type 2B von Willebrand's disease can be hazardous, as it is likely to cause thrombocytopenia (2). The use of desmopressin in bleeding disorders has been reviewed (3). Tachyphylaxis develops if desmopressin is used for prolonged periods to control bleeding disorders, because desmopressin causes release of stored factor VIII and von Willebrand factor, after which it takes time for them to accumulate again.

Intravenous injection is the most common route although subcutaneous injection may also be used. A concentrated nasal spray formulation has been proved to be efficient for home treatment of patients with bleeding episodes or even minor surgical procedures and has also been used prophylacticly (4). The nasal spray used to treat diabetes insipidus (Desmospray) is too dilute for use in disorders of hemostasis. Similarly, desmopressin in tablet form (Desmotabs) is intended for treatment of nocturnal enuresis in children and is of no use in the treatment of hemostatic disorders.

Desmopressin also shortens the prolonged skin bleeding time in patients with renal insufficiency (5,6), hepatic cirrhosis (7,8), and congenital or acquired defects of platelet function (9–11), including aspirin-induced platelet dysfunction (12).

Desmopressin reduces blood loss in patients without bleeding disorders during surgical procedures, including cardiac surgery (13,14). However, similar benefits have also been observed with other agents, including aprotinin, tranexamic acid, and aminocaproic acid. Meta-analyses have confirmed the efficacy of these agents and have shown that aprotinin is the most effective of these agents in reducing blood loss, while desmopressin was the least effective (15,16).

Children with nocturnal enuresis treated with desmopressin have fewer wet nights per week, but this effect does not persist after therapy is stopped. A meta-analysis showed an overall rate of 7.1 adverse events per 100 children (17). These were almost all local nasal reactions, including nasal irritation and epistaxis.

In an open trial of high-dose desmopressin 1.5 mg intranasally to control bleeding in 278 patients with congenital bleeding disorders, headache occurred in 3.6% and flushing in 3.2% of patients (18). Dizziness and nausea were reported in 1–1.5% and edema in 0.3% of patients.

General adverse effects

The adverse effects of desmopressin include headache, tachycardia, facial flushing, abdominal pain, tremor, and sweating during or shortly after intravenous administration (1). These symptoms are quite common but are usually simply the consequence of rapid intravenous infusion, and symptoms usually quickly subside after slowing, or even temporarily stopping, the infusion. The incidence of these relatively minor adverse effects increases with the dose of desmopressin.

Organs and Systems

Cardiovascular

Facial flushing occurred in two of 25 children with either hemophilia or von Willebrand disease given high-dose intranasal desmopressin (150 micrograms) in a single-dose open study (19).

Marked hypotension with circulatory collapse has occasionally been reported with desmopressin (20,21), although both of these reports related to patients with pre-existing cardiac conditions.

Thrombotic disorders

Desmopressin stimulates the release from endothelial cells of all the multimeric forms of von Willebrand factor found in normal plasma, including large forms that are not normally present (22). These abnormal multimers can aggregate platelets, particularly at the high levels of fluid shear stress that occur at sites of arterial stenosis.

Myocardial thrombosis

There have been several reports of arterial thrombosis associated with the use of desmopressin, including myocardial infarction (23–27). One of these reports concerned a case of fatal myocardial infarction in a blood donor in excellent health, with no risk factors and no signs of vascular disease (25).

- A 59-year-old woman with hemolytic–uremic syndrome and a recent history of atypical chest pain was given prophylactic desmopressin 0.4 micrograms/kg immediately before a renal biopsy (28). Within 30 minutes she developed chest pain and bradycardia due to myocardial infarction.

Three other cases of myocardial infarction in the absence of desmopressin have been reported in patients with hemolytic–uremic syndrome, who already have an increased risk of thrombosis.

A meta-analysis of placebo-controlled trials of desmopressin in 702 cardiac surgery patients showed a significantly increased risk of myocardial infarction in treated patients (RR = 2.39, CI = 1.02, 5.60) (29). Overall mortality was not different from placebo. Desmopressin was less efficacious in reducing perioperative blood loss than either aprotinin or lysine analogues.

Cerebral thrombosis

Cerebral infarction has also been reported in association with the use of desmopressin in children (30,31). One of these cases involved a 7-month-old child with congenital nephrotic syndrome who developed a cerebral infarction after surgery (30). One child developed cerebral ischemia after *Varicella* infection and desmopressin for enuresis (31).

Thromboembolism

There are isolated reports of thromboembolic complications in recipients of desmopressin; most occurred in patients with pre-existing vascular disease. However, in nine trials of the hemostatic efficacy of desmopressin in reducing blood and transfusion requirements in 763 patients, there were no significant differences between the frequencies of thromboembolism in subjects treated with desmopressin and controls (32). An analysis of 31 clinical trials of desmopressin in patients undergoing cardiac, vascular, orthopedic, or other major surgery showed that desmopressin did not increase the incidence of thrombosis (33).

Most of the reported thromboembolic complications occurred in elderly patients and desmopressin should not be used in patients with documented arterial disease or even in elderly patients, in whom some degree of latent arterial disease may be assumed to be present (33). Concomitant use of antifibrinolytic agents, such as tranexamic acid, should also be avoided.

Ear, nose, throat

Nasal irritation and rhinitis are common adverse effects of nasal desmopressin: treatment does not normally have to be altered as a result (34,35).

Fluid balance

A potential risk of desmopressin is of water intoxication with resultant hyponatremia (36), and rapid falls in serum sodium concentration can result in seizures. The risk is increased in infants and patients receiving hypotonic intravenous fluids, and such patients need to be carefully monitored.

- A 37-year-old woman with primary enuresis continued her customary daily fluid intake (2 liters) when she started intranasal desmopressin 30 micrograms at night. Within 2 days she became severely hyponatremic, with loss of consciousness, generalized seizures, and cerebral edema.
- An 80-year-old woman with a high baseline fluid intake developed severe hyponatremia, with loss of consciousness and seizures, after a single dose of desmopressin 0.2 mg (37).
- An 89-year-old woman, who had previously been stable on desmopressin, developed severe hyponatremia and became confused and unresponsive after an increase in fluid intake (37).
- A 47-year-old woman with von Willebrand disease, who was given desmopressin and intravenous fluids perioperatively, developed hyponatremia and seizures, which resolved after water restriction (38).

In a double-blind study of desmopressin, 10 of 224 adult men had serum sodium concentrations below 130 mmol/l during a 3-week, open, dose-titration period. Men aged

65 years and over were more likely to develop hyponatremia (39).

In another open study of elderly men and women, one of 30 subjects developed generalized weakness in association with a serum sodium concentration of 125 mmol/l and a serum potassium concentration of 3.1 mmol/l (40).

In a double-blind, crossover study, 20 men aged 52–80 years were given desmopressin for nocturia. Three of them had symptoms due to fluid retention, particularly bloating, headache, and reversible weight gain, and two of these had a significant fall in plasma sodium (41). In a meta-analysis of 14 studies of serum sodium in 529 patients treated with desmopressin there was mild asymptomatic hyponatremia in up to 10% of patients (42).

Fluid balance and plasma electrolytes should be monitored to prevent this complication, particularly if repeated doses are required. Children seem to be particularly vulnerable to this complication (43). In a long-term, open study of 245 Swedish children given intranasal desmopressin 20–40 micrograms at night for enuresis, five had an asymptomatic fall in plasma sodium (34). Mild hyponatremia, which did not cause symptoms, was found in five of 399 children in an open, multicenter trial (44).

Convulsions have been reported after desmopressin administration, some associated with excessive fluid intake.

- In a 12-year-old boy taking desmopressin for nocturnal enuresis, hyponatremia and cerebral edema developed after high fluid intake before a urodynamic procedure (45).
- A 13 kg 3-year-old boy given 40 micrograms of desmopressin intravenously and 1.6 liters of hypotonic fluid over 12 hours had convulsions and a respiratory arrest: his plasma sodium fell to 114 mmol/l (46).

There have been several reports of seizures in association with hyponatremia after intravenous administration of desmopressin to cover surgery in young children with congenital bleeding disorders such as mild hemophilia A or von Willebrand's disease (46–48). Hyponatremia and convulsions have occurred in children without congenital bleeding disorders who received desmopressin for urine concentration tests or to treat nocturnal enuresis (42,49,50).

Pulmonary edema associated with fluid retention occurred in a 27-year-old man after the administration of desmopressin to reduce blood loss during surgery (51).

Excess water intake during desmopressin therapy was implicated in seven cases of cerebral edema in children, which occurred over a 5-year period in the Czech Republic (52). A non-metered dropper was used for the desmopressin, so overdosage may have contributed.

Hematologic

Thrombocytopenia is rarely reported in patients who receive desmopressin, and is probably due to increased platelet aggregation (SEDA-13, 1310) (53).

- In a 50-year-old woman with uremia the platelet count fell from 149×10^9/l to 45×10^9/l after an abdominal hysterectomy with prophylactic desmopressin, and she developed a fatal subdural hemorrhage (53).
- A 38-year-old man with von Willebrand disease type 2B developed severe thrombocytopenia after a single dose of desmopressin (54).

Desmopressin also stimulates fibrinolysis (55), and this may have contributed to the outcome in the first patient.

In four patients with von Willebrand disease, desmopressin caused a significant but transient reduction in platelet count without an increase in plasma glycocalicin concentrations nor enhanced expression of P selectin, suggesting that acute thrombocytopenia after the administration of desmopressin in type 2B von Willebrand disease is not related to platelet activation and consumption (56).

In 224 adult men, mean age 65 (range 37–88) years, thrombocytopenia developed in one man during a 1-week washout period after dose titration to up to 0.4 mg of oral desmopressin daily over the preceding 3 weeks; thrombocytopenia did not recur on rechallenge (39).

Second-Generation Effects

Pregnancy

There is growing evidence that desmopressin can be used safely in pregnant women and no adverse effects have been reported in either mothers with diabetes insipidus or their babies (57), or in women with clotting factor deficiencies (58). However, the manufacturers advise that it should be used with caution in women with bleeding disorders, who require high doses.

One report described adverse reactions in two pregnant women with von Willebrand disease (59). One went into premature labor after a single dose (attributed to the oxytocic effect of desmopressin) and the other had severe hyponatremia associated with seizures after repeated administration of desmopressin to cover a cesarean section.

Lactation

Insignificant quantities of desmopressin pass into breast milk (60), and so breastfeeding is not contraindicated in association with desmopressin administration to a nursing mother.

Drug–Drug Interactions

Carbamazepine

Carbamazepine increases the release of endogenous antidiuretic hormone and can therefore potentiate the antidiuretic effect of desmopressin. Of 103 children with cranial diabetes insipidus included in a retrospective analysis, 10% became hyponatremic (61). The risk of hyponatremia was three-fold higher when desmopressin and carbamazepine were given in combination.

Chlorpromazine

Chlorpromazine increases the release of endogenous antidiuretic hormone and can therefore potentiate the antidiuretic effect of desmopressin (62).

Lamotrigine

In 103 children with cranial diabetes insipidus, 3 children who started or had an increase in dose of lamotrigine needed a larger dose of desmopressin, suggesting an effect on the renal tubule or on drug clearance (61). Lamotrigine also increased desmopressin dosage requirements in two other children with cranial diabetes insipidus (63).

Tricyclic antidepressants

Tricyclic antidepressants increase the release of endogenous antidiuretic hormone and can therefore potentiate the antidiuretic effect of desmopressin. A hyponatremic convulsion occurred in a child who was given desmopressin and imipramine (64).

References

1. Mannucci PM. Desmopressin (DDAVP) in the treatment of bleeding disorders: the first 20 years. Blood 1997;90(7):2515–21.
2. Holmberg L, Nilsson IM, Borge L, Gunnarsson M, Sjorin E. Platelet aggregation induced by 1-desamino-8-D-arginine vasopressin (DDAVP) in Type IIB von Willebrand's disease. N Engl J Med 1983;309(14):816–21.
3. Sutor AH. Desmopressin (DDAVP) in bleeding disorders of childhood. Semin Thromb Hemost 1998;24(6):555–66.
4. Lethagen S, Ragnarson Tennvall G. Self-treatment with desmopressin intranasal spray in patients with bleeding disorders: effect on bleeding symptoms and socioeconomic factors. Ann Hematol 1993;66(5):257–60.
5. Mannucci PM, Remuzzi G, Pusineri F, Lombardi R, Valsecchi C, Mecca G, Zimmerman TS. Deamino-8-D-arginine vasopressin shortens the bleeding time in uremia. N Engl J Med 1983;308(1):8–12.
6. Watson AJ, Keogh JA. 1-Deamino-8-D-arginine vasopressin as a therapy for the bleeding diathesis of renal failure. Am J Nephrol 1984;4(1):49–51.
7. Burroughs AK, Matthews K, Qadiri M, Thomas N, Kernoff P, Tuddenham E, McIntyre N. Desmopressin and bleeding time in patients with cirrhosis. BMJ (Clin Res Ed) 1985;291(6506):1377–81.
8. Mannucci PM, Vicente V, Vianello L, Cattaneo M, Alberca I, Coccato MP, Faioni E, Mari D. Controlled trial of desmopressin in liver cirrhosis and other conditions associated with a prolonged bleeding time. Blood 1986;67(4):1148–53.
9. Kobrinsky NL, Israels ED, Gerrard JM, Cheang MS, Watson CM, Bishop AJ, Schroeder ML. Shortening of bleeding time by 1-deamino-8-D-arginine vasopressin in various bleeding disorders. Lancet 1984;1(8387):1145–8.
10. Schulman S, Johnsson H, Egberg N, Blomback M. DDAVP-induced correction of prolonged bleeding time in patients with congenital platelet function defects. Thromb Res 1987;45(2):165–74.
11. DiMichele DM, Hathaway WE. Use of DDAVP in inherited and acquired platelet dysfunction. Am J Hematol 1990;33(1):39–45.
12. Chard RB, Kam CA, Nunn GR, Johnson DC, Meldrum-Hanna W. Use of desmopressin in the management of aspirin-related and intractable haemorrhage after cardiopulmonary bypass. Aust NZ J Surg 1990;60(2):125–8.
13. Salzman EW, Weinstein MJ, Weintraub RM, Ware JA, Thurer RL, Robertson L, Donovan A, Gaffney T, Bertele V, Troll J, et al Treatment with desmopressin acetate to reduce blood loss after cardiac surgery. A double-blind randomized trial. N Engl J Med 1986;314(22):1402–6.
14. Cattaneo M, Mannucci PM. Desmopressin and blood loss after cardiac surgery. Lancet 1993;342(8874):812.
15. Fremes SE, Wong BI, Lee E, Mai R, Christakis GT, McLean RF, Goldman BS, Naylor CD. Metaanalysis of prophylactic drug treatment in the prevention of postoperative bleeding. Ann Thorac Surg 1994;58(6):1580–8.
16. Laupacis A, Fergusson D. Drugs to minimize perioperative blood loss in cardiac surgery: meta-analyses using perioperative blood transfusion as the outcome. The International Study of Peri-operative Transfusion (ISPOT) Investigators. Anesth Analg 1997;85(6):1258–67.
17. Glazener CM, Evans JH. Desmopressin for nocturnal enuresis in children. Cochrane Database Syst Rev 2000;(2):CD002112.
18. Leissinger C, Becton D, Cornell C Jr, Cox Gill J. High-dose DDAVP intranasal spray (Stimate) for the prevention and treatment of bleeding in patients with mild haemophilia A, mild or moderate type 1 von Willebrand disease and symptomatic carriers of haemophilia A. Haemophilia 2001;7(3):258–66.
19. Gill JC, Ottum M, Schwartz B. Evaluation of high concentration intranasal and intravenous desmopressin in pediatric patients with mild hemophilia A or mild-to-moderate type 1 von Willebrand disease. J Pediatr 2002;140(5):595–9.
20. D'Alauro FS, Johns RA. Hypotension related to desmopressin administration following cardiopulmonary bypass. Anesthesiology 1988;69(6):962–3.
21. Israels SJ, Kobrinsky NL. Serious reaction to desmopressin in a child with cyanotic heart disease. N Engl J Med 1989;320(23):1563–4.
22. Ruggeri ZM, Mannucci PM, Lombardi R, Federici AB, Zimmerman TS. Multimeric composition of factor VIII/von Willebrand factor following administration of DDAVP: implications for pathophysiology and therapy of von Willebrand's disease subtypes. Blood 1982; 59(6):1272–8.
23. Bond L, Bevan D. Myocardial infarction in a patient with hemophilia treated with DDAVP. N Engl J Med 1988;318(2):121.
24. van Dantzig JM, Duren DR, Ten Cate JW. Desmopressin and myocardial infarction. Lancet 1989;1(8639):664–5.
25. McLeod BC. Myocardial infarction in a blood donor after administration of desmopressin. Lancet 1990;336(8723): 1137–8.
26. Hartmann S, Reinhart W. Fatal complication of desmopressin. Lancet 1995;345(8960):1302–3.
27. Anonymous. Desmopressin and arterial thrombosis. Lancet 1989;1(8644):938–9.
28. Stratton J, Warwicker P, Watkins S, Farrington K. Desmopressin may be hazardous in thrombotic microangiopathy. Nephrol Dial Transplant 2001;16(1):161–2.
29. Levi M, Cromheecke ME, de Jonge E, Prins MH, de Mol BJ, Briet E, Buller HR. Pharmacological strategies to decrease excessive blood loss in cardiac surgery: a meta-analysis of clinically relevant endpoints. Lancet 1999;354(9194):1940–7.
30. Grunwald Z, Sather SD. Intraoperative cerebral infarction after desmopressin administration in infant with end-stage renal disease. Lancet 1995;345(8961):1364–5.
31. Wieting JM, Dykstra DD, Ruggiero MP, Robbins GB, Galusha K. Central nervous system ischemia after *Varicella* infection and desmopressin therapy for enuresis. J Am Osteopath Assoc 1997;97(5):293–5.
32. Mannucci PM, Lusher JM. Desmopressin and thrombosis. Lancet 1989;2(8664):675–6.
33. Mannucci PM, Carlsson S, Harris AS. Desmopressin, surgery and thrombosis. Thromb Haemost 1994;71(1):154–5.
34. Tullus K, Bergstrom R, Fosdal I, Winnergard I, Hjalmas K. Efficacy and safety during long-term treatment of primary

monosymptomatic nocturnal enuresis with desmopressin. Swedish Enuresis Trial Group. Acta Paediatr 1999;88(11):1274–8.
35. Chiozza ML, del Gado R, di Toro R, Ferrara P, Fois A, Giorgi P, Giovannini M, Rottoli A, Segni G, Biraghi M. Italian multicentre open trial on DDAVP spray in nocturnal enuresis. Scand J Urol Nephrol 1999;33(1):42–8.
36. Odeh M, Oliven A. Coma and seizures due to severe hyponatremia and water intoxication in an adult with intranasal desmopressin therapy for nocturnal enuresis. J Clin Pharmacol 2001;41(5):582–4.
37. Shindel A, Tobin G, Klutke C. Hyponatremia associated with desmopressin for the treatment of nocturnal polyuria. Urology 2002;60(2):344.
38. Pruthi RS, Kang J, Vick R. Desmopressin induced hyponatremia and seizures after laparoscopic radical nephrectomy. J Urol 2002;168(1):187.
39. Mattiasson A, Abrams P, Van Kerrebroeck P, Walter S, Weiss J. Efficacy of desmopressin in the treatment of nocturia: a double-blind placebo-controlled study in men. BJU Int 2002;89(9):855–62.
40. Kuo HC. Efficacy of desmopressin in treatment of refractory nocturia in patients older than 65 years. Urology 2002;59(4):485–9.
41. Cannon A, Carter PG, McConnell AA, Abrams P. Desmopressin in the treatment of nocturnal polyuria in the male. BJU Int 1999;84(1):20–4.
42. Robson WL, Norgaard JP, Leung AK. Hyponatremia in patients with nocturnal enuresis treated with DDAVP. Eur J Pediatr 1996;155(11):959–62.
43. Sutor AH. DDAVP is not a panacea for children with bleeding disorders. Br J Haematol 2000;108(2):217–27.
44. Hjalmas K, Hanson E, Hellstrom AL, Kruse S, Sillen U. Long-term treatment with desmopressin in children with primary monosymptomatic nocturnal enuresis: an open multicentre study. Swedish Enuresis Trial (SWEET) Group. Br J Urol 1998;82(5):704–9.
45. Brodzikowska-Pytel A, Giembicki J. Hyponatremia as a complication of nocturnal enuresis treatment with desmopressin in a child. Pediatr Pol 1999;74:79–83.
46. Francis JD, Leary T, Niblett DJ. Convulsions and respiratory arrest in association with desmopressin administration for the treatment of a bleeding tonsil in a child with borderline haemophilia. Acta Anaesthesiol Scand 1999;43(8):870–3.
47. Shepherd LL, Hutchinson RJ, Worden EK, Koopmann CF, Coran A. Hyponatremia and seizures after intravenous administration of desmopressin acetate for surgical hemostasis. J Pediatr 1989;114(3):470–2.
48. Smith TJ, Gill JC, Ambruso DR, Hathaway WE. Hyponatremia and seizures in young children given DDAVP. Am J Hematol 1989;31(3):199–202.
49. Apakama DC, Bleetman A. Hyponatraemic convulsion secondary to desmopressin treatment for primary enuresis. J Accid Emerg Med 1999;16(3):229–30.
50. Schwab M, Ruder H. Hyponatraemia and cerebral convulsion due to DDAVP administration in patients with enuresis nocturna or urine concentration testing. Eur J Pediatr 1997;156(8):668.
51. Cone A, Riley R. DDAVP and pulmonary oedema. Anaesth Intensive Care 1994;22(4):502–3.
52. Lebl J, Kolska M, Zavacka A, Eliasek J, Gut J, Biolek J. Cerebral oedema in enuretic children during low-dose desmopressin treatment: a preventable complication. Eur J Pediatr 2001;160(3):159–62.
53. Sun HL, Chien CC. Thrombocytopenia and subdural hemorrhage after desmopressin administration. Anesthesiology 1998;88(4):1115–17.
54. Gomez Garcia EB, Brouwers GJ, Kappers-Klunne MC, Leebeek FW, van Vliet HH. Intermitterende trombocytopenie als uiting van de ziekte van von Willebrand. [Intermittent thrombocytopenia as a manifestation of Von Willebrand's disease.] Ned Tijdschr Geneeskd 2002;146(25):1192–5.
55. Burroughs AK, Planas R, Svoboda P. Optimizing emergency care of upper gastrointestinal bleeding in cirrhotic patients. Scand J Gastroenterol Suppl 1998;226:14–24.
56. Casonato A, Steffan A, Pontara E, Zucchetto A, Rossi C, De Marco L, Girolami A. Post-DDAVP thrombocytopenia in type 2B von Willebrand disease is not associated with platelet consumption: failure to demonstrate glycocalicin increase or platelet activation. Thromb Haemost 1999;81(2):224–8.
57. Ray JG. DDAVP use during pregnancy: an analysis of its safety for mother and child. Obstet Gynecol Surv 1998;53(7):450–5.
58. Mannucci PM. Use of desmopressin (DDAVP) during early pregnancy in factor VIII-deficient women. Blood 2005;105(8):3382.
59. Chediak JR, Alban GM, Maxey B. von Willebrand's disease and pregnancy: management during delivery and outcome of offspring. Am J Obstet Gynecol 1986;155(3):618–24.
60. Burrow GN, Wassenaar W, Robertson GL, Sehl H. DDAVP treatment of diabetes insipidus during pregnancy and the postpartum period. Acta Endocrinol (Copenh) 1981;97(1):23–5.
61. Rizzo V, Albanese A, Stanhope R. Morbidity and mortality associated with vasopressin replacement therapy in children. J Pediatr Endocrinol Metab 2001;14(7):861–7.
62. Wilke RA. Posterior pituitary sigma receptors and drug-induced syndrome of inappropriate antidiuretic hormone release. Ann Intern Med 1999;131(10):799.
63. Mewasingh L, Aylett S, Kirkham F, Stanhope R. Hyponatraemia associated with lamotrigine in cranial diabetes insipidus. Lancet 2000;356(9230):656.
64. Hamed M, Mitchell H, Clow DJ. Hyponatraemic convulsion associated with desmopressin and imipramine treatment. BMJ 1993;306(6886):1169.

Dexamfetamine

See also Amphetamines

General Information

Dexamfetamine or (+)-amfetamine is significantly more potent than (−)-amfetamine. The use of dexamfetamine as an appetite suppressant has rapidly declined, because of appreciation of its potential for abuse and addiction. These arise mainly from euphoria, which may be followed by depression as the effect of the drug wears off. Stimulant effects were reported in 23% of 347 patients using dexamfetamine as an appetite suppressant (SED-9, 10).

Dexamfetamine is extremely variable in its effects, and can even produce drowsiness in a small proportion of subjects. Postmenopausal women are more prone to drowsiness, anger, and sadness than euphoria (1). Adverse effects due to sympathetic overactivity are fairly common but not usually serious. However, in view of dexamfetamine's addiction potential, other anorectic drugs should be considered first.

When it was first introduced, one of the most frequent uses of amfetamine was as an anorexigenic agent in the treatment of obesity. A number of anorectic agents, many of them related to amfetamine, have since been manufactured. Most are stimulants of the central nervous system. In descending order of approximate stimulatory potency, they are dexamfetamine, phentermine, chlorphentermine, mazindol, diethylpropion, and fenfluramine. The last of these has a stimulatory effect only in overdosage. One of the problems that has concerned clinicians over the use of anorectic drugs for the treatment of weight reduction is that despite 6 weeks to 3 months of weight reduction efficacy, the effect begins to wear off and on withdrawal weight gain rebounds.

The anorectic agents produce adverse effects mainly of the central nervous system sympathomimetic type. Therapy should therefore only be allowed under strict medical supervision, to ensure the earliest possible detection of any signs of drug abuse. Long-term drug treatment of obesity should be avoided altogether.

Organs and Systems

Metabolism

Hyperinsulinemia secondary to chronic administration of dexamfetamine, with a fall in fasting blood sugar after a few weeks of use, has been described (SED-9, 10).

Drug Administration

Drug formulations

Introduction of modified-release formulations has provided some improvement in the use of anorectic drugs. Steady release of the drug permits a constant concentration in the blood throughout the entire day. Thus, a sudden excess of physiological hunger is prevented, and adverse effects involving the central nervous system are diminished.

Reference

1. Halbreich U, Asnis G, Ross D, Endicott J. Amphetamine-induced dysphoria in postmenopausal women. Br J Psychiatry 1981;138:470–3.

Dexbrompheniramine

See also Antihistamines

General Information

Dexbrompheniramine is the dextrorotatory isomer of the first-generation antihistamine brompheniramine.

Drug Administration

Drug overdose

Marked dyskinesia in an 18-month-old girl followed an overdose of a combination of dexbrompheniramine and pseudoephedrine (1).

Reference

1. Barone DA, Raniolo J. Facial dyskinesia from overdose of an antihistamine. N Engl J Med 1980;303(2):107.

Dexchlorpheniramine

See also Antihistamines

General Information

Dexchlorpheniramine maleate (SED-13, 417) is the dextrorotatory isomer of chlorphenamine.

Organs and Systems

Sensory systems

In healthy volunteers dexchlorpheniramine caused impaired selective auditory attention in the absence of subjective awareness of this impairment (1).

Hematologic

Dexchlorpheniramine caused hemolytic anemia in a 47-year-old woman who took 4 mg/day for 3 days. The direct antiglobulin test was positive, and circulating antibodies were detected in the serum, which reacted in vitro with other antihistamines as well (2).

References

1. Serra-Grabulosa JM, Grau C, Escera C, Sanchez-Turet M. The H_1-receptor antagonist dextro-chlorpheniramine impairs selective auditory attention in the absence of subjective awareness of this impairment. J Clin Psychopharmacol 2001;21(6):599–602.
2. Duran-Suarez JR, Martin-Vega C, Argelagues E, Massuet L, Ribera A, Vilaseca J, Arnau JM, Triginer J. The I antigen as an immune complex receptor in a case of haemolytic anaemia induced by an antihistaminic agent. Br J Haematol 1981;49(1):153–4.

Dexibuprofen

See also Non-steroidal anti-inflammatory drugs

General Information

Dexibuprofen is the dextrorotatory isomer of ibuprofen.

Organs and Systems

Nervous system

Meningoencephalitis has been attributed to dexibuprofen in a 22-year-old woman with systemic lupus erythematosus (1). Patients with systemic lupus erythematosus have increased susceptibility to NSAID-induced aseptic meningitis or encephalitis.

Reference

1. Obermoser G, Bellmann R, Pfausler B, Schmutzhard E, Sepp N. Aseptic meningo-encephalitis related to dexibuprofen use in a patient with systemic lupus erythematosus: a case report with MR findings. Lupus 2002;11(7):451–3.

Dexindoprofen

See also Non-steroidal anti-inflammatory drugs

General Information

The NSAID dexindoprofen has a similar adverse effect pattern to the parent drug, indoprofen. Gastrointestinal, nervous system, and skin reactions are the most frequent (1).

Reference

1. Fornasari PA, Mattara L. Efficacia e tollerabilità del dexindoprofen in confronto con il diclofenac sodico nel trattamento di patienti osteoartrosici. [Efficacy and tolerance of dexindoprofen compared with diclofenac sodium in the treatment of osteoarthrosis patients.] Clin Ter 1985;113(2):125–33.

Dextrans

General Information

Dextrans are mixtures of polymerized glucose molecules, mostly alpha-1,6-glucans, of variable molecular weight from 1 to 110 kDa. Infused dextran is mainly eliminated unmodified by the kidney at a rate of 50% in the first 24 hours and 20% in the following 48 hours. The remaining 30%, which is made up of the molecules with the highest molecular weights, is partly eliminated by the gastrointestinal tract, where it is thought to be hydrolysed by coliform bacteria, and partly metabolized by splenic and hepatic dextranase (dextrano-alpha-1,6-glucosidase).

Uses

Dextran 70, so-called because its molecules have an average weight of 70 kDa, is used as a plasma substitute, as is dextran 40. Dextran 40 has been used to improve blood flow in ischemic limbs. Dextran 40 and dextran 70 have been used to prevent deep venous thrombosis. Dextran 1 is used as a desensitizer to prevent allergic reactions to dextrans of larger molecular weight. After reproductive surgery 32% dextran 70 is sometimes administered intraperitoneally in an attempt to reduce the formation of adhesions.

Dextran deposition in tissues

In biopsy and autopsy studies 32 patients treated with regular hemodialysis for an average of 61 months, who had also received dextran 40 as a plasma expander because of hypotension during hemodialysis, were compared with a control group of 11 hemodialysed patients who were given other plasma expanders. In 11 of the former who had received the largest dose of dextran 40 (0.38 g/kg/week), particles were found in the cytoplasm of macrophages in various organs, which were PAS-positive and diastase-resistant on light microscopy and birefringent on polarization. Electron microscopy showed a fibrillar structure, but ionic analysis by electronic sampler on scanning electron microscopy excluded silicone. No intracellular inclusions were observed in the control group, or in the patients given dextran 40 in doses lower than 0.08 g/kg/week. There was a linear relation between the number of particles and dose of dextran 40 that had been given, leading the authors to suggest that the material demonstrated in the macrophages was dextran that had been structurally modified and conglomerated by macrophage activity to a water-insoluble form (1).

Organs and Systems

Cardiovascular

High output left ventricular failure has been described after hysteroscopic lysis of adhesions using dextran as a distension medium. Prolonged surgical dissection of the uterine wall (the precise duration of the operation was not stated in the report) and the large volume of dextran and fluid (2 liters of 5% dextrose and an additional 800 ml of dextran) probably caused the dextran to enter into the systemic circulation, inducing a significant shift of fluid into the intravascular compartment (2).

Respiratory

Pulmonary edema and coagulopathy following intrauterine instillation of 700 ml of 32% dextran 70 has been reported (3). The volume exceeded that recommended by the manufacturer (500 ml), and the installation time (2 hours) was in excess of that recommended (45 minutes). The authors pointed out that hyperosmolarity of the agent is such that if it enters the intravascular compartment, volume overload can result, since 100 ml of intravascular dextran 70 will osmotically expand the intravascular volume by 860 ml, by drawing interstitial fluid into the central compartment. This can further aggravate the risks of pulmonary edema and dilutional coagulopathy.

Dextrans can also cause non-cardiogenic pulmonary edema and/or respiratory distress syndrome.

- Adult respiratory distress syndrome occurred after the intravenous infusion of dextran 40 in a 30-year-old woman, a smoker with a history of insulin-dependent diabetes mellitus, who had sustained an acute inferior myocardial infarction; the dextran was given in preparation for possible stent placement after angioplasty of the right coronary artery (4).

- A 43-year-old woman underwent delayed breast reconstruction 9 months after modified radical mastectomy and received 4 liters of crystalloid intraoperatively (5). Postoperatively she was given an infusion of dextran 40 preceded by a small dose of dextran 1. On the next 2 days she was febrile, with no respiratory symptoms, although her oxygen saturation was 83%. On the third day, she was febrile and dyspneic, with a respiratory rate of 29 breaths per minute. Her oxygen saturation fell to 70%. A chest X-ray showed diffuse alveolar infiltration. Dextran was withdrawn. Her lungs worsened, and on day 6 she required intubation for worsening hypoxia, dyspnea, and tachypnea. A chest X-ray showed bilateral alveolar consolidation and other signs consistent with respiratory distress syndrome. Her oxygenation slowly improved and extubation was possible on day 11.
- Acute pulmonary edema developed in a healthy patient after elective microsurgery for treatment of a malignant tumor of the forearm (6). The patient was in good physical condition before the operation, and there was no sign of volume overload perioperatively. Cardiac enzymes, electrocardiogram, and echocardiogram were normal. No other medications were likely to have caused the pulmonary edema. The gradual response to diuretics suggested a non-cardiogenic cause.

Although thromboprophylaxis of microvascular anastomoses seems advisable theoretically, there is little clinical evidence to support the use of dextran for this purpose. The pulmonary edema in these cases was thought to be non-cardiogenic, similar to that caused by heroin, methadone, propoxyphene, and salicylates, due to a direct adverse effect on the pulmonary vasculature, rather than anaphylaxis, cardiac pump failure, or volume overload.

Severe pulmonary edema developed in a patient who underwent breast reconstruction in whom dextran was used to improve the deterioration of flap perfusion during the postoperative period (7).

- A 48-year-old white woman underwent right modified radical mastectomy for infiltrative ductal carcinoma. She was given dextran 40, 10 ml/kg, on the second postoperative day because of partial ischemic changes in the flap. She then had nausea, vomiting, and fever, and 10 hours later developed dyspnea and chest pain, which worsened on the following day. Chest radiography showed bilateral pleural effusions and bilateral reticulonodular opacities that were interpreted as pneumonic infiltration. She did not have hemoptysis or pleuritic chest pain, and there were no signs of heart failure. She had a leukocytosis (16.4×10^9/l). Cultures of sputum and fluid aspirate were negative. On postoperative day 4, her dyspnea worsened, her PO_2 fell, and her pH rose to 7.53. Lymphangitic carcinomatosis was considered, but this was not supported by cytology of the effusion fluid or tumor markers. Her history of allergic reactions suggested the possibility of dextran-induced severe pulmonary edema leading to respiratory distress syndrome. Dextran was withdrawn and she was given an intravenous bolus dose of prednisolone 250 mg. Her symptoms rapidly improved and she recovered gradually over the following week.

Although severe pulmonary edema with respiratory failure is not a typical allergic reaction to dextrans, this case illustrates that it cannot be discounted.

Acid–base balance

Arterial blood gases and acid–base balance were evaluated in 50 patients with dextran-induced anaphylactic reactions. Metabolic acidosis was consistently present in severe cases, leading to cardiac arrest. Acidosis was also found in patients with less severe reactions and only slight impairment of the circulation. Bronchospastic respiratory signs were common, but acidosis also developed in the absence of these symptoms and in patients with mild or no circulatory problems. The severity of the acidosis was often underestimated during treatment. Arterial PO_2 and PCO_2 were not significantly affected during these reactions. It was suggested from this study that the circulation is unlikely to be normalized until the metabolic acidosis is corrected, despite other therapeutic efforts that may be made (8).

Liver

In a retrospective study of the adverse effects of various drugs in 197 patients who underwent infertility surgery under general anesthesia and simultaneous intraperitoneal administration of 32% dextran 70, there were increases in postoperative transaminases in 86. The use of 32% dextran 70 in combination with glucocorticoids or halothane (or other halogenized drugs) resulted in an increased risk of temporarily disturbed liver function. Of 31 patients followed after discharge from hospital, the transaminases returned to normal within 6 months in 29. The authors suggested that hepatocytes may be damaged by enhanced glycogen deposition and/or lipid accumulation in patients who receive dextran. Glucocorticoids potentially increase the risk of liver function disturbance (9).

Urinary tract

Of 207 patients with ischemic stroke, stages III or IV, treated with an intravenous infusion of dextran 40 over 4 days, 9 (4.3%) developed acute renal insufficiency attributable to the dextran. Oliguria occurred after a mean time of 4 (range 3–6) days. The incidence of dextran-induced renal insufficiency was higher in patients with pre-existing impaired kidney function. The high risk of death in the patients who developed renal insufficiency was due to non-renal complications, notably pneumonia and pulmonary embolism (10).

Of 211 patients with acute ischemic stroke, stages III or IV, treated with daily intravenous dextran 40, 500–1000 ml for 4 days, 10 (4.7%) developed acute renal insufficiency associated with dextran infusion (11). Oliguria developed after a mean time of 4 (range 3–6) days. The incidence of dextran-induced acute renal insufficiency was significantly higher in patients with pre-existing reduction of glomerular filtration rate below 30 ml/minute/1.73 m^2. Five of the patients with acute renal insufficiency died within 4–12 days after hemodilution therapy with dextran 40; this high mortality was attributable to non-renal complications.

In a report of two cases of anuric acute renal insufficiency induced by dextran 40, diuresis and renal function were quickly restored to normal after plasmapheresis (12). Renal biopsy showed normal kidneys, except for swelling and vacuolation of renal tubules suggestive of osmotic nephrosis.

Cases of acute renal insufficiency, apparently representing a hypersensitivity reaction, have been reported from Australia (SED-11, 726) (13), and elsewhere (14,15). On the basis of these observations it has been suggested that the pathogenesis of renal dysfunction during treatment with dextran 40 involves mainly intraluminal hyperviscosity, reduced tubular flow, and pinocytic uptake of colloid into tubular cells (16). Direct injury to the renal tubular epithelium cannot be ruled out (17).

- During surgery for an avulsed pinna, an 18-year-old Chinese man was given 500 ml of 10% dextran 40 infused over 2 hours at 12-hourly intervals (18). On day 3 he developed nausea and abdominal pain. The dextran infusion was stopped. His serum creatinine was 1092 μmol/l. Total anuria followed within 24 hours and he developed acute pulmonary edema. Renal biopsy was compatible with osmotic nephrosis caused by dextran.

Dextran is widely used in plastic surgery, but acute renal insufficiency is rare; according to one source only 60 cases have been reported (19). These patients were usually either critically ill or had pre-existing renal impairment. The authors presumed that acute renal insufficiency had occurred as a result of increased plasma oncotic pressure, reducing the filtration pressure in the glomerulus; alternatively, some dextran 40 polymers may have been filtered into the tubules, causing obstruction. The amount of dextran required before acute renal insufficiency develops varies from 50 to 1000 g. One patient received 300 g over 3 days, although renal function deterioration was not recognized until uremia developed. The authors suggested that care be taken when using dextran 40, especially in patients with pre-existing renal impairment or vascular disease. Regular monitoring of urine output, electrolytes, and renal function in all dextran recipients is recommended. Administering replacement fluids before checking renal function could lead to life-threatening fluid overload. Withdrawal of dextran should be considered if there is persistent oliguria or a rise in creatinine or urea concentrations. Treatment of dextran-induced acute renal insufficiency should comprise temporary hemodialysis alternating with plasmapheresis, to remove dextran molecules from the blood.

- A 45-year-old man with insulin-dependent diabetes associated with nephropathy, neuropathy, and retinopathy was given dextran 40 (25 ml/hour) after orthopedic surgery (20). His urine output fell from 2 to 3 liters on postoperative day, 1–40 ml/day on day 2, and his creatinine clearance fell from 54 to 32 ml/minute. There were many casts in the urine. Dextran was withdrawn, but his creatinine clearance fell to 12 ml/minute on day 5. On day 6 a large hematoma in the rectus sheath was drained, followed by plasmapheresis (to remove dextran) and hemodialysis. Over the next 24 hours, his urine output increased to 2.2 l/day and his creatinine clearance increased to 20 ml/minute. Plasmapheresis was repeated. Nine days later, his renal function had improved.

This is another case of dextran-induced renal insufficiency in a patient with pre-existing renal insufficiency, in this case caused by insulin-dependent diabetes mellitus of more than 30 years duration. The authors recommended that dextran should not be used in patients with chronic renal insufficiency and a creatinine clearance below 40 ml/minute. If dextran-induced renal insufficiency develops, dextran should be withdrawn and if renal function does not recover, plasmapheresis should be used to remove the dextran load.

Acute renal insufficiency due to dextran has rarely been reported after microsurgery (21).

- An 81-year-old woman underwent commando resection and supraomohyoidal lymphadenectomy for recurrent squamous cell carcinoma of the right inferior alveolar process. Preoperatively, she was given intravenous gentamicin 120 mg and clindamycin to be continued twice-daily postoperatively. During surgery and the first 5 postoperative days, she was given dextran 40, 1 l/day, as an antithrombotic and rheological agent. On the second postoperative day she became increasingly dyspneic. Despite furosemide her urine production fell and she became anuric on day 4. Gentamicin was stopped on day 3. On day 5, she was reintubated and artificially ventilated; thrice-weekly plasmapheresis was started. Three days later spontaneous diuresis recurred and she was extubated on postoperative day 10. On day 25, she refused further plasmapheresis and diuresis returned to normal.
- A 69-year-old man underwent radical resection, supraomohyoidal lymphadenectomy, and radial forearm flap reconstruction for squamous cell carcinoma of the oropharynx. Preoperatively, he was given intravenous gentamicin 320 mg/day and clindamycin 600 mg bd, to be continued for 5 days. He was given dextran 50, 500 ml/day. Despite extra intravenous hydration combined with dopamine and furosemide, his urine output fell to 40 ml/hour on the first postoperative day and he became anuric on day 2. Gentamicin and dextran were withdrawn, he was artificially ventilated, and thrice-weekly plasmapheresis was started. Renal biopsy showed hydropic swelling and vacuolation of the tubular epithelium and narrowing of the tubular lumen. After 6 days, he was extubated and his renal function recovered only marginally. One month after surgery, he died of respiratory failure.

The authors suggested that acute renal insufficiency had been caused by dextran rather than gentamicin, because both patients developed anuria, which is commonly present in dextran-induced acute renal insufficiency, rather than the initial non-oliguric course characteristic of aminoglycosides. Further evidence for this conclusion was the renal biopsy in the second patient, while negative immunofluorescence and the rapid return of kidney function in the first patient suggested a non-structural effect of dextran on the kidney. The authors have stopped using dextran as an antithrombotic agent in microsurgery.

Immunologic

Anaphylactic reactions to dextrans have been reported, for example within 10 minutes after exposure to dextran in hysteroscopy (22). It can be fatal (23).

- A 54-year-old man developed generalized pruritus, dyspnea, and sudden hemodynamic shock, with cardiac and respiratory arrest 8 hours after the resection of a hepatic hydatid cyst, while being given dextran 40. He had no prior history of atopy or adverse drug reactions. Despite intensive resuscitation he remained unconscious and hemodynamically unstable. During the succeeding days he became septic with progressive renal function impairment and died on day 5. A range of serum tests for antibodies detected dextran-reactive antibodies. In addition, there was evidence of complement protein consumption within 6–24 hours of the clinical reaction.

The authors suggested that dextran-reactive antibodies had formed immune complexes with dextran, leading to complement activation and release of mediators of anaphylaxis. There was also evidence of mast cell degranulation. They therefore recommended that titration of dextran-reactive antibodies before administration of dextrans could provide a method of identifying those who are at risk of dextran-induced anaphylactic reactions.

- A 24-year-old healthy volunteer was given 10 ml of 6% dextran 60 during a preliminary examination (24). After about 5 minutes the first clinical symptoms of anaphylactic shock were evident, with a reduction in systolic blood pressure to 90 mmHg and an increased heart rate to over 90/minute. These returned to normal after therapy in the head-down position with clemastine 2 ml (2 mg), hydrocortisone 200 mg, and etherified starch 500 ml over about 8 minutes. During this period, responsiveness was unsatisfactory although he complained of warming of the skin, paresthesia, and nausea.

The authors suggested that this reaction had been due to a dextran-induced anaphylactic reaction, but were uncertain as to the cause of these observations, as they were not accompanied by immediate symptoms of shock. It is unclear if this case was caused by an antibody reaction.

Frequency and susceptibility factors

A large-scale prospective study was carried out in 49 public and private hospitals throughout France between June 1991 and October 1992, aimed at discovering the frequency and severity of anaphylactoid reactions to colloid plasma substitutes, looking for possible risk factors, and determining the mechanisms involved (25). In all, 19 593 patients were evaluated; 48% were given gelatins, 27% starches, 16% albumin, and 9% dextrans. There were 43 anaphylactoid reactions, an overall frequency of 0.22%, or one reaction per 456 patients. The frequency differed according to the plasma substitute used: 0.35% for gelatins, 0.27% for dextrans, 0.10% for albumin, and 0.06% for starches. The reactions were serious (grades III and IV) in 20% of cases.

Multivariate analysis showed four independent susceptibility factors: the administration of gelatins (OR = 4.81), the administration of dextrans (OR = 3.83), a history of drug allergy (OR = 3.16), and being male (OR = 1.98). The relative risks of anaphylactoid reactions due to one type of plasma substitute with respect to another were estimated to be six times less with starches than with gelatins and 4.7 times less than with dextrans. The relative risk of albumin was 3.4 times less than that of gelatins, and almost identical to that of the starches. An immunological assessment was carried out in 15 patients who had been given a gelatin (Plasmion); in seven cases an IgE-dependent reaction was proved. It was concluded that gelatins and dextrans should be avoided in patients with a known history of drug allergy; when a reaction does occur, an immunological assessment should be carried out, as the reaction may be due to specific antibodies, in which case that particular plasma substitute would be contraindicated for the rest of the patient's life.

Prevention

Severe anaphylactic reactions only occur in patients with preformed dextran-reactive antibodies. Infusion of dextran causes the formation of large immune complexes that trigger activation of a cascade of enzyme systems, leukocytes, and platelets. It is possible to prevent or minimize these effects by blocking the reactive sites on the antibodies with small dextran fragments; this is hapten inhibition. The method used is to inject very low-molecular weight dextran (dextran 1, molecular weight 1 kDa) intravenously before an infusion of dextran is started; this blocks access to the antigen-combining sites by preformed circulating dextran-reactive antibodies.

In Sweden, there was a reduction in the reports of severe reactions to dextran from 22 per 100 000 units of dextran administered between 1975 and 1979 to 1.2 per 100 000 units between 1983 and 1985 (26). The number of reported fatal reactions fell over the same period from 23 to 1. More than 600 000 units of dextran were used during each period. This represented a nearly 20-fold reduction in the reported incidence of severe dextran-induced adverse reactions in the country in the 3 years following the introduction of dextran 1 for the purpose of desensitization. During the same periods the incidence of grade I reactions (which are not considered to be antibody-mediated) did not change, suggesting that the reduced incidence of severe reactions after introduction of dextran-1 was not explained by a general reduction in the reporting of adverse reactions. It was emphasized that pre-injection of dextran 1 does not eliminate completely the risk of severe reactions to dextran.

The incidence of anaphylactoid reactions to dextran was studied in 5745 patients over 63 months from January 1981 to March 1986 (27). A total of 12 646 half-liter units of dextran 70 had been administered to these patients. The average number of dextran units transfused was 2.2 per patient. There were 15 reactions, a rate of one reaction per 383 patients treated (0.26%). Seven of these reactions were potentially life-threatening (grade III or IV), giving a combined incidence of severe reactions of one in 821 patients treated (0.12%). The remaining eight reactions were less severe (grade I or II), and the combined incidence of the milder reactions was 1:718 patients treated (0.14%).

Pre- and post-reaction titers of dextran-reactive antibodies have been analysed in most Scandinavian studies (28). The incidence of severe dextran-induced anaphylactic reactions to clinical dextran after the prophylactic use of hapten inhibition was approximately 1/200 000 patients receiving dextran 1. In Sweden, where reporting of severe adverse drug reactions is mandatory, the incidence was about one in 70 000, indicating a 35-fold reduction. Only two fatal reactions were reported, an incidence of one per 2.5 million doses, indicating a 90-fold reduction. Both occurred in patients with extremely high titers of dextran-reactive antibodies. Adverse reactions to dextran 1, mostly mild, were reported in about one per 100 000 doses. These adverse effects were not antibody-mediated. The author concluded that dextran with hapten inhibition has arguably become the safest plasma substitute in current clinical practice. These conclusions were reached on the basis of a postmarketing surveillance study, and were confirmed in another publication from the same center (29).

It is possible for a severe dextran-induced anaphylactic/anaphylactoid reaction to develop despite prophylaxis with monovalent hapten dextran (30). This has been reported in a 60-year-old patient with multiple trauma, who received a dextran infusion for prophylaxis of thrombosis due to severe thrombocytosis in the late postoperative period. The causal relation to dextran was considered likely, although no serum sample was taken before the reaction, due to the close time relation to the infusion of dextran 60. In addition, there were high titers of dextran-reactive antibodies in the blood drawn immediately after the reaction occurred.

Second-Generation Effects

Pregnancy

Three cases of severe allergic reactions to dextran 70 (including one pregnant woman at the time of delivery) have been reported (31). All three had received previous hapten prophylaxis. Although the pregnant woman recovered, the baby had evidence of serious brain damage at birth. Another patient with a very high titer of dextran-reactive antibodies died from myocardial infarction, which happened at the same time. The third patient recovered without sequelae. The authors concluded that dextran 70 should be avoided in pregnancy until the baby is born, and that even in the presence of immune prophylaxis, these complications of dextran 70 can develop. Vigilant observation and resuscitation facilities are necessary in all cases.

An anaphylactoid reaction in a pregnant woman occurred immediately after the administration of dextran 40 solution (32). The baby was delivered rapidly by cesarean section after the event, and was apparently dead at birth but successfully resuscitated. The case has prompted Barbier and colleagues to report on the safety in general of dextran administered during pregnancy (32). They found information on 32 moderate anaphylactoid reactions associated with severe fetal distress and they advised avoiding preventive fluid preload with dextran in pregnancy.

Drug Administration

Drug administration route

After reproductive surgery 32% dextran 70 is sometimes administered intraperitoneally as adjuvant treatment for reducing adhesion formation. Dextran is thought to keep the raw peritoneal surfaces apart and prevent adhesion formation. However, the scientific evidence in support of the use of intraperitoneal dextran as an anti-adhesion adjuvant is scant. The complications of this procedure have been described in five patients (33). In one, a right pleural effusion was detected on the third postoperative day and resolved within 4 days. In the other four cases bilateral vulvar edema developed on the first or second postoperative day, and resolved in each case at 5–9 days after surgery. One patient had combined vulvar and leg edema, not previously reported. It is thought that this edema is due to extravasation of dextran along fascial planes, increasing the colloid-oncotic pressure in these spaces and promoting movement of a large amount of fluid from the vascular into the extravascular space. The right pleural effusion was thought to be due to movement of dextran through the diaphragmatic lymphatics or through small openings in the diaphragm, the majority of which are in the right hemidiaphragm.

In 139 consecutive patients who underwent major gynecological surgery and in whom 32% dextran 70 had been used as an anti-adhesion adjuvant (the mean amount of dextran used was 183 ml), there was an acceptably low rate of complications (34). Adverse effects involved 11 patients and included postoperative ileus (2.9%), pleural effusion (2.2%), allergic reactions (1.4%), wound infection (1.4%), and labial swelling (0.7%). There was no evidence of an increased infection rate.

The complications of repeated postoperative intraperitoneal instillation of 6% dextran 60 (given for 5 days to 32 patients) have been monitored and compared with the outcome in 15 control patients. In the dextran-treated subjects abdominal pain and dyspnea occurred significantly and more frequently than in the controls. During intraperitoneal irrigation with dextran there was a significant increase in body weight and an increased central venous pressure. Bradycardia developed between the third and sixth postoperative days. Blood pressure remained unchanged. Of the patients given dextran, 75% developed pleural effusions containing dextran by the fifth postoperative day. It was concluded that the uncertain advantages of dextran in the prevention of adhesions do not offset undesired adverse effects (35).

The syndrome of acute hypotension, adult respiratory distress syndrome, non-cardiogenic pulmonary edema, anemia, coagulopathy, and anaphylactic reactions after the administration of dextran 70 is referred to as the "dextran syndrome" (36–39). Factors other than acute volume overload due to intravascular absorption of dextran are thought to account for the syndrome. A combination of diverse pathophysiological factors may be responsible, namely direct pulmonary toxicity, activation of the coagulation cascade, release of vasoactive mediators, hypotension, pulmonary edema, intravascular intravasation of fluids, dilution of blood, and impaired renal and hepatic clearance. Cases of pulmonary edema are described under the section Respiratory.

Pulmonary hemorrhage after dextran use has also been described in hysteroscopy (40).

Drug–Drug Interactions

Radiocontrast media

- Acute anuric renal insufficiency has been described after administration of dextran 40 and radiocontrast to a 59-year-old woman (41).

Radiocontrast-induced renal ischemia may have contributed to the pathogenesis of the dextran-induced renal insufficiency, as has been shown in animal studies. The mechanism of dextran-induced acute renal insufficiency may be multifactorial, with elements of hyperoncotic acute renal insufficiency, tubular obstruction, and direct tubular toxicity. Radiocontrast-induced acute renal insufficiency is unusual in patients with normal baseline creatinine concentrations. The ischemic effect of radiocontrast seemed to be important in this case. Renal function should be carefully monitored if the simultaneous administration of dextran and radiocontrast is necessary. If renal function deteriorates and oliguria or anuria occurs, plasmapheresis may be an appropriate and effective approach for clearing dextran.

Three cases of acute renal insufficiency occurred after low molecular weight dextran infusion; two of the patients had only received standard therapeutic doses (total 450 and 650 g) (42). In both of these cases a contrast medium was co-administered, and the authors suggested that this could have predisposed to acute renal insufficiency.

References

1. Bergonzi G, Paties C, Vassallo G, Zangrandi A, Poisetti PG, Ballocchi S, Fontana F, Scarpioni L. Dextran deposits in tissues of patients undergoing haemodialysis. Nephrol Dial Transplant 1990;5(1):54–8.
2. Golan A, Siedner M, Bahar M, Ron-El R, Herman A, Caspi E. High-output left ventricular failure after dextran use in an operative hysteroscopy. Fertil Steril 1990;54(5):939–41.
3. Choban MJ, Kalhan SB, Anderson RJ, Collins R. Pulmonary edema and coagulopathy following intrauterine instillation of 32% dextran-70 (Hyskon). J Clin Anesth 1991;3(4):317–19.
4. Taylor MA, DiBlasi SL, Bender RM, Santoian EC, Cha SD, Dennis CA. Adult respiratory distress syndrome complicating intravenous infusion of low-molecular weight dextran. Cathet Cardiovasc Diagn 1994;32(3):249–53.
5. Hein KD, Wechsler ME, Schwartzstein RM, Morris DJ. The adult respiratory distress syndrome after dextran infusion as an antithrombotic agent in free TRAM flap breast reconstruction. Plast Reconstr Surg 1999;103(6):1706–8.
6. Kitziger KJ, Sanders WE, Andrews CP. Acute pulmonary edema associated with use of low-molecular weight dextran for prevention of microvascular thrombosis. J Hand Surg [Am] 1990;15(6):902–5.
7. Demirkan F, Unal S, Arslan E, Calikoglu M, Kandemir O. Severe pulmonary edema related to dextran 40. Ann Plast Surg 2002;49(2):221–2.
8. Ljungstrom KG, Renck H. Metabolic acidosis in dextran-induced anaphylactic reactions. Acta Anaesthesiol Scand 1987;31(2):157–60.
9. Weinans MJ, Kauer FM, Klompmaker IJ, Wijma J. Transient liver function disturbances after the intraperitoneal use of 32% dextran 70 as adhesion prophylaxis in infertility surgery. Fertil Steril 1990;53(1):159–61.
10. Biesenbach G, Kaiser W, Zazgornik J. Häufigkeit des akuten Nierenversagens nach Infusion von niedermolekulärem Dexran bei Patienten mit ischämischen Insult. Intensivmedizin 1990;27:133–7.
11. Biesenbach G, Kaiser W, Zazgornik J. Incidence of acute oligoanuric renal failure in dextran 40 treated patients with acute ischemic stroke stage III or IV. Ren Fail 1997;19(1):69–75.
12. Ferraboli R, Malheiro PS, Abdulkader RC, Yu L, Sabbaga E, Burdmann EA. Anuric acute renal failure caused by dextran 40 administration. Ren Fail 1997;19(2):303–6.
13. Schwarz J, Ihle B, Dowling J. Acute renal failure induced by low molecular weight dextran. Aust NZ J Med 1984;14(5):688–9.
14. Moran M, Kapsner C. Acute renal failure associated with elevated plasma oncotic pressure. N Engl J Med 1987;317(3):150–3.
15. Stein HD. Dextran-40, acute renal failure, and elevated plasma oncotic pressure. N Engl J Med 1988;318(4):253.
16. Druml W, Pölzleitner D, Laggner AN, Leuz X, Ulrich W Dextran-40, acute renal failure, and elevated plasma oncotic pressure. N Engl J Med 1988;318(4):252.
17. Moran M, Kapsner C. Dextran-40, acute renal failure, and elevated plasma oncotic pressure. N Engl J Med 1988;318(4):253–4.
18. Tsang RK, Mok JS, Poon YS, van Hasselt A. Acute renal failure in a healthy young adult after dextran 40 infusion for external-ear reattachment surgery. Br J Plast Surg 2000;53(8):701–3.
19. Türköz A, Gülcan Ö, But AK, Hazar A, Ersoy Ö. Dekstran 40 sonrasi kalp durmasi (oglu sunumu). Turk Anesteziyol Reanim Cem Mecmuasi 2000;28:105–6.
20. Brooks D, Okeefe P, Buncke HJ. Dextran-induced acute renal failure after microvascular muscle transplantation. Plast Reconstr Surg 2001;108(7):2057–60.
21. Vos SC, Hage JJ, Woerdeman LA, Noordanus RP. Acute renal failure during dextran-40 antithrombotic prophylaxis: report of two microsurgical cases. Ann Plast Surg 2002;48(2):193–6.
22. Ahmed N, Falcone T, Tulandi T, Houle G. Anaphylactic reaction because of intrauterine 32% dextran-70 instillation. Fertil Steril 1991;55(5):1014–16.
23. Hernandez D, de Rojas F, Martinez Escribano C, Arriaga F, Cuellar J, Molins J, Barber L. Fatal dextran-induced allergic anaphylaxis. Allergy 2002;57(9):862.
24. Lehmann G, Asskali F, Forster H. Schwerer Zwischen fall nach I.V. – Applikation von 10 ml (0.6 g) 6% igem Dextran60 bei einem gesunden probanden. [Severe adverse event following iv administration of 10 ml 6% Dextran 60 (0.6 g) in a healthy volunteer.] Anaesthesist 2002;51(10):820–4.
25. Laxenaire MC, Charpentier C, Feldman L. Réactions anaphylactoïdes aux substituts colloidaux du plasma: incidence, facteurs de risque, mécanismes. Enquete prospective multicentrique française. Groupe Français d'Etude de la Tolerance des Substituts Plasmatiques. [Anaphylactoid reactions to colloid plasma substitutes: incidence, risk factors, mechanisms. A French multicenter prospective study.] Ann Fr Anesth Reanim 1994; 13(3):301–10.
26. Ljungstrom KG. The antithrombotic efficacy of dextran. Acta Chir Scand Suppl 1988;543:26–30.
27. Paull J. A prospective study of dextran-induced anaphylactoid reactions in 5745 patients. Anaesth Intensive Care 1987;15(2):163–7.
28. Ljungstrom KG. Safety of dextran in relation to other colloids—ten years experience with hapten inhibition. Infusionsther Transfusionsmed 1993;20(5):206–10.
29. Ljungstrom KG, Willman B, Hedin H. Hapten inhibition of dextran anaphylaxis. Nine years of post-marketing surveillance of dextran 1. Ann Fr Anesth Reanim 1993;12(2):219–22.

30. Allhoff T, Lenhart FP. Schwere dextraninduzierte anaphylactische/anaphylactoide Reaktion (DIAR) trotz Haptenprophylaxe. [Severe dextran-induced anaphylactic/anaphylactoid reaction despite preventive hapten administration.] Infusionsther Transfusionsmed 1993; 20(6):301–6.
31. Berg EM, Fasting S, Sellevold OF. Serious complications with dextran-70 despite hapten prophylaxis. Is it best avoided prior to delivery? Anaesthesia 1991;46(12):1033–5.
32. Barbier P, Jonville AP, Autret E, Coureau C. Fetal risks with dextrans during delivery. Drug Saf 1992;7(1):71–3.
33. Tulandi T. Transient edema after intraperitoneal instillation of 32% dextran 70. A report of five cases. J Reprod Med 1987;32(6):472–4.
34. Ricaurte E, Hilgers TW. Safety of intraperitoneal 32% dextran 70 as an antiadhesion adjuvant. J Reprod Med 1989;34(8):535–9.
35. Gauwerky JF, Heinrich D, Kubli F. Complications of intraperitoneal dextran application for prevention of adhesions. Biol Res Pregnancy Perinatol 1986;7(3):93–7.
36. Ellingson TL, Aboulafia DM. Dextran syndrome. Acute hypotension, noncardiogenic pulmonary edema, anemia, and coagulopathy following hysteroscopic surgery using 32% dextran 70. Chest 1997;111(2):513–18.
37. Mangar D, Gerson JI, Constantine RM, Lenzi V. Pulmonary edema and coagulopathy due to Hyskon (32% dextran-70) administration. Anesth Analg 1989;68(5):686–7.
38. Jedeikin R, Olsfanger D, Kessler I. Disseminated intravascular coagulopathy and adult respiratory distress syndrome: life-threatening complications of hysteroscopy. Am J Obstet Gynecol 1990;162(1):44–5.
39. Schinco MA, Hughes D, Santora TA. Complications of 32% dextran-70 in 10% dextrose. A case report. J Reprod Med 1996;41(6):455–8.
40. Romero RM, Kreitzer JM, Gabrielson GV. Hyskon induced pulmonary hemorrhage. J Clin Anesth 1995;7(4):323–5.
41. Kurnik BR, Singer F, Groh WC. Case report: dextran-induced acute anuric renal failure. Am J Med Sci 1991;302(1):28–30.
42. Kato A, Yonemura K, Matsushima H, Ikegaya N, Hishida A. Complication of oliguric acute renal failure in patients treated with low-molecular weight dextran. Ren Fail 2001;23(5):679–84.

Dextromethorphan

General Information

Dextromethorphan is the dextrorotatory isomer of the synthetic opioid levorphanol and is thought to act as a central nervous system antitussive (1). It binds to CNS sigma opioid binding sites and increases 5-HT concentrations by inhibiting uptake and by enhancing the release of 5-HT. It is also an antagonist at NMDA receptors.

Dextromethorphan is metabolized by CYP2D6 to dextrorphan, which binds to phencyclidine receptors and is thought to account for the toxic effects of hallucinations, tachycardia, hypertension, ataxia, and nystagmus (2,3).

Drug studies

Pain relief

The role of dextromethorphan in acute and chronic pain control has been reviewed (4). There is a clear beneficial role of oral dextromethorphan (in doses of 30–90 mg) in acute pain management; it has no or few adverse effects and even reduces the need for analgesic adjuncts.

Three double-blind, crossover, randomized, placebo-controlled studies of the role of dextromethorphan in neurological pain conditions in 40 adults with diabetic neuropathy, postherpetic neuralgia, and non-specific neuropathic pain syndromes have been reviewed (5). Dextromethorphan dosages varied from 13.5 mg tds on alternate days to 120 mg qds. High-dose dextromethorphan significantly reduced pain in diabetic neuropathy with no effect in postherpetic neuralgia. Sedation (58%) and dizziness (25%) were the most commonly reported adverse effects.

In a randomized, placebo-controlled study in 60 patients given dextromethorphan 10, 20, or 40 mg intramuscularly before abdominal surgery, there was a dose-dependent effective postoperative analgesic effect, with lower total consumption of rescue morphine during the 3-day observation period (6). There were no opioid-related adverse effects in those who were given dextromethorphan 40 mg.

The effect of dextromethorphan premedication on postoperative analgesic requirements, pain scores, and adverse effects has been examined in two double-blind, randomized studies (7,8). In the first study, 60 adults scheduled for elective upper abdominal surgery were randomly allocated to three equal groups (7). One group received intramuscular dextromethorphan 120 mg 30 minutes before skin incision (preincisional group); the second group received placebo (intramuscular saline) 30 minutes before skin incision and intramuscular dextromethorphan 120 mg 30 minutes before the end of surgery (postincisional group); and the third group received placebo 30 minutes before skin incision and 30 minutes before the end of surgery (control group). Preincisional intramuscular dextromethorphan 120 mg provided pre-emptive analgesia, reduced the need for postoperative analgesic supplements, and had a minimal and non-significant adverse effects profile. In the second study, oral dextromethorphan 90 mg was compared with placebo given 90 minutes preoperatively to patients undergoing laparoscopic cholecystectomy or inguinal hernioplasty under general anesthesia (8). Pain intensity and sedation were significantly reduced in the experimental group, with sparing of postoperative analgesics for up to 24 hours. Dextromethorphan 90 mg also abolished postoperative thermal-induced hyperalgesia and hyperpathia. No adverse effects were recorded in either group.

A randomized, double-blind, placebo-controlled study of oral dextromethorphan and PCA morphine has been performed in 66 patients undergoing knee surgery (9). The study was in two parts. The first was a dose escalation study in 25 postoperative patients to determine the maximum tolerated oral dose of dextromethorphan. The second involved giving less than the maximum tolerated dose divided into three increments at 8-hour intervals. The maximum tolerated dose of dextromethorphan was 750 mg. One patient, who was given 800 mg of dextromethorphan, had adverse effects, including severe slurred speech and light-headedness followed by deep sedation. In the second part of the study 66 patients were intended to receive dextromethorphan 800 mg in three doses of 400, 200, and 200 mg. The treatment group was subsequently reduced to 22 patients, compared with 34 in the placebo group, because of unexpected nausea and vomiting in five patients given dextromethorphan 400 mg. Dextromethorphan 200 mg 8-hourly caused a significant increase in nausea 2–24 hours after the first dose. One patient given dextromethorphan had mild hallucinations on one occasion only. There was an associated modest reduction in postoperative morphine consumption (29%), with no other benefits. The study failed to provide evidence that the maximum tolerated dose of dextromethorphan 200 mg 8-hourly is useful in the treatment of postoperative pain after knee surgery.

Neuropathic pain

In a double-blind, placebo-controlled, crossover pilot study in three patients with cancer-associated postamputation phantom limb pain, oral dextromethorphan 60–90 mg bd or placebo were given for 1 week each, followed by dextromethorphan or placebo again (10). Dextromethorphan satisfactorily improved phantom limb pain at a dosage of 60 mg bd in two patients and 90 mg bd in the third. Even though a relatively high total dose of dextromethorphan was used, there were no adverse effects.

There have been two randomized, placebo-controlled, double-blind trials in 19 patients with painful diabetic neuropathy and 17 with postherpetic neuralgia (11). In the first trial dextromethorphan was compared with memantine and/or lorazepam. Among the patients with diabetic neuropathy, dextromethorphan (median dose 400 mg/day) reduced pain intensity by a mean of 33% from baseline; memantine reduced pain by a mean of 17% and lorazepam by 16%, showing no significant difference to placebo. Among the patients with postherpetic neuralgia, dextromethorphan (median dose 400 mg/day) reduced pain intensity by a mean of 6.5%, which was not different from the effects of memantine and lorazepam. In the second trial the 10 patients with diabetic neuropathy who had responded to dextromethorphan shared a significant dose–response effect on pain intensity; the highest dose was significantly better than that of lorazepam. The median dose was 520 (range 240–920) mg/day. The adverse effects profiles were uneventful. These results confirm the long-term safety of high-dose dextromethorphan for selected patients with painful diabetic neuropathy (5).

Non-ketotic hyperglycinemia

A review of *N*-methyl-D-aspartic acid (NMDA) antagonist interventions in the treatment of non-ketotic hyperglycinemia included six cases in which dextromethorphan was used (3). Non-ketotic hyperglycinemia is an autosomal recessive disorder in which there is failure of the glycine cleavage enzyme system, leading to impaired oxidative decarboxylation of glycine and a toxic accumulation of this amino acid. Antagonism at NMDA receptors is hypothesized to offer partial relief to the effects of this inborn error of metabolism. Of the six cases, adverse effects were described in three. Patient 1 had profound sedation in response to a dose of 7.5 mg/kg of dextromethorphan administered as a single dose when the infant was 5 days old. The same daily dosage split into three doses relieved symptoms without sedation, but doses in excess of 7.5 mg/kg resulted in somnolence, agitation, and involuntary movements. Patient 4 developed apnea, hypotonia, nystagmus, and seizures at 38 days of age and was given dextromethorphan 1 mg/kg/day at the age of 10 months, resulting in anorexia. In patient 5 an increase in dextromethorphan dosage to 10 mg/kg/day was associated with lethargy, apnea, and a return of seizure activity. Further trials are required for clarification of the use of dextromethorphan in the treatment of non-ketotic hyperglycinemia.

Parkinson's disease

In a trial of dextromethorphan in Parkinson's disease only one-third of the initial sample entered the double-blind, placebo-controlled phase (12). One-third of the sample had a reduction in the benefits of levodopa when dextromethorphan 30 mg/day was given. A further one-third withdrew because of failure to gain clinical benefit from the highest tolerated dose of dextromethorphan. Adverse effects included drowsiness, increased dystonia, increased impotence, light-headedness, sweating, and nausea.

Huntington's disease

Of 11 patients with Huntington's disease adverse effects were reported in seven. These included eczematoid rash, clumsiness, dysarthria, drowsiness, and worsening rigidity (13).

Organs and Systems

Nervous system

Although generally safe, dextromethorphan can in some individuals cause nervous system adverse effects, including hyperexcitability, increased muscle tone, and ataxia. Respiratory depression can occur with excessive doses.

Dextromethorphan has been implicated in a case of movement disorder (14).

- An 8-year-old boy complained of abnormal facial movements and hallucinations. One day before these symptoms, he had been given his sister's Cordec DM droplets (carbinoxamine maleate 2 mg, pseudoephedrine hydrochloride 25 mg, and dextromethorphan 4 mg) for a cold. He had facial dyskinesia, dilated pupils, pyrexia, tachycardia, and reduced bowel sounds and responded to a benzodiazepine.

Psychological, psychiatric

Dextromethorphan-induced psychotic and/or manic-like symptoms have been reported.

- A 2-year-old child developed hyperirritability, incoherent babbling, and ataxia after being over-medicated with a pseudoephedrine/dextromethorphan over-the-counter combination cough formulation for upper respiratory symptoms (15). The symptoms abated after withdrawal of the product.

In another three cases (girls aged 10, 13, and 15 years) severe acute psychosis was associated with the use of an over-the-counter formulation containing ephedrine or pseudoephedrine and dextromethorphan combined with other compounds (16). The psychopathology included agitation, depressed mood, flat affect, pressure of speech, visual and auditory hallucinations, and paranoia. All three improved dramatically, with residual symptoms of irritability, 2–4 days after withdrawal of the mixture and treatment with risperidone 0.5–2.0 mg/day.

- An 18-year-old student had dissociative phenomenon, nihilistic and paranoid delusions, vivid visual hallucinations, thought insertion, and broadcasting after having consumed 1–2 bottles of cough syrup (dextromethorphan 711 mg per bottle) every day for several days (17). The psychotic symptoms remitted completely without any treatment 4 days after withdrawal of dextromethorphan. He was hospitalized twice more over the next 2 months with similar symptoms; each time he had consumed large doses of dextromethorphan.

Cautious use of over-the-counter formulations is recommended in patients with a predisposition to affective illness (SEDA-21, 87).

Cognitive deterioration has been reported from prolonged use of dextromethorphan (18).

Endocrine

During a double-blind, placebo-controlled study of the effect of high doses of dextromethorphan in children with bacterial meningitis, two of four patients developed type 1 diabetes mellitus; they had received dextromethorphan and the other two placebo (19).

- A 10-year-old boy received dextromethorphan 36 mg/kg/day by nasogastric tube. He developed hyperglycemia with ketoacidosis after 5 days and required insulin. The dose of dextromethorphan was reduced over the next 4 days and withdrawn. Insulin was withdrawn 4 days later.
- A 14-year-old girl received dextromethorphan 26 mg/kg/day by nasogastric tube. She developed hyperglycemia after 2 days and needed insulin for 6 days. A later glucose tolerance test was normal.

Pancreatic beta cells in rats express NMDA receptors, stimulation of which leads to insulin secretion (20). The authors postulated that dextromethorphan inhibits insulin secretion by blocking NMDA receptors and thus impairs glucose tolerance. Both patients had reduced insulin concentrations, implying that peripheral insulin resistance was unlikely to have been the cause of diabetes.

Skin

On two occasions, a fixed drug eruption occurred on the arm of a 45-year-old woman after using dextromethorphan as an antitussive (SEDA-16, 79). Worsening of urticaria pigmentosa has been attributed to dextromethorphan (SEDA-21, 87).

Sexual function

Spontaneous ejaculation occurred in a 64-year-old man who took dextromethorphan for a common cold (21). His sexual activity normalized 7 days after stopping the dextromethorphan. He had had a similar episode 5 months before, when spontaneous ejaculation had started 3 days after he took dextromethorphan and abated 4 days after withdrawal of the drug.

Immunologic

Dextromethorphan-induced anaphylactic symptoms have been reported (22).

- A 40-year-old woman suffered repeated hives, lip swelling, and shortness of breath on taking cough suppressants containing dextromethorphan. None was sufficient to require emergency medical intervention. On challenge with dextromethorphan 1 mg, mild transient pruritus occurred. After dextromethorphan 30 mg, hives and nasal and conjunctival congestion occurred. Vital signs and peak flow remained stable. There was no bronchospasm or angioedema. No reaction occurred to hydrocodone or codeine.

The authors noted that many opioids are potent histamine releasers and most reactions to opioids are anaphylactoid rather than IgE-mediated. It was of particular interest that the patient was able to tolerate the opioids hydrocodone and codeine.

Second-Generation Effects

Teratogenicity

In 184 pregnancies exposed to dextromethorphan (128 exposures in the first trimester) there were 172 live births, 10 spontaneous abortions, one therapeutic abortion, and one stillbirth (23). There were three major malformations and seven minor malformations in the children of women who had used dextromethorphan in the first trimester. In the control group there were 174 live births, 8 spontaneous abortions, and 2 therapeutic abortions; there were 5 major and 18 minor malformations. This small study did not show that dextromethorphan used during pregnancy increases the rates of major malformations above the expected baseline rate of 1–3%.

Susceptibility Factors

Genetic factors

Individuals who are poor CYP2D6 metabolizers are at increased risk of serotonergic adverse effects, as well as the narcotic adverse effects of coma and respiratory depression (24).

Other features of the patient

Individuals who take long-acting dextromethorphan formulations are at increased risk of adverse effects.

Drug Administration

Drug formulations

Individuals who take long-acting dextromethorphan formulations are at increased risk of serotonergic adverse effects, as well as the narcotic adverse effects of coma and respiratory depression (24).

Drug overdose

Intentional dextromethorphan overdose has caused two deaths (SEDA-17, 210). Dextromethorphan toxicity occurred in a 3-year-old child who ingested up to 270 mg. The effects were reversed by naloxone (2).

Drug–Drug Interactions

Monoamine oxidase inhibitors

A possible interaction between dextromethorphan and the monoamine oxidase inhibitor isocarboxazid has been described, with myoclonic jerks, choreoathetoid movements, and marked urinary retention (25).

Individuals who take monoamine oxidase inhibitors are at increased risk of serotonergic adverse effects, as well as the narcotic adverse effects of coma and respiratory depression (25,26)

Four subjects had markedly reduced *O*-demethylation of dextromethorphan after they had taken moclobemide 300 mg bd for 9 days (27). *N*-demethylation was not affected. This result supports the hypothesis that moclobemide or a metabolite reduces the activity of the cytochrome enzyme CYP2D6. The clinical implications of this particular interaction remain to be clarified.

Morphine sulfate

Morphi Dex contains morphine sulfate and dextromethorphan in a 1:1 ratio. Double-blind, single-dose analgesic efficacy studies in over 800 patients with post-surgical pain have shown superior analgesic activity for the combination (60:60 mg) than separate doses of the individual components (28,29). In double-blind, multiple-dose studies in 321 patients with chronic pain the combination provided satisfactory pain control with a significantly lower mean daily dose of morphine sulfate. Other studies have shown similar responses (28) and an adverse events profile similar to that of a similar dose of morphine sulfate (30). The most common adverse events seen in a multiple-dose, non-placebo-controlled study in 1400 subjects were nausea, dizziness, vomiting, somnolence, confusion, and pruritus. There was a significant trend toward lower incidence of constipation with the combination than with morphine sulfate alone (31,32).

Quinidine (sulfate)

The effects of quinidine sulfate, 50 mg orally, an inhibitor of cytochrome CYP2D6, on the metabolism of dextromethorphan 50 mg have been studied in seven healthy volunteers in a randomized, double-blind, crossover, placebo-controlled study (24). Quinidine suppressed the conversion of dextromethorphan to dextrorphan in extensive metabolizers to the extent seen in poor metabolizers. The increased concentrations of dextromethorphan increased subjective and objective pain thresholds by 35 and 45% respectively. This result suggests that debrisoquine/sparteine-type polymorphisms account for important differences in the effect of dextromethorphan and the balance between the analgesic effect of dextromethorphan and the hallucinogenic effect of dextrorphan. Concomitant use of quinidine or other inhibitors of CYP2D6 could further affect this balance, increasing the risk of serotonergic- and narcotic-related adverse effects.

Serotonin reuptake inhibitors

Those who take serotonin reuptake inhibitors are at increased risk of adverse effects because of inhibition of CYP2D6 and pharmacodynamic potentiation; hallucinations and the serotonin syndrome have been reported (33,34).

References

1. Shaul WL, Wandell M, Robertson WO. Dextromethorphan toxicity: reversal by naloxone. Pediatrics 1977;59(1):117–18.
2. Katona B, Wason S. Dextromethorphan danger. N Engl J Med 1986;314(15):993.
3. Deutsch SI, Rosse RB, Mastropaolo J. Current status of NMDA antagonist interventions in the treatment of nonketotic hyperglycinemia. Clin Neuropharmacol 1998;21(2):71–9.
4. Weinbroum AA, Rudick V, Paret G, Ben-Abraham R. The role of dextromethorphan in pain control. Can J Anaesth 2000;47(6):585–96.
5. Generali J, Cada DJ. Dextromethorphan: neuropathy. Hosp Pharm 2001;36:421–5.
6. Wu CT, Yu JC, Liu ST, Yeh CC, Li CY, Wong CS. Preincisional dextromethorphan treatment for postoperative pain management after upper abdominal surgery. World J Surg 2000;24(5):512–17.
7. Helmy SA, Bali A. The effect of the preemptive use of the NMDA receptor antagonist dextromethorphan on postoperative analgesic requirements. Anesth Analg 2001;92(3):739–44.
8. Weinbroum AA, Gorodezky A, Niv D, Ben-Abraham R, Rudick V, Szold A. Dextromethorphan attenuation of postoperative pain and primary and secondary thermal hyperalgesia. Can J Anaesth 2001;48(2):167–74.
9. Wadhwa A, Clarke D, Goodchild CS, Young D. Large-dose oral dextromethorphan as an adjunct to patient-controlled analgesia with morphine after knee surgery. Anesth Analg 2001;92(2):448–54.
10. Ben Abraham R, Marouani N, Kollender Y, Meller I, Weinbroum AA. Dextromethorphan for phantom pain attenuation in cancer amputees: a double-blind crossover trial involving three patients. Clin J Pain 2002;18(5):282–5.
11. Sang CN, Booher S, Gilron I, Parada S, Max MB. Dextromethorphan and memantine in painful diabetic neuropathy and postherpetic neuralgia: efficacy and dose-response trials. Anesthesiology 2002;96(5):1053–61.
12. Verhagen, Metman L, Blanchet PJ, van den Munckhof P, Del Dotto P, Natte R, Chase TN. A trial of dextromethorphan in parkinsonian patients with motor response complications. Mov Disord 1998;13(3):414–17.
13. Walker FO, Hunt VP. An open label trial of dextromethorphan in Huntington's disease. Clin Neuropharmacol 1989;12(4):322–30.
14. Nairn SJ, Diaz JE. Cold-syrup induced movement disorder. Pediatr Emerg Care 2001;17(3):191–2.
15. Roberge RJ, Hirani KH, Rowland PL 3rd, Berkeley R, Krenzelok EP. Dextromethorphan- and pseudoephedrine-induced agitated psychosis and ataxia: case report. J Emerg Med 1999;17(2):285–8.
16. Soutullo CA, Cottingham EM, Keck PE Jr. Psychosis associated with pseudoephedrine and dextromethorphan. J Am Acad Child Adolesc Psychiatry 1999;38(12):1471–2.

17. Price LH, Lebel J. Dextromethorphan-induced psychosis. Am J Psychiatry 2000;157(2):304.
18. Hinsberger A, Sharma V, Mazmanian D. Cognitive deterioration from long-term abuse of dextromethorphan: a case report. J Psychiatry Neurosci 1994;19(5):375–7.
19. Konrad D, Sobetzko D, Schmitt B, Schoenle EJ. Insulin-dependent diabetes mellitus induced by the antitussive agent dextromethorphan. Diabetologia 2000;43(2):261–2.
20. Molnar E, Varadi A, McIlhinney RA, Ashcroft SJ. Identification of functional ionotropic glutamate receptor proteins in pancreatic beta-cells and in islets of Langerhans. FEBS Lett 1995;371(3):253–7.
21. Rafols A, Garcia Vicente JA, Farre M, Mas M. Disfuncion sexual por dextrometorfang. [Dextromethorphan-induced sexual dysfunction.] Aten Primaria 1999;24(8):495–7.
22. Knowles SR, Weber E. Dextromethorphan anaphylaxis. J Allergy Clin Immunol 1998;102(2):316–17.
23. Einarson A, Lyszkiewicz D, Koren G. The safety of dextromethorphan in pregnancy: results of a controlled study. Chest 2001;119(2):466–9.
24. Desmeules JA, Oestreicher MK, Piguet V, Allaz AF, Dayer P. Contribution of cytochrome P-450 2D6 phenotype to the neuromodulatory effects of dextromethorphan. J Pharmacol Exp Ther 1999;288(2):607–12.
25. Sovner R, Wolfe J. Interaction between dextromethorphan and monoamine oxidase inhibitor therapy with isocarboxazid. N Engl J Med 1988;319(25):1671.
26. Anonymous. High-dose fentanyl. Lancet 1979;1(8107):81–2.
27. Hartter S, Dingemanse J, Baier D, Ziegler G, Hiemke C. Inhibition of dextromethorphan metabolism by moclobemide. Psychopharmacology (Berl) 1998;135(1):22–6.
28. Caruso FS, Goldblum R. Dextromethorphan, an NMDA receptor antagonist, enhances the analgesic properties of morphine. Inflammopharmacology 2000;8:161–73.
29. Caruso FS. MorphiDex pharmacokinetic studies and single-dose analgesic efficacy studies in patients with postoperative pain. J Pain Symptom Manage 2000;19(Suppl 1):S31–6.
30. Katz NP. MorphiDex (MS:DM) double-blind, multiple-dose studies in chronic pain patients. J Pain Symptom Manage 2000;19(Suppl 1):S37–41.
31. Goldblum R. Long-term safety of MorphiDex. J Pain Symptom Manage 2000;19(Suppl 1):S50–6.
32. Chevlen E. Morphine with dextromethorphan: conversion from other opioid analgesics. J Pain Symptom Manage 2000;19(Suppl 1):S42–9.
33. Achamallah NS. Visual hallucinations after combining fluoxetine and dextromethorphan. Am J Psychiatry 1992;149(10):1406.
34. Skop BP, Finkelstein JA, Mareth TR, Magoon MR, Brown TM. The serotonin syndrome associated with paroxetine, an over-the-counter cold remedy, and vascular disease. Am J Emerg Med 1994;12(6):642–4.

Dextropropoxyphene

General Information

The most frequent adverse effects of dextropropoxyphene are dizziness, sedation, and nausea and vomiting. Other reported effects include constipation, abdominal pain, skin rashes, light-headedness, headache, weakness, euphoria, dysphoria, minor reversible visual disturbances, and liver dysfunction (1).

A systematic review of single-dose dextropropoxyphene for postoperative pain identified 130 published articles (2). Of these, 11 placebo-controlled studies met the inclusion criteria for the review, 6 of dextropropoxyphene (65 mg) and five of the same dose of dextropropoxyphene plus paracetamol (650 mg) (co-proxamol). Pooled data from the studies showed that the incidence of nausea, drowsiness, and headache with dextropropoxyphene alone was not significantly different from placebo. Previous reports have suggested that dextropropoxyphene is significantly associated with dizziness, sedation, and nausea and vomiting. However, co-proxamol caused significantly increased dizziness (relative risk 2.2, 95% CI = 1.1, 4.3) and drowsiness (2.1, 1.5, 2.9). The relative risk of headache was reduced to 0.5 (0.3, 0.9). Analgesic effect was greater with co-proxamol than with dextropropoxyphene alone.

Organs and Systems

Cardiovascular

Dextropropoxyphene-induced cardiogenic shock has been described (3).

- A 32-year-old man became deeply comatose, with intraventricular conduction disturbances, after taking dextropropoxyphene 4.6 g. Treatment-resistant seizures lasted for hours. He was treated with an intra-aortic balloon pump and a continuous infusion of milrinone for 7 days and recovered fully.

The mechanism of cardiotoxicity of dextropropoxyphene is unknown, but the membrane-stabilizing effect of its major metabolite, norpropoxyphene, seems to play a central part. The cardiac effects are not reversed by naloxone (4), but dopamine may be effective.

Respiratory

Hypersensitivity pneumonitis has been associated with co-proxamol (paracetamol plus dextropropoxyphene) (5).

- A 61-year-old man, who was taking prednisolone 20 mg and co-proxamol as required for cranial arteritis, presented with a 2-month history of increasing breathlessness. His chest X-ray showed vague shadowing in both lower zones, consistent with an interstitial abnormality, and a lung biopsy confirmed focal interstitial hypersensitivity pneumonitis. After a diffuse rash appeared, the co-proxamol was withdrawn and then reintroduced. The rash recurred and the breathlessness deteriorated. A subsequent challenge with paracetamol did not produce the same symptoms. The dosage of prednisolone was not altered.

Sensory systems

Nerve deafness in a 44-year-old woman, dependent on co-proxamol (dextropropoxyphene plus paracetamol), has been reported (SEDA-17, 80).

Metabolism

Severe hypoglycemia has been reported in the elderly (SEDA-17, 80).

Hematologic

Hemolytic anemia has been attributed to dextropropoxyphene (6).

Gastrointestinal

Four cases each of necrotizing anorectitis and proctitis have been reported after long-term (2–24 months) use of suppositories containing dextropropoxyphene and paracetamol (SEDA-10, 62). Perineal ulceration can also occur (7).

Liver

Various forms of hepatotoxicity, sometimes involving jaundice or mimicking biliary tract disease, have been reported by the UK Committee on Safety of Medicines (8). In most, but not all, cases the drug had been taken with paracetamol. In some cases, rechallenge caused hepatotoxicity within a few hours, and an immunologically based mechanism has been suggested.

Dextropropoxyphene has been implicated in hepatic injury in four patients taking co-proxamol (dextropropoxyphene plus paracetamol) (9). The cases were recorded at the Regional Centre of Pharmacovigilance in St Etienne, France between 1985 and 2000 and were similar to 29 cases published in the international literature between 1971 and 1994. The risk factors identified in the confirmed cases included age over 50 years, female sex, and a history of excessive alcohol consumption or previous pathology that might have caused liver damage. Drug withdrawal produced good outcomes.

Skin

Acute generalized pustulosis attributed to dextropropoxyphene has been reported (10).

- A 43-year-old woman, who had taken antibiotics and analgesics, including dextropropoxyphene, for parotitis, developed generalized erythema with numerous pustules on the trunk followed by a pyrexia. Patch testing was positive with dextropropoxyphene only and negative with paracetamol, spiramycin, aspirin, and tenoxicam.

Musculoskeletal

Fibrous myopathy has been reported after long-term dextropropoxyphene injections (SEDA-18, 85).

Long-Term Effects

Drug dependence

In common with other opioids, dextropropoxyphene can produce dependence (11). However, it has also been used to withdraw patients from morphine (12).

Susceptibility Factors

Age

Acute respiratory failure predominated in patients under 30 years of age whilst cardiotoxic effects predominated in the elderly.

Renal disease

Severe hypoglycemia has been reported in a patient with chronic renal insufficiency (13).

Drug Administration

Drug overdose

Dextropropoxyphene is widely prescribed in combination with aspirin or paracetamol. It is particularly dangerous when taken in overdose (14). A mortality rate of 8% was described in a series of 222 self-harm patients (15).

Drug–Drug Interactions

Alcohol

Cardiorespiratory arrest can occur only 15 minutes after drug ingestion (16). This risk is enhanced if ethanol is taken concomitantly.

Alprazolam

Inhibition of alprazolam metabolism by dextropropoxyphene has been reported (17).

Carbamazepine

Dextropropoxyphene inhibits the oxidative metabolism of carbamazepine, leading to clinically significant rises in carbamazepine concentrations (18).

Severe carbamazepine toxicity can occur if dextropropoxyphene is taken concurrently (19).

Nortriptyline

Inhibition of nortriptyline metabolism by dextropropoxyphene has been reported (20).

Warfarin

Prolongation of the prothrombin time was observed in a patient concurrently taking warfarin and a compound analgesic containing dextropropoxyphene (21).

Smoking

Heavy smoking can increase the elimination of dextropropoxyphene (22).

References

1. Grover H. Propoxyphene. J Indian Med Assoc 1988;86(1):21–3.
2. Collins SL, Edwards JE, Moore RA, McQuay HJ. Single-dose dextropropoxyphene in post-operative pain: a quantitative systematic review. Eur J Clin Pharmacol 1998;54(2):107–12.
3. Gillard P, Laurent M. Dextropropoxyphene-induced cardiogenic shock: treatment with intra-aortic balloon pump and milrinone. Intensive Care Med 1999;25(3):335.
4. Pickar D, Dubois M, Cohen MR. Behavioral change in a cancer patient following intrathecal beta-endorphin administration. Am J Psychiatry 1984;141(1):103–4.
5. Matusiewicz SP, Wallace WA, Crompton GK. Hypersensitivity pneumonitis associated with co-proxamol

(paracetamol + dextropropoxyphene) therapy Postgrad Med J 1999;75(886):475–6.
6. Fulton JD, McGonigal G. Steroid responsive haemolytic anaemia due to dextropropoxyphene paracetamol combination. J R Soc Med 1989;82(4):228.
7. Bosisio OA, Gonzales AU, Bravard JD, et al Ulcera medicamentosa de ano. Prensa Med Argent 1986;73:437.
8. Committee on Safety of Medicines. Hepatotoxicity with dextropropoxyphene. Curr Probl 1986;17.
9. Bergeron L, Guy C, Ratrema M, Beyens MN, Mounier G, Ollagnier M. Dextropropoxyphène et atteintes hépatiques: à propos de 4 cas et revue de literature. [Dextropropoxyphene hepatotoxicity: four cases and literature review.] Thérapie 2002;57(5):464–72.
10. Machet L, Martin L, Machet MC, Lorette G, Vaillant L. Acute generalized exanthematous pustulosis induced by dextropropoxyphene and confirmed by patch testing. Acta Derm Venereol 2000;80(3):224–5.
11. Strode SW. Propoxyphene dependence and withdrawal. Am Fam Physician 1985;32(3):105–8.
12. Hasday JD, Weintraub M. Propoxyphene in children with iatrogenic morphine dependence. Am J Dis Child 1983;137(8):745–8.
13. Almirall J, Montoliu J, Torras A, Revert L. Propoxyphene-induced hypoglycemia in a patient with chronic renal failure. Nephron 1989;53(3):273–5.
14. Proudfoot AT. Clinical features and management of Distalgesic overdose. Hum Toxicol 1984;3(Suppl):S85–94.
15. Sloth Madsen P, Strom J, Reiz S, Bredgaard Sorensen M. Acute propoxyphene self-poisoning in 222 consecutive patients. Acta Anaesthesiol Scand 1984;28(6):661–5.
16. Young RJ. Dextropropoxyphene overdosage. Pharmacological considerations and clinical management. Drugs 1983;26(1):70–9.
17. Abernethy DR, Greenblatt DJ, Morse DS, Shader RI. Interaction of propoxyphene with diazepam, alprazolam and lorazepam. Br J Clin Pharmacol 1985;19(1):51–7.
18. Hansen BS, Dam M, Brandt J, Hvidberg EF, Angelo H, Christensen JM, Lous P. Influence of dextropropoxyphene on steady state serum levels and protein binding of three anti-epileptic drugs in man. Acta Neurol Scand 1980;61(6):357–67.
19. Yu YL, Huang CY, Chin D, Woo E, Chang CM. Interaction between carbamazepine and dextropropoxyphene. Postgrad Med J 1986;62(725):231–3.
20. Jerling M, Bertilsson L, Sjoqvist F. The use of therapeutic drug monitoring data to document kinetic drug interactions: an example with amitriptyline and nortriptyline. Ther Drug Monit 1994;16(1):1–12.
21. Smith R, Prudden D, Hawkes C. Propoxyphene and warfarin interaction. Drug Intell Clin Pharm 1984;18(10):822.
22. D'Arcy PF. Tobacco smoking and drugs: a clinically important interaction? Drug Intell Clin Pharm 1984;18(4):302–7.

Dezocine

General Information

Dezocine is structurally related to pentazocine (1). It reacts primarily with OP_3 (μ) receptors, but also has some affinity for OP_1 (δ) and OP_2 (κ) receptors. It is slightly more potent than morphine, but with similar adverse effects at effective doses (2.5–10 mg). The most common adverse effects (3–9%) are nausea and vomiting, sedation, or local injection site reactions; dizziness/vertigo have also been reported (1–3%) (SEDA-16, 88). However, in some trials nausea and/or vomiting were reported in 5–22%, while headache was the most common CNS complaint (16–35%). Other adverse effects reported in 1% of patients involve the cardiovascular system, respiratory system, urogenital system, CNS, gastrointestinal system, and visual senses.

Reference

1. O'Brien JJ, Benfield P. Dezocine. A preliminary review of its pharmacodynamic and pharmacokinectic properties, and therapeutic efficacy. Drugs 1989;38(2):226–48.

Diacerein

General Information

Diacerein (diacetylrhein), an anthraquinone derivative, is said to be effective in the treatment of osteoarthritis. Its active metabolite is rhein, about which there are very few clinical data. Diacerein does not affect arachidonic acid metabolism and might be better tolerated than other NSAIDs with regards to renal and gastric toxicity. Epigastric or abdominal pain and diarrhea are the most frequent adverse effects. Diarrhea occurred in 37% of patients with osteoarthritis taking diacerein (1). Acute hepatitis has been described (SEDA-22, 119), as have skin reactions.

Reference

1. Nguyen M, Dougados M, Berdah L, Amor B. Diacerhein in the treatment of osteoarthritis of the hip. Arthritis Rheum 1994;37(4):529–36.

Dialysis fluids

General Information

Dialysis fluids are solutions of electrolytes formulated in concentrations similar to those of extracellular fluid or plasma. They contain, or may contain:

- sodium
- chloride
- bicarbonate or lactate
- calcium
- magnesium
- potassium
- glucose
- amino acids
- icodextrin

Dialysis fluids are provided in a sterile concentrated form for dilution with water before use; the water used need not be sterile.

Icodextrin

Icodextrin (rINN) is a maltodextrin glucose polymer with a mean molecular weight of 20 kDa, which is broken down to maltose. It is used as an alternative to glucose as the active osmotic agent for peritoneal dialysis. Icodextrin is similar in structure to dextran, but has improved ultrafiltration properties, because it is less well absorbed than glucose.

Organs and Systems

Skin

The manufacturers have reported from pharmacovigilance data that the incidence rate of all skin reactions with icodextrin is of the order of 2.5%; in most cases the symptoms are mild, often not requiring withdrawal (1).

The adverse effects associated with icodextrin in patients with renal insufficiency over 12 months have been reviewed (2). There were three cases of exfoliative skin reactions in 102 patients. Each was acute and started within 3 days of icodextrin exposure. All resolved promptly on withdrawal. There were two acute blistering reactions on sun-exposed areas, occurring within 3–6 months after icodextrin. Both responded slowly to withdrawal, taking 6–8 weeks to resolve completely. Nine further patients reported some form of minor skin problem (itching, dryness, rash, and blistering).

- A 48-year-old woman with a long history of insulin-dependent diabetes mellitus developed a severe cutaneous reaction to icodextrin (3). This happened 10 days after changing over to 7.5% icodextrin in order to improve ultrafiltration. The rash was maculopapular and it affected most parts of her body. It was associated with severe pruritus. By the 13th day after it first appeared the rash had become exfoliative and erythrodermic. There was rapid improvement in the first few days after the icodextrin dialysate had been withdrawn and she reverted to conventional glucose peritoneal dialysate.

Allergy to icodextrin was the most likely explanation for the severe cutaneous reaction. The epitope(s) for allergic reactions to dextrans have not been defined, although they are undoubtedly immunogenic. It is possible that the same or a similar epitope may be responsible for allergic reactions to icodextrin.

- A 50-year-old woman with insulin-dependent diabetes developed end-stage renal insufficiency secondary to diabetic nephropathy, and was treated with standard CAPD containing glucose (4). About 20 months later she was given 2 liters of icodextrin 7.5% postoperatively and 11 days later complained of pruritus on the lateral aspects of the thigh with erythroderma, which quickly spread to the back, abdomen, arms, hands, and head, followed by a widespread pruritic erythematous maculopapular rash, which became exfoliated and psoriasiform. Icodextrin was withdrawn 5 days later and there was rapid healing of the dermatitis, almost completely within 7 days. Rechallenge resulted in recurrence within 2 days.

The authors pointed out that in previous cases scaly and exfoliative rashes occurred several days after starting icodextrin but regressed without the need to withdraw icodextrin, except in one case. They concluded that, given the therapeutic advances made possible by icodextrin, and the extreme rarity of such adverse events, there should be no hesitation in using it in CAPD. The possibility of cutaneous adverse events 10–12 days after starting peritoneal exchange should be borne in mind, although the normal transient nature of such reactions rarely requires withdrawal.

Serosae

Giant and atypical mesothelial cells can develop in the peritoneum in response to irritation caused by peritoneal dialysis solutions. Mesothelial hyperplasia without an increase in mesothelial cell size, cytological atypia in mesothelial cells, polynucleate cells with nucleoles, and enlarged mesothelial cells with a flat small nucleus and without evident nucleoles have all been described (5). These giant cells are not found unless there is peritonitis. During peritonitis mesothelial cells detach en masse from the basal lamina.

Continual exposure of the peritoneum over a period of years to conventional peritoneal dialysis fluids contributes to loss of membrane function in two ways: (i) by compromising peritoneal host defences mediated by resident and infiltrating leukocytes and the resident cells of the peritoneal membrane and (ii) by directly contributing to structural changes in the peritoneal membrane (6). Peritoneal dialysis fluids have significant modulatory and, in some cases, toxic effects on peripheral and peritoneal cell functions. The impact of long-term exposure of the peritoneum to peritoneal dialysis fluids and how its function as a dialysing organ is affected are less well understood. From a comprehensive review of the literature it has emerged that lactate-buffered peritoneal dialysis fluids inhibit many leukocyte and peritoneal cell functions, even when exposure times are short. This suggests the need for more biocompatible peritoneal dialysis fluids. Neutral pH bicarbonate- or bicarbonate/lactate-buffered fluids are superior in all test systems to lactate-buffered fluids, irrespective of the concentration of glucose present in the solution. The cell inhibitory and stimulatory effects of high glucose concentrations remain, and this issue will have to be addressed before the perfect biocompatible alternative is produced. It is not clear whether long-term use of bicarbonate-containing fluids will improve patient outcome by reducing infection rates and better preserving the integrity of the peritoneal membrane.

The adverse effects of peritoneal dialysis fluids on the peritoneum have been succinctly summarized by authors arguing the case for a new, less toxic, and less acidic fluid for peritoneal dialysis (7). A low pH, high osmolality and lactate concentration, and the presence of several toxic contaminants may all contribute to impaired cellular function in the peritoneal membrane. In conventional peritoneal dialysis pH is deliberately lowered to 5.0–5.6

in order to prevent caramelization of the glucose (that is the production of glucose degradation products) during heat sterilization and storage. Low pH, especially in combination with tissue fluid hyperosmolality and high lactate concentrations, will cause vasodilatation and recruitment of capillaries in microvascular beds. In the peritoneal membrane, acidic solutions cause an increased "effective" vascular surface area and more rapid loss of glucose gradient than a neutral solution. Thus, a neutral solution would theoretically behave more favorably with regard to transperitoneal ultrafiltration (glucose-induced osmosis) than a conventional acidic solution. This is because the glucose osmotic gradient will be better preserved over time with neutral solutions. Even neutralized peritoneal dialysis solutions seem to be cytotoxic in vitro. This cytotoxicity is related less to hyperosmolality and the presence of lactate in the fluid than the toxicity occurring at a low pH. Glucose degradation products formed during heat sterilization and storage include acetaldehyde, methylglyoxal, 2-furaldehyde, formaldehyde, 5-hydroxymethylfurfural, and formic acid. All may, in the long term, affect the peritoneum adversely and lead to a deterioration of peritoneal membrane function. The risk of losing ultrafiltration capacity after 6 years of continuous ambulatory peritoneal dialysis is as high as 31%. Glucose degradation products can also cause abdominal discomfort and pain, and can be responsible for acute losses in ultrafiltration capacity.

Infection risk

Infectious peritonitis contributes to death in 5% of patients receiving peritoneal dialysis (8). The common organisms that cause peritonitis are *Staphylococcus epidermidis*, *Staphylococcus aureus*, streptococci, Gram-negative bacilli, and fungi. Predisposing factors are exit-site infections leading to tunnel infections, catheter infections, and nasal carriage of *S. aureus*, which is associated with exit-site and tunnel infections and peritonitis. Coagulase-negative staphylococci are often resistant to methicillin, and methicillin-resistant *S. aureus* was the cause of 13% of all peritonitis episodes and 30% of catheter infections in one study (8). Vancomycin is required for treatment (but not prophylaxis) of such cases.

References

1. Divino Fiho JC. Allergic reactions to icodextrin in patients with renal failure. Lancet 2000;355(9212):1364–5.
2. Goldsmith D, Jayawardene S, Sabharwal N, Cooney K. Allergic reactions to the polymeric glucose-based peritoneal dialysis fluid icodextrin in patients with renal failure. Lancet 2000;355(9207):897.
3. Lam-Po-Tang MK, Bending MR, Kwan JT. Icodextrin hypersensitivity in a CAPD patient. Perit Dial Int 1997;17(1):82–4.
4. Queffeulou G, Bernard M, Vrtovsnik F, Skhiri H, Lebrun-Vigne B, Hufnagel G, Michel C, Mignon F. Severe cutaneous hypersensitivity requiring permanent icodextrin withdrawal in a CAPD patient. Clin Nephrol 1999;51(3):184–6.
5. Di Paolo N, Garosi G, Monaci G, Brardi S. Biocompatibility of peritoneal dialysis treatment. Nephrol Dial Transplant 1997;12(Suppl 1):78–83.
6. Jorres A, Williams JD, Topley N. Peritoneal dialysis solution biocompatibility: inhibitory mechanisms and recent studies with bicarbonate-buffered solutions. Perit Dial Int 1997;17(Suppl 2):S42–6.
7. Rippe B, Simonsen O, Wieslander A, Landgren C. Clinical and physiological effects of a new, less toxic and less acidic fluid for peritoneal dialysis. Perit Dial Int 1997;17(1):27–34.
8. Piraino B. Infectious complications of peritoneal dialysis. Perit Dial Int 1997;17(Suppl 3):S15–18.

Diamorphine

See also Opioid analgesics

General Information

Heroin is a potent opioid that offers no substantial advantages over morphine. In the UK it is the preferred parenteral opioid for subcutaneous administration to cachectic cancer patients, because of its high solubility.

In a randomized, double-blind study, 14 patients who underwent elective surgery for correction of bilateral arthritic deformities of the feet received 15 ml of 0.9% saline containing diamorphine 2.5 mg into the cannula in one foot and 15 ml of saline into the other foot (1). Intravenous regional diamorphine did not improve postoperative pain relief or secondary hyperalgesia. There were no significant adverse effects.

High-dose diamorphine has been compared with morphine in a double-blind, crossover, randomized study in 39 intravenous opioid users who were allocated to either morphine 3% solution or diamorphine 2% solution, gradually increasing up to an individual maintenance dose adjusted to meet the patient's subjective needs (2). Those who started with diamorphine and subsequently switched to morphine terminated prematurely owing to excessive histamine reactions, all of which occurred during crossover to morphine. Symptoms included severe pruritus, flushing, swelling, urticaria, severe headaches, nausea, general malaise, hypotension, and tachycardia. Only 44% of the original cohort finished the 6-week study (14 getting diamorphine at the end and three getting morphine). Average daily doses were 491 mg for diamorphine and 597 mg for morphine. These results suggest that diamorphine produces fewer adverse effects than morphine and may be preferable for high-dose maintenance prescription. However, the study was very small and the subject selection was biased, as were the variables used to determine a successful outcome. The result was contrary to all the well-established pharmacological facts, and the authors did not mention the risks associated with high doses of short-acting opioids.

In a randomized, double-blind study, 64 patients undergoing total knee arthroplasty received either intrathecal morphine 0.3 mg or intrathecal diamorphine, 0.3 mg in 0.3 ml, with 2–2.5 ml of 0.5% heavy spinal bupivacaine (3). The patients given morphine had significantly greater analgesia at 4, 8, and 12 hours postoperatively. The incidence of opioid-related adverse effects was not significantly different between the groups.

In a single-blind, randomized, controlled study, 70 patients scheduled for elective cesarean section under spinal anesthesia using hyperbaric bupivacaine 0.5% received intrathecal fentanyl 20 μg, intrathecal diamorphine 300 μg, or 0.9% saline (4). Significantly less intraoperative and postoperative "analgesic control" was required in the opioid groups, especially in those given diamorphine. Diamorphine produced longer-lasting analgesia than fentanyl (12 hours versus 1 hour). Nausea, vomiting, and pruritus occurred relatively infrequently, with no differences between the groups; sedation was more frequent with fentanyl.

Organs and Systems

Respiratory

"Chasing the dragon," or inhaling heroin vapor through a straw, is a technique by which heroin users avoid the risks of injection. In Amsterdam, 85% of heroin users smoke or chase the drug. Pulmonary function can be affected by heroin inhalation. It can depress the respiratory center, release histamine (which can trigger asthma), result in septic emboli, and increase susceptibility to infectious diseases, such as tuberculosis and pneumonia. In 100 methadone maintenance users, lung function and shortness of breath were evaluated using spirometry and clinical history (5). Impaired lung function and shortness of breath correlated with chronic heroin smoking.

Heroin-induced pulmonary edema, or "heroin lung" (SEDA-19, 29) (SEDA-25, 39), is a serious complication, which may be due to release of histamine, with increased pulmonary lymph flow and capillary permeability. There have been 27 reports of non-fatal heroin overdose associated with non-cardiogenic pulmonary edema (6). In a retrospective case-control study there were 23 heroin fatalities and 12 controls with sudden cardiac deaths (7). The authors tried to verify that defects of the alveolar capillary membranes and/or an acute anaphylactic reaction can lead to pulmonary congestion, edema, and hemorrhages. There were defects of the epithelial and endothelial basal laminae of the alveoli in both groups. There was an insignificant increase in IgE-positive cells in the heroin group. The findings suggested that heroin-associated lung edema is generally not caused by an anaphylactic reaction.

Bilateral pulmonary edema associated with heroin abuse has been reported several times (8). Bronchospasm has been noted following the use of street heroin, perhaps due to contaminants (9).

Nervous system

Delayed onset oculogyric crisis and generalized dystonia occurred in a 19-year-old man after intranasal heroin use, possibly due to bilateral hypoxic infarction of the pallidum and pallidothalamic tracts (10).

There has been one report of mixed transcortical aphasia attributed to heroin (11).

Myoclonic spasm has been reported about 24 hours after withdrawal of an epidural infusion of diamorphine (SEDA-16, 81).

Demyelination has been attributed to diamorphine (12).

- A 41-year-old chronic diamorphine user developed an unsteady gait and dysarthria over 2 weeks, followed by severe cerebellar ataxia and moderate dysmetria of the arms and legs. An MRI scan suggested myelin damage, with symmetrical involvement of the cerebellar hemispheres and decussation of the superior cerebellar peduncles, the corticospinal tracts, and the centrum semiovale, suggesting spongiform leukoencephalopathy. Two years later having taken no more diamorphine he was improved, with minor regression of the MRI lesions, especially the white matter lesions.

Myelopathy has been reported after intranasal insufflation of diamorphine (13).

- A 52-year-old man with a history of diamorphine abuse presented with sudden paraplegia a few hours after intranasal insufflation. He had flaccid paralysis of both legs, acute urinary retention, and reduced rectal tone. Deep tendon reflexes were absent and plantar responses were extensor. An MRI scan of the spine and an immunoglobulin profile supported the conclusion that this was a case of acute myelopathy with an immunopathological cause, involving a protein specific to spinal cord parenchyma, triggering acute local inflammation, ischemia, and tissue damage. Seven weeks later he recovered normal neurological function.

This case of heroin myelopathy is similar to other reported cases, except that this case occurred with intranasal rather than intravenous use. The MRI findings were consistent with a transverse myelitis. The authors suggested that hypersensitivity and an immune-mediated attack on the spinal cord was the likely mechanism of injury.

Reflex sympathetic dystrophy, in which there is an excessive or abnormal sympathetic nervous system response in a limb, has been associated with rhabdomyolysis secondary to heroin abuse (14).

- A 37-year-old male heroin smoker developed tea-colored urine and pain, swelling, and tenderness in both feet. He had acute renal insufficiency and rhabdomyolysis and was treated with hemodialysis. Urine toxicology was negative. He also had persistent, burning pain in both feet, with cool, pale, thin skin on both legs, a mild reduction in sensation on the lateral aspects of the lower legs and diminished bilateral knee and ankle reflexes. Walking was restricted, with limited range of movement owing to the severe pain. His feet would swell and redden after a 5-meter walk, suggesting loss of sympathetic regulation. Nerve conduction velocity studies of the tibial, peroneal, and sural nerves were abnormal. Radiographs showed mildly reduced bone mineralization in the legs. Three-phase bone scintigraphy showed diffusely increased radiotracer accumulation over both feet in all three phases, as found in reflex sympathetic dystrophy. The diagnosis was confirmed by local anesthetic sympathetic blockade. Nasal calcitonin spray led to pain relief 2 months later. A follow-up three-phase bone scintigram showed less radiotracer uptake, consistent with a good response to calcitonin therapy.

Progressive spongiform leukoencephalopathy

A rare consequence of inhaling heated heroin ("chasing the dragon") is a progressive spongiform leukoencephalopathy. The first three cases in the USA were reported in 1996 (SEDA-22, 35). The presentation includes apathy, bradyphrenia, motor restlessness, and progressive cerebellar ataxia. Another report has provided more details from physical assessments and laboratory and radiological (MRI and MRS) data, and more information about the course of this heroin-related effect (15). The three cases showed raised concentrations of intracerebral lactate (reflecting mitochondrial dysfunction), which suggests a conversion of aerobic to anaerobic metabolism seen in hypoxic-ischemic conditions, including stroke. One patient recovered quite well after antioxidant therapy, supporting a metabolic effect of the heroin-related toxin; a similar response to co-enzyme Q has been found in other mitochondrial disorders with a high CSF lactate. Thus, the authors recommended that although the role of antioxidant therapy in this condition is unclear, it may be prudent to administer oral co-enzyme Q supplemented with vitamins C and E to patients with this syndrome.

Intravenous administration of pure heroin did not cause a leukoencephalopathy in a patient in whom inhalation had caused it (16), and toxicity in these cases may have been due to the heating of the heroin. This might have implications for young heroin users who, because of the known increased risk of HIV infection, prefer to "chase" (smoke) the drug, rather than to inject it intravenously.

- A 23-year-old pregnant woman at 39 weeks of gestation developed tonic-clonic seizures and hypothermia after taking excessive heroin intravenously (17). She developed Cheyne-Stokes respiration needing intubation and a cesarean section was performed, after which she developed inappropriate secretion of antidiuretic hormone and acute renal insufficiency. She made a complete recovery.

The etiology of this leukoencephalopathy is unclear. Because cases occur in clusters, even though many others who inhale heroin do not get this effect, there is suspicion about the possible role of contaminants of small batches of drug by an unknown substance. In addition, some have suggested that heating could be important, since leukoencephalopathy has not been reported with other means of heroin use (until this year, as reported in the next case). The authors of the report postulated that there might be a relation between the amount of heroin inhaled and the severity of the illness. Once symptoms develop, progression continues, usually for 2–3 weeks, but in some individuals it progresses for up to 6 months after exposure. "Coasting," or the phenomenon of symptom progression after cessation of exposure to toxins, has been observed with other toxins, and it is proposed to result from the storage of toxin in lipid-rich neural or non-neural body tissues, with subsequent release into the bloodstream. Although the "toxin" involved in this condition is unknown, progression could be due to "coasting." Alternatively, oxidative damage could be initiated by the toxin and produce persistent metabolic changes in the affected white matter. Whatever the mechanism, the illness is extremely grave, with no known treatment and with progression to akinetic mutism and death in about 20% of reported cases.

- A 37-year-old male cocaine abuser was admitted with intoxication, mutism, and substupor (18). His toxicological screening was positive for heroin and cocaine. There was spasticity of all limbs and Babinski reflexes. The CSF contained some erythrocytes. The electroencephalogram showed generalized slowing, and a CT scan showed bifrontal confluent hypodensities in the deep white matter. The cranial MRI scan showed diffuse bihemispheric white matter lesions dominantly in the frontal lobe on T2-weighted images. There were abnormal hyperintense lesions in the pyramidal tracts and the corpus callosum. He gradually improved and made a complete recovery within 6 months, as confirmed by neurological and neuropsychological examination.

The findings of toxic leukoencephalopathy in this patient's brain-imaging studies were similar to those reported in patients who have inhaled impure heroin. However, he had used intravenous heroin and cocaine. This is therefore the first case report of leukoencephalopathy after intravenous use of these drugs. However, it should be noted that the authors did not indicate how the route of drug use was confirmed. They noted that lipophilic substances, such as hexachlorophene or triethylthin, were likely impurities in the abused substances.

- A 53-year-old man with a 7-year history of heroin abuse presented with confused speech and unsteady gait (19). A CT scan showed low attenuation in the white matter tracts and an MRI scan showed increased signal intensity in the white matter tracts extending from the centrum semiovale, corpus callosum, corona radiata, posterior limbs of the internal capsules, cerebral and cerebellar peduncles, and pyramidal tracts, suggestive of spongiform demyelination. He became bed-bound and tetraplegic and died of a chest infection.
- A 37-year-old man, with a short history of heroin and cocaine use, presented with spasticity of all limbs, a confusional state, and mutism (18). The electroencephalogram, CT scan, and MRI scan showed predominantly positive frontal pathology, with other lesions in the pyramidal tracts and corpus callosum. The diagnosis was leukoencephalopathy. The symptoms gradually abated after 4 weeks, and repeat tests after 6 months shown to be normal.

Three cases of toxic and progressive spongiform leukoencephalopathy have also been reported as a result of vapor inhalation of heroin (15). There were generalized white matter abnormalities and pathology in the cerebellum, internal capsule, corpus callosum, and brain stem.

Heroin-induced leuckoencephalopathy has been misdiagnosed as psychiatric illness (20).

- A 47-year-old woman, with a history of amphetamine abuse, depression, and paranoia, smoked heroin for 4 weeks after stopping amphetamines, and 10 days later became drowsy and confused with increased paranoia and depression. She was disoriented and restless. Her speech was garbled. She had frequent non-purposeful movements and an unsteady gait. A CT brain scan was normal. She was given chlorpromazine, doxepin, and diazepam, but her ataxia and incontinence worsened, her speech and all her movements slowed, with increased tone in all limbs and cogwheel rigidity. Her power and sensation were normal. Truncal ataxia impaired walking. An MRI brain scan showed diffuse high-intensity signals in both cerebral hemispheres, and review of the CT scan showed hypodensities in the same regions. She was treated with co-enzyme Q and regained mobility and continence, but with no improvement in cognitive impairment.

Sensory systems

Profound reversible deafness with vestibular dysfunction has been attributed to heroin abuse (21).

- A 47-year-old intravenous opiate user, after a period of abstinence, injected about 0.25 g of illicit diamorphine during a period of 24 hours and developed bilateral symmetrical sensorineural hearing loss, ear fullness, and loud tinnitus 20 minutes later. His symptoms gradually subsided with no sequelae after 3 weeks.

The authors pointed out that bilateral deafness after heroin relapse after prolonged abstinence had been reported in previous two cases, suggesting resensitization of a tolerized opioid system or prolonged hypersensitization of a system in withdrawal.

Endocrine

The syndrome of inappropriate secretion of antidiuretic hormone (SIADH) has been attributed to heroin (17).

- A 23-year-old pregnant woman developed antepartum bleeding at 35 weeks and a tonic-clonic convulsion and hypothermia at 39 weeks, having used heroin 4 hours before. She had further tonic-clonic seizures, became obtunded, and required intubation. She had occasional runs of ventricular bigeminy. A cesarean section was performed. The neonate had poor respiratory effort and required ventilation. Blood chemistry suggested inappropriate secretion of antidiuretic hormone, acute renal insufficiency, and acute pancreatitis. She and the baby recovered after 2 weeks.

Urinary tract

Following an observation that many patients develop acute renal insufficiency after using heroin, the authors identified 27 patients (mostly men, average age 29 years) who developed renal insufficiency after intravenous heroin use (22). Rhabdomyolysis was the likely cause of renal insufficiency in all cases. Twelve had a history of polydrug abuse and all had a history of intravenous diamorphine use in the 24 hours before presentation. Eight patients required renal dialysis for an average of 14 days. Patients who required dialysis had a higher admission creatine kinase, a higher peak creatine kinase, and a lower urine output in the initial 24 hours. They also had a longer hospital stay. Some had positive tests for hepatitis B (10%), hepatitis C (74%) and HIV (5%); viral infections can compound rhabdomyolysis and subsequent renal impairment through glomerulonephritis. No patient died and all patients recovered normal renal function. Rhabdomyolysis is a recognized cause of renal insufficiency, but its pathogenesis after heroin use is not fully understood.

In most of 19 renal specimens from autopsies of intravenous diamorphine users there was severe lymphomonocytic glomerulonephritis as a result of activation of the classical pathway of the complement binding system (23). This could have been a result of diamorphine itself, adulterants, or active hepatitis B and/or C infection.

Heroin was presumed to be the cause of reversible nephrotic syndrome in patients dependent on heroin (24).

Renal amyloidosis can be a late effect (24).

Skin

A traumatic skin lesion with blisters and sweat gland necrosis was described in a 24-year-old man who was comatose as a result of heroin overdose; immunofluorescence showed deposits of immunoglobulin and C3 in dermal vessels (25).

Musculoskeletal

Focal myopathy has been reported after intramuscular diamorphine (26).

- A 36-year-old man developed progressive, painless stiffness of both knee joints over 3 months. It had started 4 weeks after he began to give himself heroin injections two to three times a day in alternate thigh muscles. He had a broad-based stiff gait, and he walked without bending his knees. Because of contractures of the quadriceps muscles, which were indurated, active and passive knee flexion was limited to an angle of 5–10 degrees. Electromyography of the right quadriceps muscle showed firm fibrous resistance to needling without insertional activity. Ultrasound showed a preserved but enlarged muscle structure and thickening of the connective tissue. A muscle biopsy showed variation in fiber size with scattered collection of atrophic fibers and perivascular and endomysial infiltrates comprised chiefly of lymphocytes and macrophages. The serum creatine kinase activity was normal. After 7 weeks of physiotherapy, MRI of the thighs showed severe fibrosis of the muscle, suggesting a possible inflammatory component. Following treatment with prednisone and D-penicillamine, he was entirely normal, except for slightly limited knee flexion on both sides.

This patient's main symptom was progressive stiffness, due to contractures of the quadriceps muscles induced by chronic heroin injections. The findings made it very likely that heroin caused a primarily vascular lesion leading to non-specific inflammatory changes and subsequent fibrosis. Clinically, weakness was minimal and there was painless contracture. This presumably reflects the predominantly fibrotic process within muscle tissue. Combination therapy with prednisone and D-penicillamine led to significant improvement. The regenerating process was confirmed by the second muscle biopsy, and electromyography showed reinnervation. The second biopsy did not show inflammatory cells, indicating absence of the inflammatory component. Thus, this case suggests that heroin-induced fibrotic myopathy is reversible.

Long-Term Effects

Drug abuse

Smoking heroin by heating the free base over tin foil and inhaling the vapors is known as "chasing the dragon," a method that probably originated in Southeast Asia. Some are using this to reverse the stimulant effects of ecstasy. In 102 patients (55 men and 47 women, mean age 21 years) interviewed at four clinics in Dublin, Ireland, three subgroups of opiate users were identified: (a) those who had ever used opiates to come off ecstasy, who were compared with those who had never used opiates for this purpose, (b) those whose first use of opiates had been to come off ecstasy, and (c) those who had started opiates by "chasing" and then did or did not move to injecting (27). Of the 102 patients, 92 reported having taken ecstasy, 68 of whom reported having taken opiates to come off it, and the remaining 24 of whom had not. The 68 patients who reported taking opiates to come off ecstasy had significantly heavier ecstasy use, in terms of the number of nights per week and number of tablets taken per night. Of 36 who reported that their first ever experience of using opiates was in the context of "chasing" to come off ecstasy, 28 reported this as their main reason for starting to use opiates and the other eight reported that they would probably have tried opiates independent of their ecstasy use. Of the 86 patients whose initial route of using heroin was "chasing," 61 reported changing to injecting, 23 continued to smoke heroin, and two switched to an oral formulation of methadone or morphine. When those who came to inject heroin were compared with those who did not (61 versus 23), the injectors had begun illicit drug use earlier, had started heroin at a younger age, were younger at the time of interview, and had been more likely to have a history of ecstasy use. Despite the younger age of onset of illicit drug use in those who came to inject, they had not been using illicit drugs for longer at the time of interview. This study confirmed the authors' previous findings that heroin smoking was associated with ecstasy use.

The Swiss government has developed a program called PROVE, which provides prescriptions of injectable opioids for the treatment of heroin-dependent patients. This program has generally been viewed to be successful in terms of retention in treatment, morbidity and mortality, legal behavior, and cost-effectiveness. However, during the 26-month observation period, epileptic seizures occurred in 11% of the 186 patients treated. This finding, along with previous reports of reduced regional blood supply to the brains of opioid users, led the authors to study cerebral deoxygenation after intravenous opioid administration in ten opioid-dependent subjects and to compare it with intravenous saline in ten matched controls using Near Infrared Spectroscopy (NIRS) (28). Heroin and methadone produced a rapid and dramatic reduction in both respiratory rate and cortical hemoglobin oxygenation, while saline had no effects. The authors suggested that opioid-induced acute deoxygenation of cortical hemoglobin was probably associated with respiratory depression. In one in three subjects, oxygen saturation after intravenous heroin fell rapidly, a finding that has not previously been described in humans.

The authors suggested two possible mechanisms for this phenomenon. They discounted the possibility that opioids increase the utilization of oxygenated hemoglobin in the CNS, because PET data from other studies suggest decreased utilization of glucose (indicating reduced brain activity) following opioids. They believed that it was more likely that the increase in cortical-reduced hemoglobin was related to opioid-induced respiratory depression, with carbon dioxide retention and resulting vasodilatation. Although preliminary, these data have potential implications for treatment programs involving intravenous opioid maintenance. The authors suggested that intravenous opioids may produce both systemic and cerebral hypoxia, which may at least in part account for the hyperexcitability (as measured by electroencephalography) found after intravenous opioids in other studies. Furthermore, hypoxia may mediate or contribute to the rush sensation, similar to that seen with high altitude or in cases of asphyxiophilia.

Drug withdrawal

The relation between the severity of opiate withdrawal and the dose, duration, and route of administration of heroin has been assessed in a retrospective analysis of heroin withdrawal in 22 patients (29). Abrupt withdrawal from opiates resulted in increased symptom severity, peaking on day 2 and then abating after that until day 7. Both the dose and the route of administration were related to the withdrawal score: intravenous heroin was linked to greater total and maximum withdrawal severity than smoking heroin. The authors speculated that the effect of the route of administration may have been due to lower systemic availability of smoked compared with injected heroin. Their data suggested that even the duration of the withdrawal symptoms seemed to increase with higher doses and intravenous use. However, there were several limitations to this study. It was retrospective and the period of observation lasted only 7 days although the withdrawal symptoms lasted much longer. In addition, many subjects took doxepin and benzodiazepines during the observation phase, which may have reduced or suppressed their withdrawal symptoms.

Second-Generation Effects

Fetotoxicity

A report of death associated with intravenous heroin use has provided insights about the distribution of heroin and its metabolites in the fetus (30).

- A 17-year-old girl with a history of heavy drug abuse for 2 years was found dead in a public restroom, with fresh needle puncture marks. She was 18–20 weeks pregnant with a male fetus, and had massive brain and lung edema from acute intoxication. Analysis of her hair showed that she had used heroin over the previous few months. Drug screening of body fluids showed only opiates (high concentrations of 6-monoacetylmorphine and morphine) in the maternal and fetal circulation at the time of death. Unexpectedly high amounts of morphine, 6-monoacetyl-morphine, and morphine-3-glucuronide were also found in the amniotic fluid. Only morphine-3-glucuronide was detected in the fetus, whereas both morphine-3-glucuronide and morphine-6-glucuronide were detected in the mother, in the body fluids, and in all investigated organ tissues except the brain.

The authors noted that heroin is considered a "prodrug," with 6-monoacetyl-morphine, morphine, and morphine-6-glucuronide accounting for most of its narcotic activity. In blood, diamorphine is rapidly converted to the active metabolite 6-monoacetyl-morphine, which is presumably converted to morphine in the liver. The majority of the morphine is converted to morphine-3-glucuronide and small amounts are converted to morphine-6-glucuronide, which is pharmacologically active. They concluded that morphine-3-glucuronide can cross the placenta and that high concentrations of heroin and its metabolites can be found in fetal compartments during heroin abuse by the mother. Lastly, heroin and its pharmacologically active metabolites appear to be present in the fetal central nervous system for much longer than in the maternal circulation, because of low fetal drug-metabolizing capacity as well as minimal drug elimination from the amniotic fluid in advancing pregnancy.

Drug Administration

Drug dosage regimens

High-dose intrathecal diamorphine for analgesia after elective cesarean section has been studied in 40 women who were randomized to diamorphine 0.5 or 1 mg (31). All also received diclofenac 100 mg at the end of the cesarean section and morphine via a patient-controlled analgesia system. Postoperative analgesia was more prolonged and reliable in those who were given diamorphine 1 mg, who needed significantly less morphine. There was postoperative nausea in just under half of the patients in each group, and most of the patients (93%) had mild to moderate pruritus. There were no cases of excessive sedation or oxygen desaturation.

Drug administration route

Nasal diamorphine is as effective as intramuscular morphine and is much better tolerated by children, with no apparent increased risk of adverse effects (32,33). In a multicenter, randomized, controlled study, 404 children aged 3–16 years with a fracture of an arm or leg were given either nasal diamorphine 0.1 mg/kg or intramuscular morphine 0.2 mg/kg. The onset of pain relief was faster with nasal diamorphine, and there were no serious adverse effects. The frequencies of opioid-related mild adverse effects were similar in the two groups.

In a randomized, placebo-controlled, double-blind study of the relative efficacies of patient-controlled analgesia (PCA) regimens (34), 60 patients undergoing elective total hip or knee replacement were randomly allocated to receive epidural diamorphine 2.5 mg followed by a PCA bolus 1 mg with a 20-minute lockout (group 1), subcutaneous diamorphine 2.5 mg followed by a PCA bolus 1 mg with a 10-minute lockout (group 2), or epidural diamorphine 2.5 mg in 4 ml of 0.125% bupivacaine followed by a PCA bolus of 1 mg diamorphine in 4 ml 0.125% bupivacaine with a 20-minute lockout (group 3). Diamorphine demands were significantly higher in group 2 in the first postoperative 24-hour period, but pain scores were only significantly higher in group 2 in the first 3 hours postoperatively compared with group 3 and group 1. There were also fewer opioid-related adverse effects in group 2, and group 3 reported higher incidences of various adverse effects. The conclusion was that PCA diamorphine given with or without bupivacaine provides analgesia of similar efficacy once adequate pain relief has been achieved. Taking the incidences of adverse effect profiles into account, diamorphine subcutaneous PCA was a simple and effective method of providing analgesia.

In 62 women who asked for regional analgesia in labor and who were randomized to an intrathecal injection of either bupivacaine 2.5 mg with fentanyl 25 μg or bupivacaine 2.5 mg with diamorphine 250 μg, the diamorphine provided longer analgesia (35). There were significant differences in adverse effects between the groups. There were no instances of nausea or vomiting, but pruritus was more common in those who received fentanyl. The dose of diamorphine was deliberately low, and more studies are needed to confirm these findings.

Drug overdose

The main life-threatening complications of heroin intoxication include acute pulmonary edema and delayed respiratory depression with coma after successful naloxone treatment. In a prospective study of the management of 160 heroin and heroin mixture intoxication cases treated in an emergency room in Switzerland between 1991 and 1992, there were no rehospitalizations after discharge from the emergency room and there was only one death outside the hospital due to pulmonary edema, which occurred at between 2.25 and 8.25 hours after intoxication (36). A literature review found only two reported cases of delayed pulmonary edema, which occurred 4 and 6 hours after hospitalization. The authors recommended surveillance of a heroin user for at least 8 hours after successful opiate antagonist treatment.

Among heroin users, the annual rate of mortality is 1–4%; overdose and HIV infection being the leading causes. The effect of the frequency and route of heroin administration on the occurrence of non-fatal heroin overdose has been studied (37). Among 2556 subjects with heroin dependence, 10% had taken overdoses requiring emergency care in the prior 12 months. The cumulative risk of overdose increased as the frequency of heroin use fell. Among daily heroin users, the risk was greater with increased frequency of heroin injection, but not among non-daily users. The risk of overdose was greater with injection than with other routes of administration.

Drug–Drug Interactions

Alcohol

Many heroin users use heroin and alcohol together. There has been an evaluation of the pharmacokinetic interaction between heroin and alcohol and the role of that interaction in the cause of 39 heroin-related deaths that were attributed to either heroin or heroin + ethanol (38). The cases were arbitrarily divided into two groups according to blood ethanol concentration (low-ethanol group, under 1000 μg/ml, and high ethanol group, over 1000 μg/ml. The high-ethanol group was associated with reduced hydrolysis of 6-acetylmorphine to morphine, and there was an inverse correlation between blood ethanol concentration and hydrolysis of 6-acetylmorphine to morphine. The concentration of total morphine was lower in the high-ethanol group. High blood ethanol concentrations were also associated with an increased ratio of unbound to total morphine and with reduced excretion of unbound and total morphine. The relative concentrations of conjugated heroin metabolites were reduced in the presence of a high blood ethanol concentration. The authors hypothesized that alcohol inhibits the glucuronidation of morphine, resulting in less conjugated morphine in the blood. Thus, in patients with high blood ethanol concentrations the additional depressant effects of unconjugated heroin metabolites may contribute to a more acute death.

Anticholinergic drugs

Combining opiates with anticholinergic drugs is a common practice in recreational abuse (SEDA-21, 34). Heroin mixed with hyoscine (scopolamine) is nicknamed "polo" and "point on point." Mixed drug toxicity, with atypical signs and symptoms of opiate abuse, has been reported (39).

- A 41-year-old woman who had taken 11 alprazolam tablets and heroin mixed with an unknown substance developed slurred speech and a staggering gait. She was also taking paroxetine. Her pupils were dilated, her skin warm and dry. Electrocardiography showed a sinus bradycardia. She was given intravenous naloxone 2.0 mg and became acutely agitated and combative. She was delirious, agitated, and disoriented, and was given an intravenous sedative and intubated. Her urine contained codeine, morphine, and atropine.

This case exemplifies the difficulty in identifying anticholinergic drugs such as atropine, and unfortunately the finding of dilated pupils did not raise the suspicion of mixed drug toxicity. The use of naloxone uncovered florid agitation due to anticholinergic drug toxicity.

Interference with Diagnostic Tests

Blood glucose

Diamorphine flattens the glucose tolerance curve and increases glycosylation of HbA_1 (40).

Antithrombin III

Diamorphine depresses the biological activity of antithrombin III (41).

References

1. Serpell MG, Anderson E, Wilson D, Dawson N. I.v. regional diamorphine for analgesia after foot surgery. Br J Anaesth 2000;84(1):95–6.
2. Haemmig RB, Tschacher W. Effects of high-dose heroin versus morphine in intravenous drug users: a randomised double-blind crossover study. J Psychoactive Drugs 2001;33(2):105–10.
3. Riad T, Williams B, Musson J, Wheatley B. Intrathecal morphine compared with diamorphine for postoperative analgesia following unilateral knee arthroplasty. Acute Pain 2002;4:5–8.
4. Cowan CM, Kendall JB, Barclay PM, Wilkes RG. Comparison of intrathecal fentanyl and diamorphine in addition to bupivacaine for caesarean section under spinal anaesthesia. Br J Anaesth 2002;89(3):452–8.
5. Buster M, Rook L, van Brussel GH, van Ree J, van den Brink W. Chasing the dragon, related to the impaired lung function among heroin users. Drug Alcohol Depend 2002;68(2):221–8.
6. Servin FS, Raeder JC, Merle JC, Wattwil M, Hanson AL, Lauwers MH, Aitkenhead A, Marty J, Reite K, Martisson S, Wostyn L. Remifentanil sedation compared with propofol during regional anaesthesia. Acta Anaesthesiol Scand 2002;46(3):309–15.
7. Dettmeyer R, Schmidt P, Musshoff F, Dreisvogt C, Madea B. Pulmonary edema in fatal heroin overdose: immunohistological investigations with IgE, collagen IV and laminin—no increase of defects of alveolar-capillary membranes. Forensic Sci Int 2000;110(2):87–96.
8. Reynes AN, Pujol JA, Baixeras RP, Fernandez B. Edema agudo de pulmon unilateral en paciente con sobredosis do heroina y tratado con naloxona intravenosa. Med Clin (Barc) 1990;94:637.
9. Anderson K. Bronchospasm and intravenous street heroin. Lancet 1986;1(8491):1208.
10. Schoser BG, Groden C. Subacute onset of oculogyric crises and generalized dystonia following intranasal administration of heroin. Addiction 1999;94(3):431–4.
11. Chenery HJ, Murdoch BE. A case of mixed transcortical aphasia following drug overdose. Br J Disord Commun 1986;21(3):381–91.
12. Koussa S, Tamraz J, Nasnas R. Leucoencephalopathy after heroin inhalation. A case with partial regression of MRI lesions. J Neuroradiol 2001;28(4):268–71.
13. McCreary M, Emerman C, Hanna J, Simon J. Acute myelopathy following intranasal insufflation of heroin: a case report. Neurology 2000;55(2):316–17.
14. Lee BF, Chiu NT, Chen WH, Liu GC, Yu HS. Heroin-induced rhabdomyolysis as a cause of reflex sympathetic dystrophy. Clin Nucl Med 2001;26(4):289–92.
15. Kriegstein AR, Shungu DC, Millar WS, Armitage BA, Brust JC, Chillrud S, Goldman J, Lynch T. Leukoencephalopathy and raised brain lactate from heroin vapor inhalation ("chasing the dragon"). Neurology 1999;53(8):1765–73.
16. Wolters EC, van Wijngaarden GK, Stam FC, Rengelink H, Lousberg RJ, Schipper ME, Verbeeten B. Leucoencephalopathy after inhaling "heroin" pyrolysate. Lancet 1982;2(8310):1233–7.
17. Cooley S, Lalchandani S, Keane D. Heroin overdose in pregnancy: an unusual case report. J Obstet Gynaecol 2002;22(2):219–20.
18. Maschke M, Fehlings T, Kastrup O, Wilhelm HW, Leonhardt G. Toxic leukoencephalopathy after intravenous consumption of heroin and cocaine with unexpected clinical recovery. J Neurol 1999;246(9):850–1.
19. Au-Yeung K, Lai C. Toxic leucoencephalopathy after heroin inhalation. Australas Radiol 2002;46(3):306–8.
20. Sayers GM, Green MC, Shaffer RE. Heroin-induced leucoencephalopathy misdiagnosed as psychiatric illness. Int J Psychiatry Clin Pract 2002;6:53–5.
21. Ishiyama A, Ishiyama G, Baloh RW, Evans CJ. Heroin-induced reversible profound deafness and vestibular dysfunction. Addiction 2001;96(9):1363–4.

22. Rice EK, Isbel NM, Becker GJ, Atkins RC, McMahon LP. Heroin overdose and myoglobinuric acute renal failure. Clin Nephrol 2000;54(6):449–54.
23. Dettmeyer R, Stojanovski G, Madea B. Pathogenesis of heroin-associated glomerulonephritis. Correlation between the inflammatory activity and renal deposits of immunoglobulin and complement? Forensic Sci Int 2000;113(1–3):227–31.
24. Llach F, Descoeudres C, Massry SG. Heroin associated nephropathy: clinical and histological studies in 19 patients. Clin Nephrol 1979;11(1):7–12.
25. Rocamora A, Matarredona J, Sendagorta E, Ledo A. Sweat gland necrosis in drug-induced coma: a light and direct immunofluorescence study. J Dermatol 1986;13(1):49–53.
26. Weber M, Diener HC, Voit T, Neuen-Jacob E. Focal myopathy induced by chronic heroin injection is reversible. Muscle Nerve 2000;23(2):274–7.
27. Gervin M, Hughes R, Bamford L, Smyth BP, Keenan E. Heroin smoking by "chasing the dragon" in young opiate users in Ireland: stability and associations with use to "come down" off "Ecstasy". J Subst Abuse Treat 2001;20(4):297–300.
28. Stohler R, Dursteler KM, Stormer R, Seifritz E, Hug I, Sattler-Mayr J, Muller-Spahn F, Ladewig D, Hock C. Rapid cortical hemoglobin deoxygenation after heroin and methadone injection in humans: a preliminary report. Drug Alcohol Depend 1999;57(1):23–8.
29. Smolka M, Schmidt LG. The influence of heroin dose and route of administration on the severity of the opiate withdrawal syndrome. Addiction 1999;94(8):1191–8.
30. Potsch L, Skopp G, Emmerich TP, Becker J, Ogbuhui S. Report on intrauterine drug exposure during second trimester of pregnancy in a heroin-associated death. Ther Drug Monit 1999;21(6):593–7.
31. Stacey R, Jones R, Kar G, Poon A. High-dose intrathecal diamorphine for analgesia after Caesarean section. Anaesthesia 2001;56(1):54–60.
32. Davies M, Crawford I. Towards evidence based emergency medicine: best BETs from the Manchester Royal Infirmary. Nasal diamorphine for acute pain relief in children. Emerg Med J 2001;18(4):271.
33. Kendall JM, Reeves BC, Latter VS; Nasal Diamorphine Trial Group. Multicentre randomised controlled trial of nasal diamorphine for analgesia in children and teenagers with clinical fractures. BMJ 2001;322(7281):261–5.
34. Gopinathan C, Sockalingham I, Fung MA, Peat S, Hanna MH. A comparative study of patient-controlled epidural diamorphine, subcutaneous diamorphine and an epidural diamorphine/bupivacaine combination for postoperative pain. Eur J Anaesthesiol 2000;17(3):189–96.
35. Vaughan DJ, Ahmad N, Lillywhite NK, Lewis N, Thomas D, Robinson PN. Choice of opioid for initiation of combined spinal epidural analgesia in labour—fentanyl or diamorphine. Br J Anaesth 2001;86(4):567–9.
36. Osterwalder JJ. Patients intoxicated with heroin or heroin mixtures: how long should they be monitored? Eur J Emerg Med 1995;2(2):97–101.
37. Brugal MT, Barrio G, De LF, Regidor E, Royuela L, Suelves JM. Factors associated with non-fatal heroin overdose: assessing the effect of frequency and route of heroin administration. Addiction 2002;97(3):319–27.
38. Polettini A, Groppi A, Montagna M. The role of alcohol abuse in the etiology of heroin-related deaths. Evidence for pharmacokinetic interactions between heroin and alcohol. J Anal Toxicol 1999;23(7):570–6.
39. Wang HE. Street drug toxicity resulting from opiates combined with anticholinergics. Prehosp Emerg Care 2002;6(3):351–4.
40. Ceriello A, Giugliano D, Dello Russo P, Sgambato S, D'Onofrio F. Increased glycosylated haemoglobin A_1 in opiate addicts: evidence for a hyperglycaemic effect of morphine. Diabetologia 1982;22(5):379.
41. Ceriello A, Dello Russo P, Curcio F, Tirelli A, Giugliano D. Depressed antithrombin III biological activity in opiate addicts. J Clin Pathol 1984;37(9):1040–2.

Diazepam

See also Benzodiazepines

General Information

Diazepam produces less sedation in cigarette smokers, and higher (not lower, as stated in SEDA-20) doses may be required for the same sedative or anxiolytic effect. Owing in part to its continued widespread use, several unusual adverse effects of diazepam continue to be reported. These include cases of urinary retention and compartment syndrome, which are not explicable by its pharmacology. On the other hand, accumulation of diazepam and attendant complications of obtundation and respiratory depression may be understood in terms of its long half-life, particularly in elderly people and medically ill patients. Caution about the intravenous use of diazepam comes from a study that showed cardiac dysrhythmias (mainly ventricular extra beats) in a quarter of oral surgery patients; midazolam and lorazepam were much safer (1).

Organs and Systems

Cardiovascular

Cases of inadvertent intra-arterial injection of diazepam have been reported.

- A 51-year-old woman with an acute claustrophobic anxiety attack developed gangrene of the fingers after she was inadvertently given diazepam 10 mg intra-arterially (2).
- Inadvertent intra-arterial injection of diazepam (2.5 mg in 0.5 ml) has been reported in an 8-year-old girl (3). Gangrene resulted and amputation of the 4th and 5th fingers was required.

Gangrene has been previously reported with intra-arterial injection of diazepam and is also well known with other classes of drugs, such as barbiturates and phenothiazines. It appears to be caused by the drug rather than the solvent used in the intravenous formulations.

Respiratory

Respiratory difficulties are a major potential adverse effect of rectal diazepam (4).

Of 94 children who presented with seizures, 11 had respiratory depression after intravenous or rectal diazepam (5). However, this finding was challenged (6,7). The authors of the second comment stated that this complication does not occur when rectal diazepam gel is used without other benzodiazepines; they also recommended that during long-term therapy families should be instructed not to give rectal diazepam more than once every 5 days or five times in 1 month.

Patients receiving intravenous benzodiazepines must be monitored for respiratory depression, which may demand artificial ventilation during intensive treatment. Diazepam may cause more respiratory depression than lorazepam at equieffective dosages (SEDA-20, 59) and is contraindicated in neonates for this reason and because it produces unacceptably prolonged sedation (8).

Nervous system

In an open study in 104 patients with acute stroke, diazepam 10 mg bd for 3 days was well tolerated (9).

In a multicenter, double-blind study, 310 patients with generalized anxiety disorder were treated for 6 weeks with abecarnil (mean daily dose 12 mg), diazepam (mean daily dose 22 mg), or placebo in divided doses for 6 weeks (10). Those who had improved at 6 weeks could volunteer to continue double-blind treatment for a total of 24 weeks. Slightly more patients who took diazepam (77%) and placebo (75%) completed the 6-week study than those who took abecarnil (66%). The major adverse events during abecarnil therapy were similar to those of diazepam, namely drowsiness, dizziness, fatigue, and difficulty in coordination. Abecarnil and diazepam both produced statistically significantly more symptom relief than placebo at 1 week, but at 6 weeks only diazepam was superior to placebo. In contrast to diazepam, abecarnil did not cause withdrawal symptoms. The absence of a placebo control makes it difficult to interpret the results of another study of the use of abecarnil and diazepam in alcohol withdrawal, which appeared to show comparable efficacy and adverse effects of the two drugs (11).

The mechanism of rare extrapyramidal effects with diazepam is unexplained (SEDA-18, 44).

Seizures

In a randomized trial, seizures occurred in 14 (16%) of 86 patients with gliomas undergoing contrast CT examinations; however, in 83 other patients with gliomas receiving diazepam prophylaxis, seizures occurred in only two patients (2.2%).

Six patients had untoward effects from excessive rectal diazepam (12). In three cases, seizures reappeared and were interrupted by rectal diazepam, followed by sedation and gradual awakening; the intervals were about 4 days. The other three patients had variable and complex symptoms, with serial seizures and alternating states of tension, apathy, and sleepiness. The plasma concentrations of diazepam and desmethyldiazepam showed rapid fluctuations.

- A 20-year-old man with complex partial seizures presented with exacerbation of his disease (13). He was taking phenytoin and sodium valproate, with plasma concentrations in the target ranges. During a video electroencephalogram recording he was given diazepam 10 mg, and the partial seizures developed into frequent generalized seizures. The same response was seen on a subsequent occasion.

The authors commented that although paradoxical reactions to benzodiazepines are rare, they should be considered in cases of refractory epilepsy.

- A 28-year old man with complex partial status, which lasted for 2 months, had a paradoxical worsening of seizure activity in response to diazepam and midazolam (13).

Neuromuscular function

Muscle rigidity after high-dose opioids can be reduced by the benzodiazepines midazolam and diazepam (SEDA-19, 82).

Psychological, psychiatric

A fugue-like state with retrograde amnesia has been associated with diazepam (14).

- A 23-year-old military officer on active duty took diazepam 5 mg tds and ibuprofen for back spasms. Three days later he was found sitting in a church, having assumed a previous role from his past life. He identified the date as 14 months before and his memory before that time was intact. However, he had no memory of events during the previous 14 months. There were no symptoms suggesting a schizophrenic disorder and his mental function was normal. His symptoms resolved within 24 hours of withdrawal of diazepam, except for amnesia of the event. He assumed his correct identity and was aware of the correct date. He had taken ibuprofen in the past with no adverse effects and this was his first exposure to a benzodiazepine. No other medications were involved and a full medical review found no cause for his symptoms other than diazepam use.

Endocrine

Gynecomastia, with raised estradiol, has been reported in men taking diazepam (15).

Skin

Cutaneous adverse effects of diazepam are rare. The incidence was 0.4 per 1000 in the Boston Collaborative Surveillance Program (16).

- A 50-year-old woman was referred to hospital for chronic depression with alcohol dependence (17). There was no history of drug allergy. She was given oral thioridazine 100 mg/day and diazepam 10 mg qds. After 2 days she noticed an erythematous eruption on her ankles. Thioridazine was withdrawn, but the eruption became more erythematous and affected both extremities and flanks within a few hours. She was given methylprednisolone 80 mg/day. The next day the eruption became bullous and she became pyrexial (39.4°C). Urea and creatinine concentrations were normal. Blood cultures were negative. A skin biopsy showed bullous vasculitis with numerous eosinophils in the dermis. Diazepam was then withdrawn, the pyrexia resolved, and the skin lesions healed, although post-inflammatory ulcers persisted on both ankles for 2 months. A lymphocyte blast transformation test was positive for diazepam.

Sweet's syndrome has been attributed to diazepam (18).

- A 70-year-old white man, with no significant preceding medical history, developed an acute painful rash, a fever (38.4°C), and severe arthralgia 5 days after starting to take diazepam 10 mg bd for lumbar muscular contracture due to hard physical exercise. He had taken no other medications. There were well-defined purple-red skin plaques, surmounted by vesicular and hemorrhagic blisters. He had a leukocytosis. Sweet's syndrome was confirmed by punch biopsy of a lesion. Diazepam was withdrawn, and prednisolone 30 mg/day was given for 2 weeks and then tapered. The patient improved quickly and the eruption cleared in 10 days.

Immunologic

Hypersensitivity reactions after diazepam are very rare and usually mild. However, some severe reactions have been reported.

- A 50-year-old woman with chronic depression or dysthymic disorder and alcohol dependence was given oral thioridazine 100 mg/day and diazepam 10 mg qds (19). She had no history of drug allergy. Two days later she noticed an erythematous eruption on her ankles. Thioridazine was withdrawn, but the eruption became more widespread over a few hours. She was given methylprednisolone 80 mg/day, but the following day the eruption progressively became bullous and her condition worsened. She developed a fever of 39.4°C, felt ill, and had a neutrophilia, but blood cultures were sterile and her renal function was normal. A skin biopsy showed bullous vasculitis with numerous eosinophils in the dermis. Diazepam was then withdrawn, which led to resolution of pyrexia and gradual healing of the skin lesions over the next 2 months. The lymphocyte blast transformation test was positive for diazepam.
- A 28-year-old nurse had generalized urticaria and collapsed while she was undergoing a gastroscopy for suspected *Helicobacter pylori* infection (20). Before the start of the procedure she was given lidocaine oral spray and intravenous diazepam 10 mg, and at the end intravenous flumazenil 1 mg. Skin prick tests and intradermal tests with diazepam 5 mg/ml produced a weal-and-flare reaction; flumazenil 0.1 mg/ml and lidocaine 2% had no effect.

Although in the second case, for safety reasons, a challenge test was not performed, it was suggested that the reaction had been IgE-mediated.

Second-Generation Effects

Fetotoxicity

Postnatal, longitudinal, somatic, neurological, mental, and behavioral development has been studied at birth and at 8, 15, and 24 months of life in children whose mothers had been treated during pregnancy with diazepam ($n = 126$) or promethazine ($n = 127$) and in children whose mothers had not been exposed (21). The children in the diazepam group weighed less at birth but not at 8 months or subsequently.

Diazepam has been reported to cause inappropriate ADH secretion in a neonate (22).

- A female infant was delivered vaginally at 41 weeks. Her 30-year-old mother had taken diazepam for epilepsy and hysterical attacks throughout the pregnancy. The pregnancy and delivery were uneventful. The baby was admitted to the neonatal ward in anticipation of neonatal drug withdrawal syndrome. On the first day of life, milk feeding was stopped because of poor sucking, vomiting, and increased gastric aspirate volume. On the same day oliguria was reported and the urine osmolality was increased. Secretion of antidiuretic hormone was suspected as the cause of the oliguria, and so fluid intake was restricted and a diuretic was given. Subsequently the urine output increased and the urine osmolality gradually fell. The baby's condition became stable and she was discharged on day 16.

Susceptibility Factors

Age

Five neonates who suffered an unexpected long period of respiratory failure, muscular hypotonia, and drowsiness were retrospectively investigated (8). Unusually high doses of diazepam had been given by intravenous bolus injection and serum concentrations of diazepam and its active metabolites were high. The authors emphasized the persistence of the very long-acting *N*-desmethyldiazepam, particularly in neonates and even more exaggeratedly in premature infants, owing to reduced capacity of hepatic uridine diphosphate glucuronyl transferase activity (8).

Drug Administration

Drug administration route

Although intravenous diazepam is the preferred route, the undiluted intravenous solution of diazepam can be given rectally, and is effective in the emergency management of seizures in children (23). Rectal gel is an alternative, and can be given by non-medical personnel (24). Adverse effects of rectal diazepam are rare and mild. Animal studies and clinical experience have not shown damage to the rectal mucosa.

Drug overdose

- A 54-year-old man took 2 g of laboratory-grade diazepam and was treated with activated charcoal, diuresis, and flumazenil infusion (25). He wakened, but had drowsiness, dysarthria, diplopia, and dizziness for 9 days. Blood concentrations of diazepam and its main metabolite, *N*-desmethyldiazepam, remained high for over 4 weeks.

Of 149 patients, 10 received an overdose of rectal diazepam indicated for acute repetitive seizures (51 overdoses in total) (26). There were no untoward events in 40 cases, and the adverse events were most often not drug-related. No patient had bradypnea or apnea.

Drug–Drug Interactions

Antihistamines

Drugs that depress the CNS, such as the benzodiazepines, have their effects increased by interaction with the classic antihistamines. However, the second-generation antihistamines have not yet been proven to interact with CNS depressants such as alcohol or diazepam (27–30).

Antiepileptic drugs

Some interactions of diazepam with antiepileptic drugs are listed in Table 2 in the monograph on antiepileptic drugs.

Beta-adrenoceptor antagonists

Lipophilic beta-adrenoceptor antagonists are metabolized to varying degrees by oxidation by liver microsomal cytochrome P450 (for example propranolol by CYP1A2 and CYP2D6 and metoprolol by CYP2D6). They can therefore reduce the clearance and increase the steady-state plasma concentrations of other drugs that undergo similar metabolism, potentiating their effects. Drugs that interact in this way include diazepam (31).

Bupivacaine

Animal studies have shown that diazepam can prolong the half-life of bupivacaine (32).

Caffeine

At least 40 drugs interact with caffeine, including benzodiazepines (for example diazepam, whose sedative effect is counteracted by caffeine) (33).

Cholinesterase inhibitors

Although diazepam does not have anticholinergic properties, it is possible to reverse diazepam-induced delirium by the use of cholinesterase inhibitors, such as physostigmine; however, physostigmine can on occasion induce severe arterial hypertension, especially if the dose exceeds 2 mg intravenously. In healthy volunteers sedated with diazepam, an increase in awareness was established with the use of physostigmine, but there was also a reduction in ventilatory drive (SEDA-10, 119).

Cisapride

Cisapride increases the absorption of diazepam (34).

Clozapine

Hypotension, collapse, and respiratory arrest occurred when low doses (12.5–25 mg) of clozapine were added to a pre-existing diazepam regimen (SEDA-22, 41).

- A 50-year-old man with symptoms of chronic paranoid schizophrenia resistant to typical neuroleptic drugs had a brief syncopal attack with significant electrocardiographic changes (sinus bradycardia and deep anteroseptal inverted T waves and minor ST segment changes) after the dosage of clozapine was increased to 300 mg/day while he was taking diazepam 30 mg/day (35).

The mechanism of this presumed interaction is unknown.

Disulfiram

Disulfiram inhibits hepatic drug metabolism and can prolong the effects of substances that are normally metabolized in the liver. This has been studied for various benzodiazepines. The clearances of chlordiazepoxide and diazepam were significantly reduced and their half-lives prolonged by disulfiram (36).

Heparin

In healthy non-fasting subjects, 100–1000 IU of heparin given intravenously caused a rapid increase in the unbound fractions of chlordiazepoxide, diazepam, and oxazepam (37,38), but no change in the case of lorazepam (37). The clinical implications of this finding are not known.

Ibuprofen

The effect of diazepam on the pharmacokinetics of ibuprofen has been studied in eight healthy subjects, who took ibuprofen or ibuprofen plus diazepam at 10.00 or 22.00 hours in a randomized, crossover study (39). Diazepam significantly prolonged the half-life of ibuprofen at 22.00 hours but not at 10.00 hours. The mean clearance of ibuprofen was therefore reduced by diazepam at night. This time-dependent effect of diazepam on the pharmacokinetics of ibuprofen may be due to circadian variation in the pattern of protein production in the liver and/or competitive protein binding of the two drugs during the night.

Lithium

There has been a well-documented case of profound hypothermia in a patient taking lithium and diazepam; it did not occur with either drug alone (40). Otherwise, benzodiazepines and lithium are compatible.

Naltrexone

The effects of naltrexone on diazepam intoxication were investigated in 26 non-drug-abusing subjects who received either naltrexone 50 mg or placebo and 90 minutes later oral diazepam 10 mg in a double-blind, crossover trial (41). Naltrexone was significantly associated with negative mood states, such as sedation, fatigue, and anxiety, compared with placebo, while positive states (friendliness, vigor, liking the effects of diazepam, feeling high from diazepam) were significantly more common with placebo. Naltrexone significantly delayed the time to peak diazepam concentrations (135 minutes) compared with placebo (75 minutes), but there were no significant differences in the concentrations of nordiazepam, the main metabolite of diazepam, at any stage in the study.

Omeprazole

In human liver microsomes, the metabolism of diazepam was mainly to 3-hydroxydiazepam (90%); omeprazole inhibited this conversion (42).

In a double blind, placebo-controlled, crossover study in eight white and seven Chinese men who were extensive metabolizers of debrisoquine and mephenytoin, omeprazole 40 mg/day reduced the oral clearance of diazepam by 38% and increased desmethyldiazepam AUC by 42%. In contrast, in the Chinese men the oral clearance of diazepam fell by only 21% and desmethyldiazepam AUC by 25%. The authors concluded that the extent of the inhibitory effect of omeprazole on diazepam metabolism depends on ethnicity (43). Differences between Caucasians and Asians may account for such effects.

Penicillamine

In one patient the use of penicillamine led to exacerbation of phlebitis that had been caused by intravenous diazepam (44).

References

1. Roelofse JA, van der Bijl P. Cardiac dysrhythmias associated with intravenous lorazepam, diazepam, and midazolam during oral surgery. J Oral Maxillofac Surg 1994;52(3):247–50.
2. Joist A, Tibesku CO, Neuber M, Frerichmann U, Joosten U. Fingergangrän nach akziden teller intraarterieller Injektion von Diazepam. [Gangrene of the fingers caused by accidental intra-arterial injection of diazepam.] Dtsch Med Wochenschr 1999;124(24):755–8.
3. Derakshan MR. Amputation due to inadvertent intra-arterial diazepam injection. Iran J Med Sci 2000;25:84–6.
4. Dooley JM. Rectal use of benzodiazepines. Epilepsia 1998;39(Suppl 1):S24–7.
5. Norris E, Marzouk O, Nunn A, McIntyre J, Choonara I. Respiratory depression in children receiving diazepam for acute seizures: a prospective study. Dev Med Child Neurol 1999;41(5):340–3.
6. Mackereth S. Use of rectal diazepam in the community. Dev Med Child Neurol 2000;42(11):785.
7. Kriel RL, Cloyd JC, Pellock JM. Respiratory depression in children receiving diazepam for acute seizures: a prospective study. Dev Med Child Neurol 2000;42(6):429–30.
8. Peinemann F, Daldrup T. Severe and prolonged sedation in five neonates due to persistence of active diazepam metabolites. Eur J Pediatr 2001;160(6):378–81.
9. Lodder J, Luijckx G, van Raak L, Kessels F. Diazepam treatment to increase the cerebral GABAergic activity in acute stroke: a feasibility study in 104 patients. Cerebrovasc Dis 2000;10(6):437–40.
10. Rickels K, DeMartinis N, Aufdembrinke B. A double-blind, placebo-controlled trial of abecarnil and diazepam in the treatment of patients with generalized anxiety disorder. J Clin Psychopharmacol 2000;20(1):12–18.
11. Anton RF, Kranzler HR, McEvoy JP, Moak DH, Bianca R. A double-blind comparison of abecarnil and diazepam in the treatment of uncomplicated alcohol withdrawal. Psychopharmacology (Berl) 1997;131(2):123–9.
12. Brodtkorb E, Aamo T, Henriksen O, Lossius R. Rectal diazepam: pitfalls of excessive use in refractory epilepsy. Epilepsy Res 1999;35(2):123–33.
13. Al Tahan A. Paradoxic response to diazepam in complex partial status epilepticus. Arch Med Res 2000;31(1):101–4.
14. Simmer ED. A fugue-like state associated with diazepam use. Mil Med 1999;164(6):442–3.
15. Bergman D, Futterweit W, Segal R, Sirota D. Increased oestradiol in diazepam-related gynaecomastia. Lancet 1981;2(8257):1225–6.
16. Bigby M, Jick S, Jick H, Arndt K. Drug-induced cutaneous reactions. A report from the Boston Collaborative Drug Surveillance Program on 15,438 consecutive inpatients, 1975 to 1982. JAMA 1986;256(24):3358–63.
17. Olcina GM, Simonart T. Severe vasculitis after therapy with diazepam. Am J Psychiatry 1999;156(6):972–3.
18. Guimera FJ, Garcia-Bustinduy M, Noda A, Saez M, Dorta S, Sanchez R, Martin-Herrera A, Garcia-Montelongo R. Diazepam-associated Sweet's syndrome. Int J Dermatol 2000;39(10):795–8.
19. Olcina GM, Simonart T. Severe vasculitis after therapy with diazepam. Am J Psychiatry 1999;156(6):972–3.
20. Asero R. Hypersensitivity to diazepam. Allergy 2002;57(12):1209.
21. Czeizel AE, Szegal BA, Joffe JM, Racz J. The effect of diazepam and promethazine treatment during pregnancy on the somatic development of human offspring. Neurotoxicol Teratol 1999;21(2):157–67.
22. Nako Y, Tachibana A, Harigaya A, Tomomasa T, Morikawa A. Syndrome of inappropriate secretion of antidiuretic hormone complicating neonatal diazepam withdrawal. Acta Paediatr 2000;89(4):488–9.
23. Seigler RS. The administration of rectal diazepam for acute management of seizures. J Emerg Med 1990;8(2):155–9.
24. Shafer PO. New therapies in the management of acute or cluster seizures and seizure emergencies. J Neurosci Nurs 1999;31(4):224–30.
25. de Haro L, Valli M, Bourdon JH, Iliadis A, Hayek-Lanthois M, Arditti J. Diazepam poisoning with one--month monitoring of diazepam and nordiazepam blood levels. Vet Hum Toxicol 2001;43(3):174–5.
26. Brown L, Bergen DC, Kotagal P, Groves L, Carson D. Safety of Diastat when given at larger-than-recommended doses for acute repetitive seizures. Neurology 2001;56(8):1112.
27. Bhatti JZ, Hindmarch I. The effects of terfenadine with and without alcohol on an aspect of car driving performance. Clin Exp Allergy 1989;19(6):609–11.
28. Moser L, Huther KJ, Koch-Weser J, Lundt PV. Effects of terfenadine and diphenhydramine alone or in combination with diazepam or alcohol on psychomotor performance and subjective feelings. Eur J Clin Pharmacol 1978;14(6):417–23.
29. Rombaut N, Heykants J, Vanden Bussche G. Potential of interaction between the H_1-antagonist astemizole and other drugs. Ann Allergy 1986;57(5):321–4.
30. Doms M, Vanhulle G, Baelde Y, Coulie P, Dupont P, Rihoux JP. Lack of potentiation by cetirizine of alcohol-induced psychomotor disturbances. Eur J Clin Pharmacol 1988;34(6):619–23.
31. Ochs HR, Greenblatt DJ, Verburg-Ochs B. Propranolol interactions with diazepam, lorazepam, and alprazolam. Clin Pharmacol Ther 1984;36(4):451–5.
32. Yan AC, Newman RD. Bupivacaine-induced seizures and ventricular fibrillation in a 13-year-old girl undergoing wound debridement. Pediatr Emerg Care 1998;14(5):354–5.
33. Mattila MJ, Nuotto E. Caffeine and theophylline counteract diazepam effects in man. Med Biol 1983;61(6):337–43.
34. Bateman DN. The action of cisapride on gastric emptying and the pharmacodynamics and pharmacokinetics of oral diazepam. Eur J Clin Pharmacol 1986;30(2):205–8.

35. Tupala E, Niskanen L, Tiihonen J. Transient syncope and ECG changes associated with the concurrent administration of clozapine and diazepam. J Clin Psychiatry 1999;60(9):619–20.
36. MacLeod SM, Sellers EM, Giles HG, Billings BJ, Martin PR, Greenblatt DJ, Marshman JA. Interaction of disulfiram with benzodiazepines. Clin Pharmacol Ther 1978;24(5):583–9.
37. Desmond PV, Roberts RK, Wood AJ, Dunn GD, Wilkinson GR, Schenker S. Effect of heparin administration on plasma binding of benzodiazepines. Br J Clin Pharmacol 1980;9(2):171–5.
38. Routledge PA, Kitchell BB, Bjornsson TD, Skinner T, Linnoila M, Shand DG. Diazepam and N-desmethyldiazepam redistribution after heparin. Clin Pharmacol Ther 1980;27(4):528–32.
39. Bapuji AT, Rambhau D, Srinivasu P, Rao BR, Apte SS. Time dependent influence of diazepam on the pharmacokinetics of ibuprofen in man. Drug Metabol Drug Interact 1999;15(1):71–81.
40. Naylor GJ, McHarg A. Profound hypothermia on combined lithium carbonate and diazepam treatment. BMJ 1977;2(6078):22.
41. Swift R, Davidson D, Rosen S, Fitz E, Camara P. Naltrexone effects on diazepam intoxication and pharmacokinetics in humans. Psychopharmacology (Berl) 1998;135(3):256–62.
42. Zomorodi K, Houston JB. Diazepam–omeprazole inhibition interaction: an in vitro investigation using human liver microsomes. Br J Clin Pharmacol 1996;42(2):157–62.
43. Caraco Y, Tateishi T, Wood AJ. Interethnic difference in omeprazole's inhibition of diazepam metabolism. Clin Pharmacol Ther 1995;58(1):62–72.
44. Brandstetter RD, Gotz VP, Mar DD, Sachs D. Exacerbation of diazepam-induced phlebitis by oral penicillamine. BMJ (Clin Res Ed) 1981;283(6290):525.

Diazoxide

General Information

Diazoxide is a direct vasodilator that acts on vascular smooth muscle to produce systemic vasodilatation. As a result there is baroreceptor-mediated activation of the sympathetic nervous system and the renin–angiotensin system.

Vasodilators (as monotherapy) are associated acutely with flushing, headache, dizziness, reflex tachycardia, and palpitation. Chronic treatment can be complicated by fluid retention.

Organs and Systems

Cardiovascular

Rapid administration of diazoxide intravenously can cause severe hypotension. In some cases this has resulted in abnormal neurological signs associated with ischemic damage (1).

Metabolism

Diazoxide can cause hyperglycemia and diabetes mellitus and has been used to treat hyperinsulinism in infancy, although its use may be hazardous (2,3).

References

1. Ledingham JG, Rajagopalan B. Cerebral complications in the treatment of accelerated hypertension. Q J Med 1979;48(189):25–41.
2. Low LC, Yu EC, Chow OK, Yeung CY, Young RT. Hyperinsulinism in infancy. Aust Paediatr J 1989; 25(3):174–7.
3. Abu-Osba YK, Manasra KB, Mathew PM. Complications of diazoxide treatment in persistent neonatal hyperinsulinism. Arch Dis Child 1989;64(10):1496–500.

Dibenzepin

See also Tricyclic antidepressants

General Information

Dibenzepin is a 6,7,6 tricyclic compound of the dibenzodiazepine type. A comparison with imipramine was said to show equal efficacy; adverse effects were comparable in type and degree (1).

Reference

1. Sim M, Armitage GH, Davies WH, Gordon EB. The treatment of depressive states: a comparative trial of dibenzepin (Noveril) with imipramine (Tofranil). Clin Trial J 1971;1:29.

Dibromopropamidine

General Information

Dibromopropamidine in a cream base is used to treat herpesvirus skin lesions.

Organs and Systems

Immunologic

Contact allergy is infrequently reported with dibromopropamidine.

- A 40-year-old man with genital herpes and an acute edematous vesicobullous dermatitis on his penile shaft had a positive patch test with dibromopropamidine and not the other ingredients of the cream (1).

Reference

1. Selvaag E. Contact allergy to dibromopropamidine cream. Contact Dermatitis 1999;40(1):58.

Dichloralphenazone

General Information

Dichloralphenazone is a complex of phenazone (antipyrine) and chloral hydrate, which dissociates in aqueous solution. It has been used as a hypnotic but is obsolete. Its adverse effects are those of its components (1,2).

Drug Interactions

Phenytoin

The phenazone component of dichloralphenazone is an enzyme inducer and hastens the metabolism of phenytoin (3).

Warfarin

The phenazone component of dichloralphenazone is an enzyme inducer and hastens the metabolism of warfarin (4).

References

1. Limb DG. Anaphylaxis after dichloralphenazone treatment. BMJ 1977;2(6100):1480.
2. Perl S. Anaphylaxis after dichloralphenazone treatment. BMJ 1977;2(6096):1187–8.
3. Riddell JG, Salem SA, McDevitt DG. Interaction between phenytoin and dichloralphenazone. Br J Clin Pharmacol 1980;9(1):118P.
4. Breckenridge A, Orme ML, Thorgeirsson S, Davies DS, Brooks RV. Drug interactions with warfarin: studies with dichloralphenazone, chloral hydrate and phenazone (antipyrine). Clin Sci 1971;40(4):351–64.

Dichlorophen

General Information

Dichlorophen is an antihelminthic drug that was used in the treatment of tapeworm infections but has been superseded by praziquantel and niclosamide. It also has antifungal and antibacterial activity and has been used topically in the treatment of fungal infections and as a germicide in soaps and cosmetics (1).

During the first few hours after taking a single oral dose one-third of patients have nausea, diarrhea, or abdominal pain, and some experience vomiting. Urticaria, contact allergic dermatitis, and photosensitivity can occur. In the past, with larger doses, jaundice and even hepatic necrosis have been described.

Reference

1. Yamarik TA. Safety assessment of dichlorophene and chlorophene. Int J Toxicol 2004;23(Suppl 1):1–27.

Diclofenac

See also Non-steroidal anti-inflammatory drugs

General Information

The overall incidence of adverse reactions to diclofenac is about 30%, but less than 1% of patients have to have treatment withdrawn for this reason. The manufacturers' analysis of 1966 adverse effects in 987 patients over about 6 years, when over 30 million patients had been treated, provided some interesting quantitative data. Of the total number of adverse reactions, 34% were gastrointestinal and 16% hematological. Worldwide experience with diclofenac showed that the incidences of serious adverse drug reactions in phase III short-term trials (1227 patients) and long-term trials (1173 patients) in the USA were respectively as follows (1):

- peptic ulcer 0.16 and 0.34%;
- gastrointestinal bleeding 0.16 and 0.17%;
- hepatitis 0 and 0.26%;
- thrombocytopenia 0 and 0.17%.

Organs and Systems

Respiratory

Diclofenac caused eosinophilic pneumonitis in a 67-year-old man (SEDA-18, 103).

Nervous system

The frequency of central nervous system adverse effects is 1–9%. Headache, dizziness, vertigo, insomnia, drowsiness, and agitation have been reported. Hallucinatory symptoms and generalized tonic-clonic seizures have also been described (SEDA-16, 109). Toxic encephalitis can be part of a general toxic reaction (2). Diclofenac provoked aseptic meningitis in patients with systemic lupus erythematosus (SEDA-17, 109).

Sensory systems

Hyperemia, burning of the eyes, eyelid allergic contact dermatitis, and conjunctivitis can occur in patients who use diclofenac eye-drops (SEDA-20, 92) (SEDA-21, 104).

Diclofenac can cause reduced corneal sensitivity, starting from 15 minutes after instillation and measurable after 1 hour (3). This corneal hypesthesia can be useful in reducing pain and discomfort in ocular inflammation and after surgery. In chronic treatment, however, the effect of diclofenac on corneal nerves can cause either increased healing time of the corneal epithelium or a neurotrophic epitheliopathy in patients with conditions that predispose to epithelial damage, such as dry eyes. In contrast, flurbiprofen, indometacin, and ketorolac tromethamine did not cause corneal hypesthesia.

Electrolyte balance

Severe hyponatremia developed in an elderly woman treated with intramuscular diclofenac (SEDA-13, 80).

NSAIDs can cause hyperkalemic acidosis and should be used with caution in the presence of renal impairment (4).

- A 76-year-old woman developed quadriparesis associated with hyperkalemia after taking diclofenac 100 mg/day for 10 months for gouty arthritis. She had a metabolic acidosis with a normal anion gap and mild renal impairment. Her weakness resolved after withdrawal of diclofenac and correction of the hyperkalemia.

Mineral balance

At least three reports of severe hyponatremia have been described (SEDA-12, 85) (SEDA-13, 80) (SEDA-18, 103). In the last case the withdrawal of diclofenac and fluid restriction led to normal fluid and electrolyte balance within 10 days, despite concomitant treatment with nabumetone.

Hematologic

In an analysis of 447 adverse effects in 194 patients worldwide (5), 20 had blood abnormalities, including two cases of agranulocytosis and one of granulocytopenia. One of these patients, who was sensitive to pyrazolone, had taken a pyrazolone compound as well. Immune-mediated agranulocytosis and thrombocytopenia have been reported (SEDA-16, 110).

Reversible hemolytic anemia (SEDA-4, 69) (6), two cases of severe immune hemolytic anemia with acute renal insufficiency (SEDA-20, 92) (SEDA-22, 115), and fatal hemolytic anemia have occurred (7).

Diclofenac can cause panmyelopathy (8). Data from the International Agranulocytosis and Aplastic Anemia Study showed an increased risk of aplastic anemia (multivariate rate-ratio 8.8) (9). Fatal aplastic anemia has also been described (SEDA-4, 69) (10), as have purpura and thrombocytopenia, although not always with certainty. Spontaneous bleeding (subcutaneous bruises, hematoma, greater wound drainage) has been associated with diclofenac (SEDA-15, 100).

Gastrointestinal

Gastrointestinal adverse effects are particularly frequent, and affect some 14–25% of patients; the incidence of the most serious, peptic ulcer and bleeding were 0.16–0.34% and 0.16–0.17%, respectively (1). A prospective 12-week endoscopic study documented better gastrointestinal tolerability with diclofenac than naproxen (SEDA-20, 92). Upper gastrointestinal hemorrhage has been associated with transdermal application of diclofenac, with massive bleeding in two of four patients (SEDA-21, 104).

Perforation of the terminal ileum occurred in one patient who had taken a high dose (400 mg/day) of modified-release diclofenac (11).

Colonic stricture, similar to ileum "diaphragm" disease, developed in a patient during prolonged administration of modified-release diclofenac (12). Pseudomembranous colitis and colonic ulceration, with or without a diaphragm-like colonic stricture, have been reported (SEDA-16, 110) (SEDA-17, 109). Dispersible diclofenac is a formulation from which absorption is more rapid than the usual formulation, but gastrointestinal adverse events still occur (SEDA-20, 92).

Rectal administration caused adverse effects in 16% of patients (13); anorectal lesions (erosions, ulcers, stenosis of the anal margin) occurred after a relatively short period of suppository use (14).

Liver

Liver function can be impaired during diclofenac treatment, and liver damage may be more common than previously thought (SEDA-10, 83) (15). The risk is the same as with the few other NSAIDs that have been adequately studied. Biopsy-proven hepatitis with positive rechallenge and dechallenge has been described (16) and confirmed (17,18). The usual clinical presentation is acute hepatitis, but chronic active hepatitis has been described (17–20). Although recovery is usually rapid in the acute form after drug withdrawal, fatal cases have occurred (SEDA-11, 93) (SEDA-12, 85) (SEDA-13, 80) (21). Diclofenac-induced fulminant hepatic failure has been successfully treated with liver transplantation (22). Patients who developed combined reversible hepatorenal damage have also been reported (23–25) (SEDA-20, 91).

In a retrospective study, two-thirds of cases were detected by symptoms (jaundice, anorexia, nausea, vomiting, with or without fever) (26). The illness developed more than 5 weeks after starting diclofenac in more than 75% of patients, and within six months in 85%. Liver injury was classified as hepatocellular in 54% of patients and the histology was acute hepatocellular injury (nine patients) and chronic hepatitis (six patients). Factors affecting the susceptibility to diclofenac liver damage were sex (female) and type of disease (osteoarthritis). The mechanism of diclofenac-induced liver injury is unknown, but since the incidence is very low an idiosyncratic mechanism rather than intrinsic toxicity of the drug seems likely. In view of the rarity of hallmarks of hypersensitivity, the delayed development of injury and the delayed response to rechallenge, a metabolic effect rather than immunological idiosyncratic mechanism seems probable in most cases. The usefulness of monitoring serum enzymes is unknown, but it might be prudent to do so in the first 6 months of treatment.

Urinary tract

Renal papillary necrosis and interstitial nephritis with the nephrotic syndrome have been documented (27,28). Other cases of the nephrotic syndrome, with or without renal insufficiency, which were apparently due to minimal-change nephropathy (which is relatively more common in NSAID users), have been reported (29,30). The unusual feature of diclofenac-associated renal interstitial mucinosis has been described (SEDA-17, 109). Functional renal insufficiency after the use of diclofenac in a patient with burns has been described (SEDA-20, 92).

Skin

Allergic skin rashes, serous bullous dermatitis with positive rechallenge, and linear IgA deposits along the basal membrane in lesional and perilesional skin have all been reported (31). A patient who developed Stevens–Johnson syndrome died (SEDA-5, 103). Contact dermatitis and a generalized maculopapular eruption caused by delayed hypersensitivity to diclofenac have been reported with topical and oral diclofenac (SEDA-18, 104). Photosensitivity after topical application has been described (SEDA-22, 115). Diclofenac triggered pemphigus vulgaris, an uncommon manifestation of NSAID toxicity (SEDA-22, 115).

- Contact dermatitis on the eyelids developed in a 70-year-old-woman after she had used eye-drops containing diclofenac. Patch tests were positive to both diclofenac and indometacin, suggesting possible cross-reactivity between the two compounds (32).
- Staphylococcal scalded skin syndrome developed in a 68-year-old man after he had taken diclofenac for knee arthritis subsequently diagnosed as septic arthritis due to *Staphylococcus aureus* (33).

NSAIDs can predispose to severe infections (SEDA-22, 112).

Nicolau syndrome (embolia cutis medicamentosa) is a very rare complication of intramuscular injections, in which there is extensive necrosis of the injected skin area, perhaps due to accidental intra-arterial and/or para-arterial injection; it usually occurs in children (34). Of the NSAIDs with which it has been reported, diclofenac is the most common (35–38).

Musculoskeletal

Massive rhabdomyolysis resulting in renal insufficiency with complete recovery after withdrawal has been described in a man who took diclofenac for 2 weeks (SEDA-21, 104).

Immunologic

Acute allergic reactions were reported in 48 patients, and included anaphylactic or anaphylactoid reactions and angioedema without shock. Two anaphylactic reactions, one fatal, to parenteral diclofenac have been reported (SEDA-18, 104). Hepatorenal damage (SEDA-15, 100), thrombocytopenia, and hemolytic anemia mediated by an immune mechanism have been reported (SEDA-16, 110).

Skin tests with diclofenac were not useful in diagnosing hypersensitivity in a series of 12 non-atopic patients who had severe symptoms of hypersensitivity (39). However, oral challenge in patients who had had only cutaneous symptoms was diagnostic.

Second-Generation Effects

Fertility

Three cases of infertility have been reported with diclofenac (SEDA-21, 104).

Fetotoxicity

As inhibitors of cyclo-oxygenase, NSAIDs given during pregnancy can cause adverse maternal and fetal effects (SEDA-22, 112).

- Premature closure of the ductus arteriosus occurred in a fetus who was exposed in utero to diclofenac at 34–35 weeks of gestation (40). Emergency cesarean section was performed and the baby girl required cardiorespiratory support and multiple medications. She gradually improved and further development was normal.

Susceptibility Factors

The Japanese Health Authority has sent a "Dear Doctor" letter warning against the use of diclofenac in patients with encephalitis or encephalopathy related to influenza, which may be associated with higher mortality (41).

Drug Administration

Drug administration route

Aseptic tissue necrosis after intramuscular injection (Nicolau syndrome) has been reported after accidental intra-arterial injection. Antirheumatic drugs are often involved in these reactions and diclofenac has also been implicated (42). Other consequences of intramuscular administration of diclofenac are asymptomatic high serum creatine kinase activity or damage to muscle, nerve, or blood vessels (SEDA-17, 109).

Necrotizing fasciitis was reported in three patients, two of whom died as a consequence of severe local reactions associated with intramuscular diclofenac (43).

If appropriately diluted and infused intravenously, diclofenac is usually well tolerated, although local venous thrombosis has been described (SEDA-17, 109).

Drug–Drug Interactions

Ciclosporin

The risk of ciclosporin-induced nephrotoxicity can be increased when NSAIDs are also used (44,45). Diclofenac in particular should be avoided, because it is more likely to cause deterioration of renal function in patients taking ciclosporin (SEDA-15, 100) (SEDA-17, 107). There is also a pharmacokinetic interaction, which may be caused by inhibition by ciclosporin of the first-pass metabolism of diclofenac (SEDA-21, 104).

In 16 healthy volunteers there were no important pharmacokinetic changes when a single dose of ciclosporin was taken during steady-state administration of aspirin, indometacin, or piroxicam, but there was an interaction with diclofenac, whose AUC was doubled in the presence of ciclosporin (46).

In patients with rheumatoid arthritis, steady-state coadministration of diclofenac with ciclosporin was associated with a significant rise in serum creatinine concentration.

Lithium

Diclofenac increases serum lithium concentrations by impairing its renal excretion (47).

Triamterene

The interaction between diclofenac and triamterene causes renal impairment (48).

Interference with Diagnostic Tests

Thyroid hormone tests

Diclofenac alters thyroid hormone tests, causing a fall in total serum triiodothyronine, principally by interfering with its serum protein binding (SEDA-19, 98).

References

1. Catalano MA. Worldwide safety experience with diclofenac. Am J Med 1986;80(4B):81–7.
2. Bandelot JB, Mihout B. Encephalopathie myoclonique au diclofénac. [Myoclonic encephalopathy due to diclofenac.] Nouv Presse Med 1978;7(16):1406.
3. Aragona P, Tripodi G, Spinella R, Lagana E, Ferreri G. The effects of the topical administration of non-steroidal anti-inflammatory drugs on corneal epithelium and corneal sensitivity in normal subjects. Eye 2000;14(Pt 2):206–10.
4. Patel P, Mandal B, Greenway MW. Hyperkalaemic quadriparesis secondary to chronic diclofenac treatment. Postgrad Med J 2001;77(903):50–1.
5. Ciucci AG. A review of spontaneously reported adverse drug reactions with diclofenac sodium (Voltarol). Rheumatol Rehabil 1979;(Suppl 2):116–21.
6. Salama A, Gottsche B, Mueller-Eckhardt C. Autoantibodies and drug- or metabolite-dependent antibodies in patients with diclofenac-induced immune haemolysis. Br J Haematol 1991;77(4):546–9.
7. Heuft HG, Postels H, Hoppe I, Weisbach V, Zeiler T, Zingsem J, Eckstein R. Eine todlich verlaufene immunhämolytische Anämie nach Applikation von Diclofenac. [Fatal course of immune hemolytic anemia following administration of diclofenac.] Beitr Infusionsther 1990;26:412–14.
8. Porzsolt F, Heit W, Heimpel H, Asbeck F. Panmyelopathie nach Einnahme von Diclofenac? [Panmyelopathy after administration of diclofenac?] Dtsch Med Wochenschr 1979;104(27):986–7.
9. The International Agranulocytosis and Aplastic Anemia Study. Risks of agranulocytosis and aplastic anemia. A first report of their relation to drug use with special reference to analgesics. JAMA 1986;256(13):1749–57.
10. Eustace S, O'Neill T, McHale S, Molony J. Fatal aplastic anaemia following prolonged diclofenac use in an elderly patient. Ir J Med Sci 1989;158(8):217.
11. Deakin M. Small bowel perforation associated with an excessive dose of slow release diclofenac sodium. BMJ 1988;297(6646):488–9.
12. Huber T, Ruchti C, Halter F. Nonsteroidal antiinflammatory drug-induced colonic strictures: a case report. Gastroenterology 1991;100(4):1119–22.
13. Baroni L, Comoglio T, Trombetta N, Cornelli U. Il diclofenac sodico nella terapia ambulatoriale dell'infiammazione o del dolore articolare. Ricerca multicentrica aperta condotta da 223 medici italiani. [Sodium diclofenac in the ambulatory therapy of joint inflammation and pain. Multicentric open-ended research performed by 223 Italian physicians.] Clin Ter 1982;100(4):383–99.
14. Gizzi G, Villani V, Brandi G, Paganelli GM, Di Febo G, Biasco G. Ano-rectal lesions in patients taking suppositories containing non-steroidal anti-inflammatory drugs (NSAID). Endoscopy 1990;22(3):146–8.
15. Tanner E, Wachter G, Lasarof I, Gaida P. Klinische Erfahrungen mit dem neuen Antirheumatikum Diclofenac. [Clinical experiences with the new antirheumatic diclo fenac.] Z Gesamte Inn Med 1982;37(1):8–12.
16. Dunk AA, Walt RP, Jenkins WJ, Sherlock SS. Diclofenac hepatitis. BMJ (Clin Res Ed) 1982;284(6329):1605–6.
17. Iveson TJ, Ryley NG, Kelly PM, Trowell JM, McGee JO, Chapman RW. Diclofenac associated hepatitis. J Hepatol 1990;10(1):85–9.
18. Strom BL, Carson JL, Schinnar R, Sim E, Morse ML. The effect of indication on the risk of hypersensitivity reactions associated with tolmetin sodium vs other nonsteroidal anti-inflammatory drugs. J Rheumatol 1988;15(4):695–9.
19. Mazeika PK, Ford MJ. Chronic active hepatitis associated with diclofenac sodium therapy. Br J Clin Pract 1989;43(3):125–6.
20. Sallie RW, McKenzie T, Reed WD, Quinlan MF, Shilkin KB. Diclofenac hepatitis. Aust NZ J Med 1991;21(2):251–5.
21. Helfgott SM, Sandberg-Cook J, Zakim D, Nestler J. Diclofenac-associated hepatotoxicity. JAMA 1990;264(20):2660–2.
22. Jones AL, Latham T, Shallcross TM, Simpson KJ. Fulminant hepatic failure due to diclofenac treated successfully by orthotopic liver transplantation. Transplant Proc 1998;30(1):192–4.
23. Diggory P, Golding RL, Lancaster R. Renal and hepatic impairment in association with diclofenac administration. Postgrad Med J 1989;65(765):507–8.
24. Hovette P, Touze JE, Debonne JM, Delmarre B, Rogier C, Schmoor P, Aubry P. Hépatite cholèstatique et insuffisance rénale aiguë au cours d'un traitement par diclofénac. [Cholestatic hepatitis and acute kidney insufficiency during treatment with diclofenac.] Ann Gastroenterol Hepatol (Paris) 1989;25(6):257–8.
25. Gray GR. Another side effect of NSAIDs. JAMA 1990;264:2677.
26. Banks AT, Zimmerman HJ, Ishak KG, Harter JG. Diclofenac-associated hepatotoxicity: analysis of 180 cases reported to the Food and Drug Administration as adverse reactions. Hepatology 1995;22(3):820–7.
27. Wolters J, van Breda Vriesman PJ. Minimal change nephropathy and interstitial nephritis associated with diclofenac. Neth J Med 1985;28(8):311–14.
28. Campistol JM, Galofre J, Botey A, Torras A, Revert L. Reversible membranous nephritis associated with diclofenac. Nephrol Dial Transplant 1989;4(5):393–5.
29. Beun GD, Leunissen KM, Van Breda Vriesman PJ, Van Hooff JP, Grave W. Isolated minimal change nephropathy associated with diclofenac. BMJ (Clin Res Ed) 1987;295(6591):182–3.
30. Yinnon AM, Moreb JS, Slotki IN. Nephrotic syndrome associated with diclofenac sodium. BMJ (Clin Res Ed) 1987;295:556.
31. Gabrielsen TO, Staerfelt F, Thune PO. Drug-induced bullous dermatosis with linear IgA deposits along the basement membrane. Acta Derm Venereol 1981;61(5):439–41.
32. Ueda K, Higashi N, Kume A, Ikushima-Fujimoto M, Ogiwara S. Allergic contact dermatitis due to diclofenac and indomethacin. Contact Dermatitis 1998;39(6):323.
33. Oono T, Kanzaki H, Yoshioka T, Arata J. Staphylococcal scalded skin syndrome in an adult. Identification of exfoliative toxin A and B genes by polymerase chain reaction. Dermatology 1997;195(3):268–70.
34. Saputo V, Bruni G. La sindrome di Nicolau da preparati di penicillina: analisi della letteratura alla ricerca di potenziali fattori di rischio. [Nicolau syndrome caused by penicillin preparations: review of the literature in search for potential risk factors.] Pediatr Med Chir 1998;20(2):105–23.
35. Stricker BH, van Kasteren BJ. Diclofenac-induced isolated myonecrosis and the Nicolau syndrome. Ann Intern Med 1992;117(12):1058.
36. Rygnestad T, Kvam AM. Streptococcal myositis and tissue necrosis with intramuscular administration of diclofenac (Voltaren). Acta Anaesthesiol Scand 1995;39(8):1128–30.

37. Forsbach Sanchez G, Eloy Tamez H. Sindrome de nicolau por la administracion intramuscular de diclofenaco. [Nicolau syndrome caused by intramuscular administration of diclofenac.] Rev Invest Clin 1999;51(1):71.
38. Ezzedine K, Vadoud-Seyedi J, Heenen M. Nicolau syndrome following diclofenac administration. Br J Dermatol 2004;150(2):385–7.
39. del Pozo MD, Lobera T, Blasco A. Selective hypersensitivity to diclofenac. Allergy 2000;55(4):412–13.
40. Mas C, Menahem S. Premature in utero closure of the ductus arteriosus following maternal ingestion of sodium diclofenac. Aust NZ J Obstet Gynaecol 1999;39(1):106–7.
41. Anonymous. Diclofenac Dear Doctor letter issue in Japan. Scrip 2000;17:2597.
42. Muller-Vahl H. Aseptische Gewebsnekrose: eine schwerwiegende Komplikation nach intramuskularer Injektion. [Aseptic tissue necrosis: a severe complication after intramuscular injections.] Dtsch Med Wochenschr 1984;109(20):786–92.
43. Pillans PI, O'Connor N. Tissue necrosis and necrotizing fasciitis after intramuscular administration of diclofenac. Ann Pharmacother 1995;29(3):264–6.
44. Deray G, Le Hoang P, Aupetit B, Achour A, Rottembourg J, Baumelou A. Enhancement of cyclosporine A nephrotoxicity by diclofenac. Clin Nephrol 1987;27(4):213–14.
45. Harris KP, Jenkins D, Walls J. Nonsteroidal antiinflammatory drugs and cyclosporine. A potentially serious adverse interaction. Transplantation 1988;46(4):598–9.
46. Kovarik JM, Mueller EA, Gerbeau C, Tarral A, Francheteau P, Guerret M. Cyclosporine and nonsteroidal antiinflammatory drugs: exploring potential drug interactions and their implications for the treatment of rheumatoid arthritis. J Clin Pharmacol 1997;37(4):336–43.
47. Reimann IW, Frolich JC. Effects of diclofenac on lithium kinetics. Clin Pharmacol Ther 1981;30(3):348–52.
48. Weinblatt ME. Drug interactions with non steroidal anti-inflammatory drugs (NSAIDs). Scand J Rheumatol Suppl 1989;83:7–10.

Dicycloverine

See also Anticholinergic drugs

General Information

Dicycloverine, in the doses generally used (up to 450 mg/day), is of disputed value. It may have a non-specific relaxant action on the gastrointestinal muscle. The evidence of its effects is meager and it seems to be an anticholinergic drug that which has been promoted in doses that are often too low to result in either a useful therapeutic effect or in adverse effects.

Second-Generation Effects

Teratogenicity

Dicycloverine was formerly combined with doxylamine succinate and sometimes with pyridoxine in Debendox (Bendectin) tablets, which were used in certain countries for the treatment of nausea and vomiting in pregnancy. There has been a widely discussed suggestion that Debendox might cause a range of fetal malformations, but numerous studies have failed to confirm this (1).

For example, in a survey of 22 977 pregnant women in Great Britain 620 of whom had been given Debendox and 743 other women had been given agents other than Debendox containing pyridoxine during the first 13 weeks of gestation, the rates for all abnormal outcomes among women given Debendox and those not given it were 5.0 and 5.4% respectively (2).

However, the sporadic reports of such problems sometimes involved women who took the product in high doses for long periods in early pregnancy and there is some doubt as to the dosage schedule used in the larger studies. Particularly since the pattern of supposed malformations was highly variable, and they were of types which tend to occur spontaneously, the point cannot be considered settled. However, any teratogenic effect must have been very slight.

References

1. Brent RL. Bendectin: review of the medical literature of a comprehensively studied human nonteratogen and the most prevalent tortogen-litigen. Reprod Toxicol 1995;9(4):337–49.
2. Fleming DM, Knox JD, Crombie DL. Debendox in early pregnancy and fetal malformation. BMJ (Clin Res Ed) 1981;283(6284):99–101.

Didanosine

See also Nucleoside analogue reverse transcriptase inhibitors (NRTIs)

General Information

Didanosine (2′,3′-dideoxyinosine, ddI) is a purine analogue reverse transcriptase inhibitor. The major clinical adverse effects reported during the first years of use of didanosine were acute pancreatitis and a painful neuropathic syndrome (due to a peripheral neuropathy), which appeared to be related to both dosage and cumulative dose (SEDA-17, 340) (1). However, the incidence of acute pancreatitis and peripheral neuropathy in these studies was lower than in earlier studies with didanosine (2,3). This may be related to the fact that treatment was started earlier or to the use of lower dosages (200–400 mg/day) in these studies compared with earlier studies. In the latter studies, gastrointestinal symptoms, most notably nausea and vomiting, were the most commonly reported adverse effects in patients taking didanosine. Minor adverse effects include insomnia, headaches, anxiety, irritability, rash, increased plasma uric acid concentration, and increased hepatic transaminase activities combined with a rash (4). There were no toxic effects of didanosine on hematological laboratory indices (5).

Observational studies

The use of didanosine 125–200 mg bd plus interferon alfa-2b in AIDS-associated Kaposi's sarcoma has been studied in 68 patients (6). Withdrawal of didanosine was required in cases of peripheral neuropathy, rises in serum amylase activity, and hypertriglyceridemia.

Organs and Systems

Sensory systems

Eyes

Retinal depigmentation has been described in children taking didanosine (7).

Ears

Hearing loss attributed to didanosine has been reported in an HIV-infected adult (8).

- A 37-year-old HIV-infected man developed bilateral deafness while taking didanosine (400 mg/day), which had been started about 4 years before. He was also taking azithromycin, ciprofloxacin, and myambutol for about 1 month for a *Mycobacterium avium* infection. Otoscopic examination and tympanometry were normal. Audiometry showed a bilateral sensorineural hearing deficit of 40–60 dB. There were no other neurological abnormalities. An MRI scan of the brain was normal. Didanosine was withdrawn and replaced by alternative antiretroviral agents. All other medications were continued. His hearing improved progressively and returned to normal after 2 months.

In the absence of rechallenge, there was no conclusive evidence for a causative role of didanosine in the development of hearing loss in this case. However, the authors argued that the improvement on discontinuation of didanosine, which is known to cause neuritis, implicated the drug.

Extensive serial audiological studies in an HIV-infected child showed high-frequency hearing loss after 19 months of combined treatment with zidovudine and didanosine (dosages unknown), which were started at 24 months of age (9). Normal tympanograms indicated that this hearing loss was sensorineural.

While no conclusive evidence was given for a causative role of either antiretroviral drug, the authors concluded that children taking antiretroviral therapy need to be monitored for possible ototoxicity.

Hematologic

Thrombocytopenia has been observed in patients using didanosine (10,11).

Musculoskeletal

There is no evidence that didanosine contributes to the development of myopathy in patients taking didanosine and zidovudine in whom this adverse event occurs (12).

Multiorgan failure

There has been a report of a patient in whom pancreatitis, fulminant hepatic failure, and persistent lactic acidosis occurred, culminating in death from liver failure (13).

References

1. Yarchoan R, Mitsuya H, Pluda JM, Marczyk KS, Thomas RV, Hartman NR, Brouwers P, Perno CF, Allain JP, Johns DG, et al The National Cancer Institute phase I study of 2′,3′-dideoxyinosine administration in adults with AIDS or AIDS-related complex: analysis of activity and toxicity profiles. Rev Infect Dis 1990;12(Suppl 5):S522–33.
2. Delta Coordinating Committee. Delta: a randomised double-blind controlled trial comparing combinations of zidovudine plus didanosine or zalcitabine with zidovudine alone in HIV-infected individuals Lancet 1996;348(9023):283–91.
3. Hammer SM, Katzenstein DA, Hughes MD, Gundacker H, Schooley RT, Haubrich RH, Henry WK, Lederman MM, Phair JP, Niu M, Hirsch MS, Merigan TC. A trial comparing nucleoside monotherapy with combination therapy in HIV-infected adults with CD4 cell counts from 200 to 500 per cubic millimeter. AIDS Clinical Trials Group Study 175 Study Team. N Engl J Med 1996;335(15):1081–90.
4. Franssen RM, Meenhorst PL, Koks CH, Beijnen JH. Didanosine, a new antiretroviral drug. A review. Pharm Weekbl Sci 1992;14(5):297–304.
5. Lambert JS, Seidlin M, Reichman RC, Plank CS, Laverty M, Morse GD, Knupp C, McLaren C, Pettinelli C, Valentine FT, et al 2′,3′-dideoxyinosine (ddI) in patients with the acquired immunodeficiency syndrome or AIDS-related complex. A phase I trial. N Engl J Med 1990;322(19):1333–40.
6. Krown SE, Li P, Von Roenn JH, Paredes J, Huang J, Testa MA. Efficacy of low-dose interferon with antiretroviral therapy in Kaposi's sarcoma: a randomized phase II AIDS clinical trials group study. J Interferon Cytokine Res 2002;22(3):295–303.
7. Pizzo PA, Wilfert C. Antiretroviral therapy for infection due to human immunodeficiency virus in children. Clin Infect Dis 1994;19(1):177–96.
8. Vogeser M, Colebunders R, Depraetere K, Van Wanzeele P, Van Gehuchten S. Deafness caused by didanosine. Eur J Clin Microbiol Infect Dis 1998;17(3):214–15.
9. Christensen LA, Morehouse CR, Powell TW, Alchediak T, Silio M. Antiviral therapy in a child with pediatric human immunodeficiency virus (HIV): case study of audiologic findings. J Am Acad Audiol 1998;9(4):292–8.
10. Yarchoan R, Perno CF, Thomas RV, Klecker RW, Allain JP, Wills RJ, McAtee N, Fischl MA, Dubinsky R, McNeely MC, et al Phase I studies of 2′,3′-dideoxycytidine in severe human immunodeficiency virus infection as a single agent and alternating with zidovudine (AZT). Lancet 1988;1(8577):76–81.
11. Dolin R, Lambert JS, Morse GD, Reichman RC, Plank CS, Reid J, Knupp C, McLaren C, Pettinelli C. 2′,3′-Dideoxyinosine in patients with AIDS or AIDS-related complex. Rev Infect Dis 1990;12(Suppl 5):S540–9.
12. Pedrol E, Masanes F, Fernandez-Sola J, Cofan M, Casademont J, Grau JM, Urbano-Marquez A. Lack of muscle toxicity with didanosine (ddI). Clinical and experimental studies. J Neurol Sci 1996;138(1-2):42–8.
13. Calegari J, Lorenzana R, Cheyer C, Gang DL, Higgins TL. Lactic acidosis and fulminant hepatic failure in a patient treated with didanosine, nelfinavir and stavudine. Clin Intensive Care 1999;10:61–3.

Diethyl sebacate

General Information

Diethyl sebacate is an emulsifier used in cosmetics and topical medicaments. In contrast to the emulsifying agents stearyl alcohol, stearic acid, and glyceryl stearate, diethyl sebacate is considered to be a rare sensitizer.

Organs and Systems

Immunologic

There were positive patch tests to diethyl sebacate (10 and 30% in ether and 1 and 10% in petrolatum) in a 48-year-old woman who had been using a topical antimycotic ointment (1).

Reference

1. Kimura M, Kawada A. Contact dermatitis due to diethyl sebacate. Contact Dermatitis 1999;40(1):48–9.

Diethylcarbamazine

General Information

Diethylcarbamazine is an antihelminthic drug used in the treatment of filarial infections. With some infecting species it is effective in both the adult and microfilarial stages, whilst with others it is active only against the microfilarial stages and does not eradicate the infection.

Pharmacokinetics

Diethylcarbamazine is extensively metabolized, the half-life being 6–12 hours; the remainder enters the urine within 48 hours. Over the initial period the dosage should be increased slowly to avoid or reduce allergic responses as a result of destruction of parasites and liberation of antigen, and then maintained at 3 mg/kg tds for 34 weeks. Not all of its adverse effects are necessarily due to destruction of the parasite; weakness, lethargy, anorexia, and nausea can be due to the drug itself.

The pharmacokinetics, safety, and tolerability of co-administered diethylcarbamazine and albendazole have been investigated in a double-blind, randomized, placebo-controlled trial in 42 subjects (aged 18–52 years, weighing 46–67 kg) living in a lymphatic filariasis endemic region but without detectable microfilariae (1). Three groups of 14 patients received diethylcarbamazine 6 mg/kg alone, albendazole 400 mg alone, or diethylcarbamazine 6 mg/kg plus albendazole 400 mg. Both diethylcarbamazine and albendazole were well tolerated alone and in combination. In contrast to a study in patients with lymphatic filariasis (2), there were no adverse events in amicrofilaremic individuals. In all three treatment groups the drugs were rapidly absorbed from the gastrointestinal tract, although there was marked interindividual variation. The pharmacokinetics of diethylcarbamazine, albendazole, and albendazole sulfoxide were similar.

Observational studies

Brugia malayi* and *Wuchereria bancrofti

When treating *Brugia malayi* and *Wuchereria bancrofti* infections, reactions include headache and fever, sometimes accompanied by malaise, nausea, and vomiting. Urticarial skin rashes can occur, and subsequently lymphangitis and lymphadenopathy often appear (SEDA-17, 357). Abscess formation can occur in association with adult worms. Major systemic complications of therapy include proteinuria and severe pruritus; proteinuria has even been seen in some patients using the drug topically. Circulating immune complexes have been found to be increased in many cases. Those with CIq binding greater than 3% are at significantly increased risk of developing visual field constriction and proteinuria.

In lymphatic filariasis diethylcarbamazine can cause systemic reactions, such as fever, arthralgia, headache, and malaise, and local reactions such as swollen and painful lymph nodes. All of these reactions are thought to be caused by an allergic reaction to antigens from the dying microfilaria and not to a toxic effect of the drug itself. This causal relation is further emphasized by a study from Indonesia, in which adverse reactions to treatment with diethylcarbamazine were studied in patients with *B. malayi* filariasis—26 microfilaria-positive patients (mean 235 mf/10 ml), 12 "endemic" controls (from the endemic area, but microfilaria counts negative), and 17 patients with elephantiasis, of whom three had with high microfilaria counts (3). Adverse effects, mainly fever, headache, and body aches, started 2–24 hours after the administration of diethylcarbamazine 6 mg/kg/day for 12 days. Of the patients with positive pretreatment microfilaria counts 15% had severe adverse reactions, 19% moderate reactions, and 65% mild reactions. There was a direct relation between the severity of the adverse effects and the height of pretreatment microfilaria counts, and the more severe adverse effects occurred in the patients with the highest pretreatment microfilaria counts. In the endemic controls there were no reactions or only mild ones. In the patients with elephantiasis there were no reactions or only mild ones in all but two patients, both of whom had moderate reactions and had high pretreatment microfilaria counts.

That diethylcarbamazine may still be the more effective drug in *B. malayi* infections, despite these adverse effects, is suggested in a study from India, in which the efficacy and safety of several single-dose drug combinations, including albendazole, diethylcarbamazine, and ivermectin were compared in 51 microfilaria-positive patients with *B. malayi* and in which diethylcarbamazine was more effective in reaching a sustained reduction in microfilaria counts after 1 year than ivermectin, although the study was small (4). Adverse reactions (fever, headache, myalgia, and chills) occurred in all of the 16 patients treated with a combination of ivermectin (200 micrograms/kg as a single dose) and diethylcarbamazine (6 mg/kg as a single dose), in 15 of the 16 patients treated with albendazole (400 mg as a single dose) and diethylcarbamazine (6 mg/kg as a single dose), and in 12 of the 16 patients treated with ivermectin and albendazole.

In order to assess the effects of re-treatment in *B. malayi* infections, 35 asymptomatic microfilaremic patients were re-treated at the end of the first year with an additional single dose of the combination they had previously received (5). Eleven patients received ivermectin 200 micrograms/kg plus diethylcarbamazine 6 mg/kg, nine patients received ivermectin 200 micrograms/kg plus albendazole 400 mg, and 15 patients received diethylcarbamazine 6 mg/kg plus albendazole 400 mg. The best suppression of brugian microfilaremia 1 year after re-treatment was obtained with combinations that included diethylcarbamazine. Whatever the drug regimen, both the frequency and intensity of adverse reactions after re-treatment were less than after initial treatment. The greatest difference was in patients who received ivermectin plus diethylcarbamazine, who also had the lowest mean microfilarial counts immediately before re-treatment. None of the adverse reactions after re-treatment was severe. Most of them, including fever, headache, and myalgia, were easily controlled with paracetamol. Postural hypotension and the "string sign" (dilated painful and inflamed lymphatic channels) did not occur with re-treatment.

In another study the cost-effectiveness of a revised mass annual single-dose regimen of diethylcarbamazine 6 mg/kg was estimated for large-scale control of lymphatic filariasis in a pilot program launched in Tamil Nadu (6). This regimen gave good coverage (90% of the population studied) and high compliance of 82%. Adverse effects occurred in 22% of patients and most were non-specific (giddiness in 54%, vomiting in 11%, nausea in 1%, fever in 14%, and headache in 20%).

Loa loa

In loiasis both adult and microfilariae are susceptible to diethylcarbamazine. However, encephalitis is a major risk in patients with heavy infestation (SEDA-17, 356) (7), and ivermectin should be preferred. Severe allergic reactions can need treatment with antihistamines and glucocorticoids. The risk of encephalitis has led to the recommendation that prophylactic use of diethylcarbamazine against *Loa loa* should only be contemplated when the chance of infection is considerable.

Onchocerca volvulus

In onchocerciasis, severe reactions can occur in the initial stages of therapy, particularly since diethylcarbamazine only kills the microfilariae of *Onchocerca volvulus* (resulting in the release of toxins) and does not eradicate the infection. The Mazzotti reaction, a Herxheimer-like response, can be severe and even fatal; it comprises a pruritic papular dermatitis, urticaria, fever, malaise, and postural hypotension; asthma and respiratory distress can occur and the hypotension can be associated with irreversible collapse. There can be painful lymphadenopathy.

Ocular complications are of particular importance: iritis can be induced by dying microfilariae and may call for topical or systemic glucocorticoid treatment. Associated complications include chorioretinitis, anterior uveitis, and punctate keratitis. Changes can also occur in the posterior segment (8), with visual field defects; there can be transient retinal pigment epithelial lesions at the posterior pole, globular infiltrates at the limbus, and optic disk leakage (9) with visible pallor. Similar ocular lesions can develop after topical diethylcarbamazine (SEDA-7, 316). Visual field defects are not reversible and they limit the clinical value of diethylcarbamazine in this disease.

Mass treatment with diethylcarbamazine is a key measure for control of the transmission of bancroftian filariasis. However, severe adverse reactions can occur in patients with onchocerciasis treated with high doses of diethylcarbamazine, which may limit the prospects for the use of common salt medicated with diethylcarbamazine in many parts of Africa. However, the daily dose of diethylcarbamazine-medicated salt is considerably lower than that of conventional tablets (25–50 mg od for the first 1 or 2 days followed by 100 mg bd for 5–7 days).

The adverse effects of diethylcarbamazine-medicated salt in patients with *O. volvulus* has been assessed in a double-blind, placebo-controlled trial in four groups of ten men (10). Groups I and II had *O. volvulus* microfilariae only, group III had both *O. volvulus* and *W. bancrofti* microfilariae, and group IV had *W. bancrofti* microfilariae only. Groups I, III, and IV received diethylcarbamazine-medicated salt. Group II served as a control group and received cooking salt. The medicated salt (0.33% w/w) originated from a batch previously produced for control trials. Each individual was given a total daily dose of 5.8 g of salt for 10 days, corresponding to the average daily salt intake for individuals aged over 15 years in the area. The salt supplement was spaced over three daily meals: 0.5 g, 2.5 g, and 2.8 g at breakfast, lunch, and dinner respectively. Hence, the daily dose of diethylcarbamazine was 19.1 mg. Diethylcarbamazine-medicated salt had no significant effect on *O. volvulus* microfilarial counts, but *W. bancrofti* microfilarial counts were significantly reduced in groups III and IV. The most pronounced adverse reactions occurred in groups I and III and were mild to moderate itching and rash. They were observed on days 3–4 and lasted for the remaining medication period, but did not interfere with normal daily activities. At day 30, all the reactions had abated. There were no severe adverse events, perhaps because of low pre-existing microfilarial counts and the short duration of therapy. There was no evidence that patients with *O. volvulus* and *W. bancrofti* double infection had a different adverse reaction pattern than individuals with *O. volvulus* infection only. Thus, diethylcarbamazine-medicated salt may be an important drug for the control of bancroftian filariasis in Africa. Salt with an even lower concentration of diethylcarbamazine may still have microfilaricidal properties in bancroftian filariasis without inducing microfilarial killing and adverse reactions in onchocerciasis, which may further improve treatment compliance and ease of use.

Wolbachia

In 15 Indonesian patients with *B. malayi* infection, the release of *Wolbachia* bacteria was studied in relation to adverse events after diethylcarbamazine treatment (6 mg/kg orally for 12 days) (11). Three patients had severe reactions and six patients had moderate reactions. In all samples from the three patients with severe reactions and in one of the six with moderate reactions, *Wolbachia* PCR products were detected from 4 hours after treatment, and persisted for 8–20 hours. These data suggest that release of *Wolbachia* bacteria into the blood may be associated with severe inflammatory reactions after diethylcarbamazine. Adverse reactions associated with increases in proinflammatory cytokines have also been reported in bancroftian filariasis and onchocerciasis, suggesting that similar events can also occur in these filarial infections.

Comparative studies

Filariasis

The efficacy of new treatment strategies for lymphatic filariasis using a single dose of diethylcarbamazine or a combination of diethylcarbamazine plus albendazole has been studied in 30 people (aged 11–52 years, weighing 25–63 kg) infected with *Brugia timori* and compared with the results of 27 people (aged 13–52 years, weighing 27–73 kg) infected with *W. bancrofti* (2). All were allocated at random to diethylcarbamazine (100 mg on day 1 and up to a total dose of 6 mg/kg on day 3) or diethylcarbamazine plus albendazole group (placebo on day 1 and diethylcarbamazine 6 mg/kg plus albendazole 400 mg on day 3). There was no difference in adverse reactions between diethylcarbamazine alone and diethylcarbamazine plus albendazole. Headache ($n = 15$), myalgia ($n = 13$), itching ($n = 8$), and adenolymphangitis ($n = 8$) were the most common adverse effects; none were severe or life-threatening. The microfilaricidal effect of the drugs was achieved more rapidly for *B. timori*, which is associated with more adverse reactions than *W. bancrofti* filariasis. As previously shown, there was a strong correlation of microfilarial density with the frequency and severity of adverse reactions. The addition of albendazole resulted in no additional adverse reactions compared with diethylcarbamazine alone.

General adverse effects

Adverse reactions to treatment with diethylcarbamazine vary with the infecting filarial species and are most severe in onchocerciasis. Minor reactions include malaise, nausea, and headache, but diethylcarbamazine also depresses the central nervous system in some individuals, resulting in dizziness and somnolence; reversible coma has been reported in patients in poor physical condition. Nicotine-like properties can produce autonomic effects. A degree of eosinophilia during treatment is usual.

Although over 120 million individuals have lymphatic filariasis, it may be eradicable. Newer strategies for the elimination of lymphatic filariasis aim at transmission control through the use of annual doses of combinations of ivermectin, diethylcarbamazine, or albendazole, and disease control through individual patient management. Mass chemotherapy appears to be essential in the control of lymphatic filariasis. However, drug availability and the co-endemicity of onchocerciasis and loiasis play crucial roles. Although a single annual dose of diethylcarbamazine may be an effective approach toward long-term suppression of brugian and bancroftian microfilaremia, repeated multidrug chemotherapy is the preferred approach for control of lymphatic filariasis, as in other chronic infections, such as tuberculosis and leprosy. In addition, combining diethylcarbamazine with albendazole has the advantage of controlling intestinal parasites.

Organs and Systems

Immunologic

Brugia malayi is more susceptible to diethylcarbamazine than *W. bancrofti*. A study of the former, undertaken to explain the very severe effects often associated with diethylcarbamazine treatment of lymphatic filariasis, provided evidence of the involvement of the cytokine interleukin-6 (IL-6), concentrations of which were raised during treatment (12).

The involvement of inflammatory mediators in the development of adverse events has recently been studied in 29 patients with *B. malayi* microfilaremia treated with diethylcarbamazine (13). Before and at serial time points after the start of treatment, plasma concentrations of the inflammatory mediators interleukin-6, interleukin-8, interleukin-10, tumor necrosis factor-alfa, and lipopolysaccharide-binding protein were measured in relation to diethylcarbamazine concentrations and adverse events. The adverse effects of diethylcarbamazine correlated well with pretreatment microfilariae counts, consistent with previous experience with diethylcarbamazine in lymphatic filariasis and onchocerciasis. Concurrent measurements of diethylcarbamazine concentrations failed to establish a clear relation between diethylcarbamazine concentrations and adverse events. Detailed kinetic studies showed the strongest association of the severity of symptoms with interleukin-6 and lipopolysaccharide-binding protein. Concentrations of interleukin-6 started to rise as early as 2–4 hours and reached a maximum after about 8 hours. Fever also occurred at 4–8 hours, consistent with the pyrogenic activity of interleukin-6. In addition, interleukin-6 plays a central role in the induction of the acute phase proteins involved in inflammatory reactions. Indeed, concentrations of the acute phase protein, lipopolysaccharide-binding protein, started to rise at 8 hours (that is after interleukin-6), and also peaked later than interleukin-6, at 24–48 hours after diethylcarbamazine. These observations suggest that the adverse effects of diethylcarbamazine result from an exaggerated host inflammatory response stimulated by a high load of antigen released from killed or degenerating microfilariae.

Susceptibility Factors

Renal disease

The clearance of diethylcarbamazine is reduced in renal insufficiency (14), and dosages should be reduced.

References

1. Shenoy RK, Suma TK, John A, Arun SR, Kumaraswami V, Fleckenstein LL, Na-Bangchang K. The pharmacokinetics, safety and tolerability of the co-administration of diethylcarbamazine and albendazole. Ann Trop Med Parasitol 2002;96(6):603–14.
2. Supali T, Ismid IS, Ruckert P, Fischer P. Treatment of *Brugia timori* and *Wuchereria bancrofti* infections in

Indonesia using DEC or a combination of DEC and albendazole: adverse reactions and short-term effects on microfilariae. Trop Med Int Health 2002;7(10):894–901.
3. Haarbrink M, Terhell AJ, Abadi GK, Mitsui Y, Yazdanbakhsh M. Adverse reactions following diethylcarbamazine (DEC) intake in "endemic normals", microfilaraemics and elephantiasis patients. Trans R Soc Trop Med Hyg 1999;93(1):91–6.
4. Shenoy RK, Dalia S, John A, Suma TK, Kumaraswami V. Treatment of the microfilaraemia of asymptomatic brugian filariasis with single doses of ivermectin, diethylcarbamazine or albendazole, in various combinations. Ann Trop Med Parasitol 1999;93(6):643–51.
5. Shenoy RK, John A, Babu BS, Suma TK, Kumaraswami V. Two-year follow-up of the microfilaraemia of asymptomatic brugian filariasis, after treatment with two, annual, single doses of ivermectin, diethylcarbamazine and albendazole, in various combinations. Ann Trop Med Parasitol 2000;94(6):607–14.
6. Krishnamoorthy K, Ramu K, Srividya A, Appavoo NC, Saxena NB, Lal S, Das PK. Cost of mass annual single dose diethylcarbamazine distribution for the large scale control of lymphatic filariasis. Indian J Med Res 2000;111:81–9.
7. Carme B, Boulesteix J, Boutes H, Puruehnce MF. Five cases of encephalitis during treatment of loiasis with diethylcarbamazine. Am J Trop Med Hyg 1991;44(6):684–90.
8. Bird AC, El-Sheikh H, Anderson J, et al Changes in visual function and in the posterior segment of the eye during treatment of loiasis with diethylcarbamazine. Am J Trop Med Hyg 1991;44:684–90.
9. Bird AC, El-Sheikh H, Anderson J, Fuglsang H. Visual loss during oral diethylcarbamazine treatment for onchocerciasis. Lancet 1979;2(8132):46.
10. Meyrowitsch DW, Simonsen PE, Magnussen P. Tolerance to diethylcarbamazine-medicated salt in individuals infected with *Onchocerca volvulus*. Trans R Soc Trop Med Hyg 2000;94(4):444–8.
11. Cross HF, Haarbrink M, Egerton G, Yazdanbakhsh M, Taylor MJ. Severe reactions to filarial chemotherapy and release of *Wolbachia* endosymbionts into blood. Lancet 2001;358(9296):1873–5.
12. Yazdanbakhsh M, Duym L, Aarden L, Partono F. Serum interleukin-6 levels and adverse reactions to diethylcarbamazine in lymphatic filariasis. J Infect Dis 1992;166(2):453–4.
13. Reuben R, Rajendran R, Sunish IP, Mani TR, Tewari SC, Hiriyan J, Gajanana A. Annual single-dose diethylcarbamazine plus ivermectin for control of bancroftian filariasis: comparative efficacy with and without vector control. Ann Trop Med Parasitol 2001;95(4):361–78.
14. Adjepon-Yamoah KK, Edwards G, Breckenridge AM, Orme ML, Ward SA. The effect of renal disease on the pharmacokinetics of diethylcarbamazine in man. Br J Clin Pharmacol 1982;13(6):829–34.

Diethylenetriamine penta-acetic acid

General Information

Diethylenetriamine penta-acetic acid (DTPA) is a chelating agent that has been used in radiolabeled form as a tracer. It has been used in the following combinations:

- DTPA: to assess iron body stores (1–3);
- ^{111}indium-DTPA: to label proteins, such as albumin (4) and monoclonal antibodies (5), for the radiodetection of cancers;
- ^{99m}technetium-DTPA: for scanning organs such as the kidneys (6), lungs (7), and brain (8);
- dysprosium-DTPA: in experimental imaging of cerebral ischemia (9);
- ^{97}ruthenium-DTPA: to label cerebrospinal fluid (10);
- gadolinium-DTPA: as a contrast agent in computed tomography (11) and magnetic resonance imaging (12).

In a study of the use of $^{117m}Sn^{4+}$-DTPA for palliative pain reduction in 15 patients with bone metastases, there were no myelotoxic or other adverse effects (13).

Organs and Systems

Hematologic

In nine patients with advanced breast carcinoma, administration of a ^{90}Y-DTPA-BrE-3 complex was associated with transient and uncomplicated thrombocytopenia in four patients and leukopenia in two patients (14).

References

1. Powell LW, Thomas MJ. Use of diethylenetriamine penta-acetic acid (D.T.P.A.) in the clinical assessment of total body iron stores. J Clin Pathol 1967; 20(6):896–904.
2. Barry M, Cartei G, Sherlock S. Quantitative measurement of iron stores with diethylenetriamine penta-acetic acid. Gut 1970;11(11):891–8.
3. Barry M, Cartei G, Sherlock S. Measurement of iron stores in cirrhosis using diethylenetriamine penta-acetic acid. Gut 1970;11(11):899–904.
4. Clorius JH, Sinn H, Manke HG, Schrenk HH, Blatter J, Werling C, Friedrich EA, Voges J, Bahner M, Sturm V, et al Serum albumin (SA) accumulation by bronchogenic tumours: a tracer technique may help with patient selection for SA-delivered chemotherapy. Eur J Nucl Med 1995;22(9):989–96.
5. Griffin TW, Brill AB, Stevens S, Collins JA, Bokhari F, Bushe H, Stochl MC, Gionet M, Rusckowski M, Stroupe SD, et al Initial clinical study of indium-111-labeled clone 110 anticarcinoembryonic antigen antibody in patients with colorectal cancer. J Clin Oncol 1991;9(4):631–40.
6. Roman MR, Gruenewald SM, Saunders CA. The incidence of left iliac fossa uptake of (99m)Tc-DTPA in renal scanning. Eur J Nucl Med 2001;28(12):1842–4.
7. Mogulkoc N, Brutsche MH, Bishop PW, Murby B, Greaves MS, Horrocks AW, Wilson M, McCullough C, Prescott M, Egan JJ; Greater Manchester Pulmonary Fibrosis Consortium. Pulmonary (99m)Tc-DTPA aerosol clearance and survival in usual interstitial pneumonia (UIP). Thorax 2001;56(12):916–23.
8. Kaufman M, Swartz BE, Mandelkern M, Ropchan J, Gee M, Blahd WH. Diagnosis of delayed cerebral radiation necrosis following proton beam therapy. Arch Neurol 1990;47(4):474–6.
9. Haraldseth O, Jones RA, Muller TB, Fahlvik AK, Oksendal AN. Comparison of dysprosium DTPA BMA and superparamagnetic iron oxide particles as susceptibility contrast agents for perfusion imaging of regional

cerebral ischemia in the rat J Magn Reson Imaging 1996;6(5):714–17.
10. Oster ZH, Som P, Gil MC, Fairchild RG, Goldman AG, Schachner ER, Sacker DF, Atkins HL, Meinken GE, Srivastava SC, Richards P, Brill AB. Ruthenium-97 DTPA: a new radiopharmaceutical for cisternography. J Nucl Med 1981;22(3):269–73.
11. Chryssidis S, Davies RP, Tie ML. Gadolinium-enhanced computed tomographic aortography. Australas Radiol 2002;46(1):97–100.
12. Muramatsu K, Hachiya Y, Morita C. Postoperative magnetic resonance imaging of lumbar disc herniation: comparison of microendoscopic discectomy and Love's method. Spine 2001;26(14):1599–605.
13. Atkins HL, Mausner LF, Srivastava SC, Meinken GE, Cabahug CJ, D'Alessandro T. Tin-117m(4+)-DTPA for palliation of pain from osseous metastases: a pilot study. J Nucl Med 1995;36(5):725–9.
14. Schrier DM, Stemmer SM, Johnson T, Kasliwal R, Lear J, Matthes S, Taffs S, Dufton C, Glenn SD, Butchko G, Ceriani RL, Rovira D, Bunn P, Shpall EJ, Bearman SI, Purdy M, Cagnoni P, Jones RB. High-dose 90Y Mx-diethylenetriaminepentaacetic acid (DTPA)-BrE-3 and autologous hematopoietic stem cell support (AHSCS) for the treatment of advanced breast cancer: a phase I trial. Cancer Res 1995;55(Suppl 23):S5921–4.

Diethylstilbestrol

General Information

For a complete account of the adverse effects of estrogens, readers should consult the following monographs as well as this one:

- Estrogens
- Hormonal contraceptives—emergency contraception
- Hormonal contraceptives—oral
- Hormone replacement therapy—estrogens
- Hormone replacement therapy—estrogens + androgens
- Hormone replacement therapy—estrogens + progestogens.

Diethylstilbestrol and other non-steroidal estrogens came into vogue at a time when the cost of producing steroidal estrogens, whether synthetic or of natural origin, was still prohibitive. They have largely fallen out of favor, in view of the association between the use of diethylstilbestrol in pregnancy and second-generation injury. There seems to be no reason for believing that the short-term acute adverse reactions to these non-steroidal compounds differ from those of estrogenic steroids.

Diethylstilbestrol continues to be recommended in some centers as one of the agents of last resort when prostate cancer proves refractory to steroid hormones or androgen deprivation therapy has done all it can (1). In a Japanese study in which 16 patients were given a daily intravenous injection of diethylstilbestrol diphosphate 250 mg for 28 days, the short-term response was favorable and the drug was well tolerated (2).

Organs and Systems

Cardiovascular

In a randomized study of men treated hormonally for prostatic cancer (3), cardiovascular adverse effects were reported more often in patients treated with diethylstilbestrol than in those treated with cyproterone acetate. The risk was highest during the first 6 months of treatment.

Mineral balance

Profound hypocalcemia occurred in a patient with osteoblastic metastatic carcinoma of the prostate after treatment with diethylstilbestrol 15 mg/day for 7 days (SED-12, 1032) (4).

Immunologic

In 13 women exposed to diethylstilbestrol in utero compared with similar control subjects with respect to the in vitro T cell response to the mitogens phytohemagglutinin, concanavalin A, and interleukin-2, incorporation of tritiated thymidine into T cells from diethylstilbestrol-exposed women was increased three-fold over a range of concentrations in response to concanavalin A, increased by 50% over a range of concentrations in response to phytohemagglutinin, and increased two-fold in response to the endogenous mitogen interleukin-2 (5). This in vitro evidence of a change in T cell-mediated immunity clearly raises questions about the clinical consequences.

Long-Term Effects

Tumorigenicity

Exposure to diethylstilbestrol during pregnancy in 4836 women has been reported to carry a relative risk of 1.27 of breast cancer later in life. However, the authors found no evidence to support the link between diethylstilbestrol exposure and ovarian, endometrial, or other cancers.

In a 25-year follow-up study there were very slightly more breast tumors in women using diethylstilbestrol in pregnancy and significantly more cancer deaths (6).

In one study there was a six-fold risk of endometrial cancer among estrogen users compared with non-users; long-term users (over 5 years) had a 15-fold risk; there were excess risks for both diethylstilbestrol and conjugated estrogens (7).

Diethylstilbestrol can cause hepatic adenomas and carcinomas in experimental animals (8), and hepatocellular carcinoma has been reported in a man who took a total of 668 g over 12 years for suspected carcinoma of the prostate (9).

Second-Generation Effects

Teratogenicity

Diethylstilbestrol was used extensively in pregnancies between 1940 and about 1975, in the belief that it could protect threatened pregnancies and counter the risk of spontaneous abortion. Toward the end of that period, increasingly clear evidence emerged that diethylstilbestrol could have an adverse effect on the second generation that did not become apparent until puberty or adulthood, and perhaps could also appear in the third generation (10). It appears to be the only estrogen with this effect, but it is naturally not excluded that some structurally related non-steroidal estrogens might carry the same risk, although these have never been used in the same way in pregnancy.

History

Diethylstilbestrol provides several illustrations of how societies cope with the risks of harm from a drug. Under different brand names diethylstilbestrol has been given to a wide range of patients over many years, mostly pregnant women and aging men with prostate cancer. The history of iatrogenic disease as a result of the use of diethylstilbestrol in pregnant women shows that patients can play an important role in securing legitimacy for research and the publication of data on the harmful effects of a drug.

Diethylstilbestrol was given to pregnant women in many countries, mainly in the 1940s to 1970s, in the mistaken belief that it would prevent miscarriage and provide strong healthy babies (11,12). The application to market diethylstilbestrol in the USA was the first new drug application submitted to the FDA shortly after the 1938 Food, Drugs, and Cosmetics Act had been passed; permission was granted, although diethylstilbestrol had already been identified as a carcinogen in animals (13). Diethylstilbestrol was especially popular in some maternity clinics in North America, serving middle-class and upper-middle class women, and in the Netherlands, where the Queen's gynecologist promoted it. In other countries it was dispensed through public health maternity centers.

In the USA, evidence showing that it was ineffective for its intended purpose appeared by the 1950s. However, conclusions based on animal experiments, as well as a major double-blind, controlled clinical trial (14), remained unheeded, partly because prescribing physicians trusted their collegial loyalty more than data that implicitly threw doubt on their practice.

In 1971, a rare form of aggressive cancer in the vagina of young girls was attributed to the girls' exposure to diethylstilbestrol in utero in a report that was based on a case-control study of eight young women, two of whom had died, at the Massachusetts General Hospital (15). It was already clear from this small study that monitoring young women exposed to diethylstilbestrol would save lives. However, months and even years were to pass before the discovery led to any public action, at different times in different countries. Only after 5 months, when the risk of cancer in patients exposed to diethylstilbestrol was featured at hearings in the US Congress, did the FDA react. The FDA's Administrator then announced that diethylstilbestrol products were to be labelled with a warning that diethylstilbestrol was contraindicated in pregnancy and should not be given to pregnant women because of risk of the cancer in the offspring (16).

Drug regulatory agencies in other countries in which diethylstilbestrol had also been commonly used in pregnancy delayed taking action. In the Netherlands, the first change of labelling to include a warning to physicians that diethylstilbestrol given to pregnant women might harm the fetus was implemented in 1972. A similar change in labelling was introduced in France in 1977. In many other countries, the news that some daughters of women who had taken diethylstilbestrol while pregnant were at risk of developing a potentially lethal cancer was passed over in silence.

In Britain, the medical community was alerted to the risks by an editorial in the British Medical Journal in 1971, but it was only in 1973 that the Committee on Safety of Medicines advised against the use of diethylstilbestrol during pregnancy (17). In Britain, drugs were commonly not labelled with information about their contents, nor with warnings of risk until well into the 1990s; thus, patients were kept in ignorance. No measures have yet been taken in Britain to alert the public to the need for medical surveillance of women who have been exposed to diethylstilbestrol in utero.

It is estimated that in the USA, the Netherlands, and France, diethylstilbestrol was given to over 5.3 million pregnant women, and it is known that it has been given to pregnant women in most parts of the world. Single cases of clear-cell vaginal carcinoma from many countries are known, but systematic studies have not been conducted everywhere.

One in a thousand young women exposed to diethylstilbestrol before birth have been estimated to be at risk of developing clear-cell vaginal adenocarcinoma (18). Exposure to diethylstilbestrol in utero also has a range of other effects on exposed women, including malformations of the reproductive organs and difficulties in conception and carrying a pregnancy to term. Some of the men exposed to diethylstilbestrol in utero have urogenital malformations and an increased risk of testicular cancer (19).

Most of the women who suspected that they had taken diethylstilbestrol were to learn of the problems from the media, and they had to guess that their daughters might be at risk of developing cancer. When they tried to discover whether they had been given diethylstilbestrol during pregnancy, many of the women found that their obstetricians were not willing to give them access to their own medical records. In a report from a nationwide US survey intended to locate pregnant women who had been given diethylstilbestrol during 1940–72, the investigators complained that at some clinics they had encountered extreme difficulties in getting access to the records (20). Women who have been exposed to diethylstilbestrol sometimes say that never have so many medical files reportedly been lost through fire and inundation, as when they asked for access to records that might document the use of diethylstilbestrol during pregnancy.

Many doctors did not notice or did not heed warnings in the early 1970s about the risks of giving diethylstilbestrol to pregnant women. As late as 1974, according to one writer, some 11 000 prescriptions for diethylstilbestrol to be used during pregnancy were written in the USA (21). In 1976, it was observed that diethylstilbestrol was given to unsuspecting pregnant women in several Latin-American countries (21). In other countries, prescribing physicians' responses to reports that linked the use of diethylstilbestrol during pregnancy with cancer risks in their daughters were even slower. The latest documented prescription of diethylstilbestrol in Europe was in Spain in 1983 (22).

The first batches of educational material for physicians, with warnings and advice regarding health care for women who had been exposed to diethylstilbestrol, were distributed in the USA in 1971, in the Netherlands in

1974, and in France in 1989. No such material has been distributed in Britain.

Mothers in the USA who had taken diethylstilbestrol formed an organization, DES Action, to inform the public about the risks and to alert exposed mothers that their daughters needed regular medical examinations, so that potential tumor development would be detected early. Through DES Action they also gave each other mutual support during litigation against the manufacturers and acted politically to ensure that health care would be available for their daughters. DES Action groups outside the USA were formed in Australia, Belgium, Canada, France, Great Britain, Italy, Ireland, and the Netherlands. DES Action was still in the 1990s a prime mover in securing resources for research and follow-up of women who had been exposed to diethylstilbestrol, and in promoting educational programs for those women and for medical professionals.

Initiatives by medical researchers, by DES Action, and by the Public Citizen's Health Research Group secured funding in the USA for medical research on the prevalence of cancer and other effects in the young women who had been exposed in utero, and eventually also the men. The US National Institute for Environmental Health Sciences (NIEHS) has been one of the centers for toxicological studies of the effects of diethylstilbestrol. A substantial amount of research on the effects of diethylstilbestrol—animal experiments as well as epidemiological studies—has produced a valuable body of knowledge about how hormones affect the development of the fetus and prime the individual for disease later in life.

As in the case of thalidomide, the emotional engagement evoked by the harm caused by diethylstilbestrol in pregnancy led to committed action. Some physicians have devoted a major part of their careers to finding out why and how diethylstilbestrol produced adverse effects. The anger over the harm caused by diethylstilbestrol inspired patients to a commitment to prevent further harm by engaging in political action and achieving an effective response from legislators and governmental administrators. Despite the abandonment of diethylstilbestrol in pregnancy for habitual or threatened abortion, its late effects continue to be reported. Essentially, the female offspring of these pregnancies tend to develop vaginal changes (adenosis, with cervical ectropion) when reaching adolescence or adulthood and these can subsequently give rise to a clear-cell adenocarcinoma. Whereas carcinomas are a late and infrequent event, even in exposed subjects, cervical vaginal adenosis is common, the incidence probably being some 30% (23). The estimated tumor risk is only 0.14–1.4 per 1000 diethylstilbestrol-exposed subjects, but since up to 6 million fetuses were exposed to diethylstilbestrol between 1940 and 1970 the total number affected in some way may be very high indeed. There is also a high incidence of fertility disturbances among these daughters, and their own pregnancies apparently stand a high chance of not going normally to term (SED-12, 1023) (24). Analogous changes were found in male offspring (25). As in the case of thalidomide, an important element in determining cause and effect was the characteristic nature of the defect: the vaginal pathology does occur spontaneously but is highly unusual. A major problem has been the fact that the defect is as a rule only recognizable so many years after birth, by which time the history of the original treatment may be difficult or impossible to reconstruct. Even today the material is not homogeneous and strict statistical analysis of some of the epidemiological data has been claimed to point to a series of shortcomings. This does not undermine the clear conclusion that the drug is indeed responsible for the effects described (26).

Epidemiological studies on the complications of the use of diethylstilbestrol in pregnancy will certainly produce new data as time goes on: most of the data will probably continue to come from the USA and the Netherlands, where diethylstilbestrol was much more widely used to treat habitual or threatened abortion than elsewhere. In France 150 000–200 000 pregnancies were involved; in the Netherlands, with a much smaller population, 180 000–380 000 pregnant women were treated with diethylstilbestrol up to 1976.

Vaginal adenosis and adenocarcinoma

Second-generation (and possible third-generation) effects of diethylstilbestrol continue to be reported (27,28). Typical is a 1987 update analysing 519 cases of clear-cell carcinoma of the vagina and cervix identified by the Registry for Research on Hormonal Transplacental Carcinogenesis of the University of Chicago (18); in 60% of all cases the patient's mother could be shown to have used diethylstilbestrol during pregnancy. The median age at diagnosis was 19 years. The authors argued that in view of the relative rarity of the tumors, even in exposed women, one could consider that diethylstilbestrol is not a complete carcinogen and that some other factor is also involved in the pathogenesis of this type of carcinoma. The particular question of third-generation injury has actually been the subject of judicial proceedings in the USA (27,28); on the balance of evidence it seems that it can occur, although the mechanism is not clear.

Evidence has also emerged on long-term survival in young women with a clear-cell adenocarcinoma of the vagina, 20% of whom had been exposed to diethylstilbestrol and 80% had not (29). The probabilities of survival at 5 and 10 years for diethylstilbestrol-associated cases were 84 and 78% respectively, compared with 69 and 60% for those not associated with diethylstilbestrol. These differences were not due to differences in clinical prognostic factors, but suggest differences in tumor behavior for as yet undetermined reasons.

Although it is more than 30 years since the full extent of the injury to offspring by the ill-advised use of diethylstilbestrol during pregnancy became clear, details of that injury are still being filled in as the individuals concerned grow older. The picture will continue to develop as long as this generation of individuals lives, and it is even possible that findings in the third generation will throw light on the persisting injury to the family.

Psychological research among "DES daughters" has shown how traumatic it can be for a woman to learn of her prenatal exposure to diethylstilbestrol, and the extent to which this creates persistent uncertainty about her health; the failure of a physician to provide reliable information and continuing support can severely undermine her faith in health care (30).

Table 1 Outcomes in pregnancies exposed and not exposed to diethylstilbestrol

Outcome	Exposed (%)	Non-exposed (%)
Full-term delivery	64	85
Spontaneous abortion	19	10
Preterm delivery	12	4.1
Ectopic pregnancy	4.2	0.8

Long-term studies of the pregnancy experiences of women exposed to diethylstilbestrol in utero, compared with unexposed women, now include one in the US National Collaborative Diethylstilbestrol Adenosis cohort and one in the Chicago cohort and their respective non-exposed comparison groups. A review of questionnaire replies from 3373 exposed daughters and from controls has confirmed that diethylstilbestrol-exposed women were less likely than unexposed women to have had full-term live births and more likely to have had premature births, spontaneous pregnancy losses, or ectopic pregnancies (31). The data are shown in Table 1. Second-trimester spontaneous pregnancy losses were much more common in diethylstilbestrol-exposed women.

Other cancers

Long-term data are also accumulating on the actual incidence of genital cancer in women exposed to diethylstilbestrol in utero (32). In the Netherlands, a country in which diethylstilbestrol was used intensively in pregnancy, there is evidence that the risk of cervical cancer in these women is trebled, rather than doubled as was previously supposed (33).

- A diethylstilbestrol-exposed woman developed concurrent primary cancers of both the vagina and the endometrium at the age of 39 (34).

However, it is important to bear in mind that cases occur in which there is no history of the mother's having taken diethylstilbestrol during pregnancy. In one such case, HIV/AIDS infection was also a predisposing factor for vaginal carcinoma and this could explain a proportion of new cases that are being reported today (35).

A further follow-up and analysis of 3879 women, taken from two earlier US studies, who had been exposed to diethylstilbestrol during pregnancy has been presented (36). The results showed a modest association between diethylstilbestrol exposure and the risk of breast cancer (RR = 1.27; 95% CI = 1.07, 1.52). The increased risk was not further aggravated by a family history of breast cancer, by use of oral contraceptives, or by HRT. There was no evidence that diethylstilbestrol was associated with a raised risk of ovarian, endometrial, or other hormone-associated cancers.

Sensory systems

A study in the USA has produced some evidence that in people with amblyopia, those who were exposed to diethylstilbestrol before birth may be more likely to develop myopia (37).

Menstrual and vaginal disturbances

The effects of in-utero exposure to diethylstilbestrol on the menstrual cycle have been studied prospectively in 198 women and in 162 unexposed controls (38). A major limitation of this study was the exclusion of women with a severe menstrual abnormality. Exposure to diethylstilbestrol was associated with a statistical significantly lower duration of menstrual bleeding but not with dysmenorrhea. For most women exposed to diethylstilbestrol, any effects on reproductive hormonal function are in all probability minor, if present at all.

Even the classic genital manifestations of diethylstilbestrol in women who have been exposed to it in fetal life may be overlooked unless one is alert to them; vaginal discharge with ectropion should cause one to enquire as to possible prenatal diethylstilbestrol exposure (39).

Autoimmune disease

During the last 15 years, various additional aspects of the diethylstilbestrol problem have given rise to concern. One emerged in 1988 from a large multicenter epidemiological cohort study established by the US National Cancer Institute (DESAD Project), in which it was found that women exposed in utero to diethylstilbestrol had a 50% increased incidence of autoimmune disease (40).

Drug Administration

Drug formulations

The parenteral formulation diethylstilbestrol diphosphate is less commonly used than the oral formulation. In Japan, 24 elderly patients with advanced relapsed prostatic cancer were treated with high doses supplemented with ethinylestradiol (doses unclear); there was some slight therapeutic effect, but there were gastrointestinal symptoms and fluid retention (41). Also in Japan, a few patients with advanced disease were treated using intravenous diethylstilbestrol diphosphate 500 mg/day for 20 consecutive days to a total dose of 10 g; the authors' conclusion was more positive but adverse events were not specified (42).

Drug contamination

Contamination of isoniazid tablets with diethylstilbestrol was the cause of several cases of precocious puberty in a children's tuberculosis ward (43).

References

1. Lonning PE, Taylor PD, Anker G, Iddon J, Wie L, Jorgensen LM, Mella O, Howell A. High-dose estrogen treatment in postmenopausal breast cancer patients heavily exposed to endocrine therapy. Breast Cancer Res Treat 2001;67(2):111–16.
2. Takezawa Y, Nakata S, Kobayashi M, Kosaku N, Fukabori Y, Yamanaka H. Moderate dose diethylstilbestrol diphosphate therapy in hormone refractory prostate cancer. Scand J Urol Nephrol 2001;35(4):283–7.

3. Pavone-Macaluso M, de Voogt HJ, Viggiano G, Barasolo E, Lardennois B, de Pauw M, Sylvester R. Comparison of diethylstilbestrol, cyproterone acetate and medroxyprogesterone acetate in the treatment of advanced prostatic cancer: final analysis of a randomized phase III trial of the European Organization for Research on Treatment of Cancer Urological Group. J Urol 1986;136(3):624–31.
4. Harley HA, Mason R, Phillips PJ. Profound hypocalcaemia associated with oestrogen treatment of carcinoma of the prostate. Med J Aust 1983;2(1):41–2.
5. Burke L, Segall-Blank M, Lorenzo C, Dynesius-Trentham R, Trentham D, Mortola JF. Altered immune response in adult women exposed to diethylstilbestrol in utero. Am J Obstet Gynecol 2001;185(1):78–81.
6. Herbst AL, editor. Intrauterine exposure to diethlystilbestrol in the human. Proceedings, "Symposium on DES". Chicago: American College of Obstetricians and Gynecologists, 1977.
7. Antunes CM, Strolley PD, Rosenshein NB, Davies JL, Tonascia JA, Brown C, Burnett L, Rutledge A, Pokempner M, Garcia R. Endometrial cancer and estrogen use. Report of a large case-control study. N Engl J Med 1979;300(1):9–13.
8. Williams GM, Iatropoulos M, Cheung R, Radi L, Wang CX. Diethylstilbestrol liver carcinogenicity and modification of DNA in rats. Cancer Lett 1993; 68(2–3):193–8.
9. Rosinus V, Maurer R. [Diättylstilböstrol-induziertes Leberzellkarzinom? Diethylstilbestrol-induced liver cancer?] Schweiz Med Wochenschr 1981;111(30):1139–42.
10. Martino MA, Nevadunsky NS, Magliaro TJ, Goldberg MI. The DES (diethylstilbestrol) years: bridging the past into the future. Prim Care Update Ob Gyns 2002;9:7–12.
11. Smith OW. Diethylstilbestrol in prevention of complications of pregnancy. Am J Obstet Gynecol 1948;56:821–34.
12. Smith OW, Smith GV. The influence of diethylstilbestrol on the progress and outcome of pregnancy as based on a comparison of treated with untreated primigravidas. Am J Obstet Gynecol 1949;58(5):994–1009.
13. Lacassagne A. Apparition d'adénocarcinomes mammaires chez des souris mâles traités par une substance oestrogène synthétique. Comptes Rend Séances Soc Biol 1938;129:641–3.
14. Dieckmann WJ, Davis ME, Rynkiewicz LM, Pottinger RE. Does the administration of diethylstilbestrol during pregnancy have therapeutic value? Am J Obstet Gynecol 1953;66(5):1062–81.
15. Herbst AL, Ulfelder H, Poskanzer DC. Adenocarcinoma of the vagina. Association of maternal stilbestrol therapy with tumor appearance in young women. N Engl J Med 1971;284(15):878–81.
16. US Department of Health, Education and Welfare, Food and Drug Administration. Certain estrogens for oral or parenteral use. Drugs for human use. Drug efficacy study implementation. Federal Register 1971;36(217):21537–8.
17. Mitchell S, producer, Wait J, presenter. Face the Facts. BBC Radio 4, 21 February 2000.
18. Melnick S, Cole P, Anderson D, Herbst A. Rates and risks of diethylstilbestrol-related clear-cell adenocarcinoma of the vagina and cervix. An update. N Engl J Med 1987;316(9):514–16.
19. Palmlund I. Exposure to a xenoestrogen before birth: the diethylstilbestrol experience. J Psychosom Obstet Gynaecol 1996;17(2):71–84.
20. Nash S, Tilley BC, Kurland LT, Gundersen J, Barnes AB, Labarthe D, Donohew PS, Kovacs L. Identifying and tracing a population at risk: the DESAD Project experience. Am J Public Health 1983;73(3):253–9.
21. Norwood C. At highest risk: environmental hazards to young and unborn children. New York: McGraw-Hill, 1980:141.
22. Direcks A, Figueroa S, Mintzes B, Banta D. DES European Study: DES Action the Netherlands for the European Commission Programme "Europe Against Cancer". Utrecht: DES Action the Netherlands, 1991:13, 25.
23. Sopena-Bonnet B. L'adénose cervico-vaginale: l'une des conséquences possibles de l'exposition in utero au DES. Contracept Fertil Sex 1989;17:461.
24. Senekjian EK, Potkul RK, Frey K, Herbst AL. Infertility among daughters either exposed or not exposed to diethylstilbestrol. Am J Obstet Gynecol 1988;158(3 Pt 1):493–8.
25. Hembree WC, Nagler HM, Fang JS, Myles EL, Jagiello GM. Infertility in a patient with abnormal spermatogenesis and in utero DES exposure. Int J Fertil 1988;33(3):173–7.
26. Buitendijk S. Diethylstilbestrol and the next generation—a challenge to the evidence? In: Dukes MNG, editor. Side Effects of Drugs, Annual 12. Amsterdam: Elsevier, 1988:346–8.
27. Lynch HT, Quinn T, Severin MJ. Diethylstilbestrol, teratogenesis and carcinogenesis: medical/legal implications of its long-term sequelae, including third-generation effects. Int J Risk Safety Med 1990;1:171.
28. Curran WJ. The DES product liability story in America: the third generation litigation. Int J Risk Safety Med 1992;3:229.
29. Waggoner SE, Mittendorf R, Biney N, Anderson D, Herbst AL. Influence of in utero diethylstilbestrol exposure on the prognosis and biologic behavior of vaginal clear-cell adenocarcinoma. Gynecol Oncol 1994;55(2):238–44.
30. Duke SS, McGraw SA, Avis NE, Sherman A. A focus group study of DES daughters: implications for health care providers. Psychooncology 2000;9(5):439–44.
31. Kaufman RH, Adam E, Hatch EE, Noller K, Herbst AL, Palmer JR, Hoover RN. Continued follow-up of pregnancy outcomes in diethylstilbestrol-exposed offspring. Obstet Gynecol 2000;96(4):483–9.
32. Herbst AL. Behavior of estrogen-associated female genital tract cancer and its relation to neoplasia following intrauterine exposure to diethylstilbestrol (DES). Gynecol Oncol 2000;76(2):147–56.
33. Verloop J, Rookus MA, van Leeuwen FE. Prevalence of gynecologic cancer in women exposed to diethylstilbestrol in utero. N Engl J Med 2000;342(24):1838–9.
34. Keller C, Nanda R, Shannon RL, Amit A, Kaplan AL. Concurrent primaries of vaginal clear cell adenocarcinoma and endometrial adenocarcinoma in a 39-year old woman with in utero diethylstilbestrol exposure. Int J Gynecol Cancer 2001;11(3):247–50.
35. Izquierdo Mendez N, Herraiz Martinez MA, Furio Bacete V, Cristobal Garcia I, Vidart Aragon JA, Escudero Fernandez M. Adenocarcinoma de celulas claras de cupula vaginal sin relacion con des (dietilestilbestrol): a proposito de un caso y revision de la literatura. Acta Ginecol 2001;58:21–6.
36. Titus-Ernstoff L, Hatch EE, Hoover RN, Palmer J, Greenberg ER, Ricker W, Kaufman R, Noller K, Herbst AL, Colton T, Hartge P. Long-term cancer risk in women given diethylstilbestrol (DES) during pregnancy. Br J Cancer 2001;84(1):126–33.
37. Lempert P. Myopia in diethylstilboestrol exposed amblyopic subjects. Br J Ophthalmol 1999;83(1):126.
38. Hornsby PP, Wilcox AJ, Weinberg CR, Herbst AL. Effects on the menstrual cycle of in utero exposure to diethylstilbestrol. Am J Obstet Gynecol 1994;170(3):709–15.
39. Wingfield M. Not just a cervical ectropion. Three case reports of diethylstilbestrol (DES) exposed women presenting with vaginal discharge and cervical ectropion. J Obstet Gynaecol 1999;19(6):649–51.

40. Noller KL, Blair PB, O'Brien PC, Melton LJ 3rd, Offord JR, Kaufman RH, Colton T. Increased occurrence of autoimmune disease among women exposed in utero to diethylstilbestrol. Fertil Steril 1988;49(6):1080–2.
41. Hisamatsu H, Sakai H, Kanetake H. High-dose intravenous diethylstilbestrol diphosphate (DES-DP) in the treatment of prostatic cancer during relapse. Nioshinihon J Urol 2002;64:199–202.
42. Michinaga S, Ariyoshi A. High-dose intravenous diethylstilbestrol diphosphate therapy for hormone-refractory prostate cancer. Nishinihon J Urol 2002;64:203–5.
43. Weber WW, Grossman M, Thom JV, Sax J, Chan JJ, Duffy M. Drug contamination with diethylstilbestrol. Outbreak of precocious puberty due to contaminated isonicocinic acid hydrazide (INH). N Engl J Med 1963;268:411–15.

Diethyltoluamide

General Information

Diethyltoluamide is an insect repellent.

Organs and Systems

Nervous system

Toxic encephalopathy has been reported in children sprayed repeatedly with diethyltoluamide 10–15% (1).

Psychological, psychiatric

Acute manic psychosis has been attributed to percutaneous absorption of diethyltoluamide (SEDA-12, 138).

Reference

1. Edwards DL, Johnson CE. Insect-repellent-induced toxic encephalopathy in a child. Clin Pharm 1987;6(6):496–8.

Difenpiramide

See also Non-steroidal anti-inflammatory drugs

General Information

Difenpiramide, a phenylacetic acid derivative, is less efficacious but has fewer adverse effects than indometacin or phenylbutazone. The most frequent reactions are in the gastrointestinal tract and skin (1). However, gastrointestinal tolerance is, as one would expect, better (2).

References

1. Jochems OB, Janbroers JM. Diphenpyramide: a review of its pharmacology and anti-inflammatory effects. Pharmatherapeutica 1986;4(7):429–41.

2. Fumagalli M, Montrone F, Vernazza M, Tirrito M, Santandrea S, Caruso I. La difenpiramide nel trattamento dell'artrite reumatoide: studio in doppio cieco a breve termine versus indometacina. [Diphenpiramide in the treatment of rheumatoid arthritis: short-time double-blind study of its comparison with indomethacin.] Clin Ter 1979;89(6):581–8.

Difetarsone

General Information

Difetarsone is a pentavalent arsenical that often causes minor adverse effects, such as rashes, nausea, vomiting, and abdominal discomfort. Transient increases in transaminase activities can occur (SEDA-13, 834) (1).

Organs and Systems

Immunologic

Generalized angioedema occurred in a patient taking difetarsone 500 mg tds for *Entamoeba histolytica* infection (SEDA-11, 597) (2).

References

1. Committee on Antimicrobial Agents, Canadian Infectious Disease Society. Treatment of parasitic infections: Canadian versus US recommendations. Can Med Assoc J 1988;139:849.
2. McIntyre L, Krajden S, Keystone JS. Angioedema due to diphetarsone and a review of its toxicity. Trop Geogr Med 1983;35(1):49–51.

Diflunisal

General Information

Diflunisal is a fluorinated salicylic acid derivative, which is absorbed unchanged from the gastrointestinal tract, reaching peak concentrations after about 2 hours, and is metabolized by glucuronidation (1). Its adverse effects and other characteristics are those of aspirin, although gastrointestinal haemorrhage may be less common (2).

References

1. Davies RO. Review of the animal and clinical pharmacology of diflunisal. Pharmacotherapy 1983;3(2 pt 2):9S–22S.
2. Turner RA, Shackleford RW, Whipple JP. Comparison of diflunisal and aspirin in long-term treatment of patients with rheumatoid arthritis. Clin Ther 1986;9 (Suppl C):37–46.

Diftalone

General Information

Because of hepatotoxicity and carcinogenicity (hepatoma) detected in preclinical studies, and hemotoxicity and gastrointestinal adverse effects in man, diftalone has been withdrawn by its manufacturer (1).

Reference

1. Anonymous. Dow Lepetit drops diftalone. Scrip 1977; October 15;22.

Dihydrocodeine

See also Opioid analgesics

General Information

Dihydrocodeine is an opioid analgesic related to codeine, in which the double bond in the 7th position is saturated. It is about one-tenth as potent as morphine and 2–3 times more potent than codeine. It is similar to codeine in other respects. The most common adverse effects are nausea, vomiting, and drowsiness (SEDA-16, 79) (SEDA-17, 80) (SEDA-18, 79).

In a randomized, double-blind comparison of the antitussive effect of dihydrocodeine 10 mg tds with levodropropizine 75 mg tds in 140 adults with primary lung cancer or metastatic cancer there was no significant difference between the two drugs as far as cough severity and the numbers of night wakings were concerned, both drugs leading to significant improvement (1). However, dihydrocodeine caused significantly more somnolence, which was reported by 11% and in some cases was continuous. Other adverse effects reported by those taking dihydrocodeine included erythema of the abdomen and epigastric pain, although constipation, a potential adverse effect of codeine derivatives, was not reported.

Organs and Systems

Sensory systems

Severe narcosis after therapeutic doses (2) has been reported.

Urinary tract

Acute renal insufficiency after therapeutic doses (2) has been reported.

Dihydrocodeine was implicated in cases of granulomatous interstitial nephritis (3).

Immunologic

Anaphylaxis has been reported with dihydrocodeine (4).

Susceptibility Factors

Age

There is a risk in giving dihydrocodeine to the elderly (2).

Renal disease

There is a risk in giving dihydrocodeine to those with renal insufficiency (2).

Drug Administration

Drug formulations

A modified-release formulation extends the duration of action of dihydrocodeine from 2–4 hours to 12 hours. In 12 volunteers who took modified-release dihydrocodeine 60 mg or 120 mg and 120 minutes later lactulose 40 mg diluted in 100 mg of water, the orocecal transit time was significantly prolonged by dihydrocodeine compared with placebo (5). Dihydrocodeine also significantly suppressed the pupillary light reflex. Both dosages caused similar adverse effects. Tiredness and dry mouth were reported in 80%, vertigo in 5%, and headache in 1%.

References

1. Luporini G, Barni S, Marchi E, Daffonchio L. Efficacy and safety of levodropropizine and dihydrocodeine on nonproductive cough in primary and metastatic lung cancer. Eur Respir J 1998;12(1):97–101.
2. Park GR, Shelly MP, Quinn K, Roberts P. Dihydrocodeine—a reversible cause of renal failure? Eur J Anaesthesiol 1989;6(4):303–14.
3. Singer DR, Simpson JG, Catto GR, Johnston AW. Drug hypersensitivity causing granulomatous interstitial nephritis. Am J Kidney Dis 1988;11(4):357–9.
4. Panos MZ, Burnett S, Gazzard BG. Use of naloxone in opioid-induced anaphylactoid reaction. Br J Anaesth 1988;61(3):371.
5. Freye E, Baranowski J, Latasch L. Dose-related effects of controlled release dihydrocodeine on oro-cecal transit and pupillary light reflex. A study in human volunteers. Arzneimittelforschung 2001;51(1):60–6.

Dilevalol

See also Beta-adrenoceptor antagonists

General Information

Dilevalol is one of the four enantiomers of labetalol. It was withdrawn from the market by its manufacturers in early 1991 because of an unacceptably high incidence of liver damage (1).

Reference

1. Harvengt C. Labetalol hepatoxicity. Ann Intern Med 1990;114:341.

Diloxanide

General Information

Diloxanide often causes flatulence and, occasionally, nausea, vomiting, diarrhea, urticaria, and pruritus. It is an excellent luminal amebicide and is indicated after treatment with the 5-nitroimidazole compounds, which have relatively weak activity on the cyst stage. Experience over 14 years has been summarized by the Centers for Disease Control and Prevention (CDC, Atlanta), confirming the minimal toxicity of diloxanide. Fewer adverse effects were reported in patients aged 20 months to 10 years than in those aged over 10 years. There is no record of interactions between diloxanide and either metronidazole or tinidazole (SEDA-13, 830) (SEDA-17, 333).

Diltiazem

See also Calcium channel blockers

General Information

Diltiazem is a benzthiazepine calcium channel blocker.

Organs and Systems

Cardiovascular

Diltiazem can be associated with heart block (1,2). In a randomized trial in patients with non-Q-wave myocardial infarction, 38 of 287 patients who took diltiazem developed some degree of atrioventricular block at some time. Of these episodes, 32 were first-degree, eight were second-degree, and only two were third-degree. In the placebo-treated group there were 10 events in 289 patients; eight were first-degree, two second-degree, and none third-degree.

Atrioventricular block has been reported in three patients taking therapeutic doses of diltiazem; one died (3).

- A 47-year-old man taking furosemide for hypertension was given diltiazem 300 mg/day to achieve better blood pressure control; 1 month later he developed atrioventricular block, resolved by atropine.
- A 62-year-old hypertensive man with renal artery stenosis, an adrenal adenoma, peripheral artery disease, and an abdominal aortic aneurysm developed a hypertensive crisis with chest pain. He was treated with nitrates, heparin, aspirin, and nicardipine, which were afterwards replaced by diltiazem 200 mg/day, because of persistent chest pain. He developed atrioventricular block 2 hours after the second dose of diltiazem, and was successfully treated with a pacemaker.
- A 59-year-old woman with a previous myocardial infarction, hypertension, diabetes, and uterine cancer developed angina. She was treated with nitrates, aspirin, and heparin; diltiazem 200 mg/day was then added because of persistent chest pain. She developed atrioventricular block 72 hours later, and despite resuscitative efforts died in electromechanical dissociation.

Following the publication of a report of heart block (4), further cases (junctional bradycardia, sinoatrial block) have been reported (5).

Nervous system

Paresthesia of the hands and feet has been reported with diltiazem (SEDA-17, 237). Akathisia has been attributed to diltiazem (6). Parkinsonism associated with diltiazem has been reported (7).

- A 53-year-old man with hypertension took diltiazem 60–120 mg/day for 5 years and then developed parkinsonism. His neurological symptoms were treated without success and only after the substitution of diltiazem with an ACE inhibitor did his parkinsonian symptoms begin to regress, with eventual complete recovery.

Urinary tract

Diltiazem was associated with the development of acute renal insufficiency in a patient being treated for severe retrosternal chest pain who had neither primary kidney disease nor urinary tract obstruction (8,9).

Acute interstitial nephritis has been attributed to diltiazem (9).

- A 53-year-old man was given diltiazem for precordial pain and about 2 hours later developed an erythematous maculopapular rash mainly on the trunk and lower limbs. Four days later he developed abdominal pain radiating to both renal angles, accompanied by dysuria and tenesmus and followed 6 days later by acute renal insufficiency associated with raised liver function test results.

In this case, the self-limiting resolution in 4–5 days without relapse, the presence of the skin rash, and the liver sequelae suggested a common immunoallergic mechanism. The clinical symptoms, the time relation between drug administration and the occurrence of the syndrome, the inability to explain the syndrome otherwise, and its disappearance on withdrawal of diltiazem support an association with the drug.

A retrospective analysis of postoperative renal function in patients undergoing cardiac operations has been conducted to evaluate whether the use of prophylactic intravenous diltiazem, in order to reduce the incidence of ischemia and dysrhythmias, was associated with increased renal dysfunction (10). The incidence of acute renal insufficiency requiring dialysis was 4.4% with diltiazem versus 0.7% in the controls. Logistic regression analysis suggested that the risk of acute renal insufficiency was strongly associated with intravenous diltiazem, age, baseline serum creatinine, the presence of left main coronary disease, and the presence of cerebrovascular disease.

Skin

Skin reactions ranging from exanthems to severe adverse events have been reported in association with diltiazem

(SED-13, 513) (SEDA-18, 215) (SEDA-22, 216). Three cases of skin reactions (hypersensitivity syndrome reaction, pruritic exanthematous eruption, and acute generalized exanthematous pustulosis) possibly induced by diltiazem have been described and the literature on skin reactions associated with calcium antagonists has been reviewed. The number of diltiazem-induced cutaneous events was significantly greater than those induced by either nifedipine or verapamil. However, there was no difference in the proportion of serious cutaneous adverse events due to any of these three drugs (11).

Cutaneous vasculitis (12) and angioedema (13,14) have been reported with diltiazem. In 1988, the Federal German Health Authorities imposed a warning of dermal hypersensitivity reactions (including erythema multiforme) with diltiazem.

- Acute generalized exanthematous pustulosis in an 82-year-old woman was confirmed as being due to diltiazem by a positive patch test (15).
- Exfoliative dermatitis with fever occurred in a 69-year-old man with ischemic heart disease treated with mexiletine and diltiazem for three weeks; the rash resolved after withdrawal of both drugs and systemic corticosteroid therapy. Patch tests with mexiletine and diltiazem were positive. In addition to this case, 39 cases of drug eruption due to diltiazem have been reported in Japan (16).
- Lichenoid purpura of 6 months' duration occurred in a 65-year-old man with hypertension who had taken diltiazem for 1 month. Topical therapy with a very potent glucocorticoid was not effective and the eruption began to regress only after diltiazem withdrawal, after which it disappeared 3 weeks later (17).

Four cases of photodistributed hyperpigmentation associated with long-term administration of a modified-release formulation of diltiazem hydrochloride have been reported (18). All the patients were African-American women, mean age 62 (range 49–72) years. The duration of diltiazem administration before the development of hyperpigmentation was 6–11 months. The hyperpigmentation was slate-gray and reticulated. Phototesting during diltiazem therapy showed a reduced minimal erythema dose to UVA in one patient. Histological examination showed lichenoid dermatitis with prominent pigmentary incontinence. Electron microscopy showed multiple melanosome complexes. Withdrawal of diltiazem resulted in gradual resolution of the hyperpigmentation.

Acute generalized exanthematous pustular dermatitis has been reported after diltiazem (19).

Drug Administration

Drug overdose

Several cases of accidental or deliberate self-poisoning with calcium antagonists have been described (SED-12, 452) (SEDA-16, 198) (SEDA-20, 186) and different approaches to the management of these patients have been proposed.

- A 52-year-old woman with essential hypertension erroneously took a 7-day supply of modified-release diltiazem, enalapril, and trichlormethiazide, and 30 minutes later complained of nausea (20). She was treated with gastric lavage, calcium gluconate, activated charcoal, and polyethylene glycol. Her blood pressure and heart rate fell progressively to 120/62 mmHg and 40/minute respectively, 14 hours after ingestion. Afterwards, her hemodynamic status gradually normalized without further treatment.
- A 54-year-old man with severe triple vessel coronary artery disease took six modified-release diltiazem tablets 180 mg following an episode of severe angina, and 10 hours later developed bradycardia, hypotension, and severe pulmonary edema, but was free of chest pain (21). After intensive hemodynamic monitoring and noradrenaline treatment, his renal, respiratory, and cardiac problems recovered to baseline over the next 48 hours. Diltiazem overdose was confirmed by a diltiazem serum concentration of 1230 ng/ml (usual target range 40–160 ng/ml).
- A 15-year-old woman intentionally took 10 modified-release tablets of diltiazem 200 mg. She developed hypertension, oliguria, pulmonary edema, and respiratory distress syndrome, and required mechanical ventilation for 3 days, besides intravenous calcium, dopamine, and noradrenaline. After 5 days in an intensive care unit, she was transferred to a psychiatric hospital in good physical condition (22).
- A 50-year-old man took 28 modified-release tablets of diltiazem 240 mg and 28 tablets of hydrochlorothiazide and 12–14 hours later became lethargic but oriented and complaining of nausea and dizziness; he had bradypnea, hypotension, and second-degree heart block with bradycardia (23). He was given activated charcoal, oxygen, atropine, glucagon, and calcium gluconate by prolonged infusion. His heart rate, blood pressure, and electrocardiogram recovered to baseline over the next 24 hours, with no further episodes of dysrhythmias or hypotension.
- A 38-year-old white man with a history of coronary artery disease, myocardial infarction, coronary artery by-pass, alcoholism, and depression took a combined massive overdose of diltiazem and atenolol (24). He underwent cardiopulmonary resuscitation because of cardiac arrest; bradycardia, hypotension, and oliguria followed and were resistant to intravenous pacing and multiple pharmacological interventions, including intravenous fluids, calcium, dopamine, dobutamine, adrenaline, prenalterol, and glucagon. Adequate mean arterial pressure and urine output were restored only after the addition of phenylephrine and transvenous pacing. He survived despite myocardial infarction and pneumonia.

Drug–Drug Interactions

Ciclosporin

Many studies have shown an interaction of ciclosporin with diltiazem: concomitant administration allows reduction of the daily dose of ciclosporin. However, according to a study in eight renal transplant recipients, the low systemic availability and high degree of variation in diltiazem metabolism within and between patients can give unpredictable results (25).

Diltiazem abolishes the acute renal hypoperfusion and vasoconstriction induced by ciclosporin in renal transplant patients. Plasma endothelin-1 may be a mediator of ciclosporin-induced renal hypoperfusion, but is not affected by diltiazem (26). This interaction has been confirmed with a new microemulsion formulation of ciclosporin in nine patients with renal transplants who took diltiazem 90–120 mg bd for 4 weeks (27). Diltiazem caused a 51% increase in the AUC of ciclosporin and a 34% increase in peak concentration, without altering the time to peak concentration. However, the ciclosporin microemulsion did not significantly affect the pharmacokinetics of diltiazem.

- Ciclosporin-induced encephalopathy was precipitated by diltiazem in a 76-year-old white woman with corticosteroid-resistant aplastic anemia and thrombocytopenia, type 2 diabetes, and coronary artery disease, who was taking diltiazem for hypertension (28). She became comatose after 13 days of therapy with ciclosporin, and clinical examination and electroencephalography showed diffuse encephalopathy of moderate severity. Ciclosporin was withdrawn and she regained consciousness after 36 hours.

Concomitant diltiazem without proper dosage adjustment of ciclosporin can cause adverse neurological events.

Methylprednisolone

Co-administration of diltiazem with methylprednisolone increased plasma concentrations of methylprednisolone and its adrenal suppressant effects in nine healthy volunteers (29). Care should be taken when these two drugs are co-administered for a long period, even if the clinical relevance of this pharmacokinetic interaction still needs to be evaluated.

Sildenafil

Sildenafil is metabolized predominantly by CYP3A4, which diltiazem inhibits. An interaction of diltiazem with sildenafil has been reported (30).

- A 72-year-old man, who regularly took aspirin, metoprolol, diltiazem, and sublingual glyceryl trinitrate for stable angina, reported chest pain during elective prognostic coronary angiography, which resolved with half of a sublingual tablet of glyceryl trinitrate. Within 2 minutes he developed severe hypotension, with an unchanged electrocardiogram and no evidence of anaphylaxis. He had taken sildenafil 50 mg 48 hours before angiography.

The interval after which even short-acting nitrates can be safely given after the use of sildenafil is likely to be substantially longer than 24 hours when elderly patients are concurrently taking a CYP3A4 inhibitor, such as diltiazem.

Sirolimus

The pharmacokinetic interaction of a single oral dose of diltiazem 120 mg with a single oral dose of sirolimus 10 mg has been studied in 18 healthy subjects, 12 men and 6 women, 20–43 years old, in an open, three-period, randomized, crossover study (31). The whole-blood sirolimus AUC increased by 60% and the C_{max} by 43% with diltiazem co-administration; the apparent oral clearance and volume of distribution of sirolimus fell by 38 and 45% respectively, consistent with the change in half-life from 79 to 67 hours. Sirolimus had no effect on the pharmacokinetics of diltiazem or on the effects of diltiazem on either diastolic or systolic blood pressures or the electrocardiogram. Single-dose diltiazem co-administration leads to higher sirolimus exposure, presumably by the inhibition of first-pass metabolism. Because of pronounced intersubject variability in this interaction, whole-blood sirolimus concentrations should be monitored closely in patients taking the two drugs.

Statins

Atorvastatin

Rhabdomyolysis and acute hepatitis have been reported in association with the co-administration of diltiazem and atorvastatin (32).

- A 60-year-old African-American man developed abdominal pain, a racing heart, and shortness of breath over 24 hours. He had also noticed increasing fatigue and reduced urine output over the previous 2–3 days. He had been taking several medications, including atorvastatin, for more than 1 year, but diltiazem had been added 3 weeks before for atrial fibrillation. On the basis of laboratory findings and physical examination, a diagnosis of acute hepatitis and rhabdomyolysis with accompanying acute renal insufficiency was made. His renal function gradually normalized and his CK activity reached a maximum of 2092 units/l on day 1 and fell to 623 units/l on discharge. His liver function tests returned to normal by 3 months.

While rhabdomyolysis from statins is rare, the risk is increased when they are used in combination with agents that share similar metabolic pathways. Atorvastatin is metabolized by CYP3A4, which is inhibited by diltiazem.

Lovastatin

The effects of co-administration of oral diltiazem, a potent inhibitor of CYP3A, on the pharmacokinetics of lovastatin have been evaluated in a randomized study in 10 healthy volunteers (33). Lovastatin is oxidized by CYP3A to active metabolites. Diltiazem significantly increased the oral AUC and maximum serum concentration of lovastatin, but did not alter its half-life. The magnitude of the increase of plasma concentration of lovastatin suggested that caution is necessary when co-administering diltiazem and lovastatin.

In another study by the same investigators, 10 healthy volunteers were randomized in a two-way, crossover study either to oral lovastatin or to intravenous diltiazem followed by oral lovastatin. Intravenous diltiazem did not significantly affect the pharmacokinetics of lovastatin (oral AUC, C_{max}, t_{max}, or half-life), suggesting that the interaction does not occur systemically and is primarily a first-pass effect (34). Drug interactions with diltiazem may therefore become evident when a patient is changed from intravenous to oral dosing.

Pravastatin

The effects of co-administration of diltiazem, a potent inhibitor of CYP3A, on the pharmacokinetics of pravastatin have been evaluated in a randomized study in 10 healthy volunteers (33). Pravastatin is active alone and is not metabolized by CYP3A. Diltiazem did not alter the oral AUC, maximum serum concentration, or half-life of pravastatin.

Simvastatin

The interaction of diltiazem with simvastatin has been investigated in 135 patients attending a hypertension clinic (35). Cholesterol reduction in the 19 patients taking diltiazem was 33% compared with 25% in the other 116 patients (median difference 8.6%; 95% CI = 1.1, 12). Multivariate analysis showed that concurrent diltiazem therapy, age, and the starting dose of simvastatin were independent predictors of percentage cholesterol response. The authors concluded that patients who take both diltiazem and simvastatin may need lower doses of simvastatin to achieve the recommended reduction in cholesterol.

Results from two clinical studies of the interaction of diltiazem with simvastatin showed that diltiazem increased the C_{max} of simvastatin (36) and enhanced its cholesterol-reducing effect (35).

In 10 healthy volunteers taking oral simvastatin 20 mg/day, diltiazem 120 mg bd for 2 weeks significantly increased the simvastatin C_{max} 3.6-fold, the AUC 5-fold, and the half-life 2.3-fold (36). There were no changes in the t_{max} of simvastatin or simvastatin acid.

Of 135 patients attending a hypertension clinic who were taking simvastatin for primary or secondary prevention of coronary heart disease, 19 were also taking diltiazem (35). The cholesterol reduction in the 19 patients taking diltiazem was significantly higher than in the other 116 (33 versus 25%), with less interindividual variability. Concurrent diltiazem therapy, age, and the starting dose of simvastatin were significant independent predictors of the percentage cholesterol response.

Rhabdomyolysis due to an interaction of simvastatin with diltiazem has been reported (37).

- A 75-year-old-man taking simvastatin 80 mg/day and diltiazem 240 mg/day developed extreme weakness and diffuse muscle pain. All drugs were withdrawn and he underwent hemodialysis. Within 3 weeks his muscle pain disappeared and he regained function in his legs. The activities of creatine kinase and transaminases gradually returned to normal, but he continued to need hemodialysis.

Tacrolimus

Diltiazem can increase the blood concentration of the macrolide immunosuppressant tacrolimus (38).

- A 68-year-old man developed diarrhea, dehydration, and atrial fibrillation 4 months after liver transplantation. He was taking tacrolimus (blood concentration 13 ng/ml) and was given a continuous infusion of diltiazem for 1 day followed by oral therapy. Three days later he became delirious, confused, and agitated, and the blood concentration of tacrolimus was 55 ng/ml. His mental status gradually improved after withdrawal of both drugs.

The mechanism of this interaction is likely to be the inhibition of tacrolimus metabolism in the intestine and liver by the inhibition of CYP3A4 and P glycoprotein.

References

1. Hossack KF. Conduction abnormalities due to diltiazem. N Engl J Med 1982;307(15):953–4.
2. Schroeder JS, Feldman RL, Giles TD, Friedman MJ, DeMaria AN, Kinney EL, Mallon SM, Pit B, Meyer R, Basta LL, Curry RC Jr, Groves BM, MacAlpin RN. Multiclinic controlled trial of diltiazem for Prinzmetal's angina. Am J Med 1982;72(2):227–32.
3. Boujnah MR, Jaafari A, Boukhris B, Boussabah I, Thameur M. Bloc sino-auriculaire induit par le diltiazem aux doses thérapeutiques. A propos de trois observations. [Sinoatrial block induced by therapeutic doses of diltiazem. Report of 3 cases.] Tunis Med 2000;78(12):735–7.
4. Waller PC, Inman WH. Diltiazem and heart block. Lancet 1989;1(8638):617.
5. Nagle RE, Low-Beer T, Horton R. Diltiazem and heart block. Lancet 1989;1(8643):907.
6. Jacobs MB. Diltiazem and akathisia. Ann Intern Med 1983;99(6):794–5.
7. Remblier C, Kassir A, Richard D, Perault MC, Guibert S. Syndrome parkinsonien sous diltiazem. [Parkinson syndrome from diltiazem.] Therapie 2001;56(1):57–9.
8. ter Wee PM, Rosman JB, van der Geest S. Acute renal failure due to diltiazem. Lancet 1984;2(8415):1337–8.
9. Abadin JA, Duran JA, Perez de Leon JA. Probable diltiazem-induced acute interstitial nephritis. Ann Pharmacother 1998;32(6):656–8.
10. Young EW, Diab A, Kirsh MM. Intravenous diltiazem and acute renal failure after cardiac operations. Ann Thorac Surg 1998;65(5):1316–19.
11. Knowles S, Gupta AK, Shear NH. The spectrum of cutaneous reactions associated with diltiazem: three cases and a review of the literature. J Am Acad Dermatol 1998;38 (2 Pt 1):201–6.
12. Sheehan-Dare RA, Goodfield MJ. Widespread cutaneous vasculitis associated with diltiazem. Postgrad Med J 1988;64(752):467–8.
13. Romano A, Pietrantonio F, Garcovich A, Rumi C, Bellocci F, Caradonna P, Barone C. Delayed hypersensitivity to diltiazem in two patients. Am Allergy 1992;69(1):31–2.
14. Sadick NS, Katz AS, Schreiber TL. Angioedema from calcium channel blockers. J Am Acad Dermatol 1989;21(1):132–3.
15. Jan V, Machet L, Gironet N, Martin L, Machet MC, Lorette G, Vaillant L. Acute generalized exanthematous pustulosis induced by diltiazem: value of patch testing. Dermatology 1998;197(3):274–5.
16. Umebayashi Y. Drug eruption due to mexiletine and diltiazem. Nishinihon J Dermatol 2000;62:80–2.
17. Inui S, Itami S, Yoshikawa K. A case of lichenoid purpura possibly caused by diltiazem hydrochloride. J Dermatol 2001;28(2):100–2.
18. Scherschun L, Lee MW, Lim HW. Diltiazem-associated photodistributed hyperpigmentation: a review of 4 cases. Arch Dermatol 2001;137(2):179–82.
19. Lambert DG, Dalac S, Beer F, Chavannet P, Portier H. Acute generalized exanthematous pustular dermatitis induced by diltiazem. Br J Dermatol 1988;118(2):308–9.
20. Morimoto S, Sasaki S, Kiyama M, Hatta T, Moriguchi J, Miki S, Kawa T, Nakamura K, Itoh H, Nakata T, Takeda K, Nakagawa M. Sustained-release diltiazem overdose. J Hum Hypertens 1999;13(9):643–4.
21. Satchithananda DK, Stone DL, Chauhan A, Ritchie AJ. Unrecognised accidental overdose with diltiazem. BMJ 2000;321(7254):160–1.

22. Quispel R, Baur HJ. Tentamen suicidii door diltiazem met gereguleerde afgifte. [Attempted suicide with sustained release diltiazem.] Ned Tijdschr Geneeskd 2001;145(19):918–22.
23. Shah SJ, Quartin AA, Schein RMH. Diltiazem overdose—a case report. JK Pract 2001;8:40–2.
24. Snook CP, Sigvaldason K, Kristinsson J. Severe atenolol and diltiazem overdose. J Toxicol Clin Toxicol 2000; 38(6):661–5.
25. Morris RG, Jones TE. Diltiazem disposition and metabolism in recipients of renal transplants. Ther Drug Monit 1998;20(4):365–70.
26. Asberg A, Christensen H, Hartmann A, Berg KJ. Diltiazem modulates cyclosporin A induced renal hemodynamic effects but not its effect on plasma endothelin-1. Clin Transplant 1998;12(5):363–70.
27. Asberg A, Christensen H, Hartmann A, Carlson E, Molden E, Berg KJ. Pharmacokinetic interactions between microemulsion formulated cyclosporine A and diltiazem in renal transplant recipients. Eur J Clin Pharmacol 1999;55(5):383–7.
28. Jiang TT, Huang W, Patel D. Cyclosporine-induced encephalopathy predisposed by diltiazem in a patient with aplastic anemia. Ann Pharmacother 1999;33(6):750–1.
29. Varis T, Backman JT, Kivisto KT, Neuvonen PJ. Diltiazem and mibefradil increase the plasma concentrations and greatly enhance the adrenal-suppressant effect of oral methylprednisolone. Clin Pharmacol Ther 2000;67(3):215–21.
30. Khoury V, Kritharides L. Diltiazem-mediated inhibition of sildenafil metabolism may promote nitrate-induced hypotension. Aust NZ J Med 2000;30(5):641–2.
31. Bottiger Y, Sawe J, Brattstrom C, Tollemar J, Burke JT, Hass G, Zimmerman JJ. Pharmacokinetic interaction between single oral doses of diltiazem and sirolimus in healthy volunteers. Clin Pharmacol Ther 2001;69(1):32–40.
32. Lewin JJ 3rd, Nappi JM, Taylor MH, Lugo SI, Larouche M. Rhabdomyolysis with concurrent atorvastatin and diltiazem. Ann Pharmacother 2002;36(10):1546–9.
33. Azie NE, Brater DC, Becker PA, Jones DR, Hall SD. The interaction of diltiazem with lovastatin and pravastatin. Clin Pharmacol Ther 1998;64(4):369–77.
34. Masica AL, Azie NE, Brater DC, Hall SD, Jones DR. Intravenous diltiazem and CYP3A-mediated metabolism. Br J Clin Pharmacol 2000;50(3):273–6.
35. Yeo KR, Yeo WW, Wallis EJ, Ramsay LE. Enhanced cholesterol reduction by simvastatin in diltiazem-treated patients. Br J Clin Pharmacol 1999;48(4):610–15.
36. Mousa O, Brater DC, Sunblad KJ, Hall SD. The interaction of diltiazem with simvastatin. Clin Pharmacol Ther 2000;67(3):267–74.
37. Peces R, Pobes A. Rhabdomyolysis associated with concurrent use of simvastatin and diltiazem. Nephron 2001;89(1):117–18.
38. Hebert MF, Lam AY. Diltiazem increases tacrolimus concentrations. Ann Pharmacother 1999;33(6):680–2.

Dimenhydrinate

See also Antihistamines

General Information

Dimenhydrinate (SEDA-21, 173) is an antihistamine, the diphenhydramine salt of 8-chlorotheophylline.

Organs and Systems

Sensory systems

Dimenhydrinate altered color discrimination, night vision, reaction time, and stereopsis in healthy volunteers (1).

Skin

Diphenhydramine has been associated with a fixed drug eruption, but only three such cases have been published with dimenhydrinate. In one such case patch tests were conducted; there was a positive response to the dimenhydrinate patch, but negative responses to separate patches containing either dimenhydrinate or 8-chlorotheophylline.

Reference

1. Luria SM, Kinney JA, McKay CL, Paulson HM, Ryan AP. Effects of aspirin and dimenhydrinate (Dramamine) on visual processes. Br J Clin Pharmacol 1979;7(6):585–93.

Dimercaprol

General Information

Dimercaprol or British Anti-Lewisite (BAL) was originally developed to counteract arsenic-containing war gases (1). It is now used for the treatment of poisoning with heavy metals, such as arsenic, gold, lead, or mercury, and is administered by intramuscular injection. Its adverse effects include nausea, vomiting, a burning sensation in the mouth, throat, eyes, and sometimes limbs, muscle pain and spasms, lacrimation, rhinorrhea, and hypersalivation. Of importance are a raised blood pressure and tachycardia. Pain in head, teeth, or abdomen can occur. The symptoms develop soon after injection and subside within about 2 hours. Injections can be painful and give rise to sterile abscesses. Fever can occur.

Susceptibility Factors

Genetic factors

Dimercaprol is contraindicated in patients with glucose-6-phosphate dehydrogenase deficiency, because of the risk of hemolysis (2,3).

References

1. Vilensky JA, Redman K. British Anti-Lewisite (dimercaprol): an amazing history. Ann Emerg Med 2003;41(3):378–83.
2. Janakiraman N, Seeler RA, Royal JE, Chen MF. Hemolysis during BAL chelation therapy for high blood lead levels in two G6PD deficient children. Clin Pediatr (Phila) 1978;17(6):485–7.
3. Glotzer DE. The current role of 2,3-dimercaptosuccinic acid (DMSA) in the management of childhood lead poisoning. Drug Saf 1993;9(2):85–92.

Dimercaptopropane sulfonate

General Information

Dimercaptopropane sulfonate (2,3-dimercapto-1-propanesulfonate) is a water-soluble and possibly less toxic derivative of dimercaprol, used in poisoning with arsenic, bismuth, mercury, and other heavy metals.

- Dimercaptopropane sulfonate is the treatment of choice for acute arsenic poisoning and has been used safely in high doses (15.25 g in 12 days, first intravenously and later orally) in a 21-year-old man who swallowed about 1000 mg or more of arsenic trioxide (1). There were no adverse effects. A modest transient increase in serum transaminases was thought to have been due to the arsenic.

In a UK study, single oral doses of dimercaptopropane sulfonic acid or succimer in different combinations with or without acetylcysteine and potassium citrate were given to 191 patients considered to have mercury toxicity from amalgam dental fillings (2). After a single dose, about 5% of patients complained of mild gastrointestinal discomfort, fatigue, mental fuzziness, headache, and diuresis. These usually cleared within 6 hours of the dose and were considered to be due to heavy metal mobilization. There were no cases of hypersensitivity.

Reported adverse effects of dimercaptopropane sulfonate include nausea, vertigo, headache, weakness, pruritus, and allergic reactions, such as rashes (3–6). Nausea can occur after both oral and intravenous administration.

References

1. Horn J, Eicher H, Mühlberg W, Platt D. Akute Arsentrioxid-Intoxikation–blander Verlauf nauch hochdosierter Chelat-Therapie. [Acute arsenic trioxide poisoning: nonserious course of illness because of high dosage chelation therapy.] Intensivmed Notallumed 2002;39:246–53.
2. Hibberd AR, Howard MA, Hunnisett AG. Mercury from dental amalgam fillings: studies on oral chelating agents for assessing and reducing mercury burdens in humans. J Nutr Environ Med 1998;8:219–31.
3. Hruby K, Donner A. 2,3-Dimercapto-1-propanesulphonate in heavy metal poisoning. Med Toxicol Adverse Drug Exp 1987;2(5):317–23.
4. Torres-Alanis O, Garza-Ocanas L, Pineyro-Lopez A. Evaluation of urinary mercury excretion after administration of 2,3-dimercapto-1-propane sulfonic acid to occupationally exposed men. J Toxicol Clin Toxicol 1995;33(6):717–20.
5. Stevens PE, Moore DF, House IM, Volans GN, Rainford DJ. Significant elimination of bismuth by haemodialysis with a new heavy-metal chelating agent. Nephrol Dial Transplant 1995;10(5):696–8.
6. Maiorino RM, Gonzalez-Ramirez D, Zuniga-Charles M, Xu Z, Hurlbut KM, Aposhian MM, Dart RC, Woods JS, Ostrosky-Wegman P, Gonsebatt ME, Aposhian HV. Sodium 2,3-dimercaptopropane-1-sulfonate challenge test for mercury in humans. III. Urinary mercury after exposure to mercurous chloride. J Pharmacol Exp Ther 1996;277(2):938–44.

Dimetacrine

See also Tricyclic antidepressants

General Information

Dimetacrine is a 6,6,6 tricyclic acridine derivative. In a double-blind study, dimetacrine was less effective than imipramine and produced more weight loss and abnormal liver function tests more often (1).

Reference

1. Abuzzahab FS. Sr. A double-blind investigation of dimethacrine versus imipramine in hospitalized depressive states. Int J Clin Pharmacol 1973;8(3):244–53.

Dimethylsulfoxide

General Information

Dimethylsulfoxide is an agent with a wide spectrum of pharmacological effects, including membrane penetration, anti-inflammatory effects, local analgesia, and weak bacteriostasis. The principal use of dimethylsulfoxide is as a vehicle for other drugs, thereby enhancing the effect of the drug, and aiding penetration of other drugs into the skin. Dimethylsulfoxide has been given orally, intravenously, or topically for a wide range of indications. It is also given by bladder instillation in the symptomatic relief of interstitial cystitis, and is used as a cryoprotectant for various human tissues.

In preparation for bone marrow transplantation, autologous hemopoietic stem cells are normally frozen in liquid nitrogen after harvesting. However, a cryoprotective agent is required, and dimethylsulfoxide is normally used. During and immediately after stem cell infusion, many adverse effects, which may be severe or life-threatening, have been reported. They include hypotension and hypertension, anaphylactic reactions, and cardiac and respiratory failure, all possibly due to dimethylsulfoxide, hemolysis induced by cryopreservation and thawing, and fluid overload.

In a retrospective study, 30 children were reviewed after bone marrow or peripheral autologous hemopoietic transplantation (1). At the time of infusion, hydrocortisone, chlorphenamine, and hyperhydration were administered to all patients, and furosemide and tropisetron to most. Vital signs and symptoms were monitored for 6 hours after the infusion. Thawing was performed rapidly at the bedside in a 42°C water-bath, and the cells were infused through a central venous catheter at 10 ml/minute. All 32 procedures were well tolerated; there were infusion-related adverse effects in 15 of 32 infusions, but none required specific therapy. There was mild bradycardia in nine patients, one reported abdominal pain, two reported headache, and three had hemoglobinuria. The authors concluded that a single-step cryopreservation technique aimed at limiting the total amount of dimethylsulfoxide is effective in avoiding most toxicity while not compromising post-thawing viability.

The efficacy and safety of dimethylsulfoxide are still relatively unclear; few studies have been performed in such a way as to permit reliable conclusions. Dimethylsulfoxide penetrates quickly through the tissues, and there are no great differences between its effects after different routes of administration. Adverse reactions are common, but can be avoided in large part by using more dilute solutions (2). Although the systemic toxicity of dimethylsulfoxide is considered to be low, it can potentiate the effect of simultaneously administered drugs. Combinations of dimethylsulfoxide with other toxic agents probably constitute its greatest toxic potential (3).

Organs and Systems

Nervous system

The infusion of dimethylsulfoxide-cryopreserved autologous peripheral blood stem cells has been associated with a number of infusion-related adverse effects (4). Severe reversible encephalopathy was experienced by two patients after infusion of peripheral blood stem cells cryopreserved in 10% dimethylsulfoxide. In one patient, reduction of the plasma dimethylsulfoxide concentration by plasmapheresis resulted in marked improvement in encephalopathy (5). The presence of renal insufficiency may have predisposed to the development of neurological toxicity by delaying the excretion of dimethylsulfoxide and its metabolites. Other cases of dimethylsulfoxide-induced encephalopathy have been described (6–8).

Sensory systems

Animal studies have documented a characteristic change in the ocular lens, resulting in myopia, which becomes more severe with long-term administration or high concentrations of dimethylsulfoxide. However, studies and clinical experience have not shown similar effects in humans (9,10)

Hematologic

Intravenous dimethylsulfoxide poses the greatest problems and causes transient systemic hemolysis with hemoglobinuria, but without gross hematuria. The hemolysis is dose-dependent and appears within several minutes after infusions of dimethylsulfoxide 20–40% (11). There was no evidence of kidney damage because of handling higher amounts of hemoglobin after hemolysis.

Sulfhemoglobinemia has been reported after transdermal administration of dimethylsulfoxide (12).

Gastrointestinal

Dimethylsulfoxide caused gastrointestinal discomfort in volunteers who used a topical 80% solution (1 g/kg/day). Nausea developed in 32%, vomiting in 6%, diarrhea in 5%, constipation in 3%, and anorexia in 2% (6).

A garlic-like breath occurs in almost all patients who use topical dimethylsulfoxide (13) and probably by any other route of administration.

Skin

Dimethylsulfoxide has also been used to treat extravasation of vesicant drugs (14). However, dimethylsulfoxide can itself cause redness and blistering at the site of application in high concentrations (90–100%); this effect can be reduced by using it sparingly or in lower concentrations (70%).

Drug Administration

Drug formulations

A formulation of dimethylsulfoxide (RIMSO 100) has introduced a problem since, when it is diluted with water, a strong exothermic reaction results. This caused thermal injury on intracystic instillation unless one waits until the mixture cools (15).

References

1. Perseghin P, Balduzzi A, Bonanomi S, Dassi M, Buscemi F, Longoni D, Rovelli A, Uderzo C. Infusion-related side-effects in children undergoing autologous hematopoietic stem cell transplantation for acute leukemia. Bone Marrow Transplant 2000;26(1):116–18.
2. Swanson BN. Medical use of dimethyl sulfoxide (DMSO). Rev Clin Basic Pharm 1985;5(1–2):1–33.
3. Brayton CF. Dimethyl sulfoxide (DMSO): a review. Cornell Vet 1986;76(1):61–90.
4. Kessinger A, Schmit-Pokorny K, Smith D, Armitage J. Cryopreservation and infusion of autologous peripheral blood stem cells. Bone Marrow Transplant 1990;5(Suppl 1):25–7.
5. Dhodapkar M, Goldberg SL, Tefferi A, Gertz MA. Reversible encephalopathy after cryopreserved peripheral blood stem cell infusion. Am J Hematol 1994;45(2):187–8.
6. Brobyn RD. The human toxicology of dimethyl sulfoxide. Ann NY Acad Sci 1975;243:497–506.
7. Bond GR, Curry SC, Dahl DW. Dimethylsulphoxide-induced encephalopathy. Lancet 1989;1(8647):1134–5.
8. Yellowlees P, Greenfield C, McIntyre N. Dimethylsulphoxide-induced toxicity. Lancet 1980;2(8202):1004–6.
9. Rubin LF. Toxicity of dimethyl sulfoxide, alone and in combination. Ann NY Acad Sci 1975;243:98–103.
10. Olson RJ. Dimethylsulfoxide and ocular involvement. J Toxicol Cut Ocul Toxicol 1982;1:147–52.
11. Muther RS, Bennett WM. Effects of dimethyl sulfoxide on renal function in man. JAMA 1980;244(18):2081–3.
12. Burgess JL, Hamner AP, Robertson WO. Sulfhemoglobinemia after dermal application of DMSO. Vet Hum Toxicol 1998;40(2):87–9.
13. John H, Laudahn G. Clinical experiences with the topical application of DMSO in orthopedic diseases: evaluation of 4180 cases. Ann NY Acad Sci 1967;141(1):506–16.
14. St Germain B, Houlihan N, D'Amato S. Dimethyl sulfoxide therapy in the treatment of vesicant extravasation: two case presentations. J Intraven Nurs 1994;17(5):261–6.
15. Albert NE. Exothermal reaction with RIMSO 100. Urology 1982;20(6):662.

Dimethyltryptamine

General Information

Dimethyltryptamine is inactive by mouth and is only used by inhalation or injection. Its effects are similar to those of lysergic acid diethylamide (LSD) (1,2).

References

1. Brimblecombe RW. Psychotomimetic drugs: biochemistry and pharmacology. Adv Drug Res 1973;7:165–206.
2. Barker SA, Monti JA, Christian ST. N,N-dimethyltryptamine: an endogenous hallucinogen. Int Rev Neurobiol 1981;22:83–110.

Dimetindene

See also Antihistamines

General Information

Dimetindene (SEDA-21, 174) is a first-generation antihistamine. The limited published material does not suggest that the adverse reactions to dimetindene when given orally are significantly different to those of others (1). It has also been used as a nasal spray in cases of allergy (2); some local irritation can occur, as is usual with this type of administration of antihistamines.

References

1. Bauer CP, Unkauf M. Efficacy and safety of intranasally applied dimetindene maleate solution. Multicenter study in children under 14 years suffering from seasonal allergic rhinitis. Arzneimittelforschung 2001;51(3):232–7.
2. Horak F, Unkauf M, Beckers C, Mittermaier EM. Efficacy and tolerability of intranasally applied dimetindene maleate solution versus placebo in the treatment of seasonal allergic rhinitis. Arzneimittelforschung 2000;50(12):1099–105.

Dinitrochlorobenzene

General Information

Dinitrochlorobenzene is a potent sensitizer that has been applied topically in the evaluation of delayed hypersensitivity. It has also been used as an immunostimulant in conditions such as leprosy, HIV infection, and some forms of cancer, and to treat alopecia and warts.

Generalized urticaria, pruritus, and dyspepsia developed in a previously healthy individual who used dinitrochlorobenzene for alopecia totalis; all the symptoms disappeared within 10 days after the drug was withdrawn, but returned after reintroduction (1).

Organs and Systems

Skin

A woman developed an itchy brownish patch on the right upper arm, in the same place where she had previously been sensitized by dinitrochlorobenzene 2% in acetone (2). A diagnosis of lymphadenosis benigna cutis was made.

References

1. McDaniel DH, Blatchley DM, Welton WA. Adverse systemic reaction to dinitrochlorobenzene. Arch Dermatol 1982;118(6):371.
2. Yoshida Y, Duan H, Nakayama J, Furue M. Lymphadenosis benigna cutis induced by iatrogenic contact dermatitis from dinitrochlorobenzene. Contact Dermatitis 2003;49(3):165–6.

Dinoprostone

See also Prostaglandins

General Information

Dinoprostone is PGE_2 available for exogenous administration.

Organs and Systems

Reproductive system

Uterine rupture occurred after labor had been induced with dinoprostone at 10 days after term; the baby was born dead (1).

- A 26-year-old woman, whose first child had been delivered by elective cesarean section at 38 weeks of gestation because of a breech presentation, was given two doses of dinoprostone vaginal gel 1 mg 6 hours apart; 8 hours after the second dose her cervix was soft, fully effaced, and dilated to 3 cm. Since her uterine contractions were only mild and irregular, she underwent amniotomy and an infusion of oxytocin was begun. Fetal tachycardia occurred 4 hours later, with recurrent decelerations. Prolonged deceleration of the fetal heart then occurred and there was fresh vaginal bleeding. Uterine rupture was suspected and the neonate was delivered by emergency cesarean section, but could not be resuscitated. The mother required a blood transfusion, but subsequently made a good recovery.

The authors commented that induction with prostaglandins in women with a previous lower segment cesarean scar is associated with a risk of symptomatic scar rupture no greater than 0.6%, and the vaginal delivery rate is about 75%, that is similar to rates quoted for spontaneous labor in women with a cesarean scar. At present, faced with the lack of comparative evidence, clinicians can only provide women with the best estimate of risk based on uncontrolled observational data.

Reference

1. Vause S, Macintosh M. Evidence based case report: use of prostaglandins to induce labour in women with a caesarean section scar. BMJ 1999;318(7190):1056–8.

Dioxium

General Information

Dioxium is obsolete. Accounts of its adverse effects will be found in earlier volumes in this series (SED-10, 213) (SEDA-6, 131).

Diphencyprone

General Information

Diphencyprone is a potent sensitizing chemical used to induce a contact dermatitis of the scalp in the topical immunotherapy of alopecia areata.

Organs and Systems

Immunologic

- Pressure-induced urticaria and widespread severe dermographism developed after the first application to the scalp of a 0.003% solution of diphencyprone in a 19-year-old Japanese man (1). Diphencyprone was withdrawn, but the symptoms persisted for almost 3 months.

An IgE-mediated hypersensitivity reaction was suggested by the authors, but skin tests were not performed and neither was specific IgE measured. A similar case has been described and the adverse events of diphencyprone reviewed (2).

References

1. Skrebova N, Nameda Y, Takiwaki H, Arase S. Severe dermographism after topical therapy with diphenylcyclopropenone for alopecia universalis. Contact Dermatitis 2000;42(4):212–15.
2. Alam M, Gross EA, Savin RC. Severe urticarial reaction to diphenylcyclopropenone therapy for alopecia areata. J Am Acad Dermatol 1999;40(1):110–12.

Diphenhydramine

See also Antihistamines

General Information

Diphenhydramine is a typically sedating first-generation antihistamine. It is still widely used, mainly in over-the-counter products, often in combination with other drugs.

Diphenhydramine inhibits CYP2D6 and can cause clinically important interactions with many CYP2D6 substrates, particularly those with a narrow therapeutic index.

Organs and Systems

Nervous system

Diphenhydramine can cause significant daytime neurological impairment comparable to intoxication with alcohol (1). In a study of injury rates in 12 106 patients taking diphenhydramine compared with 24 968 patients taking loratadine, using a health-care claims database that included employees, dependents, and retirees who filed claims from January 1991 to December 1998, there was a strong association between the use of diphenhydramine and the occurrence of injuries: 55% of all injuries were associated with its use. The loratadine and diphenhydramine groups had similar predrug intake injury rates. The authors concluded that a substantial number of excess injuries and costs had been incurred as the result of the use of diphenhydramine (2).

Neuroleptic malignant syndrome has been attributed to diphenhydramine (3).

- A 39-year-old man presented with a gait disturbance confusion, hyperthermia (38.2°C), and hyperhidrosis after massive ingestion of a formulation containing diphenhydramine. With intensive support, including bromocriptine, he recovered within 12 days. The estimated dose of diphenhydramine was 40 mg × 60 tablets, and each tablet included 26 mg of diprophylline, a xanthine derivative.

The genesis of this case was not clear. Atropine-like effects occur with diphenhydramine, although signs such as muscle rigidity, akinesia, and hyperhidrosis, cannot be ascribed to anticholinergic activity. However, the patient had also taken sulpiride, which is a potent dopamine receptor antagonist.

Diphenhydramine can cause extrapyramidal symptoms as part of an acute dystonic reaction (SEDA-19, 173).

Psychological, psychiatric

Use of diphenhydramine, mainly as a sleeping aid, has been associated with cognitive impairment in elderly people without dementia (4).

Diphenhydramine has been associated with acute delirium in elderly patients with mild dementia, even in single doses of 25 mg (SEDA-19, 173).

Children and adolescents who are given diphenhydramine as premedication, often intravenously as a bolus, to prevent the adverse effects of blood transfusion, can develop drug-seeking behavior. It is recommended that in these circumstances antihistamines should be given orally or infused slowly (5).

Skin

- A 56-year-old woman developed itchy erythematous lesions on sun-exposed areas when she used diphenhydramine ointment 1% for 6 months; the condition gradually subsided with a glucocorticoid ointment (6).

Long-Term Effects

Drug abuse

Abuse of antihistamines in Scandinavia has been found in schoolchildren, and particularly involved diphenhydramine (alone or in combination with caffeine). As a consequence such formulations were changed from over-the-counter to prescription-only status (7,8). Abuse of diphenhydramine with drug-seeking behavior and anticholinergic adverse effects have been reported in five children and adolescents with chronic hematological or oncological diseases (5).

Reinforcing, subjective, and performance effects have been compared between oral diphenhydramine and the benzodiazepine lorazepam in men with a history of recreational abuse, and the results suggested that the two drugs have similar abuse potential (SEDA-21, 174).

Drug tolerance

In 15 healthy men tolerance to diphenhydramine developed rapidly in a randomized, placebo-controlled, crossover study (9). Diphenhydramine 50 mg or placebo was given twice a day for 4 days and tests of objective and subjective sleepiness together with computer-based tests of psychomotor performance were carried out. Compared with placebo on day 1, diphenhydramine caused significant impairment. However, by day 4 sleepiness and impairment of performance were indistinguishable from placebo.

Drug Administration

Drug administration route

Topical application of diphenhydramine can cause systemic toxicity.

- Acute anticholinergic toxicity with fever, hallucinations, and tachycardia occurred in a 2.5-year-old boy from applications of calamine + diphenhydramine lotion (10).
- A 5-year-old child who used a topical lotion containing 1% diphenhydramine for pruritic vesicular exanthema developed disorientation, agitation, dilated pupils, and ataxia (SEDA-13, 132).

Drug overdose

A total of 136 cases of self-poisoning with diphenhydramine (with suicidal intent) have been evaluated. The most common symptom was impaired consciousness, followed by psychotic behavior resembling catatonic stupor. Other symptoms included hallucinations, mydriasis, tachycardia, and less often diplopia, respiratory insufficiency, and seizures (SEDA-13, 132).

Although the clinical features of diphenhydramine overdose are well known, information about dose-dependent toxicity is still scarce. This has been investigated in patients with acute diphenhydramine poisoning in retrospective and prospective studies in 232 and 50 patients respectively (11). Mild symptoms (somnolence, anticholinergic signs, tachycardia, nausea/vomiting) occurred in 55–64% of patients, moderate symptoms (isolated and spontaneously resolving agitation, confusion, hallucinations, and electrocardiographic disturbances) in 22–27%, and severe symptoms (delirium/psychosis, seizures, coma) in 14–18%. Moderate symptoms occurred at doses over 0.3 g. For severe symptoms the critical dose limit was 1.0 g. Coma and seizures were significantly more frequent in those who took over 1.5 g compared with those who took 1.0–1.5 g. These data showed clear dose-dependent acute toxicity of diphenhydramine and suggested that only patients who take over 1.0 g are at risk of severe symptoms.

- A 35-year-old woman took diphenhydramine 16 g and developed hypertension and QRS prolongation; charcoal hemoperfusion and hemodialysis were used successfully (12).
- A 28-year-old died after an overdose of diphenhydramine. He developed hyperpyrexia and tachycardia and died from a cardiac arrest (13). Hemorrhagic pulmonary edema and renal shock were the most prominent findings. At the time of death, the plasma concentration of diphenhydramine was 5 μg/ml and there were particularly high concentrations in the lungs (55 mg/kg) and kidneys (50 mg/kg).

Rhabdomyolysis has been reported after overdose with diphenhydramine (SEDA-21, 175).

Drug–Drug Interactions

Metoprolol

Diphenhydramine inhibits the metabolism of metoprolol in extensive metabolizers, thereby prolonging its negative chronotropic and inotropic effects (14).

Prolintane

- Visual hallucinations occurred in an otherwise healthy 19-year-old man who took the stimulant prolintane and diphenhydramine (15). The psychiatric complications occurred 2 months after he started to take the two drugs and resolved quickly once they were withdrawn.

Venlafaxine

CYP2D6 is the major enzyme involved in the metabolism of venlafaxine, and diphenhydramine alters the disposition of venlafaxine, increasing plasma concentrations and predisposing to cardiovascular adverse effects (16).

References

1. O'Hanlon JF, Ramaekers JG. Antihistamine effects on actual driving performance in a standard test: a summary of Dutch experience, 1989–94. Allergy 1995;50(3):234–42.
2. Finkle WD, Adams JL, Greenland S, Melmon KL. Increased risk of serious injury following an initial prescription for diphenhydramine. Ann Allergy Asthma Immunol 2002;89(3):244–50.
3. Park-Matsumoto YC, Tazawa T. Neuroleptic malignant syndrome associated with diphenhydramine and diprophyllin overdose in a depressed patient. J Neurol Sci 1999;162(1):108–9.
4. Basu R, Dodge H, Stoehr GP, Ganguli M. Sedative-hypnotic use of diphenhydramine in a rural, older adult, community-based cohort: effects on cognition. Am J Geriatr Psychiatry 2003;11(2):205–13.
5. Dinndorf PA, McCabe MA, Frierdich S. Risk of abuse of diphenhydramine in children and adolescents with chronic illnesses. J Pediatr 1998;133(2):293–5.
6. Yamada S, Tanaka M, Kawahara Y, Inada M, Ohata Y. Photoallergic contact dermatitis due to diphenhydramine hydrochloride. Contact Dermatitis 1998;38(5):282.
7. Bjaeldager PA, Jensen K, Nielsen K, Skovgaard-Petersen K. Forgiftningstilfaelde med antihistaminer. [Poisoning with antihistaminics. Increasing abuse among young.] Ugeskr Laeger 1980;142(18):1147–9.
8. Gulmann NC, Petersen E, Nielsen U. En epidemi af antihistaminmisbrug pa en psykiatrisk afdeling. [Epidemic of antihistamine abuse in a psychiatric unit.] Ugeskr Laeger 1980;142(39):2542–6.
9. Richardson GS, Roehrs TA, Rosenthal L, Koshorek G, Roth T. Tolerance to daytime sedative effects of H_1 antihistamines. J Clin Psychopharmacol 2002;22(5):511–15.
10. Reilly JF Jr, Weisse ME. Topically induced diphenhydramine toxicity. J Emerg Med 1990;8(1):59–61.
11. Radovanovic D, Meier PJ, Guirguis M, Lorent JP, Kupferschmidt H. Dose-dependent toxicity of diphenhydramine overdose. Hum Exp Toxicol 2000;19(9):489–95.
12. Mullins ME, Pinnick RV, Terhes JM. Life-threatening diphenhydramine overdose treated with charcoal hemoperfusion and hemodialysis. Ann Emerg Med 1999;33(1):104–7.
13. Hausmann E, Wewer H, Wellhoner HH, Weller JP. Lethal intoxication with diphenhydramine. Report of a case with analytical follow-up. Arch Toxicol 1983;53(1):33–9.
14. Hamelin BA, Bouayad A, Methot J, Jobin J, Desgagnes P, Poirier P, Allaire J, Dumesnil J, Turgeon J. Significant interaction between the nonprescription antihistamine diphenhydramine and the CYP2D6 substrate metoprolol in healthy men with high or low CYP2D6 activity. Clin Pharmacol Ther 2000;67(5):466–77.
15. Paya B, Guisado JA, Vaz FJ, Crespo-Facorro B. Visual hallucinations induced by the combination of prolintane and diphenhydramine. Pharmacopsychiatry 2002;35(1):24–5.
16. Lessard E, Yessine MA, Hamelin BA, Gauvin C, Labbe L, O'Hara G, LeBlanc J, Turgeon J. Diphenhydramine alters the disposition of venlafaxine through inhibition of CYP2D6 activity in humans. J Clin Psychopharmacol 2001;21(2):175–84.

Diphenoxylate

General Information

Diphenoxylate is a synthetic compound designed to have the antidiarrheal effects of the opiates, but it also retains some less desirable opiate effects. It is generally combined with atropine, as co-phenotrope, which was originally added to the formulation in the hope of preventing misuse, although it can itself cause problems, especially if the combination is intentionally or accidentally used to excess.

In one instance keratoconjunctivitis occurred in a patient taking co-phenotrope, confirmed by rechallenge but not with diphenoxylate alone (SEDA-16, 425). Adverse effects are rare during ordinary use in adults, but children can be particularly sensitive to the adverse effects of both components, and in cases of poisoning complex and prompt measures may be needed, particularly since respiratory depression can be delayed until a day after ingestion and can recur even after a good response to opioid antagonists.

Drug Administration

Drug overdose

Only six of 36 children who took overdoses of co-phenotrope had signs of atropine overdose (central nervous system excitement, hypertension, fever, flushed dry skin) (1). Opioid overdose (central nervous system and respiratory depression with miosis) predominated or occurred without any signs of atropine toxicity in 33 cases (92%). Diphenoxylate-induced hypoxia was the major problem and was associated with slow or fast respiration, hypotonia or rigidity, cardiac arrest, and in three cases cerebral edema and death. Respiratory depression recurred 13–24 hours after the ingestion in seven cases and was probably due to accumulation of difenoxine, an active metabolite of diphenoxylate. Recommended treatment is an intravenous bolus dose of naloxone, followed by a continuous intravenous infusion, prompt gastric lavage, repeated administration of activated charcoal, and close monitoring for 24 hours.

Drug–Drug Interactions

Nitrofurantoin

Co-phenotrope, and other drugs that reduce intestinal motility, can interact with other drugs by affecting their absorption. For example, the absorption of nitrofurantoin can be doubled (2).

References

1. McCarron MM, Challoner KR, Thompson GA. Diphenoxylate–atropine (Lomotil) overdose in children: an update (report of eight cases and review of the literature) Pediatrics 1991;87(5):694–700.
2. Anonymous. Lomotil/nitrofurantoin Interaction. Oxford–New York–Tokyo: Oxford University Press, 1981.

Diphenylpyraline

See also Antihistamines

General Information

Diphenylpyraline is an antihistamine, a piperadine derivative, with antimuscarinic and sedative properties.

Organs and Systems

Skin

Cutaneous reactions have been reported with diphenylpyraline hydrochloride (1).

Reference

1. Mori Y, Sugihara K, Noda T, Yudate T, Aragane Y, Tezuka T. A case of fixed drug eruption due to diphenylpyraline hydrochloride. Skin Res 1999;41:25–9.

Diphtheria vaccine

See also Vaccines

General Information

Diphtheria vaccine contains diphtheria toxoid carried on aluminium hydroxide or calcium phosphate. Single antigen products are available only for cases in which combined antigens should not be used. The formulations used in most countries are a childhood formulation containing 25–30 Lf (flocculating units) of diphtheria toxoid (D) and an adult formulation containing 2 Lf of diphtheria toxoid (d). The formulations of choice in routine immunization are DTP (diphtheria and tetanus toxoids combined with pertussis vaccine), DT (diphtheria and tetanus toxoids) for pediatric use, and Td (tetanus and diphtheria toxoids with a limited amount of diphtheria antigen) for use in older children and adults.

Combined diphtheria + tetanus immunization

In a prospective cohort study in Italy, 380 children aged 6 years were randomly assigned to receive either the DT or the Td vaccine as a booster dose in order to determine whether a booster dose of Td (diphtheria–tetanus vaccine with a reduced amount of diphtheria toxoid, adult formulation) would produce comparable diphtheria antibody titers but lower reactogenicity than DT (childhood formulation). The frequencies of symptoms within 3 days of vaccine administration were similar in the two groups, except for local redness and swelling, which were significantly more common in the children who received DT vaccine: redness 31% versus 16%, and swelling 36% versus 26%. The mean duration of local symptoms was 3.3 days in the diphtheria–tetanus group and 2.6 days in the Td group. After booster immunization, 97% of children in the DT group and 91% of those in the Td group had antibody concentrations of at least 1 IU/ml ("long-term" protection titer) (1).

There have been comparisons of the immunogenicity and reactogenicity of different diphtheria vaccines. They have involved single or combined administration of diphtheria and/or tetanus toxoids (SEDA-13, 279) (SEDA-15, 345), booster immunization using Td vaccines including either aluminium hydroxide or calcium phosphate as adjuvant (SEDA-20, 288), or either plain or adsorbed formulations (SEDA-21, 328).

Adverse events after diphtheria–tetanus vaccine in the USA in 1982–84 have been reviewed in detail (SEDA-13, 273). The usual types of local intolerance can be seen. For example, some 5% of schoolchildren develop redness and swelling, whilst some older children develop enlargement of the regional lymph nodes. Such reactions are much less common in young children, and much more common in children given combined vaccines.

General reactions (seen in some older children and adults) are usually limited to brief fever; sustained fever and other systemic reactions are uncommon unless the person has been hyperimmunized. After the administration of DT vaccine, local reactions, generally erythema and induration, with or without tenderness, can occur. In hyperimmunized cases, Arthus-type hypersensitivity reactions can occur. These characteristically severe local reactions generally start 2–8 hours after an injection. People who have such reactions usually have very high serum antitoxin concentrations and one should be careful not to administer a booster more than once every 10 years.

The occurrence of epidemic diphtheria in Eastern Europe led to the recommendation in the UK that those aged 15–18 years should receive a combined tetanus and low-dose diphtheria toxoid vaccine instead of a tetanus booster alone. In March 1995, 220 children aged 14–16 years were inadvertently given high-dose diphtheria and tetanus toxoid vaccine, and their parents were sent a questionnaire; 153 replied. A total of 141 (92%) of adolescents reported one or more reactions, most of which were classified as mild or moderate and lasted less than 1 week. However, 47 (31%) reported at least one severe local or systemic reaction (2).

In a study of adverse events after immunization in New Zealand in 1990–95 (3), reactions at the injection site after adult tetanus–diphtheria vaccine (68 reports per 100 000 immunizations) were reported five times more often than with tetanus vaccine.

Combined diphtheria + tetanus + pertussis immunization

An overview of clinical trials with a special diphtheria and tetanus toxoids and acellular pertussis (DTaP) vaccine has been published (4). The vaccine contains as pertussis components purified filamentous hemagglutinin, pertactin, and genetically engineered pertussis toxin. The vaccine induces high and long-lasting immunity and is at least as efficacious as most whole-cell pertussis vaccines and similar in efficacy to the most efficacious DTaP vaccines that contain three pertussis antigens. The vaccine is better tolerated than whole-cell vaccines and has a similar reactogenicity profile to other acellular vaccines.

A vaccine containing diphtheria and tetanus toxoids and DTaP with reduced antigen content for diphtheria and pertussis (TdaP) has been compared with a licensed reduced adult-type diphtheria–tetanus vaccine and with an experimental candidate monovalent DTaP vaccine with reduced antigen content (ap) (5). A total of 299 healthy adults (mean age 30 years) were randomized into three groups to receive one dose of the study vaccines. The antibody responses (antidiphtheria, antitetanus, antipertussis toxin, antipertactin, antifilamentous hemagglutinin) were similar in all groups. The most frequently reported local symptom was pain at the injection site (62–94%), but there were no reports of severe pain; redness and swelling with a diameter of 5 cm or more occurred in up to 13%. The incidence of local symptoms was similar after TdaP and Td immunization. The most frequently reported general symptoms were headache and fatigue (20–50%). The incidence of general symptoms was similar in the TdaP and Td groups. There were no reports of fever over 39°C. No serious adverse events were reported.

Data from the Third National Health and Nutrition Survey (1988–94) have been used to analyse the possible effects of DTP or tetanus immunization on allergies and allergy-related symptoms among 13 944 infants, children, and adolescents aged 2 months to 16 years in the USA (6). The authors concluded that DTP or tetanus immunization increases the risk of allergies and related respiratory symptoms in children and adolescents. However, the small number of non-immunized individuals and the study design limited their ability to make firm causal inferences about the true magnitude of effect.

Tetravalent, pentavalent, and hexavalent immunization

DTaP or DTwP vaccine can be combined with other antigens, such as *Haemophilus influenzae* type b (Hib), inactivated poliovaccine (IPV), and hepatitis B vaccine. In children DTaP or DTwP vaccines are the basis for such combinations, while in adults it is mostly Td or Tdap vaccine combined with inactivated poliovaccine (IPV). Current safety concerns regarding combination vaccines have been defined and reviewed (7). The author concluded that there is no evidence that adding vaccines to combination products increases the burden on the immune system, which can respond to many millions of antigens. Combining antigens usually does not increase adverse effects, but it can lead to an overall reduction in adverse events. Before licensure, combination vaccines undergo extensive testing to assure that the new products are safe and effective.

The frequency, severity, and types of adverse reactions after DTP-Hib immunization in very preterm babies have been studied (8). Adverse reactions were noted in 17 of 45 babies: nine had major events (apnea, bradycardia, or desaturation) and eight had minor reactions (increased oxygen requirements, temperature instability, poor handling, and feeding intolerance). Babies who had major adverse reactions were significantly younger at the time of immunization than the babies who did not have major reactions. Of 27 babies immunized at 70 days or less, nine developed major reactions compared with none of those who were immunized at over 70 days.

The Hexavalent Study Group has compared the immunogenicity and safety of a new liquid hexavalent vaccine against diphtheria, tetanus, pertussis, poliomyelitis, hepatitis B, and Hib (DTP + IPV + HB + Hib vaccine, manufactured by Aventis Pasteur MSD, Lyon, France) with two reference vaccines, the pentavalent DTP + IPV + Hib vaccine and the monovalent hepatitis B vaccine, administrated separately at the same visit (9). Infants were randomized to receive either the hexavalent vaccine ($n = 423$) or (administered at different local sites) the pentavalent and the HB vaccine ($n = 425$) at 2, 4, and 6 months of age. The hexavalent vaccine was well tolerated (for details, see the monograph on Pertussis vaccines). At least one local reaction was reported in 20% of injections with hexavalent vaccine compared with 16% after the receipt of pentavalent vaccine or 3.8% after the receipt of hepatitis B vaccine. These reactions were generally mild and transient. At least one systemic reaction was reported in 46% of injections with hexavalent vaccine, whereas the respective rate for the recipients of pentavalent and HB vaccine was 42%. No vaccine-related serious adverse event occurred during the study. The hexavalent vaccine provided immune responses adequate for protection against the six diseases.

Organs and Systems

Cardiovascular

Myopericarditis has been attributed to Td-IPV vaccine (10).

- A 31-year-old man developed arthralgia and chest pain 2 days after Td-IPV immunization and had an acute myopericarditis. He recovered within a few days with high-dose aspirin.

The authors discussed two possible causal mechanisms, natural infection or an immune complex-mediated mechanism. Infection was excluded by negative bacterial and viral serology and the favorable outcome within a few days without antimicrobial treatment.

Nervous system

Supposed neurological adverse effects of diphtheria immunization have been reported, but a causal connection was unclear (11). Of five cases of neurological complications after diphtheria or diphtheria-tetanus immunizations two were classified as vaccine-induced poliomyelitis; the other three could be traced back to a hyperergic reaction to diphtheria toxoids in the cerebral vessels (12).

Guillain–Barré syndrome (13) and polyradiculoneuritis (14,15) have rarely been reported. In a national surveillance study of Guillain–Barré syndrome in the USA, 31 of 998 cases developed the illness within 8 weeks after immunization. Of these 31 cases, 5 had been immunized with DT or DPT vaccine (16).

The bioelectric activity of the brain after DT immunization was studied in healthy children. Electroencephalography showed significant changes in 13 of 17 children, which resolved within 3 weeks (17). The question has arisen of whether this is of more than experimental significance: between 1980 and 1982 in the

Campana region of Italy, several cases of encephalopathy in children who had been given DT immunization 1 week before were reported to the health authorities. However, summarizing the results of a case-control study, Greco pointed out that the statistical association that he found between the incidence of encephalopathy and DT administration did not imply a causal association (18).

Sensory systems

Optic neuritis has been attributed to Td-IPV vaccine (19).

- Ten days after receiving Td-IPV vaccine a 56-year-old woman developed acute unilateral optic neuritis. Complete remission occurred within 6 weeks of prednisolone treatment. No other causes were found.

Skin

Erythema multiforme developed 8 hours after diphtheria–tetanus immunization in a 9-month-old infant (20). There have also been reports of erythema multiforme after hepatitis B vaccine, MMR vaccine, and DPT vaccine.

Bullous pemphigoid has been attributed to DTP-IPV vaccine (21).

A previous healthy 3.5-month-old infant developed bullous pemphigoid 3 days after receiving a first dose of DTP-IPV vaccine. *Staphylococcus aureus* was isolated from purulent bullae. The lesions resolved rapidly after treatment with antibiotics and methylprednisolone.

The authors mentioned 12 other cases of bullous pemphigoid, reported during the last 5 years, that had possibly been triggered by vaccines (influenza, tetanus toxoid booster, and DTP-IPV vaccine).

Immunologic

- A six-year-old child had anaphylaxis 30 minutes after a fifth dose of DT vaccine (22). Skin tests, in vitro determination of specific IgE antibodies, and immunoblotting assays showed that the IgE response was directed against tetanus and diphtheria toxoids. Cross-reactivity between the two toxoids was not demonstrated, indicating the presence of co-existing but non-cross-reacting IgE and IgG antibodies.

Susceptibility Factors

Other features of the patient

The only contraindication to administering single diphtheria toxoid or combined diphtheria and tetanus toxoids is a history of a severe hypersensitivity or neurological reaction after a previous dose.

References

1. Ciofi degli Atti ML, Salmaso S, Cotter B, Gallo G, Alfarone G, Pinto A, Bella A, von Hunolstein C. Reactogenicity and immunogenicity of adult versus paediatric diphtheria and tetanus booster dose at 6 years of age. Vaccine 2001;20(1–2):74–9.
2. Sidebotham PD, Lenton SW. Incidence of adverse reactions after administration of high dose diphtheria with tetanus vaccine to school leavers: retrospective questionnaire study. BMJ 1996;313(7056):533–4.
3. Mansoor O, Pillans PI. Vaccine adverse events reported in New Zealand 1990–5. NZ Med J 1997;110(1048):270–2.
4. Matheson AJ, Goa KL. Diphtheria-tetanus-acellular pertussis vaccine adsorbed (Triacelluvax; DTaP3-CB): a review of its use in the prevention of *Bordetella pertussis* infection. Paediatr Drugs 2000;2(2):139–59.
5. Van der Wielen M, Van Damme P. Tetanus–diphtheria booster in non-responding tetanus–diphtheria vaccinees. Vaccine 2000;19(9–10):1005–6.
6. Hurwitz EL, Morgenstern H. Effects of diphtheria-tetanus-pertussis or tetanus vaccination on allergies and allergy-related respiratory symptoms among children and adolescents in the United States. J Manipulative Physiol Ther 2000;23(2):81–90.
7. Halsey NA. Combination vaccines: defining and addressing current safety concerns. Clin Infect Dis 2001;33(Suppl 4):S312–18.
8. Sen S, Cloete Y, Hassan K, Buss P. Adverse events following vaccination in premature infants. Acta Paediatr 2001;90(8):916–20.
9. Mallet E, Fabre P, Pines E, Salomon H, Staub T, Schodel F, Mendelman P, Hessel L, Chryssomalis G, Vidor E, Hoffenbach A, Abeille A, Amar R, Arsene JP, Aurand JM, Azoulay L, Badescou E, Barrois S, Baudino N, Beal M, Beaude-Chervet V, Berlier P, Billard E, Billet L, Blanc B, Blanc JP, Bohu D, Bonardo C, Bossu C; Hexavalent Vaccine Trial Study Group. Immunogenicity and safety of a new liquid hexavalent combined vaccine compared with separate administration of reference licensed vaccines in infants. Pediatr Infect Dis J 2000;19(12):1119–27.
10. Boccara F, Benhaiem-Sigaux N, Cohen A. Acute myopericarditis after diphtheria, tetanus, and polio vaccination. Chest 2001;120(2):671–2.
11. Van Ramshorst JD, Ehrengut W. Die Diphtherieschutzimpfung. In: Herrlich A, editor. Handbuch der Schutzimpfungen. Berlin: Springer, 1965:394.
12. Ehrengut W. Komplikationen nach Diphtherieschutzimpfung und Impfungen mit Diphtherietoxoid-Mischimpfstoffen. [Neural complications after diphtheria vaccination and inoculations with diphtheria toxoid-mixed vaccines. Observations on their etiopathogenesis.] Dtsch Med Wochenschr 1986;111(24):939–42.
13. Onisawa S, Sekine I, Ichimura T, Homma N. Guillain–Barré syndrome secondary to immunization with diphtheria toxoid. Dokkyo J Med Sci 1985;12:227.
14. Holliday PL, Bauer RB. Polyradiculoneuritis secondary to immunization with tetanus and diphtheria toxoids. Arch Neurol 1983;40(1):56–7.
15. Immunization Practices Advisory committee (ACIP). Diphtheria, tetanus, and pertussis: recommendations for vaccine use and other preventive measures. MMWR Recomm Rep 1991;40(RR-10):1–28.
16. Hurwitz ES, Holman RC, Nelson DB, Schonberger LB. National surveillance for Guillain–Barré syndrome: January 1978–March 1979. Neurology 1983;33(2):150–7.
17. Wstepne D. Prophylactic vaccinations and seizure activity in EEG. Neurol Neurochir Pol 1981;5:553.
18. Greco D. Case-control study on encephalopathy associated with diphtheria–tetanus immunization in Campania, Italy. Bull World Health Organ 1985;63(5):919–25.
19. Burkhard C, Choi M, Wilhelm H. Optikusneuritis als Komplikaton einer Tetanus–Diphtherie–Poliomyelitis–Schutzimpfung: ein Fallbericht. [Optic neuritis as a

complication in preventive tetanus–diphtheria–poliomyelitis vaccination: a case report.] Klin Monatsbl Augenheilkd 2001;218(1):51–4.
20. Griffith RD, Miller OF 3rd. Erythema multiforme following diphtheria and tetanus toxoid vaccination. J Am Acad Dermatol 1988;19(4):758–9.
21. Baykal C, Okan G, Sarica R. Childhood bullous pemphigoid developed after the first vaccination. J Am Acad Dermatol 2001;44(Suppl 2):348–50.
22. Martin-Munoz MF, Pereira MJ, Posadas S, Sanchez-Sabate E, Blanca M, Alvarez J. Anaphylactic reaction to diphtheria–tetanus vaccine in a child: specific IgE/IgG determinations and cross-reactivity studies. Vaccine 2002;20(27–28):3409–12.

Dipyridamole

General Information

Dipyridamole inhibits platelet aggregation by inhibiting platelet cyclic AMP phosphodiesterase, potentiating adenosine inhibition of platelet function by blocking adenosine reuptake by vascular and blood cells and breakdown of adenosine, and by potentiating prostaglandin I_2 antiaggregatory activity and enhancement of its synthesis. These independent processes inhibit platelet aggregation by increasing platelet cyclic AMP through a reduction in enzymatic breakdown of cyclic AMP and stimulation of cyclic AMP formation by activation of adenyl cyclase by adenosine and possibly prostaglandin I_2 (1).

Dipyridamole is also a potent coronary arteriolar vasodilator, perhaps by opening of vascular K_{ATP} channels (2). However, the Food and Drug Administration withdrew conditional approval for certain drug products containing dipyridamole, because of a lack of sufficient evidence of effectiveness in the long-term therapy of angina pectoris (3).

Observational studies

The incidence of major adverse reactions to dipyridamole was determined in a multicenter retrospective study, involving 73 806 patients who underwent intravenous dipyridamole stress imaging in 59 hospitals and 19 countries (4). The main conclusion was that the risk of serious dipyridamole-induced adverse effects is very low, a conclusion that is in line with other reports (5), and comparable to that reported for exercise testing in a similar patient population. Combined major adverse events among the entire patient population included 7 cardiac deaths (0.95 per 10 000), 13 non-fatal myocardial infarctions (1.76 per 10 000), 6 non-fatal sustained ventricular dysrhythmias (0.81 per 10 000) (ventricular tachycardia in 2 and ventricular fibrillation in 4), 9 transient cerebral ischemic attacks (1.22 per 10 000), 1 stroke, and 9 severe cases of bronchospasm (1.22 per 10 000). Minor non-cardiac adverse effects were less frequent among the elderly and more frequent in women and patients taking maintenance aspirin.

Placebo-controlled studies

The efficacy and safety of dipyridamole have been assessed in patients with chronic stable angina in a large-scale, international, randomized, placebo-controlled, parallel-group study, in which 400 patients with chronic stable angina pectoris and a positive treadmill exercise test were randomized to receive either modified-release dipyridamole (200 mg bd orally; $n = 198$) or placebo ($n = 202$) for 24 weeks as an add-on to conventional anti-anginal therapy and for 4 additional weeks as monotherapy, the latter after withdrawal of standard treatment with calcium channel blockers and/or beta-blockers and/or long-acting (prophylactic) nitrates (6). Of the 198 patients randomized to dipyridamole, 134 completed the add-on phase but only 12 completed the monotherapy phase. Of the 202 patients randomized to placebo, 162 reached the add-on phase but only 12 reached the monotherapy phase. There were serious adverse events in 15 patients who took dipyridamole and 12 who took placebo (7.6 versus 6.0%). These included chest pain, angina pectoris, and non-cardiac adverse effects, such as diarrhea, nausea, and headache.

Organs and Systems

Cardiovascular

Dipyridamole is used with ^{201}thallium imaging in the detection of coronary artery disease, but can cause dysrhythmias.

- A 41-year-old man with hypertension was investigated for chest tightness by dipyridamole–thallium single-photon emission computed tomography (7). A standard dose of dipyridamole (0.56 mg/kg) was infused intravenously over 4 minutes, during which his heart rate increased from 68 to 88/minute and his blood pressure fell slightly (from 160/80 to 140/76 mmHg). He had no subjective symptoms, such as palpitation, dizziness, or chest tightness, but had ventricular extra beats 40 seconds after completion of the dipyridamole infusion, followed 1 minute later by a sustained ventricular tachycardia. His blood pressure fell to 80/50 mmHg and he complained of dizziness. Intravenous aminophylline 125 mg was given immediately. About 30 seconds later, the ventricular tachycardia terminated and his hemodynamics stabilized. The ventricular extra beats persisted for another 30 seconds.
- Two cases of severe bradydysrhythmias (one complete heart block, one sinus bradycardia) occurred after intravenous dipyridamole (8).

Dipyridamole can also cause myocardial ischemia.

- A 43-year-old man had an acute myocardial infarction immediately after exercise and pharmacological stress echocardiography with dipyridamole + atropine 1 month after successful stent implantation (9).
- A 59-year-old man developed unstable angina 1 month after coronary artery bypass surgery (10). During dipyridamole scintigraphy, 2 minutes after the beginning of dipyridamole infusion, ST segment elevation occurred in the inferior electrocardiographic leads and there

were two marked anteroseptal and inferior defects on myocardial scintigraphy.

A patient with aorto-iliac occlusive vascular disease and hypertension suffered a stroke 6.5 minutes after administration of intravenous dipyridamole during a ^{201}thallium myocardial study (11). Aminophylline did not reverse its progression.

Respiratory

The practicability of dipyridamole ^{13}N-ammonia myocardial positron emission tomography for perioperative risk assessment of coronary artery disease in patients with severe chronic obstructive pulmonary disease undergoing lung volume reduction surgery has been studied in 13 men and 7 women (mean age 57 years) without symptoms of coronary artery disease (12). Nine patients had intolerable dyspnea due to bronchoconstriction and required intravenous aminophylline. Dipyridamole cannot be recommended as a pharmacological stress in this setting.

Fatal respiratory insufficiency after dipyridamole–thallium imaging has been described in patients with a history of chronic obstructive lung disease (13,14). The authors of these reports concluded that patients with a history of chronic obstructive lung disease may have an increased risk of bronchospasm after dipyridamole infusion, and caution is advised in such patients.

Nervous system

Dipyridamole in combination with aspirin was more effective in preventing secondary stroke than low-dose aspirin or dipyridamole alone in only one of several studies (15). There is some evidence that dipyridamole can sometimes cause transient ischemic attacks (16).

- A 74-year-old woman had a 3-year history of mild dysarthria, dizziness, and gait ataxia, accompanied by two transient ischemic attacks with involuntary ballistic movements of her left arm lasting several seconds each, and another transient ischemic attack with a right homonymous hemianopia lasting 30 minutes. About 45 minutes after her first-ever oral administration of dipyridamole plus aspirin she developed a transient cerebellar deficit that reproduced features of previous vertebrobasilar ischemic events, as well as severe headache, flushing, and diarrhea.

The acute onset, the pattern of the cerebellar deficit, and the absence of features of epilepsy suggested that the episode was a transient ischemic attack. Aspirin is not known to cause transient ischemic attacks, and only rarely causes headache, flushing, and diarrhea. Since headache, flushing, and diarrhea, which can be caused by dipyridamole, occurred at the same time as the transient ischemic attacks and did not recur after withdrawal, dipyridamole may have caused the transient ischemic attacks. However, it was not clear whether the attacks occurred despite treatment rather than because of it.

In the Second European Stroke Prevention Study, headaches associated with dipyridamole (in 8% of patients taking dipyridamole or dipyridamole + aspirin versus 2% of patients taking aspirin alone or placebo) often led to withdrawal of therapy.

The predictive factors for headaches were explored in a study of the bioequivalence of two formulations of dipyridamole 200 mg in a modified-release combination with aspirin 25 mg (17). The conclusion was that the rapid fall in the incidence of headaches over time implied that most patients quickly develop tolerance to dipyridamole-associated headaches. However, in the European Stroke Prevention Study 2, headache was the most common adverse event, and it occurred more often in dipyridamole-treated patients (18).

Biliary tract

Recurrent drug-containing gallstones, 18 months after a previous stone had been removed endoscopically, were attributed to dipyridamole (19).

Immunologic

Infusion of dipyridamole caused an acute allergic reaction during myocardial scintigraphy (20).

- A 56-year old man with a history of allergy to aspirin, tetracycline, and penicillin, including angioedema and dyspnea, was given a dipyridamole stress test. About 1 minute after the infusion was started he reported periorbital pruritus. The infusion was completed uneventfully with the administration of ^{99m}technetium sestamibi at 7 minutes. Twenty minutes later he had tightness in the neck, dyspnea, and generalized facial swelling. He was given oxygen and intravenous promethazine hydrochloride and hydrocortisone. He improved over the next 2 hours, with residual periorbital edema but complete recovery from the respiratory symptoms. The cardiac study was completed without further events. The result was normal.

References

1. Harker LA, Kadatz RA. Mechanism of action of dipyridamole. Thromb Res Suppl 1983;4:39–46.
2. Bijlstra P, van Ginneken EE, Huls M, van Dijk R, Smits P, Rongen GA. Glyburide inhibits dipyridamole-induced forearm vasodilation but not adenosine-induced forearm vasodilation. Clin Pharmacol Ther 2004;75(3):147–56.
3. Anonymous. Dipyridamole—withdrawn. WHO Pharm Newslett 1999;5/6:2.
4. Lette J, Tatum JL, Fraser S, Miller DD, Waters DD, Heller G, Stanton EB, Bom HS, Leppo J, Nattel S. Safety of dipyridamole testing in 73,806 patients: the Multicenter Dipyridamole Safety Study. J Nucl Cardiol 1995;2(1):3–17.
5. Beller GA. Pharmacologic stress imaging. JAMA 1991;265(5):633–8.
6. Picano E; PISA (Persantin In Stable Angina) study group. Dipyridamole in chronic stable angina pectoris; a randomized, double blind, placebo-controlled, parallel group study. Eur Heart J 2001;22(19):1785–93.
7. Chang WT, Lin LC, Yen RF, Huang PJ. Persistent myocardial ischemia after termination of dipyridamole-induced ventricular tachycardia by intravenous aminophylline: scintigraphic demonstration. J Formos Med Assoc 2000;99(3):264–6.
8. Bielen M, Karsera D, Melon P, Kulbertus H. Bradyarythmies sevères au cours d'ure scintigraphie myocardique de perfusion avec injection de dipyridamole

(persantine). [Severe bradyarrhythmia during myocardial perfusion scintigraphy with injection of dipyridamole (Persantine).] Rev Med Liege 1999;54(2):105–8.
9. Nedeljkovic MA, Ostojic M, Beleslin B, Nedeljkovic IP, Stankovic G, Stojkovic S, Saponjski J, Babic R, Vukcevic V, Ristic AD, Orlic D. Dipyridamole–atropine-induced myocardial infarction in a patient with patent epicardial coronary arteries. Herz 2001;26(7):485–8.
10. Wartski M, Caussin C, Lancelin B. Spasme coronaire plurifocal declenche par l'injection de dipyridamole. Med Nucl 2001;25:153–9.
11. Whiting JH Jr, Datz FL, Gabor FV, Jones SR, Morton KA. Cerebrovascular accident associated with dipyridamole thallium-201 myocardial imaging: case report. J Nucl Med 1993;34(1):128–30.
12. Thurnheer R, Laube I, Kaufmann PA, Stumpe KD, Stammberger U, Bloch KE, Weder W, Russi EW. Practicability and safety of dipyridamole cardiac imaging in patients with severe chronic obstructive pulmonary disease. Eur J Nucl Med 1999;26(8):812–17.
13. Ottervanger JP, Haan D, Gans SJ, Hoorntje JC, Stricker BH. Bronchospasme, apnoe en hartstilstand na een dipyridamol-perfusiescintigrafie. [Bronchospasm, apnea and heart arrest following dipyridamole perfusion scintigraphy.] Ned Tijdschr Geneeskd 1993;137(3):142–3.
14. Hillis GS, al-Mohammad A, Jennings KP. Respiratory arrest during dipyridamole stress testing. Postgrad Med J 1997;73(859):301–2.
15. Diener HC, Cunha L, Forbes C, Sivenius J, Smets P, Lowenthal A; European Stroke Prevention Study. 2. Dipyridamole and acetylsalicylic acid in the secondary prevention of stroke. J Neurol Sci 1996;143(1–2):1–13.
16. Siegel AM, Sandor P, Kollias SS, Baumgartner RW. Transient ischemic attacks after dipyridamole–aspirin therapy. J Neurol 2000;247(10):807–8.
17. Theis JG, Deichsel G, Marshall S. Rapid development of tolerance to dipyridamole-associated headaches. Br J Clin Pharmacol 1999;48(5):750–5.
18. Diener H, Cunha L, Forbes C, Sirenius J, Smets P, Lowenthal A. European stroke prevention study 2. Nervenheilkunde 1999;18:380–90.
19. Sautereau D, Moesch C, Letard JC, Cessot F, Gainant A, Pillegand B. Recurrence of biliary drug lithiasis due to dipyridamole. Endoscopy 1997;29(5):421–3.
20. Angelides S, Van der Wall H, Freedman SB. Acute reaction to dipyridamole during myocardial scintigraphy. N Engl J Med 1999;340(5):394.

Direct thrombin inhibitors

General Information

The class of direct thrombin inhibitors includes the hirudins, lepirudin and bivalirudin, and the tripeptide or peptidomimetic compounds argatroban, efegatran, inogatran, napsagatran, melagatran, and ximelagatran. They act by binding to the active site on thrombin and inhibiting its enzymatic activity. They thus inhibit fibrin formation, activation of anticoagulant factors V, VIII, and XIII, and protein C, and platelet aggregation. The antithrombin action occurs rapidly and is quickly reversible.

In a meta-analysis of individual patients' data from 11 randomized comparisons of direct thrombin inhibitors (hirudin, bivalirudin, argatroban, efegatran, or inogatran) with heparin, 35 970 patients were treated for up to 7 days and followed for at least 30 days (1). Compared with heparin, the direct thrombin inhibitors were associated with a lower risk of death or myocardial infarction at the end of treatment (OR = 0.85; 95% CI = 0.77, 0.94) and at 30 days (OR = 0.91; CI = 0.84, 0.99). There was no excess of intracranial hemorrhages with the direct thrombin inhibitors.

Hirudin

Hirudin is the principal anticoagulant of the medicinal leech (*Hirudo medicinalis*). Though long known in its natural form, this is now produced by recombinant DNA techniques and characterized by a high affinity for thrombin, whether it is free in the plasma or absorbed onto the fibrin clot. The high incidence of hemorrhagic strokes in patients treated with both thrombolytic drugs and hirudin led to the redesign of three major trials (GUSTO-IIA, TIMI-9A, HIT III) of the effect of these antithrombotic agents in myocardial infarction (2–4). Hirudin is now regarded as the treatment of choice for heparin-induced thrombocytopenia. It is not recommended for use in pregnancy as it can cross the placenta; however, its safe use has been reported (5).

There is no specific antidote for the direct thrombin inhibitors: they are not neutralized by protamine sulfate.

Desirudin

Desirudin, similarly produced by recombinant techniques, has been used to prevent venous thromboembolism. It has been investigated in studies in patients with total hip replacements. In a large comparison of desirudin and low molecular weight heparin (enoxaparin), desirudin produced better prophylaxis against proximal deep vein thrombosis after total hip replacement (6) with no differences between the two groups with respect to perioperative, postoperative, and total blood loss. There were no cases of thrombocytopenia associated with desirudin.

Argatroban

Argatroban has been approved in the USA and Canada for the prophylaxis and treatment of thrombosis in patients with heparin-induced thrombocytopenia, and in Japan and Korea for various thrombotic disorders. Its effects can be monitored using the activated partial thromboplastin time for low doses and the activated clotting time for high doses. Its pharmacology, clinical pharmacology, and uses have been reviewed (7–14).

Organs and Systems

Immunologic

The effects on activated partial thromboplastin time and the incidence and clinical relevance of antihirudin antibodies in patients treated with lepirudin have been studied using data from two prospective multicenter studies, in which patients with heparin-induced thrombocytopenia received one of four intravenous lepirudin dosage regimens (15). Of 196 evaluable patients, 87 (44%) had IgG antihirudin antibodies. The development of antihirudin antibodies depended on the duration of treatment (antibody-positive patients 18.6 days versus antibody-negative patients 11.6 days). Antihirudin antibodies were not associated with increases in clinical endpoints (limb amputation, new thromboembolic complications, or major bleeding). In 23 of 51 evaluable patients in whom antihirudin antibodies developed during treatment with lepirudin, the antibodies enhanced the anticoagulatory effect of lepirudin. During prolonged treatment with lepirudin, anticoagulatory activity should be monitored daily.

Desirudin has a very low immunogenic potential. During repeated administration to 263 healthy volunteers, there were no signs or symptoms directly attributable to desirudin and only three volunteers exposed to a second course had allergic reactions with pruritic erythema attributable to desirudin in one case (16). In this study, specific antibodies directed against desirudin were detected in only one subject.

Drug–Drug Interactions

Digoxin

The pharmacokinetics of intravenous argatroban 1.5–2.0 μg/kg/minute were unaffected by co-administration of oral digoxin in healthy volunteers (17).

Erythromycin

Argatroban is metabolized by CYP3A4/5, and its pharmacokinetics might therefore be expected to be altered by inhibitors of CYP3A. However, in 14 healthy men erythromycin 500 mg qds had no effects on the pharmacokinetics of argatroban 1 μg/kg/minute infused over 5 hours (18).

Lidocaine

The pharmacokinetics of intravenous argatroban 1.5–2.0 μg/kg/minute were unaffected by co-administration of intravenous lidocaine in healthy volunteers (17).

Paracetamol

The pharmacokinetics of intravenous argatroban 1.5–2.0 μg/kg/minute were unaffected by co-administration of oral paracetamol in healthy volunteers (17).

References

1. Direct Thrombin Inhibitor Trialists' Collaborative Group. Direct thrombin inhibitors in acute coronary syndromes: principal results of a meta-analysis based on individual patients' data. Lancet 2002;359(9303):294–302.
2. Antman EM. Hirudin in acute myocardial infarction. Safety report from the Thrombolysis and Thrombin Inhibition in Myocardial Infarction (TIMI) 9A Trial. Circulation 1994;90(4):1624–30.
3. Neuhaus KL, von Essen R, Tebbe U, Jessel A, Heinrichs H, Maurer W, Doring W, Harmjanz D, Kotter V, Kalhammer E, et al Safety observations from the pilot phase of the randomized r-Hirudin for Improvement of Thrombolysis (HIT-III) study. A study of the Arbeitsgemeinschaft Leitender Kardiologischer Krankenhausarzte (ALKK). Circulation 1994;90(4):1638–42.
4. The Global Use of Strategies to Open Occluded Coronary Arteries (GUSTO) IIa Investigators. Randomized trial of intravenous heparin versus recombinant hirudin for acute coronary syndromes. Circulation 1994;90(4):1631–7.
5. Huhle G, Geberth M, Hoffmann U, Heene DL, Harenberg J. Management of heparin-associated thrombocytopenia in pregnancy with subcutaneous r-hirudin. Gynecol Obstet Invest 2000;49(1):67–9.
6. Eriksson BI, Wille-Jorgensen P, Kalebo P, Mouret P, Rosencher N, Bosch P, Baur M, Ekman S, Bach D, Lindbratt S, Close P. A comparison of recombinant hirudin with a low-molecular-weight heparin to prevent thromboembolic complications after total hip replacement. N Engl J Med 1997;337(19):1329–35.
7. Hursting MJ, Alford KL, Becker JC, Brooks RL, Joffrion JL, Knappenberger GD, Kogan PW, Kogan TP, McKinney AA, Schwarz RP Jr. Novastan (brand of argatroban): a small-molecule, direct thrombin inhibitor. Semin Thromb Hemost 1997;23(6):503–16.
8. Walenga JM. An overview of the direct thrombin inhibitor argatroban. Pathophysiol Haemost Thromb 2002;32(Suppl 3):9–14.
9. Ikoma H. Development of argatroban as an anticoagulant and antithrombin agent in Japan. Pathophysiol Haemost Thromb 2002;32(Suppl 3):23–8.
10. Fareed J, Hoppensteadt D, Iqbal O, Tobu M, Lewis BE. Practical issues in the development of argatroban: a perspective. Pathophysiol Haemost Thromb 2002;32(Suppl 3):56–65.
11. Hauptmann J. Pharmacokinetics of an emerging new class of anticoagulant/antithrombotic drugs. A review of small-molecule thrombin inhibitors. Eur J Clin Pharmacol 2002;57(11):751–8.
12. Kathiresan S, Shiomura J, Jang IK. Argatroban. J Thromb Thrombolysis 2002;13(1):41–7.
13. Kaplan KL, Francis CW. Direct thrombin inhibitors. Semin Hematol 2002;39(3):187–96.
14. Breddin HK. Experimentelle und klinische Befunde mit dem Thrombinhemmer Argatroban. [Experimental and clinical results with the thrombin inhibitor Argatroban.] Hämostaseologie 2002;22(3):55–9.
15. Eichler P, Friesen HJ, Lubenow N, Jaeger B, Greinacher A. Antihirudin antibodies in patients with heparin-induced thrombocytopenia treated with lepirudin: incidence, effects on aPTT, and clinical relevance. Blood 2000;96(7):2373–8.
16. Close P, Bichler J, Kerry R, Ekman S, Bueller HR, Kienast J, Marbet GA, Schramm W, Verstraete M. Weak allergenicity of recombinant hirudin CGP 39393 (REVASC) in immunocompetent volunteers. The European Hirudin in Thrombosis Group (HIT Group). Coron Artery Dis. 1994;5(11):943–9.
17. Inglis AM, Sheth SB, Hursting MJ, Tenero DM, Graham AM, DiCicco RA. Investigation of the interaction between argatroban and acetaminophen, lidocaine, or digoxin. Am J Health Syst Pharm 2002;59(13):1258–66.
18. Tran JQ, Di Cicco RA, Sheth SB, Tucci M, Peng L, Jorkasky DK, Hursting MJ, Benincosa LJ. Assessment of the potential pharmacokinetic and pharmacodynamic interactions between erythromycin and argatroban. J Clin Pharmacol 1999;39(5):513–19.

Dirithromycin

See also Macrolide antibiotics

General Information

Adverse effects of dirithromycin were studied in 4263 patients (1). There was abdominal pain in 5.6%, diarrhea in 5.0%, and nausea in 4.9%. Headache was relatively common (4.5%). In 63% of cases the adverse events were considered mild, in 31% moderate, and in 6.3% severe. Adverse events resulted in withdrawal in 3.1%, mainly because of gastrointestinal symptoms such as nausea and abdominal pain.

Organs and Systems

Respiratory

Adverse events involving the respiratory system (dyspnea, increased cough, or asthma) were reported in about 2% of patients taking dirithromycin (1).

Drug–Drug Interactions

Ciclosporin

Dirithromycin has a small effect on ciclosporin concentrations but to a clinically insignificant extent (2).

Oral contraceptives

Oral dirithromycin reduced the mean ethinylestradiol 24-hour AUC and increased its oral clearance in women using an oral contraceptive (3). However, since there was no effect on inhibition of ovulation, the clinical importance of this interaction may be negligible.

Theophylline and other xanthines

Drug interactions with dirithromycin have rarely been reported, since it does not interact with cytochrome P450. Nevertheless, in 13 healthy volunteers 500 mg/day for 10 days caused a significant 18% fall in the average steady-state plasma theophylline concentration and a 26% fall in peak concentration, with a 14–15% increase in clearance (4). In contrast, the steady-state pharmacokinetics of theophylline did not change in 14 patients with chronic obstructive airways disease who took dirithromycin for 10 days (5).

References

1. Brogden RN, Peters DH. Dirithromycin. A review of its antimicrobial activity, pharmacokinetic properties and therapeutic efficacy. Drugs 1994;48(4):599–616.
2. Bachmann K, Sullivan TJ, Reese JH, Jauregui L, Miller K, Scott M, Sides GD, Shapiro R. The influence of dirithromycin on the pharmacokinetics of cyclosporine in healthy subjects and in renal transplant patients. Am J Ther 1995;2(7):490–8.
3. Wermeling DP, Chandler MH, Sides GD, Collins D, Muse KN. Dirithromycin increases ethinyl estradiol clearance without allowing ovulation. Obstet Gynecol 1995;86(1):78–84.
4. Bachmann K, Nunlee M, Martin M, Sullivan T, Jauregui L, DeSante K, Sides GD. Changes in the steady-state pharmacokinetics of theophylline during treatment with dirithromycin. J Clin Pharmacol 1990;30(11):1001–5.
5. Bachmann K, Jauregui L, Sides G, Sullivan TJ. Steady-state pharmacokinetics of theophylline in COPD patients treated with dirithromycin. J Clin Pharmacol 1993;33(9):861–5.

Disinfectants and antiseptics

See also Individual agents

General Information

Antimicrobial drugs are widely used in topical medicaments, cosmetics, household products, and industrial biocides. Depending on their concentrations, they can function as disinfectants, antiseptics, or preservatives. The prevalence and rank order of sensitization to antimicrobial allergens in Europe have been reviewed (1,2). The most frequent antimicrobial allergens in 8521 patients who were patch-tested between 1985 and 1997 in Belgium are given in Table 1 (2).

In the multicenter study of the Information Network of Departments of Dermatology, sensitization rates of preservatives in the standard series were all over 1% in the test population of 11 485 patients. Thiomersal was rating highest (5.3%), chloromethyl-isothiazolinone/methyisothiazolinone, formaldehyde, and methyl-dibromoglutaronitrile/phenoxyethanol were next at about 2%, and parabens rating lowest at 1.6%. Glutaral, a biocide

Table 1 Most frequent antimicrobial allergens in Belgium out of 8521 patients in 1985–97

Rank	Allergen	Number
1	Methyl(chloro)isothiazolinone	143*
2	Thiomersal	136
3	Merbromine	94
4	Iodine	89
5	Cetrimide	88
6	Formaldehyde	80
7	Parabens	71
8	Chloramine	43
9	Quaternium-15	32
10	Nitrofurazone	29
11	Quinoline mix	28
12	Benzyl alcohol	25
	Benzoic acid	25
	Thiocyanomethylbenzothiazole	25
	Chlorhexidine	25
13	Glutaral (glutaraldehyde)	22
	Methyldibromoglutaronitrile + phenoxyethanol	22
14	Chloroacetamide	20
	Diazolidinyl urea	20

*Methyl (chloro) isothiazolinone was not tested until 1987

mainly used as a disinfectant, showed a remarkable increase in sensitization from less than 1% in 1990 up to more than 4% at the end of 1994. Health personnel and cleaning personnel were often affected and showed a sensitization rate of 10% (1,3).

The individual compounds that are covered in separate monographs are:

- Acrisorcin
- Aliphatic alcohols
- Benzalkonium
- Benzethonium
- Benzoxonium
- Benzyl alcohol
- Boric acid
- Cetrimonium bromide and cetrimide
- Chlorhexidine
- Chloroxylenol
- Ethacridine
- Ethylene oxide
- Formaldehyde
- Glutaral (glutaraldehyde)
- Hexachlorophene
- Hexetidine
- Parabens
- Peroxides
- Phenols
- Polyhexanide
- Polyvidone
- Salicylanilides
- Sodium hypochlorite
- Sulfites
- Tosylchloramide
- Triclocarban.

References

1. Schnuch A, Geier J, Uter W, Frosch PJ. Patch testing with preservatives, antimicrobials and industrial biocides. Results from a multicentre study. Br J Dermatol 1998;138(3):467–76.
2. Goossens A, Claes L, Drieghe J, Put E. Antimicrobials: preservatives, antiseptics and disinfectants. Contact Dermatitis 1998;39(3):133–4.
3. Schnuch A, Uter W, Geier J, Frosch PJ, Rustemeyer T. Contact allergies in healthcare workers. Results from the IVDK. Acta Dermatol Venereol 1998;78(5):358–63.

Disopyramide

See also Antidysrhythmic drugs

General Information

The use, clinical pharmacology, and adverse effects of disopyramide have been reviewed thoroughly (1,2).

Comparative studies

Disopyramide (by intravenous infusion of 2 mg/kg/minute up to a maximum total dose of 100 mg) has been compared with pilsicainide (in a single oral dose of 100–150 mg) in the treatment of paroxysmal atrial fibrillation in 72 patients (3). Conversion to sinus rhythm occurred in 29 of the 40 patients given pilsicainide and 18 of 32 patients given disopyramide, a non-significant difference. However, the mean time to conversion was faster with disopyramide (23 versus 60 minutes). No adverse effects were observed with either drug.

General adverse reactions

The adverse effects of disopyramide are mostly mediated by its effects on the cardiovascular system and by its anticholinergic effects. Disopyramide has a strong negative inotropic effect on the myocardium and can cause heart failure and hypotension. It prolongs the QT interval and can cause serious ventricular tachydysrhythmias. Anticholinergic effects can cause dry mouth, blurred vision, urinary retention, glaucoma, and erectile impotence. Hypoglycemia can also occur. Disopyramide can cause uterine contractions and should not be used during pregnancy. Angioedema has been reported rarely. Tumor-inducing effects have not been reported.

Organs and Systems

Cardiovascular

Disopyramide has three effects that can lead to cardiovascular complications (4).

1. *Anticholinergic* The anticholinergic effects of disopyramide on the vagus have been reported to cause tachycardia with bundle branch block or conversion to 1:1 conduction of a supraventricular tachycardia with block.
2. *QTc interval prolongation* There have been several reports of ventricular dysrhythmias (for example polymorphous ventricular tachycardia, ventricular fibrillation, ventricular tachycardia) in association with a prolonged QTc interval (SEDA-5, 180).
3. *Negative inotropic effect* Disopyramide can worsen cardiac failure and occasionally causes hypotension.

The risk of adverse cardiac effects of disopyramide during intravenous administration relates to the speed of its administration rather than to the total dose given (SEDA-10, 149).

Torsade de pointes due to disopyramide is well described (SEDA-4, 180). This effect is associated with prolongation of the QT interval. There has been a study of the effects of disopyramide on the QT interval in patients with pre-existing QT interval prolongation (5). In eight patients with QT interval prolongation during bradycardia and five patients without QT interval prolongation, disopyramide significantly prolonged the QT interval; however, the change was more pronounced in those with pre-existing bradycardia (78 versus 35 ms). The authors proposed that this difference might be due to an underlying abnormality of potassium channels in those with pre-existing bradycardia. Thus, those who are genetically predisposed to cardiac dysrhythmias may be at greater risk of the prodysrhythmic effects of antidysrhythmic drugs.

The risk of myocardial depression with consequent hypotension is greatest when disopyramide is infused rapidly intravenously (SEDA-10, 149). Loading doses of disopyramide should therefore be infused slowly (over 30–60 minutes).

Respiratory

- Pneumonitis has been attributed to disopyramide in a 72-year-old man; the symptoms began soon after the first dose (6). Bronchoalveolar lavage fluid contained a high percentage of lymphocytes (65%) and a high CD4:CD8 ratio (69:1).

The results of a lymphocyte stimulation test suggested that disopyramide had been responsible.

Nervous system

Through its anticholinergic effects disopyramide causes dry mouth and blurred vision and can occasionally cause serious adverse effects, including glaucoma and acute urinary retention (1).

Neuropathy has rarely been attributed to disopyramide (7).

- A 71-year-old woman, who had taken disopyramide 500 mg/day for 4 years, developed fatigue, paresthesia, pain, and cramps in her legs (8). She had proximal weakness in all four limbs and an unsteady gait. Electrophysiology showed a sensorimotor polyneuropathy, with reduced motor conduction velocity and muscle denervation. All antibodies were negative. The symptoms did not respond to prednisone but improved in the months after disopyramide withdrawal.

Psychological, psychiatric

Acute psychosis has been attributed to disopyramide (9,10).

Metabolism

Disopyramide can cause hypoglycemia (SEDA-6, 180) (SEDA-17, 222) (11), perhaps due to increased secretion of insulin, and can also potentiate the effects of conventional hypoglycemic drugs (12). This effect may be due to its chief metabolite mono-*N*-dealkyldisopyramide, since many of the reported cases of hypoglycemia have been in patients with renal impairment, in which the metabolite accumulates. In six subjects who were being considered for treatment with disopyramide, serum glucose concentrations were measured at 13, 15, 17, and 19 hours after supper, with no further food, with and without the added administration of two modified-released tablets of disopyramide 150 mg with supper and 12 hours later (13). Disopyramide significantly reduced the serum glucose concentration at all measurement times by an average of 0.54 mmol/l. The fall in serum glucose concentration was not related to the serum concentration of disopyramide or the serum creatinine concentration; it was greater in older patients and in underweight patients.

- Hypoglycemia has also been reported in a 70-year-old woman with type 2 diabetes mellitus taking disopyramide (14).

Hematologic

Disopyramide has caused neutropenia (15) and a coagulopathy (16).

Liver

Liver damage was reported in 22 (0.35%) of 6294 patients given disopyramide, with jaundice in 6 (0.09%) (17). Liver damage due to disopyramide can be associated with direct hepatocellular damage (18) and intrahepatic cholestasis (19,20). However, it can also occur indirectly, because of heart failure and hepatic congestion (21). Thus, the incidence of direct liver damage quoted above may be an overestimate.

Sexual function

Erectile impotence has been attributed to disopyramide (22,23).

Immunologic

Angioedema has been attributed to disopyramide (24).

Second-Generation Effects

Pregnancy

Disopyramide can cause uterine contractions (SEDA-3, 156) (25), and has been reported to have caused the onset of uterine contractions in eight of 10 patients at term (25).

- A 26-year-old woman with Wolff–Parkinson–White syndrome was given two doses of disopyramide at 36 weeks and shortly afterwards went into active labor with prepartum hemorrhage (26). The child was delivered by cesarean section and the woman made a full recovery.

In view of these reports disopyramide should be avoided in pregnancy.

Lactation

Although disopyramide and its *N*-monodesalkyl metabolite are both excreted in breast milk, the amounts are probably too small to be of importance (27).

Susceptibility Factors

Renal disease

In renal insufficiency there are complex changes in the pharmacokinetics of disopyramide, but the overall effect is accumulation of it and its active metabolite, due to reduced renal clearance (28).

Other features of the patient

Because of the anticholinergic effects of disopyramide, care should be taken both in patients with symptoms of prostatic hyperplasia (because of the risk of urinary retention) and in patients with glaucoma.

Disopyramide is highly bound to plasma proteins and this binding is saturable within the therapeutic range. Thus, at high dosages there may be an increase in the unbound fraction of drug in the plasma with proportionately greater effects. However, this is probably of no clinical relevance.

Drug Administration

Drug overdose

Overdosage of disopyramide is associated with apnea, loss of consciousness, loss of spontaneous respiration, hypotension, and cardiac dysrhythmias (29,30). Suggested treatment (31) includes arterial blood pressure monitoring, correction of acidosis and hypokalemia, and the intravenous infusion of a pressor agent for severe hypotension. Cardiac depressant drugs (for example class I antidysrhythmic drugs) should not be used to treat dysrhythmias, and the use of pyridostigmine to reverse the anticholinergic effects of disopyramide (32) is not recommended (SEDA-10, 149).

Drug–Drug Interactions

Class I antidysrhythmic drugs

There is an increased risk of dysrhythmias if disopyramide is used in conjunction with other drugs that prolong the QT interval, for example class I or class III antidysrhythmic drugs (33).

Macrolide antibiotics

Some of the macrolide antibiotics have been reported to inhibit the clearance of disopyramide (SEDA-21, 200) (SEDA-22, 207), resulting in serious dysrhythmias or hypoglycemia. The mechanism of this interaction is presumed to be inhibition of dealkylation of disopyramide to its major metabolite, mono-*N*-dealkyldisopyramide. For example, in human liver microsomes the macrolide antibiotic troleandomycin significantly inhibited the mono-*N*-dealkylation of disopyramide enantiomers by inhibition of CYP3A4 (34). This interaction can result in serious dysrhythmias or other adverse effects of disopyramide.

- A 76-year-old woman developed torsade de pointes 5 days after starting to take clarithromycin 200 mg bd in addition to disopyramide 100 mg tds (35). Her serum potassium concentration was 2.8 mmol/l and the QT_c interval was prolonged to 0.71 seconds. The plasma disopyramide concentration was in the usual target range (3.2 μg/ml). The disopyramide and clarithromycin were withheld and potassium was given; 14 hours later the serum potassium concentration was 4.3 mmol/l and there was no further dysrhythmia, despite prolongation of the QT_c interval to 0.67 seconds, falling to 0.45 seconds 10 days later.
- A 35-year-old woman taking disopyramide phosphate modified-release capsules 150 mg qds was given azithromycin 500 mg initially and 250 mg/day thereafter (36). In 11 days she developed malaise, light-headedness, and urinary retention. After the insertion of a urinary catheter she developed a monomorphic ventricular tachycardia with left bundle branch block. She was successfully cardioverted and the electrocardiogram showed a markedly prolonged QT interval of 560 ms and T wave inversion in the anterolateral leads. Her serum disopyramide concentration, which had previously been 2.6 μg/ml, was 11 μg/ml.
- In a 59-year-old man taking disopyramide 50 mg/day the addition of clarithromycin 600 mg/day caused hypoglycemia, and the serum disopyramide concentration rose from 1.5 to 8.0 μg/ml (37). The ratio of plasma insulin concentration to blood glucose concentration was greatly increased, suggesting that hypersecretion of insulin was responsible, confirming the likelihood that the hypoglycemia was due to disopyramide intoxication secondary to inhibition of its metabolism by clarithromycin. There was also slight prolongation of the QT_c interval, but no cardiac dysrhythmias. After withdrawal of clarithromycin and disopyramide both the blood glucose concentration and the QT_c interval returned to normal.
- An 86-year-old woman presented with severe hypoglycemia after clarithromycin 500 mg/day had been added for 3 days to her other therapy, which included disopyramide 500 mg/day (38). The hypoglycemia resolved completely after withdrawal of disopyramide.

Potassium-sparing drugs

Hyperkalemia has been reported to increase the risk of dysrhythmias in patients taking disopyramide (39), and disopyramide should therefore be used with caution in patients who are taking drugs that can increase body potassium, such as potassium-sparing diuretics and ACE inhibitors.

Practolol

The combination of disopyramide and practolol can cause profound sinus bradycardia and asystole (40,41).

Warfarin

Disopyramide can potentiate the effects of warfarin (42), although it is not known whether this is of any importance (43).

References

1. Heel RC, Brogden RN, Speight TM, Avery GS. Disopyramide: a review of its pharmacological properties and therapeutic use in treating cardiac arrhythmias. Drugs 1978;15(5):331–68.
2. Koch-Weser J. Disopyramide. N Engl J Med 1979;300(17):957–62.
3. Kumagai K, Abe H, Hiraki T, Nakashima H, Oginosawa Y, Ikeda H, Nakashima Y, Imaizumi T, Saku K. Single oral administration of pilsicainide versus infusion of disopyramide for termination of paroxysmal atrial fibrillation: a multicenter trial. Pacing Clin Electrophysiol 2000;23(11 Pt 2):1880–2.
4. Warrington SJ, Hamer J. Some cardiovascular problems with disopyramide. Postgrad Med J 1980;56(654):229–33.
5. Furushima H, Niwano S, Chinushi M, Ohhira K, Abe A, Aizawa Y. Relation between bradycardia dependent long QT syndrome and QT prolongation by disopyramide in humans. Heart 1998;79(1):56–8.
6. Yamamoto Y, Narasaki F, Futsuki Y, Fukushima K, Tomono K, Kadota J, Kohno S. Disopyramide-induced

pneumonitis, diagnosed by lymphocyte stimulation test using bronchoalveolar lavage fluid. Intern Med 2001;40(8):775–8.
7. Dawkins KD, Gibson J. Peripheral neuropathy with disopyramide. Lancet 1978;1(8059):329.
8. Briani C, Zara G, Negrin P. Disopyramide-induced neuropathy. Neurology 2002;58(4):663.
9. Falk RH, Nisbet PA, Gray TJ. Mental distress in patient on disopyramide. Lancet 1977;1(8016):858–9.
10. Padfield PL, Smith DA, Fitzsimons EJ, McCruden DC. Disopyramide and acute psychosis. Lancet 1977;1(8022):1152.
11. Otsu T, Ito T, Inagaki Y, Amano I, Masamoto S, Niwa M. [Accumulation of a disopyramide metabolite in renal failure.] Nippon Jinzo Gakkai Shi 1993;35(9):1065–71; Asaio J 1993;39:M609–13.
12. Series C. Hypoglycémie induite ou favorisée par le disopyramide. [Hypoglycemia induced or facilitated by disopyramide.] Rev Med Interne 1988;9(5):528–9.
13. Hasegawa J, Mori A, Yamamoto R, Kinugawa T, Morisawa T, Kishimoto Y. Disopyramide decreases the fasting serum glucose level in man. Cardiovasc Drugs Ther 1999;13(4):325–7.
14. Reynolds RM, Walker JD. Hypoglycaemia induced by disopyramide in a patient with Type 2 diabetes mellitus. Diabet Med 2001;18(12):1009–10.
15. Conrad ME, Cumbie WG, Thrasher DR, Carpenter JT. Agranulocytosis associated with disopyramide therapy. JAMA 1978;240(17):1857–8.
16. Handa SP. Disopyramide-induced toxic cutaneous blisters and coagulopathy. Dialysis Transplant 1982;11:706–7.
17. Anonymous. Hepatic damage due to disopyramide. Jpn Med Gaz 1981;June 20:11.
18. Doody PT. Disopyramide hepatotoxicity and disseminated intravascular coagulation. South Med J 1982;75(4):496–8.
19. Meinertz T, Langer KH, Kasper W, Just H. Disopyramide-induced intrahepatic cholestasis. Lancet 1977;2(8042):828–9.
20. Riccioni N, Bozzi L, Susini N, Roni P. Disopyramide-induced intrahepatic cholestasis. Lancet 1977;2(8052–8053):1362–3.
21. Scheinman SJ, Poll DS, Wolfson S. Acute cardiac failure and hepatic ischemia induced by disopyramide phosphate. Yale J Biol Med 1980;53(5):361–6.
22. McHaffie DJ, Guz A, Johnston A. Impotence in patient on disopyramide. Lancet 1977;1(8016):859.
23. Hasegawa J, Mashiba H. Transient sexual dysfunction observed during antiarrhythmic therapy by long-acting disopyramide in a male Wolff–Parkinson–White patient. Cardiovasc Drugs Ther 1994;8(2):277.
24. Porterfield JG, Antman EM, Lown B. Respiratory difficulty after use of disopyramide. N Engl J Med 1980;303(10):584.
25. Tadmor OP, Keren A, Rosenak D, Gal M, Shaia M, Hornstein E, Yaffe H, Graff E, Stern S, Diamant YZ. The effect of disopyramide on uterine contractions during pregnancy. Am J Obstet Gynecol 1990;162(2):482–6.
26. Abbi M, Kriplani A, Singh B. Preterm labor and accidental hemorrhage after disopyramide therapy in pregnancy. A case report. J Reprod Med 1999;44(7):653–5.
27. Barnett DB, Hudson SA, McBurney A. Disopyramide and its N-monodesalkyl metabolite in breast milk. Br J Clin Pharmacol 1982;14(2):310–12.
28. Perlman PE, Adams WG Jr, Ridgeway NA. Extreme pyrexia during bretylium administration. Postgrad Med 1989;85(1):111–14.
29. Hayler AM, Holt DW, Volans GN. Fatal overdosage with disopyramide. Lancet 1978;1(8071):968–9.
30. Larcan A, Lambert H, Laprevote-Heully MC, Delorme N, Royer MJ, Guillet J. Les intoxications aiguës volontaires au disopyramide: à propos de 20 observations. Ann Med Nancy 1981;20:901–17.
31. Hayler AM, Medd RK, Holt DW, O'Keefe BD. Treatment of disopyramide overdosage. Vet Hum Toxicol 1979;21(Suppl):93–5.
32. Teichman SL, Fisher JD, Matos JA, Kim SG. Disopyramide–pyridostigmine: report of a beneficial drug interaction. J Cardiovasc Pharmacol 1985;7(1):108–13.
33. Ellrodt G, Singh BN. Adverse effects of disopyramide (Norpace): toxic interactions with other antiarrhythmic agents. Heart Lung 1980;9(3):469–74.
34. Echizen H, Tanizaki M, Tatsuno J, Chiba K, Berwick T, Tani M, Gonzalez FJ, Ishizaki T. Identification of CYP3A4 as the enzyme involved in the mono-N-dealkylation of disopyramide enantiomers in humans. Drug Metab Dispos 2000;28(8):937–44.
35. Hayashi Y, Ikeda U, Hashimoto T, Watanabe T, Mitsuhashi T, Shimada K. Torsades de pointes ventricular tachycardia induced by clarithromycin and disopyramide in the presence of hypokalemia. Pacing Clin Electrophysiol 1999;22(4 Pt 1):672–4.
36. Granowitz EV, Tabor KJ, Kirchhoffer JB. Potentially fatal interaction between azithromycin and disopyramide. Pacing Clin Electrophysiol 2000;23(9):1433–5.
37. Iida H, Morita T, Suzuki E, Iwasawa K, Toyo-oka T, Nakajima T. Hypoglycemia induced by interaction between clarithromycin and disopyramide. Jpn Heart J 1999;40(1):91–6.
38. Morlet-Barla N, Narbonne H, Vialettes B. Hypoglycémie grave et récidivante secondaire à l'interaction disopyramide–clarithromicine. [Severe hypoglycemia and recurrence caused by disopyramide–clarithromycin interaction.] Presse Méd 2000;29(24):1351.
39. Maddux BD, Whiting RB. Toxic synergism of disopyramide and hyperkalemia. Chest 1980;78(4):654–6.
40. Cumming AD, Robertson C. Interaction between disopyramide and practolol. BMJ 1979;2(6200):1264.
41. Gelipter D, Hazell M. Interaction between disopyramide and practolol. BMJ 1980;280:52.
42. Haworth E, Burroughs AK. Disopyramide and warfarin interaction. BMJ 1977;2(6091):866–7.
43. Sylven C, Anderson P. Evidence that disopyramide does not interact with warfarin. BMJ (Clin Res Ed) 1983;286(6372):1181.

Disulfiram

General Information

Disulfiram (tetraethylthiuram) has been widely used since the late 1940s to facilitate abstinence from alcohol (1). Concomitant use of alcohol during disulfiram therapy results in an autonomic symptom complex that can involve headache, flushing, nausea and vomiting, sweating, tachycardia, hypotension, and confusion. The mechanism of action of disulfiram is inhibition of aldehyde dehydrogenase; alcohol is metabolized to acetaldehyde, which accumulates (2).

Sulfiram

Sulfiram is similar in structure to disulfiram, but has one less sulfur atom in its central chain. It is a much weaker inhibitor of aldehyde dehydrogenase than disulfiram and is used in the topical treatment of scabies.

General adverse effects

Several adverse effects of disulfiram itself (as opposed to the aldehyde that it allows to accumulate) have been described. They include neurological reactions and skin reactions, but hepatotoxicity is the only previously reported life-threatening reaction, and it is rare (3).

Disulfiram modifies the metabolism of many drugs by inhibiting the cytochrome CYP2E1. Adverse reactions to disulfiram occur with a frequency of 1 in 200 to 1 in 2000 per treatment-year (4). The death rate is about one per 25 000 patients per year, and hepatic failure accounts for most of these (4). Allergic reactions can occur. Tumor-inducing effects have not been described.

Organs and Systems

Cardiovascular

Disulfiram in a dose of 250–300 mg/day does not affect pulse rate, blood pressure, or plasma noradrenaline concentrations, but 500 mg/day causes an increase in plasma noradrenaline, increased systolic blood pressure both recumbent and erect, and an increased erect pulse rate. The raised blood pressure does not reach hypertensive values, but the results suggest increased sympathetic nervous system activity in patients who take disulfiram. Caution should therefore be exercised in using disulfiram in hypertensive patients. Close monitoring of blood pressure is advised, and the dose of disulfiram should preferably be reduced to 250 mg/day (5).

Cardiac dysrhythmias occurred during a disulfiram + alcohol test in a 48-year-old man who had been an alcoholic for 5 years (6). After drinking a test amount of alcohol, he developed flushing, nausea, vomiting, sweating, dyspnea, and hyperventilation, palpitation, tremor, confusion, and syncope. The electrocardiogram showed atrial fibrillation and non-sustained bouts of ventricular tachycardia of 7–8/minute. He also had severe hypotension.

Nervous system

Disulfiram can cause a polyneuritis (7), which can occasionally be fulminant and irreversible.

- A 39-year-old woman developed a severe sensori motor polyneuritis after taking ethanol and disulfiram in high doses (8). The disorder was similar to other cases of disulfiram neuropathy, but was acute and more severe.

The neurotoxic effects of disulfiram have been compared with those of carbon disulfide, a disulfiram metabolite (9). The results suggested that carbon disulfide may be responsible for the behavioural and neurological adverse effects of disulfiram. If so, other toxic effects of carbon disulfide might follow administration of high doses of disulfiram, such as parkinsonism, psychotic behaviour, and encephalopathy.

Disulfiram-induced neurotoxicity caused parkinsonism in a man who had been an alcoholic for 10 years (10).

- A 52-year-old alcoholic stopped drinking in August 1996 and started to take disulfiram 500 mg/day. His usual medications had been aspirin 300 mg/day and levothyroxine 100 μg/day. He had had severe loss of visual acuity (2/10) in the left eye 3 months before admission. He was admitted to hospital because of drowsiness. Neurological examination showed severe hypophonia, difficulty in swallowing, and mild rigidity of the limbs. Disulfiram was withdrawn but the other medications were maintained. His drowsiness improved over 5 days, but he remained bradykinetic, with extrapyramidal hypertonia, facial hypomobility, and abnormal posture. His gait was slow and shuffling.
- A 20-year-old woman was referred for implantation of an intrathecal baclofen pump (11). She had had severe dystonia and spasticity following a suicide attempt with disulfiram at age 14 years. T1-weighted MRI scanning of her brain showed bilateral globus pallidus infarction. She had profound relief of spasticity after intrathecal test injections of baclofen and underwent implantation of an intrathecal baclofen pump. Her spasticity subsequently improved.

Sensory systems

Retrobulbar neuritis can be part of a disulfiram-induced polyneuritis, with dramatic reduction in visual acuity and impaired colour perception (SEDA-10, 349) (12). This complication is rare but serious. It occurs at dosages of 500 mg/day, and there is a latent period of 2–36 months. Tobacco abuse is thought to be a predisposing factor.

Disulfiram can cause optic neuropathy (13,14).

Psychological, psychiatric

Disulfiram can cause distressing neuropsychiatric effects including paranoia, impaired memory and concentration, ataxia, dysarthria, and frontal release signs (signs that can be indicative of permanent structural damage or temporary metabolic or infectious changes to the brain's frontal lobes), such as snout and grasp reflexes (2,15). The mechanisms are not properly understood, but adverse effects develop more frequently in subjects with low plasma dopamine beta-hydroxylase activity. In one study, a research subject with low dopamine beta-hydroxylase activity developed a schizophrenic reaction to disulfiram; it would be useful to know whether determining blood dopamine beta-hydroxylase activities predicts the risk of adverse reactions to disulfiram (16).

Of 52 patients with alcohol dependence/abuse who were given disulfiram 250 mg bd after food, six developed psychotic symptoms; all had a mood disorder but no thought disorder (17). The psychotic symptoms remitted completely after withdrawal and a short course of antipsychotic therapy, except in one patient who had to be given lithium.

- A 47-year-old man with alcohol abuse took disulfiram (18). He developed a psychosis while taking it and for 2 weeks after. He stated that he had not taken alcohol. He was successfully treated with antipsychotic drugs. Afterwards it was discovered that his family history was positive for schizophrenia; it is therefore possible that he was more vulnerable to develop psychosis due to disulfiram.

Prolonged toxic delirium related to disulfiram and alcohol intake has been reported (19). The predominant presenting feature was neuropsychiatric rather than autonomic symptoms.

- A 50-year-old woman with a history of bipolar disorder type I and alcohol dependence taking disulfiram had a 4-day history of a change in mental status, including visual hallucinations and deficits in orientation and concentration. Other features included a tachycardia and non-focal neurological signs. Extensive metabolic, infectious, and neurological investigations revealed no abnormalities that alone could explain her acute confusional state. It was subsequently discovered that she had drunk alcohol on at least two separate occasions while taking disulfiram before her change in mental status, and that a similar, although shorter, episode had occurred previously.

Gastrointestinal

In a colostomy patient, the smell of the colostomy was present only so long as disulfiram exposure continued (20). The cause was obscure.

Liver

About 25 cases of disulfiram-induced liver damage (apparently as a result of an immunological mechanism) have been reported, some fatal. The cause is not known, since many alcoholic patients who use disulfiram have pre-existing liver damage. Nevertheless, it is believed that disulfiram does sometimes trigger serious liver damage (SEDA-10, 438); severe hepatitis, sometimes fatal, has been reported (21–24). Liver function should be checked before giving disulfiram, especially since there may be a long history of alcohol abuse (25).

The Swedish adverse drug reactions register, SWEDIS, received 149 case reports of 157 adverse reactions associated with disulfiram from 1971 to 1999, of which 63 cited disorders of the liver and biliary tract (26). Of these 63 reports, seven were classified as serious. In three cases of severe liver damage with a fatal outcome, disulfiram was suspected to have caused the reaction. If signs of liver damage appear, it is recommended that disulfiram be withdrawn and liver function tests performed.

Skin

A fatal rash has been attributed to disulfiram.

- A 47-year-old man developed a generalized rash and malaise (27). He had chronic alcoholism and had taken disulfiram 250 mg/day for 1 month. He denied previous liver disease, blood transfusions, or having taken hepatotoxic drugs or alcohol. He was given clarithromycin 500 mg bd and paracetamol 500 mg tds and 1 week later noticed non-pruritic cutaneous maculopapular lesions on the legs, which spread to the rest of his body, excluding the palms and soles. His temperature was 41°C, his blood pressure 90/60 mmHg, and his heart rate 130/minute. There were no signs of encephalopathy. His conjunctivae were yellow. There was furfuraceous desquamation on his face and confluent erythematous annular lesions with a purpuric component on the groins, thighs, and the undersides of his arms. There was edema of the hands and feet. During the next several days the skin lesions worsened. He developed blisters, initially covering less than 10% of the body surface, but then extending all over the body. He developed septic shock and, despite supportive measures, died.
- A 49-year-old woman developed pruritic erythema 2 weeks after the implantation of a modified-release formulation of disulfiram, Esperal, in her left buttock (28). Three months later she started drinking alcohol and developed generalized erythema with numerous papules on her face and limbs; the dermatitis at the site of the implant became more severe. The serum ethanol concentration was 270 mg/dl. Methanol was not detected.
- A 55-year-old man developed yellow palms and soles while taking disulfiram (29).

The authors speculated that the mechanism was inhibition of carotene metabolism by disulfiram.

Immunologic

Allergic reactions to disulfiram tend to be limited (30). However, the possibility of hypersensitivity should be borne in mind in patients who have had allergic reactions in the past, regardless of the allergen concerned.

Second-Generation Effects

Pregnancy

Disulfiram should not be used in women who may become pregnant because of potential teratogenicity (31).

Drug–Drug Interactions

Alcohol

The interaction of disulfiram with alcohol, the metabolism of which is interfered with at the aldehyde stage, is the basis for its therapeutic use; disulfiram renders alcohol intake unpleasant, and dangerous if much alcohol is taken.

Sulfiram is related to disulfiram, and after repeated topical treatment the ingestion of alcohol can rarely cause a similar reaction, with generalized flushing, malaise, and rhinorrhea (32).

Amitriptyline

Amitriptyline potentiates the disulfiram reaction (33).

Benzodiazepines

Disulfiram inhibits the hepatic metabolism of other drugs and can prolong their effects. The half-lives of chlordiazepoxide and diazepam increase significantly after disulfiram, while the clearances are reduced, with accumulation. No change in half-life or clearance has been noted for oxazepam (which is not metabolized in the liver) (34). The benzodiazepines reduce the disulfiram reaction to alcohol.

Caffeine

Disulfiram reduces caffeine clearance (35).

Cocaine

Simultaneous abuse of cocaine and alcohol is common and alcohol reduces negative stimulant effects and potentiates "highs." Disulfiram has therefore also been used to treat cocaine dependence, with the rationale that an inability to modulate the effects of cocaine with alcohol may reduce cocaine use.

Six volunteers with cocaine dependence and alcohol abuse or dependence, mean age 32 years, took disulfiram 250 mg/day or placebo (36). After 3 days they participated in cocaine administration sessions (one session daily for 3 days). The study drugs were separated by at least 5 days, based on the time needed for enzyme regeneration (37). After disulfiram, cocaine significantly increased heart rate and blood pressure, and they remained high when plasma cocaine concentrations were falling at later times, and were greatest for cocaine 2 mg/kg. These findings contrast with those obtained when multiple doses of cocaine alone have been given to healthy volunteers, in whom there was evidence of acute tolerance to the cardiovascular effects of cocaine (38,39). Disulfiram therefore has potential as a treatment for cocaine + alcohol abuse, but could also increase the risk of toxicity as a result of its pharmacokinetic interaction with cocaine.

Warfarin

Bad breath has been reported in patients taking disulfiram concurrently with warfarin (40).

References

1. Wright C, Moore RD. Disulfiram treatment of alcoholism. Am J Med 1990;88(6):647–55.
2. Peachey JE, Brien JF, Roach CA, Loomis CW. A comparative review of the pharmacological and toxicological properties of disulfiram and calcium carbimide. J Clin Psychopharmacol 1981;1(1):21–6.
3. Rabkin JM, Corless CL, Orloff SL, Benner KG, Flora KD, Rosen HR, Olyaei AJ. Liver transplantation for disulfiram-induced hepatic failure. Am J Gastroenterol 1998; 93(5):830–1.
4. Enghusen Poulsen H, Loft S, Andersen JR, Andersen M. Disulfiram therapy—adverse drug reactions and interactions. Acta Psychiatr Scand Suppl 1992;369:59–66.
5. Lake CR, Major LF, Ziegler MG, Kopin IJ. Increased sympathetic nervous system activity in alcoholic patients treated with disulfiram. Am J Psychiatry 1977;134(12):1411–14.
6. Savas MC, Gullu IH. Disulfiram–ethanol test reaction: significance of supervision. Ann Pharmacother 1997; 31(3):374–5.
7. Dupuy O, Flocard F, Vial C, Rode G, Charles N, Boisson D, Flechaire A. Toxicité du disulfirame (Esperal). A propos de trois observations originales. [Disulfiram (Esperal) toxicity. Apropos of 3 original cases.] Rev Med Interne 1995;16(1):67–72.
8. Rothrock JF, Johnson PC, Rothrock SM, Merkley R. Fulminant polyneuritis after overdose of disulfiram and ethanol. Neurology 1984;34(3):357–9.
9. Rainey JM Jr. Disulfiram toxicity and carbon disulfide poisoning. Am J Psychiatry 1977;134(4):371–8.
10. Boukriche Y, Weisser I, Aubert P, Masson C. MRI findings in a case of late onset disulfiram-induced neurotoxicity. J Neurol 2000;247(9):714–15.
11. Mesiwala AH, Loeser JD. Bilateral globus pallidus infarction secondary to disulfiram ingestion. Pediatr Neurosurg 2001;34(4):224.
12. Frisoni GB, Di Monda V. Disulfiram neuropathy: a review (1971-1988) and report of a case. Alcohol Alcohol 1989;24(5):429–37.
13. Palliyath S, Schwartz BD. Disulfiram neuropathy: electrophysiological study. Electromyogr Clin Neurophysiol 1988;28(5):245–7.
14. Acheson JF, Howard RS. Reversible optic neuropathy associated with disulfiram. Neuroophthalmology 1988;8:175.
15. Gostout CJ. Patient assessment and resuscitation. Gastrointest Endosc Clin N Am 1999;9(2):175–87.
16. Ewing JA, Rouse BA, Mueller RA, Silver D. Can dopamine beta-hydroxylase levels predict adverse reactions to disulfiram? Alcohol Clin Exp Res 1978;2(1):93–4.
17. Murthy KK. Psychosis during disulfiram therapy for alcoholism. J Indian Med Assoc 1997;95(3):80–1.
18. Verbon H, de Jong CA. Psychose tijdens en na disulfiram-gebruik. [Psychosis during and after disulfiram use.] Ned Tijdschr Geneeskd 2002;146(12):571–3.
19. Park CW, Riggio S. Disulfiram–ethanol induced delirium. Ann Pharmacother 2001;35(1):32–5.
20. Miller SI. Disulfiram: an unusual side effect. JAMA 1977;237(24):2602–3.
21. Kerkhof SC, de Doelder PF, Harinck HI, Stricker BH. Leverbeschadiging toegeschreven aan het gebruik van disulfiram. [Liver damage attributed to the use of disulfiram.] Ned Tijdschr Geneeskd 1995;139(46):2378–81.
22. Knudsen TE, Nielsen-Kudsk JE. Letalt forlobende hepatitis efter disulfiram. [Fatal hepatitis caused by disulfiram.] Ugeskr Laeger 1990;152(20):1457–8.
23. Vanjak D, Samuel D, Gosset F, Derrida S, Moreau R, Soupison T, Soulier A, Bismuth H, Sicot C. Hépatite fulminante au disulfirame chez un malade atteint de cirrhose alcoolique. Survie après transplantation hépatique. [Fulminant hepatitis induced by disulfiram in a patient with alcoholic cirrhosis. Survival after liver transplantation.] Gastroenterol Clin Biol 1989;13(12):1075–8.
24. Mason NA. Disulfiram-induced hepatitis: case report and review of the literature. DICP 1989;23(11):872–5.
25. Bartle WR, Fisher MM, Kerenyi N. Disulfiram-induced hepatitis. Report of two cases and review of the literature. Dig Dis Sci 1985;30(9):834–7.
26. Anonymous. Disulfiram. Liver reactions. WHO Newslett 2000;4:11.
27. Masia M, Gutierrez F, Jimeno A, Navarro A, Borras J, Matarredona J, Martin-Hidalgo A. Fulminant hepatitis and fatal toxic epidermal necrolysis (Lyell disease) coincident with clarithromycin administration in an alcoholic patient receiving disulfiram therapy. Arch Intern Med 2002;162(4):474–6.
28. Kiec-Swierczynska M, Krecisz B, Fabicka B. Systemic contact dermatitis from implanted disulfiram. Contact Dermatitis 2000;43(4):246–7.
29. Santonastaso M, Cecchetti E, Pace M, Piccolo D. Yellow palms with disulfiram. Lancet 1997;350(9073):266.
30. Minet A, Frankart M, Eggers S, Lachapelle JM, Bourlond A. Réactions allergiques aux implants de disulfirame. [Allergic reactions to disulfiram implants.] Ann Dermatol Venereol 1989;116(8):543–5.
31. Nora AH, Nora JJ, Blu J. Limb-reduction anomalies in infants born to disulfiram-treated alcoholic mothers. Lancet 1977;2(8039):664.

32. Blanc D, Deprez P. Unusual adverse reaction to an acaricide. Lancet 1990;335(8700):1291–2.
33. Maany I, Hayashida M, Pfeffer SL, Kron RE. Possible toxic interaction between disulfiram and amitriptyline. Arch Gen Psychiatry 1982;39(6):743–4.
34. MacLeod SM, Sellers EM, Giles HG, Billings BJ, Martin PR, Greenblatt DJ, Marshman JA. Interaction of disulfiram with benzodiazepines. Clin Pharmacol Ther 1978;24(5):583–9.
35. Beach CA, Mays DC, Guiler RC, Jacober CH, Gerber N. Inhibition of elimination of caffeine by disulfiram in normal subjects and recovering alcoholics. Clin Pharmacol Ther 1986;39(3):265–70.
36. McCance-Katz EF, Kosten TR, Jatlow P. Chronic disulfiram treatment effects on intranasal cocaine administration: initial results. Biol Psychiatry 1998;43(7):540–3.
37. Helander A, Carlsson S. Use of leukocyte aldehyde dehydrogenase activity to monitor inhibitory effect of disulfiram treatment. Alcohol Clin Exp Res 1990;14(1):48–52.
38. Fischman MW, Schuster CR, Hatano Y. A comparison of the subjective and cardiovascular effects of cocaine and lidocaine in humans. Pharmacol Biochem Behav 1983;18(1):123–7.
39. Foltin RW, Fischman MW. Smoked and intravenous cocaine in humans: acute tolerance, cardiovascular and subjective effects. J Pharmacol Exp Ther 1991;257(1):247–61.
40. O'Reilly RA, Motley CH. Breath odor after disulfiram. JAMA 1977;238(24):2600.

Diuretics

See also Individual agents

General Information

Diuretics are among the most widely used drugs, particularly for the treatment of hypertension and of various conditions associated with sodium retention.

Considering the widespread use of diuretics over a long period (chlorothiazide was introduced in 1957) their safety record is remarkable, and reports of adverse effects of any significance with the best-known drugs of this type are uncommon.

When problems do arise they usually reflect either interactions, which with caution could have been avoided, or relative overdosage. In the course of time the recommended antihypertensive doses of diuretics have been reduced, and some adverse effects that were noted in the early years are now of less significance; these include hypotension, dehydration, reduction of the glomerular filtration rate, and severe hypokalemia. Continued use of thiazides in excessive doses may reflect ignorance of their very flat dose–response curve (1). At currently recommended low doses, diuretics improve overall quality of life, even in asymptomatic patients with mild hypertension (2). The large HANE study (3) provided no evidence of superior efficacy or tolerability of new classes of antihypertensive drugs.

Uses

Hypertension

The popularity of thiazide diuretics in the management of hypertension reflects three major factors (4):

- recognition of the effectiveness of much lower dosages than those used previously, thereby providing good antihypertensive efficacy with fewer adverse effects (SED-13, 558);
- the excellent reductions in morbidity and mortality that have been achieved by low-dosage diuretic-based therapy in multiple randomized, controlled trials (SED-13, 558);
- the increasing awareness that some diuretic-induced shrinkage of effective blood volume is essential for adequate treatment of most patients with hypertension.

The Seventh Joint Committee Report on Detection, Evaluation, and Treatment of High Blood Pressure (5) concluded that a diuretic should be the first-step drug of choice, unless there are specific indications for other drugs. Although there may be theoretical advantages of certain newer types of drugs, the data thus far have not consistently shown that these drugs are more effective in reducing morbidity and mortality than therapy based on diuretics or beta-blockers (6). Emphasis is correctly placed on the important role of ACE inhibitors in retarding progression of renal insufficiency in diabetic and other nephropathies (7). However, in these circumstances, ACE inhibitors are added to a background of other antihypertensive therapies, commonly including a diuretic. Therefore, the renal protective action of ACE inhibitors is in the context of combination regimens. The ability of low doses of diuretics to enhance efficacy has been demonstrated for all other classes of drugs (8). Moreover, the tendency for increased retention of sodium by the hypertensive kidney when non-diuretic drugs cause the blood pressure to fall has long been recognized to contribute to loss of antihypertensive efficacy, which can be restored immediately by the addition of a diuretic.

Clinical trials

The LIVE (Left ventricular regression, Indapamide Versus Enalapril) study was a 1-year, prospective, randomized, double-blind comparison of modified-release indapamide 1.5 mg and enalapril 20 mg in reducing left ventricular mass in 411 hypertensive patients with left ventricular hypertrophy (9). For equivalent reductions in blood pressure, indapamide was significantly more effective than enalapril in reducing left ventricular mass index.

The effectiveness of specific first-line antihypertensive drugs in lowering blood pressure and preventing adverse outcomes has been systematically quantified in a meta-analysis of randomized controlled trials that lasted at least 1 year, and compared one of six possible first-line antihypertensive therapies either with another of the six drug therapies or with no treatment (10). Of 38 trials identified, 23 in 50 853 patients met the inclusion criteria. Four drug classes were evaluated: thiazides (21 trials), beta-blockers (5 trials), calcium antagonists (4 trials), and ACE inhibitors (1 trial). In five comparisons of thiazides with beta-blockers, thiazides were associated with a significantly lower rate of withdrawal because of adverse effects (RR = 0.69; 95% CI = 0.63, 0.76). In the trials that had an untreated control group, low-dose thiazide therapy was associated with a significant reduction in the risk of death (RR = 0.89; CI = 0.81, 0.99), stroke (RR = 0.66; CI = 0.56, 0.79), coronary heart disease (RR = 0.71, CI = 0.60, 0.84), and cardiovascular events (RR = 0.68; CI = 0.62, 0.75). Low-dose thiazide therapy reduced the absolute risk of cardiovascular events by 5.7% (CI = 4.2, 7.2); the number needed to treat (NNT) for approximately 5 years to prevent one event was 18. High-dose thiazide, beta-blocker, and calcium antagonist therapy did not significantly reduce the risk of death or coronary heart disease. Thiazides were significantly better than the other drugs in reducing systolic pressure, but antihypertensive efficacy did not differ between the high- and low-dose thiazide trials.

In the UK Medical Research Council (MRC) trial, the outcome of antihypertensive treatment based on diuretics was compared with placebo in a very large number of hypertensive subjects (11). Treatment based on a thiazide did not increase the incidence of coronary events or sudden death; indeed, thiazide-based treatment reduced the incidence of strokes by 67% and of all cardiovascular complications by 20%. It should be noted that the dose of bendroflumethiazide used in the MRC trial (10 mg/day) is now known to be unnecessarily high and that it was used without prophylaxis against hypokalemia. Even so, a subgroup analysis of data from the MRC Trial provided no evidence that the association between major electrocardiographic abnormalities and an increased likelihood of a clinical event was strengthened by bendroflumethiazide treatment (12).

A series of trials in elderly hypertensive subjects has shown a very pronounced reduction in cardiac events as a result of treatment based on thiazide diuretics. In the European Working Party on Hypertension in the Elderly (EWPHE) trial (13), total cardiovascular deaths were reduced by 38%, all cardiac deaths by 43%, and deaths due to myocardial infarction by 60%. Benefits in the Systolic Hypertension in the Elderly Program (SHEP) included a reduction in fatal and non-fatal myocardial infarction of 25% and major cardiovascular events of 32% (14) and were seen in those with and without electrocardiographic abnormalities at entry. The risk of heart failure was also reduced in patients taking chlortalidone-based therapy (15). Relative risk was similar in patients with and without non-insulin dependent diabetes mellitus; absolute risk reduction was twice as great in the diabetic subjects (16). The Swedish Trial of Old Patients with Hypertension (STOP-Hypertension) reported a significant reduction in myocardial infarction and all-cause mortality (17). In the MRC Trial in elderly adults (18), diuretic treatment reduced coronary events by 44% and fatal cardiovascular events by 35%.

In the MRC trials (11,18), the IPPPSH trial (19), and the HAPPHY trial (20), antihypertensive treatment based on a thiazide diuretic was compared with treatment based on a beta-blocker. The results with diuretic treatment were no less favorable as regards cardiac events than those when using a "cardioprotective" beta-blocker (20). In the IPPPSH trial, the group using no beta-blockers (but with a higher incidence of diuretic use and of hypokalemia) showed no excess of cardiac events, even in patients who had an abnormal electrocardiogram when they entered the study. The MRC trial in elderly adults (18) showed a significantly lower risk of cardiovascular events with the diuretic compared with the beta-blocker, raising the possibility that diuretics confer benefit through a mechanism other than the reduction of blood pressure.

In the MAPHY study (21), total mortality was significantly lower for metoprolol than for thiazide, because of fewer deaths from coronary heart disease and stroke. However, the MAPHY study population comprised a subgroup of about half of the patients from the HAPPHY trial followed for an extended period. The difference in mortality between metoprolol and diuretics did not emerge during this extended follow-up, but was present during the first period of observation (that is during the HAPPHY trial), when there was no overall difference between beta-blockers and thiazides. Therefore, patients treated with atenolol in the HAPPHY trial must have fared worse than those treated with thiazides and much worse than those treated with metoprolol. Since there was no prior hypothesis for a difference between atenolol and metoprolol (and no plausible explanation for it), it seems reasonable to conclude that the apparent advantage of metoprolol was a chance finding produced by post-hoc subgroup analysis. The MAPHY study should be interpreted with extreme caution.

A review of the large trials has shown that the reduction in the incidence of events with usual thiazide-based treatment is 16% (95% CI = 8, 23%) against the prediction from epidemiological studies of 20–25% (22). This shortfall in benefit could easily be due to chance.

In the Antihypertensive and Lipid-Lowering Treatment to Prevent Heart Attack Trial (ALLHAT), over 40 000 participants aged 55 years or older with hypertension and at least one other risk factor for coronary heart disease were randomized to chlortalidone, amlodipine, doxazosin, or lisinopril (23,24). Doxazosin was discontinued prematurely because chlortalidone was clearly superior in preventing cardiovascular events, particularly heart failure (24). Otherwise, mean follow-up was 4.9 years. There were no differences between chlortalidone, amlodipine, and lisinopril in the primary combined outcome or all-cause mortality. Compared with chlortalidone heart failure was more common with amlodipine and lisinopril, and chlortalidone was better than lisinopril at preventing stroke. The authors concluded that diuretics are superior to other antihypertensive drugs in preventing one or more major form of cardiovascular disease and are less expensive. They should therefore be used as the preferred first-step treatment of hypertension. Although the design, conduct, and analyses of ALLHAT can be criticized (25), it was a huge, prospective, randomized study and its results suggest that diuretic-based therapy is unsurpassed in the management of hypertension.

Adverse effects

The frequencies and the profile of adverse effects of five major classes of antihypertensive agents have been assessed in an unselected group of 2586 chronically drug-treated hypertensive patients (26). This was accompanied by a questionnaire-based survey among patients attending a general practitioner. The percentages of patients who reported adverse effects spontaneously, on general inquiry, and on specific questioning were 16, 24, and 62% respectively. The percentage of patients in whom discontinuation was due to adverse effects with diuretics was 2.8%. The authors did not find a significant effect of age on the pattern of adverse effects. Women reported more effects and effects that were less related to the pharmacological treatment.

Heart failure

Loop and thiazide diuretics

Loop and thiazide diuretics have been the mainstay of treatment for symptomatic heart failure (27), relieving symptoms and improving cardiovascular hemodynamics. However, despite their widespread use, they have not been shown to improve survival in patients with heart failure. As it is not feasible to conduct such a trial in patients with pulmonary edema due to heart failure, the place of diuretic therapy in the management of heart failure appears secure.

Aldosterone receptor antagonists

Although they are widely used in the management of heart failure, loop and thiazide diuretics have not been shown to prolong survival. However, spironolactone and eplerenone must be added to the list of medications that offer improved survival for patients with heart failure.

In the Randomized Aldactone Evaluation Study (RALES) in 1663 patients with New York Heart Association (NYHA) class III (70%) or IV (30%) symptoms and an ejection fraction less than 35%, the addition of spironolactone 25 mg/day to conventional treatment (an ACE inhibitor, a loop diuretic, in most cases digoxin, and in 11% a beta-blocker) for an average of 24 months lowered the risk of all-cause mortality by 30% (from 46% to 35%), death from progressive heart failure, and sudden death (28). There were similar reductions in hospital admissions for worsening heart failure and for all cardiac causes. The magnitude of the overall effect was similar and additional to the proven benefit from ACE inhibition in severe heart failure.

In the Eplerenone Post-Acute Myocardial Infarction Heart Failure Efficacy and Survival Study (EPHESUS), in 6632 patients with an acute myocardial infarction complicated by left ventricular dysfunction and heart failure, the addition of eplerenone 25–50 mg/day to optimal medical therapy significantly reduced all-cause mortality by 15% and cardiovascular mortality by 17% over a mean follow-up period of 16 months; hospitalization rates were also reduced (29).

Mechanisms

Several mechanisms have been postulated to underlie the benefits of aldosterone receptor antagonists in heart failure (30). Aldosterone-induced cardiac fibrosis may reduce systolic function, impair diastolic function, and promote intracardiac conduction defects, with the potential for serious dysrhythmias. Aldosterone may also increase vulnerability to serious dysrhythmias by other mechanisms. The diuretic and hemodynamic effects of spironolactone in RALES and EPHESUS were subtle, and there were no significant changes in body weight, sodium retention, or systemic blood pressure.

Clinical use

The safe and effective dose of spironolactone remains uncertain (30). Pilot data from RALES showed that the frequency of hyperkalemia and uremia increased with doses of spironolactone above 50 mg/day (SEDA-20, 202). Doses up to 50 mg/day are appropriate, with adequate monitoring of serum electrolytes and renal function. The optimum strategy in the face of hyperkalemia, uremia, or symptomatic hypotension (reduction in frequency of spironolactone to alternate-day dosing, reduction in dose of ACE inhibitor, and/or increased dose of loop diuretics) is unclear, and how frequent such dose adjustments were necessary in RALES was not stated (28).

Adverse effects

The only frequent adverse effects were gynecomastia, breast pain, or both in 10% of men. The rate of discontinuation because of these events was 2%. The risk of gynecomastia should not be an argument against the use of spironolactone in men with severe heart failure, since it reduces both morbidity and death.

At the dose of spironolactone used in RALES (28), there was serious hyperkalemia, defined as a serum potassium concentration over 6.0 mmol/l, in 2% (compared with 1% of controls) and uremia was rare. However, a serum potassium concentration over 5 mmol/l and a serum creatinine concentration over 220 μmol/l were exclusion criteria. Although 29% of patients in the spironolactone group used potassium supplements, the benefit of spironolactone in these patients was similar to that in patients who did not.

In EPHESUS, as in RALES, the exclusion criteria included a serum potassium concentration over 5 mmol/l and a serum creatinine concentration over 220 μmol/l. There was serious hyperkalemia (a serum potassium concentration of 6.0 mmol/l or over) in 5.5% of those who took eplerenone and in 3.9% of those who took placebo. In each treatment group the incidence of hyperkalemia was higher among patients with the lowest baseline creatinine clearances.

The use of diuretics in patients with renal insufficiency

About 84% of the patients in the Reduction of Endpoints in NIDDM with the Angiotensin II Antagonist Losartan Study (RENAAL) required diuretic therapy to effect blood pressure control (31). Although not specifically reported, a similarly high proportion of patients were likely to have required diuretic therapy to reach the target blood pressure in the Irbesartan Diabetic Nephropathy Trial (IDNT) (32). These studies remind us once again of the importance of targeting volume control in order to reduce blood pressure in patients with chronic renal insufficiency.

In a cohort study of 552 patients with acute renal insufficiency studied from 1989 to 1995 diuretic use was associated with a significant increase in the risk of death or non-recovery of renal function (33). This increased risk was largely borne by patients who were relatively unresponsive to diuretics. Although this study was observational, which prohibits causal inference, it is unlikely that diuretics afford any material benefit in the setting of acute renal insufficiency.

Thiazide and loop diuretics

Various factors influence the choice of a diuretic in patients with renal insufficiency. First, it is widely believed that thiazide diuretics are ineffective once renal function falls below a creatinine clearance of 40–50 ml/minute. Diuretics need to enter the renal tubule to reach their luminal sites of action. In renal insufficiency, higher diuretic doses are required to overcome disease-related impediments to drug delivery to their sites of action. In the case of the loop diuretics the common practice is to titrate the dose of the diuretic until the desired response occurs (34). No such titration generally occurs with thiazide-type diuretics; consequently they are likely to fail, although for no reason other than their not being titrated to a truly effective dose. The true basis for "failure" of thiazide-type diuretics in patients with renal insufficiency resides in the fact that these diuretics are not of sufficient maximal efficacy to produce adequate volume control in these typically volume-expanded patients (35).

However, resistance to loop diuretics can occur by various mechanisms (36). These include poor adherence to therapy, poor absorption, progressive worsening of heart failure, excess volume loss, renal insufficiency, secondary hyperaldosteronism, and hypertrophy of the tubular cells of the distal nephron. Resistance due to inadequate drug absorption—either its speed or extent—is common with furosemide, which is poorly absorbed (34). Once recognized, this hurdle to response can be overcome by using loop diuretics that are predictably well absorbed, such as bumetanide and torasemide or by giving intravenous furosemide (37).

If loop diuretics fail to produce the desired diuretic response, combination diuretic therapy can be considered by adding a thiazide or a thiazide-like diuretic, such as metolazone. Such combinations are generally quite successful in both advanced congestive heart failure and late-stage chronic renal insufficiency, although excessive diuresis is a constant risk with such combinations. An excess diuresis with combination loop plus thiazide diuretic therapy is best managed by temporarily withdrawing both diuretics. Generally, diuretic doses are reduced when therapy is resumed (38).

An alternative in the diuretic-resistant patient is the use of continuous infusions of loop diuretics rather than bolus diuretic therapy. Such infusions can also be given with a small volume of hypertonic saline, with good effect (39). The reasons why continuous infusions of loop diuretics work when bolus doses have failed may relate to a more efficient time-course of diuretic delivery and/or less activation of the renin–angiotensin system (40). Furosemide and torasemide may be the safest loop diuretics to be given as infusions, in that infusion of bumetanide has been associated with severe musculoskeletal symptoms (41).

The importance of volume control in patients with renal insufficiency extends beyond its effect on blood pressure. Accordingly, the addition of hydrochlorothiazide can overcome the blunting by a high sodium intake of the therapeutic efficacy of ACE inhibition on proteinuria (42). This presumably relates to volume-related activation of the renin–angiotensin system.

Finally, loop diuretics reduce the metabolic demand of tubular cells, reducing oxygen requirements and thereby, in theory, increasing resistance to ischemic insults and perhaps other toxic circumstances. This property has been advanced as the basis for using diuretics in acute renal insufficiency. Although an attractive hypothesis to date, there is no compelling evidence to suggest any benefit from loop diuretics in established acute renal insufficiency. Alternatively, loop diuretics can convert oliguric to non-oliguric acute renal insufficiency, thereby easing the fluid restriction that would otherwise be necessary in such patients (43).

Aldosterone receptor antagonists

It is no longer appropriate to consider the endocrine or paracrine properties of aldosterone as being restricted to the classical target cells. Hemodynamic and humoral actions of aldosterone have important clinical implications for the pathogenesis of progressive renal disease, and may therefore affect future antihypertensive strategies. Initially, one might anticipate that the adverse effects of aldosterone could be attenuated merely by blocking aldosterone release with either an ACE inhibitor or angiotensin-II receptor antagonists. However, this appears not to be the case. Several investigators have now shown that ACE inhibitors acutely reduce aldosterone concentrations, but that with continued use this suppression fades. Thus, the presumption that ACE inhibitors would suppress the production of both aldosterone and angiotensin-II was incorrect. So, although ACE inhibitors and angiotensin-II receptor antagonists are individually very effective in retarding disease progression, additional benefit may be realized with a concurrent aldosterone receptor antagonist. As observed in clinical studies of congestive heart failure, as well as in animals with renal disease, antagonism of aldosterone receptors protects against end-organ damage through a combination of both hemodynamic and direct cellular actions (44).

An important consideration regarding the feasibility of aldosterone receptor antagonist therapy in chronic renal insufficiency is the risk of provoking hyperkalemia. Many patients with chronic renal insufficiency are already taking an ACE inhibitor or an angiotensin-II receptor antagonist, with the attendant risk of hyperkalemia. Despite such concerns, the results of the RALES and EPHESUS trials have been reassuring (28). In those studies, patients taking an ACE inhibitor who were randomized to spironolactone or eplerenone 25–50 mg/day had only small increases in potassium concentrations. Although the differences between those who took aldosterone receptor antagonists and those who took placebo were statistically significant, the mean increases were not clinically important, and serious hyperkalemia was uncommon. However, in clinical practice the risk of hyperkalemia may be greater (45), and close laboratory monitoring and judicious use of these drugs is necessary to minimize the risk.

Although it is an effective aldosterone receptor antagonist, spironolactone is limited by its tendency to cause undesirable sexual adverse effects. At standard doses, impotence and gynecomastia can occur in men, and premenopausal women can have menstrual disturbances. These adverse effects, caused by the binding of spironolactone to progesterone and androgen receptors, are substantial causes of drug withdrawal. In the RALES study there was a 10% incidence of gynecomastia or breast pain in men, compared with 1% with placebo, and significantly more patients discontinued treatment (2 versus 0.2%).

Although troublesome, these adverse effects are reversible and dose-related. The advent of selective aldosterone receptor antagonists, such as eplerenone, should reduce these adverse effects and thereby improve patient compliance. In EPHESUS there was no increase in the incidence of gynecomastia, breast pain, or impotence in men or menstrual irregularities in women who took eplerenone.

Organs and Systems

Cardiovascular

Cardiac dysrhythmias

Changes in potassium metabolism supposedly cause electrical instability in the heart, cardiac dysrhythmias, and increased mortality; replacement of potassium has been said to eliminate the risk of dysrhythmias (46–48). Mild hypokalemia might be expected to cause dysrhythmias in patients with serious organic heart disease (cardiomegaly, an abnormal electrocardiogram, frequent ventricular extra beats before treatment). However, the evidence suggests that hypokalemia after myocardial infarction is not the cause of dysrhythmias, but that both are the result of excess catecholamines. Furthermore, although hypertensive patients with left ventricular hypertrophy have an increased frequency of ventricular dysrhythmias, extra beats do not increase in frequency during diuretic treatment, even in the face of profound hypokalemia (49).

Early evidence linking thiazide-induced hypokalemia with dysrhythmias and sudden death was indirect and tenuous at best (50,51). One study suggested that diuretics are not responsible for the relation between hypokalemia and ventricular fibrillation in acute myocardial infarction (50). Chronic preoperative hypokalemia due to diuretics was not a risk factor for intraoperative dysrhythmias (52). Two large studies using 24-hour electrocardiographic monitoring failed to show a relation between diuretic-induced hypokalemia and ventricular dysrhythmias (53,54).

However, a retrospective analysis of 6797 patients with ejection fractions below 0.36 enrolled in the Studies Of Left Ventricular Dysfunction (SOLVD) was conducted to assess the relation between diuretic use at baseline and the subsequent risk of dysrhythmic death (54). Patients who were taking a diuretic at baseline ($n = 2901$) were significantly more likely to have such an event than those not taking a diuretic ($n = 2896$): 3.1 versus 1.7 per 1000 person-years. On univariate analysis and after controlling for important co-variates, the relation remained significant (relative risks 1.85 and 1.37 respectively). However, the association was seen only with non-potassium-sparing diuretics ($n = 2495$; relative risk 1.33); for potassium-sparing diuretics, alone or in combination with a non-potassium-sparing diuretic ($n = 406$), the relative risk was 0.90.

These data suggest that diuretic-induced potassium disturbances can cause fatal dysrhythmias in patients with left ventricular systolic dysfunction. SOLVD were not randomized trials of the risk of dysrhythmic death caused by diuretics. On average, patients retaking diuretics not only had lower serum potassium concentrations, but were also older, had more severe heart failure and were more likely to be taking antidysrhythmic drugs at baseline, although they had fewer indicators of ischemic heart disease. Even controlling for bias in multivariate analysis does not exclude the influence of unrecognized confounders. It is unknown whether diuretics were continued or changed during the 3 years of the trial. Thus, it remains uncertain that diuretic therapy is related to a risk of sudden dysrhythmic death in patients with heart failure.

Diuretic-induced hypokalemia is undoubtedly associated with a risk of serious ventricular dysrhythmias if diuretics are co-administered with drugs that prolong the QT interval (SED-13, 563). Diuretics increase the risk of torsade de pointes during antidysrhythmic drug therapy, independent of serum potassium concentration (54). The list of cardiac and non-cardiac drugs that prolong the QT interval continues to lengthen (54). It includes various antidysrhythmic drugs, including ibutilide, almokalant, and dofetilide; antimicrobial drugs, including clarithromycin, clindamycin, co-trimoxazole, pentamidine, imidazoles (such as ketoconazole), some fluoroquinolones, and antimalarial drugs (quinine, halofantrine); histamine H_1 receptor antagonists (terfenadine and astemizole); the antidepressant zimeldine; antipsychotic drugs (pimozide and sertindole); tricyclic/tetracyclic antidepressants; and cisapride. Particular care should be taken to avoid diuretic-induced hypokalemia when any of these agents is co-prescribed.

Coronary heart disease

There is no valid evidence that diuretics contribute to myocardial infarction, sudden death, or a failure of antihypertensive treatment or other risk factor interventions to prevent coronary deaths (50). An association between diuretics and sudden death has been suggested only in selected subset analyses, which allow no valid conclusions. Even in subjects with electrocardiographic abnormalities before treatment, there is no sound or consistent evidence to support the suggestion that diuretics predispose to sudden death.

Two retrospective case-control studies have reported an increased risk of cardiac arrest in hypertensive patients treated with thiazide-type diuretics (55,56). The risk was less among those treated with low-dose thiazides (equivalent to hydrochlorothiazide 25 mg/day) or with thiazides plus potassium-sparing drugs. The case-control design lacks one of the major advantages of randomized clinical trials, a tendency to equalize unknown, but important, differences between the comparison groups. Underadjustment is usual in case-control studies; for example, patients with more severe hypertension were more likely to have been treated with higher doses and less likely to have received potassium-sparing drugs because of renal dysfunction. Failure to randomize treatment tends to exaggerate differences between groups. Data from the prospective observational Gothenburg study suggested that metabolic changes during long-term treatment with antihypertensive drugs (predominantly beta-blockers and thiazides) are not associated with increased risk of coronary heart disease (57).

Metabolism

Despite their safety record, speculation persists that the metabolic effects of long-term diuretic treatment predispose to myocardial infarction or sudden death, and that diuretic treatment may therefore be hazardous. It is worth noting that much of this speculation is found outside the columns of the legitimate medical press (SEDA-10, 185). The supposed risks of diuretics are broadcast in countless symposium proceedings, monographs, and such like, sponsored by pharmaceutical companies with a vested interest in diverting prescriptions from diuretics to other drugs. Needless to say, these publications do not present a balanced view. Studies of dubious quality are published repeatedly without ever appearing in refereed journals, and eventually come to be cited in independent reviews and articles. There can be no doubt that these publications have a large impact on prescribing practices.

It is relatively easy to foster these concerns, particularly since antihypertensive therapy would be expected to prevent myocardial infarction and sudden death, but in selected studies does not appear to do so. To explain this, it is suggested that the beneficial effects of lowering blood pressure are offset in part by adverse effects related to thiazide-induced biochemical disturbances. Hypokalemia and hypomagnesemia might, for example, be dysrhythmogenic and cause sudden death; or hyperlipidemia and impaired glucose tolerance might be atherogenic and promote myocardial infarction. Some authors have suggested that thiazides should certainly be avoided in left ventricular hypertrophy and coronary heart disease, because of an increased risk of ventricular extra beats (58,59), and that diuretics are not appropriate options in those who already have hyperglycemia, hyperuricemia, or hyperlipidemia (60). The argument has been taken ad absurdum by a suggestion that the use of diuretics as first-line treatment of hypertension is illogical (27). Others have argued effectively that we should not be impressed by such speculations and that treatment should be based on long-term experience (61), a conclusion similar to that reached in volumes of SEDA, from SEDA-9 to SEDA-19.

Impaired glucose tolerance and insulin resistance

There is little doubt that high dosages of diuretics carry an appreciable risk of impairing diabetic control in patients with established diabetes mellitus. However, their role in causing de novo glucose intolerance is not clear (63). Long-acting diuretics are more likely to alter glucose metabolism. Impaired glucose tolerance is a relatively rare complication with loop diuretics, although isolated cases of non-ketotic hyperglycemia in diabetics have been described (SED-9, 350).

The effects of thiazide-type diuretics on carbohydrate tolerance cannot be ignored (50). There is a definite relation between diuretic treatment, impaired glucose tolerance, and biochemical diabetes, and a possible relation with insulin resistance (64). It is well established that the effect of thiazides on blood glucose is dose-related, probably linearly, while the antihypertensive effect has little relation to dose (65–67). There is relatively little information on the time-course; numerous short-term studies have shown that the blood glucose concentration increases in 4–8 weeks (68). The evidence that current low dosages impair glucose tolerance in the long term is not entirely consistent, perhaps because of differences between studies in dosages, diuretics used, durations of treatment, and types of patient (68,69). In SHEP, low-dosage chlortalidone in elderly patients for 3 years resulted in a non-significant excess of diabetes (8.6 versus 7.5%) compared with placebo (70). The apparent differences between diuretics may be due to comparisons of dosages that are not equivalent (71). Important differences between individual diuretics will be established only when their complete dose–response relations for metabolic variables and blood pressure have been defined (68).

In contrast to the wealth of evidence on impaired glucose tolerance in diabetics, sound clinical trials of the effect on insulin resistance are difficult to find, considering the amount of comment and speculation on the topic (SEDA-15, 216). It is not known whether insulin resistance is completely or even partly responsible for the changes in glucose tolerance that occur during long-term thiazide treatment; impaired insulin secretion may also have a role (72). Hypokalemia or potassium depletion may contribute to impaired glucose tolerance, by inhibiting insulin secretion rather than by causing insulin resistance, but is not the only or even the main cause of impaired glucose tolerance during long-term diuretic treatment (68,69). The routine use of potassium-sparing diuretics with relatively low dosages of thiazides does not prevent impaired glucose tolerance.

Diuretics worsen metabolic control in established diabetes, but it is not known whether this adversely affects prognosis (68). Disturbances of carbohydrate homeostasis have been detected by detailed biochemical testing, but their clinical importance is uncertain (64). The major clinical trials have not shown a major risk of diabetes mellitus. The incidence of diabetes mellitus in diuretic-treated subjects is only about 1%, even when large dosages are used (73). In ALLHAT, among patients classified as non-diabetic at baseline, the incidence of diabetes after more than 4 years was 12% with chlortalidone compared with 9.8% (amlodipine) and 8.1% (lisinopril). Despite these trends, there was no excess of cardiovascular events or mortality from chlortalidone in the entire population or among patients with diabetes. Although these data are reassuring, observational data suggest that diuretic-induced new-onset diabetes carries an increased risk of cardiovascular morbidity and mortality, but that this may take 10–15 years to become fully apparent (74).

Since changes in glucose balance after diuretics tend to be reversible on withdrawal, measures of carbohydrate homeostasis should be assessed after several months of thiazide treatment to detect those few patients who experience significant glucose intolerance (75). With this approach, the small risk of diabetes mellitus secondary to diuretic therapy can be minimized.

Hyperuricemia

Most diuretics cause hyperuricemia. Increased reabsorption of uric acid (along with other solutes) in the proximal tubule as a consequence of volume depletion is one reason; however, diuretics also compete with uric acid for excretory transport mechanisms. There is a small increased risk of acute gout in susceptible subjects (73). In the large outcome trials, about 3–5% of subjects treated with diuretics for hypertension developed clinical gout

(76). In those with acute gout during diuretic treatment, attacks were more strongly related to loop diuretics than to thiazides (77). Gout was significantly associated with obesity and a high alcohol intake in the subgroup taking only a thiazide diuretic. About 40% of cases of acute gout may have been prevented by avoiding thiazides in those 20% of men who weighed over 90 kg and/or who consumed more than 56 units of alcohol per week.

Well-conducted studies have shown that diuretic-induced changes in serum uric acid are dose-related (66,78). In low-dosage regimens, as currently recommended, alterations are minor, and other than the risk of gout the long-term consequences of an increased serum uric acid are unknown.

The issues of whether hyperuricemia is an independent risk factor for cardiovascular disease and the clinical relevance of the rise in serum uric acid caused by diuretic treatment are controversial (SED-14, 660) (50). In the Systolic Hypertension in the Elderly Program (SHEP), diuretic-based treatment in 4327 men and women, aged 60 years or more, with isolated systolic hypertension was associated with significant reduction in cardiovascular events (SED-14, 657). Serum uric acid independently predicted cardiovascular events in these patients (79). The benefit of active treatment was not affected by baseline serum uric acid. After randomization, however, an increase in serum uric acid of less than 0.06 mmol/l (median change) in the active treatment group was associated with a hazard ratio (HR) of 0.58 (CI = 0.37, 0.92) for coronary heart disease compared with those whose serum uric acid rose by 0.6 mmol/l or more. This was despite a slight but significantly greater reduction in both systolic and diastolic blood pressures in the latter. Those with serum uric acid increases of 0.6 mmol/l or more in the active group had a similar risk of coronary events as those in the placebo group.

This analysis of the SHEP database confirms the findings of a systematic worksite hypertension program (80). In 7978 treated patients with mild to moderate hypertension, cardiovascular disease was significantly associated with serum uric acid (HR = 1.22; CI = 1.11, 1.35), controlling for known cardiovascular risk factors. The cardioprotective effect of diuretics increased from 31% to 38% after adjustment for serum uric acid.

These observations suggest that persistent elevation of serum uric acid during diuretic-based antihypertensive therapy may detract from the benefit of blood pressure reduction. However, the relation between serum uric acid and cardiovascular disease was independent of the effects of diuretics. Furthermore, low-dose thiazide regimens have a smaller impact on serum uric acid (SED-14, 660).

Lipid metabolism

Reviews of the influence of diuretics on serum lipids (81–84) are in broad agreement as regards short-term effects. Thiazide and loop diuretics increase low-density lipoprotein (LDL) cholesterol, very-low-density lipoprotein (VLDL) cholesterol, total cholesterol, and triglycerides. The effect on high-density lipoprotein (HDL) cholesterol has been variable. The ratio of LDL/HDL or total cholesterol/HDL is generally increased, but not in all studies. Spironolactone 50 mg bd caused modest falls in HDL cholesterol and triglycerides (85). The effects of other potassium-sparing drugs on lipid metabolism have not been well documented. The possible mechanisms of these various short-term effects have been discussed (84).

Diuretic-induced effects on lipid metabolism are dose-related (66,67): at low dosages of thiazides, changes are very slight while antihypertensive efficacy is well maintained. Diuretic-induced lipid changes have not been prominent in studies lasting one year or longer (11,20,81,84,86). An association between thiazide use or antihypertensive treatment and changes in serum lipids has been shown in some population surveys (87,88) but not in others (89).

Most studies of the effects of diuretics on serum lipids have lacked a placebo control to allow identification of time-dependent or environmental changes, or have been confounded intentionally or unknowingly by life-style interventions, including weight loss, diet, and exercise (69). The argument that the effects of diuretics on lipids may limit the beneficial effect of blood pressure reduction is difficult to sustain (50). The effect of thiazides is largely transient, and in the long term total cholesterol and LDL cholesterol are raised only slightly and HDL cholesterol is unchanged. It is not known whether diuretic-induced changes in cholesterol carry the same prognostic significance as naturally occurring hyperlipidemia (50,90). Attempts to calculate a potential impact of diuretic-induced increases in total cholesterol and LDL cholesterol on coronary prognosis are premature. Observations have so far been limited largely to serum concentrations. However, binding of lipids to vascular cells, rather than in the bloodstream, is decisive for atherogenesis, and the effect at the cellular level remains to be investigated.

It has been suggested that even small changes in lipids might be clinically significant (91). However, the study was underpowered to show statistical significance of minor effects. Since under 50% of the patients in each group were followed for 1 year, selection bias may also have been introduced. It should be remembered that lipid changes are subsidiary to mortality. In this respect, diuretics are the best established of the antihypertensive drug classes.

There is little or no evidence that thiazides should be avoided in patients with hyperlipidemia (75), although some physicians continue to make this recommendation. Serum lipids should be checked within 3–6 months of starting thiazides to detect the very few patients who have an increase in total cholesterol or LDL cholesterol. This should not add to the cost of care, since serum chemistry need only be obtained once or twice a year and is no reason to avoid the use of these drugs as initial monotherapy.

Electrolyte balance

Potassium-wasting diuretics can cause sodium and potassium depletion with hyponatremia and hypokalemia. Potassium-retaining diuretics can cause hyperkalemia.

Hyponatremia

Treatment with thiazide diuretics is one of the most common causes of hyponatremia (92). Patients can present with variable hypovolemia or apparent euvolemia, depending on the magnitude of sodium loss and water retention.

Two major surveys have reviewed the features of diuretic-induced hyponatremia (93,94). Thiazide-like diuretics alone or in combination with potassium-sparing diuretics are responsible for more than 90% of cases. Hyponatremia occurs mainly in elderly women, although the relation with age probably merely reflects the widespread use of diuretics in older subjects. In most cases, the interval between starting thiazide and clinical presentation is less than 2 weeks; serum sodium may fall by 5 mmol/l or more in 24 hours or less in patients who develop severe hyponatremia. In contrast, when loop diuretics cause hyponatremia, the lag period is usually several months. Hypertension is the indication for diuretics in over 80% of cases. The patient is clinically euvolumic, but in the majority excess antidiuretic hormone (ADH) activity, hypokalemia, excess water intake, and increased free water clearance singly or together appear to contribute to the development of hyponatremia. The urine is inappropriately concentrated and contains moderately large amounts of sodium. The findings may be clinically indistinguishable from those of the syndrome of inappropriate ADH secretion. Severe neurological complications are seen in about 60%; seizures (30%), stupor or coma (30%), and death (5–10%). The extent of irreversible loss of intellectual function is unknown. Serum sodium concentration is usually in the range 105–120 mmol/l. If diuretics are withdrawn, the serum sodium concentration returns to normal, but hyponatremia is reproducible on rechallenge.

Comprehensive accounts of the pathophysiology, etiology, and management of hyponatremia have stressed the care required in correction of symptomatic hyponatremia (95). Neurological signs are an indication for active sodium replacement using hypertonic saline. Correction should be planned over 24–48 hours to increase serum sodium by 1 mmol/l each hour with a target increase of 20–25 mmol/l, a serum sodium concentration of 130 mmol/l or abolition of symptoms. If onset is within 24 hours of starting diuretics, correction should be rapid but within a total increase of 20 mmol/l in the first 24 hours. If the onset is over several days or longer, correction should be slower, aiming for 12–15 mmol/l in 24 hours. There is concern that rapid correction of hyponatremia and a relatively high total correction (more than 20 mmol/l in the first 24 hours) can be associated with higher morbidity or a demyelinating syndrome (94), but the rate of correction does not appear to be important to the outcome if the absolute increase is limited to 25 mmol/l over 48 hours (95). An extensive review of the literature suggested that rate of correction is not a factor in the genesis of hyponatremic brain syndrome (95).

The use of fixed combination of a thiazide and a potassium-sparing drug, often Moduretic (hydrochlorothiazide 50 mg with amiloride 5 mg), has been consistently implicated in diuretic-induced hyponatremia. Treatment with chlorpropamide (200–800 mg/day) along with Moduretic has precipitated hyponatremia in several cases (96). Simultaneous use of Moduretic with trimethoprim has also been reported to increase the risk (97). The mechanism appears to be impairment of the clearance of free water, resulting in dilutional hyponatremia. Whether data such as these point to a special risk of Moduretic as a product or merely reflect its extraordinarily widespread use in old people is not clear. In a survey of electrolyte disturbances in 1000 geriatric admissions, the incidence of hyponatremia with the combination of hydrochlorothiazide and amiloride was twice that with other diuretics, although the difference failed to reach statistical significance (98).

Management

There is no consensus about the optimal treatment of symptomatic hyponatremia. The authors of a comprehensive review recommended a targeted rate of correction that does not exceed 8 mmol/l on any day of treatment (92). Remaining within this target, the initial rate of correction can still be 1–2 mmol/l/hour for several hours in patients with severe symptoms (SED-13, 562). They suggested the following formulae for calculating the effect of giving 1 liter of infusate on serum sodium.

- Solutions containing sodium only:
  Change in serum sodium concentration (mmol/l) = (infusate Na^+ – serum Na^+)/(total body water + 1)
- Solutions containing sodium and potassium:
  Change in serum sodium concentration (mmol/l) = (infusate Na^+ + infusate K^+ – serum Na^+)/(total body water + 1)

Estimated total body water (in liters) is calculated as a function of body weight: 0.6 l/kg in children; 0.6 and 0.5 l/kg in non-elderly men and women respectively; 0.5 and 0.45 l/kg in elderly men and women respectively.

Loop diuretics can cause hypernatremia by increasing free water clearance (net water loss in the form of hypotonic fluid) (99). Over-rapid correction should be avoided.

Hypokalemia

The loss of potassium caused by diuretics is their most intensively debated adverse effect, and the extent and significance of the problem has long been disputed. The effect of diuretics on potassium balance and their clinical consequences have been reviewed extensively (50–52,65,100–102). The risks of diuretic-induced hypokalemia have been greatly exaggerated (50,65,102). A fall in plasma potassium is common, but sound studies have consistently showed that diuretics do not deplete body potassium or cause potassium deficiency during long-term therapy in hypertensive patients (50).

Susceptibility factors

In most patients, routine monitoring of serum potassium and routine administration of potassium-sparing diuretics is unnecessary (65,102), although patients at special risk require particular attention. Routine administration of potassium-sparing diuretics may have some justification in such patients. The following postulates seem to summarize the present position:

- When there is severe hypokalemia, it should not be attributed immediately to diuretic treatment. It may well be due to primary hyperaldosteronism, occult chronic liver disease, or abuse of licorice or laxatives.

- Relatively mild degrees of hypokalemia can be dangerous in patients taking cardiac glycosides, because their effects on the myocardium are potentiated in the absence of potassium (51).
- Diuretic-induced hypokalemia should also be avoided in patients taking drugs that prolong the QT interval, for example some antidysrhythmic drugs (quinidine, procainamide, disopyramide, encainide, sotalol, amiodarone), some psychotropic drugs (thioridazine, imipramine, phenothiazines), the lipid lowering drug probucol, the antibiotic erythromycin, and the 5-HT_2 receptor antagonist ketanserin.
- The risk of a clinically important degree of hypokalemia is increased in patients with liver cirrhosis and those with severe cardiac failure complicated by secondary hyperaldosteronism.
- In heart failure, depletion of potassium can provoke fatigue and lethargy and can cause ventricular dysrhythmias in the failing heart (102). Potassium depletion can occur in cardiac failure when neurohumoral systems are stimulated by diuretics and can be especially profound when skeletal muscle wasting is advanced (101). However, since heart failure itself, independent of diuretic treatment, is associated with loss of total body potassium, it is difficult to assess the independent contribution of diuretic treatment to this potassium deficit.

Critical reviews have concluded that in most patients (that is in the absence of the occasional risk factors listed above) diuretics can be prescribed alone, and that there is no need to take precautions against hypokalemia (63,103). Precautions, including the monitoring of serum potassium, have to be taken when there are risk factors or when symptoms (for example muscle pain) occur, or in patients who require aggressive treatment with both a thiazide and a loop diuretic; such a combination is indeed likely to provoke considerable falls in serum potassium, even to concentrations below 2.5 mmol/l (104). An observational study in 43 738 American men aged 40–75 years and without cardiovascular disease or diabetes showed that stroke was less likely in those with high potassium intake and that use of potassium supplements was related inversely to stroke in men taking diuretics (105). Diuretic-based treatment was associated with a significant mean reduction in serum potassium in SHEP (70). Although there were notable reductions in stroke in SHEP (14), potassium supplements were used if the serum potassium fell below 3.5 mmol/l. Therefore, avoidance of hypokalemia may be important in ensuring the cardiovascular benefits of thiazides in the management of hypertension.

Well-conducted studies (66,78) have underlined the fact that the dose–response curves for lowering blood pressure and lowering plasma potassium during diuretic treatment are dissociated. There is little if any loss of antihypertensive effect with low doses of diuretics, whereas hypokalemia is much less prominent. Although low dosages of diuretics are to be preferred in uncomplicated hypertension, very low dosages of thiazides may not be as effective as higher dosages (106).

Management

In patients in whom hypokalemia needs to be prevented or corrected, potassium-sparing diuretics should be preferred to potassium supplements, which are relatively ineffective, even in high dosages (SEDA-14, 180) (SEDA-15, 214).

The National Council on Potassium in Clinical Practice has provided guidelines on potassium replacement (107). In hypertensive patients with drug-induced hypokalemia, an effort should be made to achieve and maintain the serum potassium concentration at 4.0 mmol/l or over. Potassium replacement should be considered routinely in patients with congestive heart failure, even if the initial potassium determination is normal. Regular monitoring of serum potassium is essential in these patients, because of the risk of hyperkalemia in patients given potassium (or potassium-sparing diuretics) and ACE inhibitors or angiotensin receptor antagonists. Maintenance of optimal potassium concentrations (4.0 mmol/l or over) is critical in patients with cardiac dysrhythmias, and again routine potassium monitoring is obligatory.

Angiotensin-converting enzyme inhibitors are widely believed to attenuate diuretic-induced falls in plasma potassium. However, captopril 25 mg bd had no effect on plasma potassium in hypertensive patients treated with bendroflumethiazide 5 mg/day (108).

Hyperkalemia

All potassium-sparing diuretics can cause hyperkalemia. Several groups of patients are at particularly high risk of developing hyperkalemia if they take potassium-sparing diuretics (109). These include patients with moderate to severe chronic renal insufficiency, hypoaldosteronism, and diseases associated with impaired response to the potassium secretory effects of aldosterone. Hypoaldosteronism is often seen in elderly patients, those with chronic renal impairment or diabetic nephropathy, those with AIDS, or those with primary adrenal disease. In addition, patients with sickle cell disease, obstructive uropathy, systemic lupus erythematosus with nephropathy, and renal transplants may have tubular resistance to the effects of mineralocorticoids. Spironolactone 300 mg can significantly increase the serum potassium concentration in hemodialysis patients, suggesting that aldosterone may affect the cellular handling and gastrointestinal excretion of potassium. Commonly forgotten is the patient for whom these diuretics are prescribed as a precautionary measure and who for many years has been flavoring a low-salt diet with "salt substitutes," which are often based on potassium chloride (110).

Life-threatening hyperkalemia has been observed in patients receiving potassium-sparing diuretics (111). The most distressing finding in this study was that these agents were far more often prescribed in patients with abnormal kidney function than were other diuretics. Combining potassium-sparing diuretics with potassium supplements borders on malpractice; regular monitoring of serum potassium is mandatory in all patients treated with potassium-sparing diuretics, particularly if they are elderly or have abnormal renal or hepatic function.

Mineral balance

Thiazide and thiazide-like diuretics reduce the renal clearance of calcium by inhibiting the tubular secretion of calcium ions. In contrast, furosemide (which does not promote reabsorption of calcium in the distal tubule) causes transient hypercalciuria, an effect that has been exploited on occasion in the treatment of hypercalcemia (SED-9, 346) (112).

Metal metabolism

Diuretic-induced magnesium loss has been heavily stressed both by some independent investigators and by those seeking for commercial reasons to discredit the diuretics; there are far more reviews on the subject than sound original studies. It has been declared (113) that diuretic-induced magnesium deficiency "positively contributes" to myocardial infarction, delayed infarct healing, coronary and cerebral arterial spasm, hyperlipidemia, and cardiac dysrhythmias, with the addition of a horrific catalog of clinical manifestations, including ataxia, delirium, convulsions, coma, and ventricular fibrillation. Ramsay has remarked that this review, and others like it, belongs to the category of science fiction rather than that of serious medical writing (SEDA-10, 187).

Most reviews of the effects of diuretics on magnesium metabolism are uncritical and extrapolate wildly from the little sound evidence that is available (50). Several uncontrolled studies and very few controlled studies have suggested that long-term thiazide treatment causes a small fall in serum magnesium within the reference range. The complex relation between intracellular free and total magnesium content remains to be clarified, and there is absolutely no evidence that diuretic treatment reduces intracellular magnesium, and the few competent investigations have suggested that it does not. Diuretic-induced disturbances of magnesium balance do not cause depletion of intracellular potassium. The clinical significance of the small diuretic-induced alterations in magnesium balance, if any, is obscure. There is no satisfactory evidence that diuretic-induced magnesium disturbances cause or predispose to cardiac dysrhythmias, either in general or specifically after myocardial infarction (114).

A balanced account (115) concluded that the controlled trials, of which there are few, do not substantiate a role of diuretics in causing magnesium deficiency. Consequently, the vast majority of patients taking conventional doses of thiazides do not need magnesium supplements. On balance, potassium-sparing diuretics tend to increase serum and intracellular magnesium content, but this should not be taken as evidence of prior magnesium deficiency. It remains theoretically possible that large doses of loop diuretics given more than once-daily for long periods could induce negative magnesium balance and magnesium deficiency. However, it is difficult to conduct appropriately controlled trials in heart failure, in which such treatment is needed, and until more reliable information becomes available no absolute recommendation can be made. Magnesium depletion should be regarded as no more than a possible, as yet unproven, risk factor for cardiovascular morbidity and mortality (116).

In ordinary practice, serum magnesium need not be monitored in patients taking diuretics, and potassium-sparing drugs should not be used to prevent non-existent magnesium problems (SEDA-10, 190).

Gastrointestinal

Potassium, given separately or in combination with a diuretic, introduces the risk of esophageal injury; attempts to provide potassium in modified-release formulations have simply transposed the site of injury from the esophagus to the small bowel (SEDA-10, 187).

Urinary tract

Since diuretics act primarily on the kidney, it is hardly surprising that renal damage can occur including interstitial nephritis (117,118). However, toxic damage is very rare in relation to the number of patients treated. Renal damage due to interstitial nephritis is more likely to occur in patients with pre-existing glomerular disease. It tends to present 4–10 weeks after starting treatment, with non-oliguric acute renal insufficiency and in some cases pyrexia and eosinophilia. This complication probably always recovers spontaneously and completely, although some consider it prudent to give high doses of glucocorticoids.

Sexual function

The adverse effects of thiazide and thiazide-like diuretics on male sexual function include reduced libido, erectile dysfunction, and difficulty in ejaculating. The exact incidence of sexual dysfunction in patients taking diuretics is poorly documented, perhaps because of the personal nature of the problem and the reluctance of patients and/or physicians to discuss it. However, these abnormalities have been reported with incidence rates of 3–32%. The true incidence of sexual dysfunction probably lies closer to the lower end of this range (119). In a meta-analysis of 13 randomized, placebo-controlled trials conducted over a mean of 4 years the NNH (number needed to harm) for erectile impotence with thiazide diuretics in hypertension was 20 and the relative risk was 5.0 (120).

The mechanisms by which thiazides affect erectile dysfunction or libido are unclear, but it has been suggested that they have a direct effect on vascular smooth muscle cells or reduce the response to catecholamines. Sexual dysfunction does not appear to be mediated by either a low serum potassium concentration or a low blood pressure. Since sexual dysfunction can adversely affect the quality of life of hypertensive patients, physicians or health-care providers should take an accurate baseline sexual history and monitor sexual status for changes during therapy. If there are significant changes in sexual function, diuretic therapy can be withdrawn and an alternative drug class substituted. However, not uncommonly sexual dysfunction will persist despite withdrawal of the diuretic, suggesting that elements of the hypertensive state itself contribute to the process.

Analysis of the risk of erectile impotence has been hampered by the fact that impotence is common in men beyond middle age and is likely to be even more common in hypertension, treated or otherwise. The UK MRC trial (11) was the first to provide quantified evidence of a link with diuretics; in men taking bendroflumethiazide 10 mg/day, the withdrawal rate for impotence was 19.6 cases per 1000 treatment years, compared with 0.9 cases with placebo. However, these figures may exaggerate the effect, since the trial was single-blind. A questionnaire pointed to a less striking difference; after 3 months impotence was noted in 16% of diuretic-treated patients and 9% of those taking placebo, and the roughly 2:1 ratio was again noted after 2 years. Later studies (16,86,121–123), pointed to a similar effect, even when low-dosage regimens were used (16,86). Some studies (123) but not others (86) have suggested that weight reduction ameliorates diuretic-induced sexual dysfunction. Erectile dysfunction occurs early and is often tolerable; onset after 2 years is unlikely (86).

Erectile impotence is particularly common in men with diabetes (16), who are likely to have difficulties because of autonomic dysfunction. It is unclear whether younger men and women are similarly affected and whether normotensive men have fewer such problems (124). Most investigations of the effects of diuretics on sexual function have been characterized by poor study design (125); the majority had no placebo control and relied on comparisons with baseline. The best studies have suggested an increase in erectile dysfunction in thiazides users compared with placebo. Bearing in mind all the confounding factors, it can be concluded that diuretics will sometimes cause impotence, but that in the population as a whole the effect is slight compared with other causes (SEDA-11, 197) (SEDA-11, 198).

Sexual problems due to diuretics are very rare in women (16,86).

Long-Term Effects

Drug abuse

When diuretics are abused it is mostly in the course of a misguided attempt to lose weight; in the past, various "slimming remedies" offered for sale outside normal trading channels have been found to contain diuretics, sometimes with components such as thyroid extract. The unnecessary use of diuretics by a healthy individual, perhaps in excessive doses, can lead to dehydration, hypokalemia, and hypotension; when furosemide is abused, even tetany can occur because of hypocalcemia (126). The weight loss achieved by using diuretics in this way is purely due to dehydration and will soon be annulled by extra fluid intake.

One complication of long-term diuretic therapy in otherwise healthy individuals is edema, and it has been suggested that surreptitious use of diuretics can explain some otherwise paradoxical cases of idiopathic edema; presumably the diuretic induces a persistent increase in plasma renin activity and secondary hyperaldosteronism, and attempts to stop the diuretic intake can at first actually aggravate the condition (127). However, three studies have furnished strong evidence that diuretic abuse is not an important cause of idiopathic edema (128–130).

In some patients the covert use of diuretics leads to a complete replica of Bartter's syndrome, characterized by hypokalemia and hyper-reninemia without hypertension (131,132). In a patient who denies having taken diuretics, the true diagnosis may only be made by finding the drug or its metabolites in the urine, although challenge with diuretic may provoke the syndrome, while withdrawal leads to weight gain and the resolution of metabolic alkalosis.

The dangers of diuretic abuse among athletes have been discussed (SEDA-21, 228). Diuretics are used illegitimately by many athletes and amount for 6% of all drugs abused. They are taken by body builders to dehydrate the tissues, giving better definition to muscle shape, as well as to offset the fluid retaining effect of concomitant anabolic steroids and growth hormone, used to increase muscle mass. Diuretics are used in other sports to reduce weight, allowing competition in lower body weight classes, and to dilute the urine, reducing its specific gravity and making difficult the detection of other banned drugs. This practice is not only unethical but also hazardous.

Tumorigenicity

There is an association between diuretic use and renal cell carcinoma (133). Some of the studies that support this association can be dismissed, since the epidemiological data on which they were based were not suitably adjusted for confounding variables, including obesity, hypertension, age, and cigarette smoking. However, other case-control studies have shown a small risk of renal cell carcinoma in patients taking long-term diuretics after adjustment of the data for potentially confounding variables.

The carcinogenic mechanism of diuretics is not known, but could be related to a carcinogenic action of *N*-nitroso metabolic derivatives of thiazide and loop diuretics or structural changes in the transporting tubular epithelia, which provoke different stages of apoptosis. Rats and mice treated with diuretics have been reported to develop nephropathies and renal adenomas. Renal cell carcinoma arises in renal tubular cells, which are the principal site of action of diuretics. Contact over years or decades may have a low-grade carcinogenic effect. However, most prospective randomized trials provide too short a period of observation to assess the potential for carcinogenicity unequivocally. Furthermore, the findings may have been confounded by other risk factors for renal cell carcinoma. Adjustment for confounders greatly attenuated the risk (to non-significance) in one study, and in another the association with diuretic use disappeared completely. Therefore, the findings from these observational studies may have resulted from uncontrolled confounding by known or unrecognized risk factors.

The relation between diuretic therapy and the risk of malignancies has been examined in a review of pertinent publications between 1966 and 1998 (134). In nine case control studies (4185 cases), the odds ratio for renal cell carcinoma in patients treated with diuretics was 1.55 (95% CI = 1.42, 1.71) compared with non-users of diuretics. In three cohort studies of 1 226 229 patients (802 cases), patients taking diuretics had a more than twofold risk of renal cell carcinoma compared with patients not taking diuretics. Women had an odds ratio of 2.01 (CI = 1.56, 1.67) compared with 1.96 (CI = 1.34, 2.13) in men. Thus, the cumulative evidence suggests that long-term use of diuretics may be associated with renal cell carcinoma.

The findings linking diuretic therapy with renal cell carcinoma need careful scrutiny. The strength of evidence provided by observational studies is limited, and such studies have yielded contradictory and controversial results in the past. An accompanying editorial (135) pointed out that some of the studies reviewed appear to have been designed to evaluate predictors of renal cell carcinoma without an a priori hypothesis that diuretics might be implicated. Statistical significance (set at $P < 0.05$) may have emerged merely by chance if 20 risk factors were examined.

Another commentary (136) emphasized the potential bias of observational studies and also publication bias in meta-analysis. The contemporary relevance of the findings is further reduced, since many of the studies included patients taking very high doses of thiazides. It is difficult to disentangle a drug-related effect from the association between hypertension and renal cell carcinoma.

Since renal cell carcinoma is rare, the practical importance of these observations is small: one extra case of renal cell carcinoma in 1500 patients treated for 20 years. If the hypothesis is correct, antihypertensive therapy with diuretics will prevent 20–40 strokes, 3–28 heart attacks, 3–10 cardiovascular deaths, and 4–14 deaths overall for every extra case of renal cell carcinoma. Even middle-aged women would be spared six strokes for each potential case of renal cell carcinoma. If a low grade carcinogen is involved, most patients will not live long enough for its effect to be expressed. The available information does not support a change in current prescription practices for diuretics in the treatment of hypertension and cardiac failure. Physicians should be more concerned about controlling blood pressure rather than concerning themselves with what at best might be a small risk of renal cell carcinoma.

Other cancer types have been evaluated for their association with diuretic therapy. The development of colon cancer has been studied in 14 166 patients aged 45–74 years with a previous myocardial infarction and/or stable angina, screened for participation in the Bezafibrate Infarction Prevention Study (137). Of these, 2153 used diuretics and 12 013 did not. Multivariate analysis identified diuretics as an independent predictor of an increased incidence of colon cancer (hazard ratio 2.0) and colon cancer mortality (hazard ratio 3.7). However, the association between diuretic therapy and a higher incidence of colon cancer was observed only among non-users of aspirin. There was a relatively lower incidence of colon cancer in furosemide users and a higher incidence in the small combined subgroup of those who took amiloride and/or hydrochlorothiazide. Further studies to test the association between diuretics and colon cancer, as well as the potential protective effects of aspirin, are needed. Until these data become available, physicians should be aware of the potential effects of diuretics, especially when choosing long-term treatment for young patients with mild hypertension.

Second-Generation Effects

Pregnancy

Diuretics have been used for the treatment of both hypertension and edema in pregnancy. While regimens including thiazides have improved the outcome in hypertension developing during the first 20 weeks of pregnancy, the situation in later pregnancy seems to be different. Some controlled studies have shown that the thiazides do not influence the development of pre-eclampsia (138) and can even aggravate it.

Edema is a relatively frequent finding in normal pregnancy. It appears to be benign and can even be associated with improved obstetric performance (139). Edema, even in the presence of hypertension or proteinuria, is not a useful predictor of obstetric complications (140). These observations are important, in view of the finding that treatment with thiazide diuretics is associated with a reduced birth weight in normotensive pregnant subjects (141).

In a review of eight large-scale trials, four well-controlled studies did not show any benefit, whereas four others, which showed some benefit, were judged to be totally unsatisfactory, either because control was not strict enough or because inclusion and exclusion criteria were either not sufficiently well-defined or were scientifically unacceptable (142). The general consensus in earlier publications was that diuretics are useless, because they reduce the already lowered cardiac output in pre-eclamptic toxemia and so further reduce placental and uterine perfusion (143,144); diuretics do not alter the incidence of pre-eclamptic toxemia and eclampsia and they do not improve perinatal mortality or birth weight. Both the maternal adverse effects (hypokalemia, metabolic acidosis, hyperglycemia, hyperuricemia, hemorrhagic pancreatitis, and even death due to abuse) and the fetal and perinatal adverse effects (hyponatremia, fetal dysrhythmias induced by hypokalemia, thrombocytopenia, and jaundice) preclude the use of diuretics in pre-eclamptic toxemia.

Nine randomized, controlled studies of the use of diuretics in pre-eclampsia have been analysed (145). There were almost 7000 subjects in whom thiazides had been compared with placebo or no treatment. In the pooled analysis, diuretic treatment was associated with a non-significant reduction in perinatal mortality (about 10%) and stillbirths (about 33%). There was no excess of serious adverse reactions, either in the mothers or the neonates. These findings thus give no support to the belief that diuretics are harmful in pregnancy. It should not be concluded that diuretics ought to be used in pre-eclampsia in preference to other well-established agents, but they certainly can be used with confidence when they are really needed, for example in patients with severe hypertension that predates pregnancy and in heart failure.

Nevertheless, substantial numbers of pregnant women use these agents during pregnancy. In a Swedish study (146), 11% of 341 women took diuretics in the third trimester, while in a Tennessee Medical study (147) diuretics were prescribed as frequently as hypnotics and minor tranquilizers (7% for each category of drug). On the other hand, a study based on a University obstetrics programme in Florida (148) found that diuretics had been prescribed for only 2.4% of the patients.

Obviously treatment with any drug during pregnancy will affect both mother and fetus, and two aspects of such therapy are important: the adverse effects of the drug and the potential for teratogenicity.

Chlorothiazide readily crosses the placenta (149), but there have been few studies of the effects of diuretic treatment on the fetus. There are case reports of abnormalities of glucose handling (150) and severe electrolyte disturbances (151) in pregnant women taking diuretics, but these reports generally do not mention the metabolic values in the neonate. There has been one report of chronic fetal bradycardia associated with a low serum potassium in the diuretic-treated mother (152). Infusion of potassium restored maternal electrolytes and fetal heart rate. Normal delivery followed later, and electrolyte values in the child were normal. With regard to glucose handling, Senior and others (153) have raised the possibility that thiazide treatment of the mother can lead to neonatal hypoglycemia. In the absence of other predisposing factors, thiazides had been given to the mothers of 57% of their affected children, and, in the general population, the risk of neonatal hyperglycaemia was increased five-fold by thiazide treatment of the mother.

Hematological effects in the neonate have also been ascribed to maternal diuretic treatment. Seven cases of neonatal thrombocytopenia attributed to chlorothiazide have been described (154) and one case in which hydrochlorothiazide may have played a role (155). None of the mothers had thrombocytopenia. There was one death among the affected infants. Neonatal hemolysis occurred in two infants and was attributed to maternal thiazide therapy (156).

There is no evidence of a teratogenic effect of diuretics in humans, although one case of teratoma has been reported in the offspring of a woman treated for the first 19 weeks of pregnancy with acetazolamide (157), which is teratogenic in experimental animals. The lack of evidence of teratogenicity is not surprising. Assuming a basic malformation rate of 0.1% and that a drug that is used by 2% of pregnant women increases the malformation rate six times, it would require more than 100 000 women to be sure of detecting such an effect (146).

Susceptibility Factors

Age

There has been much discussion about the safety or risks of diuretics in elderly people. Although diuretic use has been implicated as a cause of urinary incontinence, no evidence has been presented to confirm this. An epidemiological survey of 1956 respondents aged at least 60 years showed no significant difference between diuretic-users and non-users in the prevalence of incontinence (158).

Orthostatic hypotension, although often loosely referred to in older literature (SED-10, 370) (159), is in fact only likely to become a problem in very old subjects, aged 90 years or more, even if a potent loop diuretic is used; this was the clear conclusion of a good prospective study published in 1978 (159). In 843 independent living men and women aged 60–87 years, postural fall in systolic blood pressure was not related to treatment with diuretics, after correction for initial blood pressure (160). At currently recommended doses, older subjects do not generally experience particular problems from hypokalemia and do not appear to be at special risk of cardiac dysrhythmias in the face of diuretic-induced hypokalemia (SEDA-15, 218).

Reviews of the age-related effects of diuretics in hypertensive subjects (161,162) have concluded that symptomatic adverse reactions are not more frequent in older patients and some trials have suggested a lower frequency than in younger subjects. Although the elderly may be susceptible to some metabolic effects of diuretics, the evidence for cardiotoxic potential is not conclusive.

The best overall evidence of the safety of diuretics in old people comes from the large-scale outcome trials in hypertensive patients (11,13,15,17,18). These studies in over 10 000 subjects aged over 60 years showed clearly that thiazide-based treatment reduces the risk of stroke, coronary heart disease events, and cardiovascular events in older hypertensive patients. A meta-analysis (163) of randomized trials lasting at least 1 year and involving 16 164 individuals aged at least 60 years showed that diuretics were superior to beta-blockers with regard to all endpoints (stroke, coronary heart disease events, cardiovascular mortality, and all-cause mortality). The beneficial effects noted in these trials should dispel any doubts about the safety and efficacy of diuretics in old people.

Drug Administration

Drug formulations

Fixed combinations of thiazides and loop diuretics with potassium and of thiazides with beta-blockers serve little useful purpose and can in fact do harm. Combinations of thiazides and loop diuretics with potassium-sparing diuretics serve the needs of the small minority of patients who develop clinically significant hypokalemia when given diuretics alone, or in whom hypokalemia is particularly risky. In fact, these combinations are much too widely used, and since individual needs vary so much there is a spectrum of risk, ranging from hypokalemia to hyperkalemia (SEDA-10, 370) (SEDA-10, 371).

Drug–Drug Interactions

Antidysrhythmic drugs

Hypokalemia due to diuretics potentiates the dysrhythmogenic actions of antidysrhythmic drugs that prolong the QT interval, such as Class I and Class III antidysrhythmic drugs, increasing the risk of torsade de pointes (164). This can also happen with other drugs that prolong the QT interval, such as phenothiazines (165).

Beta-blockers

Interaction of thiazides with beta-blockers can cause a greater risk of hyperglycemia than if either component is given separately (166,167).

Cardiac glycosides

Hypokalemia due to diuretics potentiates the actions of cardiac glycosides and can result in digitalis toxicity. In 67 patients taking a maintenance dose of digoxin, 42 with digoxin toxicity and 25 without, the mean serum digoxin concentration was significantly higher in the former and the mean serum potassium concentration was significantly lower (168). Among the patients with toxicity, 24% had hypokalemia due to diuretics. The mean serum digoxin concentration in those with hypokalemia and toxicity was significantly lower than in those with normokalemia and toxicity.

References

1. Cranston WI, Juel-Jensen BE, Semmence AM, Jones RP, Forbes JA, Mutch LM. Effects of oral diuretics on raised arterial pressure. Lancet 1963;186:966–70.
2. Grimm RH Jr, Grandits GA, Cutler JA, Stewart AL, McDonald RH, Svendsen K, Prineas RJ, Liebson PR. Relationships of quality-of-life measures to long-term lifestyle and drug treatment in the Treatment of Mild Hypertension Study. Arch Intern Med 1997;157(6):638–48.
3. Philipp T, Anlauf M, Distler A, Holzgreve H, Michaelis J, Wellek S. Randomised, double blind, multicentre comparison of hydrochlorothiazide, atenolol, nitrendipine, and enalapril in antihypertensive treatment: results of the HANE study. HANE Trial Research Group. BMJ 1997;315(7101):154–9.
4. Kaplan NM. Diuretics as a basis of antihypertensive therapy. An overview. Drugs 2000;59(Suppl 2):21–5.
5. Chobanian AV, Bakris GL, Black HR, Cushman WC, Green LA, Izzo JL J Jr, Jones DW, Materson BJ, Oparil S, Wright JT Jr, Roccella EJ, Joint National Committee on Prevention, Detection, Evaluation, and Treatment of High Blood Pressure. National Heart, Lung, and Blood Institute; National High Blood Pressure Education Program Coordinating Committee. Seventh report of the Joint National Committee on Prevention, Detection, Evaluation, and Treatment of High Blood Pressure. Hypertension 2003;42(6):1206–52.
6. Moser M. National recommendations for the pharmacological treatment of hypertension: should they be revised? Arch Intern Med 1999;159(13):1403–6.
7. Zanchetti A. Contribution of fixed low-dose combinations to initial therapy in hypertension. Eur Heart J 1999;1(Suppl L):L5–9.
8. Kaplan N. Low dose combinations in the treatment of hypertension: theory and practice. J Hum Hypertens 1999;13(10):707–10.
9. Gosse P, Sheridan DJ, Zannad F, Dubourg O, Gueret P, Karpov Y, de Leeuw PW, Palma-Gamiz JL, Pessina A, Motz W, Degaute JP, Chastang C. Regression of left ventricular hypertrophy in hypertensive patients treated with indapamide SR 1.5 mg versus enalapril 20 mg: the LIVE study. J Hypertens 2000;18(10):1465–75.
10. Wright JM, Lee CH, Chambers GK. Systematic review of antihypertensive therapies: does the evidence assist in choosing a first-line drug? CMAJ 1999;161(1):25–32.
11. Medical Research Council Working Party. MRC trial of treatment of mild hypertension: principal results. BMJ (Clin Res Ed) 1985;291(6488):97–104.
12. Medical Research Council Working Party on Mild Hypertension. Coronary heart disease in the Medical Research Council trial of treatment of mild hypertension. Br Heart J 1988;59(3):364–78.
13. Amery A, Birkenhager W, Brixko P, Bulpitt C, Clement D, Deruyttere M, De Schaepdryver A, Dollery C, Fagard R, Forette F, et al. Mortality and morbidity results from the European Working Party on High Blood Pressure in the Elderly trial. Lancet 1985;1(8442):1349–54.
14. SHEP Cooperative Research Group. Prevention of stroke by antihypertensive drug treatment in older persons with isolated systolic hypertension. Final results of the Systolic Hypertension in the Elderly Program (SHEP). JAMA 1991;265(24):3255–64.
15. Kostis JB, Davis BR, Cutler J, Grimm RH Jr, Berge KG, Cohen JD, Lacy CR, Perry HM Jr, Blaufox MD, Wassertheil-Smoller S, Black HR, Schron E, Berkson DM, Curb JD, Smith WM, McDonald R, Applegate WB. Prevention of heart failure by antihypertensive drug treatment in older persons with isolated systolic hypertension. SHEP Cooperative Research Group. JAMA 1997;278(3):212–6.
16. Curb JD, Pressel SL, Cutler JA, Savage PJ, Applegate WB, Black H, Camel G, Davis BR, Frost PH, Gonzalez N, Guthrie G, Oberman A, Rutan GH, Stamler J. Effect of diuretic-based antihypertensive treatment on cardiovascular disease risk in older diabetic patients with isolated systolic hypertension. Systolic Hypertension in the Elderly Program Cooperative Research Group. JAMA 1996;276(23):1886–92.
17. Dahlof B, Lindholm LH, Hansson L, Schersten B, Ekbom T, Wester PO. Morbidity and mortality in the Swedish Trial in Old Patients with Hypertension (STOP-Hypertension). Lancet 1991;338(8778):1281–5.
18. MRC Working Party. Medical Research Council trial of treatment of hypertension in older adults: principal results. BMJ 1992;304(6824):405–12.
19. The IPPPSH Collaborative Group. Cardiovascular risk and risk factors in a randomized trial of treatment based on the beta-blocker oxprenolol: the International Prospective Primary Prevention Study in Hypertension (IPPPSH). J Hypertens 1985;3(4):379–92.
20. Wilhelmsen L, Berglund G, Elmfeldt D, Fitzsimons T, Holzgreve H, Hosie J, Hornkvist PE, Pennert K, Tuomilehto J, Wedel H. Beta-blockers versus diuretics in hypertensive men: main results from the HAPPHY trial. J Hypertens 1987;5(5):561–72.
21. Wikstrand J, Warnold I, Olsson G, Tuomilehto J, Elmfeldt D, Berglund G. Primary prevention with metoprolol in patients with hypertension. Mortality results from the MAPHY study. JAMA 1988;259(13):1976–82.
22. Collins R, MacMahon S. Blood pressure, antihypertensive drug treatment and the risks of stroke and of coronary heart disease. Br Med Bull 1994;50(2):272–98.
23. ALLHAT Collaborative Research Group. Major cardiovascular events in hypertensive patients randomized to doxazosin vs chlorthalidone: the antihypertensive and lipid-lowering treatment to prevent heart attack trial (ALLHAT). JAMA 2000;283(15):1967–75.
24. ALLHAT Officers and Coordinators for the ALLHAT Collaborative Research Group. The Antihypertensive and Lipid-Lowering Treatment to Prevent Heart Attack Trial. Major outcomes in high-risk hypertensive patients randomized to angiotensin-converting enzyme inhibitor or calcium channel blocker vs diuretic: The Antihypertensive and Lipid-Lowering Treatment to Prevent Heart Attack Trial (ALLHAT). JAMA 2002;288(23):2981–97.
25. McInnes GT. Size isn't everything—ALLHAT in perspective. J Hypertens 2003;21(3):459–61.
26. Olsen H, Klemetsrud T, Stokke HP, Tretli S, Westheim A. Adverse drug reactions in current antihypertensive therapy: a general practice survey of 2586 patients in Norway. Blood Press 1999;8(2):94–101.
27. Kramer BK, Schweda F, Riegger GA. Diuretic treatment and diuretic resistance in heart failure. Am J Med 1999;106(1):90–6.
28. Pitt B, Zannad F, Remme WJ, Cody R, Castaigne A, Perez A, Palensky J, Wittes J. The effect of spironolactone on morbidity and mortality in patients with severe heart failure. Randomized Aldactone Evaluation Study Investigators. N Engl J Med 1999;341(10):709–17.
29. Pitt B, Remme W, Zannad F, Neaton J, Martinez F, Roniker B, Bittman R, Hurley S, Kleiman J, Gatlin M, Eplerenone Post-Acute Myocardial Infarction Heart Failure Efficacy and Survival Study Investigators. Eplerenone, a selective aldosterone blocker, in patients with left ventricular dysfunction after myocardial infarction. N Engl J Med 2003;348(14):1309–21.

30. Richards AM, Nicholls MG. Aldosterone antagonism in heart failure. Lancet 1999;354(9181):789–90.
31. Brenner BM, Cooper ME, de Zeeuw D, Keane WF, Mitch WE, Parving HH, Remuzzi G, Snapinn SM, Zhang Z, Shahinfar S, RENAAL Study Investigators. Effects of losartan on renal and cardiovascular outcomes in patients with type 2 diabetes and nephropathy. N Engl J Med 2001;345(12):861–9.
32. Lewis EJ, Hunsicker LG, Clarke WR, Berl T, Pohl MA, Lewis JB, Ritz E, Atkins RC, Rohde R, Raz I; Collaborative Study Group. Renoprotective effect of the angiotensin-receptor antagonist irbesartan in patients with nephropathy due to type 2 diabetes. N Engl J Med 2001;345(12):851–60.
33. Mehta RL, Pascual MT, Soroko S, Chertow GM; PICARD Study Group. Diuretics, mortality, and nonrecovery of renal function in acute renal failure. JAMA 2002;288(20):2547–53.
34. Brater DC. Diuretic therapy. N Engl J Med 1998;339(6):387–95.
35. Schwenger V, Zeier M, Ritz E. Antihypertensive therapy in renal patients—benefits and difficulties. Nephron 1999;83(3):202–13.
36. Grahame-Smith DG. The Lilly Prize Lecture. 1996 "Keep on taking the tablets": pharmacological adaptation during long-term drug therapy. Br J Clin Pharmacol 1997;44(3):227–38.
37. Knauf H, Mutschler E. Clinical pharmacokinetics and pharmacodynamics of torasemide. Clin Pharmacokinet 1998;34(1):1–24.
38. Sica DA, Gehr TW. Diuretic combinations in refractory oedema states: pharmacokinetic–pharmacodynamic relationships. Clin Pharmacokinet 1996;30(3):229–49.
39. Paterna S, Di Pasquale P, Parrinello G, Amato P, Cardinale A, Follone G, Giubilato A, Licata G. Effects of high-dose furosemide and small-volume hypertonic saline solution infusion in comparison with a high dose of furosemide as a bolus, in refractory congestive heart failure. Eur J Heart Fail 2000;2(3): 305–313.
40. Ravnan SL, Ravnan MC. Management of adult heart failure: bolus versus continuous infusion loop diuretics, a review of the literature. Hosp Pharm 2000;35:832–6.
41. Howard PA, Dunn MI. Severe musculoskeletal symptoms during continuous infusion of bumetanide. Chest 1997;111(2):359–64.
42. Buter H, Hemmelder MH, Navis G, de Jong PE, de Zeeuw D. The blunting of the antiproteinuric efficacy of ACE inhibition by high sodium intake can be restored by hydrochlorothiazide. Nephrol Dial Transplant 1998;13(7):1682–5.
43. Dishart MK, Kellum JA. An evaluation of pharmacological strategies for the prevention and treatment of acute renal failure. Drugs 2000;59(1):79–91.
44. Epstein M. Aldosterone as a mediator of progressive renal disease: pathogenetic and clinical implications. Am J Kidney Dis 2001;37(4):677–88.
45. Juurlink DN, Mamdani MM, Lee DS, Kopp A, Austin PC, Laupacis A, Redelmeier DA. Rates of hyperkalemia after publication of the Randomized Aldactone Evaluation Study. N Engl J Med 2004;351(6):543–51.
46. Andersson OK, Gudbrandsson T, Jamerson K. Metabolic adverse effects of thiazide diuretics: the importance of normokalaemia. J Intern Med Suppl 1991;735:89–96.
47. Dyckner T. Relation of cardiovascular disease to potassium and magnesium deficiencies. Am J Cardiol 1990;65(23):K44–6.
48. Schulman M, Narins RG. Hypokalemia and cardiovascular disease. Am J Cardiol 1990;65(10):E4–9.
49. Papademetriou V, Burris JF, Notargiacomo A, Fletcher RD, Freis ED. Thiazide therapy is not a cause of arrhythmia in patients with systemic hypertension. Arch Intern Med 1988;148(6):1272–6.
50. McInnes GT, Yeo WW, Ramsay LE, Moser M. Cardiotoxicity and diuretics: much speculation—little substance. J Hypertens 1992;10(4):317–35.
51. Papademetriou V. Diuretics in hypertension: clinical experiences. Eur Heart J 1992;13(Suppl G):92–5.
52. Restrick LJ, Huddy N, Hoffbrand BI. Diuretic-induced hypokalaemia and surgery: much ado about nothing? Postgrad Med J 1992;68(799):318–20.
53. Kostis JB, Lacy CR, Hall WD, Wilson AC, Borhani NO, Krieger SD, Cosgrove NM. The effect of chlorthalidone on ventricular ectopic activity in patients with isolated systolic hypertension. The SHEP Study Group. Am J Cardiol 1994;74(5):464–7.
54. Neaton JD, Grimm RH Jr, Prineas RJ, Stamler J, Grandits GA, Elmer PJ, Cutler JA, Flack JM, Schoenberger JA, McDonald R, Lewis CE, Liebson PR; Treatment of Mild Hypertension Study. Final results. Treatment of Mild Hypertension Study Research Group. JAMA 1993;270(6):713–24.
55. Cooper HA, Dries DL, Davis CE, Shen YL, Domanski MJ. Diuretics and risk of arrhythmic death in patients with left ventricular dysfunction. Circulation 1999;100(12):1311–5.
56. Viskin S. Long QT syndromes and torsade de pointes. Lancet 1999;354(9190):1625–33.
57. Yap YG, Camm J. Risk of torsades de pointes with non-cardiac drugs. Doctors need to be aware that many drugs can cause QT prolongation. BMJ 2000;320(7243):1158–9.
58. Hoes AW, Grobbee DE, Lubsen J, Man in't Veld AJ, van der Does E, Hofman A. Diuretics, beta-blockers, and the risk for sudden cardiac death in hypertensive patients. Ann Intern Med 1995;123(7):481–7.
59. Siscovick DS, Raghunathan TE, Psaty BM, Koepsell TD, Wicklund KG, Lin X, Cobb L, Rautaharju PM, Copass MK, Wagner EH. Diuretic therapy for hypertension and the risk of primary cardiac arrest. N Engl J Med 1994;330(26):1852–7.
60. Samuelsson O, Pennert K, Andersson O, Berglund G, Hedner T, Persson B, Wedel H, Wilhelmsen L. Diabetes mellitus and raised serum triglyceride concentration in treated hypertension—are they of prognostic importance? Observational study. BMJ 1996;313(7058):660–3.
61. Kaplan NM. How bad are diuretic-induced hypokalemia and hypercholesterolemia? Arch Intern Med 1989;149(12):2649.
62. Lipsitz LA. Hypertension in the elderly. Hosp Pract (Off Ed) 1989;24(4):119–26133, 137–8 passim.
63. Weinberger MH. Selection of drugs for initial treatment of hypertension. Pract Cardiol 1989;15:81.
64. Moser M. In defense of traditional antihypertensive therapy. Hypertension 1988;12(3):324–6.
65. Thompson WG. An assault on old friends: thiazide diuretics under siege. Am J Med Sci 1990;300(3):152–8.
66. Anonymous. Potassium-sparing diuretics—when are they really needed. Drug Ther Bull 1985;23(5):17–20.
67. Ramsay LE, Yeo WW, Jackson PR. Diabetes, impaired glucose tolerance and insulin resistance with diuretics. Eur Heart J 1992;13(Suppl G):68–71.
68. Saunders A, Wilson SM. Do diuretics differ in degree of hypokalaemia, and does it matter? Aust J Hosp Pharm 1991;21:120–1.
69. Carlsen JE, Kober L, Torp-Pedersen C, Johansen P. Relation between dose of bendrofluazide, antihypertensive effect, and adverse biochemical effects. BMJ 1990;300(6730):975–8.

70. McVeigh GE, Dulie EB, Ravenscroft A, Galloway DB, Johnston GD. Low and conventional dose cyclopenthiazide on glucose and lipid metabolism in mild hypertension. Br J Clin Pharmacol 1989;27(4):523–6.
71. Ramsay LE, Yeo WW, Jackson PR. Influence of diuretics, calcium antagonists, and alpha-blockers on insulin sensitivity and glucose tolerance in hypertensive patients. J Cardiovasc Pharmacol 1992;20(Suppl 11):S49–54.
72. Weinberger MH. Mechanisms of diuretic effects on carbohydrate tolerance, insulin sensitivity and lipid levels. Eur Heart J 1992;13(Suppl G):5–9.
73. Savage PJ, Pressel SL, Curb JD, Schron EB, Applegate WB, Black HR, Cohen J, Davis BR, Frost P, Smith W, Gonzalez N, Guthrie GP, Oberman A, Rutan G, Probstfield JL, Stamler J. Influence of long-term, low-dose, diuretic-based, antihypertensive therapy on glucose, lipid, uric acid, and potassium levels in older men and women with isolated systolic hypertension: The Systolic Hypertension in the Elderly Program. SHEP Cooperative Research Group. Arch Intern Med 1998;158(7):741–51.
74. Green TP, Johnson DE, Bass JL, Landrum BG, Ferrara TB, Thompson TR. Prophylactic furosemide in severe respiratory distress syndrome: blinded prospective study. J Pediatr 1988;112(4):605–12.
75. Johnston GD. Treatment of hypertension in older adults. BMJ 1992;304:639.
76. Moser M. Diuretics and cardiovascular risk factors. Eur Heart J 1992;13(Suppl G):72–80.
77. Verdecchia P, Reboldi G, Angeli F, Borgioni C, Gattobigio R, Filippucci L, Norgiolini S, Bracco C, Porcellati C. Adverse prognostic significance of new diabetes in treated hypertensive subjects. Hypertension 2004;43(5):963–9.
78. Moser M. Diuretics should continue to be recommended as initial therapy in the treatment of hypertension. In: Puschett JB, Greenberg A, editors. Diuretics IV: Chemistry, Pharmacology and Clinical Applications. Amsterdam: Elsevier, 1993:465–76.
79. Moser M. Do different hemodynamic effects of antihypertensive drugs translate into different safety profiles? Eur J Clin Pharmacol 1990;38(Suppl 2):S134–8.
80. Waller PC, Ramsay LE. Predicting acute gout in diuretic-treated hypertensive patients. J Hum Hypertens 1989;3(6):457–61.
81. McVeigh G, Galloway D, Johnston D. The case for low dose diuretics in hypertension: comparison of low and conventional doses of cyclopenthiazide. BMJ 1988;297(6641):95–8.
82. Franse LV, Pahor M, Di Bari M, Shorr RI, Wan JY, Somes GW, Applegate WB. Serum uric acid, diuretic treatment and risk of cardiovascular events in the Systolic Hypertension in the Elderly Program (SHEP). J Hypertens 2000;18(8):1149–54.
83. Alderman MH, Cohen H, Madhavan S, Kivlighn S. Serum uric acid and cardiovascular events in successfully treated hypertensive patients. Hypertension 1999;34(1):144–50.
84. Freis ED, Papademetriou V. How dangerous are diuretics? Drugs 1985;30(6):469–74.
85. Spence JD. Effects of antihypertensive drugs on atherogenic factors: possible importance of drug selection in prevention of atherosclerosis. J Cardiovasc Pharmacol 1985;7(Suppl 2):S121–5.
86. Weinberger MH. Antihypertensive therapy and lipids. Evidence, mechanisms, and implications. Arch Intern Med 1985;145(6):1102–5.
87. Weidmann P, Ferrier C, Saxenhofer H, Uehlinger DE, Trost BN. Serum lipoproteins during treatment with antihypertensive drugs. Drugs 1988;35(Suppl 6):118–34.
88. Falch DK, Schreiner A. The effect of spironolactone on lipid, glucose and uric acid levels in blood during long-term administration to hypertensives. Acta Med Scand 1983;213(1):27–30.
89. Grimm RH Jr, Grandits GA, Prineas RJ, McDonald RH, Lewis CE, Flack JM, Yunis C, Svendsen K, Liebson PR, Elmer PJ, Stamler J. Long-term effects on sexual function of five antihypertensive drugs and nutritional hygienic treatment in hypertensive men and women. Treatment of Mild Hypertension Study (TOMHS). Hypertension 1997;29(1 Pt 1):8–14.
90. MacMahon SW, Macdonald GJ, Blacket RB. Plasma lipoprotein levels in treated and untreated hypertensive men and women. The National Heart Foundation of Australia Risk Factor Prevalence Study. Arteriosclerosis 1985;5(4):391–6.
91. Wallace RB, Hunninghake DB, Chambless LE, Heiss G, Wahl P, Barrett-Connor E. A screening survey of dyslipoproteinemias associated with prescription drug use. The Lipid Research Clinics Program Prevalence Study. Circulation 1986;73(1 Pt 2):I70–9.
92. Tuomilehto J, Salonen JT, Nissinen A. Factors associated with changes in serum cholesterol during a community-based hypertension programme. Acta Med Scand 1985;217(3):243–52.
93. Weidmann P, de Courten M, Ferrari P. Effect of diuretics on the plasma lipid profile. Eur Heart J 1992;13(Suppl G):61–7.
94. Golomb BA, Criqui MH. Antihypertensives: much ado about lipids. Arch Intern Med 1999;159(6):535–7.
95. Adrogué HJ, Madias NE. Hyponatremia. N Engl J Med 2000;342(21):1581–9.
96. Fernandez P, Choi M. Thiazide-induced hyponatraemia. In: Puschett JB, Greenberg A, editors. Diuretics IV: Chemistry, Pharmacology and Clinical Applications. Amsterdam: Elsevier, 1993;199–209.
97. Sonnenblick M, Friedlander Y, Rosin AJ. Diuretic-induced severe hyponatremia. Review and analysis of 129 reported patients. Chest 1993;103(2):601–6.
98. Arieff AI. Management of hyponatraemia. BMJ 1993;307(6899):305–8.
99. Zalin AM, Hutchinson CE, Jong M, Matthews K. Hyponatraemia during treatment with chlorpropamide and Moduretic (amiloride plus hydrochlorothiazide). BMJ (Clin Res Ed) 1984;289(6446):659.
100. Hart TJ, Johnston LJ, Edmonds MW, Brownscombe L. Hyponatraemia secondary to thiazide–trimethoprim interaction. Can J Hosp Pharm 1989;42:243–6.
101. Byatt CM, Millard PH, Levin GE. Diuretics and electrolyte disturbances in 1000 consecutive geriatric admissions. J R Soc Med 1990;83(11):704–8.
102. Adrogue HJ, Madias NE. Hypernatremia. N Engl J Med 2000;342(20):1493–9.
103. Frohlich ED. Current issues in hypertension. Old questions with new answers and new questions. Med Clin North Am 1992;76(5):1043–56.
104. Nicholls MG. Interaction of diuretics and electrolytes in congestive heart failure. Am J Cardiol 1990;65(10):E17–21.
105. McInnes GT. Potassium and diuretics—when does it matter? Med Resource 1992;6:21–4.
106. Kassirer JP. Does the benefit of aggressive potassium replacement in diuretic-treated patients outweigh the risk? J Cardiovasc Pharmacol 1984;6(Suppl 3):S488–92.
107. Shintani S, Shiigai T, Tsukagoshi H. Marked hypokalemic rhabdomyolysis with myoglobinuria due to diuretic treatment. Eur Neurol 1991;31(6):396–8.
108. Ascherio A, Rimm EB, Hernan MA, Giovannucci EL, Kawachi I, Stampfer MJ, Willett WC. Intake of potassium, magnesium, calcium, and fiber and risk of stroke among US men. Circulation 1998;98(12):1198–204.

109. Harper R, Ennis CN, Sheridan B, Atkinson AB, Johnston GD, Bell PM. Effects of low dose versus conventional dose thiazide diuretic on insulin action in essential hypertension. BMJ 1994;309(6949):226–30.
110. Cohn JN, Kowey PR, Whelton PK, Prisant LM. New guidelines for potassium replacement in clinical practice: a contemporary review by the National Council on Potassium in Clinical Practice. Arch Intern Med 2000;160(16):2429–36.
111. Murdoch DL, Gillen GJ, Morton JJ, Leckie B, Murray GD, Davies DL, McInnes GT. Twice-daily low-dose captopril in diuretic-treated hypertensives. J Hum Hypertens 1989;3(1):29–33.
112. Perazella MA. Drug-induced hyperkalemia: old culprits and new offenders. Am J Med 2000;109(4):307–14.
113. McCaughan D. Hazards of non-prescription potassium supplements. Lancet 1984;1(8375):513–14.
114. Lawson DH, O'Connor PC, Jick H. Drug attributed alterations in potassium handling in congestive cardiac failure. Eur J Clin Pharmacol 1982;23(1):21–5.
115. Suki WN, Yium JJ, Von Minden M, Saller-Hebert C, Eknoyan G, Martinez-Maldonado M. Actue treatment of hypercalcemia with furosemide. N Engl J Med 1970;283(16):836–40.
116. Reyes AJ, Leary WP. Cardiovascular toxicity of diuretics related to magnesium depletion. Hum Toxicol 1984;3(5):351–71.
117. Gettes LS. Electrolyte abnormalities underlying lethal and ventricular arrhythmias. Circulation 1992;85(Suppl 1):I70–6.
118. Davies DL, Fraser R. Do diuretics cause magnesium deficiency? Br J Clin Pharmacol 1993;36(1):1–10.
119. Leary WP. Diuretics and increase in urinary magnesium excretion: possible clinical relevance. In: Puschett JB, Greenberg A, editors. Diuretics IV: Chemistry, Pharmacology and Clinical Applications. Amsterdam: Elsevier, 1993:261–5.
120. Jennings M, Shortland JR, Maddocks JL. Interstitial nephritis associated with frusemide. J R Soc Med 1986;79(4):239–40.
121. Magil AB. Drug-induced acute interstitial nephritis with granulomas. Hum Pathol 1983;14(1):36–41.
122. Fogari R, Zoppi A. Effects of antihypertensive therapy on sexual activity in hypertensive men. Curr Hypertens Rep 2002;4(3):202–10.
123. Loke Y. A systematic review of the benefits and harms of antihypertensive drug therapy. European Council for Blood Pressure and Cardiovascular Research Meeting, Holland 9–11 Oct 1999. Hypertension 1999;34(4):710.
124. Grimm RH Jr, Cohen JD, Smith WM, Falvo-Gerard L, Neaton JD. Hypertension management in the Multiple Risk Factor Intervention Trial (MRFIT). Six-year intervention results for men in special intervention and usual care groups. Arch Intern Med 1985;145(7):1191–9.
125. Helgeland A, Strommen R, Hagelund CH, Tretli S. Enalapril, atenolol, and hydrochlorothiazide in mild to moderate hypertension. A comparative multicentre study in general practice in Norway. Lancet 1986;1(8486):872–5.
126. Wassertheil-Smoller S, Blaufox MD, Oberman A, Davis BR, Swencionis C, Knerr MO, Hawkins CM, Langford HG. Effect of antihypertensives on sexual function and quality of life: the TAIM Study. Ann Intern Med 1991;114(8):613–20.
127. Smith PJ, Talbert RL. Sexual dysfunction with antihypertensive and antipsychotic agents. Clin Pharm 1986;5(5):373–84.
128. Prisant LM, Carr AA, Bottini PB, Solursh DS, Solursh LP. Sexual dysfunction with antihypertensive drugs. Arch Intern Med 1994;154(7):730–6.
129. Kaufmann H, Elijovich F, Yahr MD. An unusual cause of tetany: surreptitious use of furosemide. Mt Sinai J Med 1984;51(5):625–8.
130. De Wardener HE. Idiopathic edema: role of diuretic abuse. Kidney Int 1981;19(6):881–91.
131. Dunnigan MG, Denning DW, Henry JA, de Wolff FA. Idiopathic oedema and diuretics. Postgrad Med J 1987;63(735):25–6.
132. Pelosi AJ, Sykes RA, Lough JR, Muir WJ, Dunnigan MG. A psychiatric study of idiopathic oedema. Lancet 1986;2(8514):999–1002.
133. Young JB, Brownjohn AM, Lee MR. Diuretics and idiopathic oedema. Nephron 1986;43(4):311–12.
134. Marty H. Pseudo-Bartter Syndrom bei Diuretika-Abusus. [Pseudo-Bartter syndrome in diuretics abuse.] Schweiz Med Wochenschr 1985;115(7):250–2.
135. Lopez Jimenez M, Barbado FJ, Mateos F, Pena JM, Gil A, Arnalich F, Tovar I, Alonso FG, Vazquez Rodriguez JJ. Sindrome de Bartter factitio inducido por la ingestion subrepticia de diureticos. [Factitious Bartter's syndrome induced by the surreptitious ingestion of diuretics.] Med Clin (Barc) 1985;84(1):23–6.
136. Schmieder RE, Delles C, Messerli FH. Diuretic therapy and the risk for renal cell carcinoma. J Nephrol 2000;13(5):343–6.
137. Grossman E, Messerli FH, Goldbourt U. Does diuretic therapy increase the risk of renal cell carcinoma? Am J Cardiol 1999;83(7):1090–3.
138. Lee IM, Hennekens CH. Diuretics and renal cell carcinoma. Am J Cardiol 1999;83(7):1094.
139. Lip GY, Ferner RE. Diuretic therapy for hypertension: a cancer risk? J Hum Hypertens 1999;13(7):421–3.
140. Tenenbaum A, Grossman E, Fisman EZ, Adler Y, Boyko V, Jonas M, Behar S, Motro M, Reicher-Reiss H. Long-term diuretic therapy in patients with coronary disease: increased colon cancer-related mortality over a 5-year follow-up. J Hum Hypertens 2001;15(6):373–9.
141. Chesley LC. Preeclampsia: Early signs and development. In: Hypertensive Disorders in Pregnancy. New York: Appleton-Century-Crofts, 1978:302–6.
142. Thomson AM, Hytten FE, Billewicz WZ. The epidemiology of oedema during pregnancy. J Obstet Gynaecol Br Commonw 1967;74(1):1–10.
143. Friedman EA, Neff RK. Pregnancy outcome as related to hypertension, edema and proteinuria. In: Hypertension in Pregnancy. New York: John Wiley and Sons, 1976.
144. Campbell DM, MacGillivray I. The effect of a low calorie diet or a thiazide diuretic on the incidence of pre-eclampsia and on birth weight. Br J Obstet Gynaecol 1975;82(7):572–7.
145. Beilin LJ, Redman CWG. The use of antihypertensive drugs in pregnancy. In: Lewis PJ, editor. Therapeutic Problems in Pregnancy. Lancaster: MTP Press, 1977:1.
146. Gant NF, Madden JD, Siteri PK, MacDonald PC. The metabolic clearance rate of dehydroisoandrosterone sulfate. III. The effect of thiazide diuretics in normal and future pre-eclamptic pregnancies. Am J Obstet Gynecol 1975;123(2):159–63.
147. Zuspan FP, Zuspan KJ, Wilson AL. Acute and chronic hypertension in pregnancy. In: Rayburn WF, Zuspan FP, editors. Drug Therapy in Obstetrics and Gynecology. Norwalk, CT: Appleton-Century-Crofts, 1982:65.
148. Collins R, Yusuf S, Peto R. Overview of randomised trials of diuretics in pregnancy. BMJ (Clin Res Ed) 1985;290(6461):17–23.
149. Boethius G. Recording of drug prescriptions in the county of Jamtland, Sweden. II. Drug exposure of pregnant women in relation to course and outcome of pregnancy. Eur J Clin Pharmacol 1977;12(1):37–43.
150. Brocklebank JC, Ray WA, Federspiel CF, Schaffner W. Drug prescribing during pregnancy. A controlled study of

Tennessee Medicaid recipients. Am J Obstet Gynecol 1978;132(3):235–44.
151. Doering PL, Stewart RB. The extent and character of drug consumption during pregnancy. JAMA 1978;239(9):843–6.
152. Garnet JD. Placental transfer of chlorothiazide. Obstet Gynecol 1963;21:123–5.
153. Goldman JA, Neri A, Ovadia J, Eckerling B, de Vries A. Effect of chlorothiazide on intravenous glucose tolerance in pregnancy. Am J Obstet Gynecol 1969;105(4):556–60.
154. Pritchard JA, Walley PJ. Severe hypokalemia due to prolonged administration of chlorothiazide during pregnancy. Am J Obstet Gynecol 1961;81:1241–4.
155. Anderson GG, Hanson TM. Chronic fetal bradycardia: possible association with hypokalemia. Obstet Gynecol 1974;44(6):896–8.
156. Senior B, Slone D, Shapiro S, Mitchell AA, Heinonen OP. Letter: Benzothiadiazides and neonatal hypoglycaemia. Lancet 1976;2(7981):377.
157. Rodriguez SU, Leikin SL, Hiller MC. Neonatal thrombocytopenia associated with ante-partum administration of thiazide drugs. N Engl J Med 1964;270:881–4.
158. Combe R. Perturbations sanguines chez un premature apres administration de guanéthidiine et hydrochloride au cours de la grossesse. [Blood disorders in a premature infant after guanethidine and hydrochlorothiazide administration during pregnancy.] Pédiatrie 1978; 33(6):599–601.
159. Harley JD, Robin H, Robertson SE. Thiazide-induced neonatal haemolysis? BMJ 1964;5384:696–7.
160. Worsham F Jr, Beckman EN, Mitchell EH. Sacrococcygeal teratoma in a neonate. Association with maternal use of acetazolamide. JAMA 1978;240(3):251–2.
161. Diokno AC, Brown MB, Herzog AR. Relationship between use of diuretics and continence status in the elderly. Urology 1991;38(1):39–42.
162. Myers MG, Kearns PM, Kennedy DS, Fisher RH. Postural hypotension and diuretic therapy in the elderly. Can Med Assoc J 1978;119(6):581–4.
163. Burke V, Beilin LJ, German R, Grosskopf S, Ritchie J, Puddey IB, Rogers P. Postural fall in blood pressure in the elderly in relation to drug treatment and other lifestyle factors. Q J Med 1992;84(304):583–91.
164. Applegate WB. Hypertension in elderly patients. Ann Intern Med 1989;110(11):901–15.
165. Nicholls MG. Age-related effects of diuretics in hypertensive subjects. J Cardiovasc Pharmacol 1988;12(Suppl 8):S51–9.
166. Messerli FH, Grossman E, Goldbourt U. Are beta-blockers efficacious as first-line therapy for hypertension in the elderly? A systematic review JAMA 1998;279(23):1903–7.
167. Moro C, Romero J, Corres Peiretti MA. Amiodarone and hypokalemia. A dangerous combination. Int J Cardiol 1986;13(3):365–8.
168. Jarchovsky J, Zamir D, Plavnik L. [Torsade de pointes and use of phenothiazine and diuretic.]Harefuah 1991;121(11):435–6.
169. Bengtsson C, Blohme G, Lapidus L, Lindquist O, Lundgren H, Nystrom E, Petersen K, Sigurdsson JA. Do antihypertensive drugs precipitate diabetes? BMJ (Clin Res Ed) 1984;289(6457):1495–7.
170. O'Rahilly S. Beta blockers, blood sugars, and thiazides. Lancet 1985;1(8427):515–16.
171. Sundar S, Burma DP, Vaish SK. Digoxin toxicity and electrolytes: a correlative study. Acta Cardiol 1983;38(2):115–23.

Dobutamine

General Information

Dobutamine is a relatively selective $beta_1$-adrenoceptor agonist with only slight $beta_2$- and alpha-adrenoceptor activity. It has been developed as a positive inotropic agent that is less vasoconstrictive than high doses of dopamine.

Organs and Systems

Cardiovascular

Dobutamine stress testing, particularly combined with echocardiography, is a very widely used tool in cardiological investigation, and its safety continues to be examined in great detail. In a review of 37 publications, each reporting on 100 or more patients, with a total of over 26 000 tests, 79 life-threatening complications were described, including acute myocardial infarction, a variety of cardiac dysrhythmias, and severe hypotension (1). The authors also referred to 29 isolated case reports of severe complications, including two deaths. They concluded that there must be a clear indication for the procedure, informed consent must be obtained, a physician should be present during the test, and patients should be carefully followed as outpatients in case of delayed problems.

An Israeli group has reviewed the hemodynamic and adverse effects of dobutamine in 400 patients, of whom 187 were aged 65–79 years and 49 were 80 years or older (2). They found a very low incidence (1.5%) of serious adverse effects, even at high doses of up to 50 micrograms/kg/minute, and noted that most problems occur transiently at a lower dose and then resolve. Hypotension and dysrhythmias were the most common adverse effects, and their incidence was not related to age.

Acute subaortic left ventricular outflow tract obstruction has been described during dobutamine infusion in a patient who had no evidence of this at rest but developed severe obstruction when his pulse rate exceeded 105/minute (3). The subaortic gradient eventually reached the very high figure of 182 mmHg, even though the patient remained asymptomatic and there was no clear reason why this occurred in this particular patient.

In 47 consecutive patients (mean age 64 years, 46 men) with three or more cardiovascular risk factors, intravenous dobutamine was given at a rate of 40 micrograms/kg/minute until the target heart rate was achieved, which took a mean of 11.6 minutes (4). Subjective sensations occurred in 49% of the patients (palpitation 21%, chest pain 6%, nausea 6%, headache 6%, dizziness 13%), while half the patients had abnormal cardiac rhythms (ventricular extra beats 38%, supraventricular tachycardia 10%, and non-sustained ventricular tachycardia 2%). The authors concluded that the safety and tolerability of this procedure is comparable to that of standard dobutamine stress testing, although its specificity and selectivity are still uncertain.

The value and safety of dobutamine stress echocardiography have been studied in 135 patients aged 70 years or older (mean age 74 years; 58% men) soon after myocardial infarction (5). A diagnostic end-point was reached in 83% of patients, a figure comparable to younger populations. No major complications were reported. The procedure was terminated prematurely because of symptomatic hypotension ($n=8$), non-sustained ventricular tachycardia ($n=2$), systolic hypertension ($n=2$), atrial fibrillation ($n=1$), or bladder discomfort ($n=1$). All of these problems resolved rapidly after the procedure was stopped. At the time of discontinuation, seven of these 16 patients had objective evidence of myocardial ischemia.

Cardiac dysrhythmias

Dobutamine increases cardiac output after acute myocardial infarction without exacerbating myocardial infarction or ventricular dysrhythmias. However, a mild increase in heart rate often occurs, and occasionally a more marked tachycardia.

Cardiac dysrhythmias of various types (including occasional ventricular dysrhythmias) when dobutamine is used as a stress-inducing agent during echocardiography have been described (SEDA-18, 158).

- A 56-year-old woman with dilated cardiomyopathy developed QT interval prolongation and torsade de pointes during infusion of dobutamine in a low dose (2.5 micrograms/kg/minute). She had no previous documented dysrhythmias (6). She was hypokalemic and when her plasma potassium concentration was restored to normal the dysrhythmia disappeared and the QT interval normalized. The authors observed that this was the first case of its kind and emphasized the importance of normokalemia in dobutamine-treated patients.
- A 55-year-old man with stable angina was admitted for dobutamine stress testing (7). He had been taking metoprolol, but this was withdrawn 2 days before the test. During the lowest dose of the dobutamine infusion (5 micrograms/kg/minute) his heart rate rose to 143/minute and he developed chest pain and ST segment depression in the lateral chest leads of the electrocardiogram. The drug was stopped and metoprolol and glyceryl trinitrate were given immediately, but a few minutes later he developed torsade de pointes followed by ventricular fibrillation. Resuscitation was unsuccessful. There was no evidence of acute myocardial infarction at autopsy.
- A 74-year-old man with idiopathic dilated cardiomyopathy was given dobutamine (5 micrograms/kg/minute) to determine whether it would produce a positive inotropic effect (8). After 14 minutes he developed asymptomatic pulsus alternans, which resolved within 20 minutes of withdrawal.

A much more serious complication of dobutamine therapy is ventricular dysrhythmias. Of 305 patients with acutely decompensated congestive heart failure, 58 were given dobutamine (although it is difficult to ascertain the dose), 44 were given other standard inotropic drugs such as milrinone, and 203 were treated with brain natriuretic peptide (nesiritide, 0.015 or 0.03 micrograms/kg/minute) (9). Of those given dobutamine 7% had sustained ventricular tachycardia, 17% had non-sustained ventricular tachycardia, and 5% had a cardiac arrest. In contrast, the figures for nesiritide were 1, 11, and 0% respectively. There was no analysis of other outcomes but these results certainly do not encourage the use of dobutamine in these very vulnerable patients.

A study from Rotterdam, has examined the consequences of adding atropine to dobutamine in 200 patients with impaired left ventricular function (ejection fraction less than 35%) (10). There were cardiac dysrhythmias in 6% of patients and significant hypotension in 11%, figures comparable to those in other published studies. In the 36 patients who required atropine to achieve target heart rates the incidence of adverse effects was not increased. The same group has studied over 1000 consecutive patients undergoing dobutamine stress scintigraphic imaging of the myocardium (11). In these patients the incidence of dysrhythmias was about 8%, of whom about half had transient ventricular tachycardia, but only about 3% had significant hypotension (defined as a fall in systolic blood pressure of 40 mmHg). Atropine was required in nearly 40% of the patients in order to achieve target heart rates, but it is difficult to determine whether this had any influence on the occurrence of adverse effects.

A report from the Mayo Clinic has described 27 elderly patients (mean age 71 years) with aortic stenosis in whom dobutamine stress hemodynamic testing was used to assess the severity of the stenosis (12). There were no severe adverse effects, but relatively minor problems occurred in 16 patients, including chest pain and ventricular extra beats ($n=9$ each) and atrial dysrhythmias ($n=4$). The authors concluded that the procedure appears to be safe in these high-risk patients, although its diagnostic value may be limited.

There are variants of the standard procedure that do not appear to be associated with increased risk. An accelerated high-dose protocol, in which a constant infusion of 50 micrograms/kg/minute was given for up to 10 minutes in 100 patients, has been compared with the standard stepwise procedure in a similar number (13). The cumulative dose was somewhat lower in the accelerated protocol, while the duration of the test was halved. Dysrhythmic adverse effects occurred in 28 patients on the accelerated protocol and in 39 of those tested by the standard method: this difference was said to be non-significant. In another study, transesophageal was compared with transthoracic dobutamine stress echocardiography in 63 and 100 patients respectively (14). Baseline pulse and blood pressure were higher in the transesophageal group. The authors noted that there were no cases of ventricular tachycardia or fibrillation in either group, or of myocardial infarction. They also stated that the incidence of less serious dysrhythmias was similar in the two groups; however, no figures were quoted.

In the PRECEDENT study, dobutamine was compared with nesiritide (B natriuretic peptide) in patients with acutely decompensated congestive heart failure (15). The primary objective of the study was to assess the risk of ventricular dysrhythmias with the two therapies. Altogether 255 patients (mean age 61 years, 67% men) were randomized to receive dobutamine 5 micrograms/kg/hour or one of two doses of nesiritide 0.015 or 0.03 micrograms/kg/hour. Dobutamine significantly increased the number of episodes of ventricular tachycardia by 48/day, ventricular extra beats by 69/hour, and overall heart rate by 5/minute. These parameters were unchanged or improved by nesiritide. Since the two drugs had similar effects on the hemodynamic features of heart failure and its symptoms, the authors concluded that nesiritide should be considered as an alternative to dobutamine in this type of patient.

Myocardial ischemia

Angina and coronary artery spasm (16) have also occurred under these and other conditions. Some 10% of patients require treatment for angina occurring during stress testing, but up to a quarter have ischemic changes on the electrocardiogram (SEDA-17, 163), while others have headache, palpitation, anxiety, nausea, tingling, and flushing.

Myocardial ischemia has also been reported in susceptible patients. A Japanese group carried out dobutamine stress echocardiography in 51 patients with a presumptive diagnosis of variant angina (17). All had coronary vasospasm in response to intracoronary acetylcholine and seven also had chest pain and reversible ST segment elevation. One must incidentally wonder whether this procedure was entirely advisable.

In 47 patients in Mannheim (mean age 61 years, 34 men) dobutamine echocardiography was carried out, with blood sampling immediately before and after the procedure and then at 1, 2, 4, 6, and 12 hours (18). Assays were carried out for creatine kinase-MB, troponins I and T, myoglobin, and fibrin monomer antigen. There were no significant increases in these markers of myocardial damage and coagulation, regardless of the outcome of the stress test. These findings have confirmed those of an earlier study, although the data do not absolutely exclude abnormal findings in a minority of individuals (19).

Hypotension

In one study 38% of patients undergoing dobutamine stress echocardiography developed hypotension. Increases in blood pressure are more in line with what one would expect. Although dobutamine does not as a rule cause a marked increase in systolic blood pressure in normotensive patients, hypertensive patients can develop marked systolic hypertension during an infusion of the drug. When stress echocardiography with dobutamine is performed in subjects who prove to be entirely healthy, an audible Still's-like vibratory systolic ejection murmur is nevertheless produced.

Severe peripheral ischemia (even leading to dermal necrosis) can occur, as with dopamine (20).

Urinary tract

Urinary urgency can occur during infusion of a relatively high dose (15 micrograms/kg/minute) of dobutamine (21).

References

1. Lattanzi F, Picano E, Adamo E, Varga A. Dobutamine stress echocardiography: safety in diagnosing coronary artery disease. Drug Saf 2000;22(4):251–62.
2. Chenzbraun A, Khoury Z, Gottlieb S, Keren A. Impact of age on the safety and the hemodynamic response pattern during high dose dobutamine echocardiography. Echocardiography 1999;16(2):135–42.
3. Roldan FJ, Vargas-Barron J, Espinola-Zavaleta N, Keirns C, Romero-Cardenas A. Severe dynamic obstruction of the left ventricular outflow tract induced by dobutamine. Echocardiography 2000;17(1):37–40.
4. Lu D, Greenberg MD, Little R, Malik Q, Fernicola DJ, Weissman NJ. Accelerated dobutamine stress testing: safety and feasibility in patients with known or suspected coronary artery disease. Clin Cardiol 2001;24(2):141–5.
5. Previtali M, Scelsi L, Sebastiani R, Lanzarini L, Raisaro A, Klersy C. Feasibility, safety, and prognostic value of dobutamine stress echocardiography in patients > or = 70 years of age early after acute myocardial infarction. Am J Cardiol 2002;90(7):792–5.
6. Vecchia L, Ometto R, Finocchi G, Vincenzi M. Torsade de pointes ventricular tachycardia during low dose intermittent dobutamine treatment in a patient with dilated cardiomyopathy and congestive heart failure. Pacing Clin Electrophysiol 1999;22(2):397–9.
7. Varga A, Picano E, Lakatos F. Fatal ventricular fibrillation during a low-dose dobutamine stress test. Am J Med 2000;108(4):352–3.
8. Kahn JH, Starling MR, Supiano MA. Transient dobutamine-mediated pulsus alternans. Can J Cardiol 2001;17(2):203–5.
9. Burger AJ, Elkayam U, Neibaur MT, Haught H, Ghali J, Horton DP, Aronson D. Comparison of the occurrence of ventricular arrhythmias in patients with acutely decompensated congestive heart failure receiving dobutamine versus nesiritide therapy. Am J Cardiol 2001;88(1):35–9.
10. Poldermans D, Rambaldi R, Bax JJ, Cornel JH, Thomson IR, Valkema R, Boersma E, Fioretti PM, Breburda CS, Roelandt JR. Safety and utility of atropine addition during dobutamine stress echocardiography for the assessment of viable myocardium in patients with severe left ventricular dysfunction. Eur Heart J 1998;19(11):1712–18.
11. Elhendy A, Valkema R, van Domburg RT, Bax JJ, Nierop PR, Cornel JH, Geleijnse ML, Reijs AE, Krenning EP, Roelandt JR. Safety of dobutamine-atropine stress myocardial perfusion scintigraphy. J Nucl Med 1998;39(10):1662–6.
12. Lin SS, Roger VL, Pascoe R, Seward JB, Pellikka PA. Dobutamine stress Doppler hemodynamics in patients with aortic stenosis: feasibility, safety, and surgical correlations. Am Heart J 1998;136(6):1010–16.
13. Burger AJ, Notarianni MP, Aronson D. Safety and efficacy of an accelerated dobutamine stress echocardiography protocol in the evaluation of coronary artery disease. Am J Cardiol 2000;86(8):825–9.
14. Garcimartin I, San Roman JA, Vilacosta I, Munoz JC, de la Torre M, Fernandez-Aviles F. Complicaciones de la ecocardíografia de estrés transesofágica con dobutamina. [Complications of transesophageal echocardiography with dobutamine.] Rev Esp Cardiol 2000;53(8):1136–9.
15. Burger AJ, Horton DP, LeJemtel T, Ghali JK, Torre G, Dennish G, Koren M, Dinerman J, Silver M, Cheng ML, Elkayam U; Prospective Randomized Evaluation of Cardiac Ectopy with Dobutamine or Natrecor Therapy. Effect of nesiritide (B-type natriuretic peptide) and dobutamine on ventricular arrhythmias in the treatment of patients with acutely decompensated congestive heart failure: the PRECEDENT study. Am Heart J 2002;144(6):1102–8.
16. Friart A, Hermans L, De Valeriola Y. Unusual side-effect of a dobutamine stress echocardiography. Am J Noninvasive Cardiol 1993;7:63–4.

17. Kawano H, Fujii H, Motoyama T, Kugiyama K, Ogawa H, Yasue H. Myocardial ischemia due to coronary artery spasm during dobutamine stress echocardiography. Am J Cardiol 2000;85(1):26–30.
18. Pfleger S, Scherhag A, Latsch A, Dempfle CE, Simonis B, Haux P, Voelker W, Gaudron P. Safety of dobutamine echocardiography: no signs of myocardial cell damage or activation of the coagulation system. Dis Manag Clin Outcomes 2001;3:15–19.
19. Beckmann S, Bocksch W, Muller C, Schartl M. Does dobutamine stress echocardiography induce damage during viability diagnosis of patients with chronic regional dysfunction after myocardial infarction? J Am Soc Echocardiogr 1998;11(2):181–7.
20. Hoff JV, Peatty PA, Wade JL. Dermal necrosis from dobutamine. N Engl J Med 1979;300(22):1280.
21. Waagstein F, Malek I, Hjalmarson AC. The use of dobutamine in myocardial infarction for reversal of the cardiodepressive effect of metoprolol. Br J Clin Pharmacol 1978;5(6):515–21.

Docetaxel

See also Cytostatic and immunosuppressant drugs

General Information

Docetaxel is a taxane that is used in combination with doxorubicin in the treatment of metastatic breast cancer and as a single agent in metastatic lung cancer.

Organs and Systems

Respiratory

Interstitial pneumonitis has been attributed to docetaxel in four cases (1). None of the patients had lung disease and they all had normal liver function. Within 8–14 days of receiving a second cycle of docetaxel (75 mg/m^2 in three cases and 60 mg/m^2 in the other), all developed acute dyspnea and fever, which progressed until they needed ventilation; two died. In contrast, in a study of 33 patients treated with paclitaxel and carboplatin, only one had reduced diffusion capacity for carbon monoxide, with no accompanying clinical or radiological changes (2).

Fluid balance

Fluid retention has previously been reported with docetaxel. Some believe that this effect depends on the dose and the duration of infusion (3,4) and that high concentrations of M4, the cyclized oxazolidinedione metabolite of docetaxel, cause more pronounced fluid retention.

Hematologic

In 46 chemotherapy-naive patients, docetaxel had an important but reversible non-specific lymphopenic effect, thought to be associated with an increased risk of non-neutropenic infections (5).

Gastrointestinal

Three of 14 patients in a phase 1 study of docetaxel plus vinorelbine for metastatic breast cancer developed colitis (6). A further three patients were identified in other studies of docetaxel.

Skin

Of 99 patients who received low-dose docetaxel (60 mg/m^2 every 3 or 4 weeks), 25 had skin toxicity, mainly erythema and nail changes (7). Of a subset of 25 patients who received irradiation before docetaxel, four had recall dermatitis during their first infusion of docetaxel. All had previously received doxorubicin, which may in part have explained some of the toxicity.

Maculopapular eruptions and desquamation of hands and/or feet occurred in 35% of patients with non-small cell lung cancers given docetaxel (8).

Four cases of fixed plaques of erythrodysesthesia have been attributed to intravenous docetaxel (9). There had been no extravasation or previous skin injury. While this was a new presentation, the authors did not explain why the lesions were not just late presentations of small-volume extravasation injuries.

Nails

Onycholysis has been reported in patients receiving docetaxel (10).

Immunologic

A 25% incidence of grade 2 or more severe immunological reactions to docetaxel has been reported after the use of oral prednisone (100 mg orally before treatment and 50 mg once on the morning of treatment and the following 2 days) in 20 patients with non-small-cell lung cancers (8). No other premedications were given routinely. If infusion-related symptoms occurred, the infusion was interrupted and diphenhydramine was given. On subsequent cycles those patients then were routinely premedicated with diphenhydramine 25 or 50 mg intravenously and cimetidine 300 mg intravenously.

References

1. Read WL, Mortimer JE, Picus J. Severe interstitial pneumonitis associated with docetaxel administration. Cancer 2002;94(3):847–53.
2. Dimopoulou I, Galani H, Dafni U, Samakovii A, Roussos C, Dimopoulos MA. A prospective study of pulmonary function in patients treated with paclitaxel and carboplatin. Cancer 2002;94(2):452–8.
3. Shin E, Ishitobi M, Hiraoia M, Kazumasa F, Hideyuki M, Nishisho I, Toshiro S, Yasunori H, Tosimasa T. Phase I study of docetaxel administered by bi-weekly infusion to patients with metastatic breast cancer. Anticancer Res 2000;20(6C):4721–6.
4. Rosing H, Lustig V, van Warmerdam LJ, Huizing MT, ten Bokkel Huinink WW, Schellens JH, Rodenhuis S, Bult A, Beijnen JH. Pharmacokinetics and metabolism of docetaxel administered as a 1-h intravenous infusion. Cancer Chemother Pharmacol 2000;45(3):213–18.
5. Kotsakis A, Sarra E, Peraki M, Koukourakis M, Apostolaki S, Souglakos J, Mavromanomakis E,

Vlachonikolis J, Georgoulias V. Docetaxel-induced lymphopenia in patients with solid tumors: a prospective phenotypic analysis. Cancer 2000;89(6):1380–6.
6. Ibrahim NK, Sahin AA, Dubrow RA, Lynch PM, Boehnke-Michaud L, Valero V, Buzdar AU, Hortobagyi GN. Colitis associated with docetaxel-based chemotherapy in patients with metastatic breast cancer. Lancet 2000;355(9200):281–3.
7. Ando M, Watanabe T, Nagata K, Narabayashi M, Adachi I, Katsumata N. Efficacy of docetaxel 60 mg/m^2 in patients with metastatic breast cancer according to the status of anthracycline resistance. J Clin Oncol 2001;19(2):336–42.
8. Miller VA, Rigas JR, Francis PA, Grant SC, Pisters KM, Venkatraman ES, Woolley K, Heelan RT, Kris MG. Phase II trial of a 75-mg/m^2 dose of docetaxel with prednisone premedication for patients with advanced non-small cell lung cancer. Cancer 1995;75(4):968–72.
9. Chu CY, Yang CH, Yang CY, Hsiao GH, Chiu HC. Fixed erythrodysaesthesia plaque due to intravenous injection of docetaxel. Br J Dermatol 2000;142(4):808–11.
10. Correia O, Azevedo C, Pinto Ferreira E, Braga Cruz F, Polonia J. Nail changes secondary to docetaxel (Taxotere). Dermatology 1999;198(3):288–90.

Dofetilide

See also Antidysrhythmic drugs

General Information

Dofetilide is a pure Class III antidysrhythmic drug, without actions of any other class. It was developed following the observation that bis(arylalkyl)amines with methanesulfonamido moieties on both aryl groups prolong the cardiac action potential without significantly altering the maximum rate of depolarization (1). The pharmacology, clinical pharmacology, uses, adverse effects, and interactions of dofetilide have been reviewed (2–8). Cardiovascular adverse effects of dofetilide are the most troublesome. Other common effects have included mild headache, dizziness, dyspepsia, nausea, and vomiting (9).

Pharmacology

Dofetilide is a highly selective blocker of the rapidly activating component of the inward rectifier potassium channel, IK_r (10–16). It therefore delays ventricular repolarization, which becomes less heterogeneous (17), and prolongs the action potential duration and effective refractory period (14,18,19); it has the same effects in ventricular muscle in dilated cardiomyopathy and chronic ischemic cardiomyopathy (10). It has greater affinity for atrial than ventricular tissues in animals (20), but probably not in man (14,18). It preferentially blocks open channels and has Group 3 actions (SEDA-25, 209), with slow-onset kinetics (21) and an increased likelihood of being prodysrhythmic at slower heart rates (22).

Dofetilide causes a dose-related and plasma concentration-related prolongation of the QT_c interval (14,18,19,23–27), and either reduces QT_c dispersion (26) or has no effect on it (28,29). The effects on the QT_c interval are rate-dependent, being greater at slower heart rates (30). Dofetilide does not usually broaden the QRS complex, but this was reported (and published twice) in a single patient with atrial fibrillation, in whom it was attributed to aberrant conduction (31,32).

During repeated oral administration of dofetilide 1.0–2.5 mg/day for 5 days the effect on the QT interval was slightly greater on day 1 than on day 5 at a range of plasma concentrations of about 1–4 ng/ml; this observation suggests the occurrence of tolerance, but in that case one would have expected a clockwise hysteresis loop in the effect concentration curve, and no hysteresis was seen either after a single dose or at steady state (25).

Dofetilide has a small positive inotropic effect in animal hearts (15,33). In a double-blind, placebo-controlled study of oral dofetilide 125, 250, or 500 mg bd for the maintenance of sinus rhythm after cardioversion of sustained atrial fibrillation or flutter in 201 patients, there were small changes in echocardiographic measures of atrial contractility, but no changes in stroke volume or cardiac output (34).

Clinical pharmacology

The pharmacokinetics of dofetilide are linear after single oral doses of 2–10 micrograms/kg (24,35) and repeated doses of 1.0–2.5 mg/day (25). Dofetilide is well absorbed (about 90%) after oral administration (24,35,36). Its absorption is relatively slow and peak concentrations are not reached for 1–2.5 hours; absorption is slower after food. It is a low clearance drug, with a clearance rate of about 6 ml/minute/kg, and has a volume of distribution of about 3 l/kg (23,36). It is mostly excreted unchanged by the kidneys, with a half-life of about 8 hours. Its clearance is therefore roughly proportional to creatinine clearance, particularly at high rates of clearance. A small proportion is metabolized in the liver by CYP3A4 to inactive metabolites (37).

In a pharmacokinetic–pharmacodynamic study in 10 healthy volunteers intravenous dofetilide 0.5 mg caused a mean maximum prolongation of the QT_c interval of 121 ms and the mean plasma concentration associated with half-maximal effect was 2.2 ng/ml (36).

Uses

Dofetilide has been used to convert atrial fibrillation and atrial flutter to sinus rhythm, in maintaining sinus rhythm thereafter, in suppressing paroxysmal supraventricular tachycardia, inducible atrioventricular nodal re-entry tachycardia, and inducible sustained ventricular tachycardia, in suppressing the dysrhythmias of the Wolff–Parkinson–White syndrome, and in facilitating conversion of ventricular fibrillation.

Open clinical studies

In 19 patients with atrial fibrillation and five with atrial flutter, dofetilide 2.5–8.0 micrograms/kg caused conversion to sinus rhythm in 14 (10 with atrial fibrillation and four with atrial flutter) (38).

In patients with sustained monomorphic ventricular tachycardia inducible by programmed electrical stimulation, who had previously been unsuccessfully treated with

0–7 other drugs, intravenous dofetilide 3–15 micrograms/kg suppressed or slowed inducible ventricular tachycardia in 17 of 41 patients, compared with none of nine patients who received only 1.5 micrograms/kg (19).

Intravenous dofetilide 2.5–5.0 micrograms/kg produced sinus rhythm in seven patients with paroxysmal atrial fibrillation of recent onset (under 7 days) and terminated paroxysmal supraventricular tachycardia in four of six patients (39).

In patients with electrically inducible atrioventricular re-entrant tachycardia intravenous dofetilide 1.5–15 micrograms/kg had no effect on tachycardia inducibility at two lower doses but prevented the re-induction of tachycardia at three higher doses in 11 of 31 patients (40).

Placebo-controlled studies

Conversion of atrial fibrillation and flutter

In a crossover, placebo-controlled study in 16 patients with recent onset atrial fibrillation, cardioversion was achieved in two of six patients who received dofetilide 8 micrograms/kg and in two of nine who received 12 micrograms/kg (41). None cardioverted with placebo. However, the average duration of atrial fibrillation was 35 days in those who cardioverted with dofetilide and 83 days in those who did not. The authors concluded that dofetilide had only limited effect in cardioverting atrial fibrillation of moderate duration.

In a double-blind, placebo-controlled study 98 patients, who developed atrial fibrillation/flutter within 1–6 days after coronary artery bypass graft surgery, were given dofetilide 4 or 8 micrograms/kg intravenously over 15 minutes (42). Eight of 33 patients converted to sinus rhythm after placebo, 12 of 33 after dofetilide 4 micrograms/kg, and 14 of 32 after dofetilide 8 micrograms/kg.

In a double-blind, placebo-controlled study in patients with sustained atrial fibrillation ($n = 75$) or atrial flutter ($n = 16$), dofetilide 8 micrograms/kg terminated the dysrhythmia in nine of 29 patients, compared with only four of 32 who received 4 micrograms/kg and none of 30 who received placebo (43). Patients with atrial flutter had a greater response to dofetilide (six of 11) than those with atrial fibrillation (five of 49).

In a placebo-controlled study in patients with atrial fibrillation or atrial flutter with a median dysrhythmia duration of 62 (range 1–180) days, there was conversion to sinus rhythm in 20 of 66 patients given dofetilide, compared with one of 30 patients given placebo (44). The conversion rate was higher in atrial flutter (seven of 11 patients) than in atrial fibrillation (13 of 55).

In a double-blind, placebo-controlled study in 325 patients with atrial fibrillation or flutter cardioversion, rates for dofetilide 125, 250, and 500 micrograms bd were 6.1, 9.8, and 30% respectively, compared with 1.2% with placebo (45). The probabilities of remaining in sinus rhythm at 1 year with dofetilide 125, 250, and 500 micrograms bd were 0.40, 0.37, and 0.58 respectively, and 0.25 for placebo.

In a double-blind, placebo-controlled study in 69 patients with atrial fibrillation or flutter, intravenous dofetilide 2–8 micrograms/kg caused conversion to sinus rhythm in 16 of 51 patients, compared with one of 18 who were given placebo; conversion of atrial flutter occurred in five of seven who were given dofetilide compared with none of three who were given placebo (46).

In a randomized, placebo-controlled, crossover study in 15 men, mean age 34 (range 18–63) years, with Wolff–Parkinson–White syndrome and atrial fibrillation or atrioventricular re-entrant tachycardia induced electrophysiologically, six of ten patients who were given dofetilide converted to sinus rhythm, compared with one of five who were given placebo (47). There were no dysrhythmias.

Ventricular tachydysrhythmias

In a placebo-controlled study, sustained ventricular tachycardia or fibrillation, reproducibly inducible electrophysiologically, was no longer inducible in eight of 18 patients who were given intravenous dofetilide 0.1–8.0 ng/ml, compared with one of six patients who received placebo (48).

In a randomized, double-blind, placebo-controlled study in 32 patients with ventricular extra beats (more than 30/hour on two consecutive 24-hour Holter recordings while drug free and more than 50/hour during 2-hour telemetric electrocardiography), dofetilide 7.5 micrograms/kg produced an 83% and placebo a 2.9% median reduction in ventricular extra beats (49).

Sudden death

The Danish Investigations of Arrhythmia and Mortality ON Dofetilide (DIAMOND) study comprised two studies in patients at high risk of sudden death: one in patients with congestive heart failure and one in patients with acute myocardial infarction within the previous 7 days (50).

In the congestive heart failure study, 1518 patients with symptomatic congestive heart failure and severe left ventricular dysfunction were recruited at 34 Danish hospitals; 762 were randomized double-blind to dofetilide and 756 to placebo (51). After 1 month, 22 of 190 patients with atrial fibrillation at baseline had sinus rhythm restored by dofetilide, compared with only three of 201 who took placebo. Dofetilide was also significantly more effective than placebo in maintaining sinus rhythm (hazard ratio for the recurrence of atrial fibrillation = 0.35; CI = 0.22, 0.57). Dofetilide significantly reduced the risk of hospitalization for worsening congestive heart failure (risk ratio = 0.75; CI = 0.63, 0.89). During a median follow-up of 18 months, 311 patients taking dofetilide and 317 patients taking placebo died (hazard ratio = 0.95; CI = 0.81, 1.11).

In the corresponding myocardial infarction study, 1510 patients with severe left ventricular dysfunction after myocardial infarction were recruited in 37 Danish coronary-care units; 749 were randomized double-blind to dofetilide and 761 to placebo (52). There were no significant differences between dofetilide and placebo in all-cause mortality or total dysrhythmic deaths. Dofetilide was significantly better than placebo at restoring sinus rhythm in patients with atrial fibrillation or flutter.

Comparative studies with other antidysrhythmic drugs

Amiodarone

In a comparison of intravenous dofetilide (8 micrograms/kg; $n = 48$), amiodarone (5 mg/kg; $n = 50$), or placebo ($n = 52$) in converting atrial fibrillation or flutter to sinus rhythm in 150 patients, sinus rhythm was restored in 35, 4, and 4% respectively (53).

Flecainide

In a non-randomized comparison of flecainide (2 mg/kg; $n = 11$) and dofetilide (8 micrograms/kg; $n = 10$) in patients with atrial flutter, only one patient given flecainide converted to sinus rhythm compared with seven of the 10 patients given dofetilide (54).

Propafenone

In a randomized, placebo-controlled, parallel-group comparison of oral dofetilide 500 micrograms bd, propafenone 150 mg tds, or placebo in preventing the recurrence of paroxysmal supraventricular tachycardia in 122 symptomatic patients, the respective probabilities of remaining free of episodes of paroxysmal supraventricular tachycardia were 50, 54, and 6%; both dofetilide and propafenone also reduced the frequency of episodes (median numbers 1, 0.5, and 5 respectively) (55).

Sotalol

In a double-blind, randomized, crossover comparison of oral dofetilide 500 micrograms bd with sotalol 160 mg bd in 128 patients with ischemic heart disease and inducible sustained ventricular tachycardia, 46 patients responded to dofetilide and 43 to sotalol; however, only 23 patients responded to both dofetilide and sotalol (9).

The hemodynamic effects of dofetilide 500 micrograms bd and sotalol 160 mg bd for 3–5 days have been studied in 12 patients with ischemic heart disease and sustained ventricular tachycardia (56). There were significant reductions in heart rate, mean systemic pressure, and cardiac index (–13%) with sotalol, but cardiac index increased significantly with dofetilide (11%) with no effect on heart rate or systemic blood pressure. The authors suggested that oral dofetilide could be useful in patients with ventricular tachydysrhythmias associated with impaired left ventricular function. One patient taking dofetilide reported mild dizziness and there were no cardiac dysrhythmias.

Organs and Systems

Cardiovascular

Because dofetilide prolongs the QT interval, there is a risk of ventricular tachydysrhythmias, which have often been reported, after both intravenous and oral administration.

In 154 patients with implantable cardioverter-defibrillators randomly assigned to dofetilide or placebo, there were pause-dependent runs of polymorphic ventricular tachycardia in 15 of the 87 patients who received dofetilide and in only five of the 87 who received placebo (57). There were five early events (at less than 3 days of therapy), all torsade de pointes in patients taking dofetilide. There were 15 late events, 10 with dofetilide and five with placebo. The median time to a late event was 22 (range 6–107) days for dofetilide and 99 (34–207) days for placebo.

In the DIAMOND study in congestive heart failure, there were 25 cases of torsade de pointes in the dofetilide group (3.3%) compared with none in the placebo group (51). In the DIAMOND myocardial infarction study there were seven cases of torsade de pointes (0.93%), all in those who were given dofetilide (52).

In a double-blind, placebo-controlled study in 325 patients with atrial fibrillation or atrial flutter randomized to dofetilide 125, 250, or 500 micrograms bd or placebo, there were two cases of torsade de pointes, one on day 2 and the other on day 3 (0.8% of all patients given the active drug); there was one sudden cardiac death, classified as prodysrhythmic, on day 8 (0.4% of all patients given the active drug). The authors recommended that dosage adjustment based on QT_c interval and renal function would minimize the small but not negligible prodysrhythmic risk of dofetilide.

In 128 patients who received dofetilide and sotalol in a crossover study, there were treatment-related adverse events in 2.3% of the patients who received dofetilide and 8.6% of those who received sotalol (9). Three patients who took dofetilide had torsade de pointes.

In a comparison of intravenous dofetilide (8 micrograms/kg; $n = 48$), amiodarone (5 mg/kg; $n = 50$), or placebo ($n = 52$) in converting atrial fibrillation or flutter to sinus rhythm in 150 patients, two patients given dofetilide had non-sustained ventricular tachycardias; four had torsade de pointes, in one case requiring electrical cardioversion (53).

- In one of 10 healthy men given intravenous dofetilide 0.5 micrograms/kg there was prolongation of the QT_c interval from 451 to 808 ms 5 minutes after the end of the infusion; this was associated with five beats of polymorphic ventricular tachycardia, several multifocal ventricular extra beats, and ventricular couplets and triplets, all within 10 minutes after the end of the infusion (24).
- In a 37-year-old woman with atrial flutter with 1:1 conduction and partial right bundle branch block, intravenous dofetilide 5 micrograms/kg given over 5 minutes not only suppressed the atrioventricular nodal block to 2:1 or 3:1 but also caused complete right bundle branch block and QT interval prolongation (58).
- Self-limiting torsade de pointes developed in a 67-year-old man who was given 12.8 micrograms/kg (plasma concentration 7.1 ng/ml) in an open study; the QT_c interval was prolonged to over 600 ms (19).

This patient had stopped taking amiodarone 1 month before the administration of dofetilide, and that may have contributed to the prolongation of the QT_c interval.

- A woman with atrial fibrillation developed torsade de pointes after receiving intravenous dofetilide 6 micrograms/kg (plasma concentration 26 ng/ml) (41).
- A patient with atrial fibrillation received intravenous dofetilide 8 micrograms/kg and developed torsade de pointes before reverting to sinus rhythm (41).
- One of 18 patients with sustained ventricular tachycardia or fibrillation, reproducibly inducible electrophysiologically, developed torsade de pointes after receiving intravenous dofetilide 8 micrograms/kg (plasma concentration 5.3 ng/ml) (48).
- Short episodes of aberrant ventricular conduction and ventricular tachycardia occurred in three of 32

patients with atrial fibrillation who were given dofetilide 8 micrograms/kg (42).

- Torsade de pointes occurred in two of 62 patients with atrial tachydysrhythmias who received dofetilide 4 or 8 micrograms/kg; two other patients had ventricular extra beats associated with prolongation of the QT_c interval (43).
- In a placebo-controlled study of the effect of dofetilide 8 micrograms/kg in converting atrial fibrillation or flutter, transient torsade de pointes occurred in two men, aged 57 and 67, with prolongation of the QT_c interval from 370 and 420 ms to 450 and 510 ms respectively (44).

- A 58-year-old woman developed torsade de pointes with prolongation of the QT_c interval to 490 ms after receiving intravenous dofetilide 4.3 micrograms/kg; she responded to intravenous magnesium sulfate plus isoprenaline (46).

Other cardiac dysrhythmias that have been reported have included episodes of junctional rhythm with bundle branch block, spontaneous atrioventricular re-entrant tachycardia, and sustained supraventricular tachycardia (40).

Hypotension occasionally occurs after intravenous dofetilide (40).

Death

The risk of death in patients with supraventricular dysrhythmias taking dofetilide has been studied in a systematic review of randomized controlled trials (59). After adjusting for the effects of dysrhythmia diagnosis, age, sex, and structural heart disease, the hazard ratio was 1.1 (CI = 0.3, 4.3).

Drug–Drug Interactions

Digoxin

In 14 healthy men dofetilide 250 micrograms bd for 5 days had no effect on the pharmacokinetics of digoxin at a steady-state trough concentration of 1.0 ng/ml (60). However, in a placebo-controlled study in patients with atrial fibrillation or atrial flutter, conversion to sinus rhythm in patients given dofetilide was more likely if they were also given digoxin (44), suggesting that there may be a pharmacodynamic interaction.

Histamine (H_2) receptor antagonists

In a randomized, placebo-controlled study of the effects of cimetidine and ranitidine on the pharmacokinetics and pharmacodynamics of a single dose of dofetilide 500 micrograms in 20 healthy men, ranitidine 150 mg bd did not affect the pharmacokinetics or pharmacodynamics of dofetilide, but there was a dose-dependent increase in exposure to dofetilide with cimetidine (61). With cimetidine 100 and 400 mg bd the AUC of dofetilide increased by 11 and 48%, the maximum plasma dofetilide concentration increased by 11 and 29%, renal clearance fell by 13 and 33%, and non-renal clearance by 5 and 21%; dofetilide-induced prolongation of the QT_c interval was increased by 22 and 33%. The authors suggested that cimetidine inhibited renal tubular dofetilide secretion, an effect that is specific to cimetidine in its class. Cimetidine should be avoided in patients taking dofetilide.

Verapamil

Pharmacokinetic and pharmacodynamic interactions between dofetilide 0.5 mg bd and verapamil 80 mg tds have been studied in 12 healthy men (62). At steady state verapamil increased the peak plasma concentration of dofetilide from 2.40 to 3.43 ng/ml, without other pharmacokinetic effects. This was accompanied by a small increase in the prolongation of the QT_c interval produced by dofetilide alone, from 20 to 26 ms. Although this small effect is unlikely to be of clinical significance, it would be wise to avoid verapamil in patients taking dofetilide.

References

1. Cross PE, Arrowsmith JE, Thomas GN, Gwilt M, Burges RA, Higgins AJ. Selective class III antiarrhythmic agents. 1 Bis(arylalkyl)amines. J Med Chem 1990; 33(4):1151–5.
2. Anonymous. Dofetilide for atrial fibrillation. Med Lett Drugs Ther 2000;42(1078):41–2.
3. Torp-Pedersen C, Moller M, Kober L, Camm AJ. Dofetilide for the treatment of atrial fibrillation in patients with congestive heart failure. Eur Heart J 2000;21(15):1204–6.
4. Al-Dashti R, Sami M. Dofetilide: a new class III antiarrhythmic agent. Can J Cardiol 2001;17(1):63–7.
5. Ansani NT. Dofetilide: a new treatment of arrhythmias. P&T 2001;26:372–8.
6. Lauer MR. Dofetilide: is the treatment worse than the disease? J Am Coll Cardiol 2001;37(4):1106–10.
7. Saoudi N, Rinaldi JP, Yaici K, Bergonzi M. Dofetilide: what role in the treatment of ventricular tachyarrhythmias? Eur Heart J 2001;22(23):2141–3.
8. Tran A, Vichiendilokkul A, Racine E, Milad A. Practical approach to the use and monitoring of dofetilide therapy. Am J Health Syst Pharm 2001;58(21):2050–9.
9. Boriani G, Lubinski A, Capucci A, Niederle R, Kornacewicz-Jack Z, Wnuk-Wojnar AM, Borggrefe M, Brachmann J, Biffi M, Butrous GS; Ventricular Arrhythmias Dofetilide Investigators. A multicentre, double-blind randomized crossover comparative study on the efficacy and safety of dofetilide vs sotalol in patients with inducible sustained ventricular tachycardia and ischaemic heart disease. Eur Heart J 2001;22(23):2180–91.
10. Sanguinetti MC, Jurkiewicz NK. Two components of cardiac delayed rectifier K^+ current. Differential sensitivity to block by class III antiarrhythmic agents. J Gen Physiol 1990;96(1):195–215.
11. Tande PM, Bjornstad H, Yang T, Refsum H. Rate-dependent class III antiarrhythmic action, negative chronotropy, and positive inotropy of a novel Ik blocking drug, UK-68,798: potent in guinea pig but no effect in rat myocardium. J Cardiovasc Pharmacol 1990;16(3):401–10.
12. Gwilt M, Arrowsmith JE, Blackburn KJ, Burges RA, Cross PE, Dalrymple HW, Higgins AJ. UK-68,798: a novel, potent and highly selective class III antiarrhythmic agent which blocks potassium channels in cardiac cells. J Pharmacol Exp Ther 1991;256(1):318–24.
13. Gwilt M, Blackburn KJ, Burges RA, Higgins AJ, Milne AA, Solca AM. Electropharmacology of dofetilide, a new class III agent, in anaesthetised dogs. Eur J Pharmacol 1992;215(2–3):137–44.

14. Sedgwick ML, Rasmussen HS, Cobbe SM. Clinical and electrophysiologic effects of intravenous dofetilide (UK-68,798), a new class III antiarrhythmic drug, in patients with angina pectoris. Am J Cardiol 1992;69(5):513–17.
15. Abrahamsson C, Duker G, Lundberg C, Carlsson L. Electrophysiological and inotropic effects of H 234/09 (almokalant) in vitro: a comparison with two other novel IK blocking drugs, UK-68,798 (dofetilide) and E-4031. Cardiovasc Res 1993;27(5):861–7.
16. Montero M, Schmitt C. Recording of transmembrane action potentials in chronic ischemic heart disease and dilated cardiomyopathy and the effects of the new class III antiarrhythmic agents D-sotalol and dofetilide. J Cardiovasc Pharmacol 1996;27(4):571–7.
17. Gwilt M, King RC, Milne AA, Solca AM. Dofetilide, a new class III antiarrhythmic agent, reduces pacing induced heterogeneity of repolarisation in vivo. Cardiovasc Res 1992;26(11):1102–8.
18. Sedgwick ML, Dalrymple I, Rae AP, Cobbe SM. Effects of the new class III antiarrhythmic drug dofetilide on the atrial and ventricular intracardiac monophasic action potential in patients with angina pectoris. Eur Heart J 1995;16(11):1641–6.
19. Yuan S, Wohlfart B, Rasmussen HS, Olsson S, Blomstrom-Lundqvist C. Effect of dofetilide on cardiac repolarization in patients with ventricular tachycardia. A study using simultaneous monophasic action potential recordings from two sites in the right ventricle. Eur Heart J 1994;15(4):514–22.
20. Baskin EP, Lynch JJ Jr. Differential atrial versus ventricular activities of class III potassium channel blockers. J Pharmacol Exp Ther 1998;285(1):135–42.
21. Snyders DJ, Chaudhary A. High affinity open channel block by dofetilide of HERG expressed in a human cell line. Mol Pharmacol 1996;49(6):949–55.
22. Sager PT. Frequency-dependent electrophysiologic effects of dofetilide in humans. Circulation 1995;92:1774.
23. Sedgwick M, Rasmussen HS, Walker D, Cobbe SM. Pharmacokinetic and pharmacodynamic effects of UK-68,798, a new potential class III antiarrhythmic drug. Br J Clin Pharmacol 1991;31(5):515–19.
24. Tham TC, MacLennan BA, Burke MT, Harron DW. Pharmacodynamics and pharmacokinetics of the class III antiarrhythmic agent dofetilide (UK-68,798) in humans. J Cardiovasc Pharmacol 1993;21(3):507–12.
25. Allen MJ, Nichols DJ, Oliver SD. The pharmacokinetics and pharmacodynamics of oral dofetilide after twice daily and three times daily dosing. Br J Clin Pharmacol 2000;50(3):247–53.
26. Boriani G, Biffi M, De Simone N, Bacchi L, Martignani C, Bitonti F, Zannoli R, Butrous G, Branzi A. Repolarization changes in a double-blind crossover study of dofetilide versus sotalol in the treatment of ventricular tachycardia. Pacing Clin Electrophysiol 2000;23(11 Pt 2):1935–8.
27. Bashir Y, Thomsen PE, Kingma JH, Moller M, Wong C, Cobbe SM, Jordaens L, Campbell RW, Rasmussen HS, Camm AJ. Electrophysiologic profile and efficacy of intravenous dofetilide (UK-68,798), a new class III antiarrhythmic drug, in patients with sustained monomorphic ventricular tachycardia. Dofetilide Arrhythmia Study Group. Am J Cardiol 1995;76(14):1040–4.
28. Sedgwick ML, Rasmussen HS, Cobbe SM. Effects of the class III antiarrhythmic drug dofetilide on ventricular monophasic action potential duration and QT interval dispersion in stable angina pectoris. Am J Cardiol 1992;70(18):1432–7.
29. Demolis JL, Funck-Brentano C, Ropers J, Ghadanfar M, Nichols DJ, Jaillon P. Influence of dofetilide on QT-interval duration and dispersion at various heart rates during exercise in humans. Circulation 1996;94(7):1592–9.
30. Lande G, Maison-Blanche P, Fayn J, Ghadanfar M, Coumel P, Funck-Brentano C. Dynamic analysis of dofetilide-induced changes in ventricular repolarization. Clin Pharmacol Ther 1998;64(3):312–21.
31. Crijns HJ, Kingma JH, Gosselink AT, Lie K. Comparison in the same patient of aberrant conduction and bundle branch reentry after dofetilide, a new selective class III antiarrhythmic agent. Pacing Clin Electrophysiol 1993;16(5 Pt 1):1006–16.
32. Crijns HJ, Kingma JH, Gosselink AT, Dalrymple HW, De Langen CD, Lie K. Sequential bilateral bundle branch block during dofetilide, a new class III antiarrhythmic agent, in a patient with atrial fibrillation. J Cardiovasc Electrophysiol 1993;4(4):459–66.
33. Doggrell SA, Nand V. Effects of dofetilide on cardiovascular tissues from normo- and hypertensive rats. J Pharm Pharmacol 2002;54(5):707–15.
34. DeCara JM, Pollak A, Dubrey S, Falk RH. Positive atrial inotropic effect of dofetilide after cardioversion of atrial fibrillation or flutter. Am J Cardiol 2000;86(6):685–8.
35. Gemmill JD, Howie CA, Meredith PA, Kelman AW, Rasmussen HS, Hillis WS, Elliott HL. A dose-ranging study of UK-68,798, a novel class III anti-arrhythmic agent, in normal volunteers. Br J Clin Pharmacol 1991;32(4):429–32.
36. Le Coz F, Funck-Brentano C, Morell T, Ghadanfar MM, Jaillon P. Pharmacokinetic and pharmacodynamic modeling of the effects of oral and intravenous administrations of dofetilide on ventricular repolarization. Clin Pharmacol Ther 1995;57(5):533–42.
37. Walker DK, Alabaster CT, Congrave GS, Hargreaves MB, Hyland R, Jones BC, Reed LJ, Smith DA. Significance of metabolism in the disposition and action of the antidysrhythmic drug, dofetilide. In vitro studies and correlation with in vivo data. Drug Metab Dispos 1996;24(4):447–55.
38. Suttorp MJ, Polak PE, van't Hof A, Rasmussen HS, Dunselman PH, Kingma JH. Efficacy and safety of a new selective class III antiarrhythmic agent dofetilide in paroxysmal atrial fibrillation or atrial flutter. Am J Cardiol 1992;69(4):417–19.
39. Kobayashi Y, Atarashi H, Ino T, Kuruma A, Nomura A, Saitoh H, Hayakawa H. Clinical and electrophysiologic effects of dofetilide in patients with supraventricular tachyarrhythmias. J Cardiovasc Pharmacol 1997;30(3):367–73.
40. Cobbe SM, Campbell RW, Camm AJ, Nathan AW, Rowland E, Bloch-Thomsen PE, Moller M, Jordaens L. Effects of intravenous dofetilide on induction of atrioventricular re-entrant tachycardia. Heart 2001;86(5):522–6.
41. Sedgwick ML, Lip G, Rae AP, Cobbe SM. Chemical cardioversion of atrial fibrillation with intravenous dofetilide. Int J Cardiol 1995;49(2):159–66.
42. Frost L, Mortensen PE, Tingleff J, Platou ES, Christiansen EH, Christiansen N. Efficacy and safety of dofetilide, a new class III antiarrhythmic agent, in acute termination of atrial fibrillation or flutter after coronary artery bypass surgery. Dofetilide Post-CABG Study Group. Int J Cardiol 1997;58(2):135–40.
43. Falk RH, Pollak A, Singh SN, Friedrich T. Intravenous dofetilide, a class III antiarrhythmic agent, for the termination of sustained atrial fibrillation or flutter. Intravenous Dofetilide Investigators. J Am Coll Cardiol 1997;29(2):385–90.
44. Norgaard BL, Wachtell K, Christensen PD, Madsen B, Johansen JB, Christiansen EH, Graff O, Simonsen EH. Efficacy and safety of intravenously administered dofetilide in acute termination of artrial fibrillation and flutter: a multicenter, randomized, double-blind, placebo-controlled trial. Danish Dofetilide in Atrial Fibrillation and Flutter Study Group. Am Heart J 1999;137(6):1062–9.
45. Singh S, Zoble RG, Yellen L, Brodsky MA, Feld GK, Berk M, Billing CB Jr. Efficacy and safety of oral dofetilide in converting to and maintaining sinus rhythm in patients

with chronic atrial fibrillation or atrial flutter: the symptomatic atrial fibrillation investigative research on dofetilide (SAFIRE-D) study. Circulation 2000;102(19):2385–90.
46. Lindeboom JE, Kingma JH, Crijns HJ, Dunselman PH. Efficacy and safety of intravenous dofetilide for rapid termination of atrial fibrillation and atrial flutter. Am J Cardiol 2000;85(8):1031–3.
47. Krahn AD, Klein GJ, Yee R. A randomized, double-blind, placebo-controlled evaluation of the efficacy and safety of intravenously administered dofetilide in patients with Wolff–Parkinson–White syndrome. Pacing Clin Electrophysiol 2001;24(8 Pt 1):1258–60.
48. Echt DS, Lee JT, Murray KT, Vorperian V, Borganelli SM, Crawford DM, Friedrich T, Roden DM. A randomized, double-blind, placebo-controlled, dose-ranging study of dofetilide in patients with inducible sustained ventricular tachyarrhythmias. J Cardiovasc Electrophysiol 1995; 6(9):687–99.
49. Pool PE, Singh SN, Friedrich T. Effects of intravenous dofetilide in patients with frequent premature ventricular contractions: a clinical trial. Clin Cardiol 2000;23(6):415–16.
50. Danish Investigations of Arrhythmia and Mortality ON Dofetilide. Dofetilide in patients with left ventricular dysfunction and either heart failure or acute myocardial infarction: rationale, design, and patient characteristics of the DIAMOND studies. Clin Cardiol 1997;20(8):704–10.
51. Torp-Pedersen C, Moller M, Bloch-Thomsen PE, Kober L, Sandoe E, Egstrup K, Agner E, Carlsen J, Videbaek J, Marchant B, Camm AJ. Dofetilide in patients with congestive heart failure and left ventricular dysfunction. Danish Investigations of Arrhythmia and Mortality on Dofetilide Study Group. N Engl J Med 1999;341(12):857–65.
52. Kober L, Bloch Thomsen PE, Moller M, Torp-Pedersen C, Carlsen J, Sandoe E, Egstrup K, Agner E, Videbaek J, Marchant B, Camm AJ; Danish Investigations of Arrhythmia and Mortality on Dofetilide (DIAMOND) Study Group. Effect of dofetilide in patients with recent myocardial infarction and left-ventricular dysfunction: a randomised trial. Lancet 2000;356(9247):2052–8.
53. Bianconi L, Castro A, Dinelli M, Alboni P, Pappalardo A, Richiardi E, Santini M. Comparison of intravenously administered dofetilide versus amiodarone in the acute termination of atrial fibrillation and flutter. A multicentre, randomized, double-blind, placebo-controlled study. Eur Heart J 2000;21(15):1265–73.
54. Crijns HJ, Van Gelder IC, Kingma JH, Dunselman PH, Gosselink AT, Lie KI. Atrial flutter can be terminated by a class III antiarrhythmic drug but not by a class IC drug. Eur Heart J 1994;15(10):1403–8.
55. Tendera M, Wnuk-Wojnar AM, Kulakowski P, Malolepszy J, Kozlowski JW, Krzeminska-Pakula M, Szechinski J, Droszcz W, Kawecka-Jaszcz K, Swiatecka G, Ruzyllo W, Graff O. Efficacy and safety of dofetilide in the prevention of symptomatic episodes of paroxysmal supraventricular tachycardia: a 6-month double-blind comparison with propafenone and placebo. Am Heart J 2001;142(1):93–8.
56. Boriani G, Biffi M, Bacchi L, Martignani C, Zannoli R, Butrous GS, Branzi A. A randomised cross-over study on the haemodynamic effects of oral dofetilide compared with oral sotalol in patients with ischaemic heart disease and sustained ventricular tachycardia. Eur J Clin Pharmacol 2002;58(3):165–9.
57. Mazur A, Anderson ME, Bonney S, Roden DM. Pause-dependent polymorphic ventricular tachycardia during long-term treatment with dofetilide: a placebo-controlled, implantable cardioverter–defibrillator-based evaluation. J Am Coll Cardiol 2001;37(4):1100–5.
58. Deal BJ, Keane JF, Gillette PC, Garson A Jr. Wolff–Parkinson–White syndrome and supraventricular tachycardia during infancy: management and follow-up. J Am Coll Cardiol 1985;5(1):130–5.
59. Pfammatter JP, Stocker FP. Re-entrant supraventricular tachycardia in infancy: current role of prophylactic digoxin treatment. Eur J Pediatr 1998;157(2):101–6.
60. Norgaard BL, Wachtell K, Christensen PD, Madsen B, Johansen JB, Christiansen EH, Graff O, Simonsen EH. Efficacy and safety of intravenously administered dofetilide in acute termination of atrial fibrillation and flutter: a multicenter, randomized, double-blind, placebo-controlled trial. Danish Dofetilide in Atrial Fibrillation and Flutter Study Group. Am Heart J 1999;137(6):1062–9.
61. Sanatani S, Saul JP, Walsh EP, Gross GJ. Spontaneously terminating apparent ventricular fibrillation during transesophageal electrophysiological testing in infants with Wolff-Parkinson-White syndrome. Pacing Clin Electrophysiol 2001;24(12):1816–18.
62. Spodick DH. Well concealed atrial tachycardia with Wenckebach (Mobitz I) atrioventricular block: digitalis toxicity. Am J Geriatr Cardiol 2001;10(1):59.

Domperidone

General Information

Domperidone is a neuroleptic antiemetic, a dopamine receptor antagonist. It produces the expected range of dystonic and extrapyramidal adverse effects (1), which seem, as with metoclopramide, to be more likely to occur in children (2). It is difficult to accept that claims for lower frequencies than with metoclopramide are justified, particularly when one reads a report of neuroleptic malignant syndrome (3). Like its congeners, domperidone has repeatedly been shown to cause symptoms attributable to hyperprolactinemia (galactorrhea, amenorrhea, and breast tenderness), despite claims that there is a lower incidence of effects on prolactin concentrations. However, a study in patients with Parkinson's disease using domperidone did not suggest that the adverse effects are especially problematical in these patients (4).

Observational studies

The mechanism of action and clinical use of domperidone and its specific use in diabetic gastroparesis have been reviewed (5,6). Domperidone is generally well tolerated and has a low incidence of adverse effects. Adverse effects after oral administration include headache, dry mouth, diarrhea, itching, muscle cramps, and anxiety. Galactorrhea, breast tenderness, and pseudopregnancy can occur in women because of a dopamine-induced increase in serum prolactin concentration.

Comparative studies

The efficacy and adverse effects of domperidone and metoclopramide have been compared in a double-blind, multicenter, randomized trial in 93 insulin-dependent diabetics with symptomatic gastroparesis (7). Domperidone 20 mg qds and metoclopramide 10 mg qds, for 4 weeks, were equally effective in alleviating symptoms of gastroparesis. Somnolence, akathisia, anxiety, and depression were more severe with metoclopramide. Of the spontaneously reported adverse effects, nausea, vomiting, headache, insomnia, and diarrhea occurred in 6–10% of patients treated with domperidone and in up to 4% of patients treated with metoclopramide. The incidence of prolactin-related adverse effects was similar in the two groups (6%).

Organs and Systems

Cardiovascular

Intravenous infusion of domperidone, withdrawn some years ago, has caused convulsions and cardiac arrest (8–10).

Nervous system

- A 9-year-old child developed dysphagia and involuntary movements of the facial muscles after being treated with domperidone 0.25 mg/kg/day (11). There was complete recovery after withdrawal.

Drug–Drug Interactions

Anticholinergic drugs

Concomitant administration of anticholinergic drugs can antagonize the beneficial effects of domperidone (12).

Azole antifungals

Because domperidone is metabolized mainly by CYP3A4, interactions of azole antifungals with domperidone can occur. In human liver microsomes domperidone underwent hydroxylation to 5-hydroxydomperidone and N-dealkylation to 2,3-dihydro-2-oxo-1H-benzimidazole-1-propionic acid and 5-chloro-4-piperidinyl-1,3-dihydrobenzimidazol-2-one (13). The rate of domperidone metabolism correlated with the activity of CYP3A. Ketoconazole 1 μmol/l inhibited the metabolism of domperidone 5 μmol/l by 87%.

Cimetidine and antacids

Since cimetidine and antacids can interfere with the systemic availability of domperidone (SEDA-22, 389), they should not be co-administered.

Troleandomycin

In human liver microsomes domperidone underwent hydroxylation to 5-hydroxydomperidone and N-dealkylation to 2,3-dihydro-2-oxo-1H-benzimidazole-1-propionic acid and 5-chloro-4-piperidinyl-1,3-dihydro-benzimidazol-2-one. The rate of domperidone metabolism correlated with the activity of CYP3A. Troleandomycin 50 μmol/l inhibited the metabolism of domperidone 5 μmol/l by 64%.

References

1. Barone JA. Domperidone: a peripherally acting dopamine2-receptor antagonist. Ann Pharmacother 1999;33(4):429–40.
2. Pellegrino M, Sacco M, Lotti F. Sindrome extrapiramidale da moderato hiperdosaggio di domperidone. Descrizione di un caso. [Extrapyramidal syndrome caused by moderate overdosage of domperidone. Description of a case.] Pediatr Med Chir 1990;12(2):205–6.
3. Spirt MJ, Chan W, Thieberg M, Sachar DB. Neuroleptic malignant syndrome induced by domperidone. Dig Dis Sci 1992;37(6):946–8.
4. Soykan I, Sarosiek I, Shifflett J, Wooten GF, McCallum RW. Effect of chronic oral domperidone therapy on gastrointestinal symptoms and gastric emptying in patients with Parkinson's disease. Mov Disord 1997;12(6): 952–7.
5. Barone JA. Domperidone: mechanism of action and clinical use. Hosp Pharm 1998;33:191–7.
6. Prakash A, Wagstaff AJ. Domperidone. A review of its use in diabetic gastropathy. Drugs 1998;56(3):429–45.
7. Patterson D, Abell T, Rothstein R, Koch K, Barnett J. A double-blind multicenter comparison of domperidone and metoclopramide in the treatment of diabetic patients with symptoms of gastroparesis. Am J Gastroenterol 1999;94(5):1230–4.
8. Roussak JB, Carey P, Parry H. Cardiac arrest after treatment with intravenous domperidone. BMJ (Clin Res Ed) 1984;289(6458):1579.
9. Osborne RJ, Slevin ML, Hunter RW, Hamer J. Cardiac arrhythmias during cytotoxic chemotherapy: role of domperidone. Hum Toxicol 1985;4(6):617–26.
10. Anonymous. Sale of drug for cancer patients suspended due to side effects. Asahi Evening News (Tokyo), 1985.
11. Perez Blanco JL, Garcia Angleu F, Caceres Espejo J, Panadero Ruz Ma D. Extrapyramidal effects as a possible adverse reaction to domperidone. Rev Esp Pediatr 2000;56:189–92.
12. Greiff JM, Rowbotham D. Pharmacokinetic drug interactions with gastrointestinal motility modifying agents. Clin Pharmacokinet 1994;27(6):447–61.
13. Ward BA, Morocho A, Kandil A, Galinsky RE, Flockhart DA, Desta Z. Characterization of human cytochrome P450 enzymes catalyzing domperidone N-dealkylation and hydroxylation in vitro. Br J Clin Pharmacol 2004;58(3):277–87.

Donepezil

General Information

The approval of donepezil in several countries in America and Europe has been hailed as a major milestone, because it has met regulatory guidelines for the approval of anti-dementia drugs (1). Donepezil belongs to a piperidine class of reversible acetylcholinesterase inhibitors, chemically unrelated to either tacrine or physostigmine. It is highly specific for acetylcholinesterase and does not inhibit butyrylcholinesterase. The incidence of adverse effects with donepezil is comparable to that of placebo in controlled trials, and unlike tacrine, liver enzyme monitoring is not required. The long-term effectiveness of donepezil in large populations is yet to be established. Moreover, while it improves cognitive symptoms, it does not alter the course of the disease. Based on a limited number of studies, support for the use of donepezil in Alzheimer's disease has emerged (2–5).

Clinical trials of donepezil were funded by the manufacturer and appear to have been methodologically sound, although the absence of caregiver quality-of-life measures and outcomes related to activities of daily living is difficult to reconcile. An earlier 12-week study showed no improvement in caregiver quality of life with donepezil (4). As with most phase 3 studies, extrapolation of these results to routine practice is hampered by the fact that study populations are likely to be healthier than patients seen in routine clinical practice. Whether the results would be any different in a more heterogeneous population remains to be seen (6).

In a more recent 12-week double-blind, placebo-controlled, parallel-group study, aimed at establishing the efficacy and safety of donepezil in patients with mild to moderately severe Alzheimer's disease, donepezil (5 and 10 mg od) was well tolerated and efficacious (7). Adverse events significantly more common with donepezil were nausea, insomnia, and diarrhea, which appeared to be dose related and did not require treatment. Seven patients treated with placebo and six in each of the donepezil groups had serious adverse events during the trial. Three had events that were considered possibly related to donepezil. These included gastric ulceration with hemorrhage, syncope and a transient ischemic attack, nausea, aphakia, tremor, and sweating. Both groups of patients treated with donepezil had falls in mean heart rate that were larger than with placebo. Two patients treated with donepezil had electrocardiographic changes: one developed an intraventricular conduction defect and ventricular extra beats, while the other had sinus arrhythmia, left axis deviation, and increased QRS voltage, possibly secondary to left ventricular enlargement. Neither reported cardiovascular adverse events. Two patients taking placebo also had electrocardiographic abnormalities: one with bundle branch block, the other with sinus bradycardia and ventricular extra beats.

The launch of donepezil has attracted intense interest among both the scientific community and the public. The debate regarding "lessons for health care policy" (8) has been summarized:

(1) Licensing trials in highly selected patients may provide insignificant information on which to base clinical decisions, especially when the effect sizes are small and comorbidity is common.
(2) All trial evidence should be published before new drugs are marketed, and medical journals should not carry advertisements referring to unpublished data.
(3) Communication of benefits and risks should emphasize clinical effect sizes rather than statistical significance.
(4) Claims about effects on populations or services should be based on evidence.
(5) Secrecy surrounding licensing should be ended, and data from trials should be available for independent analysis.
(6) Overvaluation of new technology could threaten funding for vital but more mundane care.

There was intense debate in response to the above publication, as reflected by several letters to the Editor of the *British Medical Journal* (9–14).

Further evidence that donepezil is effective and well tolerated in treating symptoms of mild to moderately severe Alzheimer's disease has emerged from a multinational trial (15). Common adverse effects were nausea, vomiting, diarrhea, anorexia, dizziness, and confusion, consistent with previous findings.

A meta-analysis of various drugs approved for treating Alzheimer's disease in the USA and Canada has suggested that donepezil can delay cognitive impairment and deterioration in global health for at least 6 months in patients with mild-to-moderate Alzheimer's disease (16). Patients taking active treatment will have more favorable Alzheimer's Disease Assessment Scale cognitive subscale (ADAS-cog) scores for at least 6 months, after which their scores will begin to converge with those who are taking placebo. The cost-effectiveness data were inconclusive.

Although once-daily donepezil is effective and well tolerated for the symptoms of mild-to-moderate Alzheimer's disease (17), two practical questions arise:

(1) Which patients are too severely affected to be treated with donepezil?
(2) At what point should donepezil be discontinued if the patient continues to deteriorate?

The current status of donepezil in the management of Alzheimer's disease has been comprehensively reviewed (18). Several recent studies have confirmed the efficacy and tolerability of donepezil using different doses, study designs, and durations of treatment (19–23). Some relevant conclusions were the following:

(1) Younger patients should be targeted for assessment and treatment (24).
(2) Of the patients 6% discontinued medication owing to adverse events (23).
(3) Sleep disturbances were more common in trials with bedtime dosing of donepezil (22).
(4) Long-term safety and realistic improvement were observed over a period of up to 4.9 years (25).
(5) The presence of the apolipoprotein E4 allele did not predict donepezil failure (20).

Seven elderly patients with psychotic or non-psychotic behavioral symptoms in Lewy body dementia had some benefit from donepezil (26). Donepezil was withdrawn prematurely in three patients owing to poor response and/or adverse events. The adverse events were sedation, somnolence, worsening of chronic obstructive pulmonary disease, syncope, sweating, and bradycardia. These results have to be confirmed in controlled trials.

In two patients with Alzheimer's disease, donepezil provided some benefit in relieving cognitive symptoms, but there were increased behavioral problems, such as anxiety, agitation, irritability, and lack of impulse control; these were then successfully controlled by adding gabapentin (27).

The adverse effects of donepezil in general practice have been evaluated in a post-marketing pharmacovigilance study in 1762 patients in the UK (28). This observational cohort study used the technique of prescription-event monitoring for a minimum period of 6 months. The commonest adverse events were nausea, diarrhea, malaise, dizziness, and insomnia. Aggression, agitation, and abnormal dreams were uncommonly associated with the drug. There were no causally associated cardiac rhythm disturbances or liver disorders. The authors suggested that the abnormal dreams and psychiatric disturbances were possible adverse drug reactions that require further confirmation.

The beneficial effect of donepezil on global ratings of dementia symptoms, cognition, and activities of daily living has been confirmed (29,30). Donepezil was to be well tolerated for periods up to 1 year, and adverse events were usually mild and transient, lasted only an initial few days, and typically resolved without the need for dosage modification. It has been suggested that patients with Alzheimer's disease do best while taking donepezil 10 mg/day and when the dosage is maintained at that level without interruption. Donepezil treatment effects that are lost after prolonged withdrawal do not fully recover when the drug is restarted (31).

Organs and Systems

Cardiovascular

Symptomatic sinus bradycardia is a possible adverse effect of treatment with donepezil in Alzheimer's disease (32).

- An 84-year-old patient with hypertensive cardiomyopathy developed bradycardia, fainting, and left-sided heart failure 3 weeks after starting treatment with donepezil. When donepezil was withdrawn, the sinus bradycardia disappeared; 24-hour electrocardiography showed no signs of sinus node disease, and no episodes of this type recurred during the next 6 months.

It is important to emphasize that disorders of cardiac rhythm associated with the use of donepezil are extremely unusual.

Nervous system

Convulsions have been reported during treatment with donepezil (33).

- A patient with mild Alzheimer's disease taking donepezil, 5 mg/day for 2 weeks and then 10 mg/day for 23 days, was admitted with convulsions. His only other medication was aspirin 100 mg/day. Blood analysis was normal, and a computerized tomographic (CT) scan showed a mild degree of cortical atrophy with no structural lesions. Donepezil was withdrawn, and no other drug treatment was given. Six weeks later, donepezil 5 mg/day was restarted. On day 52, he developed loss of consciousness and convulsions, necessitating withdrawal of donepezil.

Convulsions in Alzheimer's disease are very rare until late in the illness, and the authors attributed this patient's convulsions to donepezil.

Restless legs, mumbling, and stuttering have been reported in a patient taking donepezil (34). According to the Naranjo probability scale, the causality was probable, since rechallenge was positive.

Extrapyramidal effects have been reported in three patients taking donepezil; in two cases, the effects disappeared when donepezil was withdrawn (35).

Psychological, psychiatric

Behavioral worsening in seven patients with Alzheimer's disease after the start of donepezil therapy has been described (36). Their mean age was 76 years, and their mean score on the Mini-Mental State Examination was 18. Five patients had had dementia-related delusions and irritability before taking donepezil, one had had a history of major depression, and another had had a history of somatization disorder. At the start of treatment with donepezil, four were taking sertraline, one paroxetine, one venlafaxine, and four risperidone. All took donepezil 5 mg/day, and after 4–6 weeks the dosage in five patients was increased to 10 mg/day. In the other two cases, donepezil was discontinued after 5 weeks: in one case because of gastrointestinal symptoms and in the other because of increasing agitation. After an average of 7.3 (range 1–13) weeks after starting donepezil, all seven patients had a recurrence of previous behavioral problems. Five became agitated, one became depressed, and the other became more anxious and somatically preoccupied. The pattern of behavioral change involves regression to an earlier behavioral problem.

Violent behavior has been described with donepezil (37).

- A 76-year-old man who was taking oxybutynin 3 mg tds for bladder instability took donepezil 5 mg/day for presumed Alzheimer's disease and 5 days later became very paranoid, believing that his wife had been stealing his money. He beat her and held her hostage in their house with a knife until their daughter intervened. He was given haloperidol 0.5 mg bd, and donepezil and oxybutynin were withdrawn. His paranoid ideation resolved within a few days and did not recur despite withdrawal of haloperidol.

Although a causal relation between this violent incident and donepezil cannot be proved, the temporal relation was suggestive.

Liver

Donepezil has not been associated with hepatotoxic effects, which is a distinct advantage over tacrine. Donepezil treatment benefit persisted over 98 weeks, with no evidence of hepatotoxicity (38).

Urinary tract

Urinary incontinence may often be disregarded as a manifestation of dementia, but it has also been attributed to donepezil.

Of 94 patients with mild-to-moderate disease treated with recommended dosages of donepezil (3 mg/day during the first week and then 5 mg/day), 7 developed urinary incontinence (39). In five of them, the incontinence was transient, and there was no need to change the prescription. Incontinence occurred in both sexes, in relatively young and old patients, and in those with very mild-to-moderate dementia. In six patients the incontinence occurred at the higher dosage of 5 mg/day, in one patient it disappeared when donepezil was withdrawn, and in another an increase in dosage caused the reappearance of incontinence, suggesting a likely causal, dose-dependent relation between donepezil and urinary incontinence.

Urinary incontinence in patients with Down syndrome treated with donepezil has been described before (40). Urinary incontinence can be a major concern and a source of distress, not only for patients but also for caregivers. Clinicians should be alert to the possibility of urinary incontinence when prescribing donepezil for individuals with Alzheimer's disease. The authors emphasized that the incontinence may often be transient and not serious, but it could limit a patient's activities and quality of life and could also affect therapeutic adherence.

Skin

A purpuric rash associated with donepezil has been reported (41).

- An 82-year-old woman with hypertension, taking long-term atenolol and doxazosin, developed moderate cognitive impairment attributed to Alzheimer's disease. She was given donepezil 5 mg/day and, after 4 days, developed diarrhea, vomiting, and a purpuric rash on her trunk, arms, and legs. Platelet counts were 119–157 × 10^9/l. Donepezil was withdrawn, with resolution of the gastrointestinal symptoms.

Donepezil was the probable cause of this rash, because of the temporal association with treatment and its recurrence on rechallenge.

Susceptibility Factors

Other features of the patient

Three patients with Alzheimer's disease associated with Down syndrome were treated with donepezil (40). One became agitated and aggressive; the other two developed urinary incontinence. In all three cases donepezil was withdrawn. These results are important, because many individuals with Down syndrome develop clinical and neuropathological evidence of Alzheimer's disease after the age of 40 years. Also, patients with Down syndrome were excluded from donepezil clinical trials. Therefore, lesser data on the efficacy or safety of donepezil are available for this population.

Drug Administration

Drug overdose

Two cases of donepezil overdose have been reported (42,43).

- A 79-year-old nursing home patient was given donepezil 50 mg in error. She developed nausea, vomiting, and persistent bradycardia—typical cholinergic adverse effects. She was treated with atropine, 0.2 mg as needed, for bradycardia (total dose 3 mg over 18 hours) and was discharged on the second day.
- A 74-year-old woman with a history of stroke, myocardial infarction, hypothyroidism, and probable multi-infarct dementia took nine donepezil tablets (a total dose of 45 mg). She developed nausea and vomiting 2 hours later. She fell asleep for 4–5 hours but remained rousable. About 9 hours after ingestion, she became flushed and had a bout of diarrhea. Donepezil was withdrawn for 3 days, and there were no adverse effects when it was reintroduced.

Drug–Drug Interactions

Neostigmine

An additive inhibitory effect of donepezil and neostigmine on acetylcholinesterase has been proposed to explain prolonged neuromuscular blockade during anesthesia in an 85-year-old woman taking donepezil (44).

Paroxetine

A possible interaction between donepezil and paroxetine has been described (45).

- Two elderly patients with Alzheimer's disease and a mood disorder were treated with donepezil 5 mg/day and paroxetine 20 mg/day. One of them became agitated, confused, and aggressive, and donepezil was withdrawn after 8 days. On reintroduction of donepezil she again became rapidly confused, irritable, and verbally aggressive. In the other case, while the patient was taking paroxetine, donepezil 5 mg/day resulted in severe diarrhea, flatulence, and insomnia. The dosage of donepezil was reduced to 5 mg on alternate days, but the diarrhea and flatulence persisted. The symptoms resolved when donepezil was stopped.

Donepezil is metabolized in the liver by CYP2D6 and CYP3A4. Selective serotonin re-uptake inhibitors (SSRIs), such as paroxetine, are potent inhibitors of CYP2D6. Mood disorders are common in patients with Alzheimer's disease, and SSRIs are used in these patients and can increase the plasma concentration of donepezil, increasing the risk of severe adverse reactions.

Risperidone

Extrapyramidal effects occurred in a patient who took donepezil and risperidone concurrently (46). Although risperidone is less likely than conventional antipsychotic drugs to cause extrapyramidal effects, and is therefore particularly useful for older patients who are very susceptible to developing extrapyramidal disturbances, an increase in brain acetylcholine resulting from donepezil, along with dopamine receptor blockade by risperidone, would have led to an imbalance between cholinergic and dopaminergic systems. Although a clinically significant interaction between donepezil and risperidone seems to be rare, clinicians should be alert to such a possibility.

Tiapride

Parkinsonism has been reported in a patient concurrently taking donepezil and tiapride, probably through a pharmacodynamic interaction (47).

References

1. Whitehouse PJ. Donepezil. Drugs Today (Barc) 1998;34(4):321–6.
2. Barner EL, Gray SL. Donepezil use in Alzheimer disease. Ann Pharmacother 1998;32(1):70–7.
3. Peruche B, Schulz M. Donepezil—a new agent against Alzheimer's disease. Pharm Ztg 1998;143:38–42.

4. Rogers SL, Friedhoff LT, Apter JT, Richter RW, Hartford JT, Walshe TM, Baumel B, Linden RD, Kinney FC, Doody RS, Borison RL, Ahem GL. The efficacy and safety of donepezil in patients with Alzheimer's disease: results of a US multicentre, randomized, double-blind, placebo-controlled trial. The Donepezil Study Group. Dementia 1996;7(6):293–303.
5. Rogers SL, Farlow MR, Doody RS, Mohs R, Friedhoff LT. A 24-week, double-blind, placebo-controlled trial of donepezil in patients with Alzheimer's disease. Donepezil Study Group. Neurology 1998;50(1):136–45.
6. Warner JP. Commentary on donepezil. Evid Based Med 1998;3:155.
7. Rogers SL, Doody RS, Mohs RC, Friedhoff LT. Donepezil improves cognition and global function in Alzheimer disease: a 15-week, double-blind, placebo-controlled study. Donepezil Study Group. Arch Intern Med 1998;158(9):1021–31.
8. Melzer D. New drug treatment for Alzheimer's disease: lessons for healthcare policy. BMJ 1998;316(7133):762–4.
9. Dening T, Lawton C. New drug treatment for Alzheimer's disease. Doctors want to offer more than sympathy. BMJ 1998;317(7163):945.
10. Levy R. New drug treatment for Alzheimer's disease. Effects of drugs can be variable. BMJ 1998;317(7163):945.
11. Evans M. New drug treatment for Alzheimer's disease. Drugs should not need to show cost effectiveness to justify their prescription. BMJ 1998;317(7163):945–6.
12. Johnstone P. New drug treatment for Alzheimer's disease. Information from unpublished trials should be made available. BMJ 1998;317(7163):946.
13. Zamar AC, Wise ME, Watson JP. New drug treatment for Alzheimer's disease. Treatment with metrifonate warrants multicentre trials. BMJ 1998;317(7163):946.
14. Baxter T, Black D, Prempeh H. New drug treatment for Alzheimer's disease. SMAC's advice on use of donepezil is contradictory. BMJ 1998;317(7163):946.
15. Burns A, Rossor M, Hecker J, Gauthier S, Petit H, Moller HJ, Rogers SL, Friedhoff LT. The effects of donepezil in Alzheimer's disease—results from a multinational trial. Dement Geriatr Cogn Disord 1999;10(3):237–44.
16. Wolfson C, Oremus M, Shukla V, Momoli F, Demers L, Perrault A, Moride Y. Donepezil and rivastigmine in the treatment of Alzheimer's disease: a best-evidence synthesis of the published data on their efficacy and cost-effectiveness. Clin Ther 2002;24(6):862–86.
17. Doody RS. Clinical profile of donepezil in the treatment of Alzheimer's disease. Gerontology 1999;45(Suppl 1):23–32.
18. Dooley M, Lamb HM. Donepezil: a review of its use in Alzheimer's disease. Drugs Aging 2000;16(3):199–226.
19. Cameron I, Curran S, Newton P, Petty D, Wattis J. Use of donepezil for the treatment of mild–moderate Alzheimer's disease: an audit of the assessment and treatment of patients in routine clinical practice. Int J Geriatr Psychiatry 2000;15(10):887–91.
20. Greenberg SM, Tennis MK, Brown LB, Gomez-Isla T, Hayden DL, Schoenfeld DA, Walsh KL, Corwin C, Daffner KR, Friedman P, Meadows ME, Sperling RA, Growdon JH. Donepezil therapy in clinical practice: a randomized crossover study. Arch Neurol 2000;57(1):94–9.
21. Homma A, Takeda M, Imai Y, Udaka F, Hasegawa K, Kameyama M, Nishimura T. Clinical efficacy and safety of donepezil on cognitive and global function in patients with Alzheimer's disease. A 24-week, multicenter, double-blind, placebo-controlled study in Japan. E2020 Study Group. Dement Geriatr Cogn Disord 2000;11(6):299–313.
22. Knopman DS. Management of cognition and function: new results from the clinical trials programme of Aricept® (donepezil HCl). Int J Neuropsychopharmacol 2000;3(7):13–20.
23. Matthews HP, Korbey J, Wilkinson DG, Rowden J. Donepezil in Alzheimer's disease: eighteen month results from Southampton Memory Clinic. Int J Geriatr Psychiatry 2000;15(8):713–20.
24. Evans M, Ellis A, Watson D, Chowdhury T. Sustained cognitive improvement following treatment of Alzheimer's disease with donepezil. Int J Geriatr Psychiatry 2000;15(1):50–3.
25. Rogers SL, Doody RS, Pratt RD, Ieni JR. Long-term efficacy and safety of donepezil in the treatment of Alzheimer's disease: final analysis of a US multicentre open-label study. Eur Neuropsychopharmacol 2000;10(3):195–203.
26. Lanctot KL, Herrmann N. Donepezil for behavioural disorders associated with Lewy bodies: a case series. Int J Geriatr Psychiatry 2000;15(4):338–45.
27. Dallocchio C, Buffa C, Mazzarello P. Combination of donepezil and gabapentin for behavioral disorders in Alzheimer's disease. J Clin Psychiatry 2000;61(1):64.
28. Dunn NR, Pearce GL, Shakir SA. Adverse effects associated with the use of donepezil in general practice in England. J Psychopharmacol 2000;14(4):406–8.
29. Mohs RC, Doody RS, Morris JC, Ieni JR, Rogers SL, Perdomo CA, Pratt RD; "312" Study Group. A 1-year, placebo-controlled preservation of function survival study of donepezil in AD patients. Neurology 2001;57(3):481–8.
30. Winblad B, Engedal K, Soininen H, Verhey F, Waldemar G, Wimo A, Wetterholm AL, Zhang R, Haglund A, Subbiah P; Donepezil Nordic Study Group. A 1-year, randomized, placebo-controlled study of donepezil in patients with mild to moderate AD. Neurology 2001;57(3):489–95.
31. Doody RS, Geldmacher DS, Gordon B, Perdomo CA, Pratt RD; Donepezil Nordic Study Group. Open-label, multicenter, phase 3 extension study of the safety and efficacy of donepezil in patients with Alzheimer disease. Arch Neurol 2001;58(3):427–33.
32. Calvo-Romero JM, Ramos-Salado JL. Bradycardia sinusal sintomatica associada a donepecilo. [Symptomatic sinus bradycardia associated with donepezil.] Rev Neurol 1999;28(11):1070–2.
33. Babic T, Zurak N. Convulsions induced by donepezil. J Neurol Neurosurg Psychiatry 1999;66(3):410.
34. Amouyal-Barkate K, Bagheri-Charabiani H, Montastruc JL, Moulias S, Vellas B. Abnormal movements with donepezil in Alzheimer disease. Ann Pharmacother 2000;34(11):1347.
35. Carcenac D, Martin-Hunyadi C, Kiesmann M, Demuynck-Roegel C, Alt M, Kuntzmann F. Syndrome extrapyramidal sous donepezil. [Extra-pyramidal syndrome induced by donepezil.] Presse Méd 2000;29(18):992–3.
36. Wengel SP, Roccaforte WH, Burke WJ, Bayer BL, McNeilly DP, Knop D. Behavioral complications associated with donepezil. Am J Psychiatry 1998;155(11):1632–3.
37. Bouman WP, Pinner G. Violent behavior associated with donepezil. Am J Psychiatry 1998;155(11):1626–7.
38. Rogers SL, Friedhoff LT. Long-term efficacy and safety of donepezil in the treatment of Alzheimer's disease: an interim analysis of the results of a US multicentre open label extension study. Eur Neuropsychopharmacol 1998;8(1):67–75.
39. Hashimoto M, Imamura T, Tanimukai S, Kazui H, Mori E. Urinary incontinence: an unrecognised adverse effect with donepezil. Lancet 2000;356(9229):568.
40. Hemingway-Eltomey JM, Lerner AJ. Adverse effects of donepezil in treating Alzheimer's disease associated with Down's syndrome. Am J Psychiatry 1999;156(9):1470.
41. Bryant CA, Ouldred E, Jackson SH, Kinirons MT. Purpuric rash with donepezil treatment. BMJ 1998;317(7161):787.

42. Shepherd G, Klein-Schwartz W, Edwards R. Donepezil overdose: a tenfold dosing error. Ann Pharmacother 1999;33(7–8):812–15.
43. Greene YM, Noviasky J, Tariot PN. Donepezil overdose. J Clin Psychiatry 1999;60(1):56–7.
44. Sprung J, Castellani WJ, Srinivasan V, Udayashankar S. The effects of donepezil and neostigmine in a patient with unusual pseudocholinesterase activity. Anesth Analg 1998;87(5):1203–5.
45. Carrier L. Donepezil and paroxetine: possible drug interaction. J Am Geriatr Soc 1999;47(8):1037.
46. Magnuson TM, Keller BK, Burke WJ. Extrapyramidal side effects in a patient treated with risperidone plus donepezil. Am J Psychiatry 1998;155(10):1458–9.
47. Arai M. Parkinsonism onset in a patient concurrently using tiapride and donepezil. Intern Med 2000;39(10):863.

Dopamine

General Information

Dopamine is a naturally occurring catecholamine and central neurotransmitter capable of raising cardiac output, reducing peripheral resistance, and specifically increasing renal blood flow. Infusions (generally up to 10 micrograms/kg/hour) have proven valuable in shock and congestive heart failure.

Common adverse reactions during infusion include extra beats, tachycardia, and palpitation. Angina pectoris, bradycardia, altered cardiac conduction, nausea and vomiting, headache, and dyspnea can occur. Piloerection and uremia have been reported and blood pressure can either rise or fall.

Organs and Systems

Cardiovascular

The major risk during dopamine treatment is that of severe peripheral ischemia, particularly in patients in whom the peripheral circulation is already impaired, since dopamine is converted to noradrenaline; gangrene has repeatedly resulted. In some of the reported cases the error lay in extravasation of dopamine from a peripheral venous infusion site; in others the dosage had been high and prolonged, or ergometrine had also been given. In cases of pre-existing vascular damage from arteriosclerosis, diabetes, Raynaud's disease, or frostbite, particular care must be taken. If discoloration appears, the infusion should be stopped and phentolamine 5–10 mg given intravenously. Nitroprusside may fail to prevent the onset of gangrene.

Nervous system

In one case, dopamine was considered to have produced myoclonic encephalopathy (1).

Hematologic

When used to treat low-output congestive heart failure, dopamine can inhibit platelet aggregation, in contrast to the platelet-aggregating properties of many catecholamines (2).

Susceptibility Factors

Other features of the patient

For obvious reasons, the use of dopamine may be dangerous in cases of coronary or peripheral vascular disorders. Dopamine used for hypotension during percutaneous transluminal angioplasty (PTCA) can be associated with diffuse coronary spasm, and it should therefore be used with caution, particularly if high doses are required. When dopamine aggravates pulmonary hypertension and right ventricular failure, isoprenaline should be considered as an alternative inotropic drug.

Drug–Drug Interactions

Alkali

Dopamine is unstable in the presence of alkalis (3). It should not be infused in bicarbonate solutions.

Cyclopropane and halogenated hydrocarbon anesthetics

In the nucleus accumbens of rats the dopamine concentration was increased by both cyclopropane and halothane anesthesia; cyclopropane, but not halothane, also increased the dopamine concentration in the caudate nucleus halothane, but not cyclopropane, significantly reduced the dopamine concentration in the ventral nucleus of the thalamus (4). It has been suggested that potentiation of the actions of dopamine could occur with cyclopropane or halogenated hydrocarbon anesthetics, but there is no direct evidence that this interaction occurs in humans.

Monoamine oxidase inhibitors

The hypertensive effect of dopamine is potentiated by monoamine oxidase inhibitors.

- A 75-year-old man who was taking selegiline 5 mg bd for Parkinson's disease was given an intravenous infusion of dopamine for reduced urine output and hypotension (5). Within minutes of starting the infusion, his systolic blood pressure rose from 105 to 228 mmHg. Similar reactions occurred during two subsequent rechallenges.

The authors proposed that selegiline may have caused this effect by inhibiting dopamine metabolism, and that selegiline may not be as specific an inhibitor of monoamine oxidase type B as previously thought.

References

1. Boudouresques G, Tafani B, Benichou M, Sarlon R. Encéphalopathie myoclonique à la dopamine. [Myoclonal encephalopathy due to dopamine.] Sem Hop 1982;58(46):2729–30.
2. Smith RE, Briggs B, Unverferth DV, Leier CV. Dobutamine-induced inhibition of platelet function. Intensive Care Med 1982;8:155.

3. Lee CY, Mauro VF, Alexander KS. Visual and spectrophotometric determination of compatibility of alteplase and streptokinase with other injectable drugs. Am J Hosp Pharm 1990;47(3):606–8.
4. Roizen MF, Kopin IJ, Zivin J, Muth EA, Jacobowitz DM. The effect of two anesthetic agents on norepinephrine and dopamine in discrete brain nuclei, fiber tracts, and terminal regions of the rat. Brain Res 1976;110(3):515–22.
5. Rose LM, Ohlinger MJ, Mauro VF. A hypertensive reaction induced by concurrent use of selegiline and dopamine. Ann Pharmacother 2000;34(9):1020–4.

Dopexamine

General Information

Dopexamine, which is related structurally to dopamine, is a potent beta$_2$-adrenoceptor agonist (1). Its reported adverse effects include cases of atrial fibrillation and single instances of supraventricular tachycardia and hypotension.

Reference

1. Fitton A, Benfield P. Dopexamine hydrochloride. A review of its pharmacodynamic and pharmacokinetic properties and therapeutic potential in acute cardiac insufficiency. Drugs 1990;39:308–30.

Dornase alfa

General Information

Dornase alfa is human recombinant deoxyribonuclease. Daily therapy with dornase alfa in patients with cystic fibrosis can reduce the frequency of respiratory infections and improve lung function in patients with bronchiectasis.

Therapeutic studies

The role of dornase alfa in modifying bronchial secretions in patients with cystic fibrosis has been evaluated in 54 subjects aged 5 years or over (1). They were treated for 12 months with mesna by nebulizer bd and oral ambroxol (30 mg bd). Dornase alfa was then given once daily by aerosol 2.5 mg for 12 months. Mesna and ambroxol caused reductions in FEV_1 and FVC (FEV_1 fell by 11%, FVC by 13%). After 12 months of dornase alfa, FEV_1 had increased by 7.7% and FVC by 5.3%. The patients found treatment with dornase alfa more acceptable than mucolytic therapy. Hemoptysis was the only reported adverse effect, but it occurred frequently in only one patient.

The effect of daily nebulized dornase for 24 weeks has been studied in a randomized, double-blind, placebo-controlled trial in 349 patients with idiopathic bronchiectasis (2). Three patients withdrew from the trial; two in the placebo group (hemoptysis and sinusitis) and one in the treatment group (increased sputum production, probably an adverse event). The primary outcome measures were the number of infective exacerbations and a fall in FEV_1. There were more exacerbations in the treatment group, with a relative risk of 1.35 (not statistically significant). The rate of fall in FEV_1 and FVC was significantly higher in the treatment group than in the placebo group, and the treatment group required more days of antibiotics and corticosteroids. Four patients died during the study, three in the treatment group. No deaths were considered to have been due to the treatment. Adverse events occurred equally in both groups, the commonest being non-specific respiratory disorders (10% in the placebo group and 15% in the treatment group). No other adverse events were detailed. These results suggest that dornase is not effective in patients with idiopathic bronchiectasis and may even be detrimental. Dornase should not be used in these patients.

References

1. Derelle J, Bertolo-Houriez E, Marchal F, Weber M, Virion JM, Vidailhet M. Evolution réspiratoire de patients atteints de mucoviscidose traités par mucofluidifiants puis par dornase alfa. [Respiratory evolution of patient with mucoviscidosis treated with mucolytic agents plus dornase alfa.] Arch Pediatr 1998;5(4):371–7.
2. O'Donnell AE, Barker AF, Ilowite JS, Fick RB. Treatment of idiopathic bronchiectasis with aerosolized recombinant human DNase I. rhDNase Study Group. Chest 1998;113(5):1329–34.

Dosulepin

See also Tricyclic antidepressants

General Information

Dosulepin (dothiepin) is a tricyclic antidepressant that has been available in Europe for over 30 years and is particularly popular in the UK. Its animal and clinical pharmacology has been described in an extensive review (1). It appears to be equivalent to amitriptyline, although few studies have reported dosages above 225 mg/day. Dosulepin is as effective and sedative as amitriptyline, with somewhat fewer anticholinergic adverse effects in several studies. However, it does not appear to have been compared with other less sedative or anticholinergic tricyclic compounds or second-generation drugs. Although it is claimed to have fewer cardiovascular effects, this has not been well substantiated in controlled comparative studies, and the cardiovascular and other effects of overdosage appear to be identical for all tricyclic compounds. Fetal tachydysrhythmias were believed to be caused by maternal ingestion of dosulepin (2).

References

1 Goldstein BJ, Claghorn JL. An overview of seventeen years of experience with dothiepin in the treatment of depression in Europe. J Clin Psychiatry 1980;41(12 Pt 2):64–70.
2 Prentice A, Brown R. Fetal tachyarrhythmia and maternal antidepressant treatment. BMJ 1989;298(6667):190.

Doxacurium chloride

See also Neuromuscular blocking drugs

General Information

Doxacurium chloride is a long-acting non-depolarizing neuromuscular blocking agent. It is a bisquaternary benzylisoquinolinium derivative (a diester). It is subject to minimal hydrolysis by plasma cholinesterase (at about 6% of the rate of hydrolysis of suxamethonium when incubated with purified pooled human plasma cholinesterase) (1). Antagonism by edrophonium (1 mg/kg) was considered inadequate in one study, whereas no difficulties were experienced with neostigmine (0.05 mg/kg) (2).

Organs and Systems

Cardiovascular

No rise in plasma histamine concentration was found with bolus doses up to 0.08 mg/kg (1), but in one case there was transient hypotension 1 minute after a bolus dose of 0.05 mg/kg via a pulmonary artery cannula, with cutaneous flushing at 2 minutes, suggesting that histamine release can occur on occasion (3). There was no tachycardia or bronchospasm, but the mean arterial pressure fell from 88 to 40 mmHg and recovered with therapy within 3 minutes, by which time the skin flushing was fading.

In a study of 54 patients, plasma histamine concentrations increased by 200% following doxacurium in two patients, but there were no changes in heart rate or blood pressure (4). Indeed, cardiovascular stability has been reported in several studies (1,4) and only minor clinically insignificant changes have been seen with doses up to 0.08 mg/kg, even in cardiac patients (AHA classes III–IV) (5,6).

Bradycardia is occasionally seen (2), but this may be due to co-administration of vagotonic drugs with atracurium, vecuronium, and pipecuronium.

Susceptibility Factors

Renal disease

Renal excretion is the main route of elimination of doxacurium, and its duration of action would be expected to be prolonged in patients with renal dysfunction. There have been two reports of the use of doxacurium in patients with chronic renal insufficiency. In the first it was reported that the action of doxacurium (0.025 mg/kg bolus dose) was "markedly but not statistically prolonged"; the mean time to 25% recovery of the twitch height was 121 minutes in the group of patients with renal insufficiency as opposed to 67 minutes in the control group, with great interindividual variation in both groups (7). The second was a study of the pharmacokinetics and pharmacodynamics of doxacurium in patients undergoing cadaveric kidney or liver transplantation (8). The duration of action of doxacurium was more variable and greatly prolonged in patients with end-stage renal insufficiency, although once again the results were clinically but not statistically significant, because of the small numbers of patients and large variability. Plasma clearance was significantly slower and mean residence time significantly greater in the renal transplant group than in control patients. In the patients with liver disease there were no significant pharmacokinetic changes, but the duration of action of the low dose used (15 mg/kg) did tend to be somewhat prolonged.

References

1. Basta SJ, Savarese JJ, Ali HH, Embree PB, Schwartz AF, Rudd GD, Wastila WB. Clinical pharmacology of doxacurium chloride. A new long-acting nondepolarizing muscle relaxant. Anesthesiology 1988;69(4):478–86.
2. Scott RP, Norman J. Doxacurium chloride: a preliminary clinical trial. Br J Anaesth 1989;62(4):373–7.
3. Reich DL. Transient systemic arterial hypotension and cutaneous flushing in response to doxacurium chloride. Anesthesiology 1989;71(5):783–5.
4. Murray DJ, Mehta MP, Choi WW, Forbes RB, Sokoll MD, Gergis SD, Rudd GD, Abou-Donia MM. The neuromuscular blocking and cardiovascular effects of doxacurium chloride in patients receiving nitrous oxide narcotic anesthesia. Anesthesiology 1988;69(4):472–7.
5. Stoops CM, Curtis CA, Kovach DA, McCammon RL, Stoelting RK, Warren TM, Miller D, Abou-Donia MM. Hemodynamic effects of doxacurium chloride in patients receiving oxygen sufentanil anesthesia for coronary artery bypass grafting or valve replacement. Anesthesiology 1988;69(3):365–70.
6. Reich DL, Konstadt SN, Thys DM, Hillel Z, Raymond R, Kaplan JA. Effects of doxacurium chloride on biventricular cardiac function in patients with cardiac disease. Br J Anaesth 1989;63(6):675–81.
7. Cashman JN, Luke JJ, Jones RM. Neuromuscular block with doxacurium (BW A938U) in patients with normal or absent renal function. Br J Anaesth 1990;64(2):186–92.
8. Cook DR, Freeman JA, Lai AA, Robertson KA, Kang Y, Stiller RL, Aggarwal S, Abou-Donia MM, Welch RM. Pharmacokinetics and pharmacodynamics of doxacurium in normal patients and in those with hepatic or renal failure. Anesth Analg 1991;72(2):145–50.

Doxapram

General Information

Generalized stimulation of the central nervous system has been observed with doxapram, particularly in large doses. Adverse reactions have included hyperactivity, tachycardia, increased deep tendon reflexes and muscle twitching, and laryngospasm. Raised blood pressure can also occur.

Doxapram is contraindicated in epilepsy and other convulsive disorders and in hypertension. Doxapram has been used to treat post-anesthetic shivering; in one study it was effective (1).

Adverse effects of doxapram are not long-lasting, because of its short half-life of 2–4 hours.

In seven patients treated with doxapram after anesthesia, the adverse effects were not serious and comprised excessive coughing, weeping, muscle tremor, nausea, and hysterical reactions to dreams. However, sweating, excessive salivation, and vomiting were noted in the control patients, and the authors concluded that recovery was smoother with doxapram.

There was a very high incidence of adverse reactions, such as hot flushes, sweating, hyperventilation, tremor, nausea, and vertigo, in postoperative analgesia combined with doxapram 1 mg/kg (2).

In a controlled study of the use of doxapram infusion for late postoperative hypoxemia (3) three of nine patients who received doxapram had an adverse event, compared with none of the placebo patients. In 18 patients there was a significant trend toward higher mean oxygen saturation in the doxapram group and a significantly higher minimum oxygen saturation and reduced number of hypoxemic events on the first postoperative night. The authors concluded that although the results were promising, continuous nocturnal postoperative doxapram infusion should be postponed until there is more information about its pharmacokinetics in this condition.

The effects of doxapram given enterally or intravenously have been studied in a prospective randomized trial in 15 infants with apnea of prematurity who had not responded to caffeine (4). Of the nine infants randomized to receive enteral treatment, five had to be changed to intravenous treatment, largely owing to doxapram-induced upper gastrointestinal symptoms (vomiting and large gastric residuals). Doxapram significantly reduced the frequency of attacks of apnea and associated bradycardia and hypoxia in 82% of the infants. The major adverse event was feeding intolerance in one-third of infants given enteral treatment. This resolved when doxapram was given intravenously. Importantly, some infants responded to and could tolerate enteral treatment, thus avoiding the need for an intravenous line.

Organs and Systems

Cardiovascular

Dysrhythmias consisting of self-limiting or single ventricular extra beats were observed after doxapram was given by injection; it was suggested that electrocardiographic dysrhythmias occurring in anesthesia could be associated with analeptic drug administration (5).

Doxapram is used to treat idiopathic apnea in premature infants. Second-degree atrioventricular heart block developed after its administration to three neonates (6).

- Thirty-six hours after an infusion of doxapram was started, the first infant developed second-degree AV block, with QT interval prolongation and an increase in the QRS interval. There was no hypotension. Sinus rhythm returned 92 hours after stopping the infusion.
- Doxapram was given orally, every 6 hours, to the second infant. After 43 hours second-degree AV block with a prolonged QT interval was noted. Echocardiography showed a normal heart. Doxapram was discontinued and 8 hours later sinus rhythm returned.
- The third infant was given aminophylline orally and doxapram by intravenous infusion; 5 days later cisapride was added to treat suspected gastro-esophageal reflux. The next day the infant had developed second-degree AV block, with a prolonged QT interval. Doxapram was withdrawn and sinus rhythm returned 36 hours later.

Heart block did not occur in the third case until cisapride, which can prolong the QT interval, was added.

There has been another report of three cases of second-degree atrioventricular block and QT interval prolongation associated with doxapram; sinus rhythm returned after withdrawal (7).

The mean pulmonary arterial pressure was significantly, but not severely, increased in 10 patients receiving intravenous infusions of doxapram (8).

There have been two studies of doxapram in very low birth weight infants before extubation. In one it was concluded that doxapram did not increase the likelihood of successful extubation. In the other there was an increase in systolic blood pressure along with much higher plasma doxapram concentrations than expected (9,10).

Nervous system

Of 20 patients, mean age 72, treated with low doses of doxapram by infusion, four developed violent restlessness, confusion, and hallucinations (SED-9, 5). Of these, three were known to drink excessive alcohol and two had abnormal liver function. The reactions were relatively brief and occurred at the beginning and end of doxapram administration.

In a controlled study of the use of doxapram infusion for late postoperative hypoxemia (3) the drug was withdrawn because of brainstem infarction in a 90-year-old woman.

In 285 surgical patients, respiratory stimulation was safely performed with doxapram, especially with small, frequently repeated doses. Adverse effects included neuromuscular signs of excessive central nervous system stimulation in a very few patients at 1 mg/kg. Seven patients had excitement and there was tremor in three and rigidity in two. Coughing, laryngospasm, and salivation are probably physiological manifestations of the return of protective reflexes secondary to arousal (11).

Liver

Reversible hepatotoxicity has been attributed to doxapram (12).

References

1. Wrench IJ, Singh P, Dennis AR, Mahajan RP, Crossley AW. The minimum effective doses of pethidine and doxapram in the treatment of post-anaesthetic shivering. Anaesthesia 1997;52(1):32–6.

2. Andersen R, Krohg K. Letter: Post-operative analgesia combined with doxapram. Anaesthesia 1976;31(1):114–15.
3. Rosenberg J, Kristensen PA, Pedersen MH, Overgaard H. Adverse events with continuous doxapram infusion against late postoperative hypoxaemia. Eur J Clin Pharmacol 1996;50(3):191–4.
4. Poets CF, Darraj S, Bohnhorst B. Effect of doxapram on episodes of apnoea, bradycardia and hypoxaemia in preterm infants. Biol Neonate 1999;76(4):207–13.
5. Stephen CR, Talton I. Effects of doxapram on the electrocardiogram during anesthesia. Anesth Analg 1966;45(6):783–9.
6. Wengel SP, Roccaforte WH, Burke WJ, Bayer BL, McNeilly DP, Knop D. Behavioral complications associated with donepezil. Am J Psychiatry 1998;155(11):1632–3.
7. De Villiers GS, Walele A, Van der Merwe PL, Kalis NN. Second-degree atrioventricular heart block after doxapram administration. J Pediatr 1998;133(1):149–50.
8. Weitzenblum E, Parini JP, Roeslin N. The effects on ventilation, gas exchange and haemodynamics of the respiratory stimulation of doxapram in cases of chronic respiratory failure. J Med Strasb 1973;4:1063.
9. Huon C, Rey E, Mussat P, Parat S, Moriette G. Low-dose doxapram for treatment of apnoea following early weaning in very low birthweight infants: a randomized, double-blind study. Acta Paediatr 1998;87(11):1180–4.
10. Barrington KJ, Muttitt SC. Randomized, controlled, blinded trial of doxapram for extubation of the very low birthweight infant. Acta Paediatr 1998;87(2):191–4.
11. Martin JL. Clinical evaluation of doxapram hydrochloride, a respiratory stimulant. J Okla State Med Assoc 1973;66(12):481–7.
12. Fancourt GJ, Ashton RJ, Talbot IC, Wales JM. Hepatic necrosis with doxapram hydrochloride. Postgrad Med J 1985;61(719):833–5.

Doxazosin

See also Alpha-adrenoceptor antagonists

General Information

The $alpha_1$-adrenoceptor antagonist doxazosin has similar adverse effects to those of prazosin. In a review of its clinical pharmacology and therapeutic uses, reports of tolerability included an update from previously unpublished pooled data on file (1). In 339 patients treated with doxazosin for hypertension compared with 336 treated with placebo, adverse effects were essentially the same as those reported in 665 patients being treated for benign prostatic hyperplasia compared with 300 treated with placebo. Dizziness (19 versus 9% and 16 versus 9%) and fatigue (12 versus 6% and 8 versus 2%) were reported significantly more often than with placebo (figures for patients with hypertension and benign prostate hyperplasia respectively, versus placebo). However, in hypertensive patients somnolence was reported more often than with placebo (5 versus 1%). In patients with benign prostatic hyperplasia the following adverse effects were reported significantly more often than with placebo: hypotension (17 versus 0%), edema (2.7 versus 0.7%), and dyspnea (2.6 versus 0.3%).

The Antihypertensive and Lipid-Lowering Treatment to Prevent Heart Attack Trial (ALLHAT) (2) was a multicenter comparison of drugs from each of three classes of antihypertensive agents (amlodipine, lisinopril, and doxazosin) with chlortalidone as an active control, in 24 335 adults with hypertension and at least one other coronary heart disease risk factor. In an interim analysis (median follow-up 3.3 years) there was no significant difference in the rates of fatal coronary heart disease or non-fatal myocardial infarction, or in total mortality between doxazosin and chlortalidone, but doxazosin was associated with higher rates of stroke (RR = 1.19; CI = 1.01, 1.40) and combined cardiovascular disease (RR = 1.24; CI = 1.17, 1.33). Considered separately, the risk of congestive heart failure was doubled (RR = 2.04; CI = 1.79, 2.32). Mean systolic blood pressure with doxazosin was about 2–3 mmHg higher than with chlortalidone and mean diastolic pressure was similar in the two groups. The authors concluded that the difference in blood pressure control did not account for the differences in cardiovascular end-points.

Doxazosin, and perhaps the whole class of alpha-blockers, should no longer be considered as first-line antihypertensive therapy. Doxazosin can still be used for symptom relief in patients with nocturia secondary to prostatic hyperplasia, although it should probably be avoided in patients with manifest or latent congestive heart failure (3). This issue has been intensely debated (4).

Phenoxybenzamine and doxazosin have been compared in 35 patients with pheochromocytoma (5). Hemodynamic, pharmacological, and biochemical indicators of alpha- and beta-adrenoceptor blockade were measured before, during, and after anesthesia and surgery in eight patients pretreated with phenoxybenzamine and in 27 patients pretreated with doxazosin. Doxazosin (2–16 mg/day) was as effective as phenoxybenzamine in controlling arterial blood pressure and heart rate before and during surgery and it caused fewer adverse effects.

Organs and Systems

Cardiovascular

Hypotension is a risk with doxazosin and has been reported to cause stroke (6).

- A 64-year-old man developed a right hemiparesis after taking one dose of doxazosin 4 mg for prostatic symptoms. A CT scan of the brain and carotid ultrasound studies were normal. He recovered most of his neurological function within a few days. Ambulatory blood pressure monitoring after treatment with doxazosin 2 mg showed striking blood pressure reduction during sleep.

Psychological, psychiatric

Doxazosin, 16 mg/day, has been reported to have caused an acute psychosis.

- A 71-year-old woman with type II diabetes and hypertension began to hear voices and to have auditory hallucinations. Doxazosin was progressively withdrawn over the next 14 days and by the time the dosage had been reduced to 8 mg a day the psychosis was much less severe; it disappeared completely after withdrawal (7).

Drug Administration

Drug formulations

Doxazosin can cause a sharp fall in blood pressure at the start of therapy, and a modified-release formulation has been developed in an attempt to obviate this. In an open, non-comparative, sequential study in primary care, the ordinary formulation (1–16 mg/day for 3–6 months) was replaced by the modified-release formulation (4–8 mg/day for 3 months) in 3537 patients (8). The most common reasons for withdrawal from the study were loss to follow-up (37%) and adverse events (28%). Blood pressure fell from 160/95 to 139/82 mmHg with the ordinary formulation and to 135/79 mmHg when the modified-release formulation was used instead. The most common adverse events were weakness, headache, dizziness, and hypotension, all of which were more common with the ordinary formulation. However, these differences could have been due to a healthy survivor effect, in which those who had an adverse event early on (that is while taking the ordinary formulation) dropped out before taking the modified-release formulation, which would therefore appear to be safer. Thus, the lack of crossover in this study makes the results hard to interpret, although it appears that the two formulations were at worst no different from each other.

Drug overdose

A case of doxazosin overdose has been reported.

- Hypotension, bradycardia, and ST segment elevation on the electrocardiogram occurred in a patient who took doxazosin 40 mg (9). His blood pressure was 90/60 mmHg and his heart rate fell to 50/minute. Eight hours after aggressive saline infusion and gastric lavage the patient was awake, but his hypotension and bradycardia were corrected only after 96 hours and the administration of intravenous atropine 0.5 mg.

References

1. Fulton B, Wagstaff AJ, Sorkin EM. Doxazosin. An update of its clinical pharmacology and therapeutic applications in hypertension and benign prostatic hyperplasia. Drugs 1995;49(2):295–320.
2. Davies BR, Furberg CD, Wright JT. Major cardiovascular events in hypertensive patients randomized to doxazosin vs chlorthalidone: the antihypertensive and lipid-lowering treatment to prevent heart attack trial (ALLHAT). ALLHAT Collaborative Research Group. JAMA 2000;283(15):1967–75.
3. Messerli FH. Implications of discontinuation of doxazosin arm of ALLHAT. Antihypertensive and Lipid-Lowering Treatment to Prevent Heart Attack Trial. Lancet 2000;355(9207):863–4.
4. Beevers DG, Lip GY. Do alpha blockers cause heart failure and stroke? Observations from ALLHAT. J Hum Hypertens 2000;14(5):287–9.
5. Prys-Roberts C, Farndon JR. Efficacy and safety of doxazosin for perioperative management of patients with pheochromocytoma. World J Surg 2002;26(8):1037–42.
6. Mansoor GA, Tendler BE. Stroke associated with alpha blocker therapy for benign prostatic hypertrophy. J Natl Med Assoc 2002;94(1):1–4.
7. Evans M, Perera PW, Donoghue J. Drug induced psychosis with doxazosin. BMJ 1997;314(7098):1869.
8. Anegon M, Esteban J, Jimenez-Garcia R, Sanz de Burgoa V, Martinez J, Gil de Miguel A. A postmarketing, open-label study to evaluate the tolerability and effectiveness of replacing standard-formulation doxazosin with doxazosin in the gastrointestinal therapeutic system formulation in adult patients with hypertension. Clin Ther 2002;24(5):786–97.
9. Gokel Y, Dokur M, Paydas S. Doxazosin overdosage. Am J Emerg Med 2000;18(5):638–9.

Doxepin

See also Tricyclic antidepressants

General Information

Doxepin is a tricyclic antidepressant that has also been used topically in the treatment of atopic dermatitis and other forms of eczematous dermatitis. It causes the adverse effects that one would expect, and systemic effects can result from absorption after topical administration.

Organs and Systems

Nervous system

Short-term treatment with 5% doxepin cream caused mild transient drowsiness in 16–28% of patients, severe enough to necessitate withdrawal in about 2% (1). In addition, 5% of treated patients noted a dry mouth. Excessive use in children can result in intoxication, with seizures, respiratory depression, electrocardiographic abnormalities, and coma (2).

References

1. Drake LA, Millikan LE. The antipruritic effect of 5% doxepin cream in patients with eczematous dermatitis. Doxepin Study Group. Arch Dermatol 1995;131(12):1403–8.
2. Vo MY, Williamsen AR, Wasserman GS, Duthie SE. Toxic reaction from topically applied doxepin in a child with eczema. Arch Dermatol 1995;131(12):1467–8.

Doxifluridine

See also Cytostatic and immunosuppressant drugs

General Information

Doxifluridine is a derivative of 5-fluorouracil. It has been used to treat a variety of solid tumors, including cancers of the breast, pancreas, stomach (1), and large bowel.

Organs and Systems

Nervous system

In a neurological evaluation of 17 patients treated with doxifluridine 3 or 5 g/m^2/day for 5 days every 4 weeks for 3 months, 10 developed symptoms of central nervous system toxicity. The neurological symptoms, cerebellar and encephalopathic, developed simultaneously and were commonly first noted during the second week of the first cycle. The neurotoxicity was dose-related and worsened during subsequent treatment. The symptoms of cerebellar disease ranged from a subjective feeling of unsteady gait to disability, while the encephalopathy resulted in difficulties with concentration and memory. Patients with marked weight loss and with generalized electrocardiographic dysrhythmias are at greatest risk of developing neurotoxicity with doxifluridine (2).

Gastrointestinal

Anorexia has been reported with doxifluridine in the absence of nausea or vomiting (3).

References

1. Nakagawa H, Kobayashi K, Tono T, Fukuda K, Shinn E, Mishima H, Yagyu T, Kobayashi T, Kikkawa N. [Combination of intra-hepatic arterial infusion of low-dose cisplatin and oral administration of high-dose doxyfluridine for patients with liver metastases of gastric cancer.] Gan To Kagaku Ryoho 1996;23(6):783–5.
2. Heier MS, Fossa SD. Wernicke–Korsakoff-like syndrome in patients with colorectal carcinoma treated with high-dose doxifluridine (5′-dFUrd). Acta Neurol Scand 1986;73(5):449–57.
3. Tamaki Y, Tono T, Kobayashi K, Yagyu T, Takatsuka Y, Shin E, Mishima H, Kikkawa N. [Combination with intra-hepatic arterial infusion of low-dose cisplatin and oral administration of high-dose doxyfluridine in patients with liver metastases of gastric cancer.] Gan To Kagaku Ryoho 1994;21(13):2140–2.

Doxycycline

See also Tetracyclines

General Information

Doxycycline and minocycline are more lipophilic tetracyclines. They are well absorbed after oral administration. Their half-lives are 16–18 hours. Their higher affinity for fatty tissues improves their effectiveness and changes their adverse effects profile. Local gastrointestinal irritation and disturbance of the intestinal bacterial flora occur less often than with the more hydrophilic drugs, which have to be given in higher oral doses for sufficient absorption.

Nevertheless, their toxic effects are similar to those of other tetracyclines and arise from accumulation in fatty tissues. Accumulation in a third compartment and the resulting long half-life may contribute to an increased incidence of various toxic adverse effects during long-term treatment, even if lower daily doses are used. This seems also to be the case for pigmentation disorders and possibly for neurological disturbances (1).

Minocycline and doxycycline are predominantly eliminated by the liver and biliary tract (70–90%). Therefore, no change in dose is needed in patients with impaired renal function. However, it should be considered that hepatic elimination of doxycycline or minocycline might be accelerated by co-administration of agents that induce hepatic enzymes.

Organs and Systems

Nervous system

Peripheral neuropathy from doxycycline has been reported (2).

- A 61-year-old doctor with recurrent bronchopneumonia took two courses of doxycycline. During the first course he had persistent numbness in his feet. During the second course, a few months later, he noticed after only 2 or 3 days that the numbness accelerated markedly and was associated with a low threshold for muscle cramps in the feet. He stopped taking doxycycline and during the following weeks noticed slight improvement. However, some symptoms persisted and he had neurological investigations. A wide range of clinical and laboratory tests showed no cause for his neuropathy.

A search for an association between doxycycline and polyneuropathy failed to identify any documented cases. An inquiry to the Swedish Adverse Drug Reactions Advisory Committee elicited information about three cases of "paresthesia," two cases of "sensitivity disturbance," and one case of "neuropathy." The last was a man who had had pain and paresthesia in the feet, arms, and face after taking doxycycline 100 mg/day for 2 weeks for prostatitis. The symptoms began to wane 1 week after treatment was stopped, and disappeared completely 1 week later.

Metabolism

Doxycycline can cause hypoglycemia.

- A 70-year-old man with type 2 diabetes mellitus presented with sudden confusion, which rapidly progressed to loss of consciousness (3). The only drug he had taken during the previous 2 months was doxycycline (100 mg/day), which he had taken for 5 days for an upper respiratory tract infection. Urine tests for sulfonylureas were negative. Routine hematological and biochemical tests and an electrocardiogram were normal. He improved with intravenous glucose and withdrawal of doxycycline and had no further episodes of hypoglycemia over the next 3 months.

Plasma insulin was not measured in this case, so the mechanism of hypoglycemia was unclear.

Hypoglycemia has also been attributed to doxycycline in a non-diabetic patient (4).

Gastrointestinal

Esophageal ulcers have been described in association with oral doxycycline or tetracycline. Acute onset of substernal burning pain and dysphagia was noted within hours of taking the drug (5–9). Remaining parts of the ingested capsule were identified by esophagoscopy.

Thirty centers for pharmacovigilance in France have reported 81 cases of esophageal damage after treatment with tetracyclines collected between 1985 and 1992 (10). There were 64 ulcers, eight cases of dysphagia, and nine of esophagitis. Most (96%) of the cases were caused by doxycycline and 73% of the patients were female, mean age 29 years. Prescriptions were for dermatological (54%), urogenital (23%), and ENT diseases. In one patient, a 71-year-old man, an esophagobronchial fistulation required esophagectomy. In 92% the drugs were not taken correctly, that is at bedtime or without a sufficient quantity of fluid. Treatment with sucralfate 1 g tds did not change the outcome of tetracycline-induced esophageal ulcers (11).

Two cases of esophagitis in children have been reported (12).

- A 12-year-old boy developed lower chest pain, having taken doxycycline for 7 days for presumed epididymitis. He had a normal chest X-ray and electrocardiogram and no signs of infection. Doxycycline was withdrawn, but the chest pain persisted. After 4 days endoscopy showed two very large ulcerated craters measuring about 5 × 12 mm in the distal esophagus.
- A 15-year-old girl developed chest pain and difficulty in swallowing after having taken five doses of doxycycline. Physical examination was normal and she had a normal chest X-ray and electrocardiogram. Doxycycline was withdrawn and she was given sucralfate 10 ml tds, omeprazole having been ineffective. Gastroscopy was not performed. Her pain began to improve 2 days later.

The authors stated that it is important to inquire about the use of tetracyclines in children with chest pain, and to consider them as a possible cause of the pain.

Esophageal ulceration occurred in two adults taking doxycycline as malaria chemoprophylaxis (13).

- A 20-year-old woman, who had been taking doxycycline malaria prophylaxis, took a doxycycline capsule (dose not given) before going to bed and awoke hours later with the feeling that the capsule was stuck in her esophagus. Over the next 4 days she developed worsening dysphagia. Esophagoscopy showed an esophageal ulcer over 20% of the esophageal surface. She was treated with ranitidine and sucralfate and improved over the next 2 days.
- A 27-year-old man with an 8-day history of dysphagia and retrosternal pain was taking doxycycline prophylaxis and occasional terfenadine (doses not stated). He recalled no problems with taking any of his doxycycline prophylaxis. He had an esophagoscopy, which showed a 1 cm esophageal ulcer. He improved with ranitidine.

Liver

Doxycycline-induced liver injury has been reported (14). The patient took oral doxycycline 200 mg/day for 8 days and had markedly altered liver function. The liver enzyme activities normalized only 109 days after withdrawal.

Skin

Fixed drug eruptions have been attributed to doxycycline (15).

Immunologic

Renal small-vessel vasculitis related to doxycycline has been reported (16).

Second-Generation Effects

Teratogenicity

Doxycycline has not been shown to be teratogenic (17).

Susceptibility Factors

Renal disease

Doxycycline is almost completely eliminated via the liver and the biliary tract and is therefore safe in patients with pre-existing renal insufficiency. However, for intravenous administration, doxycycline is solubilized with polyvinylpyrrolidone, the clearance of which is less than that of doxycycline. In patients with a serum creatinine concentration of more than 250 μmol/l (3 mg/dl), it is therefore advisable to limit the duration of treatment to a few days.

Drug Administration

Drug administration route

When intravenous tetracycline became no longer available, many centers began to use doxycycline as a sclerosant. In one review (18), chest pain was the most frequent adverse event with doxycycline, occurring in about 40% of the 60 patients in whom it had been used, and fever occurred in about 7%. In a more recent controlled trial in 106 patients treated with either doxycycline or bleomycin, there was chest pain in 20% of the patients treated with doxycycline, and nausea in one patient (19).

Drug–Drug Interactions

Methotrexate

Doxycycline can be added to the long list of drugs (SEDA-18, 262) (SEDA-23, 253) that can interact with methotrexate (20).

- A 17-year-old girl with a femoral osteosarcoma received her 11th cycle of methotrexate and simultaneously oral doxycycline 100 mg bd for a palpebral abscess. As in previous cycles, pharmacokinetic monitoring of methotrexate was performed. On this occasion the half-life of methotrexate was more than doubled. She developed hematological and gastroenterological toxicity.

The authors recommended that in patients receiving methotrexate an alternative to doxycycline should be used.

Warfarin

There has been a report of bleeding and prolonged international normalized ratio in a 69-year-old man given warfarin and doxycycline (21).

References

1. Lander CM. Minocycline-induced benign intracranial hypertension. Clin Exp Neurol 1989;26:161–7.
2. Olsson R. Can doxycycline cause polyneuropathy? J Intern Med 2002;251(4):361–2.
3. Odeh M, Oliven A. Doxycycline-induced hypoglycemia. J Clin Pharmacol 2000;40(10):1173–4.
4. Basaria S, Braga M, Moore WT. Doxycycline-induced hypoglycemia in a nondiabetic young man. South Med J 2002;95(11):1353–4.
5. Baeriswyl G, Bengoa J, de Peyer R, Loizeau E. Importance des ulcérations médicamenteuses dans les lésions endoscopiques de l'oesophage. [Importance of drug-induced ulceration in endoscopic lesions of the esophagus.] Schweiz Med Wochenschr Suppl 1985;19:6–9.
6. Bonavina L, DeMeester TR, McChesney L, Schwizer W, Albertucci M, Bailey RT. Drug-induced esophageal strictures. Ann Surg 1987;206(2):173–83.
7. Zijnen-Suyker MP, Hazenberg BP. Oesophagusbeschadiging door doxycycline. [Esophageal lesions caused by doxycycline.] Ned Tijdschr Geneeskd 1981;125(35):1407–10.
8. Schneider R. Doxycycline esophageal ulcers. Am J Dig Dis 1977;22(9):805–7.
9. Crowson TD, Head LH, Ferrante WA. Esophageal ulcers associated with tetracycline therapy. JAMA 1976;235(25):2747–8.
10. Champel V, Jonville-Bera AP, Bera F, Autret E. Les tétracyclines peuvent être responsables d'ulcérations oesophagiennes si leur prise est incorrecte. Rev Prat Med Gen 1998;12:9–10.
11. Huizar JF, Podolsky I, Goldberg J. Ulceras esofagicas inducidas por doxiciclina. [Doxycycline-induced esophageal ulcers.] Rev Gastroenterol Mex 1998;63(2):101–5.
12. Palmer KM, Selbst SM, Shaffer S, Proujansky R. Pediatric chest pain induced by tetracycline ingestion. Pediatr Emerg Care 1999;15(3):200–1.
13. Morris TJ, Davis TP. Doxycycline-induced esophageal ulceration in the U.S. Military service. Mil Med 2000;165(4):316–19.
14. Bjornsson E, Lindberg J, Olsson R. Liver reactions to oral low-dose tetracyclines. Scand J Gastroenterol 1997;32(4):390–5.
15. Alanko K. Topical provocation of fixed drug eruption. A study of 30 patients. Contact Dermatitis 1994;31(1):25–7.
16. Goland S, Kazarsky R, Kagan A, Huszar M, Abend I, Malnick SDH. Renal vasculitis associated with doxycycline. J Pharm Technol 2001;17:220–2.
17. Czeizel AE, Rockenbauer M. Teratogenic study of doxycycline. Obstet Gynecol 1997;89(4):524–8.
18. Walker-Renard PB, Vaughan LM, Sahn SA. Chemical pleurodesis for malignant pleural effusions. Ann Intern Med 1994;120(1):56–64.
19. Patz EF Jr, McAdams HP, Erasmus JJ, Goodman PC, Culhane DK, Gilkeson RC, Herndon J. Sclerotherapy for malignant pleural effusions: a prospective randomized trial of bleomycin vs doxycycline with small-bore catheter drainage. Chest 1998;113(5):1305–11.
20. Tortajada-Ituren JJ, Ordovas-Baines JP, Llopis-Salvia P, Jimenez-Torres NV. High-dose methotrexate–doxycycline interaction. Ann Pharmacother 1999;33(7–8):804–8.
21. Baciewicz AM, Bal BS. Bleeding associated with doxycycline and warfarin treatment. Arch Intern Med 2001;161(9):1231.

Doxylamine

See also Antihistamines

General Information

Doxylamine is an antihistamine, a monoethanolamine derivative, with antimuscarinic and pronounced sedative effects.

Second-Generation Effects

Teratogenicity

The mixture of doxylamine succinate and pyridoxine (at one time combined with dicycloverine), known under the brand names of Bendectin and Debendox, was withdrawn after a campaign had incriminated it as a teratogen. Used mainly in some English-speaking countries, it was used primarily to treat nausea and vomiting during pregnancy in circumstances in which, in other countries, dietary measures and/or low doses of antihistamines alone are more customary. No consistent picture of the congenital defects that it was alleged to produce (for example pyloric stenosis) ever emerged, and reviews have never concluded otherwise than that it was at most a low-grade teratogen (SEDA-9, 311) or entirely innocent. A review of the literature (1) and a meta-analysis failed to detect any evidence that Bendectin has a teratogenic effect (2).

References

1. Brent RL. Bendectin: review of the medical literature of a comprehensively studied human nonteratogen and the most prevalent tortogen-litigen. Reprod Toxicol 1995;9(4):337–49.
2. McKeigue PM, Lamm SH, Linn S, Kutcher JS. Bendectin and birth defects: I. A meta-analysis of the epidemiologic studies. Teratology 1994;50(1):27–37.

Droperidol

See also Neuroleptic drugs

General Information

Droperidol is a butyrophenone with actions similar to those of haloperidol.

Of 20 volunteers who took droperidol 5 mg orally in orange juice, none had a neutral or pleasant experience (1). All reported restlessness, 17 felt sedated, and 11 reported dysphoria, the onset being relatively immediate; one subject broke down in tears within an hour of taking droperidol. Suicidal feelings emerged acutely in two subjects and were entertained in two more subjects. Among other adverse events were skin hypersensitivity ($n = 5$), aching in the muscles ($n = 6$), wheezing consistent with respiratory dyskinesia ($n = 1$), change in voice quality ($n = 1$), and marked rhinorrhea ($n = 1$). Mental effort was difficult, and all subjects reported some problems with concentration.

Droperidol 5–7.5 mg given during induction of anesthesia was associated with impaired well-being scores 6 hours postoperatively in a randomized double-blind comparison of similar doses of droperidol ($n = 78$) and midazolam ($n = 72$) for preventing postoperative nausea and vomiting (2).

Organs and Systems

Cardiovascular

Droperidol has been associated with QT interval prolongation (SED-14, 141) (3–5) and torsade de pointes has been reported (6).

- A 59-year-old woman with no history of cardiac problems, except for hypertension, who was taking amlodipine 5 mg qds, cyclobenzaprine 10 mg qds, and co-triamterzide 37.5 + 25 mg qds, and who had a QT_c interval of 497 ms, was given intravenous droperidol 0.625 mg and metoclopramide 10 mg 45 minutes before surgery. About 1.75 hours after surgery she developed a polymorphic ventricular tachycardia with findings consistent with torsade de pointes, which resolved with defibrillation.

Nervous system

Intramuscular droperidol 2.5 mg was used to treat 23 consecutive patients with acute migraine who had not responded to other drugs (7). If no relief was achieved by 30–60 minutes after treatment, and no significant adverse effects were reported, a second dose of droperidol 2.5 mg was given. Varying degrees of akathisia after treatment were reported by six patients. Similarly, in a retrospective series of 37 patients who received droperidol 2.5 mg for migraine, 3 developed mild akathisia and 5 had drowsiness (8).

Balance disturbances have been described with droperidol in 120 women undergoing gynecological dilatation and curettage, who were randomly assigned to receive either 0.9% saline (placebo) or droperidol 0.625 mg intravenously before surgery (9). The change in body sway from the baseline before anesthesia was significantly greater after droperidol (61%) than after placebo (33%).

Drug–Drug Interactions

Fentanyl

An exception to the relatively safe use of high-potency agents has been noted in the combination of droperidol with the narcotic fentanyl, which can cause marked hypotension (10).

Neuromuscular blocking agents

Animal studies suggest that large doses of pethidine and droperidol can augment the myoneural effects of neuromuscular blocking agents (11).

References

1. Healy D, Farquhar G. Immediate effects of droperidol. Human Psychopharmacol 1998;13:113–20.
2. Eberhart LH, Seeling W. Droperidol-supplemented anaesthesia decreases post-operative nausea and vomiting but impairs post-operative mood and well-being. Eur J Anaesthesiol 1999;16(5):290–7.
3. Warner JP, Barnes TR, Henry JA. Electrocardiographic changes in patients receiving neuroleptic medication. Acta Psychiatr Scand 1996;93(4):311–13.
4. Iwahashi K. Significantly higher plasma haloperidol level during cotreatment with carbamazepine may herald cardiac change. Clin Neuropharmacol 1996;19(3):267–70.
5. Reilly JG, Ayis SA, Ferrier IN, Jones SJ, Thomas SH. QTc-interval abnormalities and psychotropic drug therapy in psychiatric patients. Lancet 2000;355(9209):1048–52.
6. Michalets EL, Smith LK, Van Tassel ED. Torsade de pointes resulting from the addition of droperidol to an existing cytochrome P450 drug interaction. Ann Pharmacother 1998;32(7–8):761–5.
7. Mendizabal JE, Watts JM, Riaz S, Rothrock JF. Open-label intramuscular droperidol for the treatment of refractory headache: a pilot study. Headache 1999;10:55–7.
8. Richman PB, Reischel U, Ostrow A, Irving C, Ritter A, Allegra J, Eskin B, Szucs P, Nashed AH. Droperidol for acute migraine headache. Am J Emerg Med 1999;17(4):398–400.
9. Song D, Chung F, Yogendran S, Wong J. Evaluation of postural stability after low-dose droperidol in outpatients undergoing gynaecological dilatation and curettage procedure. Br J Anaesth 2002;88(6):819–23.
10. Mandelstam JP. An inquiry into the use of Innovar for pediatric premedication. Anesth Analg 1970; 49(5):746–50.
11. Boros M, Chaudhry IA, Nagashima H, Duncalf RM, Sherman EH, Foldes FF. Myoneural effects of pethidine and droperidol. Br J Anaesth 1984;56(2):195–202.

Droseraceae

See also Herbal medicines

General Information

The family of Droseraceae contains two genera:

1. *Dionaea* (Venus flytrap)
2. *Drosera* (sundew).

Dionaea muscipula

The expressed sap of *Dionaea muscipula*, a fly-catching plant (Venus flytrap), was once available in Germany as an herbal oncolytic in the form of ampoules and oral drops (1). However, when it became apparent that intramuscular administration could produce shivers, fever, and anaphylactic shock, the health authorities banned the ampoules. They also ruled that the product information on the oral drops should warn against use in pregnancy and should list reddening of the face, headache, dyspnea, nausea, and vomiting as adverse effects.

Reference

1. Anonymous. Carnivorsa–Phytothexapeutikum zur Behandlung maligner Erkrankungen. Dokumentation Nr. 15. [Carnivora–phytotherapeutic agent for the treatment of malignant diseases. Documentation No. 15.] Schweiz Rundsch Med Prax 1988;77(11):283–7.

Droxicam

See also Non-steroidal anti-inflammatory drugs

General Information

Droxicam, a piroxicam prodrug, has similar adverse effects (SEDA-16, 113) (1). Because of many Spanish reports of non-fatal liver damage, according to the CPMP the Summary of Product Characteristics should state that serious hepatic damage can occur (SEDA-17, 113). Owing to its hepatotoxicity, droxicam has been withdrawn in many countries (SEDA-19, 99).

Reference

1. Jane F, Rodriguez de la Serna A. Droxicam: a pharmacological and clinical review of a new NSAID. Eur J Rheumatol Inflamm 1991;11(4):3–9.

Dryopteraceae

See also Herbal medicines

General Information

The genera in the family of Dryopteraceae (Table 1) include various types of fern.

Table 1 The genera of Dryopteraceae

Arachniodes (holly fern)
Athyrium (ladyfern)
Bolbitis (creeping fern)
Ctenitis (lacefern)
Cyclopeltis (cyclopeltis)
Cyrtomium (netvein hollyfern)
Cystopteris (bladderfern)
Deparia (false spleenwort)
Diplazium (twinsorus fern)
Dryopteris (wood fern)
Elaphoglossum (tongue fern)
Fadyenia (dotted fern)
Gymnocarpium (oak fern)
Hemidictyum (hemidictyum)
Hypoderris (hypoderris)
Lastreopsis (shield fern)
Lomagramma (lomagramma)
Lomariopsis (fringed fern)
Matteuccia (ostrich fern)
Megalastrum (megalastrum)
Nephrolepis (sword fern)
Nothoperanema (island lace fern)
Oleandra (oleander fern)
Olfersia (island fern)
Onoclea (sensitive fern)
Phanerophlebia (phanerophlebia)
Polystichum (holly fern)
Rumohra (rumohra)
Tectaria (halberd fern)
Triplophyllum (triplophyllum)
Woodsia (cliff fern)

Dryopteris filix-mas

The rhizome of *Dryopteris filix-mas* (male fern) was formerly used as an antihelminthic drug (1), but it is highly toxic and has been superseded by other less-dangerous agents. In spite of poor absorption, serious poisoning can occur, for example when absorption is increased by the presence of fatty foods. Poisoning is characterized by vomiting, diarrhea, vertigo, headache, tremor, cold sweats, dyspnea, cyanosis, convulsions, mental disturbances, disturbed vision, and even blindness, which in a few instances is permanent.

Reference

1. Vinkenborg J. [The male fern as a medicinal plant.] Pharm Weekbl 1961;96:726–36.